W9-DHJ-152

	Hydroxyzine	Meperidine	Metoclopramide	Midazolam	Morphine	Nalbuphine	Pentazocine	Pentobarbital	Perphenazine	Prochlorperazine	Promazine	Promethazine	Ranitidine	Scopolamine Hbr	Secobarbital	Thiethylperazine
	C	C	C	C	C	C	C	C	C	C	C	C	C	C	I	
	C	C	C	C	C		C	I	C	C		C		C	I	C
	C	C	C	C	C		C	I	C	C	C	C	C	C	I	
								I								I
	I	I	I		I	I	I	I	I	I	I	I	I		I	I
	I	C	C	I	C		C	I	C	I	I	I		C	C	I
	C	C	C		C	C	C	I	C	C	C	C	C		C	I
	C	C	C		C		C	I	C	C	C	C	C	C	I	
	C	C			C		I	I			C	C	C	C	I	
		I			I		I						I			
		C	C		C	C	C	I			C	C	C	I	C	I
	C		C		I		C	I	C	I	I	I	C	C	I	
	C	C		C			C			C	C	C	C	C	I	
	C		C		C	C		I	I	I	C	C	I	C		C
	C	I	C			C	I	C	C	C	C	C	C	I		
	C						I			C		*	C	C	I	C
	C	C	C		C		I	C	C	C	C	C	C	I		
	I	I			I	I	I	I		I	I	I	I		C	I
		C	C		C		C	I			C		C	C	I	I
	C	C	C		C	C	C	I	C		C	C	C	C	I	
	C	C	C		C		C	I		C		C		C	I	
	C	C	C		C	C	C	I	C	C	C	C		C	I	
		C	C	I	C	C	C			C	C		C		C	
	C	C	C		C	C	C	C	C	C	C	C	C		I	
	I	I	I		I	I	I	I	I	I	I	I	I		I	I
					C				I				C		I	

Parenteral compatibility occurs when two or more drugs are successfully mixed without liquefaction, deliquescence, or precipitation.

≡ 2003 ≡

Mosby's
Nursing
Drug
Reference

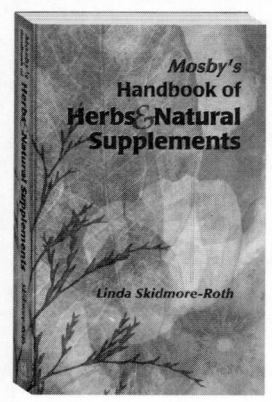

2003

Mosby's
Nursing
Drug
Reference

Linda Skidmore-Roth, RN, MSN, NP

Consultant
Littleton, Colorado

Formerly, Nursing Faculty,
New Mexico State University,
Las Cruces, New Mexico;
El Paso Community College,
El Paso, Texas

An Affiliate of Elsevier Science

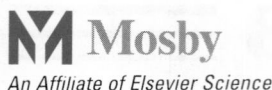
Mosby

An Affiliate of Elsevier Science

11830 Westline Drive
St. Louis, Missouri 63146

MOSBY'S 2003 NURSING DRUG REFERENCE   ISSN 1044-8470
Copyright © 2003, Mosby, Inc. All rights reserved. ISBN 0-323-00983-2

Notice

Pharmacology is an ever-changing field. Standard safety precautions must be followed, but as new research and clinical experience broaden our knowledge, changes in treatment and drug therapy may become necessary or appropriate. Readers are advised to check the most current product information provided by the manufacturer of each drug to be administered to verify the recommended dose, the method and duration of administration, and contraindications. It is the responsibility of the treating physician, relying on experience and knowledge of the patient, to determine dosages and the best treatment for each individual patient. Neither the Publisher nor the author assume any liability for any injury and/or damage to persons or property arising from this publication.

The Publisher

Vice President, Publishing Director: Sally Schrefer
Executive Editor, Nursing: Darlene Como
Senior Developmental Editor: Tamara A. Myers
Publishing Services Manager: Deborah L. Vogel
Design Manager: Bill Drone

GW/RDC

Printed in the United States of America

Last digit is the print number: 9 8 7 6 5 4 3 2

Consultants

Jean Krajicek Bartek, PhD, APRN
Associate Professor
University of Nebraska Medical
  Center
Colleges of Nursing and Medicine
  (Pharmacology)
Omaha, Nebraska

Rita Hanover Berdan, MS, RN, C
Nursing Faculty
St. Joseph's Hospital Health Center
  School of Nursing
Syracuse, New York

Barbara L. Cary, MSN, RN
Adjunct Faculty
University of Maine
Augusta, Maine

Tamara Conroy, RMA, CPT, SPN
Pittston, Pennsylvania

Henry B. Geiter, Jr, RN, C, CCRN
Vencor Hospital
St. Petersburg Junior College
St. Petersburg, Florida

F. James Grogan, PharmD
Executive Director
Grogan Communications
Swansea, Illinois

Jennifer L. Gudeman, PharmD
Product Surveillance Specialist
Corporate Product Monitoring
Mallinckrodt/Tyco Healthcare
St. Louis, Missouri

Scott Harrington, PharmD, RPh
Harrington Health Informatics
Tucson, Arizona

Phyllis Howard, RN, BSN
Associate Professor of Practical
  Nursing
Ashland Technical College
Ashland, Kentucky

Joan Ann Leach, RNC, MS, ME
Professor of Nursing
Capital Community College
Hartford, Connecticut

Mary Jo Mattocks, PhD, MN, BSN
Assistant Professor
Montana State University
Northern Great Falls Campus
Great Falls, Montana

Jennifer L. McQuade, PharmD
Medical Information Consultant
Douglasville, Georgia

Michelle M. Montpas, RN, MSN, OCN
CS Mott Community College
Flint, Michigan

Janet Rentfro, RN, ADN, ACLS
Medical Supervisor
Ascension Island
South Atlantic Ocean

Becky A. Ridenhour, PharmD
St. Louis College of Pharmacy
St. Louis, Missouri

Roberta Secrest, PharmD, PhD
Global Scientific Information and
  Communication
Eli Lilly and Company
Indianapolis, Indiana

Patricia R. Teasley, MSN, RN, CS
Central Texas College
Killeen, Texas

Brenda L. Thompson, PharmD
Assistant Professor
Pharmacy Practice Division
St. Louis College of Pharmacy
St. Louis, Missouri

Joyce S. Willens, PhD, RN
Assistant Professor
College of Nursing
Villanova University
Villanova, Pennsylvania

Preface

Since the first publication of *Mosby's Nursing Drug Reference* in 1988, more than 100 U.S. and Canadian pharmacists and consultants have reviewed the book's content closely. Today, *Mosby's 2003 Nursing Drug Reference* is more up-to-date than ever—with features that make it easy to find critical information fast!

New facts
This edition features more than 2000 new drug facts, including:
- new drugs and new dosage information
- newly researched side effects and adverse reactions
- the latest precautions, interactions, and contraindications
- IV therapy updates
- revised nursing considerations
- updated patient/family teaching guidelines

New features
- Monographs for 118 "high-alert" medications are highlighted with a blue background in the A-Z section to remind you to use extra care in administering these drugs. Appendix I provides a complete list of "high-alert" drugs most capable of causing significant harm to patients.
- "Research notes" heading that describes current key studies on drug uses, doses, and interactions for 40 drugs.
- Appendix A, "Selected new drugs," provides detailed monographs for 24 drugs recently approved by the FDA. (See Table of Contents for complete list.) Included are monographs for:
  - frovatriptan (Frova) for treatment of migraines
  - bosentan (Tracleer) for treatment of pulmonary arterial hypertension
  - dutasteride (Duagen) for treatment of benign prostatic hyperplasia
  - valdecoxib (Bextra) for treatment of rheumatoid arthritis and osteoarthritis
- Appendix B, "Recent FDA drug approvals," lists generic/trade names and uses for 3 of the most recently approved drugs.

Organization
This reference is organized into four main sections:
- Drug categories
- Individual drug monographs (in alphabetical order by generic name)
- Drug Identification Guide
- Appendixes (identified by the wide dark blue thumb tabs on the edge)

The guiding principle behind this book is to provide fast, easy access to drug information and nursing considerations. Every detail—from the paper, typeface, cover, binding, use of color, and appendixes—has been carefully chosen with the user in mind.

Individual Drug Monographs

This book includes monographs for more than 1300 generic and 4500 trade medications. Common trade names are given for all drugs regularly used in the United States and Canada, with drugs available only in Canada identified by an asterisk.

The following information is provided, whenever possible, for safe, effective administration of each drug:

High-alert status: Identifies high-alert drugs; screened light-blue for easy identification.

Pronunciation: Helps the nurse master complex generic names.

℞/OTC: Identifies prescription or over-the-counter drugs.

Functional and chemical classifications: Allows the nurse to see similarities and dissimilarities among drugs in the same functional but different chemical classes.

Controlled-substance schedule: Includes schedules for the United States (I, II, III, IV, V) and Canada (F, G).

Action: Describes pharmacologic properties concisely.

Uses: Lists the conditions the drug is used to treat.

Investigational uses: Describes drug uses that may be encountered in practice but are not yet FDA-approved.

Research notes: Describes key studies on new drug uses, doses, and interactions with specific references.

Dosages and routes: Lists all available and approved dosages and routes for adult, pediatric, and geriatric patients.

Available forms: Includes tablets, capsules, extended-release, injectables (IV, IM, SC), solutions, creams, ointments, lotions, gels, shampoos, elixirs, suspensions, suppositories, sprays, aerosols, and lozenges.

Side effects/adverse reactions: Groups these reactions by body system, with common side effects *italicized* and life-threatening reactions in **_bold italic type_** for emphasis.

Contraindications: Lists conditions under which the drug absolutely should not be given, including FDA pregnancy safety categories D or X.

Precautions: Lists conditions that require special consideration when the drug is prescribed, including FDA pregnancy safety categories A, B, and C.

Pharmacokinetics: Outlines metabolism, distribution, and elimination.

Interactions: Includes confirmed drug and food interactions, followed by the drug or nutrient causing that interaction, when applicable.

"Herb-Drug Interaction" icon (🌿): Highlights more than 400 potential interactions between herbal products and prescription or OTC drugs.

Do not confuse: Presents drug names that might easily be confused, within each appropriate monograph.

Lab test interferences: Identifies how the drug may affect lab test results.

Nursing considerations: Identifies key nursing considerations for each step of the nursing process: Assess, Administer, Perform/provide, Evaluate, and Teach patient/family. Instructions for giving drugs by various routes (e.g., IV, IM, PO) are included, with route subheadings in bold.

Compatibilities: Lists syringe, Y-site, and additive compatibilities and incompatibilities. If no compatibilities are listed for a drug, the necessary compatibility testing has not been done and that compatibility information is unknown. To ensure safety, assume that the drug may not be mixed with other drugs unless specifically stated.

"Nursing Alert" icon ($\Leftrightarrow$): Highlights a critical consideration.

"Do Not Crush" icon ($\bigcirc$): Denotes drugs that may not be administered in crushed form.

Treatment of overdose: Provides drugs and treatment for overdoses where appropriate.

Appendixes
Selected new drugs: Includes comprehensive information on 24 key drugs approved by the FDA during the last 12 months.

Recent FDA drug approvals: Summarizes basic information, such as generic name, trade name and uses, for drugs so recently approved by the FDA that complete information was not yet available when this book went to press.

Ophthalmic, otic, nasal, and topical products: Provides monographs for more than 140 ophthalmic, otic, nasal, and topical products commonly used today, grouped by chemical drug class.

Commonly used antiinfectives in adults and children: Presents at-a-glance adult and pediatric dosage information for common antiinfectives.

Vaccines and toxoids: Features an easy-to-use table with generic and trade names, uses, dosages and routes, and contraindications for 32 key vaccines and toxoids.

Antitoxins and antivenins: Provides dosages and contraindications.

Combination products: Provides details on the forms and uses of more than 700 combination products.

Less frequently used antihistamines: Includes names, uses, doses, forms, interactions and contraindications.

High-alert drugs: Lists the 118 drugs in *Mosby's Nursing Drug Reference* that are considered high-alert because of their potential to cause significant harm to patients.

Look-alike/sound-alike drug names: Includes 200 pairs of generic and trade drug names that are easily confused.

Herbal products: Features basic usage information on more than 70 common herbs and natural supplements.

FDA pregnancy categories: Explains the 5 FDA pregnancy categories.

Controlled substance chart: Covers both United States and Canadian drug schedules, with examples.

Abbreviations: Lists abbreviations alphabetically with their meanings.

Weights and equivalents: Provides the conversion for weight and volume among the metric, apothecary, and avoirdupois systems.

Formulas for drug calculations: Lists some of the most common and useful drug calculation formulas.

Nomogram for calculation of body surface area: Provides a quick, handy chart for calculating body surface area for patient drug calculations.

Bibliography: Lists key resources used in creating and updating *Mosby's 2003 Nursing Drug Reference*.

I am indebted to the nursing and pharmacology consultants who reviewed the manuscript and galley pages and thank them for their criticism and encouragement. I would also like to thank Darlene Como and Tamara Myers, my editors, whose active encouragement and enthusiasm have made this book better than it might otherwise have been. I am likewise grateful to Deborah Vogel, Carol O'Connell, and Graphic World, Inc., for the coordination of the production process, and to Dana Knighten for assistance with the development of the new edition.

Linda Skidmore-Roth

Contents

Drug Monographs New to This Edition (Appendix A)

alemtuzumab
almotriptan
anakinra
bosentan
cefditoren pivoxil
darbepoetin alfa
desloratadine
dexmethylphenidate
drotrecogin alfa
dutasteride
eprosartan mesylate/
    hydrochlorothiazide
ertapenem

esomeprazole
fondaparinux
formoterol fumarate
frovatriptan
galantamine
imatinib
nesiritide
perflutren lipid microsphere
tenofovir disoproxil fumarate
valdecoxib
valganciclovir
zoledronic acid

ALPHA-ADRENERGIC BLOCKERS

Action: Acts by binding to α-adrenergic receptors, causing dilation of peripheral blood vessels. Lowers peripheral resistance, resulting in decreased blood pressure.

Uses: Used for pheochromocytoma, prevention of tissue necrosis and sloughing associated with extravasation of IV vasopressors.

Side effects/adverse reactions: The most common side effects are hypotension, tachycardia, nasal stuffiness, nausea, vomiting, and diarrhea.

Contraindications: Hypersensitive reactions may occur, and allergies should be identified before these products are given. Patients with myocardial infarction, coronary insufficiency, angina, or other evidence of coronary artery disease should not use these products.

Pharmacokinetics: Onset, peak, and duration vary among products.

Interactions: Vasoconstrictive and hypertensive effects of epinephrine are antagonized by α-adrenergic blockers.

Possible nursing diagnoses:
• Altered tissue perfusion *[uses]*
• Risk for injury *[adverse reactions]*
• Sleep pattern disturbance *[adverse reactions]*

NURSING CONSIDERATIONS

Assess:
• Electrolytes: K, Na, Cl, CO_2
• Weight daily, I&O
• B/P lying, standing before starting treatment, q4h thereafter
• Nausea, vomiting, diarrhea
• Skin turgor, dryness of mucous membranes for hydration status

Administer:
• Starting with low dose, gradually increasing to prevent side effects
• With food or milk for GI symptoms

Evaluate:
• Therapeutic response: decreased B/P, increased peripheral pulses

Teach patient/family:
• To avoid alcoholic beverages
• To report dizziness, palpitations, fainting
• To change position slowly or fainting may occur
• To take drug exactly as prescribed
• To avoid all OTC products (cough, cold, allergy) unless directed by prescriber

---

Selected generic names
phentolamine

ANESTHETICS—GENERAL/LOCAL

Action: Anesthetics (general) act on the CNS to produce tranquilization and sleep before invasive procedures. Anesthetics (local) inhibit conduction of nerve impulses from sensory nerves.

Uses: General anesthetics are used to premedicate for surgery, induction and maintenance in general anesthesia. For local anesthetics, refer to individual product listing for indications.

Side effects/adverse reactions: The most common side effects are dystonia, akathisia, flexion of arms, fine tremors, drowsiness, restlessness, and hypotension. Also common are chills, respiratory depression, and laryngospasm.

Contraindications: Persons with CVA, increased intracranial pressure, severe hypertension, cardiac decompensation should not use these products, since severe adverse reactions can occur.

Precautions: Anesthetics (general) should be used with caution in the elderly, cardiovascular disease (hypotension, bradydysrhythmias), renal disease, liver disease, Parkinson's disease, children <2 yr. The precaution for anesthetics (local) is pregnancy.

Pharmacokinetics: Onset, peak, and duration vary widely among products. Most products are metabolized in the liver and excreted in urine.

Interactions: MAOIs, tricyclics, phenothiazines may cause severe hypotension or hypertension when used with local anesthetics. CNS depressants will potentiate general and local anesthetics.

Possible nursing diagnoses:

General:
• Risk for injury *[adverse reactions]*
• Knowledge deficit *[teaching]*

Local:
• Pain *[uses]*
• Knowledge deficit *[teaching]*

NURSING CONSIDERATIONS

Assess:
• VS q10min during IV administration, q30min after IM dose

Administer:
• Anticholinergic preoperatively to decrease secretions
• Only with crash cart, resuscitative equipment nearby

Perform/provide:
• Quiet environment for recovery to decrease psychotic symptoms

Evaluate:
• Therapeutic response: maintenance of anesthesia, decreased pain

Selected generic names (Injectables only)

General anesthetics
droperidol
etomidate
fentanyl
fentanyl/droperidol
fentanyl transdermal
ketamine
methohexital
midazolam
propofol
thiopental

Local anesthetics
lidocaine
procaine
ropivacaine
tetracaine

ANTACIDS

Action: Antacids are basic compounds that neutralize gastric acidity and decrease the rate of gastric emptying. Products are divided into those containing aluminum, magnesium, calcium, or a combination of these.

Uses: Hyperacidity is decreased by antacids in conditions such as peptic ulcer disease, reflux esophagitis, gastritis, and hiatal hernia.

Side effects/adverse reactions: The most common side effect caused by aluminum-containing antacids is constipation, which may lead to fecal impaction and bowel obstruction. Diarrhea occurs often when magnesium products are given. Alkalosis may occur when systemic products are used. Constipation occurs more frequently than laxation with calcium carbonate. The release of CO_2 from carbonate-containing antacids causes belching, abdominal distention, and flatulence. Sodium bicarbonate may act as a systemic antacid and produce systemic electrolyte disturbances and alkalosis. Calcium carbonate and sodium bicarbonate may cause rebound hyperacidity and milk-alkali syndrome. Alkaluria may occur when products are used on a long-term basis, particularly in persons with abnormal renal function.

Contraindications: Sensitivity to aluminum or magnesium products may cause hypersensitive reactions. Aluminum products should not be used by persons sensitive to aluminum; magnesium products should not be used by persons sensitive to magnesium. Check for sensitivity before administering.

Precautions: Magnesium products should be given cautiously to patients with renal insufficiency and during pregnancy and lactation. Sodium content of antacids may be significant; use with caution for patients with hypertension, CHF, or those on a low-sodium diet.

Pharmacokinetics: Duration is 20-40 min. If ingested 1 hr after meals, acidity is reduced for at least 3 hr.

Interactions: Drugs whose effects may be increased by some antacids: quinidine, amphetamines, pseudoephedrine, levodopa, valproic acid, dicumarol. Drugs whose effects may be decreased by some antacids: cimetadine, corticosteroids, ranitidine, iron salts, phenothiazines, phenytoin, digoxin, tetracyclines, ketoconazole, salicylates, isoniazid.

Possible nursing diagnoses:
• Pain *[uses]*
• Constipation *[adverse reactions]*
• Diarrhea *[adverse reactions]*

NURSING CONSIDERATIONS

Assess:
• Aggravating and alleviating factors of epigastric pain or hyperacidity; identify the location, duration, and characteristics of epigastric pain
• GI symptoms, including constipation, diarrhea, abdominal pain; if severe abdominal pain with fever occurs, these drugs should not be given
• Renal symptoms, including increasing urinary pH, electrolytes

Administer:
• All products with an 8-oz glass of water to ensure absorption in the stomach
• Another antacid if constipation occurs with aluminum products

Evaluate:
• The therapeutic effectiveness of the drug; absence of epigastric pain and decreased acidity should occur

Teach patient/family:
• Not to take other drugs within 1-2 hr of antacid administration, since antacids may impair absorption of other drugs

---

Selected generic names

aluminum hydroxide
bismuth subsalicylate
calcium carbonate
dihydroxyaluminum
   sodium carbonate

magaldrate
magnesium oxide
sodium bicarbonate

ANTIANGINALS

Action: The antianginals are divided into the nitrates, calcium channel blockers, and β-adrenergic blockers. The nitrates dilate coronary arteries, causing decreased preload, and dilate systemic arteries, causing decreased afterload. Calcium channel blockers dilate coronary arteries, decrease SA/AV node conduction. β-Adrenergic blockers decrease heart rate so that myocardial O_2 use is decreased. Dipyridamole selectively dilates coronary arteries to increase coronary blood flow.

Uses: Antianginals are used in chronic stable angina pectoris, unstable angina, vasospastic angina. Some (i.e., calcium channel blockers and β-blockers) may be used for dysrhythmias and in hypertension.

Side effects/adverse reactions: The most common side effects are postural hypotension, headache, flushing, dizziness, nausea, edema, and drowsiness. Also common are rash, dysrhythmias, and fatigue.

Contraindications: Persons with known hypersensitivity, increased intracranial pressure, or cerebral hemorrhage should not use some of these products.

Precautions: Antianginals should be used with caution in postural hypotension, pregnancy, lactation, children, renal disease, and hepatic injury.

Pharmacokinetics: Onset, peak, and duration vary widely among coronary products. Most products are metabolized in the liver and excreted in urine.

Interactions: Please check individual monographs since interactions vary widely among products.

Possible nursing diagnoses:
• Altered tissue perfusion: cardiopulmonary *[uses]*
• Pain *[uses]*
• Risk for injury *[uses]*
• Knowledge deficit *[teaching]*
• Decreased cardiac output *[adverse reactions]*

NURSING CONSIDERATIONS

Assess:
• Orthostatic B/P, pulse
• Pain: duration, time started, activity being performed, character
• Tolerance if taken over long period
• Headache, light-headedness, decreased B/P; may indicate a need for decreased dosage

Perform/provide:
• Storage protected from light, moisture; place in cool environment

Evaluate:
• Therapeutic response: decrease, prevention of anginal pain
Teach patient/family:
• To keep tabs in original container
• Not to use OTC products unless directed by prescriber
• To report bradycardia, dizziness, confusion, depression, fever
• To take pulse at home, advise when to notify prescriber
• To avoid alcohol, smoking, sodium intake
• To comply with weight control, dietary adjustments, modified exercise program
• To carry Medic Alert ID to identify drug that you are taking, allergies
• To make position changes slowly to prevent fainting

Selected generic names

Nitrates
amyl nitrite
isosorbide
nitroglycerin

β-*Adrenergic blockers*
atenolol
dipyridamole
metoprolol
nadolol
propranolol

Calcium channel blockers
amlodipine
bepridil
diltiazem
nicardipine
nifedipine
verapamil

ANTICHOLINERGICS

Action: Anticholinergics inhibit the muscarinic actions of acetylcholine at receptor sites in the autonomic nervous system; anticholinergics are also known as antimuscarinic drugs.

Uses: Anticholinergics are used for a variety of conditions: gastrointestinal anticholinergics are used to decrease motility (smooth muscle tone) in the GI, biliary, and urinary tracts and for their ability to decrease gastric secretions (propantheline, glycopyrrolate); decreasing involuntary movements in parkinsonism (benztropine, trihexyphenidyl); bradydysrhythmias (atropine); nausea and vomiting (scopolamine); and as cycloplegic mydriatics (atropine, hematropine, scopolamine, cyclopentolate, tropicamide).

Side effects/adverse reactions: The most common side effects are dry mouth, constipation, urinary retention, urinary hesitancy, headache, and dizziness. Also common is paralytic ileus.

Contraindications: Persons with narrow-angle glaucoma, myasthenia gravis, or GI/GU obstruction should not use some of these products.

Precautions: Anticholinergics should be used with caution in patients who are elderly, pregnant, or lactating or in those with prostatic hypertrophy, CHF, or hypertension; use with caution in presence of high environmental temp.

Pharmacokinetics: Onset, peak, and duration vary widely among products. Most products are metabolized in the liver and excreted in urine.

Interactions: Increased anticholinergic effects may occur when used with MAOIs and tricyclic antidepressants and amantadine. Anticholinergics may cause a decreased effect of phenothiazines and levodopa.

Possible nursing diagnoses:
• Decreased cardiac output [uses]
• Constipation [adverse reactions]
• Knowledge deficit [teaching]

NURSING CONSIDERATIONS
Assess:
• I&O ratio; retention commonly causes decreased urinary output
• Urinary hesitancy, retention; palpate bladder if retention occurs
• Constipation; increase fluids, bulk, exercise if this occurs
• For tolerance over long-term therapy, dose may need to be increased or changed
• Mental status: affect, mood, CNS depression, worsening of mental symptoms during early therapy
Administer:
• Parenteral dose with patient recumbent to prevent postural hypotension
• With or after meals to prevent GI upset; may give with fluids other than water
• Parenteral dose slowly; keep in bed for at least 1 hr after dose; monitor vital signs
• After checking dose carefully; even slight overdose can lead to toxicity
Perform/provide:
• Storage at room temp
• Hard candy, frequent drinks, sugarless gum to relieve dry mouth
Evaluate:
• Therapeutic response: decreased secretions, absence of nausea and vomiting
Teach patient/family:
• To avoid driving or other hazardous activities; drowsiness may occur

• To avoid OTC medication: cough, cold preparations with alcohol, antihistamines unless directed by prescriber

---

Selected generic names

atropine	hyoscyamine
benztropine	propantheline
biperiden	scopolamine (transdermal)
dicyclomine	trihexyphenidyl
glycopyrrolate	

ANTICOAGULANTS

Action: Anticoagulants interfere with blood clotting by preventing clot formation.

Uses: Anticoagulants are used for deep-vein thrombosis, pulmonary emboli, myocardial infarction, open-heart surgery, disseminated intravascular clotting syndrome, atrial fibrillation with embolization, transfusion, and dialysis.

Side effects/adverse reactions: The most serious adverse reactions are hemorrhage, agranulocytosis, leukopenia, eosinophilia, and thrombocytopenia, depending on the specific product. The most common side effects are diarrhea, rash, and fever.

Contraindications: Persons with hemophilia, leukemia with bleeding, peptic ulcer disease, thrombocytopenic purpura, blood dyscrasias, acute nephritis, and subacute bacterial endocarditis should not use these products.

Precautions: Anticoagulants should be used with caution in alcoholism, elderly, and pregnancy.

Pharmacokinetics: Onset, peak, and duration vary widely among products. Most products are metabolized in the liver and excreted in urine.

Interactions: Salicylates, steroids, and nonsteroidal antiinflammatories will potentiate the action of anticoagulants. Anticoagulants may cause serious effects; please check individual monographs.

Possible nursing diagnoses:

• Altered tissue perfusion *[uses]*
• Risk for injury *[side effects]*
• Knowledge deficit *[teaching]*

NURSING CONSIDERATIONS
Assess:
- Blood studies (Hct, platelets, occult blood in stools) q3mo
- Partial prothrombin time, which should be 1½-2 × control PPT qd, also APTT, ACT
- B/P, watch for increasing signs of hypertension
- Bleeding gums, petechiae, ecchymosis; black, tarry stools; hematuria
- Fever, skin rash, urticaria
- Needed dosage change q1-2wk

Administer:
- At same time each day to maintain steady blood levels
- Do not massage area or aspirate when giving SC injection; give in abdomen between pelvic bone, rotate sites; do not pull back on plunger; leave in for 10 sec; apply gentle pressure for 1 min
- Without changing needles
- Avoiding all IM injections that may cause bleeding

Perform/provide:
- Storage in tight container

Evaluate:
- Therapeutic response: decrease of deep-vein thrombosis

Teach patient/family:
- To avoid OTC preparations that may cause serious drug interactions unless directed by prescriber
- That drug may be held during active bleeding (menstruation), depending on condition
- To use soft-bristle toothbrush to avoid bleeding gums, avoid contact sports, use electric razor
- To carry a Medic Alert ID identifying drug taken
- To report any signs of bleeding: gums, under skin, urine, stools

---

Selected generic names

ardeparin
argatroban (Appx A)
dalteparin
danaparoid
enoxaparin

fondaparinux (Appx A)
heparin
lepirudin
tinzaparin
warfarin

ANTICONVULSANTS

Action: Anticonvulsants are divided into the barbiturates (p. 35), benzodiazepines (p. 37), hydantoins, succinimides, and miscellaneous products. Barbiturates and benzodiazepines are discussed in separate sections. Hydantoins act by inhibiting the spread of seizure activity in the motor cortex. Succinimides act by inhibiting spike and wave formation; they also decrease amplitude, frequency, duration, and spread of discharge in seizures.

Uses: Hydantoins are used in generalized tonic-clonic seizures, status epilepticus, and psychomotor seizures. Succinimides are used for absence (petit mal) seizures. Barbiturates are used in generalized tonic-clonic and cortical focal seizures.

Side effects/adverse reactions: Bone marrow depression is the most life-threatening adverse reaction associated with hydantoins or succinimides. The most common side effects are GI symptoms. Other common side effects for hydantoins are gingival hyperplasia and CNS effects such as nystagmus, ataxia, slurred speech, and mental confusion.

Contraindications: Hypersensitive reactions may occur, and allergies should be identified before these products are given.

Precautions: Persons with renal or hepatic disease should be watched closely.

Pharmacokinetics: Onset, peak, and duration vary widely among products. Most products are metabolized in the liver and excreted in urine, bile, and feces.

Interactions: Decreased effects of estrogens, oral contraceptives (hydantoins).

Possible nursing diagnoses:
- Risk for injury *[uses]*
- Noncompliance *[teaching]*
- Sleep pattern disturbance *[adverse reactions]*

NURSING CONSIDERATIONS
Assess:
- Renal function studies, including BUN, creatinine, serum uric acid, urine creatinine clearance before and during therapy
- Blood studies: RBC, Hct, Hgb, reticulocyte counts qwk for 4 wk then qmo
- Hepatic studies: AST, ALT, bilirubin, creatinine
- Mental status, including mood, sensorium, affect, behavorial changes; if mental status changes, notify prescriber
- Eye problems, including need for ophthalmic exam before, during, and after treatment (slit lamp, fundoscopy, tonometry)

• Allergic reactions, including red, raised rash; if this occurs, drug should be discontinued
• Blood dyscrasia, including fever, sore throat, bruising, rash, jaundice
• Toxicity, including bone marrow depression, nausea, vomiting, ataxia, diplopia, cardiovascular collapse, Stevens-Johnson syndrome
Administer:
• With food, milk to decrease GI symptoms
Perform/provide:
• Good oral hygiene is important for hydantoins
Evaluate:
• Therapeutic response, including decreased seizure activity; document on patient's chart
Teach patient/family:
• To carry ID card or Medic Alert bracelet stating drugs taken, condition, prescriber's name, phone number
• To avoid driving, other activities that require alertness

Selected generic names

Hydantoins	gabapentin
fosphenytoin	lamotrigine
phenytoin	magnesium sulfate
	paraldehyde
Succinimides	paramethadione
ethosuximide	phenacemide
methsuximide	phenobarbital
	primidone
Miscellaneous	tiagabine
acetazolamide	topiramate
carbamazepine	valproate/valproic acid,
clonazepam	divalproex sodium
diazepam	zonisamide
felbamate	

ANTIDEPRESSANTS

Action: Antidepressants are divided into the tricyclics, MAOIs, and miscellaneous antidepressants. The tricyclics work by blocking reuptake of norepinephrine and serotonin into nerve endings and increasing action of norepinephrine and serotonin in nerve cells. MAOIs act by increasing concentrations of endogenous epinephrine, norepinephrine, serotonin, dopamine in storage sites in CNS by inhibition of MAO; increased concentration reduces depression.

Uses: Antidepressants are used for depression and, in some cases, enuresis in children.

Side effects/adverse reactions: The most serious adverse reactions are paralytic ileus, acute renal failure, hypertension, and hypertensive crisis, depending on the specific product. Common side effects are dizziness, drowsiness, diarrhea, dry mouth, retention, and orthostatic hypotension.

Contraindications: The contraindications to antidepressants are convulsive disorders, prostatic hypertrophy, severe renal, hepatic, cardiac disease depending on the type of medication.

Precautions: Antidepressants should be used cautiously in suicidal patients, severe depression, schizophrenia, hyperactivity, diabetes mellitus, pregnancy, and the elderly.

Pharmacokinetics: Onset, peak, and duration vary widely among products. Most products are metabolized in the liver and excreted in urine.

Interactions: Please check individual monographs since interactions vary widely among products.

Possible nursing diagnoses:
• Ineffective individual coping *[uses]*
• Risk for injury *[uses/adverse reactions]*
• Knowledge deficit *[teaching]*

NURSING CONSIDERATIONS
Assess:
• B/P (lying, standing), pulse q4h; if systolic B/P drops 20 mm Hg, hold drug, notify prescriber; take vital signs q4h in patients with cardiovascular disease
• Blood studies: CBC, leukocytes, differential, cardiac enzymes if patient is receiving long-term therapy
• Hepatic studies: AST, ALT, bilirubin, creatinine
• Weight qwk; appetite may increase with drug
• EPS, primarily in elderly: rigidity, dystonia, akathisia
• Mental status: mood, sensorium, affect, suicidal tendencies, increase in psychiatric symptoms: depression, panic
• Urinary retention, constipation; constipation is more likely to occur in children, elderly
• Withdrawal symptoms: headache, nausea, vomiting, muscle pain, weakness; do not usually occur unless drug was discontinued abruptly
• Alcohol consumption; if alcohol is consumed, hold dose until morning
Administer:
• Increased fluids, bulk in diet if urinary retention, constipation occur
• With food or milk for GI symptoms
• Gum, hard candy, or frequent sips of water for dry mouth

Perform/provide:
- Storage in tight container at room temp; do not refreeze
- Assistance with ambulation during beginning therapy, since drowsiness, dizziness occur
- Safety measures including side rails primarily in elderly
- Checking to see PO medication swallowed

Evaluate:
- Therapeutic response: decreased depression

Teach patient/family:
- That therapeutic effects may take 2-3 wk
- To use caution in driving, other activities requiring alertness because of drowsiness, dizziness, blurred vision
- To avoid alcohol ingestion, other CNS depressants
- Not to discontinue medication quickly after long-term use; may cause nausea, headache, malaise
- To wear sunscreen or wide-brimmed hat, since photosensitivity may occur

---

Selected generic names

Tetracyclics	*Miscellaneous*	*SSRIs*
mirtazapine	bupropion	citalopram
	nefazodone	fluoxetine
Tricyclics	trazodone	fluvoxamine
amitriptyline	venlafaxine	paroxetine
amoxapine		sertraline
clomipramine	*MAOIs*	
desipramine	phenelzine	
doxepin	tranylcypromine	
imipramine		
nortriptyline		
trimipramine		

ANTIDIABETICS

Action: Antidiabetics are divided into the insulins that decrease blood sugar, phosphate, and potassium and increase blood pyruvate and lactate; and oral antidiabetics that cause functioning β-cells in the pancreas to release insulin, improve the effect of endogenous and exogenous insulin.
Uses: Insulins are used for ketoacidosis and diabetes mellitus types I (IDDM) and II (NIDDM); oral antidiabetics are used for stable adult-onset diabetes mellitus type II (NIDDM).

Side effects/adverse reactions: The most common side effect of insulin and oral antidiabetics is hypoglycemia. Other adverse reactions to oral antidiabetics include blood dyscrasias, hepatotoxicity, and rarely, cholestatic jaundice. Adverse reactions to insulin products include allergic responses and more rarely, anaphylaxis.

Contraindications: Hypersensitive reactions may occur, and allergies should be identified before these products are given. Oral antidiabetics should not be used in juvenile or brittle diabetes, diabetic ketoacidosis, severe renal disease, or severe hepatic disease.

Precautions: Oral antidiabetics should be used with caution in the elderly, in cardiac disease, pregnancy, lactation, and in the presence of alcohol.

Pharmacokinetics: Onset, peak, and duration vary widely among products. Oral antidiabetics are metabolized in the liver, with metabolites excreted in urine, bile, and feces.

Interactions: Interactions vary widely among products. Check individual monographs for specific information.

Possible nursing diagnoses:
• Altered nutrition: more than body requirements *[uses]*

NURSING CONSIDERATIONS
Assess:
• Blood, urine glucose levels during treatment to determine diabetes control (oral products)
• Fasting blood glucose, 2 hr PP (60-100 mg/dl normal fasting level) (70-130 mg/dl normal 2-hr level)
• Hypoglycemic reaction that can occur during peak time
Administer:
• Insulin after warming to room temp by rotating in palms to prevent lipodystrophy from injecting cold insulin
• Human insulin to those allergic to beef or pork
• Oral antidiabetic 30 min before meals
Perform/provide:
• Rotation of injection sites when giving insulin; use abdomen, upper back, thighs, upper arm, buttocks; rotate sites within one of these regions; keep a record of sites
Evaluate:
• Therapeutic response, including decrease in polyuria, polydipsia, polyphagia, clear sensorium, absence of dizziness, stable gait
Teach patient/family:
• To avoid alcohol and salicylates except on advice of prescriber
• Symptoms of ketoacidosis: nausea, thirst, polyuria, dry mouth, decreased B/P; dry, flushed skin; acetone breath, drossiness, Kussmaul respiration

- Symptoms of hypoglycemia: headache, tremors, fatigue, weakness; and that candy or sugar should be carried to treat hypoglycemia
- To test urine for glucose/ketones tid if this drug is replacing insulin
- To continue weight control, dietary restrictions, exercise, hygiene

Selected generic names

chlorpropamide
glipizide
glyburide
insulin aspart
insulin glargine
insulin lispro
insulin, regular
insulin, regular concentrated
insulin, zinc suspension
  (Lente)

insulin, zinc suspension
  extended (Ultralente)
insulin, zinc suspension,
  prompt (Semilente)
metformin
miglitol
pioglitazone
repaglinide
rosiglitazone
tolbutamide

ANTIDIARRHEALS

Action: Antidiarrheals work by various actions, including direct action on intestinal muscles to decrease GI peristalsis; by inhibiting prostaglandin synthesis responsible for GI hypermotility; by acting on mucosal receptors responsible for peristalsis; or by decreasing water content of stools.

Uses: Antidiarrheals are used for diarrhea of undetermined causes.

Side effects/adverse reactions: The most serious adverse reactions of some products are paralytic ileus, toxic megacolon, and angioneurotic edema. The most common side effects are constipation, nausea, dry mouth, and abdominal pain.

Contraindications: Persons with severe ulcerative colitis, pseudomembranous colitis with some products.

Precautions: Antidiarrheals should be used with caution in the elderly, pregnancy, lactation, children, dehydration.

Pharmacokinetics: Onset, peak, and duration vary widely among products. Most products are metabolized in the liver and excreted in urine.

Interactions: Please check individual monographs, since interactions vary widely among products.

Possible nursing diagnoses:
- Diarrhea *[uses]*
- Constipation *[adverse reactions]*
- Fluid volume deficit *[adverse reactions]*
- Knowledge deficit *[teaching]*

NURSING CONSIDERATIONS
Assess:
• Electrolytes (K, Na, Cl) if on long-term therapy
• Bowel pattern before; for rebound constipation after termination of medication
• Response after 48 hr; if no response, drug should be discontinued
• Dehydration in children
Administer:
• For 48 hr only
Evaluate:
• Therapeutic response: decreased diarrhea
Teach patient/family:
• To avoid OTC products
• Not to exceed recommended dose

Selected generic names

bismuth subsalicylate	loperamide
difenoxin	opium tincture
kaolin/pectin	

ANTIDYSRHYTHMICS

Action: Antidysrhythmics are divided into four classes and miscellaneous antidysrhythmics:
• Class I increases the duration of action potential and effective refractory period and reduces disparity in the refractory period between a normal and infarcted myocardium; further subclasses include Ia, Ib, Ic
• Class II decreases the rate of SA node discharge, increases recovery time, slows conduction through the AV node, and decreases heart rate, which decreases O_2 consumption in the myocardium
• Class III increases the duration of action potential and the effective refractory period
• Class IV inhibits calcium ion influx across the cell membrane during cardiac depolarization; decreases SA node discharge, decreases conduction velocity through the AV node
• Miscellaneous antidysrhythmics include those such as adenosine, which slows conduction through the AV node, and digoxin, which decreases conduction velocity and prolongs the effective refractory period in the AV node
Uses: These products are used for PVCs, tachycardia, hypertension, atrial fibrillation, angina pectoris.

Side effects/adverse reactions: Side effects and adverse reactions vary widely among products.
Contraindications: Contraindications vary widely among products.
Precautions: Precautions vary widely among products.
Pharmacokinetics: Onset, peak, and duration vary widely among products.
Interactions: Interactions vary widely among products; check individual monographs for specific information.
Possible nursing diagnoses:
* Decreased cardiac output *[uses]*
* Altered tissue perfusion: cardiopulmonary *[uses]*
* Diarrhea *[adverse reactions]*
* Impaired gas exchange *[adverse reactions]*

NURSING CONSIDERATIONS
Assess:
* ECG continuously to determine drug effectiveness, PVCs, or other dysrhythmias
* IV infusion rate to avoid causing nausea, vomiting
* For dehydration or hypovolemia
* B/P continuously for hypotension, hypertension
* I&O ratio
* Serum potassium
* Edema in feet and legs daily
Evaluate:
* Therapeutic response, including decrease in B/P in hypertension; decreased B/P, edema, moist rales in CHF
Teach patient/family:
* To comply with dosage schedule, even if patient is feeling better
* To report bradycardia, dizziness, confusion, depression, fever

Selected generic names

Class I	*Class II*
moricizine	acebutolol
	esmolol
Class Ia	propranolol
disopyramide	sotalol
procainamide	
quinidine	*Class III*
	amiodarone
Class Ib	bretylium
lidocaine	ibutilide
mexiletine	
phenytoin	*Class IV*
tocainide	verapamil
Class Ic	*Miscellaneous*
flecainide	adenosine
indecainide	atropine
propafenone	digoxin

ANTIFUNGALS (SYSTEMIC)

Action: Antifungals act by increasing cell membrane permeability in susceptible organisms by binding sterols and decreasing potassium, sodium, and nutrients in the cell.

Uses: Antifungals are used for infections of histoplasmosis, blastomycosis, coccidiomycosis, cryptococcosis, aspergillosis, phycomycosis, candidiasis, sporotrichosis causing severe meningitis, septicemia, and skin infections.

Side effects/adverse reactions: The most serious adverse reactions include renal tubular acidosis, permanent renal impairment, anuria, oliguria, hemorrhagic gastroenteritis, acute liver failure, and blood dyscrasias. Some common side effects include hypokalemia, nausea, vomiting, anorexia, headache, fever, and chills.

Contraindications: Persons with severe bone depression or hypersensitivity should not use these products.

Precautions: Antifungals should be used with caution in renal disease, pregnancy, and hepatic disease.

Pharmacokinetics: Onset, peak, and duration vary widely among products. Most products are metabolized in the liver and excreted in urine.

Interactions: Please check individual monographs since interactions vary widely among products.

Possible nursing diagnoses:
• Risk for infection *[uses]*
• Risk for injury *[adverse reactions]*
• Knowledge deficit *[teaching]*

NURSING CONSIDERATIONS

Assess:
• VS q15-30min during first infusion; note changes in pulse, B/P
• I&O ratio; watch for decreasing urinary output, change in specific gravity; discontinue drug to prevent permanent damage to renal tubules
• Blood studies: CBC, K, Na, Ca, Mg q2wk
• Weight weekly; if weight increases over 2 lb/wk, edema is present; renal damage should be considered
• For renal toxicity: increasing BUN, if >40 mg/dl or if serum creatinine >3 mg/dl; drug may be discontinued or dosage reduced
• For hepatotoxicity: increasing AST, ALT, alk phosphatase, bilirubin
• For allergic reaction: dermatitis, rash; drug should be discontinued, antihistamines (mild reaction) or epinephrine (severe reaction) administered
• For hypokalemia: anorexia, drowsiness, weakness, decreased reflexes, dizziness, increased urinary output, increased thirst, paresthesias
• For ototoxicity: tinnitus (ringing, roaring in ears), vertigo, loss of hearing (rare)

Administer:
• IV using in-line filter (mean pore diameter >1 μm) using distal veins; check for extravasation, necrosis q8h
• Drug only after C&S confirms organism, drug needed to treat condition; make sure drug is used in life-threatening infections

Perform/provide:
• Protection from light during infusion, cover with foil
• Symptomatic treatment as ordered for adverse reactions: aspirin, antihistamines, antiemetics, antispasmodics
• Storage protected from moisture and light; diluted sol is stable for 24 hr

Evaluate:
• Therapeutic response: decreased fever, malaise, rash, negative C&S for infecting organism

Teach patient/family:
• That long-term therapy may be needed to clear infection (2 wk-3 mo depending on type of infection)

Selected generic names

amphotericin B	itraconazole
fluconazole	ketoconazole
griseofulvin	nystatin

ANTIHISTAMINES

Action: Antihistamines compete with histamines for H_1-receptor sites. They antagonize in varying degrees most of the pharmacologic effects of histamines.

Uses: Products are used to control the symptoms of allergies, rhinitis, and pruritus.

Side effects/adverse reactions: Most products cause drowsiness; however, two of the newer products, astemizole and terfenadine, produce little, if any, drowsiness. Other common side effects are headache and thickening of bronchial secretions. Serious blood dyscrasias may occur, but are rare. Urinary retention, GI effects occur with many of these products.

Contraindications: Hypersensitivity to H_1-receptor antagonists occurs rarely. Patients with acute asthma and lower respiratory tract disease should not use these products since thick secretions may result. Other contraindications include narrow-angle glaucoma, bladder neck obstruction, stenosing peptic ulcer, symptomatic prostatic hypertrophy, newborn, lactation.

Precautions: These products must be used cautiously in conjunction with intraocular pressure since they increase intraocular pressure. Caution should also be used in patients with renal and cardiac disease, hypertension, seizure disorders, pregnancy, lactation, and in the elderly.

Pharmacokinetics: Onset varies from 20-60 min, with duration lasting 4-12 hr. In general, pharmacokinetics vary widely among products.

Interactions: Barbiturates, narcotics, hypnotics, tricyclic antidepressants, or alcohol can increase CNS depression when taken with antihistamines.

Possible nursing diagnoses:

• Ineffective airway clearance [uses]

NURSING CONSIDERATIONS

Assess:

• I&O ratio; be alert for urinary retention, frequency, dysuria; drug should be discontinued if these occur

• CBC during long-term therapy, since hemolytic anemia, although rare, may occur

- Blood dyscrasias: thrombocytopenia, agranulocytosis (rare)
- Respiratory status, including rate, rhythm, increase in bronchial secretions, wheezing, chest tightness
- Cardiac status, including palpitations, increased pulse, hypotension

Administer:
- With food or milk to decrease GI symptoms; absorption may be decreased slightly
- Whole (sustained release tabs)

Perform/provide:
- Hard candy, gum, frequent rinsing of mouth for dryness

Evaluate:
- Therapeutic response, including absence of allergy symptoms, itching

Teach patient/family:
- To notify prescriber if confusion, sedation, hypotension occur
- To avoid driving, other hazardous activity if drowsiness occurs
- To avoid concurrent use of alcohol, other CNS depressants
- To discontinue a few days before skin testing

Selected generic names

acrivastine/pseudoephedrine	diphenhydramine
azatadine	fexofenadine
brompheniramine	loratadine
budesonide	promethazine
cetirizine	trimeprazine
chlorpheniramine	tripelennamine
cyproheptadine	triprolidine
desloratadine (Appx A)	
dexchlorpheniramine	

ANTIHYPERTENSIVES

Action: Antihypertensives are divided into angiotensin-converting enzyme (ACE) inhibitors, β-adrenergic blockers, calcium channel blockers, centrally acting adrenergics, diuretics, peripherally acting antiadrenergics, and vasodilators. β-Blockers, calcium channel blockers, and diuretics are discussed in separate sections. Angiotensin-converting enzyme inhibitors act by selectively suppressing renin-angiotensin I to angiotensin II; dilation of arterial and venous vessels occurs. Centrally acting adrenergics act by inhibiting the sympathetic vasomotor center in the CNS that reduces impulses in the sympathetic nervous system; blood pressure, pulse rate, and cardiac output decrease. Peripherally acting antiadrenergics inhibit sympathetic vasoconstriction by inhibiting release of norepinephrine and/or depleting norepinephrine stores in adrenergic nerve endings. Vasodilators act on arteriolar smooth muscle by producing direct relaxation or vaso-dilation; a reduction in blood pressure, with concomitant increases in heart rate and cardiac output, occurs.

Uses: Used for hypertension and for heart failure not responsive to conventional therapy. Some products are used in hypertensive crisis, angina, and for some cardiac dysrhythmias.

Side effects/adverse reactions: The most common side effects are marked hypotension, bradycardia, tachycardia, headache, nausea, and vomiting. Side effects and adverse reactions may vary widely between classes and specific products.

Contraindications: Hypersensitive reactions may occur, and allergies should be identified before these products are given. Antihypertensives should not be used in patients with heart block or in children.

Precautions: Antihypertensives should be used with caution in the elderly, in dialysis patients, and in the presence of hypovolemia, leukemia, and electrolyte imbalances.

Pharmacokinetics: Onset, peak, and duration vary widely among products. Most products are metabolized in the liver, with metabolites excreted in urine, bile, and feces.

Interactions: Interactions vary widely among products; check individual monographs for specific information.

Possible nursing diagnoses:
• Altered tissue perfusion *[uses]*
• Decreased cardiac output *[uses]*
• Diarrhea *[adverse reactions]*
• Impaired gas exchange *[adverse reactions]*

NURSING CONSIDERATIONS
Assess:
• Blood studies: neutrophil; decreased platelets occur with many of the products
• Renal studies: protein, BUN, creatinine; watch for increased levels that may indicate nephrotic syndrome; obtain baselines in renal and liver function studies before beginning treatment
• Edema in feet and legs daily
• Allergic reaction, including rash, fever, pruritus, urticaria: drug should be discontinued if antihistamines fail to help
• Symptoms of CHF: edema, dyspnea, wet rales, B/P
• Renal symptoms: polyuria, oliguria, frequency
Perform/provide:
• Supine or Trendelenburg position for severe hypotension

Evaluate:
• Therapeutic response, including decrease in B/P in hypotension; decreased B/P, edema, moist rales in CHF

Teach patient/family:
• To comply with dosage schedule, even if feeling better
• To rise slowly to sitting or standing position to minimize orthostatic hypotension

Selected generic names

Angiotensin-converting enzyme inhibitors
benazepril
enalapril
fosinopril
quinapril
ramipril
trandolapril

Angiotensin II receptor blocker
candesartan
eprosartan (Appx A)
irbesartan
losartan
telmisartan
valsartan

Centrally acting adrenergics
clonidine
guanabenz

guanfacine
methyldopa

Peripherally acting antiadrenergics
guanadrel
guanethidine
prazosin
reserpine
terazosin

Vasodilators
diazoxide
fenoldopam
hydralazine
minoxidil
nitroprusside

Antiadrenergic combined
α-/β-*blocker*
labetalol

ANTIINFECTIVES

Action: Antiinfectives are divided into several groups, which include but are not limited to penicillins, cephalosporins, aminoglycosides, sulfonamides, tetracyclines, monobactam, erythromycins, and quinolones. These drugs act by inhibiting the growth and replication of susceptible bacterial organisms.

Uses: Used for infections of susceptible organisms. These products are effective against bacterial, rickettsial, and spirochete infections.

Side effects/adverse reactions: The most common side effects are nausea, vomiting, and diarrhea. Adverse reactions include bone marrow depression and anaphylaxis.

Contraindications: Hypersensitivity reactions may occur, and allergies should be identified before these products are given. Cross-sensitivity can occur between products of different classes (penicillins or cephalosporins). Many persons allergic to penicillins are also allergic to cephalosporins.

Precautions: Antiinfectives should be used with caution in persons with renal and liver disease.

Pharmacokinetics: Onset, peak, and duration vary widely among products. Most products are metabolized in the liver, and metabolites are excreted in urine, bile, and feces.

Interactions: Interactions vary widely among products; check individual monographs for specific information.

Possible nursing diagnoses:
• Risk for infection *[uses]*
• Diarrhea *[adverse reactions]*

NURSING CONSIDERATIONS

Assess:
• Nephrotoxicity, including increased BUN, creatinine
• Blood studies: AST, ALT, CBC, Hct, bilirubin; test monthly if patient is on long-term therapy
• Bowel pattern qd; if severe diarrhea occurs, drug should be discontinued
• Urine output; if decreasing, notify prescriber; may indicate nephrotoxicity
• Allergic reaction, including rash, fever, pruritus, urticaria; drug should be discontinued
• Bleeding: ecchymosis, bleeding gums, hematuria, stool guaiac daily
• Overgrowth of infection: perineal itching, fever, malaise, redness, pain, swelling, drainage, rash, diarrhea, change in cough, sputum

Administer:
• For 10-14 days to ensure organism death, prevention of superinfection
• After C&S completed; drug may be taken as soon as culture is taken

Evaluate:
• Therapeutic response, including absence of fever, fatigue, malaise, draining wounds

Teach patient/family:
• To comply with dosage schedule, even if feeling better
• To report sore throat, bruising, bleeding, joint pain; may indicate blood dyscrasias (rare)

Selected generic names

Aminoglycosides
amikacin
azithromycin
clarithromycin
gentamicin
kanamycin
neomycin
streptomycin
tobramycin

Cephalosporins
cefaclor
cefadroxil
cefamandole
cefazolin
cefdinir
cefditoren (Appx A)
cefepime
cefixime
cefmetazole
cefonicid
cefoperazone
ceforanide
cefotaxime
cefprozil
ceftibuten
cefuroxime
cephalexin
cephalothin
cephapirin
cephradine
moxalactam

Fluoroquinolones
alatrofloxacin/trovafloxacin
ciprofloxacin
enoxacin
levofloxacin

lomefloxacin
nalidixic acid
norfloxacin
ofloxacin
sparfloxacin

Miscellaneous
ertapenem (Appx A)
meropenem

Penicillins
amoxicillin/clavulanate
ampicillin/sulbactam
cloxacillin
dicloxacillin
imipenem/cilastatin
mezlocillin
nafcillin
oxacillin
penicillin G benzathine
penicillin G potassium
penicillin G procaine
penicillin G sodium
penicillin V potassium
piperacillin
ticarcillin
ticarcillin/clavulanate

Sulfonamides
sulfasalazine
sulfisoxazole

Tetracyclines
demeclocycline
doxycycline
minocycline
tetracycline

ANTINEOPLASTICS

Action: Antineoplastics are divided into alkylating agents, antimetabolites, antibiotic agents, hormonal agents, and miscellaneous agents. Alkylating agents act by cross-linking strands of DNA. Antimetabolites act by inhibiting DNA synthesis. Antibiotic agents act by inhibiting RNA synthesis and by delaying or inhibiting mitosis. Hormones alter the effects of androgens, luteinizing hormone, follicle-stimulating hormone, and estrogen by changing the hormonal environment.

Uses: Uses vary widely among products and classes of drugs. They are used to treat leukemia, Hodgkin's disease, lymphomas, and other tumors throughout the body.

Side effects/adverse reactions: Most products cause thrombocytopenia, leukopenia, and anemia, and if these reactions occur, the drug may have to be stopped until the problem is corrected. Other side effects include nausea, vomiting, glossitis, and hair loss. Some products also cause hepatotoxicity, nephrotoxicity, and cardiotoxicity.

Contraindications: Hypersensitive reactions may occur, and allergies should be identified before these products are given. Also, persons with severe liver and kidney disease should not use these products unless the benefits outweigh the risks.

Precautions: Persons with bleeding, severe bone marrow depression, or renal or hepatic disease should be watched closely.

Pharmacokinetics: Onset, peak, and duration vary widely among products. Most products cross the placenta and are excreted in breast milk and in urine.

Interactions: Toxicity may occur when used with other antineoplastics or radiation.

Possible nursing diagnoses:
• Risk for infection [adverse reactions]
• Altered nutrition: less than body requirements [adverse reactions]
• Altered oral mucous membrane [adverse reactions]

NURSING CONSIDERATIONS
Assess:
• CBC, differential, platelet count weekly; withhold drug if WBC is <4000/mm^3 or platelet count is <75,000/mm^3; notify prescriber of results
• Renal function studies, including BUN, creatinine, serum uric acid, and urine creatinine clearance before and during therapy
• I&O ratio; report fall in urine output of 30 ml/hr
• Monitor temp q4h (may indicate beginning infection)
• Liver function tests before and during therapy (bilirubin, AST, ALT, LDH) as needed or monthly
• Bleeding, including hematuria, guaiac, bruising or petechiae, mucosa, or orifices q8h; obtain prescription for viscous Xylocaine (lidocaine)
• Yellowing of skin, sclera, dark urine, clay-colored stools, itchy skin, abdominal pain, fever, diarrhea
• Edema in feet, joint pain, stomach pain, shaking
• Inflammation of mucosa, breaks in skin

Administer:
• Checking IV site for irritation; phlebitis
• Epinephrine for hypersensitivity reaction
• Antibiotics for prophylaxis of infection
Perform/provide:
• Strict asepsis, protective isolation if WBC levels are low
• Comprehensive oral hygiene, using careful technique and soft-bristle brush
Evaluate:
• Therapeutic response, including decreased tumor size
Teach patient/family:
• To report signs of infection, including increased temp, sore throat, malaise
• To report signs of anemia, including fatigue, headache, faintness, shortness of breath, irritability
• To report bleeding and avoid use of razors or commercial mouthwash

Selected generic names

Alkylating agents
busulfan
carboplatin
carmustine
chlorambucil
cisplatin
cyclophosphamide
dacarbazine
lomustine
mechlorethamine
melphalan
streptozocin
thiotepa

Antimetabolites
capecitabine
cytarabine
doxorubicin
etoposide
fludarabine
fluorouracil
mercaptopurine
thioguanine (6-TG)

Antibiotic agents
bleomycin
dactinomycin
daunorubicin
epirubicin
methotrexate
mitomycin
mitoxantrone
plicamycin

Hormonal agents
aminoglutethimide
estramustine
flutamide
goserelin
irinotecan
leuprolide
megestrol
mitotane
nilutamide
tamoxifen
testolactone
topotecan

Miscellaneous
altretamine
anastrozole
arsenic trioxide
asparaginase
cladribine
gemcitabine
interferon alfa-2A
interferon alfa-2B
irinotecan
pentostatin
porfimer
procarbazine
rituximab
vinblastine
vincristine
vinorelbine

ANTIPARKINSON AGENTS

Action: Antiparkinson agents are divided into cholinergics and dopamine agonists. Cholinergics work by blocking or competing at central acetylcholine receptors; dopamine agonists work by decarboxylation to dopamine or by activation of dopamine receptors; monoamine oxidase type B inhibitors work by increasing dopamine activity by inhibiting MAO type B activity.

Uses: Antiparkinson agents are used alone or in combination for patients with Parkinson's disease.

Side effects/adverse reactions: Side effects and adverse reactions vary widely among products. The most common side effects include involuntary movements, headache, numbness, insomnia, nightmares, nausea, vomiting, dry mouth, and orthostatic hypotension.

Contraindications: Persons with hypersensitivity, narrow-angle glaucoma, and undiagnosed skin lesions should not use these products.

Precautions: Antiparkinson agents should be used with caution in pregnancy, lactation, children, renal, cardiac, hepatic disease, and affective disorder.

Pharmacokinetics: Onset, peak, and duration vary widely among products. Most products are metabolized in the liver and excreted in urine.

Interactions: Please check individual monographs since interactions vary widely among products.

Possible nursing diagnoses:
- Risk for injury [uses]
- Risk for impaired physical mobility [uses]
- Knowledge deficit [teaching]

NURSING CONSIDERATIONS

Assess:
- B/P, respiration
- Mental status: affect, mood, behavioral changes, depression, complete suicide assessment

Administer:
- Drug up until NPO before surgery
- Adjust dosage depending on patient response
- With meals; limit protein taken with drug
- Only after MAOIs have been discontinued for 2 wk

Perform/provide:
- Assistance with ambulation, during beginning therapy
- Testing for diabetes mellitus, acromegaly if on long-term therapy

Evaluate:
• Therapeutic response: decrease in akathisia, increased mood
Teach patient/family:
• To change positions slowly to prevent orthostatic hypotension
• To report side effects: twitching, eye spasm; indicate overdose
• To use drug exactly as prescribed; if drug is discontinued abruptly, parkinsonian crisis may occur

Selected generic names

amantadine	levodopa
benztropine	pramipexole
biperiden	selegiline
bromocriptine	tolcapone
cabergoline	trihexyphenidyl
carbidopa-levodopa	

ANTIPSYCHOTICS

Action: Antipsychotics/neuroleptics are divided into several subgroups: phenothiazines, thioxanthenes, butyrophenones, dibenzoxazepines, dibenzodiazepines, and indolones and other heterocyclic compounds. Although chemically different, these subgroups share many pharmacologic and clinical properties. All antipsychotics work to block postsynaptic dopamine receptors in the brain that are responsible for psychotic behavior, including hallucinations, delusions, and paranoia.

Uses: Antipsychotic behavior is decreased in conditions such as schizophrenia, paranoia, and mania. These agents are also effective for severe anxiety, intractable hiccups, nausea, vomiting, behavioral problems in children, and for relaxation before surgery.

Side effects/adverse reactions: The most common side effects include EPS such as pseudoparkinsonism, akathisia, dystonia, and tardive dyskinesia, which may be controlled by use of antiparkinsonian agents. Serious adverse reactions such as hypotension, agranulocytosis, cardiac arrest, and laryngospasm have occurred. Other common side effects include dry mouth and photosensitivity.

Contraindications: Persons with liver damage, severe hypertension or coronary disease, cerebral arteriosclerosis, blood dyscrasias, bone marrow depression, parkinsonism, severe depression, narrow-angle glaucoma, children <12 yr, or persons withdrawing from alcohol or barbiturates should not use antipsychotics until these conditions are corrected.

Precautions: Caution must be used when antipsychotics are given to the elderly since metabolism is slowed and adverse reactions can occur rapidly. Hepatic and renal disease may cause poor metabolism and excretion of the drug. Seizure threshold is decreased with these products; increases in the dose of anticonvulsants may be required. Persons with diabetes mellitus, prostatic hypertrophy, chronic respiratory disease, and peptic ulcer disease should be monitored closely.

Pharmacokinetics: Onset, peak, and duration vary widely with different products and routes. Products are metabolized by the liver, are excreted in urine as metabolites, are highly bound to plasma proteins, cross the placenta, and enter breast milk. Half-life can be extended over 3 days.

Interactions: Because other CNS depressants can cause oversedation, these combinations should be used carefully. Anticholinergics may decrease the therapeutic actions of phenothiazines and also cause increased anticholinergic effects.

Possible nursing diagnoses:
• Altered thought processes *[uses]*
• Sensory/perceptual alterations *[uses]*

NURSING CONSIDERATIONS
Assess:
• Bilirubin, CBC, liver function studies qmo, since these drugs are metabolized in the liver and excreted in urine
• I&O ratio: palpate bladder if low urinary output occurs, since urinary retention occurs with many of these products
• Affect, orientation, LOC, reflexes, gait, coordination, sleep pattern disturbances
• Dizziness, faintness, palpitations, tachycardia on rising
• B/P lying and standing; wide fluctuations between lying and standing B/P may require dosage or product change, since orthostatic hypotension is occurring
• EPS, including akathisia, tardive dyskinesia, pseudoparkinsonism
Administer:
• Antiparkinsonian agent if EPS occur
• Liquid concentrates mixed in glass of juice or cola, since taste is unpleasant; avoid contact with skin when preparing liquid concentrate or parenteral medications
Perform/provide:
• Supervised ambulation until stabilized on medication; do not involve in strenuous exercise program because fainting is possible; patient should not stand still for long periods
• Increased fluids to prevent constipation
• Sips of water, candy, gum for dry mouth

Evaluate:
• Therapeutic response: decrease in excitement, hallucinations, delusions, paranoia, reorganization of thought patterns, speech

Teach patient/family:
• To rise from sitting or lying position gradually, since fainting may occur
• To remain lying down for at least 30 min after IM injections
• To avoid hot tubs, hot showers, or tub baths, since hypotension may occur
• To wear a sunscreen or protective clothing to prevent burns
• To take extra precautions during hot weather to stay cool; heat stroke can occur
• To avoid driving, other activities requiring alertness until response to medication is known
• That drowsiness or impaired mental/motor activity is evident the first 2 wk, but tends to decrease over time

---

Selected generic names

Phenothiazines	*Butyrophenone*
chlorpromazine	haloperidol
fluphenazine	
mesoridazine	*Miscellaneous*
perphenazine	loxapine
prochlorperazine	molindone
thioridazine	olanzapine
thiothixene	quetiapine
trifluoperazine	risperidone

ANTITUBERCULARS

Action: Antituberculars act by inhibiting RNA or DNA, or interfering with lipid and protein synthesis, thereby decreasing tubercle bacilli replication.

Uses: Antituberculars are used for pulmonary tuberculosis.

Side effects/adverse reactions: They vary widely among products. Most products can cause nausea, vomiting, anorexia, and rash. Serious adverse reactions include renal failure, nephrotoxicity, ototoxicity, and hepatic necrosis.

Contraindications: Persons with severe renal disease or hypersensitivity should not use these products.

Precautions: Antituberculars should be used with caution with pregnancy, lactation, and hepatic disease.

Pharmacokinetics: Onset, peak, and duration vary widely among products. Most products are metabolized in the liver and excreted in urine.

Interactions: Please check individual monographs since interactions vary widely among products.

Possible nursing diagnoses:
• Risk for infection *[uses]*
• Risk for injury *[adverse reactions]*
• Knowledge deficit *[teaching]*
• Noncompliance *[teaching]*

NURSING CONSIDERATIONS

Assess:
• Signs of anemia: Hct, Hgb, fatigue
• Liver studies qwk: ALT, AST, bilirubin
• Renal status before, qmo: BUN, creatinine, output, specific gravity, urinalysis
• Hepatic status: decreased appetite, jaundice, dark urine, fatigue

Administer:
• For some of these agents on empty stomach, 1 hr ac (only for isoniazid and rifampin) or 2 hr pc
• Antiemetic if vomiting occurs
• After C&S is completed; qmo to detect resistance

Evaluate:
• Therapeutic response: decreased symptoms of TB, culture negative

Teach patient/family:
• That compliance with dosage schedule, duration is necessary
• That scheduled appointments must be kept; relapse may occur
• To avoid alcohol while taking drug
• To report flulike symptoms: excessive fatigue, anorexia, vomiting, sore throat; unusual bleeding, yellowish discoloration of skin/eyes

---

Selected generic names

ethambutol	rifabutin
isoniazid	rifampin
pyrazinamide	streptomycin

ANTITUSSIVES/EXPECTORANTS

Action: Antitussives act by suppressing the cough reflex by direct action on the cough center in the medulla. Expectorants act by liquefying and reducing the viscosity of thick, tenacious secretions.

Uses: Antitussives/expectorants are used to treat cough occurring in pneumonia, bronchitis, TB, cystic fibrosis, and emphysema; as an adjunct in atelectasis (expectorants); and nonproductive cough (antitussives).

Side effects/adverse reactions: The most common side effects are drowsiness, dizziness, and nausea.

Contraindications: Some products are contraindicated in hypothyroidism, iodine sensitivity, pregnancy, and lactation.

Precautions: Some products should be used cautiously in asthmatic, elderly, and debilitated patients.

Pharmacokinetics: Onset, peak, and duration vary widely among products. Some products are metabolized in the liver and excreted in urine.

Interactions: Please check individual monographs since interactions vary widely among products.

Possible nursing diagnoses:
• Ineffective breathing pattern *[uses]*
• Ineffective airway clearance *[uses]*
• Knowledge deficit *[teaching]*

NURSING CONSIDERATIONS

Assess:
• Cough: type, frequency, character (including sputum)

Administer:
• Decreased dose to elderly patients; their metabolism may be slowed

Perform/provide:
• Increased fluids to liquefy secretions
• Humidification of patient's room

Evaluate:
• Therapeutic response: absence of cough

Teach patient/family:
• To avoid driving, other hazardous activities until patient is stabilized on this medication
• To avoid smoking, smoke-filled rooms, perfumes, dust, environmental pollutants, cleaners that increase cough

---

Selected generic names

acetylcysteine	dextromethorphan
ammonium chloride	guaifenesin
benzonatate	hydrocodone
codeine	

ANTIVIRALS/ANTIRETROVIRALS

Action: Antivirals act by interfering with DNA synthesis that is needed for viral replication.

Uses: Antivirals are used for mucocutaneous herpes simplex virus, herpes genitalis (HSV_1, HSV_2), advanced HIV infections, herpes simplex virus encephalitis, varicella-zoster encephalomyelitis.

Side effects/adverse reactions: Serious adverse reactions are fatal metabolic encephalopathy, blood dyscrasias, and acute renal failure. Common side effects are nausea, vomiting, anorexia, diarrhea, headache, vaginitis, and moniliasis.

Contraindications: Persons with hypersensitivity, or immunosuppressed individuals with herpes zoster should not use these products.

Precautions: Antivirals should be used with caution in renal disease, liver disease, lactation, pregnancy, and dehydration.

Pharmacokinetics: Onset, peak, and duration vary widely among products. Most products are metabolized in the liver and excreted in urine.

Interactions: Please check individual monographs since interactions vary widely among products.

Possible nursing diagnoses:

- Risk for infection *[uses]*
- Risk for injury *[adverse reactions]*
- Knowledge deficit *[teaching]*

NURSING CONSIDERATIONS

Assess:

- Signs of infection, anemia
- I&O ratio; report hematuria, oliguria, fatigue, weakness; may indicate nephrotoxicity; check for protein in urine during treatment
- Any patient with compromised renal system, since drug is excreted slowly in poor renal system function; toxicity may occur rapidly
- Liver studies: AST, ALT
- Blood studies: WBC, RBC, Hct, Hgb, bleeding time; blood dyscrasias may occur; drug should be discontinued
- Renal studies: urinalysis, protein, BUN, creatinine, CrCl
- C&S before drug therapy; drug may be taken as soon as culture is taken; repeat C&S after treatment
- Bowel pattern before, during treatment; if severe abdominal pain with bleeding occurs, drug should be discontinued
- Skin eruptions: rash, urticaria, itching
- Allergies before treatment, reaction of each medication; record allergies on chart in bright red letters

Administer:
• Increased fluids to 3 L/day to decrease crystalluria when given IV
Perform/provide:
• Storage at room temp for up to 12 hr after reconstitution
• Adequate intake of fluids (2 L) to prevent deposit in kidneys
Evaluate:
• Therapeutic response: absence or control of infection
Teach patient/family:
• That drug does not cure infection, just controls symptoms
• To report sore throat, fever, fatigue; could indicate superinfection
• That drug must be taken in equal intervals around the clock to maintain blood levels for duration of therapy
• To notify prescriber of side effects of bruising, bleeding, fatigue, malaise; may indicate blood dyscrasias

Selected generic names

abacavir	nelfinavir
acyclovir	nevirapine
amantadine	rimantadine
cidofovir	ritonavir
delavirdine	saquinavir
didanosine	stavudine
famciclovir	tenofovir (Appx A)
foscarnet	valganciclovir (Appx A)
ganciclovir	zalcitabine
indinavir	zidovudine

BARBITURATES

Action: Barbiturates act by decreasing impulse transmission to the cerebral cortex.

Uses: All forms of epilepsy can be controlled, since the seizure threshold is increased. Uses also include febrile seizures in children, sedation, insomnia, hyperbilirubinemia, chronic cholestasis with some of these products. Ultra-short-acting barbiturates are used as anesthetics.

Side effects/adverse reactions: The most common side effects are drowsiness and nausea. Serious adverse reactions such as Stevens-Johnson syndrome and blood dyscrasias may occur with high doses and long-term treatment.

Contraindications: Hypersensitivity may occur, and allergies should be identified before administering. Barbiturates are identified as pregnancy category D and should not be used in pregnancy. Other contraindications include porphyria and marked impairment of liver function.

Precautions: Caution must be used when these products are given to the elderly or debilitated; usually smaller doses are needed since metabolism is slowed. Persons with renal and hepatic disease may show delayed excretion. Barbiturates may produce excitability in children.

Pharmacokinetics: Onset of action can be slow, up to 1 hr, with a peak of 8 hr and a duration of 3-10 hr. These drugs are metabolized by the liver, excreted by the kidneys, cross the placenta, and enter breast milk.

Interactions: Increased CNS depressant effect may occur with alcohol, MAOIs, sedatives, or narcotics. These products should be used together cautiously. Oral anticoagulants, corticosteroids, griseofulvin, quinidine, oral contraceptives, and theophylline may show a decreased effect when used with barbiturates.

Possible nursing diagnoses:
• Sleep pattern disturbance *[uses]*
• Risk for injury *[adverse reactions]*

NURSING CONSIDERATIONS
Assess:
• Hepatic and renal studies: AST, ALT, bilirubin, creatinine, LDH, alkaline phosphatase, BUN if patient is on long-term therapy, since these products are metabolized and excreted by the liver and kidneys
• Blood studies: CBC, hematocrit, hemoglobin, and prothrombin time if patient is on long-term therapy, since these products increase the possibility of bleeding and blood dyscrasias
• Barbiturate toxicity: hypotension, pulmonary constriction; cold, clammy skin; cyanosis of lips, insomnia, nausea, vomiting, hallucinations, delirium, weakness
Evaluate:
• Therapeutic response, including appropriate sedation or seizure control
Teach patient/family:
• That physical dependency may result when used for extended periods (45-90 days, depending on dose)
• To avoid driving, activities that require alertness since drowsiness and dizziness may occur
• To abstain from alcohol or other psychotropic medications unless directed by prescriber
• Not to discontinue medication abruptly after long-term use; withdrawal symptoms will occur

---

Selected generic names

pentobarbital	secobarbital
phenobarbital	thiopental

BENZODIAZEPINES

Action: Benzodiazepines potentiate the effects of γ-aminobutyric acid (GABA), including any other inhibitory transmitters in the CNS, resulting in decreased anxiety.

Uses: Anxiety is relieved in conditions such as phobic disorders. Benzodiazepines are also used for acute alcohol withdrawal to relieve the possibility of delirium tremens, and some products are used for relaxation before surgery.

Side effects/adverse reactions: The most common side effects are dizziness, drowsiness, blurred vision, and orthostatic hypotension. Most adverse effects are mediated through the CNS. There is a risk of physical dependence and abuse.

Contraindications: Hypersensitivity, acute narrow-angle glaucoma, children <6 mo, liver disease (clonazepam), lactation (diazepam).

Precautions: Caution must be used when these products are given to the elderly or debilitated; usually smaller doses are needed, since metabolism is slowed. Persons with renal and hepatic disease may show delayed excretion. Clonazepam may increase incidence of seizures.

Pharmacokinetics: Onset of action is ½-1 hr, with a peak of 1-2 hr and a duration of 4-6 hr. These drugs are metabolized by the liver, excreted by the kidneys, cross the placenta, and enter breast milk.

Interactions: Increased CNS depressant effect may occur with other CNS depressants. These products should be used together cautiously. Alcohol should not be used; fatal reactions can occur. The serum concentration and toxicity of digoxin may be increased.

Possible nursing diagnoses:
• Anxiety *[uses]*
• Risk for injury *[adverse reactions]*

NURSING CONSIDERATIONS
Assess:
• B/P (lying, standing), pulse; if systolic B/P drops 20 mm Hg, hold drug, notify prescriber; orthostatic hypotension is severe
• Hepatic and renal studies: AST, ALT, bilirubin, creatinine, LDH, alkaline phosphatase
• Physical dependency, withdrawal symptoms, including headache, nausea, vomiting, muscle pain, weakness after long-term use
Administer:
• With food or milk for GI symptoms; may give crushed if patient is unable to swallow medication whole

Evaluate:
• Therapeutic response, including relaxation or decreased anxiety
Teach patient/family:
• That drug should not be used for everyday stress or long-term; not to take more than prescribed amount since drug is habit-forming
• To avoid driving and activities that require alertness since drowsiness and dizziness occur
• To abstain from alcohol, other psychotropic medications unless directed by prescriber
• Not to discontinue medication abruptly after long-term use; withdrawal symptoms will occur

---

Selected generic names

alprazolam	lorazepam
chlordiazepoxide	midazolam
clonazepam	oxazepam
diazepam	temazepam
flurazepam	triazolam

BETA-ADRENERGIC BLOCKERS

Action: β-Blockers are divided into selective and nonselective blockers. Nonselective blockers produce a fall in blood pressure without reflex tachycardia or reduction in heart rate through a mixture of β-blocking effects; elevated plasma renins are reduced. Selective β-blockers competitively block stimulation of β_1-receptors in cardiac smooth muscle; these drugs produce chronotropic and inotropic effects.

Uses: β-Blockers are used for hypertension, ventricular dysrhythmias, and prophylaxis of angina pectoris.

Side effects/adverse reactions: The most common side effects are orthostatic hypotension, bradycardia, diarrhea, nausea, vomiting. Serious adverse reactions include blood dyscrasias, bronchospasm, and CHF.

Contraindications: Hypersensitive reactions may occur, and allergies should be identified before these products are given. β-Adrenergic blockers should not be used in heart block, CHF, or cardiogenic shock.

Precautions: β-Blockers should be used with caution in the elderly or in renal and thyroid disease, COPD, CAD, diabetes mellitus, pregnancy, or asthma.

Pharmacokinetics: Onset, peak, and duration vary widely among products. Most products are metabolized in the liver, with metabolites excreted in urine, bile, and feces.

Interactions: Interactions vary widely among products; check individual monographs for specific information.

Possible nursing diagnoses:
• Altered tissue perfusion *[uses]*
• Decreased cardiac output *[uses]*
• Diarrhea *[adverse reactions]*
• Impaired gas exchange *[adverse reactions]*

NURSING CONSIDERATIONS

Assess:
• Renal studies, including protein, BUN, creatinine; watch for increased levels that may indicate nephrotic syndrome; obtain baselines in renal and liver function studies before beginning treatment
• I&O, weight daily
• B/P during beginning treatment and periodically thereafter; pulse q4h, note rate, rhythm, quality
• Apical/radial pulse before administration; notify prescriber of significant changes
• Edema in feet and legs daily

Administer:
• PO ac, hs; tablets may be crushed or swallowed whole
• Reduced dosage in renal dysfunction

Evaluate:
• Therapeutic response, including decrease in B/P in hypertension, decreased B/P, edema, moist rales in CHF

Teach patient/family:
• To comply with dosage schedule, even if feeling better
• To rise slowly to sitting or standing position to minimize orthostatic hypotension
• To report bradycardia, dizziness, confusion, depression, fever
• To take pulse at home; advise when to notify prescriber
• To comply with weight control, dietary adjustment, modified exercise program
• To wear support hose to minimize effects of orthostatic hypotension
• Not to discontinue drug abruptly; taper over 2 wk; may precipitate angina

Selected generic names

Selective β_1-receptor blockers
acebutolol
atenolol
esmolol
metoprolol

Combined α_1-, β_1-, and β_2-receptor blocker
labetalol

Nonselective β_1- and β_2-blockers
carteolol
nadolol
pindolol
propranolol
timolol

BRONCHODILATORS

Action: Bronchodilators are divided into anticholinergics, α/β-adrenergic agonists, β-adrenergic agonists, and phosphodiesterase inhibitors. Anticholinergics act by inhibiting interaction of acetylcholine at receptor sites on bronchial smooth muscle; α/β-adrenergic agonists by relaxing bronchial smooth muscle and increasing diameter of nasal passages; β-adrenergic agonists by action on β_2-receptors, which relaxes bronchial smooth muscle; phosphodiesterase inhibitors by blocking phosphodiesterase increase cAMP, which mediates smooth muscle relaxation in the respiratory system.

Uses: Bronchodilators are used for bronchial asthma, bronchospasm associated with bronchitis, emphysema, or other obstructive pulmonary diseases, Cheyne-Stokes respirations, prevention of exercise-induced asthma.

Side effects/adverse reactions: The most common side effects are tremors, anxiety, nausea, vomiting, and irritation in throat. The most serious adverse reactions include bronchospasm and dyspnea.

Contraindications: Persons with hypersensitivity, narrow-angle glaucoma, tachydysrhythmias, and severe cardiac disease should not use some of these products.

Precautions: Bronchodilators should be used with caution in lactation, pregnancy, hyperthyroidism, hypertension, prostatic hypertrophy, and seizure disorders.

Pharmacokinetics: Onset, peak, and duration vary widely among products. Most products are metabolized in the liver and excreted in urine.

Interactions: Please check individual monographs since interactions vary widely among products.

Possible nursing diagnoses:
- Ineffective airway clearance *[uses]*
- Activity intolerance *[uses]*

• Risk for injury *[adverse reactions]*
• Knowledge deficit *[teaching]*

NURSING CONSIDERATIONS
Assess:
• Respiratory function: vital capacity, forced expiratory volume, ABGs, lung sounds, heart rate and rhythm
Administer:
• After shaking, exhale, place mouthpiece in mouth, inhale slowly, hold breath, remove, exhale slowly
• Gum, sips of water for dry mouth
• PO with meals to decrease gastric irritation
Perform/provide:
• Storage in light-resistant container, do not expose to temps over 86° F (30° C)
Evaluate:
• Therapeutic response: absence of dyspnea, wheezing
Teach patient/family:
• Not to use OTC medications; extra stimulation may occur
• Use of inhaler; review package insert with patient
• To avoid getting aerosol in eyes
• To wash inhaler in warm water qd and dry
• To avoid smoking, smoke-filled rooms, persons with respiratory infections

Selected generic names

albuterol	ipratropium
aminophylline	isoproterenol
atropine	levalbuterol
bitolterol	metaproterenol
dyphylline	oxtriphylline
ephedrine	pirbuterol
epinephrine	terbutaline
formoterol (Appx A)	theophylline

CALCIUM CHANNEL BLOCKERS

Action: These products act by inhibiting calcium ion influx across the cell membrane in cardiac and vascular smooth muscle. This action produces relaxation of coronary vascular smooth muscle, dilates coronary arteries, slows SA/AV node conduction, and dilates peripheral arteries.

Uses: These products are used for chronic stable angina pectoris, vasospastic angina, dysrhythmias, hypertension, and unstable angina.

Side effects/adverse reactions: The most common side effects are dysrhythmias and edema. Also common are headache, fatigue, drowsiness, and flushing.

Contraindications: Persons with 2nd or 3rd degree heart block, sick sinus syndrome, hypotension of <90 mm Hg systolic, Wolff-Parkinson-White syndrome, or cardiogenic shock should not use these products since worsening of those conditions may occur.

Precautions: CHF may worsen since edema may be increased. Hypotension may worsen since B/P is decreased. Patients with renal and liver disease should use these products cautiously since they are metabolized in the liver and excreted by the kidneys.

Pharmacokinetics: Onset, peak, and duration vary widely with route of administration. Drugs are metabolized by the liver and excreted in the urine primarily as metabolites.

Interactions: Increased levels of digoxin and theophylline may occur when used with these products. Increased effects of β-blockers and antihypertensives may occur with calcium channel blockers.

Possible nursing diagnoses:
• Altered tissue perfusion: cardiopulmonary *[uses]*
• Decreased cardiac output *[adverse reactions]*

NURSING CONSIDERATIONS
Assess:
• Cardiac system, including B/P, pulse, respirations, ECG intervals (PR, QRS, QT)
Administer:
• PO before meals and hs
Evaluate:
• Therapeutic response, including decreased anginal pain, decreased B/P, dysrhythmias
Teach patient/family:
• How to take pulse before taking drug; patient should record or graph pulses to identify changes
• To avoid hazardous activities until stabilized on this drug, since dizziness commonly occurs
• Need for compliance in all areas of medical regimen, including diet, exercise, stress reduction, drug therapy

Selected generic names

diltiazem   nifedipine
felodipine   verapamil
nicardipine

CARDIAC GLYCOSIDES

Action: Products act by inhibiting sodium and potassium ATPase and then making more calcium available to activate contracted proteins. Cardiac contractility and cardiac output are increased.

Uses: These products are used for CHF, atrial fibrillation, atrial flutter, atrial tachycardia, and rapid digitalization in these disorders.

Side effects/adverse reactions: The most common side effects are cardiac disturbances, headache, hypotension, GI symptoms. Also common are blurred vision and yellow-green halos.

Contraindications: Hypersensitive reactions may occur, and allergies should be identified before these products are given. Also, persons with ventricular tachycardia, ventricular fibrillation, and carotid sinus syndrome should not use these products.

Precautions: Persons with acute MI and those who have or may develop serum potassium, calcium, or magnesium imbalances should use these products cautiously. Also, persons with AV block, severe respiratory disease, hypothyroidism, renal and liver disease, and the elderly should exercise caution when these drugs are prescribed.

Pharmacokinetics: Onset, peak, and duration vary widely with the route of administration. Digitoxin is inactivated by the liver, and inactive metabolites are excreted in urine. Digoxin is excreted in urine mainly as the parent drug and metabolites.

Interactions: Toxicity may occur when used with diuretics, succinylcholine, quinidine, and thioamines. Increased blood levels may occur with propantheline bromide, spironolactone, quinidine, verapamil, aminoglycosides (PO), amiodarone, anticholinergics, and quinine. Diuretics may increase toxicity.

Possible nursing diagnoses:
• Altered tissue perfusion: cardiopulmonary *[uses]*
• Decreased cardiac output *[adverse reactions]*

NURSING CONSIDERATIONS
Assess:
• Cardiac system, including B/P, pulse, respirations, and increased urine output

• Apical pulse for 1 min before giving drug; if pulse <60 bpm, take again in 1 hr; if still <60 bpm, notify prescriber
• Electrolytes, including K, Na, Cl, Mg; renal function studies, including BUN and creatinine; and blood studies, including AST, ALT, bilirubin
• I&O ratio, daily weights
• Monitor therapeutic drug levels

Administer:
• K supplements if ordered for K levels <3 mg/dl

Evaluate:
• Therapeutic response, including decreased weight, edema, pulse, respiration, and increased urine output

Teach patient/family:
• How to take pulse before taking drug; patient should record or graph pulse to identify changes
• To avoid hazardous activities until stabilized on this drug, since dizziness commonly occurs
• Need for compliance in all areas of medical regimen, including diet, exercise, stress reduction, drug therapy

---

Selected generic names
digoxin

CHOLINERGICS

Action: Cholinergics act by preventing destruction of acetylcholine, which increases concentration at sites where acetylcholine is released; this exaggerates the effects of acetylcholine and facilitates transmission of impulses across the myoneural junction. Cholinergics may also act by stimulating receptors for acetylcholine.

Uses: Cholinergics are used for myasthenia gravis, as antagonists of nondepolarizing neuromuscular blockade, postoperative bladder distention and urinary distention, and postoperative ileus.

Side effects/adverse reactions: The most serious adverse reactions are respiratory depression, bronchospasm, constriction, laryngospasm, respiratory arrest, convulsions, and paralysis. The most common side effects are nausea, diarrhea, and vomiting.

Contraindications: Persons with obstruction of the intestine or renal system should not use these products.

Precautions: Caution should be used in patients with bradycardia, hypotension, seizure disorders, bronchial asthma, coronary occlusion, hyperthyroidism, lactation, and in children.

Pharmacokinetics: Onset, peak, and duration vary widely among products. Most products are metabolized in the liver and excreted in urine.

Interactions: Please check individual monographs since interactions vary widely among products.

Possible nursing diagnoses:
• Altered urinary elimination *[uses]*
• Ineffective breathing pattern *[uses]*
• Knowledge deficit *[teaching]*
• Noncompliance *[teaching]*

NURSING CONSIDERATIONS

Assess:
• VS, respiration q8h
• I&O ratio; check for urinary retention or incontinence
• Bradycardia, hypotension, bronchospasm, headache, dizziness, convulsions, respiratory depression; drug should be discontinued if toxicity occurs

Administer:
• Only with atropine sulfate available for cholinergic crisis
• Only after all other cholinergics have been discontinued
• Increased doses if tolerance occurs
• Larger doses after exercise or fatigue
• On empty stomach for better absorption

Perform/provide:
• Storage at room temp

Evaluate:
• Therapeutic response: increased muscle strength, hand grasp, improved muscle gait, absence of labored breathing (if severe)

Teach patient/family:
• That drug is not a cure; it only relieves symptoms (myasthenia gravis)
• To wear Medic Alert ID specifying myasthenia gravis, drugs taken

---

Selected generic names

bethanechol	physostigmine
edrophonium	pyridostigmine
neostigmine	

CHOLINERGIC BLOCKERS

Action: Cholinergic blockers inhibit or block acetylcholine at receptor sites in the autonomic nervous system.

Uses: Many products are used to decrease secretions before surgery, to reverse neuromuscular blockade, and to decrease motility of GI, biliary, urinary tracts. Other products are used for parkinsonian symptoms, including dystonia associated with neuroleptic drugs.

Side effects/adverse reactions: The most common side effects are dryness of the mouth and constipation, which can be prevented by frequent rinsing of the mouth and by increasing water and bulk in the diet.

Contraindications: Hypersensitivity can occur, and allergies should be identified before administering these products. Persons with GI and GU obstruction should not use these products since constipation and urinary retention may occur. They are also contraindicated in angle-closure glaucoma and myasthenia gravis.

Precautions: Caution must be used when these products are given to the elderly, since metabolism is slowed. Also, persons with tachycardia or prostatic hypertrophy should use these products with caution.

Pharmacokinetics: Onset, peak, and duration vary with route.

Interactions: Increase in anticholinergic effect occurs when used with narcotics, barbiturates, antihistamines, MAOIs, phenothiazines, and amantadine.

Possible nursing diagnoses:
• Impaired physical mobility *[uses]*
• Pain *[uses]*

NURSING CONSIDERATIONS
Assess:
• I&O ratio; be alert for urinary retention, frequency, dysuria; drug should be discontinued if these occur
• Urinary hesitancy, retention; palpate bladder if retention occurs
• Constipation; increase fluids, bulk, exercise
• For tolerance over long-term therapy, dose may have to be increased or changed
• Mental status: affect, mood, CNS depression, worsening of mental symptoms during early therapy

Administer:
• With food or milk to decrease GI symptoms
• Parenteral dose with patient recumbent to prevent postural hypotension; give parenteral dose slowly, monitoring vital signs

Perform/provide:
• Hard candy, gum, frequent rinsing of mouth for dryness
Evaluate:
• Therapeutic response, including absence of cramps and EPS
Teach patient/family:
• To avoid driving, other hazardous activity if drowsiness occurs
• To avoid concurrent use of cough, cold preparations with alcohol, antihistamines unless directed by prescriber
• To use with caution in hot weather since medication may increase susceptibility to heat stroke

---

Selected generic names

atropine	glycopyrrolate
benztropine	scopolamine
biperiden	trihexyphenidyl

CORTICOSTEROIDS

Action: Corticosteroids are divided into glucocorticoids and mineralocorticoids. Glucocorticoids decrease inflammation by the suppression of migration of polymorphonuclear leukocytes, fibroblasts, increased capillary permeability, and lysosomal stabilization. They also have varied metabolic effects and modify the body's immune responses to many stimuli. Mineralocorticoids act by increasing resorption of sodium by increasing hydrogen and potassium excretion in the distal tubule.

Uses: Glucocorticoids are used to decrease inflammation and for immunosuppression. In addition, some products may be given for allergy, adrenal insufficiency, or cerebral edema. Mineralocorticoids are given for adrenal insufficiency or adrenogenital syndrome.

Side effects/adverse reactions: The most common side effects include change in behavior, including insomnia and euphoria; GI irritation, including peptic ulcer; metabolic reactions, including hypokalemia, hyperglycemia, and carbohydrate intolerance; and sodium and fluid retention. Most adverse reactions are dose dependent.

Contraindications: Hypersensitivity may occur and should be identified before administering. Since these products mask infection, they should not be used in systemic fungal infections or amebiasis. Mothers taking pharmacologic doses of corticosteroids should not nurse.

Precautions: Caution must be used when these products are prescribed for diabetic patients since hyperglycemia may occur. Also, patients with glaucoma, seizure disorders, peptic ulcer, impaired renal function, CHF, hypertension, ulcerative colitis, or myasthenia gravis should be monitored closely if corticosteroids are given. Use with caution in children and the elderly and during pregnancy.

Pharmacokinetics: For oral preparations, the onset of action occurs between 1 and 2 hr, and duration can be up to 2 days, with a half-life of 2-4 days. Pharmacokinetics vary widely among products. These products cross the placenta and appear in breast milk.

Interactions: Decreased corticosteroid effect may occur with barbiturates, rifampin, phenytoin; corticosteroid dose may have to be increased. There is a possibility of GI bleeding when used with salicylates, indomethacin. Steroids may reduce salicylate levels. When using with digitalis glycosides, potassium-depleting diuretics, and amphotericin, serum potassium levels should be monitored.

Possible nursing diagnoses:
• Risk for infection *[adverse reactions]*
• Body image disturbance *[adverse reactions]*
• Risk for violence: self-directed (suicide) *[adverse reactions]*

NURSING CONSIDERATIONS
Assess:
• Potassium, blood sugar, urine glucose while on long-term therapy; hypokalemia and hyperglycemia are common
• Weight daily; notify prescriber of weekly gain >5 lb, since these products alter fluid and electrolyte balance
• I&O ratio; be alert for decreasing urinary output and increasing edema
• Plasma cortisol levels during long-term therapy (normal level is 138-635 nmol/L SI U when drawn at 8 AM)
• Infection, including increased temp, WBC, even after withdrawal of medication; drug masks symptoms of infection
• Adrenal insufficiency: nausea, anorexia, fatigue, dizziness, dyspnea, weakness, joint pain
• Potassium depletion, including paresthesias, fatigue, nausea, vomiting, depression, polyuria, dysrhythmias, weakness
• Mental status, including affect, mood, behavioral changes, aggression; if severe personality changes occur, including depression, drug may have to be tapered and then discontinued
Administer:
• With food or milk to decrease GI symptoms
Evaluate:
• Therapeutic response, including decreased inflammation

Teach patient/family:
- That ID as steroid user should be carried
- Not to discontinue this medication abruptly, or adrenal crisis can result
- Teach patient all aspects of drug use, including cushingoid symptoms
- That single daily or alternate-day doses should be taken in the morning before 9 AM (for replacement therapy)
- To take with meals or a snack

Selected generic names

Glucocorticoids	methylprednisolone
beclomethasone	prednisolone
betamethasone	prednisone
cortisone	triamcinolone
dexamethasone	
hydrocortisone	*Mineralocorticoid*
hydrocortisone sodium phosphate	fludrocortisone

DIURETICS

Action: Diuretics are divided into subgroups: thiazides and thiazide-like diuretics, loop diuretics, carbonic anhydrase inhibitors, osmotic diuretics, and potassium-sparing diuretics. Each one of these subgroups has its own mechanism of action. Thiazides and thiazide-like diuretics increase excretion of water and sodium by inhibiting resorption in the early distal tubule. Loop diuretics inhibit resorption of sodium and chloride in the thick ascending limb of the loop of Henle. Carbonic anhydrase inhibitors increase sodium excretion by decreasing sodium-hydrogen ion exchange throughout the renal tubule. Carbonic anhydrase inhibitors also decrease secretion of aqueous humor in the eye and thus decrease intraocular pressure. Osmotic diuretics increase the osmotic pressure of glomerular filtrate, thus decreasing net absorption of sodium. The potassium-sparing diuretics interfere with sodium resorption at the distal tubule, thus decreasing potassium excretion.

Uses: Blood pressure is reduced in hypertension; edema is reduced in CHF; intraocular pressure is decreased in glaucoma.

Side effects/adverse reactions: Hypokalemia, hyperuricemia, and hyperglycemia occur most frequently with thiazide diuretics. Aplastic anemia, blood dyscrasias, volume depletion, and dehydration may occur when thiazide-like diuretics, loop diuretics, or carbonic anhydrase inhibitors are given. Side effects and adverse reactions vary widely for the miscellaneous products.

Contraindications: Persons with electrolyte imbalances (Na, Cl, K), dehydration, or anuria should not be given these products until the problem is corrected.

Precautions: Caution must be used when diuretics are given to the elderly, since electrolyte disturbances and dehydration can occur rapidly. Hepatic and renal disease may cause poor metabolism and excretion of the drug.

Pharmacokinetics: Onset, peak, and duration vary widely among the different subgroups of these drugs.

Interactions: Cholestyramine and colestipol will decrease the absorption of thiazide diuretics. Concurrent use of thiazides with diazoxide may increase hyperuricemia, hyperglycemia, and antihypertensive effects of thiazides. Ototoxicity may occur when loop diuretics are used with aminoglycosides. Thiazide and loop diuretics may increase therapeutic and toxic effects of lithium.

Possible nursing diagnoses:
• Fluid volume excess *[uses]*
• Decreased cardiac output *[adverse reactions]*

NURSING CONSIDERATIONS

Assess:
• Weight, I&O daily to determine fluid loss; check skin turgor for dehydration
• Electrolytes: K, Na, Cl; include BUN, blood sugar, CBC, serum creatinine, blood pH, ABGs, uric acid, Ca; electrolyte imbalances may occur quickly
• B/P lying, standing; postural hypotension may occur since fluid loss occurs first from intravascular spaces
• Signs of metabolic alkalosis, including drowsiness and restlessness
• Signs of hypokalemia with some products, including postural hypotension, malaise, fatigue, tachycardia, leg cramps, weakness

Administer:
• In AM to avoid interference with sleep if using drug as a diuretic
• K replacement if K is less than 3 mg/dl

Evaluate:
• Therapeutic response: improvement in edema of feet, legs, sacral area daily if medication is being used in CHF; improvement in B/P if medication is being used as a diuretic; improvement in intraocular pressure if medication is being used to decrease aqueous humor in the eye

Teach patient/family:
• To take drug early in the day (diuretic) to prevent nocturia

Selected generic names

Thiazides
chlorothiazide
hydrochlorothiazide

Thiazide-like
chlorthalidone
indapamide
metolazone

Loop
bumetanide
furosemide
torsemide

Carbonic anhydrase inhibitors
acetazolamide

Potassium-sparing
amiloride
spironolactone
triamterene

Osmotic
mannitol
urea

HISTAMINE H$_2$ ANTAGONISTS

Action: Histamine H$_2$ antagonists act by inhibiting histamine at the H$_2$-receptor site in parietal cells, which inhibits gastric acid secretion.

Uses: Histamine H$_2$ antagonists are used for short-term treatment of duodenal and gastric ulcers and maintenance therapy for duodenal ulcer; gastroesophageal reflux disease.

Side effects/adverse reactions: The most serious adverse reactions are agranulocytosis, thrombocytopenia, neutropenia, aplastic anemia, exfoliative dermatitis. The most common side effects are confusion (not with ranitidine), headache, and diarrhea.

Contraindications: Persons with hypersensitivity should not use these products.

Precautions: Caution should be used in pregnancy, lactation, child <16 yr, organic brain syndrome, hepatic disease, renal disease.

Pharmacokinetics: Onset, peak, and duration vary widely among products. Most products are metabolized in the liver and excreted in urine.

Interactions: Antacids interfere with absorption of histamine H$_2$ antagonists. Check individual monographs for other interactions.

Possible nursing diagnoses:
• Pain *[uses]*
• Risk for injury *[bleeding]*
• Knowledge deficit *[teaching]*

NURSING CONSIDERATIONS

Assess:

• Gastric pH (>5 should be maintained)
• I&O ratio, BUN, creatinine

Administer:

• With meals for prolonged drug effect
• Antacids 1 hr before or 1 hr after cimetidine
• IV slowly; bradycardia may occur; give over 30 min

Perform/provide:

• Storage of diluted sol at room temp for up to 48 hr

Evaluate:

• Therapeutic response: decreased pain in abdomen

Teach patient/family:

• That gynecomastia, impotence may occur, but are reversible
• To avoid driving, other hazardous activities until patient is stabilized on this medication
• To avoid black pepper, caffeine, alcohol, harsh spices, extremes in temp of food
• To avoid OTC preparations: aspirin, cough, cold preparations
• That drug must be continued for prescribed time to be effective
• To report bruising, fatigue, malaise; blood dyscrasias may occur

---

Selected generic names

cimetidine   ranitidine
famotidine

IMMUNOSUPPRESSANTS

Action: Immunosuppressants act by inhibiting lymphocytes (T).
Uses: Most products are used for organ transplants to prevent rejection.
Side effects/adverse reactions: The most serious adverse reactions are albuminuria, hematuria, proteinuria, renal failure, and hepatotoxicity. The most common side effects are overgrowth of oral *Candida,* gum hyperplasia, tremors, and headache. The most serious adverse reactions for azathioprine are hematologic (leukopenia and thrombocytopenia) and GI (nausea and vomiting). There is a risk of secondary infection.
Contraindications: Products are contraindicated in hypersensitivity.
Precautions: Caution should be used in severe renal disease, severe hepatic disease, and pregnancy.
Pharmacokinetics: Onset, peak, and duration vary widely among products. Most products are metabolized in the liver and excreted in urine.

Interactions: Please check individual monographs since interactions vary widely among products.

Possible nursing diagnoses:

• Risk for infection *[adverse reactions]*
• Risk for injury *[uses]*
• Knowledge deficit *[teaching]*

NURSING CONSIDERATIONS

Assess:

• Renal studies: BUN, creatinine at least qmo during treatment, 3 mo after treatment
• Liver function studies: alk phosphatase, AST (SGOT), ALT (SGPT), bilirubin
• Drug blood levels during treatment
• Hepatotoxicity: dark urine, jaundice, itching, light-colored stools; drug should be discontinued

Administer:

• For several days before transplant surgery
• With meals for GI upset or drug mixed with chocolate milk
• With oral antifungal for *Candida* infections

Evaluate:

• Therapeutic response: absence of rejection

Teach patient/family:

• To report fever, chills, sore throat, fatigue, since serious infections may occur
• To use contraceptive measures during treatment, for 12 wk after ending therapy

---

Selected generic names

azathioprine	muromonab-CD3
basiliximab	sirolimus
cyclosporine	tacrolimus

LAXATIVES

Action: Laxatives are divided into bulk products, lubricants, osmotics, saline laxative stimulants, and stool softeners. Bulk laxatives work by absorbing water and expanding to increase moisture content and bulk in the stool. Lubricants increase water retention in the stool, causing reabsorption of water in the bowel. Stimulants act by increasing peristalsis by direct effect on the intestine. Saline draws water into the intestinal lumen.

Osmotics increase distention and promote peristalsis. Stool softeners reduce surface tension of liquids of the bowel.

Uses: Laxatives are used as a preparation for bowel and rectal exam, constipation, and stool softener.

Side effects/adverse reactions: The most common side effects are nausea, abdominal cramps, and diarrhea.

Contraindications: Persons with GI obstruction, perforation, gastric retention, toxic colitis, megacolon, abdominal pain, nausea, vomiting, or fecal impaction should not use these products.

Precautions: Caution should be used in rectal bleeding, large hemorrhoids, and anal excoriation.

Pharmacokinetics: Onset, peak, and duration vary among products.

Interactions: Please check individual monographs since interactions vary widely among products.

Possible nursing diagnoses:
• Constipation *[uses]*
• Diarrhea *[adverse reactions]*
• Knowledge deficit *[teaching]*

NURSING CONSIDERATIONS
Assess:
• Blood, urine electrolytes if drug is used often by patient
• I&O ratio: to identify fluid loss
• Cause of constipation; identify whether fluids, bulk, or exercise is missing from lifestyle
• Cramping, rectal bleeding, nausea, vomiting; if these symptoms occur, drug should be discontinued
Administer:
• Alone only with water for better absorption; do not take within 1 hr of antacids, milk, or cimetidine
Evaluate:
• Therapeutic response: decrease in constipation
Teach patient/family:
• To swallow tabs whole; not to chew
• Not to use laxatives for long-term therapy; bowel tone will be lost
• That normal bowel movements do not always occur daily
• Not to use in presence of abdominal pain, nausea, vomiting
• To notify prescriber of abdominal pain, nausea, vomiting
• To notify prescriber if constipation is unrelieved or if symptoms of electrolyte imbalance: muscle cramps, pain, weakness, dizziness

Selected generic names

Bulk laxatives
calcium polycarbophil
methylcellulose
psyllium

Lubricants
mineral oil

Osmotic agents
glycerin
lactulose

Saline laxatives
magnesium salts
sodium biphosphate/phosphate

Stimulants
bisacodyl
cascara sagrada
senna

Stool softeners
docusate

NEUROMUSCULAR BLOCKING AGENTS

Action: Neuromuscular blocking agents are divided into depolarizing and nondepolarizing blockers. They act by inhibiting transmission of nerve impulses by binding with cholinergic receptor sites.

Uses: Neuromuscular blocking agents are used to facilitate endotracheal intubation and skeletal muscle relaxation during mechanical ventilation, surgery, or general anesthesia.

Side effects/adverse reactions: The most serious adverse reactions are prolonged apnea, bronchospasm, cyanosis, respiratory depression, and malignant hyperthermia. The most common side effects are bradycardia and decreased motility.

Contraindications: Persons who are hypersensitive should not be given this product.

Precautions: Caution should be used in pregnancy, thyroid disease, collagen disease, cardiac disease, lactation, children <2 yr, electrolyte imbalances, dehydration, neuromuscular disease (myasthenia gravis), and respiratory disease.

Pharmacokinetics: Onset, peak, and duration vary widely among products. Most products are metabolized in the liver and excreted in urine.

Interactions: Aminoglycosides potentiate neuromuscular blockade. See individual monographs.

Possible nursing diagnoses:
- Ineffective breathing pattern *[uses]*
- Risk for injury *[adverse reactions]*
- Knowledge deficit *[teaching]*

NURSING CONSIDERATIONS

Assess:

• For electrolyte imbalances (K, Mg); may lead to increased action of this drug
• Vital signs (B/P, pulse, respirations, airway) q15min until fully recovered; rate, depth, pattern of respirations, strength of hand grip
• I&O ratio; check for urinary retention, frequency, hesitancy
• Recovery: decreased paralysis of face, diaphragm, leg, arm, rest of body
• Allergic reactions: rash, fever, respiratory distress, pruritus; drug should be discontinued

Administer:

• Using nerve stimulator by anesthesiologist to determine neuromuscular blockade
• Anticholinesterase to reverse neuromuscular blockade
• IV undiluted over 1-2 min (only by qualified person, usually an anesthesiologist)

Perform/provide:

• Storage in light-resistant container, cool area
• Reassurance if communication is difficult during recovery from neuromuscular blockade

Evaluate:

• Therapeutic response: paralysis of jaw, eyelid, head, neck, rest of body

---

Selected generic names

atracurium	pipecuronium
doxacurium	succinylcholine
gallamine	tubocurarine
mivacurium	vecuronium
pancuronium	

NONSTEROIDAL ANTIINFLAMMATORIES

Action: Nonsteroidals decrease prostaglandin synthesis by inhibiting an enzyme needed for biosynthesis.

Uses: Nonsteroidal antiinflammatories are used to treat mild to moderate pain, osteoarthritis, rheumatoid arthritis, and dysmenorrhea.

Side effects/adverse reactions: The most serious adverse reactions are nephrotoxicity (dysuria, hematuria, oliguria, azotemia), blood dyscrasias, and cholestatic hepatitis. The most common side effects are nausea, abdominal pain, anorexia, dizziness, and drowsiness.

Contraindications: Persons with hypersensitivity, asthma, severe renal disease, and severe hepatic disease should not use these products.

Precautions: Caution should be used in pregnancy, lactation, children, bleeding disorders, GI disorders, cardiac disorders, hypersensitivity to other antiinflammatory agents, and the elderly.

Pharmacokinetics: Onset, peak, and duration vary widely among products. Most products are metabolized in the liver and excreted in urine.

Interactions: Please check individual monographs since interactions vary widely among products.

Possible nursing diagnoses:
• Chronic pain *[uses]*
• Impaired physical mobility *[uses]*
• Knowledge deficit *[teaching]*
• Noncompliance *[teaching]*

NURSING CONSIDERATIONS

Assess:
• Renal, liver, blood studies: BUN, creatinine, AST, ALT, Hgb, before treatment, periodically thereafter
• Audiometric, ophthalmic examination before, during, and after treatment
• For eye, ear problems: blurred vision, tinnitus; may indicate toxicity

Administer:
• With food to decrease GI symptoms; however, best to take on empty stomach to facilitate absorption

Perform/provide:
• Storage at room temp

Evaluate:
• Therapeutic response: decreased pain, stiffness in joints, decreased swelling in joints, ability to move more easily

Teach patient/family:
• To report blurred vision, ringing, roaring in ears; may indicate toxicity
• To avoid driving, other hazardous activities if dizziness, drowsiness occur, especially elderly
• To report change in urine pattern, increased weight, edema, increased pain in joints, fever, blood in urine; indicate nephrotoxicity
• That therapeutic effects may take up to 1 mo

Selected generic names

celecoxib

diclofenac

etodolac

fenoprofen

flurbiprofen (Appx C)

ibuprofen

indomethacin

ketoprofen

ketorolac

mefenamic acid (Appx F)

nabumetone

naproxen

piroxicam

sulindac

tolmetin

valdecoxib (Appx A)

OPIOID ANALGESICS

Action: Opioid analgesics act by depressing pain impulse transmission at the spinal cord level by interacting with opioid receptors. Products are divided into opiates and nonopiates.

Uses: Most products are used to control moderate to severe pain and are used before and after surgery.

Side effects/adverse reactions: GI symptoms, including nausea, vomiting, anorexia, constipation, and cramps are the most common side effects. Other common side effects include light-headedness, dizziness, sedation. Serious adverse reactions such as respiratory depression, respiratory arrest, circulatory depression, and increased intracranial pressure may result but are less common and usually dose dependent.

Contraindications: Hypersensitive reactions occur frequently. Check for sensitivity before administering. These drugs should not be used if narcotic addiction is suspected, and they are also contraindicated in acute bronchial asthma and upper airway obstruction.

Precautions: Caution must be used when these products are given to a person with an addictive personality since the possibility of addiction is so great. Also, they may worsen intracranial pressure. Persons with severe heart disease, hepatic or renal disease, respiratory conditions, or seizure disorders should be monitored closely for worsening condition.

Pharmacokinetics: Onset of action is immediate by IV route and rapid by IM and PO routes. Peak occurs from 1-2 hr, depending on route, with a duration of 2-8 hr. These agents cross the placenta and appear in breast milk.

Interactions: Barbiturates, other narcotics, hypnotics, antipsychotics, or alcohol can increase CNS depression when taken with narcotics.

Possible nursing diagnoses:

• Pain *[uses]*

• Impaired gas exchange *[adverse reactions]*

NURSING CONSIDERATIONS

Assess:

• I&O ratio; be alert for urinary retention, frequency, dysuria; drug should be discontinued if these occur

• Respiratory dysfunction, including respiratory depression, rate, rhythm, character; notify prescriber if respirations are <12/min

• CNS changes: dizziness, drowsiness, hallucinations, euphoria, LOC, pupil reaction

• Allergic reactions: rash, urticaria

• Need for pain medication; use pain scoring

Administer:

• With antiemetic if nausea or vomiting occurs

• When pain is beginning to return; determine dosage interval by response

Perform/provide:

• Assistance with ambulation; patient should not be ambulating during drug peak

Evaluate:

• Therapeutic response, including decrease in pain

Teach patient/family:

• To report any symptoms of CNS changes, allergic reactions, or shortness of breath

• That physical dependency may result when used for extended periods

• That withdrawal symptoms may occur, including nausea, vomiting, cramps, fever, faintness, anorexia

• To avoid alcohol and other CNS depressants

Selected generic names

alfentanil	meperidine
buprenorphine	methadone
butorphanol	morphine
codeine	nalbuphine
dezocine	oxycodone
fentanyl	oxymorphone
fentanyl transdermal	pentazocine
hydromorphone	propoxyphene
levorphanol	remifentanil

SALICYLATES

Action: Salicylates have analgesic, antipyretic, and antiinflammatory effects. The antiinflammatory and analgesic activities may be mediated through the inhibition of prostaglandin synthesis. Antipyretic action results from inhibition of the hypothalamic heat-regulating center.

Uses: The primary uses of salicylates are relief of mild to moderate pain and fever and in inflammatory conditions such as arthritis, thromboembolic disorders, and rheumatic fever.

Side effects/adverse reactions: The most common side effects are GI symptoms and rash. Serious blood dyscrasias and hepatotoxicity may result when used for long periods at high doses. Tinnitus or impaired hearing may indicate that blood salicylate levels are reaching or exceeding the upper limit of the therapeutic range.

Contraindications: Hypersensitivity to salicylates is common. Check for sensitivity before administering. Persons with bleeding disorders, GI bleeding, and vit K deficiency should not use these products since salicylates increase prothrombin time. Children should not use these products since salicylates have been associated with Reye's syndrome.

Precautions: Caution is needed when salicylates are given to patients with anemia, hepatic or renal disease, or Hodgkin's disease. Caution should also be exercised in pregnancy and lactation.

Pharmacokinetics: Onset of action occurs in 15-30 min, with a peak of 1-2 hr and a duration up to 6 hr. These drugs are metabolized by the liver and excreted by the kidneys.

Interactions: Increased effects of anticoagulants, insulin, methotrexate, heparin, valproic acid, and oral sulfonylureas may occur when used with salicylates. Aspirin may decrease serum concentrations of nonsteroidal antiinflammatory agents.

Possible nursing diagnoses:
- Pain *[uses]*
- Impaired physical mobility *[uses]*
- Activity intolerance *[uses]*
- Sensory/perceptual alterations: auditory *[adverse reactions]*
- Ineffective thermoregulation *[uses]*

NURSING CONSIDERATIONS

Assess:
- Hepatic and renal studies: AST, ALT, bilirubin, creatinine, LDH, alk phosphatase, BUN if patient is on long-term therapy, since these products are metabolized and excreted by the liver and kidney
- Blood studies: CBC, hematocrit, hemoglobin, and prothrombin time if

patient is on long-term therapy, since these products increase the possibility of bleeding and blood dyscrasias
• Hepatotoxicity: dark urine, clay-colored stools; yellowing of skin, sclera; itching, abdominal pain, fever, diarrhea, which may occur with long-term use
• Ototoxicity: tinnitus; ringing, roaring in ears; audiometric testing is needed before and after long-term therapy
Administer:
• With food or milk to decrease gastric irritation; give 30 min before or 1 hr after meals with a full glass of water
Evaluate:
• Therapeutic response, including decreased pain, fever
Teach patient/family:
• That blood sugar levels should be monitored closely if patient is diabetic
• Not to exceed recommended dosage; acute poisoning may result
• That therapeutic response takes 2 wk in arthritis
• To avoid use of alcohol, since GI bleeding may result
• To notify prescriber of ringing in the ears or persistent GI pain
• To take with full glass of water to reduce risk of lodging in esophagus

---

Selected generic names

aspirin	magnesium salicylate
choline salicylate	salsalate

THROMBOLYTICS

Action: Thrombolytics act by activating conversion of plasminogen to plasmin (fibrinolysin): plasmin is able to break down clots (fibrin).
Uses: Thrombolytics are used to treat deep-vein thrombosis, pulmonary embolism, arterial thrombosis, arterial embolism, arteriovenous cannula occlusion, lysis of coronary artery thrombi after MI, and acute, evolving transmural MI.
Side effects/adverse reactions: Serious adverse reactions include GI, GU, intracranial retroperitoneal bleeding, and anaphylaxis. The most common side effects are decreased Hct, urticaria, headache, and nausea.
Contraindications: Persons with hypersensitivity, active bleeding, intraspinal surgery, neoplasms of the CNS, ulcerative colitis/enteritis, severe hypertension, renal disease, hepatic disease, hypocoagulation, COPD, subacute bacterial endocarditis, rheumatic valvular disease, cerebral embolism/thrombosis/hemorrhage, recent intraarterial diagnostic procedure or surgery (10 days), and recent major surgery should not use these products.

Precautions: Caution should be used in arterial emboli from left side of heart and pregnancy.

Pharmacokinetics: Onset, peak, and duration vary widely among products. Most products are metabolized in the liver and excreted in urine.

Interactions: Please check individual monographs since interactions vary widely among products.

Possible nursing diagnoses:
• Risk for injury *[uses]*

NURSING CONSIDERATIONS
Assess:
• VS, B/P, pulse, resp, neuro signs, temp at least q4h; temp >104° F (40° C) indicator of internal bleeding; cardiac rhythm following intracoronary administration; systolic pressure increase of >25 mm Hg should be reported to prescriber
• For neurologic changes that may indicate intracranial bleeding
• Retroperitoneal bleeding: back pain, leg weakness, diminished pulses
• Allergy: fever, rash, itching, chill; mild reaction may be treated with antihistamines
• For bleeding during 1st hr of treatment: hematuria, hematemesis, bleeding from mucous membranes, epistaxis, ecchymosis
• Blood studies (Hct, platelets, PTT, PT, TT, APTT) before starting therapy; PT or APTT must be less than ×2 control before starting therapy; TT or PT q3-4h during treatment

Administer:
• As soon as thrombi identified; not useful for thrombi over 1 wk old
• Cryoprecipitate or fresh, frozen plasma if bleeding occurs
• Loading dose at beginning of therapy; may require increased loading doses
• Heparin after fibrinogen level is over 100 mg/dl. Heparin infusion to increase PTT to 1.5-2 × baseline for 3-7 days
• About 10% of patients have high streptococcal antibody titers requiring increased loading doses
• IV therapy using 0.8 µm filter

Perform/provide:
• Storage of reconstituted drug in refrigerator; discard after 24 hr
• Bed rest during entire course of treatment
• Avoidance of venous or arterial puncture, inj, rectal temp
• Treatment of fever with acetaminophen or aspirin
• Pressure for 30 sec to minor bleeding sites; inform prescriber if this does not attain hemostasis; apply pressure dressing

Evaluate:
• Therapeutic response: resolution of thrombosis, embolism

Selected generic names

alteplase	streptokinase
anistreplase	tenecteplase
drotrecogin alfa (Appx A)	urokinase

THYROID HORMONES

Action: Acts by increasing metabolic rates, resulting in increased cardiac output, O_2 consumption, body temp, blood volume, growth, development at cellular level, respiratory rate, enzyme system activity.

Uses: Products are used for thyroid replacement.

Side effects/adverse reactions: The most common side effects include insomnia, tremors, tachycardia, palpitations, angina, dysrhythmias, weight loss, and changes in appetite. Serious adverse reactions include thyroid storm.

Contraindications: Persons with adrenal insufficiency, myocardial infarction, or thyrotoxicosis should not use these products.

Precautions: The elderly and patients with angina pectoris, hypertension, ischemia, cardiac disease, or diabetes mellitus or insipidus should be watched closely when using these products. Caution should be used in pregnancy (A) and lactation.

Pharmacokinetics: Pharmacokinetics vary widely among products; check specific monographs.

Interactions:
• Impaired absorption of thyroid products may occur when administered with cholestyramine (separate by 4-5 hr)
• Increased effects of anticoagulants, sympathomimetics, tricyclic antidepressants, catecholamines may occur
• Decreased effects of digitalis, glycosides, insulin, hypoglycemics may occur
• Decreased effects of thyroid products may occur with estrogens

Possible nursing diagnoses:
• Knowledge deficit *[teaching]*
• Noncompliance *[teaching]*
• Body image disturbance *[adverse reactions]*

NURSING CONSIDERATIONS
Assess:
• B/P, pulse before each dose
• I&O ratio
• Weight qd in same clothing, using same scale, at same time of day

- Height, growth rate if given to a child
- T_3, T_4, which are decreased; radioimmunoassay of TSH, which is increased; ratio uptake, which is decreased if patient is on too low a dosage of medication
- Increased nervousness, excitability, irritability; may indicate overdosage, usually after 1-3 wk of treatment
- Cardiac status: angina, palpitation, chest pain, change in VS

Administer:
- At same time each day to maintain drug level
- Only for hormone imbalances, not to be used for obesity, male infertility, menstrual conditions, lethargy

Perform/provide:
- Removal of medication 4 wk before RAIU test

Evaluate:
- Therapeutic response: absence of depression; increased weight loss; diuresis; pulse; appetite; absence of constipation; peripheral edema; cold intolerance; pale, cool, dry skin; brittle nails; alopecia; coarse hair; menorrhagia; night blindness; paresthesias; syncope; stupor; coma; rosy cheeks

Teach patient/family:
- That hair loss will occur in child and is temporary
- To report excitability, irritability, anxiety; indicates overdose
- Not to switch brands unless directed by prescriber
- That hypothyroid child will show almost immediate behavior/personality change
- That treatment drug is not to be taken to reduce weight
- To avoid OTC preparations with iodine; read labels
- To avoid iodine in food, iodinized salt, soybeans, tofu, turnips, some seafood, some bread

---

Selected generic names

levothyroxine (T_4)   liotrix
liothyronine (T_3)   thyroid USP

VASODILATORS

Action: Vasodilators have various modes of action. Please check individual monographs for specific action.

Uses: Vasodilators are used to treat intermittent claudication, arteriosclerosis obliterans, vasospasm and muscular ischemia, ischemic cerebral vascular disease, hypertension, and angina.

Side effects/adverse reactions: The most common side effects are headache, nausea, hypotension or hypertension, and ECG changes.

Contraindications: Some drugs are contraindicated in acute MI, paroxysmal tachycardia, and thyrotoxicosis.

Precautions: Caution should be used in uncompensated heart disease or peptic ulcer disease.

Pharmacokinetics: Onset, peak, and duration vary widely among products. Most products are metabolized in the liver and excreted in urine.

Interactions: Please check individual monographs since interactions vary widely among products.

Possible nursing diagnoses:
• Decreased cardiac output [uses]
• Altered tissue perfusion: cardiopulmonary [uses]
• Knowledge deficit [teaching]

NURSING CONSIDERATIONS
Assess:
• Bleeding time in individuals with bleeding disorders
• Cardiac status: B/P, pulse, rate, rhythm, character; watch for increasing pulse

Administer:
• With meals to reduce GI symptoms

Perform/provide:
• Storage in tight container at room temp

Evaluate:
• Therapeutic response: ability to walk without pain, increased temp in extremities, increased pulse volume

Teach patient/family:
• That medication is not cure; may need to be taken continuously
• That it is necessary to quit smoking to prevent excessive vasoconstriction
• That improvement may be sudden, but usually occurs gradually over several wk
• To report headache, weakness, increased pulse, as drug may have to be decreased or discontinued
• To avoid hazardous activities until stabilized on medication; dizziness may occur

---

Selected generic names

amyl nitrite
bosentan (Appx A)
dipyridamole
hydralazine

isoxsuprine
minoxidil
nesiritide (Appx A)
papaverine

VITAMINS

Action: Action varies widely among products and classes; check specific monographs.

Uses: Vitamins are used to correct and prevent vitamin deficiencies.

Side effects/adverse reactions: There are no side effects or adverse reactions with the water-soluble vitamins (C, B). However, fat-soluble vitamins (A, D, E, K) may accumulate in the body and cause adverse reactions (see specific monographs).

Contraindications: Hypersensitive reactions may occur, and allergies should be identified before these products are given.

Pharmacokinetics: Onset, peak, and duration vary widely among products; check individual monographs for specific information.

Possible nursing diagnoses:
• Altered nutrition: less than body requirements [uses]

NURSING CONSIDERATIONS
Administer:
• PO with food for better absorption
Perform/provide:
• Storage in tight, light-resistant container
Evaluate:
• Therapeutic response: no vitamin deficiency
Teach patient/family:
• Not to take more than prescribed amount

Selected generic names

Fat-soluble
phytonadione (vita-
  min K_1)
vitamin A
vitamin D
vitamin E

Water-soluble
ascorbic acid (C)

cyanocobalamin B_{12}/hydroxo-
  cobalamin (B_{12}a)
pyridoxine (B_6)
riboflavin (B_2)
thiamine (B_1)

Miscellaneous
  multivitamins

abacavir (℞)

(ah-bak'ah-veer)
Ziagen
Func. class.: Antiviral
Chem. class.: Nucleoside ana-
log

Action: A synthetic nucleoside analog with inhibitory action against
HIV. Inhibits replication of the virus
by incorporating into cellular DNA
by viral reverse transcriptase, thereby
terminating the cellular DNA chain
Uses: In combination with other antiretroviral agents for HIV-1 infection

Research note: One study has reported a reduced viral load in adults
and children with HIV when abciximab is combined with lamivudine,
zidovudine, abacavir[1]

Dosage and routes:
• *Adult:* **PO** 300 mg bid with other
antiretrovirals
• *Adolescents and child ≥3 mo:* 8
mg/kg bid, max 300 mg bid with
other antiretrovirals
Available forms: Tabs 300 mg; oral
sol 20 mg/ml

Side effects/adverse reactions:
*HEMA: **Granulocytopenia, anemia,
lymphopenia***
*CNS: Fever, headache, malaise, in-
somnia,* paresthesia
*GI: Nausea, vomiting, diarrhea, an-
orexia,* cramps, abdominal pain, in-
creased AST, ALT
RESP: Dyspnea
*INTEG: Rash, **fatal hypersensitivity
reactions,*** urticaria
*META: **Lactic acidosis***
OTHER: Increased CPK

Contraindications: Hypersensitivity

Precautions: Granulocyte count
<1000/mm³ or Hgb <9.5 g/dl, preg-
nancy (C), lactation, children, se-

vere renal disease, impaired hepatic
function

Pharmacokinetics: 50% plasma
protein binding, metabolized to
inactive metabolites, half-life 1½-
2 hr

Interactions:
• Increased abacavir levels: alcohol

**NURSING CONSIDERATIONS
Assess:**
◆For lactic acidosis and severe hepatomegaly with steatosis
◆ For fatal hypersensitivity reactions: fever, rash, nausea, vomiting,
diarrhea, abdominal discomfort;
treatment should be discontinued and
not restarted
• For blood dyscrasias (anemia,
granulocytopenia): bruising, fatigue,
bleeding, poor healing
• For increased temp, may indicate
beginning infection
• Renal function studies: BUN, serum uric acid, CrCl before, during
therapy; these may be elevated
throughout treatment
• Liver function tests before and during therapy: bilirubin, AST, ALT,
amylase, alk phosphatase q mo
• Blood counts q2wk; watch for decreasing granulocytes, Hgb; if low,
therapy may have to be discontinued and restarted after hematologic
recovery; blood transfusions may be
required

Administer:
• Give in combination with other
antiretrovirals with food

Perform/provide:
• Storage in cool environment; protect from light

Teach patient/family:
• That drug is not cure for AIDS but
will control symptoms
• To notify prescriber of sore throat,
swollen lymph nodes, malaise, fever; other infections may occur; to
stop drug if skin rash, fever, cough,
shortness of breath, GI symptoms,

notify prescriber immediately; advise all health care providers that allergic reaction has occurred with abacavir

• That patient is still infective, may pass AIDS virus on to others

• That follow-up visits must be continued since serious toxicity may occur; blood counts must be done

• To use contraception during treatment

• Give patient Medication Guide and Warning Card, discuss points on guide

• That other drugs may be necessary to prevent other infections

---

RARELY USED

abciximab (℞)
(ab-six'i-mab)
ReoPro
Func. class.: Platelet aggregation inhibitor

Uses: Used with heparin and aspirin to prevent acute cardiac ischemia following percutaneous transluminal angioplasty (PTCA) in patients at high risk for reclosure of affected arteries

Dosage and routes:
• *Adult:* IV 250 µg (0.25 mg)/kg bolus 10-60 min prior to PTCA, followed by 10 µg/min **CONT INF** for 12 hr

Contraindications: Hypersensitivity to this drug or murine protein; GI, GU bleeding; CVA within 2 yr, bleeding disorders, intracranial neoplasm, intracranial arteriovenous malformations, intracranial aneurysm, platelet count >100,000/mm^3, recent surgery, aneurysm, uncontrolled severe hypertension, vasculitis

acarbose (℞)
(ay-car'bose)
Prandese*, Precose
Func. class.: Oral antidiabetic
Chem. class.: α-Glucosidase inhibitor

Action: Delays digestion of ingested carbohydrates, results in smaller rise in blood glucose after meals; does not increase insulin production

Uses: Non–insulin-dependent diabetes mellitus (NIDDM) type II, alone or in combination with a sulfonylurea

Dosage and routes:
• *Adult:* PO 25 mg tid initially, with first bite of meal; maintenance dose may be increased to 50-100 mg tid; dosage adjustment at 4-8 wk intervals

• *Adult <60 kg:* Not to exceed 100 mg PO tid

• *Available forms:* Tabs 50, 100 mg
Side effects/adverse reactions:
GI: Abdominal pain, diarrhea, flatulence, increased serum transaminase level

Contraindications: Hypersensitivity, diabetic ketoacidosis, cirrhosis, inflammatory bowel disease, colonic ulceration, partial intestinal obstruction, chronic intestinal disease, serum creatinine >2 mg/dl

Precautions: Pregnancy (B), renal disease, lactation, children, hepatic disease

Pharmacokinetics: Metabolized in GI tract, excreted as intact drug in urine, half-life 2 hr

Interactions:
• Effect of acarbose may be decreased: digestive enzymes, intestinal absorbents

• Increased hypoglycemia: sulfonylureas, insulin, calcium channel blockers, corticosteroids, estrogen,

---

◆ = Nursing alert   ∥ = Herb-drug interaction   ⊘ = Do not crush

oral contraceptives, phenothiazines, phenytoin, sympathomimetics, diuretics, thyroid, isoniazid, nicotinic acid

Lab test interferences:
Decrease: Calcium, vit B_6
Increase: AST, bilirubin

NURSING CONSIDERATIONS
Assess:
• Hypoglycemia, hyperglycemia; even though drug does not cause hypoglycemia, if patient is on sulfonylureas or insulin, hypoglycemia may be additive; if hypoglycemia occurs, treat with dextrose, or if severe, IV glucose or glucagon.
• 1 hr postprandial for establishing effectiveness, then glycosylated Hgb q3mo
• Monitor AST q3mo × 1 yr and periodically thereafter

Administer:
PO
• Tid with first bite of each meal
Perform/provide:
• Storage in tight container in cool environment
Evaluate:
• Therapeutic response: improved signs/symptoms of diabetes mellitus (decreased polyuria, polydipsia, polyphagia; clear sensorium, absence of dizziness, stable gait)
Teach patient/family:
• The symptoms of hypo/hyperglycemia, what to do about each
• That medication must be taken as prescribed; explain consequences of discontinuing medication abruptly
• To avoid OTC medications, herbal supplements unless approved by health-care provider
• That diabetes is lifelong illness; that this drug is not a cure
• To carry a Medic Alert ID for emergency purposes
• That diet and exercise regimen must be followed

acebutolol (℞)
(a-se-byoo'toe-lole)
Monitan*, Sectral
Func. class.: Antihypertensive, β_1-blocker, antidysrhythmic (II)

Action: Competitively blocks stimulation of β-adrenergic receptors within vascular smooth muscle; decreases rate of SA node discharge, increases recovery time, slows conduction of AV node resulting in decreased heart rate (negative chronotropic effect), which decreases O_2 consumption in myocardium due to β_1-receptor antagonism; also decreases renin-aldosterone-angiotensin system at high doses, inhibits β_2-receptors in bronchial system (high doses)

Uses: Mild to moderate hypertension, sinus tachycardia, persistent atrial extrasystoles, tachydysrhythmias

Investigational uses: Prophylaxis of MI, treatment of angina pectoris, tremor, mitral valve prolapse, thyrotoxicosis, idiopathic hypertrophic subaortic stenosis

Dosage and routes:
Hypertension
• *Adult:* **PO** 400 mg qd or in 2 divided doses; may be increased to desired response; maintenance 200-1200 mg/qd in 2 divided doses
Ventricular dysrhythmia
• *Adult:* **PO** 200 mg bid, may increase gradually, usual range 600-1200 mg daily; should be tapered over 2 wk before discontinuing
• *Geriatric:* not to exceed 800 mg qd
• **Renal dose:** CrCl 25-50 ml/min, reduce dose by 50%; if <25 ml/min reduce dose by 75%
Available forms: Caps 200, 400 mg; tabs 100, 200, 400 mg*

Side effects/adverse reactions:

*CV: **Profound hypotension, bradycardia, CHF,** cold extremities, postural hypotension, **2nd- or 3rd-degree heart block***

CNS: Insomnia, fatigue, dizziness, mental changes, memory loss, hallucinations, depression, lethargy, drowsiness, strange dreams, catatonia

*GI: Nausea, diarrhea, vomiting, **mesenteric arterial thrombosis, ischemic colitis***

INTEG: Rash, fever, alopecia, dry skin

*HEMA: **Agranulocytosis, thrombocytopenia, purpura***

EENT: Sore throat; dry, burning eyes

GU: Impotence, decreased libido, dysuria, nocturia

ENDO: Increased hypoglycemic response to insulin

*RESP: **Bronchospasm,** dyspnea, wheezing, cough*

MS: Joint pain, cramping

Contraindications: Hypersensitivity to β-blockers, cardiogenic shock, heart block (2nd-, 3rd-degree), sinus bradycardia, CHF, cardiac failure

Precautions: Major surgery, pregnancy (B), lactation, diabetes mellitus, renal disease, thyroid disease, COPD, asthma, well-compensated heart failure, aortic, mitral valve, hepatic disease

Pharmacokinetics:

PO: Onset 1-1½ hr, peak 2-4 hr, duration 10-12 hr, half-life 6-7 hr, excreted unchanged in urine, protein binding 5%-15%

Interactions:

• Increased hypotension, bradycardia: reserpine, hydralazine, methyldopa, prazosin, anticholinergics, cardiac glycosides, diltiazem, verapamil, diuretics, other antihypertensives

• Decreased antihypertensive effects: NSAIDs

• Increased hypoglycemic effect: insulin, oral antidiabetics

• Decreased bronchodilation: theophyllines, β₂-agonists

// May increase acebutolol effect: buckthorn bark/berry, aloe, rhubarb root, senna leaf/fruits, cascara sagrada bark

// Dysrhythmia: Ephedra

Lab test interferences:

Positive: ANA titer

Increased: Serum lipoprotein levels

NURSING CONSIDERATIONS

Assess:

• B/P during beginning treatment, periodically thereafter; pulse q4h; note rate, rhythm, quality

• Apical/radial pulse before administration; notify prescriber of any significant changes (pulse <50 bpm); signs of CHF (dyspnea, crackles, weight gain, jugular vein distension)

• Baselines in renal, liver function tests before therapy begins

• Edema in feet, legs daily: monitor I&O

• Skin turgor, dryness of mucous membranes for hydration status, especially elderly

Administer:

PO

• Drug ac, hs, tablet may be crushed or swallowed whole; give with food to prevent GI upset

Perform/provide:

• Storage protected from light, moisture; place in cool environment

Evaluate:

• Therapeutic response: decreased B/P after 1-2 wk; decreased dysrhythmias

Teach patient/family:

◆Not to discontinue drug abruptly, severe cardiac reactions may occur, taper over 2 wk; do not double dose; if a dose is missed, take as soon as

◆ = Nursing alert   // = Herb-drug interaction   ⊘ = Do not crush remembered up to 4 hr before next dose

• Not to use OTC products containing α-adrenergic stimulants (such as nasal decongestants, OTC cold preparations) unless directed by prescriber

• To report low pulse, dizziness, confusion, depression, fever

• To take pulse, B/P at home, advise when to notify prescriber

• To comply with weight control, dietary adjustments, modified exercise program

• To carry Medic Alert ID to identify drug, allergies

• To avoid hazardous activities if dizziness, drowsiness is present

• To report symptoms of CHF: difficult breathing, especially on exertion or when lying down, night cough, swelling of extremities

• To carry ID listing condition, medications taken

• To continue with required lifestyle changes (exercise, diet, weight loss, stress reduction)

Treatment of overdose: Lavage, IV atropine for bradycardia, IV theophylline for bronchospasm, digitalis, O_2, diuretic for cardiac failure, IV glucose for hypoglycemia, IV diazepam (or phenytoin) for seizures

acetaminophen (OTC)

(a-seat-a-mee′noe-fen)
Abenol*, Acephen, Aceta, Actimol, Aminofen, Apacet, APAP, Apo-Acetaminophen*, Arthritis Foundation Pain Reliever Aspirin-Free, Aspirin Free Anacin, Aspirin Free Pain Relief, Atasol*, Banesin, Children's Feverall, Dapa, Dapacin, Datril, Exdol*, FemEtts, Genapap, Genebs, Halenol, Liquiprin, Mapap, Maranox, Meda, Neopap, Oraphen-PD, Panadol, Redutemp, Robigesic*, Rounax*, Silapap, Tapanol, Tempra, Tylenol

Func. class.: Nonopioid analgesic, antipyretic

Chem. class.: Nonsalicylate, paraaminophenol derivative

Action: May block pain impulses peripherally that occur in response to inhibition of prostaglandin synthesis; does not possess antiinflammatory properties; antipyretic action results from inhibition of prostaglandins in the CNS (hypothalamic heat-regulating center)

Uses: Mild pain or fever

Dosage and routes:

• *Adult and child >12 yr:* **PO/RECT** 325-650 mg q4h prn, max 4 g/day

• *Child:* **PO** 10-15 mg/kg q4h

• *Child 6-12 yr:* **RECT** 325 mg q4-6h, max 2.6 g/day

• *Child 3-6 yr:* **RECT** 125 mg q4-6h, max 720 mg/day

• *Child 1-3 yr:* **RECT** 80 mg q4h

• *Child 3-11 mo:* **RECT** 80 mg q6h

Available forms: Rect supp 120, 125, 325, 600, 650 mg; soft chew tabs 80, 160 mg; caps 500 mg; elix 120, 160, 325 mg/5 ml; liq 160 mg/5 ml, 500 mg/15 ml; sol 100 mg/1 ml,

---

Side effects: *italics* = common; ***bold italics*** = life-threatening

120 mg/2.5 ml; granules 80 mg/
packet, 80 mg/cap; tabs 160, 325,
500, 650 mg

Side effects/adverse reactions:
SYST: Hypersensitivity
*HEMA: **Leukopenia, neutropenia,
hemolytic anemia (long-term use),
thrombocytopenia, pancytopenia***
CNS: Stimulation, drowsiness
GI: Nausea, vomiting, abdominal
pain; *hepatotoxicity, hepatic seizure (overdose)*
INTEG: Rash, urticaria
*TOXICITY: **Cyanosis, anemia, neutropenia, jaundice, pancytopenia,
CNS stimulation, delirium followed
by vascular collapse, convulsions,
coma, death***
*GU: **Renal failure (high, prolonged
doses)***

Contraindications: Hypersensitivity, intolerance to tartrazine (yellow
dye #5), alcohol, table sugar, sac-
charin, depending on product

Precautions: Anemia, hepatic disease, renal disease, chronic alcoholism, pregnancy (B), elderly, lactation

Pharmacokinetics: Well absorbed
PO, rectal absorption varies; 85%-
90% metabolized by liver, excreted
by kidneys; metabolites may be toxic
if overdose occurs; widely distributed, crosses placenta in low concentrations, excreted in breast milk,
half-life 1-4 hr
PO: Onset 10-30 min, peak ½-2 hr,
duration 3-4 hr
RECT: Onset slow, peak 1-2 hr, duration 3-4 hr

Interactions:
• Decreased effect, increased hepatotoxicity: barbiturates, alcohol, carbamazepine, hydantoins, rifampin,
rifabutin, isoniazid, diflunisal, sulfinpyrazone
• Hypoprothrombinemia: warfarin,
long-term use, high doses of acetaminophen

• Bone marrow suppression: zidovudine
• Decreased absorption: colestipol,
cholestyramine
• Renal adverse reactions: NSAIDs,
salicylates

Lab test interferences:
Interference: Chemstrip G, Dex-
trostix, Visidex II, 5-HIAA

NURSING CONSIDERATIONS
Assess:
• Liver function studies: AST, ALT,
bilirubin, creatinine prior to therapy
if long-term therapy is anticipated;
may cause hepatic toxicity at doses
>4 g/day with chronic use
• Renal function studies: BUN, urine
creatinine, occult blood, albumin, if
patient is on long-term therapy; presence of blood or albumin indicates
nephritis
• Blood studies: CBC, PT if patient
is on long-term therapy
• I&O ratio; decreasing output may
indicate renal failure (long-term therapy)
• For fever and pain: type of pain,
location, intensity, duration
• For chronic poisoning: rapid, weak
pulse; dyspnea; cold, clammy extremities; report immediately to prescriber
• Hepatotoxicity: dark urine; clay-
colored stools; yellowing of skin,
sclera; itching, abdominal pain; fever; diarrhea if patient is on long-
term therapy
• Allergic reactions: rash, urticaria;
if these occur, drug may have to be
discontinued

Administer:
PO
• Crushed or whole; chewable tablets may be chewed; give with full
glass of water
• With food or milk to decrease gastric symptoms if needed

◆ = Nursing alert   ⬦ = Herb-drug interaction   ⊘ = Do not crush

Perform/provide:
• Storage of suppositories <80° F (27° C)
Evaluate:
• Therapeutic response: absence of pain, fever
Teach patient/family:
◆ Not to exceed recommended dosage; acute poisoning with liver damage may result
◆ That acute toxicity includes symptoms of nausea, vomiting, abdominal pain; prescriber should be notified immediately
• To read label on other OTC drugs; many contain acetaminophen and may cause toxicity if taken concurrently
• To recognize signs of chronic overdose: bleeding, bruising, malaise, fever, sore throat
• To notify prescriber of pain or fever lasting over 3 days
Treatment of overdose: Drug level, gastric lavage, activated charcoal; administer oral acetylcysteine to prevent hepatic damage *(see acetylcysteine monograph)*, monitor for bleeding

---

acetazolamide (R)

(a-set-a-zole′a-mide)
acetazolamide, Apo-Acetazolamide*, Dazamide, Diamox, Diamox Sequels
Func. class.: Diuretic, carbonic anhydrase inhibitor, antiglaucoma agent, antiepileptic
Chem. class.: Sulfonamide derivative

Action: Inhibits carbonic anhydrase activity in proximal renal tubules to decrease reabsorption of water, sodium, potassium, bicarbonate; decreases carbonic anhydrase in CNS, increasing seizure threshold; able to decrease aqueous humor in eye, which lowers intraocular pressure
Uses: Open-angle glaucoma, narrow-angle glaucoma (preoperatively, if surgery delayed), epilepsy (petit mal, grand mal, mixed), edema in CHF, drug-induced edema, acute mountain sickness
Investigational uses: Prevention of uric acid/cystine renal stones, decrease CSF production in infants with hydrocephalus
Dosage and routes:
Closed-angle glaucoma
• *Adult:* **PO/IM/IV** 250 mg q4h or 250 mg bid, to be used for short-term therapy
Open-angle glaucoma
• *Adult:* **PO/IM/IV** 250 mg-1 g/day in divided doses for amounts over 250 mg or 500 mg SR bid
Edema in CHF
• *Adult:* **IM/IV** 250-375 mg/day in AM
• *Child:* **IM/IV** 5 mg/kg/day in AM
Seizures
• *Adult:* **PO/IM/IV** 4-30 mg/kg/day, in 1-4 divided doses usual range 375-1000 mg/day
• *Child:* **PO/IM/IV** 8-30 mg/kg/day in divided doses tid or qid, or 300-900 mg/m^2/day, not to exceed 1 g/day
Mountain sickness
• *Adult:* **PO** 250 mg q8-12h
Renal stones
• *Adult:* **PO** 250 mg hs
Infants with hydrocephalus
• *Infant:* **IV** 5 mg/kg/dose q6h, may be increased up to 100 mg/kg/day if tolerated
Available forms: Tabs 125, 250 mg; caps sust rel 500 mg; inj 500 mg
Side effects/adverse reactions:
GU: Frequency, polyuria, **uremia,** glucosuria, hematuria, dysuria, crystalluria, renal calculi
CNS: Drowsiness, paresthesia, anxiety, depression, headache, dizzi-

ness, confusion, stimulation, fatigue, *convulsions,* sedation, nervousness

GI: Nausea, vomiting, anorexia, constipation, diarrhea, melena, weight loss, *hepatic insufficiency,* taste alterations

EENT: Myopia, tinnitus

INTEG: Rash, pruritus, urticaria, fever, *Stevens-Johnson syndrome,* photosensitivity

ENDO: Hyperglycemia

HEMA: Aplastic anemia, hemolytic anemia, leukopenia, agranulocytosis, thrombocytopenia, purpura, pancytopenia

META: Hypokalemia, hyperchloremic acidosis

Contraindications: Hypersensitivity to sulfonamides, severe renal disease, severe hepatic disease, electrolyte imbalances (hyponatremia, hypokalemia), hyperchloremic acidosis, Addison's disease, long-term use in narrow-angle glaucoma, COPD

Precautions: Hypercalciuria, pregnancy (C), lactation

Do not confuse:

acetazolamide/acetohexamide

Diamox/Trimox

Diamox/Dobutrex

Pharmacokinetics:

PO: Onset 1-1½ hr, peak 2-4 hr, duration 8-12 hr

PO-SUS REL: Onset 2 hr, peak 3-6 hr, duration 18-24 hr

IV: Onset 2 min, peak 15 min, duration 4-5 hr, 65% absorbed if fasting (oral), 75% absorbed if given with food; half-life 2½-5½ hr; excreted unchanged by kidneys (80% within 24 hr), crosses placenta

Interactions:

• Increased action of amphetamines, procainamide, quinidine, anticholinergics

• Increased excretion of lithium

• Increased toxicity: salicylates

• Toxicity: cyclosporine

• Decreased acetazolamide effect: methenamine

• Increased side effects: diflunisal

• Decreased primidone levels

Lab test interferences:

False positive: Urinary protein, 17 hydroxysteroid

Decrease: Thyroid iodine uptake

NURSING CONSIDERATIONS

Assess:

• Weight daily, I&O daily to determine fluid loss; effect of drug may be decreased if used qd; monitor the elderly for dehydration

• For cross-sensitivity between other sulfonamides and this drug

• B/P lying, standing; postural hypotension may occur

• Electrolytes: K, Na, chloride; also BUN, blood sugar, CBC, serum creatinine, blood pH, ABGs, liver function tests; I&O, glucose, patient may need to be on a high-K diet

Administer:

• In AM to avoid interference with sleep if using drug as diuretic

• K replacement if K level is less than 3.0 mg/dl

PO

• With food if nausea occurs; absorption may be decreased slightly

🚫 Do not break, crush, or chew sus rel caps

IV

• After diluting 500 mg in >5 ml sterile H_2O for injection; direct IV— give at 100-500 mg/min; may be diluted further in LR, D_5W, $D_{10}W$, 0.45% NaCl, 0.9% NaCl, or Ringer's sol and infused over 4-8 hr; use within 24 hr of dilution

Additive compatibilities: Cimetidine, ranitidine

Perform/provide:

• Storage in dark, cool area; use reconstituted solution within 24 hr

Evaluate:

• Therapeutic response: improvement in edema of feet, legs, sacral

---

◆◆ = Nursing alert   💉 = Herb-drug interaction   🚫 = Do not crush area daily if medication is being used in CHF; or decrease in aqueous humor if medication is being used in glaucoma

Teach patient/family:
• To take exactly as prescribed; if dose is missed, take as soon as remembered; do not double dose
• To notify prescriber if sore throat, unusual bleeding, bruising, paresthesias, tremors, flank pain, or skin rash occurs
• To use sunscreen to prevent photosensitivity; to monitor blood glucose and urine for sugar
• To avoid hazardous activities if drowsiness occurs
• Increase fluids to 2-3 L/day if not contraindicated
• Report nausea, vertigo, rapid weight gain, change in stools

Treatment of overdose: Lavage if taken orally; monitor electrolytes; administer dextrose in saline; monitor hydration, CV, renal status

---

acetylcysteine (℞)

(a-se-teel-sis′tay-een)
Mucomyst*, Mucosil, Parvolex*

Func. class.: Mucolytic; antidote—acetaminophen

Chem. class.: Amino acid L-cysteine

Action: Decreases viscosity of secretions by breaking disulfide links of mucoproteins; increases hepatic glutathione, which is necessary to inactivate toxic metabolites in acetaminophen overdose

Uses: Acetaminophen toxicity; bronchitis; pneumonia; cystic fibrosis; emphysema; atelectasis; tuberculosis; complications of thoracic, cardiovascular surgery; diagnosis in bronchial lab tests

Investigational uses: Prevention of contrast medium nephrotoxicity

Dosage and routes:
Mucolytic
• *Adult and child:* **INSTILL** 1-2 ml (10%-20% sol) q1-4h prn or 3-5 ml (20% sol) or 6-10 ml (10% sol) tid or qid

Acetaminophen toxicity
• *Adult and child:* **PO** 140 mg/kg, then 70 mg/kg q4h × 17 doses to total of 1330 mg/kg

Available forms: Sol 10%, 20%

Side effects/adverse reactions:
CNS: Dizziness, drowsiness, headache, fever, chills
GI: Nausea, stomatitis, constipation, vomiting, anorexia, ***hepatotoxicity***
EENT: Rhinorrhea, tooth damage
CV: Hypotension
INTEG: Urticaria, rash, fever, clamminess
*RESP: **Bronchospasm,*** burning, ***hemoptysis,*** chest tightness

Contraindications: Hypersensitivity, increased intracranial pressure, status asthmaticus

Precautions: Hypothyroidism, Addison's disease, CNS depression, brain tumor, asthma, hepatic disease, renal disease, COPD, psychosis, alcoholism, convulsive disorders, lactation, pregnancy (B)

Pharmacokinetics:
INH/INSTILL: Onset 1 min, duration 5-10 min, metabolized by liver, excreted in urine

Interactions:
• Do not use with iron, copper, rubber
• Do not mix with antibiotics: tetracycline, chlortetracycline, oxytetracycline, erythromycin lactobionate, amphotericin B, sodium ampicillin; iodized oil, chymotrypsin, trypsin, hydrogen peroxide

---

Side effects: *italics* = common; **bold italics** = life-threatening

NURSING CONSIDERATIONS
Assess:
• Cough: type, frequency, character, including sputum
• Rate, rhythm of respirations, increased dyspnea; sputum; discontinue if bronchospasm occurs
• VS, cardiac status including checking for dysrhythmias, increased rate, palpitations
• ABGs for increased CO_2 retention in asthma patients
• Antidotal use: liver function tests, PT, BUN, glucose, electrolytes, acetaminophen levels; inform prescriber if dose is vomited or vomiting is persistent
• Nausea, vomiting, rash; notify prescriber if these occur

Administer:
PO
• Antidotal use: give within 24 hr; give with cola or soft drink to disguise taste; can be given with H_2O through tubes; use within 1 hr
INSTILL
• By syringe 2-3 doses of 1-2 ml of 20% or 2-4 ml of 10% solution
• Decreased dose to elderly patients; their metabolisms may be slowed
• Only if suction machine is available
• Before meals ½-1 hr for better absorption, to decrease nausea
• 20% solutions diluted with NS or water for injection; may give 10% solution undiluted
• Only after patient clears airway by deep breathing, coughing

Perform/provide:
• Storage in refrigerator; use within 96 hr of opening
• Assistance with inhaled dose: bronchodilator if bronchospasm occurs
• Mechanical suction if cough insufficient to remove excess bronchial secretions
• Gum, hard candy, frequent rinsing of mouth for dryness of oral cavity

Evaluate:
• Therapeutic response: absence of purulent secretions when coughing; absence of hepatic damage in acetaminophen toxicity

Teach patient/family:
• About mucolytic use
• That unpleasant odor will decrease after repeated use
• That discoloration of solution after bottle is opened does not impair its effectiveness

---

activated charcoal (OTC)
Actidose-Aqua, CharcoAid, CharcoAid 2000, Liqui-Char
Func. class.: Antiflatulent; antidote

Action: Binds poisons, toxins, irritants; increases adsorption in GI tract; inactivates toxins and binds until excreted

Uses: Poisoning

Dosage and routes:
• Children should not get more than 1 dose of products with sorbitol
Poisoning
• *Adult and child:* PO 30-100 g or 1 g/kg, minimum dose 30 g/250 ml of water, may give 20-40 g q6h for 1-2 days in severe poisoning

Available forms: Powder 15, 25*, 30, 40, 120, 125, 240 g/container; oral susp 12.5 g/60 ml, 15 g/72 ml, 15 g/120 ml, 25 g/120 ml, 30 g/120 ml, 50 g/240 ml; Canada 15 g/120 ml, 25 g/125 ml, 50 g/225 ml, 50 g/250 ml

Side effects/adverse reactions:
GI: Nausea, black stools, vomiting, constipation, diarrhea

Contraindications: Hypersensitivity to this drug, unconsciousness, semiconsciousness, poisoning of cyanide, mineral acids, alkalis

---

◆ = Nursing alert   ∥ = Herb-drug interaction   ⃠ = Do not crush

A

Pharmacokinetics:
PO: Excreted in feces
Interactions:
• Inactivation of: ipecac, acetylcysteine
NURSING CONSIDERATIONS
Assess:
• Respiration, pulse, B/P to determine charcoal effectiveness if taken for barbiturate/opiate poisoning
Administer:
PO
• After inducing vomiting unless vomiting contraindicated (i.e., cyanide or alkalis)
• After mixing with water or fruit juice to form thick syrup; do not use dairy products to mix charcoal
• Repeat dose if vomiting occurs soon after dose; give with a laxative to promote elimination; alone, do not administer with ipecac
• After spacing at least 1 hr before or after other drugs, or absorption will be decreased
Perform/provide:
• Container closed tightly to prevent absorption of gases
NG
• Through a nasogastric tube if patient unable to swallow
Evaluate:
• Therapeutic response: LOC-alert (poisoning)
Teach patient/family:
• That stools will be black
• How to prevent further poisonings

---

acyclovir (Ŗ)

(ay-sye′kloe-ver)

Avirax*, Zovirax

Func. class.: Antiviral

Chem. class.: Acyclic purine nucleoside analog

See Topical Appendix for Topical Product

Action: Interferes with DNA synthesis by conversion to acyclovir triphosphate, causing decreased viral replication, time of lesional healing
Uses: Mucocutaneous herpes simplex virus, herpes genitalis (HSV-1, HSV-2), varicella infections, herpes zoster, herpes simplex encephalitis
Investigational uses: Cytomegalovirus, HSV after transplant, mononucleosis, herpes simplex
Dosage and routes:
Renal dose: CrCl >50 ml/min dose q8h, CrCl 25-50 ml/min dose q12h, CrCl 10-25 ml/min dose q24h, CrCl 0-10 ml/min 50% of dose q24h
Herpes simplex
• *Adult and child >12 yr:* **IV INF** 5 mg/kg over 1 hr q8h × 5 days
• *Child <12 yr:* **IV INF** 250 mg/m^2 or 30 mg/kg/day divided q8h over 1 hr × 5 days
Genital herpes
• *Adult:* **PO** 200 mg q4h (5×/day while awake) for 5 days to 6 mo depending on whether initial, recurrent, or chronic
Herpes simplex encephalitis
• *Adult:* **IV** 10 mg/kg over 1 hr q8h × 10 days
• *Child 3 mo-12 yr:* **IV** 20 mg/kg q8h × 10 days
• *Child birth-3 mo:* **IV** 10 mg/kg q8h × 10 days
Herpes zoster
• *Adult:* **PO** 800 mg q4h while awake × 7-10 days; **IV** 5 mg/kg q8h
Varicella-zoster
• *Adult:* **PO** 1000 mg q6h × 5 days or 600-800 mg q4h (5×/day while awake); **IV** 500 mg/m^2 q8h or 10 mg/kg q8h × 7 days
• *Child:* **PO** 10-20 mg/kg (max 800 mg) qid × 5 days; **IV** 500 mg/m^2 q8h or 10 mg/kg q8h × 7 days
Chickenpox
• *Adult and child:* **PO** 20 mg/kg qid × 5 days, max 800 mg/dose

---

Available forms: Caps 200 mg; inj
500 mg, oral susp, tabs 400, 800 mg
Side effects/adverse reactions:

CNS: Tremors, confusion, lethargy,
hallucinations, ***convulsions,*** dizziness, *headache,* encephalopathic
changes
GI: Nausea, vomiting, diarrhea, increased ALT, AST, abdominal pain,
glossitis, colitis
GU: ***Oliguria, proteinuria, hematuria,*** vaginitis, moniliasis, ***glomerulonephritis, acute renal failure,***
changes in menses, polydipsia
EENT: Gingival hyperplasia
INTEG: Rash, urticaria, pruritus, pain
or phlebitis at IV site, unusual sweating, alopecia
MS: Joint pain, leg pain, muscle
cramps
Contraindications: Hypersensitivity
Precautions: Lactation, hepatic disease, renal disease, electrolyte imbalance, dehydration, pregnancy (B)
Pharmacokinetics:

Distributed widely; crosses placenta,
CSF concentrations are 50% plasma
IV: Onset immediate, peak immediate, duration unknown, half-life
20 min-3 hr (terminal); metabolized
by liver, excreted by kidneys as unchanged drug (95%)
PO: Absorbed minimally; onset unknown, peak 1½-2 hr, terminal half-
life 3½ hr
Interactions:

• Increased levels, toxicity: proben-
ecid
• Synergistic effect: interferon
• CNS side effects: zidovudine
NURSING CONSIDERATIONS
Assess:

• Signs of infection, anemia
◆ Any patient with compromised
renal system, since drug is excreted slowly in poor renal system function; toxicity may occur
rapidly

• Liver studies: AST, ALT
• Blood studies: WBC, RBC, Hct,
Hgb, bleeding time; blood dyscrasias may occur; drug should be discontinued
• Renal studies: urinalysis, protein,
BUN, creatinine, CrCl, watch for
increasing BUN and serum creati-
tine or decreased CrCl, may indicate nephrotoxicity; I&O ratio; report hematuria, oliguria, fatigue,
weakness; may indicate nephrotoxicity; check for protein in urine during treatment
• C&S before drug therapy; drug
may be taken as soon as culture is
taken; repeat C&S after treatment;
determine the presence of other sexually transmitted diseases
• Bowel pattern before, during treatment; if severe abdominal pain with
bleeding occurs, drug should be discontinued
• Skin eruptions: rash, urticaria, itching
• Allergies before treatment, reaction of each medication; place allergies on chart in bright red letters
Administer:
PO
🚫 Do not break, crush, or chew
caps
• May give without regard to meals,
with 8 oz of water
• Shake suspension before use
• Lower dose in acute or chronic
renal failure
IV
• Increased fluids to 3 L/day to decrease crystalluria
• After reconstituting with 10 ml
compatible sol/500 mg of drug, concentration of 50 mg/ml, shake, further dilute in 50-100 ml compatible
sol; use within 12 hr; give over at
least 1 hr (constant rate) by infusion
pump to prevent nephrotoxicity; do
not reconstitute with sol containing
benzyl alcohol in neonates

◆ = Nursing alert   ⫽ = Herb-drug interaction   🚫 = Do not crush

Additive compatibilities: Fluconazole

Solution compatibilities: D$_5$W, LR, or NaCl (D$_5$ 0.9% NaCl, 0.9% NaCl) solutions

Y-site compatibilities: Allopurinol, amikacin, ampicillin, amphotericin B, cefamandole, cefazolin, cefonicid, cefoperazone, cefotaxime, cefoxitin, ceftazidime, ceftizoxime, ceftriaxone, cefuroxime, cephapirin, chloramphenicol, cholesteryl sulfate complex, cimetidine, clindamycin, dexamethasone sodium phosphate, dimenhydrinate, diphenhydramine, doxorubicin, doxycycline, erythromycin, famotidine, filgrastim, fluconazole, gallium, gentamicin, granisetron, heparin, hydrocortisone sodium succinate, hydromorphone, imipenem/cilastatin, lorazepam, magnesium sulfate, melphalan, methylprednisolone sodium succinate, metoclopramide, metronidazole, multivitamin, nafcillin, oxacillin, paclitaxel, penicillin G potassium, pentobarbital, perphenazine, piperacillin, potassium chloride, propofol, ranitidine, remifentanil, sodium bicarbonate, tacrolimus, teniposide, theophylline, thiotepa, ticarcillin, tobramycin, trimethoprim - sulfamethoxazole, vancomycin, zidovudine

Perform/provide:

• Storage at room temperature for up to 12 hr after reconstitution; if refrigerated, sol may show a precipitate that clears at room temperature, yellow discoloration does not affect potency

• Adequate intake of fluids (2 L) to prevent deposit in kidneys

Evaluate:

• Therapeutic response: absence of itching, painful lesions; crusting and healed lesions; decreased symptoms of chickenpox

Teach patient/family:

• To take as prescribed; if dose is missed, take as soon as remembered up to 1 hr before next dose; do not double dose; that drug does not cure the condition

• That drug may be taken orally before infection occurs; drug should be taken when itching or pain occurs, usually before eruptions

• That sexual partners need to be told that patient has herpes; they can become infected; condoms must be worn to prevent reinfections

• Not to touch lesions to avoid spreading infection to new sites

• That drug does not cure infection, just controls symptoms and does not prevent infecting others

◆ To report sore throat, fever, fatigue (may indicate superinfection)

• That drug must be taken in equal intervals around the clock to maintain blood levels for duration of therapy

• To notify prescriber of side effects of bruising, bleeding, fatigue, malaise; may indicate blood dyscrasias

• To seek dental care during treatment to prevent gingival hyperplasia

• That women with genital herpes are more likely to develop cervical cancer; to keep all gynecologic appointments

Treatment of overdose: Discontinue drug, hemodialysis, resuscitate if needed

---

adenosine (℞)

(a-den'oh-seen)
Adenocard, Adenoscan
Func. class.: Antidysrhythmic
Chem. class.: Endogenous nucleoside

Action: Slows conduction through AV node, can interrupt reentry path-

---

Side effects: *italics* = common; ***bold italics*** = life-threatening

ways through AV node, and can restore normal sinus rhythm in patients with supraventricular tachycardia (SVT)

Uses: SVT, as a diagnostic aid to assess myocardial perfusion defects in CAD

Dosage and routes:

Antidysrhythmic
• *Adult:* IV BOL 6 mg; if conversion to normal sinus rhythm does not occur within 1-2 min, give 12 mg by rapid **IV BOL;** may repeat 12 mg dose again in 1-2 min
• *Infants and children:* 0.05 mg/kg, if not effective, increase dose by 0.05 mg/kg q2min to a max of 0.25 mg/kg or 12 mg

Diagnostic use
• *Adult:* 140 µg/kg/min × 6 min

Available forms: Inj 3 mg/ml vial, 6 mg/2 ml vial

Side effects/adverse reactions:
GI: Nausea, metallic taste, throat tightness, groin pressure
RESP: Dyspnea, chest pressure, hyperventilation
CNS: Lightheadedness, dizziness, arm tingling, numbness, apprehension, blurred vision, headache
CV: Chest pain, pressure, ***atrial tachydysrhythmias,*** sweating, palpitations, hypotension, *facial flushing*

Contraindications: Hypersensitivity, 2nd- or 3rd-degree heart block, AV block, sick sinus syndrome, atrial flutter, atrial fibrillation

Precautions: Pregnancy (C), lactation, children, asthma, elderly

Do not confuse:
Adenocard/adenosine

Pharmacokinetics: Cleared from plasma in <30 sec, half-life 10 sec

Interactions:
• Increased effects of adenosine: dipyridamole

• Decreased activity of adenosine: theophylline or other methylxanthines (caffeine)
• Higher degree of heart block: carbamazepine
• Possible ventricular fibrillation: digoxin
• Smoking: increased tachycardia
  ✦ May cause increased adenosine effect: aloe, buckthorn bark/berry, cascara sagrada bark, rhubarb root, senna leaf/fruits
  ✦ Decreased adenosine effect: guarana

NURSING CONSIDERATIONS
Assess:
• I&O ratio, electrolytes (K, Na, Cl)
• Cardiopulmonary status: B/P, pulse, respiration, ECG intervals (PR, QRS, QT); check for transient dysrhythmias (PVCs, PACs, sinus tachycardia, AV block)
• Respiratory status: rate, rhythm, lung fields for rales, watch for respiratory depression; bilateral rales may occur in CHF patient; increased respiration, increased pulse, drug should be discontinued
• CNS effects: dizziness, confusion, psychosis, paresthesias, convulsions; drug should be discontinued

Administer:
IV BOLUS
• Undiluted; give 6 mg or less by rapid inj; if using an IV line, use port near insertion site, flush with normal saline (50 ml)
CONT INF
• Give 30 ml vial, undiluted, by peripheral vein

Solution compatibilities: D₅LR, D₅W, LR, 0.9% NaCl

Perform/provide:
• Storage at room temperature; sol should be clear; discard unused drug

Evaluate:
• Therapeutic response: normal sinus rhythm or diagnosis of perfusion defect

---

✦ = Nursing alert   ✦ = Herb-drug interaction   ⊘ = Do not crush

Teach patient/family:
• To report facial flushing, dizziness, sweating, palpitations, chest pain
• To rise from sitting or standing slowly to prevent orthostatic hypotension
Treatment of overdose: Defibrillation, vasopressor for hypotension

---

alatrofloxacin (R)
(ah-lat-troh-floks'ah-sin)
Trovan IV
trovafloxacin (R)
(tro-vah-floks'ah-sin)
Trovan
Func. class.: Antiinfective
Chem. class.: Fluoroquinolone

Action: Interferes with conversion of intermediate DNA fragments into high-molecular-weight DNA in bacteria; DNA gyrase inhibitor

Uses: Nosocomial pneumonia; *Escherichia coli, Proteus aeruginosa, Haemophilus influenzae, Staphylococcus aureus;* community-acquired pneumonia: *Streptococcus pneumoniae, H. influenzae, S. aureus, Klebsiella pneumoniae, Mycoplasma pneumoniae, Moraxella catarrhalis, Legionella pneumophila, Citrobacter pneumoniae;* chronic bronchitis, acute sinusitis, complicated intraabdominal infections, gyn/pelvic infections, skin/skin structure infections, UTIs, chronic bacterial prostatitis, urethral gonorrhea in males, PID, cervicitis caused by susceptible organisms

Dosage and routes:
Alatrofloxacin—serious infections
• *Adult:* IV 300 mg q24h
Other infections
• *Adult:* IV 200 mg q24h

Perioperative prophylaxis
• *Adult:* IV 200 mg ½-4 hr prior to surgery
Trovafloxacin—gonorrhea
• *Adult:* PO 100 mg as a single dose
Other infections
• *Adult:* PO 100-200 mg q24h
Perioperative prophylaxis
• *Adult:* PO 200 mg ½-4 hr prior to surgery
Available forms: Conc sol for inj 5 mg/ml (200 mg/40 ml, 300 mg/60 ml) (alatrofloxacin); tabs 100, 200 mg (trovafloxacin)
Side effects/adverse reactions:
CNS: Headache, *dizziness,* insomnia, anxiety, psychosis, **seizures**
HEMA: Anemia, **thrombocytopenia, leukopenia,** decreased Hgb; Hct, increased platelets
GI: Nausea, flatulence, vomiting, diarrhea, abdominal pain, **pseudomembranous colitis, hepatotoxicity, fatal hepatitis**
MS: Arthralgia, myalgia
GU: Vaginitis, crystalluria, increased BUN, creatinine
INTEG: Rash, pruritus, photosensitivity
SYST: **Anaphylaxis, Stevens-Johnson syndrome**
Contraindications: Hypersensitivity to quinolones, seizure disorders, cerebral atherosclerosis, photosensitivity
Precautions: Pregnancy (C), lactation, children
Pharmacokinetics: Metabolized in liver, excreted in urine unchanged
Interactions:
• May increase theophylline level, lead to toxicity
• May increase warfarin level
• Nephrotoxicity may occur with cyclosporine
• Decreased absorption of trovafloxacin: IV morphine
• Decreased absorption: antacids with aluminum, magnesium, citric

---

acid buffered with sodium citrate, sucralfate, iron products, IV morphine

Solution compatibilities: D_5, ½NaCl, D_5 ½NaCl, D_5/0.2% NaCl

NURSING CONSIDERATIONS
Assess:

• For hepatic toxicity, use only for serious or life-threatening infections

• For previous sensitivity reaction to fluoroquinolones

• For signs and symptoms of infection: characteristics of sputum, WBC >10,000, fever; obtain baseline information before and during treatment

• For CNS disorders, since other quinolones can cause CNS stimulation, seizures

• C&S before beginning drug therapy to identify if correct treatment has been initiated

• For allergic reactions and anaphylaxis: rash, urticaria, pruritus, chills, fever, joint pain; may occur a few days after therapy begins; epinephrine and resuscitation equipment should be available for anaphylactic reaction

• Bowel pattern qd; if severe diarrhea occurs, drug should be discontinued

• For overgrowth of infection, perineal itching, fever, malaise, redness, pain, swelling, drainage, rash, diarrhea, change in cough, sputum

◆Liver function tests: AST; ALT, alk phosphatase, bilirubin; identify hepatotoxicity, fatal hepatitis

Evaluate:

• Therapeutic response: absence of signs/symptoms of infection (WBC <10,000/mm³, temp WNL)

Teach patient/family:

• To avoid hazardous activities until response is known

• To contact prescriber if vaginal itching, loose foul-smelling stools, or furry tongue occurs (may indicate superinfection); to report itching, rash, pruritus, urticaria, tendon pain

• To use frequent rinsing of mouth, sugarless candy or gum for dry mouth

• To avoid other medication unless approved by prescriber

• Not to use theophylline with this product, will cause toxicity; contact prescriber if taking theophylline

• To take as prescribed, not to double or miss doses

• To notify prescriber of diarrhea with blood or pus, may indicate pseudomembranous colitis

• To prevent sun exposure or use sunscreen to prevent phototoxicity

• That drug may be taken without regard to meals; separate aluminum, magnesium, iron, or sucralfate by 4 hr; to increase fluid intake to 2 L/day to prevent crystalluria

---

albumin, normal serum 5%/25% (℞)

(al-byoo′min)
Albuminar 5%, Albuminar 25%, Albutein 5%, Albutein 25%, Buminate 5%, Buminate 25%, Plasbumin 5%, Plasbumin-25%

Func. class.: Blood derivative
Chem. class.: Placental human plasma

Action: Exerts oncotic pressure, which expands volume of circulating blood and maintains cardiac output

Uses: Restores plasma volume in burns, hyperbilirubinemia, shock, hypoproteinemia, prevention of cerebral edema, cardiopulmonary bypass procedures, ARDS

◆= Nursing alert   ▌= Herb-drug interaction   ⊘= Do not crush

Dosage and routes:

Burns

• *Adult:* **IV** dose to maintain plasma albumin at 30-50 g/L, use 5% sol initially, then 25% sol after 24 hr

Shock

• *Adult:* **IV** 500 ml of 5% sol q30 min, as needed

• *Child:* 0.5-1 g/kg/dose

Hypoproteinemia

• *Adult:* **IV** 1000-2000 ml of 5% sol qd, not to exceed 5-10 ml/min or 25-100 g of 25% sol qd, not to exceed 3 ml/min, titrated to patient response

Hyperbilirubinemia/erythroblastosis fetalis

• *Infant:* **IV** 1 g of 25% sol/kg before transfusion

Available forms: Inj 50, 250 mg/ml (5%, 25%)

Side effects/adverse reactions:

GI: Nausea, vomiting, increased salivation

INTEG: Rash, urticaria

CNS: Fever, chills, flushing, headache

RESP: Altered respirations, **_pulmonary edema_**

CV: Fluid overload, hypotension, erratic pulse, tachycardia

Contraindications: Hypersensitivity, CHF, severe anemia, renal insufficiency

Precautions: Decreased salt intake, decreased cardiac reserve, lack of albumin deficiency, hepatic disease, renal disease, pregnancy (C)

Pharmacokinetics: In hyponutrition states, metabolized as protein/energy source

Lab test interferences:

False increase: Alk phosphatase

NURSING CONSIDERATIONS

Assess:

• Blood studies Hct, Hgb; if serum protein declines, dyspnea, hypoxemia can result

• Decreased B/P, erratic pulse, respiration

• I&O ratio: urinary output may decrease

◆CVP, pulmonary wedge pressure will increase if overload occurs

• Allergy: fever, rash, itching, chills, flushing, urticaria, nausea, vomiting, hypotension, requires discontinuation of infusion, use of new lot if therapy reinstituted; premedicate with diphenhydramine

• CVP reading: distended neck veins indicate circulatory overload; shortness of breath, anxiety, insomnia, expiratory rales, frothy blood-tinged cough, cyanosis indicate pulmonary overload

Administer:

IV

• Slowly, to prevent fluid overload; dilute with NS for injection or D_5W; 5% may be given undiluted; 25% may be given diluted or undiluted, give over 4 hr, use infusion pump

Solution compatibilities: LR, NaCl, Ringer's, D_5W, $D_{10}W$, $D_{2\frac{1}{2}}W$, dextrose/saline, dextran$_6$ D_5, dextran$_6$ NaCl 0.9%, dextrose/Ringer's, dextrose/LR

Y-site compatibilities: Diltiazem, lorazepam

Perform/provide:

• Adequate hydration before, during administration

• Check type of albumin; some stored at room temperature, some need to be refrigerated

Evaluate:

• Therapeutic response: increased B/P, decreased edema, increased serum albumin levels, increased plasma protein

albuterol (℞)

(al-byoo'ter-ole)

Airet, albuterol, Gen-Salbutamol*, Novo-Salmol*, Proventil, Salbutamol, Ventodisk, Ventolin, Volmax

Func. class.: Adrenergic β_2-agonist, sympathomimetic, bronchodilator

Action: Causes bronchodilation by action on β_2 (pulmonary) receptors by increasing levels of cAMP, which relaxes smooth muscle; produces bronchodilation, CNS, cardiac stimulation, as well as increased diuresis and gastric acid secretion; longer acting than isoproterenol

Uses: Prevention of exercise-induced asthma, acute bronchospasm, bronchitis, emphysema, bronchiectasis, or other reversible airway obstruction

Investigational uses: Hyperkalemia in dialysis patients

Dosage and routes:

To prevent exercise-induced bronchospasm

• *Adult:* **INH** (metered dose inhaler) 2 puffs 15 min before exercising

Other respiratory conditions

• *Adult and child ≥12 yr:* **INH** (metered dose inhaler) 2 puffs q4h; **PO** 2-4 mg tid-qid, not to exceed 8 mg; Volmax ext rel 8 mg q12h; Repetabs 4-8 mg q12h; **NEB/IPPB** 2.5 mg tid-qid

• *Geriatric:* **PO** 2 mg tid-qid, may increase gradually to 8 mg tid-qid

• *Child 2-12 yr:* **INH** (metered dose inhaler) 0.1 mg/kg tid (max 2.5 mg tid-qid); **NEB/IPPB** 0.1-0.15 mg/kg/dose tid-qid or 1.25 mg tid-qid for child 10-15 kg or 2.5 mg tid-qid >15 kg

• *Adult and child > 4 yr:* **INH CAP** (Rotahaler inhalation) 200 µg cap inhaled q4-6h; may use 15 min before exercise

Available forms: Aerosol 90 µg/actuation; oral sol 2 mg/5 ml; tabs 2, 4 mg; ext rel 4, 8 mg; inh sol 0.83, 0.5, 1, 2, 5 mg/ml; powder for inh (RotaCaps) 200, 400 µg; powder for inh (Ventodisk) 200, 400 µg; inh cap 200 µg; 100 µg/spray, 80 inh/canister, 200 inh/canister

Side effects/adverse reactions:

CNS: *Tremors, anxiety,* insomnia, headache, dizziness, stimulation, *restlessness,* hallucinations, flushing, irritability

CV: Palpitations, tachycardia, hypertension, angina, hypotension, dysrhythmias

EENT: Dry nose, irritation of nose and throat

GI: Heartburn, nausea, vomiting

MISC: Flushing, sweating, anorexia, bad taste/smell changes

MS: Muscle cramps

RESP: Cough, wheezing, dyspnea, *bronchospasm,* dry throat

Contraindications: Hypersensitivity to sympathomimetics, tachydysrhythmias, severe cardiac disease, heart block

Precautions: Lactation, pregnancy (C), cardiac disorders, hyperthyroidism, diabetes mellitus, hypertension, prostatic hypertrophy, narrow-angle glaucoma, seizures, exercise-induced bronchospasm (aerosol) in children <12 years

Do not confuse:

albuterol/atenolol

Ventolin/Vantin

Proventil/Prinivil

Pharmacokinetics: Well absorbed PO, extensively metabolized in the liver and tissues, crosses placenta, breast milk, blood-brain barrier

PO: Onset ½ hr, peak 2½ hr, duration 4-6 hr, half-life 2½ hr

PO-ER: Onset ½ hour; peak 2-3 hr; duration 12 hr

⬧ = Nursing alert   ⦸ = Herb-drug interaction   ⊘ = Do not crush

INH: Onset 5 min, peak 1-1½ hr, duration 4-6 hr, half-life 4 hr

Interactions:

• Increased action of aerosol bronchodilators

• Increased action of albuterol: tricyclic antidepressants, MAOIs, other adrenergics; do not use together

• May inhibit action of albuterol: other β-blockers

• Severe hypotension: oxytoxics

• Toxicity: theophylline

• ECG changes/hypokalemia: potassium-losing diuretics

NURSING CONSIDERATIONS

Assess:

• Respiratory function: vital capacity, forced expiratory volume, ABGs; lung sounds, heart rate and rhythm, B/P, sputum (baseline and peak)

• That patient has not received theophylline therapy before giving dose

• Patient's ability to self-medicate

• For evidence of allergic reactions

• Paradoxical bronchospasm, hold medication, notify prescriber if bronchospasm occurs

Administer:

Inhalation

• In geriatric patients, a spacing device is advised

• After shaking metered dose inhaler, exhale, place mouthpiece in mouth, inhale slowly, hold breath, remove, exhale slowly; give INH at least 1 min apart

• NEB/IPPB diluting 5 mg/ml sol/ 2.5 ml 0.9% NaCl for INH; other sol do not require dilution; for neb O_2 flow or compressed air 6-10 L/min

• Gum, sips of water for dry mouth

PO

• With meals to decrease gastric irritation

• Oral solution to children (no alcohol, sugar)

🚫 Do not crush, break, or chew ext rel tabs

Perform/provide:

• Storage in light-resistant container, do not expose to temperatures over 86° F (30° C)

Evaluate:

• Therapeutic response: absence of dyspnea, wheezing after 1 hr, improved airway exchange, improved ABGs

Teach patient/family:

• To use exactly as prescribed; take missed dose when remembered, alter dosing schedule

• Not to use OTC medications; excess stimulation may occur

• Use of inhaler; review package insert with patient; use demonstration, return demonstration

• To avoid getting aerosol in eyes; blurring of vision may result

• To wash inhaler in warm water qd and dry

• To avoid smoking, smoke-filled rooms, persons with respiratory infections

◆ That paradoxic bronchospasm may occur and to stop drug immediately, call prescriber

• To limit caffeine products such as chocolate, coffee, tea, and colas

Treatment of overdose: Administer a β_1-adrenergic blocker

---

aldesleukin (℞)

(al-dess-loo'ken)
Interleukin-2, IL-2, Proleukin

Func. class.: Miscellaneous antineoplastic

Chem. class.: Interleukin-2, human recombinant (cytokine)

Action: Enhancement of lymphocyte mitogenesis and stimulation of IL-2–dependent cell lines; enhancement of lymphocyte cytotoxicity; induction of killer cell activity; induction of interferon-γ production;

results in activation of cellular immunity, cytokines, and inhibition of tumor growth

Uses: Metastatic renal cell carcinoma in adults, phase II for HIV in combination with zidovudine, melanoma

Investigational uses: Kaposi's sarcoma given with zidovudine, metastatic melanoma given with cyclophosphamide, non-Hodgkin's lymphoma given with lymphokine-activated killer cells, AIDS (phase I) given with zidovudine

Dosage and routes:
• *Adult:* **IV INF** 600,000 IU/kg (0.037 mg/kg) over 15 min q8h × 14 doses; off 9 days, repeat schedule for another 14 doses, for a max of 28 doses/course

Available forms: Powder for inj 22 million IU/vial

Side effects/adverse reactions:
CV: Hypotension, sinus tachycardia, dysrhythmias, bradycardia, PVCs, PACs, myocardial ischemia, *myocardial infarction, cardiac arrest, capillary leak syndrome, CVA*
RESP: Pulmonary congestion, dyspnea, *pulmonary edema, respiratory failure, apnea,* tachypnea, pleural effusion, wheezing
GI: Nausea, vomiting, *diarrhea,* stomatitis, anorexia, GI bleeding, dyspepsia, constipation, *intestinal perforation*/ileus, jaundice, ascites
HEMA: Anemia, *thrombocytopenia, leukopenia, coagulation disorders, leukocytosis, eosinophilia*
CNS: Mental status changes, dizziness, sensory dysfunction, syncope, motor dysfunction, fever, chills, headache, impaired memory, depression, sleep disturbances, hallucinations, rigors
GU: Oliguria/anuria, proteinuria, hematuria, dysuria, *renal failure*
INTEG: Pruritus, *erythema, rash,* dry skin, *exfoliative dermatitis,* purpura, petechiae, urticaria
MS: Arthralgia, myalgia
SYST: Infection
EENT: Reversible visual changes

Contraindications: Hypersensitivity, abnormal thallium stress test or pulmonary function tests, organ allografts

Precautions: CNS metastases, bacterial infections, renal/hepatic/cardiac/pulmonary disease, pregnancy (C), lactation, children, anemia, thrombocytopenia

Do not confuse:
Proleukin/Prokine

Pharmacokinetics: Renal elimination half-life 85 min; onset 4 wk, duration ≤12 mo

Interactions:
• Potentiate hypotension: antihypertensives
• Reduced antitumor effectiveness: glucocorticoids
• Increased toxicity: aminoglycosides, indomethacin, cytotoxic chemotherapy, methotrexate, asparaginase, doxorubicin
• Unpredictable reactions: psychotropics

Lab test interferences:
Increase: Bilirubin, BUN, serum creatinine, transaminase, alk phosphatase; hypomagnesemia, acidosis hypocalcemia, hypophosphatemia, hypokalemia, hyperuricemia, hypoalbuminemia, hypoproteinemia, hyponatremia, hyperkalemia, alkalosis (toxic effect of drug)

NURSING CONSIDERATIONS
Assess:
• CBC, differential, platelet count weekly; withhold drug if WBC is <2000/mm^3 or platelet count is <75,000/mm^3; notify prescriber of these results
⬥Capillary leak syndrome including a drop in mean arterial pressure (2-12 hr after initiating therapy); hy-

potension and hypoperfusion will occur; if B/P < 90 mm Hg, use CVP, ECG, VS
• Renal function studies: BUN, serum uric acid, urine CrCl, electrolytes before, during therapy; I&O ratio; report fall in urine output to <30 ml/hr
• Monitor temp q4h; fever may indicate beginning infection
• Liver function tests before, during therapy: bilirubin, AST, ALT, alk phosphatase, LDH as needed or monthly
• ECG; watch for ST-T wave changes, low QRS and T, possible dysrhythmias (sinus tachycardia, PVCs)
➤ Baselines in pulmonary function; document FEV >2 L or ≥75% prior to therapy; check daily VS, pulse oximetry, dyspnea, rales, ABGs; watch for respiratory failure, intubate if necessary
• Stress thallium study prior to therapy; document normal ejection fraction, unimpaired wall motion
• Bleeding: hematuria, guaiac, bruising or petechiae, mucosa or orifices q8h
• Buccal cavity q8h for dryness, sores, ulceration, white patches, oral pain, bleeding, dysphagia
• Local irritation, pain, burning at injection site
• GI symptoms: frequency of stools, cramping; acidosis, signs of dehydration: rapid respirations, poor skin turgor, decreased urine output, dry skin, restlessness, weakness

Administer:
IV, INT INF
• Hydrocortisone, dexamethasone or sodium bicarbonate (1 mEq/1 ml) for extravasation, apply ice compresses
• Antiemetic 30-60 min before giving drug to prevent vomiting
• IV after diluting 22 million IU (1.3 mg)/1.2 ml sterile H_2O for inj at site of vial and swirl, do not shake: dilute dose with 50 ml D_5W and give over 15 min; use plastic bag; do not use an in-line filter, give through Y-tube or 3-way stopcock
• Dopamine 1-5 kg/min before onset of hypotension; decreased dose preserves kidney output

Y-site compatibilities: Amikacin, amphotericin B, calcium gluconate, diphenhydramine, dopamine, fluconazole, foscarnet, gentamicin, heparin, IV fat emulsion, magnesium sulfate, metoclopramide, morphine, ondansetron, piperacillin, potassium chloride, ranitidine, ticarcillin, tobramycin, TPN #145, trimethoprim-sulfamethoxazole

Perform/provide:
• Liquid diet: carbonated beverage, gelatin (Jell-O) may be added if patient is not nauseated or vomiting
• Rinsing of mouth tid-qid with water, club soda; brushing of teeth bid-tid with soft brush or cotton-tipped applicators for stomatitis; use unwaxed dental floss
• Storage in refrigerator of diluted drug; do not freeze; administer within 48 hr; bring to room temperature before infusing; discard unused portion

Evaluate:
• Therapeutic response: decreased tumor size, spread of malignancy

Teach patient/family:
• To use a nonhormonal contraceptive method during therapy
• To report any complaints, side effects to nurse or prescriber
• To avoid foods with citric acid, hot or rough texture
• To avoid alcohol, NSAIDs, salicylates; GI bleeding may occur
• To report any bleeding, white spots, ulcerations in mouth to prescriber; tell patient to examine mouth qd

---

• To avoid crowds and persons with infections when granulocyte count is low

• Visual problems may occur, but are reversible

alemtuzumab
See appendix a—selected new drugs

alendronate (℞)
(al-en-drone'ate)
Fosamax
Func. class.: Bone-resorption inhibitor
Chem. class.: Biphosphonate

Action: Absorbs calcium phosphate crystal in bone and may directly block dissolution of hydroxyapatite crystals of bone; inhibits bone resorption, apparently without inhibiting bone formation, mineralization

Uses: Osteoporosis in postmenopausal women, treatment of osteoporosis in men, Paget's disease, prevention of osteoporosis, treatment of corticosteroid-induced osteoporosis in postmenopausal women not receiving estrogen

Dosage and routes:
Osteoporosis in postmenopausal women
• *Adult and elderly:* **PO** 10 mg qd
Paget's disease
• *Adult and elderly:* **PO** 40 mg qd × 6 mo
Prevention of osteoporosis
• *Adult:* **PO** 5 mg qd
Corticosteroid-induced osteoporosis
• *Adult:* **PO** 10 mg qd
Available forms: Tabs 5, 10, 35, 40, 70 mg

Side effects/adverse reactions:
CNS: Headache
META: Anemia, hypokalemia, hypomagnesemia, hypophosphatemia
GI: Abdominal pain, anorexia, constipation, nausea, vomiting, esophageal ulceration
MS: Bone pain
CV: Hypertension
GU: UTI, fluid overload

Contraindications: Hypersensitivity to biphosphonates, hypocalcemia

Precautions: Children, lactation, pregnancy (C), CrCl <35 ml/min, esophageal disease, ulcers, gastritis

Pharmacokinetics: Rapidly cleared from circulation, taken up mainly by bones, eliminated primarily through kidneys

Interactions:
• Decreased absorption: antacids, calcium supplements
• GI reactions: NSAIDs, salicylates
• Increased alendronate effect: ranitidine
• Drug/food: decreased absorption

NURSING CONSIDERATIONS
Assess:
• Electrolytes; renal function studies; Ca, P, Mg, K; confirm osteoporosis with bone density test before use
• For hypercalcemia: paresthesia, twitching, laryngospasm, Chvostek's, Trousseau's signs
• Alk phosphatase levels, baseline and periodically, 2 × upper limit of normal are indicative of Paget's disease

Administer:
PO
• For 6 months to be effective in Paget's disease; take with 8 oz of water 30 min ac

Perform/provide:
• Storage in cool environment, out of direct sunlight

◆ = Nursing alert   ✦ = Herb-drug interaction   ⊘ = Do not crush

Evaluate:
• Therapeutic response: increased bone mass, absence of fractures
Teach patient/family:
• To remain upright for 30 min after dose to prevent esophageal irritation, if dose is missed, skip dose, do not double doses or take later in day
• To take in AM before food, other meds, take with 6-8 oz of water only (no mineral water)
• To take calcium, vit D if instructed by health care provider
• To use weight-bearing exercise to increase bone density
• To let health care provider know if pregnant or if pregnancy is planned or if nursing

---

RARELY USED

alfentanil (℞)
(al-fen′ta-nil)
Alfenta, Rapifen*
Func. class.: Opioid analgesic

Controlled Substance Schedule II
Uses: In combination with other drugs in general anesthesia, as a primary anesthetic in general surgery, monitored anesthesia care (MAC)
Dosage and routes:
Anesthesia <30 min
Combination
• *Adult:* IV 8-50 µg/kg, may increase by 3-15 µg/kg
Anesthetic induction
• *Adult:* IV 3-5 µg/kg, then 0.5-1.5 µg/kg/min; total dose is 8-40 µg/kg
Anesthesia 30-60 min
Induction
• *Adult:* IV 20-50 µg/kg
Maintenance
• *Adult:* IV 5-15 µg/kg; may give up to 75 µg/kg total dose
Continuous anesthesia >45 min
Induction
• *Adult:* IV 50-75 µg/kg

Maintenance
• *Adult:* IV 0.5-3.0 µg/kg/min; rate should be decreased by 30%-50% after 1 hr maintenance **INF;** may be increased to 4 µg/kg/min or **BOL** doses of 7 µg/kg
Induction of anesthesia >45 min
• *Adult:* IV 130-245 µg/kg, then 0.5-1.5 µg/kg/min
MAC
Induction
• *Adult:* IV duration ≤½ hr 3-8 µg/kg
Maintenance
• *Adult:* 3-5 µg/kg q5-20min to 1 µg/kg/min, total dose 3-40 µg/kg
Contraindications: Child <12 yr, hypersensitivity

---

alitretinoin (℞)
(a-li-tret′i-noyn)
Panretin
Func. class.: Retinoid, 2nd generation

Action: Controls cellular differentiation and proliferation of neoplastic and healthy cells by binding to retinoid receptors
Uses: Kaposi's sarcoma cutaneous lesions
Dosage and routes:
• *Adult:* TOP Apply enough gel to cover lesions with a generous coating, allow to dry for 3-5 min, before covering with clothing, do not apply near mucosal areas, apply as long as benefit occurs
Available forms: Gel 0.1%
Side effects/adverse reactions:
INTEG: Rash, stinging, warmth, redness, erythema, blistering, crusting, peeling, contact dermatitis, *pain*
Contraindications: Hypersensitivity to retinoids, pregnancy (D)
Precautions: Lactation, eczema, sunburn, elderly, cutaneous T-cell lymphoma

---

Pharmacokinetics:
TOP: Poor systemic absorption
Interactions:
• Do not use around DEET (an insect repellant agent)

NURSING CONSIDERATIONS
Assess:
• Area of body involved, what helps or aggravates condition; cysts, dryness, itching; lesions may worsen at beginning of treatment
• Dermal toxicity that may start as erythema, then edema, may need to be discontinued and restarted
Administer:
• Bid initially to lesions, can be increased to tid-qid according to tolerance
Perform/provide:
• Storage at room temperature
• Hand washing after application
Evaluate:
• Therapeutic response: decrease in size and number of lesions
Teach patient/family:
• To avoid application on normal skin, getting cream in eyes, nose, other mucous membranes
• To avoid sunlight, sunlamps, or use protective clothing, sunscreen
• That treatment may cause warmth, stinging, dryness, peeling will occur
• That drug does not cure condition; only relieves symptoms
• That therapeutic results may be seen in 2-3 wk but may not be optimal until after 6 wk

---

allopurinol (R̶)
(al-oh-pure'i-nole)
allopurinol, Aloprim, Apo-Allopurinol*, Lopurin*, Purimol*, Zyloprim
Func. class.: Antigout drug
Chem. class.: Xanthene oxidase inhibitor

Action: Inhibits the enzyme xanthine oxidase, reducing uric acid synthesis
Uses: Chronic gout, hyperuricemia associated with malignancies, recurrent calcium oxalate calculi, Chagas' disease, cutaneous/visceral leishmaniasis
Investigational uses: Stomatitis (mouthwash)
Dosage and routes:
Increased uric acid levels in malignancies
• *Adult:* **IV INF** 200-400 mg/m^2/day, max 600 mg/day
• *Child:* **IV INF** 200 mg/m^2/day, initially
Gout/hyperuricemia
• *Adult:* **PO** 200-600 mg qd depending on severity, not to exceed 800 mg/day
• *Child 6-10 yr:* 300 mg qd
• *Child <6 yr:* 150 mg qd
Impaired renal function
• *Adult:* **PO** 200 mg qd (CrCl is 20 to 30 ml/min)
• *Adult:* **PO** 100 mg qd (CrCl <20 ml/min)
Recurrent calculi
• *Adult:* **PO** 200-300 mg qd
Uric acid nephropathy prevention
• *Adult and child >10 yr:* **PO** 600-800 mg qd × 2-3 days
Stomatitis
• *Adult:* Mouthwash dose varies, do not swallow
Available forms: Tabs, scored 100,

---

300 mg; powder for inj, lyophilized 500 mg

Side effects/adverse reactions:

*HEMA: **Agranulocytosis, thrombocytopenia, aplastic anemia, pancytopenia, leukopenia, bone marrow suppression, eosinophilia***

CNS: Headache, drowsiness, neuritis, paresthesia

GI: Nausea, vomiting, anorexia, malaise, metallic taste, cramps, peptic ulcer, diarrhea, stomatitis

MISC: Myopathy, arthralgia, hepatomegaly, ***cholestatic jaundice, renal failure, exfoliative dermatitis***

EENT: Retinopathy, cataracts, epistaxis

INTEG: Fever, chills, dermatitis, pruritus, purpura, erythema, ecchymosis, alopecia

Contraindications: Hypersensitivity

Precautions: Pregnancy (C), lactation, renal disease, hepatic disease, children

Do not confuse:

allopurinol/apresoline

Lopurin/Lupron

Pharmacokinetics:

PO: Peak 2-4 hr; excreted in feces, urine; half-life 2-3 hr, terminal half-life 18-30 hr

IV: Half-life 1 hr

Interactions:

• Increased action of oral anticoagulants, chlorpropamide, cyclophosphamide, hydantoin, theophylline, vidarabine, ACE inhibitors, mercaptopurine, azathioprine

• Possible kidney stone formation: ammonium chloride, vit C, potassium/sodium phosphate

• Decreased effects of probenecid

• Rash: ampicillin, amoxicillin, bacampicillin

• Increased allopurinol toxicity: thiazide diuretics

• Decreased effects of allopurinol: aluminum salts

• Increased bone marrow depression: antineoplastics

NURSING CONSIDERATIONS

Assess:

• Uric acid levels q2wk; uric acid levels should be 6 mg/dl or less

• CBC, AST, BUN, creatinine before starting treatment, monthly

• I&O ratio; increase fluids to 2 L/day to prevent stone formation

• Nutritional status: discourage organ meat, sardines, salmon, legumes, gravies (high-purine foods), alcohol

Administer:

PO

• With meals, to prevent GI symptoms

• A few days before antineoplastic therapy

IV INF

• Reconstitute of 30 ml vial with 25 ml of sterile water for inj; dilute to desired conc with 0.9% NaCl for inj or D$_5$ for inj, begin inf within 10 hr

Solution incompatibilities:

Amikacin, amphotericin B, carmustine, cefotaxime, chlorpromazine, cimetidine, clindamycin, cytarabine, dacarbazine, daunorubicin, diphenhydramine, doxorubicin, doxycycline, droperidol, floxuridine, gentamicin, haloperidol, hydroxyzine, idarubicin, imipenem, cilastatin, mechlorethamine, meperidine, metoclopramide, methylprednisolone, minocycline, nalbuphine, netilmicin, ondansetron, prochlorperazine, promethazine, sodium bicarbonate, streptozocin, tobramycin, vinorelbine

Evaluate:

• Therapeutic response: decreased pain in joints, decreased stone formation in kidneys

Teach patient/family:

• That tabs may be crushed

• To take as prescribed; if dose is

missed, take as soon as remembered; do not double dose
• To increase fluid intake to 2 L/day
• To report skin rash, stomatitis, malaise, fever, aching; drug should be discontinued
• To avoid hazardous activities if drowsiness or dizziness occurs
• To avoid alcohol, caffeine; will increase uric acid levels
• To avoid large doses of vit C; kidney stone formation may occur
• To maintain a diet enhancing urine alkalinity, e.g., dairy products
• To reduce dairy products, refined sugars, sodium, meat if taking for calcium oxalate stones

---

almotriptan

See appendix a—selected new drugs

---

alprazolam (℞)

(al-pray′zoe-lam)
Apo-Alpraz*, Novo-Alprazol*, Nu-Alpraz*, Xanax
Func. class.: Antianxiety; sedative/hypnotic
Chem. class.: Benzodiazepine

Controlled Substance Schedule IV
Action: Depresses subcortical levels of CNS, including limbic system, reticular formation
Uses: Anxiety, panic disorders, anxiety with depressive symptoms
Investigational uses: Depression, social phobia, premenstrual dysphoric disorders
Dosage and routes:
Anxiety disorder
• *Adult:* **PO** 0.25-0.5 mg tid, not to exceed 4 mg/day in divided doses
• *Elderly:* **PO** 0.125-0.25 mg bid; increase by 0.125 as needed

Panic disorder
• *Adult:* **PO** 0.5 mg tid may increase, max 10 mg/day
Premenstrual dysphoric disorders
• *Adult:* **PO** 0.25 mg bid-qid, starting on day 16-18 of menses, taper over 2-3 days when menses occurs
Social phobia
• *Adult:* **PO** 2-8 mg/day
Hepatic dose
Reduce dose by 50%
Available forms: Tabs 0.25, 0.5, 1, 2 mg; oral sol 0.1, 1 mg/ml
Side effects/adverse reactions:
CNS: Dizziness, drowsiness, confusion, headache, anxiety, tremors, stimulation, fatigue, depression, insomnia, hallucinations
GI: Constipation, dry mouth, nausea, vomiting, anorexia, diarrhea
INTEG: Rash, dermatitis, itching
*CV: Orthostatic hypotension, **ECG changes, tachycardia,*** hypotension
EENT: Blurred vision, tinnitus, mydriasis
Contraindications: Hypersensitivity to benzodiazepines, narrow-angle glaucoma, psychosis, pregnancy (D), lactation, addiction
Precautions: Elderly, debilitated, hepatic disease
Do not confuse:
alprazolam/lorazepam
Xanax/Lanoxin
Xanax/Tylox
Xanax/Zantac
Pharmacokinetics:
PO: Onset 30 min, peak 1-2 hr, duration 4-6 hr, therapeutic response 2-3 days; metabolized by liver, excreted by kidneys; crosses placenta, breast milk; half-life 12-15 hr
Interactions:
• Decreased sedation: xanthines
• Decreased alprazolam action: barbiturates, rifampin
• A substrate of CYP 3A4

 = Nursing alert　　🍃 = Herb-drug interaction　　🚫 = Do not crush

• Increased alprazolam action: cimetidine, disulfiram, erythromycin, fluoxetine, isoniazid, ketoconazole, metoprolol, propoxyphene, propanolol, valproic acid

• Increased CNS depression: anticonvulsants, alcohol, antihistamines, sedative/hypnotics

• Decreased action of levodopa

• Drug/food: increased drug level; grapefruit juice

🚫 Increased CNS depression, coma: kava

Lab test interferences:
Increase: AST/ALT, alk phosphatase

NURSING CONSIDERATIONS
Assess:

• Mental status: anxiety, mood, sensorium, affect, sleeping pattern, drowsiness, dizziness, especially in elderly

• B/P lying, standing; pulse; if systolic B/P drops 20 mm Hg, hold drug, notify prescriber

• Hepatic studies: AST, ALT, bilirubin, creatinine, LDH, alk phosphatase

• For indications of increasing tolerance and abuse

◆Physical dependency, withdrawal symptoms: anxiety, panic attacks, agitation, convulsions, headache, nausea, vomiting, muscle pain, weakness; withdrawal seizures may occur after rapid decrease in dose or abrupt discontinuation; since duration of action is short, considered to be the drug of choice in the elderly

Administer:
PO

• With food or milk for GI symptoms

• Crushed, mixed with food or fluids if patient is unable to swallow medication whole

• May divide total daily doses into more times/day, if anxiety occurs between doses

Evaluate:
• Therapeutic response: decreased anxiety, restlessness, sleeplessness

Teach patient/family:
• Not to double doses; take exactly as prescribed; if dose is missed, take within 1 hr as scheduled

• That drug may be taken with food

• Not to use for everyday stress or longer than 4 mo unless directed by prescriber; not to take more than prescribed amount; may be habit forming; memory impairment is a sign of long-term use

• To avoid OTC preparations unless approved by prescriber

• To avoid driving, activities that require alertness, since drowsiness may occur

• To avoid alcohol ingestion or other psychotropic medications unless directed by prescriber

• Not to discontinue medication abruptly after long-term use

• To rise slowly or fainting may occur, especially elderly

• That drowsiness may worsen at beginning of treatment

Treatment of overdose: Lavage, VS, supportive care, flumazenil

---

RARELY USED

alprostadil (℞)
(al-pros'ta-dil)
Caverject, Edex, Muse, PGEI, prostaglandin E₁, Prostin VR*, Prostin VR Pediatric
Func. class.: Hormone

Uses: To maintain patent ductus arteriosus (temporary treatment), erectile dysfunction

Dosage and routes:
Patent ductus arteriosus
• *Infants:* IV INF 0.1 µg/kg/min, until desired response, then reduce

to lowest effective amount, 0.4 µg/kg/min not likely to produce greater beneficial effects

Erectile dysfunction of vasculogenic or mixed etiology, psychogenic

• *Men:* **INTRACAVERNOSAL** 2.5 µg may increase by 2.5 µg; may then increase by 5-10 µg until adequate response occurs; **INTRA-URETHRAL:** administer as needed to achieve erection

Contraindications: Hypersensitivity, respiratory distress syndrome (RDS)

---

alteplase (℞)

(al-ti-plaze')

Activase, Activase rt-PA*, Cathflo, Lysatec-rt-PA*, tissue plasminogen activator, t-PA

Func. class.: Thrombolytic enzyme

Chem. class.: Tissue plasminogen activator (TPA)

Action: Produces fibrin conversion of plasminogen to plasmin; able to bind to fibrin, convert plasminogen in thrombus to plasmin, which leads to local fibrinolysis, limited systemic proteolysis

Uses: Lysis of obstructing thrombi associated with acute MI, ischemic conditions requiring thrombolysis, i.e., PE, DVT, unclotting arteriovenous shunts, acute ischemic CVA

Investigational uses: Unstable angina, occluded catheters

Dosage and routes:

Standard INF

• *Adult >65 kg:* **IV** a total of 100 mg; 6-10 mg given **IV BOL** over 1-2 min, 60 mg given over first hour, 20 mg given over second hour, 20 mg given over third hour; or 1.25 mg/kg given over 3 hr for smaller patients

• *Adult <65 kg:* **IV** 0.75 mg over 1st hr, 0.075-0.125 mg/kg given **IV BOL** over 1st 1-2 min; 0.25 mg/kg over 2nd hr, 0.25 mg/kg over 3rd hr to a total dose of 1.25 mg/kg, max 100 mg total

Accelerated INF

• *Adult:* **IV BOL** 15 mg; then 0.75 mg/kg over ½ hr; 0.5 mg/kg over 1 hr

Pulmonary embolism

• *Adult:* **IV** 100 mg over 2 hr, then heparin

Acute ischemic stroke

• *Adult:* **IV** 0.9 mg/kg, max 90 mg; give as **INF** over 1 hr, give 10% of dose **IV BOL** over 1st min

Occluded catheters

• *Adult:* 2 mg/2 ml infused in each port of dual-lumen catheter, dwell time varies widely

Available forms: Powder for inj 20 mg (11.6 million IU/vial), 50 mg (29 million IU/vial); 2 mg single-patient vial

Side effects/adverse reactions:

SYST: GI, GU, intracranial, retroperitoneal bleeding, surface bleeding, anaphylaxis

CV: Sinus bradycardia, ventricular tachycardia, accelerated idioventricular rhythm

INTEG: Urticaria, rash

Contraindications: Hypersensitivity, active internal bleeding, recent CVA, severe uncontrolled hypertension, intracranial/intraspinal surgery/trauma, aneurysm

Precautions: Pregnancy (C), lactation, children

Do not confuse:

alteplace/Altace

Pharmacokinetics: Cleared by liver, 80% cleared within 10 min of drug termination, onset immediate, peak 45 min, duration 4 hr

---

Interactions:
• Increased bleeding: anticoagulants, salicylates, dipyridamole, other NSAIDs, abciximab, eptifibatide, tirofiban, clopidogrel, ticlopidine, some cephalosporins, plicamycin, valproic acid

Lab test interferences:
Increase: PT, APTT, TT

NURSING CONSIDERATIONS

Assess:
• VS, B/P, pulse, respirations, neurologic signs, temperature at least q4h; temp >104° F (40° C) indicates internal bleeding; monitor rhythm closely; ventricular dysrhythmias may occur with hyperfusion; monitor heart, breath sounds, neurologic status, peripheral pulses; assess neurologic status, neurologic change may indicate intracranial bleeding

⬥For bleeding during first hour of treatment and 24 hr after procedure: hematuria, hematemesis, bleeding from mucous membranes, epistaxis, ecchymosis; guaiac all body fluids, stools. Do not use 150 mg or more total dose; intracranial bleeding may occur

⬥ Hypersensitivity: fever, rash, itching, chills, facial swelling, dyspnea, notify prescriber immediately; stop drug, keep resusciatative equipment nearby; mild reaction may be treated with antihistamines

• Blood studies (Hct, platelets, PTT, PT, TT, APTT) before starting therapy; PT or APTT must be less than 2 × control before starting therapy TT or PT q3-4h during treatment

• ECG continuously, cardiac enzymes, radionuclide myocardial scanning/coronary angiography

Administer:

Intermittent IV inf
• After reconstituting with provided diluent, add appropriate amount of sterile water for injection (no preservatives) 20 mg vial/20 ml or 50 mg vial/50 ml to make 1 mg/ml, mix by slow inversion or dilute with NaCl, D_5W to a concentration of 0.5 mg/ml; 1.5 to <0.5 mg/ml may result in precipitation of drug; use 18 G needle; flush line with NaCl after administration, give over 3 hr for MI, 2 hr for pulmonary embolism

Heparin therapy after thrombolytic therapy is discontinued, TT, ACT, or APTT less than 2 × control (about 3-4 hr)

Reconstituted IV solution within 8 hr or discard

Within 6 hr of coronary occlusion for best results

Additive compatibilities: Lidocaine, morphine, nitroglycerin

Y-site compatibilities: Lidocaine, metoprolol, propranolol

Perform/provide:
• Avoidance of invasive procedures, injection, rectal temp
• Pressure for 30 sec to minor bleeding sites; 30 min to sites of atrial puncture, followed by pressure dressing; inform prescriber if this does not attain hemostasis; apply pressure dressing
• Storage of powder at room temperature or refrigerate; protect from excessive light

Evaluate:
• Therapeutic response: lysis of thrombi

Teach patient/family:
• The purpose and expected results of the treatment; to report adverse reactions

altretamine (℞)

(al-tret'a-meen)
Hexalen, hexamethylmela-
mine, Hexastat*
Func. class.: Misc. antineoplastic
Chem. class.: S-triazine derivative (formerly known as hexa-
methylmelamine)

Action: Products of metabolism form covalent adducts with tissue macromolecules including DNA, which may be responsible for cytotoxicity; activity is not cell cycle phase specific

Uses: Palliative treatment of recurrent, persistent ovarian cancer following first-line treatment with cisplatin or alkylating agent–based combination

Dosage and routes:
• *Adult:* **PO** 260 mg/m²/day for 14 or 21 days in a 28-day cycle; give in 4 divided doses after meals and at hs

Available forms: Caps 50, 100 mg

Side effects/adverse reactions:

GI: Nausea, anorexia, vomiting, increased alk phosphatase, **hepatic toxicity,** cramping

CNS: Peripheral sensory neuropathy, fatigue, **seizures,** mood disorders, disorders of consciousness, ataxia, dizziness, vertigo, Parkinson-like tremors

*HEMA: **Leukopenia, thrombocytopenia, anemia***

GU: Increased BUN, serum creatinine

INTEG: Rash, pruritus, alopecia, eczema

Contraindications: Hypersensitivity, severe bone marrow depression, severe neurologic toxicity, pregnancy (D)

Precautions: Lactation, children

Pharmacokinetics:

PO: Well absorbed orally, rapidly metabolized in liver, metabolites excreted in urine; peak ½-3 hr, half-life 4½-10 hr

Interactions:
• Possible increased toxicity of altretamine: cimetidine
• Severe orthostatic hypotension: MAOI
• Increased bone marrow depression: radiation, antineoplastic agents
• Decreased antibody reaction: live virus vaccines

NURSING CONSIDERATIONS

Assess:
• Bone marrow depression: fever, chills, sore throat, cough, fatigue, bleeding; notify prescriber
• Neurotoxicity: anxiety, dizziness, depression
• CBC, differential, platelet count weekly, withhold drug if WBC is <2000 or platelet count is <75,000 or granulocyte count is <1000/mm³; notify prescriber of results
• Renal function studies: BUN, serum uric acid, urine CrCl before, during therapy
• I&O ratio; report fall in urine output of 30 ml/hr
• Temp q4h; may indicate beginning infection
• Liver function tests before, during therapy (bilirubin, AST, ALT, LDH) as needed or monthly

Administer:

PO
• Give pc and hs to lessen nausea
• Antacid before oral agent, give drug after meals, at hs
• Antiemetic 30-60 min before giving drug to prevent vomiting

Perform/provide:
• Strict medical asepsis, protective isolation if WBC levels are low
• All medications PO, no rectal

 = Nursing alert   = Herb-drug interaction   = Do not crush

temp, apply pressure to venipuncture sites for 10 min
Evaluate:
• Therapeutic response: decreased tumor size, spread of malignancy
Teach patient/family:
• To report signs of infection: increased temp, sore throat, flu symptoms
• To report signs of anemia: fatigue, headache, faintness, shortness of breath, irritability
• To report bleeding; avoid use of razors, commercial mouthwash
• To avoid use of aspirin products, ibuprofen
• That hair may be lost during therapy; a wig or hairpiece may make patient feel better; new hair may be different in color, texture (rare)
• To use contraception during and 4 mo after treatment
• Not to receive vaccines during treatment
• To report numbness in extremities

aluminum hydroxide (OTC)

AlternaGEL, Alu-Cap, Alugel*, aluminum hydroxide, Aluminet, Alu-Tab, Amphojel, Basal gel, Dialume

Func. class.: Antacid, hypophosphatemic, antiulcer

Chem. class.: Aluminum product

Action: Neutralizes gastric acidity, binds phosphates in GI tract; these phosphates are excreted
Uses: Antacid, hyperphosphatemia in chronic renal failure; adjunct in gastric, peptic, duodenal ulcers; hyperacidity, reflux esophagitis, heartburn
Investigational uses: Stress ulcer, GI bleeding

Dosage and routes:
Antacid
• *Adult:* SUSP 5-10 ml 1 hr pc, hs; PO 600 mg 1 hr pc, hs, chewed with milk or water
Hyperphosphatemia in renal failure
• *Adult:* SUSP 500 mg-2 g bid-qid
GI bleeding
• *Infant:* 2-5 ml/dose q1-2h
• *Child:* PO 5-15 ml/dose q1-2h
Available forms: Caps 475, 500 mg; tabs 300, 500, 600 mg; susp 450 mg/5 ml, 600 mg/5 ml; liq 320 mg/5 ml, 600 mg/5 ml, 675 mg/5 ml
Side effects/adverse reactions:
GI: Constipation, anorexia, **obstruction,** fecal impaction
META: Hypophosphatemia, hypercalciuria
Contraindications: Hypersensitivity to this drug or aluminum products
Precautions: Elderly, fluid restriction, decreased GI motility, GI obstruction, dehydration, renal disease, sodium-restricted diets, pregnancy (C), lactation
Pharmacokinetics:
PO: Onset 20-40 min, duration ½-1½ hr, excreted in feces
Interactions:
• Decreased effectiveness of tetracyclines, allopurinol, corticosteroids, diflunisal, H_2-antagonists, penicillamine, thyroid hormones, ticlopidine anticholinergics, phenothiazines, isoniazid, quinidine, phenytoin, digitalis, iron salts, warfarin, ketoconazole, ciprofloxacin; separate by at least 2 hr
NURSING CONSIDERATIONS
Assess:
• Pain: location, intensity, duration, character
• Phosphate levels, since drug is bound in GI system

• Hypophosphatemia: anorexia, weakness, fatigue, bone pain, hyporeflexia
• Constipation; increase bulk in diet if needed
• Urinary pH, Ca^{++}, electrolytes
Administer:
PO
• Give with 8 oz water for hyperphosphatemia, unless contraindicated
• Tablets must be chewed well, then give 8 oz water
• Laxatives or stool softeners if constipation occurs, especially elderly
• After shaking liquid
• With small amount of water or milk
NG
• By nasogastric tube if patient unable to swallow
Evaluate:
• Therapeutic response: absence of pain, decreased acidity, healed ulcers
Teach patient/family:
• To increase fluids to 2 L/day unless contraindicated; measures to prevent constipation
• To avoid phosphate foods (most dairy products, eggs, fruits, carbonated beverages) during drug therapy for hyperphosphatemia
• Not to use for prolonged periods in patients with low serum phosphate or if on a low-sodium diet
• To add cheese, corn, pasta, plums, prunes, lentils after drug is discontinued
• That stools may appear white or speckled
• To check with prescriber after 2 wk of self-prescribed antacid use
• To separate other medications by 2 hr

RARELY USED

amantadine (℞)
(a-man'ta-deen)
amantadine HCl, Symadine, Symmetrel
Func. class.: Antiviral, antiparkinsonian agent
Chem. class.: Tricyclic amine

Uses: Prophylaxis or treatment of influenza type A, extrapyramidal reactions, parkinsonism, respiratory tract infections
Dosage and routes:
Influenza type A
• *Adult and child >12 yr:* **PO** 200 mg/day in single dose or divided bid
• *Child 9-12 yr:* **PO** 100 mg bid
• *Child 1-9 yr:* **PO** 4.4-8.8 mg/kg/day divided bid-tid, not to exceed 200 mg/day
Extrapyramidal reaction/parkinsonism
• *Adult:* **PO** 100 mg bid, up to 400 mg/day in EPS; give for 1 wk, then 100 mg as needed up to 400 mg in parkinsonism; CrCl 40-50 ml/min 100 mg/day; CrCl 30 ml/min 200 mg 2×/wk; CrCl 20 ml/min 100 mg 3×/wk; CrCl <10 ml/min 100 mg alternating with 200 mg q7days
Contraindications: Hypersensitivity, lactation, child <1 yr, eczematic rash
Do not confuse:
amantadine/ranitidine
amantadine/rimantidine
Symmetrel/Synthroid

amifostine (R)

(a-mi-foss′teen)

Ethyol

Func. class.: Cytoprotective agent for cisplatin

Action: Binds and detoxifies damaging metabolites of cisplatin by converting this drug by alkaline phosphatase in tissue to an active free thiol compound

Uses: Used to reduce renal toxicity when cisplatin is given in ovarian cancer; reduces xerostomia in radiation therapy for head, neck cancer

Dosage and routes:

• *Adult:* IV 910 mg/m² qd, within ½ hr before chemotherapy; may reduce dose to 740 mg/m² if higher dose is poorly tolerated

Xerostomia

• *Adult:* IV 200 mg/m² qd over 3 min as an infusion 15-30 min before radiation therapy

Available forms: Powder for inj 500 mg/vial with 500 mg mannitol

Side effects/adverse reactions:

CNS: Dizziness, somnolence

EENT: Sneezing

INTEG: Flushing, feeling of warmth

CV: Hypotension

GI: Nausea, vomiting, hiccups

MISC: Hypocalcemia, rash, chills

Contraindications: Hypersensitivity to mannitol, aminothiol; hypotension, dehydration, lactation

Precautions: Elderly, CV disease, pregnancy (C), children

Pharmacokinetics: Metabolized to free thiol compound, half-life 8 min, onset 5-8 min

Interactions:

• Increased hypotension: antihypertensives

NURSING CONSIDERATIONS

Assess:

• Fluid status before administration; administer antiemetic prior to administration to prevent severe nausea and vomiting; also, dexamethasone 20 mg IV and a serotonin antagonist such as ondansetron, dolasetron, or granisetron

• Calcium levels before and during treatment; calcium supplements may be given for low calcium levels

• B/P prior to and q5min during infusion; if severe hypotension occurs, give IV 0.9% NaCl to expand fluid volume, place in Trendelenburg position

Administer:

Intermittent IV inf

• Intermittent inf after reconstituting with 9.5 ml of sterile 0.9% NaCl, further dilute with 0.9% NaCl to a concentration of 5-40 mg/ml, give at a rate over 15 min within ½ hr of chemotherapy

Y-site compatibilities: Amikacin, aminophylline, ampicillin, ampicillin/sulbactam, aztreonam, bleomycin, bumetanide, buprenorphine, butorphanol, calcium gluconate, carboplatin, carmustine, cefazolin, cefonicid, cefotaxime, cefotetan, cefoxitin, ceftazidime, ceftizoxime, ceftriaxone, cefuroxime, cimetidine, ciprofloxacin, clindamycin, cyclophosphamide, cytarabine, dacarbazine, dactinomycin, daunorubicin, dexamethasone, diphenhydramine, dobutamine, dopamine, doxorubicin, doxycycline, droperidol, enalaprilat, etoposide, famotidine, floxuridine, fluconazole, fludarabine, fluorouracil, furosemide, gallium, gentamicin, granisetron, haloperidol, heparin, hydrocortisone, hydromorphone, idarubicin, ifosfamide, imipenem-cilastatin, leucovorin, lorazepam, magnesium sulfate, mannitol, mechlorethamine, meperidine, mesna, methotrexate, methylprednisolone, metoclopramide, metronidazole, mezlocillin, mitomycin, mitoxantrone, morphine, nalbuphine, netilmicin, ondansetron, piperacillin, plicamycin, potassium chloride, promethazine, ranitidine, sodium bicarbonate, streptozocin, teniposide, thiotepa, ticarcillin, ticarcillin/clavulanate, tobramycin, trimethoprim-sulfamethoxazole, trimetrexate, vancomycin, vinblastine, vincristine, zidovudine

Additive incompatibilities: Do not mix with other drugs or solutions

Evaluate:
• Therapeutic response: prevention of renal toxicity associated with cisplatin therapy; decreased xerostomia associated with radiation therapy of head, neck cancer

Teach patient/family:
• The reason for the medication and expected results; supine position during infusion
• That side effects may cause severe nausea, vomiting, decreased B/P, chills, dizziness, somnolence, hiccups, sneezing

---

amikacin (R)

(am-i-kay'sin)
amikacin sulfate, Amikin
Func. class.: Antiinfective
Chem. class.: Aminoglycoside

Action: Interferes with protein synthesis in bacterial cell by binding to ribosomal subunit, which causes misreading of genetic code; inaccurate peptide sequence forms in protein chain, causing bacterial death
Uses: Severe systemic infections of CNS, respiratory, GI, urinary tract, bone, skin, soft tissues caused by *Staphylococcus, Proteus aeruginosa, Escherichia coli, Enterobacter, Acinetobacter, Providencia, Citrobacter, Serratia, Proteus, Klebsiella* pneumonia
Investigational uses: *Mycobacterium avium* complex (intrathecal or intraventricular) in combination; aerosolization

Dosage and routes:
Severe systemic infections
• *Adult and child:* **IV INF** 15 mg/kg/day in 2-3 divided doses q8-12h in 100-200 ml D_5W over 30-60 min, not to exceed 1.5 g; decreased doses are needed in poor renal function as determined by blood levels, renal function studies; **IM** 15 mg/kg/day in divided doses q8-12h; qd or extended interval dosing as an alternative dosing regimen
• *Infant:* **IV/IM** 5 mg/kg q8h or 7.5 mg/kg q12h
• *Neonate:* **IV/IM** 10 mg/kg, initially, 7.5 mg/kg q12h
• *Premature neonate:* 10 mg/kg initially, then 7.5 mg/kg q8-12h
Severe urinary tract infections
• *Adult:* **IM** 250 mg q12h
Adult with poor renal function:
5-7.5 mg/kg initially, then increased as determined by blood levels, renal function studies
Aerosolization
• *Adult:* Aerosol varies widely, 250 mg q12h-400 mg q8h
Available forms: Inj 50, 250 mg/ml
Side effects/adverse reactions:
GU: **Oliguria, hematuria, renal damage, azotemia, renal failure, nephrotoxicity**
CNS: Confusion, depression, numbness, tremors, **convulsions,** muscle twitching, **neurotoxicity,** dizziness, vertigo, tinnitus
EENT: **Ototoxicity,** deafness, visual disturbances
HEMA: **Agranulocytosis, thrombocytopenia,** leukopenia, eosinophilia, anemia
GI: Nausea, vomiting, anorexia; increased ALT, AST, bilirubin; hepatomegaly, **hepatic necrosis,** splenomegaly

---

◆ = Nursing alert　　🌿 = Herb-drug interaction　　🚫 = Do not crush

CV: Hypotension or hypertension, palpitations

INTEG: Rash, burning, urticaria, dermatitis, alopecia

Contraindications: Mild to moderate infections, hypersensitivity to aminoglycosides, sulfites

Precautions: Neonates, mild renal disease, pregnancy (D), myasthenia gravis, lactation, hearing deficits, Parkinson's disease, elderly

Do not confuse:
Amikin/Amicar

Pharmacokinetics:

IM: Onset rapid, peak 1-2 hr

IV: Onset immediate, peak 15-30 min; plasma half-life 2-3 hr, prolonged up to 7 hr in infants; not metabolized, excreted unchanged in urine, crosses placental barrier, poor penetration into CSF, removed by hemodialysis

Interactions:

• Increased neuromuscular blockade, respiratory depression: anesthetics, nondepolarizing neuromuscular blockers

• Inactivation of amikacin: parenteral penicillins; cephalosporins; do not use together

• May increase serum trough and peak: indomethacin

• Mask ototoxicity: dimenhydrinate, ethracrynic acid

• Nephrotoxicity: cephalosporins

Lab test interferences:

Increased: BUN, ALT, AST, bilirubin, LDH, alk phosphatase, creatinine

Decreased: Calcium, sodium, potassium, magnesium

NURSING CONSIDERATIONS
Assess:

• Weight before treatment; calculation of dosage is usually based on ideal body weight but may be calculated on actual body weight

• I&O ratio; urinalysis daily for proteinuria, cells, casts; report sudden change in urine output

• VS during infusion; watch for hypotension, change in pulse

• IV site for thrombophlebitis including pain, redness, swelling q30 min; change site if needed; apply warm compresses to discontinued site

• Serum peak, drawn at 30-60 min after IV infusion or 60 min after IM injection, trough level drawn just before next dose; peak 20-30 μg/ml, trough 4-8 μg/ml; adjust dosage per levels

• Urine pH if drug is used for UTI; urine should be kept alkaline

• Renal impairment by securing urine for CrCl, BUN, serum creatinine; lower dosage should be given in renal impairment (CrCl <80 ml/min); nephrotoxicity may be reversible if drug stopped at first sign

◆Deafness by audiometric testing, ringing, roaring in ears, vertigo; assess hearing before, during, after treatment

• Dehydration: high specific gravity, decrease in skin turgor, dry mucous membranes, dark urine

• Overgrowth of infection, including increased temp, malaise, redness, pain, swelling, perineal itching, diarrhea, stomatitis, change in cough, sputum

• C&S before starting treatment to identify organism

• Vestibular dysfunction: nausea, vomiting, dizziness, headache; drug should be discontinued if severe

• Injection sites for redness, swelling, abscesses; use warm compresses at site

Administer:
IM

• Injection in large muscle mass; rotate injection sites

• Bicarbonate to alkalinize urine if ordered for UTI because drug is most active in alkaline environment

Intermittent IV inf

• Dilute 500 mg of drug/100-200 ml of IV D_5W, D_5RL, D_5NaCl, or 0.9% NaCl and give over ½-1 hr; flush after administration with D_5W or 0.9% NaCl; solution is clear or pale yellow; discard if precipitate or dark color develop

• In evenly spaced doses to maintain blood level

Additive compatibilities:

• Avoid admixing

Syringe compatibilities: Clindamycin, doxapram

Y-site compatibilities: Acyclovir, amifostine, amiodarone, amsacrine, aztreonam, cefepime, cisatracurium, cyclophosphamide, dexamethasone, diltiazem, enalaprilat, esmolol, filgrastim, fluconazole, fludarabine, foscarnet, furosemide, granisetron, idarubicin, IL-2, labetalol, lorazepam, magnesium sulfate, melphalan, midazolam, morphine, ondansetron, paclitaxel, perphenazine, remifentanil, sargramostim, teniposide, thiotepa, TPN #54, #61, #91, #203, #204, #212, vinorelbine, warfarin, zidovudine

Perform/provide:

• Adequate fluids of 2-3 L/day, unless contraindicated, to prevent irritation of tubules

• Flush of IV line with NS or D_5W after infusion

• Supervised ambulation, other safety measures with vestibular dysfunction

Evaluate:

• Therapeutic response: absence of fever, draining wounds, negative C&S after treatment

Teach patient/family:

• To report headache, dizziness, symptoms for overgrowth of infection, renal impairment

◆ To report loss of hearing, ringing, roaring in ears or feeling of fullness in head

• To report hypersensitivity: rash, itching, trouble breathing, facial edema and notify health care provider

Treatment of hypersensitivity: Hemodialysis, exchange transfusion in the newborn, monitor serum levels of drug, may give ticarcillin or carbenicillin

---

amiloride (R)

(a-mill'oh-ride)
amiloride HCl, Midamor
Func. class.: Potassium-sparing diuretic
Chem. class.: Pyrazine

Action: Acts primarily on proximal distal tubule by inhibiting reabsorption of sodium, H_2O, and increasing potassium retention

Uses: Edema in CHF in combination with other diuretics, for hypertension, adjunct with other diuretics to maintain potassium

Dosage and routes:

• *Adult:* **PO** 5 mg qd, may be increased to 10-20 mg qd if needed

Available forms: Tabs 5 mg

Side effects/adverse reactions:

GU: Polyuria, dysuria, urinary frequency, impotence

ELECT: Hyperkalemia

RESP: Cough, dyspnea, shortness of breath

CNS: Headache, dizziness, fatigue, weakness, paresthesias, tremor, depression, anxiety

GI: Nausea, diarrhea, dry mouth, *vomiting, anorexia,* cramps, constipation, abdominal pain, jaundice, bleeding

---

◆ = Nursing alert   ∥ = Herb-drug interaction   ⊘ = Do not crush

EENT: Loss of hearing, tinnitus, blurred vision, nasal congestion, increased intraocular pressure

INTEG: Rash, pruritus, alopecia, urticaria

MS: Cramps, joint pain

CV: Orthostatic hypotension, dysrhythmias, angina

*HEMA: **Aplastic anemia, neutropenia***

Contraindications: Anuria, hypersensitivity, hyperkalemia, impaired renal function

Precautions: Dehydration, pregnancy (B), diabetes, acidosis, lactation

Pharmacokinetics:

PO: Onset 2 hr, peak 6-10 hr, duration 24 hr; excreted in urine, feces, half-life 6-9 hr

Interactions:

• Enhanced action of antihypertensives

• Hyperkalemia: other potassium-sparing diuretics, potassium products, ACE inhibitors, salt substitutes

• Decreased effect of amiloride: NSAIDs

• Lithium toxicity: lithium

• Drug/food: possible hyperkalemia: foods high in potassium

Lab test interferences:

Interference: GTT

NURSING CONSIDERATIONS

Assess:

• Weight, I&O daily to determine fluid loss; effect of drug may be decreased if used qd

• B/P lying, standing; postural hypotension may occur

• Electrolytes: K, Na, Cl; glucose (serum), BUN, CBC, serum creatinine, blood pH, ABGs

• Improvement in CVP q8h

• Rashes, temp elevation qd

• Confusion, especially in elderly; take safety precautions if needed

Administer:

PO

• In AM to avoid interference with sleep if using drug as a diuretic

• With food; if nausea occurs, absorption may be decreased slightly

Evaluate:

• Therapeutic response: improvement in edema of feet, legs, sacral area daily if medication is being used in CHF

Teach patient/family:

• To take as prescribed; if dose is missed, take when remembered within 1 hr of next dose

• About adverse reactions: muscle cramps, weakness, nausea, dizziness, blurred vision

• To take with food or milk for GI symptoms

• To take early in day to prevent nocturia

• To avoid potassium-rich foods: oranges, bananas; salt substitutes, dried fruits

Treatment of overdose: Lavage if taken orally, monitor electrolytes, administer sodium bicarbonate for $K^+ > 6.5$ mEq/L, monitor hydration, CV, renal status

---

amino acid injection (R)

(a-mee′noe)

FreAmine, HepatAmine

Func. class.: Nitrogen product

Action: Needed for anabolism to maintain structure, decrease catabolism, promote healing

Uses: Hepatic encephalopathy, cirrhosis, hepatitis, nutritional support in cancer

Dosage and routes:

• *Adult:* IV 80-120 g/day; 500 ml of amino acids/500 ml D_{50} given over 24 hr

Available forms: Inj; many strengths, types

Side effects/adverse reactions:

CNS: Dizziness, headache, confusion, ***loss of consciousness***

CV: Hypertension, ***CHF, pulmonary edema***

GI: Nausea, vomiting, liver fat deposits, abdominal pain

GU: Glycosuria, osmotic diuresis

ENDO: Hyperglycemia, rebound hypoglycemia, electrolyte imbalances, hyperosmolar syndrome, hyperosmolar hyperglycemic nonketotic syndrome, alkalosis, acidosis, hypophosphatemia, hyperammonemia, dehydration, hypocalcemia

INTEG: Chills, flushing, warm feeling, rash, urticaria, extravasation necrosis, phlebitis at injection site

Contraindications: Hypersensitivity, severe electrolyte imbalances, anuria, severe liver damage, maple syrup urine disease, PKU

Precautions: Renal disease, pregnancy (C), lactation, children, diabetes mellitus, CHF

NURSING CONSIDERATIONS

Assess:

• Electrolytes (K$^+$, Na, Ca, Cl, Mg), blood glucose, ammonia, phosphate, ketones

• Renal, liver function studies: BUN, creatinine, ALT, AST, bilirubin

• Injection site for extravasation: redness along vein, edema at site, necrosis, pain, hard tender area; site should be changed immediately

• Respiratory function q4h: auscultate lung fields bilaterally for crackles, respirations, quality, rate, rhythm

• Temp q4h for increased fever, indicating infection; if infection suspected, infusion is discontinued, tubing and solution cultured

◆ For impending hepatic coma: asterixis, confusion, uremic fetor, lethargy

• Hyperammonemia: nausea, vom-

iting, malaise, tremors, anorexia, convulsions

Administer:

Continuous IV

• Up to 40% protein and dextrose (up to 12.5%) via peripheral vein; stronger solutions require central IV administration

• TPN only mixed with dextrose to promote protein synthesis

• Immediately after mixing under strict aseptic technique, use infusion pump, in-line filter (0.22 μm) unless mixed with fat emulsion and dextrose (3 in 1)

◆ Using careful monitoring technique; do not speed up infusion; pulmonary edema, glucose overload will result

Additive compatibilities: Amikacin, aminophylline, aztreonam, calcium gluconate, cefamandole, cefazolin, cefepime, cefotaxime, cefoxitin, cefsulodin, ceftazidime, ceftriaxone, cefuroxime, cimetidine, clindamycin, cyanocobalamin, cyclophosphamide, cyclosporine, cytarabine, dopamine, epoetin, erythromycin, famotidine, folic acid, fosphenytoin, furosemide, heparin, insulin (regular), isoproterenol, lidocaine, meperidine, metaraminol, methicillin, methotrexate, methyldopate, methylprednisolone, metoclopramide, morphine, nafcillin, netilmicin, nizatidine, norepinephrine, ondansetron, oxacillin, penicillin G potassium, penicillin G sodium, phytonadione, polymyxin B, sodium bicarbonate, tacrolimus, tobramycin, vancomycin

Y-site compatibilities: Amikacin, aminophylline, amoxicillin, ampicillin, ascorbic acid inj, atracurium, azlocillin, aztreonam, bumetanide, buprenorphine, calcium gluconate, carboplatin, cefamandole, cefonicid, cefoperazone, cefotaxime, cefotetan, cefoxitin, ceftazidime, ceftizoxime,

◆ = Nursing alert   / = Herb-drug interaction   ⊘ = Do not crush

ceftriaxone, cefuroxime, cephalothin, cephapirin, chloramphenicol, chlorpromazine, cimetidine, clindamycin, clonazepam, dexamethasone, diazepam, digoxin, diphenhydramine, dobutamine, dopamine, doxycycline, droperidol, enalaprilat, epinephrine, erythromycin, famotidine, fentanyl, flucloxacillin, fluconazole, folic acid, foscarnet, gentamicin, granisetron, haloperidol, heparin, hydrocortisone, hydromorphone, hydroxyzine, idarubicin, ifosfamide, IL-2, imipenem/cilastatin, insulin (regular), isoproterenol, kanamycin, lidocaine, meperidine, methicillin, metronidazole, mezlocillin, miconazole, leucovorin, levorphanol, lorazepam, magnesium sulfate, mannitol, mesna, morphine, moxalactam, multivitamins, nafcillin, netilmicin, nitroglycerin, nitroprusside, norepinephrine, octreotide, ofloxacin, ondansetron, oxacillin, paclitaxel, penicillin G, penicillin G potassium, pentobarbital, phenobarbital, piperacillin, potassium chloride, prochlorperazine, ranitidine, salbutamol, sargramostim, tacrolimus, thiotepa, ticarcillin, ticarcillin/clavulanate, tobramycin, trimethoprim-sulfamethoxazole, urokinase, vancomycin, vecuronium, zidovudine

Perform/provide:

• Storage depends on type of solution; consult manufacturer

• Changing dressing and IV tubing to prevent infection q24-48h

Evaluate:

• Therapeutic response: weight gain, decrease in jaundice in liver disorders, increased LOC

Teach patient/family:

• The reason for use of TPN

• If chills, sweating are experienced, report at once

• About infusion pump and blood glucose monitoring

amino acid solution (℞)

Aminees, Aminosyn, Branch Amin, FreAmine III, NeprAmine, Novamine, ProcalAmine, Ren Amin, Travasol, Troph Amine

Func. class.: Nitrogen product

Action: Needed for anabolism to maintain structure, decrease catabolism, promote healing

Uses: Nutritional support in cancer, trauma, intestinal obstruction, short bowel syndrome, severe malabsorption

Dosage and routes:

• *Adult:* IV 1-1.5 g/kg/day titrated to patient's needs

• *Child:* IV 2-3 g/kg/day titrated to patient's needs

Available forms: Inj, many types, strengths

Side effects/adverse reactions:

CNS: Dizziness, headache, confusion, *loss of consciousness*

CV: Hypertension, *CHF, pulmonary edema*

GI: Nausea, vomiting, liver fat deposits, abdominal pain, jaundice

GU: Glycosuria, osmotic diuresis

ENDO: Hyperglycemia, rebound hypoglycemia, electrolyte imbalances, hyperosmolar syndrome, hyperosmolar hyperglycemic nonketotic syndrome, alkalosis, acidosis, hypophosphatemia, hyperammonemia, dehydration, hypocalcemia

INTEG: Chills, flushing, warm feeling, rash, urticaria, extravasation necrosis, phlebitis at injection site

Contraindications: Hypersensitivity, severe electrolyte imbalances, anuria, severe liver damage, maple syrup urine disease, PKU

Precautions: Renal disease, preg-

---

nancy (C), lactation, children, diabetes mellitus, CHF

NURSING CONSIDERATIONS
Assess:

• Electrolytes (K, Na, Ca, Cl, Mg), blood glucose, ammonia, phosphate

• Renal, liver function studies: BUN, creatinine, ALT, AST, bilirubin

• Injection site for extravasation: redness along vein, edema at site, necrosis, pain, hard tender area; site should be changed immediately

• Monitor respiratory function q4h: auscultate lung fields bilaterally for crackles, respirations, quality, rate, rhythm

• Monitor temp q4h for increased fever, indicating infection; if infection suspected, discontinue infusion, culture tubing, bottle

• Urine glucose q6h using Tes-Tape, Clinistix, which are not affected by infusion substances; blood glucose is preferred testing method

• Hyperammonemia: nausea, vomiting, malaise, tremors, anorexia, convulsions

Administer:
Continuous IV

• Up to 40% protein and dextrose (up to 12.5%) via peripheral vein; stronger solutions require central IV administration, use infusion pump

• TPN only mixed with dextrose to promote protein synthesis

• Immediately after mixing in pharmacy under strict aseptic technique using laminar flow hood, use infusion pump, in-line filter (0.22 μm) unless mixed with fat emulsion and dextrose (3 in 1)

◆ Using careful monitoring technique; do not speed up infusion; pulmonary edema, glucose overload will result

Y-site compatibilities: Cefamandole, cefazolin, cefoperazone, cefotaxime, cefoxitin, cephalothin, cephapirin, chloramphenicol, clin-

damycin, digoxin, dobutamine, dopamine, doxycycline, erythromycin lactobionate, fat emulsion, foscarnet, furosemide, gentamicin, isoproterenol, kanamycin, lidocaine, meperidine, methicillin, mezlocillin, miconazole, morphine, nafcillin, netilmicin, norepinephrine, oxacillin, penicillin G potassium, piperacillin, sargramostim, ticarcillin, tobramycin, urokinase, vancomycin

Perform/provide:

• Storage depends on type of solution; consult label

• Dressing and IV tubing change q24-48h to prevent infection

Evaluate:

• Therapeutic response: weight gain, decrease in jaundice in liver disorders, increased serum albumin

Teach patient/family:

• The reason for use of TPN

• That any chills, sweating should be reported at once

• About infusion pump and blood glucose monitoring

RARELY USED

aminocaproic acid (℞)

(a-mee-noe-ka-proe′ik)
Amicar, aminocaproic acid, EACA
Func. class.: Hemostatic

Uses: Hemorrhage from hyperfibrinolysis, adjunctive therapy in hemophilia

Dosage and routes:

• *Adult:* **PO/IV** 5 g loading dose, then 1-1.25 g q1h

Contraindications: Hypersensitivity, abnormal bleeding, postpartum bleeding, DIC, upper urinary tract bleeding, new burns

---

aminoglutethimide (℞)

(a-meen-oh-gloo-teth'i-mide)

Cytadren

Func. class.: Antineoplastic, adrenal steroid inhibitor

Chem. class.: Hormone

Dosage and routes:
• *Adult:* **PO** 250 mg qid at 6 hr intervals, may increase by 250 mg/day q1-2wk, not to exceed 2 g/day

Uses: Suppression of adrenal function in Cushing's syndrome, adrenal cancer

Contraindications: Hypersensitivity, hypothyroidism, pregnancy (D)

aminolevulinic acid (℞)

Levulan Kerastick

Func. class.: Photochemotherapy

Uses: Face/scalp nonhyperkeratotic actinic keratoses

Dosage and routes:
• *Adult:* **TOP** 1 application of solution and 1 dose of illumination/treatment site × 8wk

Contraindications: Hypersensitivity to porphyrins

aminophylline (℞)

(am-in-off'i-lin)

Phyllocontin, Truphylline

Func. class.: Bronchodilator, spasmolytic

Chem. class.: Xanthine, ethylenediamide

Action: Relaxes smooth muscle of respiratory system by blocking phosphodiesterase, which increases cAMP; increased cAMP alters intracellular calcium ion movements; produces bronchodilation, increased pulmonary blood flow, relaxation of respiratory tract

Uses: Bronchial asthma, bronchospasm, Cheyne-Stokes respirations

Investigational uses: Apnea in infancy for respiratory/myocardial stimulation

Dosage and routes:
• *Adult:* **PO** 6 mg/kg, then 3 mg/kg q6h × 2 doses, then 3 mg/kg q8h maintenance, max 900 mg/day or 13 mg/kg; **PO** in CHF 6 mg/kg, then 2 mg/kg q8h × 2 doses, then 1-2 mg/kg q12h maintenance; **IV** 4.7 mg/kg, then 0.55 mg/kg/hr × 12 hr, then 0.36/kg/hr maintenance; **IV** in CHF 4.7 mg/kg, then 0.39 mg/kg/hr × 12 hr, then 0.08-0.16 mg/kg/hr maintenance

• *Geriatric and in cor pulmonale:* **PO** 6 mg/kg, then 2 mg/kg q6h × 2 doses, then 2 mg/kg q8h maintenance; **IV** 4.7 mg/kg, then 0.47 mg/kg/hr × 12 hr, then 0.24 mg/kg/hr maintenance

• *Child 9-16 yr:* **PO** 6 mg/kg, then 3 mg/kg q4h × 3 doses, then 3 mg/kg q6h maintenance, max 18 mg/kg/day 12-16 yr, or 20 mg/kg/day 9-12 yr; **IV** 4.7 mg/kg, then 0.79 mg/kg/hr × 12 hr, then 0.63 mg/kg/hr maintenance

• *Child 6 mo-9 yr:* **PO** 4 mg/kg q4h × 3 doses, then 4 mg/kg q6h maintenance, max 24 mg/kg/day; **IV** 4.7 mg/kg, then 0.95 mg/kg/hr × 12 hr, then 0.79 mg/kg/hr maintenance

• *Neonate—up to 40 wk premature postconception age:* **PO/IV** 1 mg/kg q12h

• *Neonate at birth or 40 wk postconception age:* **PO/IV** Over 8 wk postnatal 1-3 mg/kg q6h; 4-8 wk postnatal 1-2 mg/kg q8h; up to 4 wk postnatal 1-2 mg/kg q12h

Hepatic disease
• *Adult:* **PO** 6 mg/kg/ then 2 mg/kg q8h × 2 doses, then 1-2 mg/kg q12h maintenance; **IV** 4.7 mg/kg, then 0.39 mg/kg/hr × 12 hr, then 0.08-0.16 mg/kg/hr maintenance

Available forms: Inj 250 mg/10 ml, 500 mg/20 ml, 100 mg/100 ml in 0.45% NaCl, 200 mg/100 ml in 0.45% NaCl; rect supp 250, 500 mg, oral liq 105 mg/5 ml; tabs 100, 200 mg, tabs con rel 225 mg

Side effects/adverse reactions:
CNS: Anxiety, restlessness, insomnia, *dizziness, seizures,* headache, light-headedness, muscle twitching
CV: Palpitations, sinus tachycardia, hypotension, flushing, **dysrhythmias,** increased respiratory rate
GI: Nausea, vomiting, anorexia, diarrhea, bitter taste, dyspepsia, anal irritation (suppositories), epigastric pain
RESP: Tachypnea
INTEG: Flushing, urticaria, *rectal irritation* (suppositories)
GU: Urinary frequency

Contraindications: Hypersensitivity to xanthines, tachydysrhythmias
Precautions: Elderly, CHF, cor pulmonale, hepatic disease, active peptic ulcer disease, diabetes mellitus, hyperthyroidism, hypertension, children, pregnancy (C), lactation, glaucoma, prostatic hypertrophy

Pharmacokinetics: Well absorbed PO; extended rel well absorbed slowly, rect supp is erratic, rect sol is absorbed quickly; metabolized by liver (caffeine); excreted in urine; crosses placenta; appears in breast milk; half-life 3-12 hr; half-life increased in geriatric patients, hepatic disease, CHF
PO: Onset ¼ hr, peak 1-2 hr, duration 6-8 hr
PO-ER: Unknown, peak 4-7 hr, duration 8-12 hr
IV: Onset rapid, duration 6-8 hr

REC: Onset erratic, peak 1-2 hr, duration 6-8 hr

Interactions:
• Increased action of aminophylline, toxicity: cimetidine, β-blockers, erythromycin, clarithromycin, oral contraceptives, corticosteroids, interferons, fluoroquinolones, disulfiram, mexiletine, fluvoxamine, high doses of allopurinol, influenza vaccines
• Dysrhythmias: halothane
• Increased elimination: smoking
• Decreased effects of lithium
• May increase or decrease aminophylline levels: carbamazepine, loop diuretics, isoniazid
• Increased adverse reactions: sympathomimetics
• Decreased effect of aminophylline: nicotine products, adrenergics, barbiturates, phenytoin, ketoconazole, rifampin
• Drug/food: increased effect: xanthines; decreased effect: charbroiled foods
🌿 Herb/drug: increased effects: ephedra, cola tree

Lab test interferences:
Increase: Plasma free fatty acids

NURSING CONSIDERATIONS
Assess:
• Theophylline blood levels (therapeutic level is 10-20 µg/ml); toxicity may occur with small increase above 20 µg/ml, especially elderly
• Monitor I&O; diuresis occurs; dehydration may occur in elderly or children
• Whether theophylline was given recently (24 hr)
• Respiratory rate, rhythm, depth; auscultate lung fields bilaterally; notify prescriber of abnormalities
• Allergic reactions: rash, urticaria; if these occur, drug should be discontinued

---

◆ = Nursing alert   🌿 = Herb-drug interaction   Ⓝ = Do not crush

Administer:
• Avoid IM injection; pain and tissue damage may occur
PO
• After meals to decrease GI symptoms; absorption may be effected with a full glass of water
🚫 Do not break, crush, or chew enteric-coated or ext rel tabs
Rectal
• If patient is unable to take PO; retain rectal dose for ½ hr
IV
• Only clear sol; flush IV line before dose
• May be diluted for IV INF in 100-200 ml in D_5W, $D_{10}W$, $D_{20}W$, 0.9% NaCl, 0.45% NaCl, LR
• Give loading dose over ½ hr; max rate of inf 25 mg/min, use infusion pump; after loading dose give by cont inf
Additive compatibilities: Amobarbital, bretylium, calcium gluconate, chloramphenicol, cibenzoline, cimetidine, dexamethasone, diphenhydramine, dopamine, erythromycin lactobionate, esmolol, floxacillin, flumazenil, furosemide, heparin, hydrocortisone, lidocaine, mephentermine, meropenem, methicillin, methyldopate, metronidazole/sodium bicarbonate, nitroglycerin, pentobarbital, phenobarbital, potassium chloride, ranitidine, secobarbital, sodium bicarbonate, terbutaline
Syringe compatibilities: Heparin, metoclopramide, pentobarbital, thiopental
Y-site compatibilities: Allopurinol, amifostine, amphotericin B, amrinone, aztreonam, ceftazidime, cholesteryl sulfate complex, cimetidine, cladribine, doxorubicin liposome, enalaprilat, esmolol, famotidine, filgrastim, fluconazole, fludarabine, foscarnet, gallium, granisetron, heparin sodium with hydrocortisone sodium succinate, labetalol, melphalan, meropenem, morphine, netilmicin, paclitaxel, pancuronium, piperacillin/tazobactam, potassium chloride, propofol, ranitidine, remifentanil, sargramostim, tacrolimus, teniposide, thiotepa, tolazoline, vecuronium, vit B/C

Perform/provide:
• Storage of diluted solution for 24 hr if refrigerated
Evaluate:
• Therapeutic response: decreased dyspnea, respiratory stimulation in infancy, clear lung fields bilaterally
Teach patient/family:
• To take doses as prescribed, not to skip dose, not to double dose
• To check OTC medications, current prescription medications for ephedrine; will increase CNS stimulation; not to drink alcohol or caffeine products (tea, coffee, chocolate, colas)
• To avoid hazardous activities; dizziness may occur
• If GI upset occurs, to take drug with 8 oz water; avoid food, since absorption may be decreased
• To remain in bed 15-20 min after rect supp is inserted to avoid removal
◆ To notify prescriber of toxicity: insomnia, anxiety, nausea, vomiting, rapid pulse, seizures, flushing, headache, diarrhea; notify prescriber immediately
• To notify prescriber of change in smoking habit; a change in dose may be required
• To increase fluids to 2 L/day to decrease secretion viscosity

---

amiodarone (R)

(a-mee-oh′da-rone)
Cordarone, Cordarone IV,
Pacerone

Func. class.: Antidysrhythmic
(class III)

Chem. class.: Iodinated benzo-
furan derivative

Action: Prolongs duration of action
potential and effective refractory
period, noncompetitive α- and
β-adrenergic inhibition; increases PR
and QT intervals, decreases sinus
rate, decreases peripheral vascular
resistance

Uses: Severe ventricular tachycardia, supraventricular tachycardia,
atrial fibrillation, ventricular fibrillation not controlled by first-line
agents, cardiac arrest

Dosage and routes:

Ventricular dysrhythmias

• *Adult:* **PO** loading dose 800-1600
mg/day for 1-3 wk; then 600-800
mg/day × 1 mo; maintenance 400
mg/day; **IV** loading dose (first rapid)
150 mg over the first 10 min then
slow 360 mg over the next 6 hr;
maintenance 540 mg given over the
remaining 18 hr, decrease rate of the
slow infusion to 0.5 mg/min

• *Child:* **PO** loading dose 10-15 mg/
kg/day in 1-2 divided doses for 4-14
days then 5 mg/kg/day (not recommended in children)

Supraventricular tachycardia

• *Adult:* **PO** 600-800 mg/day × 7
days or until desired response, then
400 mg/day × 21 days, then 200-
400 mg/day maintenance

• *Child:* **PO** 10 mg/kg/day (800 mg/
1.72 m^2/day) × 10 days or until desired response, then 5 mg/kg/day
(400 mg/1.72 m^2/day) × 21-28 days,
then 2.5 mg/kg/day (200 mg/1.72

m^2/day) (not recommended in children)

Available forms: Tabs 200, 400 mg;
inj 50 mg/ml

Side effects/adverse reactions:

CNS: Headache, dizziness, involuntary movement, tremors, peripheral
neuropathy, malaise, fatigue, ataxia,
paresthesias, insomnia

GI: Nausea, vomiting, diarrhea, abdominal pain, anorexia, constipation, *hepatotoxicity*

*CV: Hypotension, bradycardia, si-
nus arrest, CHF, dysrhythmias, SA
node dysfunction*

INTEG: Rash, photosensitivity, blue-
gray skin discoloration, alopecia,
spontaneous ecchymosis, *toxic epidermal necrolysis*

EENT: Blurred vision, halos, photophobia, *corneal microdeposits,* dry
eyes

ENDO: Hyperthyroidism or hypothyroidism

MS: Weakness, pain in extremities

RESP: Pulmonary fibrosis, pulmonary inflammation, *ARDS; gasping
syndrome if used in neonates*

MISC: Flushing, abnormal taste or
smell, edema, abnormal salivation,
coagulation abnormalities

Contraindications: Pregnancy (D),
lactation, 2nd-, 3rd-degree AV block,
bradycardia, severe sinus node dysfunction, neonates, infants

Precautions: Goiter, Hashimoto's
thyroiditis, electrolyte imbalances,
CHF, severe hepatic, respiratory disease, children

Do not confuse:

amiodarone/amrinone
Cordarone/Inocor

Pharmacokinetics:

PO: Onset 1-3 wk, peak 2-10 hr;
half-life 15-100 days; metabolized
by liver, excreted by kidneys

Interactions:

• Bradycardia: β-blockers, calcium
channel blockers

◆ = Nursing alert   ∥ = Herb-drug interaction   ⊘ = Do not crush

• Increased levels of digoxin, quinidine, procainamide, flecainide, disopyramide, phenytoin, theophylline, cyclosporine, dextromethorphan, methotrexate
• Increased anticoagulant effects: warfarin

🖊 May increase amiodarone effect: aloe, buckthorn bark/berry, cascara sagrada bark, rhubarb root, senna leaf/fruits

Lab test interferences:
Increase: T_4

NURSING CONSIDERATIONS
Assess:
• I&O ratio; electrolytes (K, Na, Cl); liver function studies: AST, ALT, bilirubin, alk phosphatase
• Chest x-ray, thyroid function tests
• ECG continuously to determine drug effectiveness, measure PR, QRS, QT intervals, check for PVCs, other dysrhythmias, B/P continuously for hypotension, hypertension
• For dehydration or hypovolemia
• For rebound hypertension after 1-2 hr
• For ARDS, pulmonary fibrosis
• CNS symptoms: confusion, psychosis, numbness, depression, involuntary movements; if these occur, drug should be discontinued
• Hypothyroidism: lethargy, dizziness, constipation, enlarged thyroid gland, edema of extremities, cool, pale skin
• Ophthalmic exams
• Hyperthyroidism: restlessness, tachycardia, eyelid puffiness, weight loss, frequent urination, menstrual irregularities, dyspnea; warm, moist skin
➤ Pulmonary toxicity: dyspnea, fatigue, cough, fever, chest pain; drug should be discontinued
• Cardiac rate, respiration: rate, rhythm, character, chest pain; start with patient hospitalized and monitored up to 1 wk

Administer:
PO
• Loading dose with food to decrease nausea

Intermittent IV inf
• 1000 mg/24 hr during loading/maintenance
• Initial loading: Add 3 ml (150 mg) 100 ml D_5W (1.5 mg/ml) give over 10 min
• Loading inf: Add 18 ml (900 mg) 500 ml D_5W (1.8 mg/ml) give over next 6 hr
• Maintenance inf: Give remainder of loading inf 540 mg over 18 hr (0.5 mg/min)

Continuous inf
• After 24 hr, give 1-6 mg/ml at 0.5 mg/ml, do not exceed 30 mg/min

Additive compatibilities: Dobutamine, lidocaine, potassium chloride, procainimide, verapamil

Y-site compatibilities: Amikacin, bretylium, clindamycin, dobutamine, dopamine, doxycycline, erythromycin, esmolol, gentamicin, insulin, isoproterenol, labetalol, lidocaine, metaraminol, metronidazole, midazolam, morphine, nitroglycerin, norepinephrine, penicillin G potassium, phentolamine, phenylephrine, potassium chloride, procainamide, tobramycin, vancomycin

Solution compatibility: D_5W, 0.9% NaCl

Evaluate:
• Therapeutic response: decrease in ventricular tachycardia, supraventricular tachycardia or fibrillation

Teach patient/family:
• To take this drug as directed; avoid missed doses
• To use sunscreen or stay out of sun to prevent burns
• To report side effects immediately
• That skin discoloration is usually reversible
• That dark glasses may be needed for photophobia

Treatment of overdose: O_2, artificial ventilation, ECG, administer dopamine for circulatory depression, administer diazepam or thiopental for convulsions, isoproterenol

---

amitriptyline (℞)

(a-mee-trip'ti-leen)
amitriptyline HCl, Apo-Amitriptyline*, Elavil, Endep, Levate*, Novotriptyn*
Func. class.: Antidepressant—tricyclic
Chem. class.: Tertiary amine

Action: Blocks reuptake of norepinephrine, serotonin into nerve endings, increasing action of norepinephrine, serotonin in nerve cells

Uses: Major depression

Investigational uses: Chronic pain management, prevention of cluster/migraine headaches, fibromyalgia

Dosage and routes:

Depression

• *Adult:* **PO** 75 mg/day in divided doses, may increase to 150 mg qd, not to exceed 300 mg/day; **IM** 20-30 mg qid, or 80-120 mg hs

• *Geriatric and adolescent:* **PO** 30 mg/day in divided doses, may be increased to 100 mg/day

Cluster/migraine headache

• *Adult:* **PO** 50-150 mg/day

Chronic pain

• *Adult:* **PO** 75-150 mg/day

Fibromyalgia

• *Adult:* **PO** 10-50 mg qhs

Available forms: Tabs 10, 25, 50, 75, 100, 150 mg; inj 10 mg/ml; syrup 10 mg/5 ml

Side effects/adverse reactions:

*HEMA: **Agranulocytosis, thrombocytopenia, eosinophilia, leukopenia***

CNS: Dizziness, drowsiness, confusion, headache, anxiety, tremors, stimulation, weakness, insomnia, nightmares, EPS (elderly), increased psychiatric symptoms, **seizures**

GI: Constipation, dry mouth, nausea, vomiting, **paralytic ileus,** increased appetite, cramps, epigastric distress, jaundice, **hepatitis,** stomatitis

GU: Retention

INTEG: Rash, urticaria, sweating, pruritus, photosensitivity

*CV: Orthostatic hypotension, **ECG changes, tachycardia, hypertension,** palpitations, **dysrhythmias***

EENT: Blurred vision, tinnitus, mydriasis, ophthalmoplegia

Contraindications: Hypersensitivity to tricyclic antidepressants, recovery phase of myocardial infarction, narrow-angle glaucoma, pregnancy (D)

Precautions: Suicidal patients, convulsive disorders, prostatic hypertrophy, schizophrenia, psychosis, severe depression, increased intraocular pressure, narrow-angle glaucoma, urinary retention, cardiac disease, hepatic disease, renal disease, hyperthyroidism, electroshock therapy, elective surgery, child <12 yr, lactation, elderly

Do not confuse:
amitriptyline/nortriptyline
Elavil/Mellaril
Elavil/Oruvail

Pharmacokinetics:

PO/IM: Onset 45 min, peak 2-12 hr, therapeutic response 4-10 days; metabolized by liver; excreted in urine, feces; crosses placenta, excreted in breast milk, half-life 10-46 hr

Interactions:

• Increased risk of agranulocytosis: Antithyroid agents

• Increased amitriptyline levels, toxicity: cimetidine, fluoxetine, phenothiazines, oral contraceptives, antidepressants, carbamazepine, IC antidysrhythmics

---

◆ = Nursing alert   ∥ = Herb-drug interaction   ⊘ = Do not crush

• Decreased effects of: guanethidine, clonidine, indirect-acting sympathomimetics (ephedrine)
• Increased effects of: direct-acting sympathomimetics (epinephrine), alcohol, barbiturates, benzodiazepines, CNS depressants, opioids, sedative/hypnotics
• Hyperpyretic crisis, convulsions, hypertensive episode: MAOIs, clonidine

🖉 Increased CNS depression: kava
🖉 Increased anticholinergic effect: belladonna leaf/root, henbane leaf
🖉 Increased action of amitriptyline: scopolia root

Lab test interferences:
Increase: Serum bilirubin, blood glucose, alk phosphatase

NURSING CONSIDERATIONS
Assess:
• B/P lying, standing; pulse q4h; if systolic B/P drops 20 mm Hg, hold drug, notify prescriber; take vital signs q4h in patients with cardiovascular disease
• Blood studies: CBC, leukocytes, differential, cardiac enzymes if patient is receiving long-term therapy
• Hepatic studies: AST, ALT, bilirubin
• Weight qwk; appetite may increase with drug
• ECG for flattening of T wave, prolongation of QTc interval, bundle branch block, AV block, dysrhythmias in cardiac patients
• EPS primarily in elderly: rigidity, dystonia, akathisia
• Mental status: mood, sensorium, affect, suicidal tendencies; increase in psychiatric symptoms: depression, panic
• Urinary retention, constipation; constipation is most likely to occur in children and elderly
• Withdrawal symptoms: headache, nausea, vomiting, muscle pain, weakness; do not usually occur unless drug was discontinued abruptly
• Alcohol consumption; if alcohol is consumed, hold dose until morning

Administer:
PO
• Increased fluids, bulk in diet if constipation, urinary retention occur, especially elderly
• With food or milk for GI symptoms
• Crushed if patient is unable to swallow medication whole
• Dosage hs if oversedation occurs during day; may take entire dose hs; elderly may not tolerate once/day dosing

Perform/provide:
• Storage at room temperature; do not freeze
• Assistance with ambulation during beginning therapy, since drowsiness/dizziness occurs
• Gum; hard, sugarless candy; or frequent sips of water for dry mouth

Evaluate:
• Therapeutic response: decrease in depression, absence of suicidal thoughts

Teach patient/family:
• To take medication as directed; do not double dose; that therapeutic effects may take 2-3 wk
• To use caution in driving, other activities requiring alertness because of drowsiness, dizziness, blurred vision; to avoid rising quickly from sitting to standing, especially elderly
• To avoid alcohol ingestion, other CNS depressants
• Not to discontinue medication quickly after long-term use: may cause nausea, headache, malaise
• To wear sunscreen or large hat, since photosensitivity occurs

---

• To use contraception during treatment

Treatment of overdose: ECG monitoring, lavage, administer anticonvulsant, sodium bicarbonate

---

amlodipine (℞)

(am-loe′di-peen)

Norvasc

Func. class.: Antianginal, antihypertensive, calcium channel blocker

Chem. class.: Dihydropyridine

Action: Inhibits calcium ion influx across cell membrane during cardiac depolarization; produces relaxation of coronary vascular smooth muscle, peripheral vascular smooth muscle; dilates coronary vascular arteries; increases myocardial oxygen delivery in patients with vasospastic angina

Uses: Chronic stable angina pectoris, hypertension, vasospastic angina (Prinzmetal's angina)

Dosage and routes:

Angina

• *Adult:* **PO** 5-10 mg qd

Hypertension

• *Adult:* **PO** 5 mg qd initially, may increase up to 10 mg/day

Hepatic dose

• *Adult:* **PO** 2.5 mg/day; may increase up to 10 mg/day (antihypertensive); 5 mg/day, may increase up to 10 mg/day (antianginal)

Available forms: Tabs 2.5, 5, 10 mg

Side effects/adverse reactions:

CV: Dysrhythmia, edema, bradycardia, hypotension, palpitations, syncope, AV block

GI: Nausea, vomiting, diarrhea, gastric upset, constipation, abdominal cramps, flatulence, anorexia, gingival hyperplasia

GU: Nocturia, polyuria

INTEG: Rash, pruritus, urticaria, hair loss

CNS: Headache, fatigue, dizziness, anxiety, depression, insomnia, paresthesia, somnolence, asthenia

OTHER: Flushing, nasal congestion, sweating, shortness of breath, sexual difficulties, muscle cramps, cough, weight gain, tinnitus, epistaxis

Contraindications: Sick sinus syndrome, 2nd- or 3rd-degree heart block, hypotension less than 90 mm Hg systolic, hypersensitivity

Precautions: CHF, hypotension, hepatic injury, pregnancy (C), lactation, children, renal disease, elderly

Do not confuse:

Norvasc/Navane

Pharmacokinetics:

PO: Onset not determined, peak 6-12 hr, half-life 30-50 hr, increased in geriatric, hepatic disease; metabolized by liver, excreted in urine (90% as metabolites), protein binding >95%

Interactions:

• Increased hypotension: alcohol, fentanyl, quinidine, antihypertensives, nitrates

• Neurotoxicity: lithium

• Decreased antihypertensive effect: NSAIDs

• Drug/food: may increase hypotensive effect: grapefruit juice

NURSING CONSIDERATIONS

Assess:

• Cardiac status: B/P, pulse, respiration, ECG; some patients have developed severe angina, acute MI after calcium channel blockers if obstructive CAD is severe

• I&O ratio, weight qd; peripheral edema, dyspnea, jugular vein distension, rales, crackles that are signs of CHF

◆ = Nursing alert   = Herb-drug interaction   ⊘ = Do not crush

Administer:
PO
• Once a day, without regard to meals
Evaluate:
• Therapeutic response: decreased anginal pain, decreased B/P, increased exercise tolerance
Teach patient/family:
• To take drug as prescribed, do not double or skip dose
• To avoid hazardous activities until stabilized on drug, dizziness is no longer a problem
• To avoid OTC drugs unless directed by prescriber
• To comply in all areas of medical regimen: diet, exercise, stress reduction, drug therapy, smoking cessation
• To notify prescriber of irregular heartbeat, shortness of breath, swelling of feet and hands, severe dizziness, constipation, nausea, hypotension
• To use protective clothing or sunscreen to prevent photosensitivity
• To use correct technique in monitoring pulse, to contact prescriber if pulse <50 bpm
• To change positions slowly, to prevent orthostatic hypotension
• To continue with good oral hygiene to prevent gingival disease
• To notify all health care providers of this drug use
Treatment of overdose: Defibrillation, β-agonists, IV calcium inotropic agents, diuretics, atropine for AV block, vasopressor for hypotension

RARELY USED

ammonium chloride (PO-OTC, IV-R̶x̶)
(ah-mohn′ee-um klor′ide)
ammonium chloride
Func. class.: Acidifier

Uses: Alkalosis (metabolic), systemic and urinary acidifier, expectorant, diuretic
Dosage and routes:
Alkalosis: Adult and child: **IV INF** 0.9-1.3 ml/min of a 2.14% sol, not to exceed 5 ml/min
Acidifier: Adult: **PO** 4-12 g/day in divided doses; *Child:* **PO** 75 mg/kg/day in divided doses
Expectorant: Adult: **PO** 250-500 mg q2-4h as needed
Contraindications: Hypersensitivity, severe hepatic disease, severe renal disease

amoxapine (R̶x̶)
(a-mox′a-peen)
amoxapine, Asendin
Func. class.: Antidepressant
Chem. class.: Dibenzoxazepine derivative—secondary amine

Action: Blocks reuptake of norepinephrine, serotonin into nerve endings, increasing action of norepinephrine, serotonin in nerve cells
Uses: Depression
Dosage and routes:
• *Adult:* **PO** 50 mg tid, may increase to 100 mg tid on 3rd day of therapy; not to exceed 300 mg/day unless lower doses have been given for at least 2 wk, may be given daily dose hs, not to exceed 600 mg/day in hospitalized patients
• *Elderly:* **PO** 25 mg hs, may in-

Side effects: *italics* = common; ***bold italics*** = life-threatening

crease by 25 mg/wk, up to 150 mg/day in divided doses

Available forms: Tabs 25, 50, 100, 150 mg

Side effects/adverse reactions:

*HEMA: **Agranulocytosis, thrombocytopenia, eosinophilia, leukopenia***

CNS: Dizziness, drowsiness, confusion, headache, anxiety, tremors, stimulation, weakness, insomnia, nightmares, EPS (elderly), increased psychiatric symptoms, paresthesia, **neuroleptic malignant syndrome,** impairment of sexual functioning

GI: Dry mouth, constipation, nausea, vomiting, ***paralytic ileus,*** increased appetite, cramps, epigastric distress, jaundice, ***hepatitis,*** stomatitis

GU: Retention, ***acute renal failure***

INTEG: Rash, urticaria, sweating, pruritus, photosensitivity

CV: Orthostatic hypotension, ECG changes, tachycardia, hypertension, palpitations

EENT: Blurred vision, tinnitus, mydriasis, ophthalmoplegia

Contraindications: Hypersensitivity to tricyclic antidepressants, recovery phase of myocardial infarction, convulsive disorders, prostatic hypertrophy, narrow-angle glaucoma

Precautions: Suicidal patients, severe depression, increased intraocular pressure, urinary retention, cardiac disease, hepatic disease, hyperthyroidism, electroshock therapy, elective surgery, elderly, pregnancy (C)

Do not confuse:

amoxapine/amoxicillin
amoxapine/Amoxil

Pharmacokinetics:

PO: Steady state 2-7 days; metabolized by liver, excreted by kidneys, crosses placenta, half-life 8 hr

Interactions:

• Increased CNS depression: CNS depressants

• Decreased amoxapine effect: barbiturates

• Increased amoxapine level: cimetidine, fluoxetine, fluvoxamine, paroxetine, sertraline

• Increased hypertensive effect: clonidine, epinephrine, norepinephrine

• Hyperpyretic crisis, convulsions, hypertensive episode: MAOIs

🖋 Increased CNS depression: kava, St. John's wort

🖋 May increase anticholinergic effects: belladonna leaf/root, henbane leaf

🖋 Increased action of amoxapine: scopolia root

Lab test interferences:

Increase: LFTs, blood glucose
Decrease: WBC, blood glucose

NURSING CONSIDERATIONS
Assess:

• B/P lying, standing; pulse q4h; if systolic B/P drops 20 mm Hg, hold drug, notify prescriber; take vital signs q4h in patients with cardiovascular disease

• Blood studies: CBC, leukocytes, differential, cardiac enzymes if patient is receiving long-term therapy

• Blood level: ther 20-100 ng/ml

• Hepatic studies: AST, ALT, bilirubin

• Weight qwk, appetite may increase with drug

• ECG for flattening of T wave, bundle branch block, AV block, dysrhythmias in cardiac patients

• EPS primarily in elderly: rigidity, dystonia, akathisia

• Mental status: mood, sensorium, affect, suicidal tendencies; increase in psychiatric symptoms: depression, panic; confusion (elderly)

• Urinary retention, constipation; constipation is more likely to occur in children, elderly

---

◆ = Nursing alert   🖋 = Herb-drug interaction   🚫 = Do not crush

• Withdrawal symptoms: headache, nausea, vomiting, muscle pain, weakness; do not usually occur unless drug is discontinued abruptly
• Alcohol consumption; if alcohol is consumed, hold dose until morning

Administer:

PO

• Increased fluids, bulk in diet if constipation, urinary retention occur, especially in elderly
• Crushed if patient is unable to swallow medication whole, with food or milk for GI symptoms
• Dosage hs if oversedation occurs during day; may take entire dose hs; elderly may not tolerate once/day dosing

Perform/provide:

• Storage at room temperature; do not freeze
• Check to see PO medication swallowed
• Gum, hard candy, or frequent sips of water for dry mouth

Evaluate:

• Therapeutic response: decreased depression, absence of suicidal thoughts

Teach patient/family:

• To take as directed, not to double dose
• That therapeutic effects may take 2-3 wk
• To use caution in driving or other activities requiring alertness because of drowsiness, dizziness, blurred vision
• To avoid alcohol ingestion, other CNS depressants
• Not to discontinue medication quickly after long-term use; may cause nausea, headache, malaise
• To wear sunscreen or large hat, since photosensitivity occurs

Treatment of overdose: ECG monitoring, induce emesis, lavage, activated charcoal, administer anticonvulsant

---

amoxicillin (℞)

(a-mox-i-sill′in)

amoxicillin, Amoxil, Apo-Amoxi*, Novamoxin*, Nu-Amoxi*, Trimox, Wymox

Func. class.: Broad-spectrum antiinfective

Chem. class.: Aminopenicillin

Action: Interferes with cell wall replication of susceptible organisms; the cell wall, rendered osmotically unstable, swells and bursts from osmotic pressure

Uses: Treatment of skin, respiratory, GI, GU infections; otitis media, gonorrhea. For gram-positive cocci *(Staphylococcus aureus, Streptococcus pyogenes, Streptococcus faecalis, Streptococcus pneumoniae),* gram-negative cocci *(Neisseria gonorrhoeae, Neisseria meningitidis),* gram-positive bacilli *(Corynebacterium diphtheriae, Listeria monocytogenes),* gram-negative bacilli *(Haemophilus influenzae, Escherichia coli, Proteus mirabilis, Salmonella);* prophylaxis of bacterial endocarditis in combination with *Helicobacter pylori*

Investigational uses: Lyme disease

Dosage and routes:

Systemic infections

• *Adult:* **PO** 750 mg-1.5 g qd in divided doses q8h
• *Child:* **PO** 20-50 mg/kg/day in divided doses q8h

Renal disease

• CrCl 10-50 ml/min dose q12h; CrCl <10 ml/min dose q24h

Gonorrhea/urinary tract infections

• *Adult:* **PO** 3 g given with 1 g probenecid as a single dose; followed by TPN or erythromycin therapy

---

Side effects: *italics* = common; ***bold italics*** = life-threatening

Chlamydia trachomatis
• *Adult:* **PO** 500 mg/day × 1 wk
Bacterial endocarditis prophylaxis
• *Child:* **PO** 50 mg/kg/hr before and 25 mg/kg 6 hr after procedure
Helicobacter pylori
• *Adult:* **PO** 1000 mg bid, given with lansoprazole 30 mg bid, clarithromycin 500 mg bid × 2 wk or 1000 mg bid given with omeprazole 20 mg bid, clarithromycin 500 mg bid × 2 wk, or 1000 mg tid given with lansoprazole 30 mg tid × 2 wk
Available forms: Caps 250, 500 mg; chew tabs 125, 200, 250, 400 mg; tabs 500, 875 mg; susp pediatric drops 50 mg/ml; susp 125, 200, 250, 400 mg/5 ml

Side effects/adverse reactions:
HEMA: Anemia, increased bleeding time, *bone marrow depression, granulocytopenia*
GI: Nausea, vomiting, diarrhea, increased AST, ALT, abdominal pain, glossitis, colitis, *pseudomembranous colitis*
CNS: Headache, *seizures*
SYST: Anaphylaxis, respiratory distress, serum sickness
INTEG: Urticaria, rash

Contraindications: Hypersensitivity to penicillins
Precautions: Pregnancy (B), lactation, hypersensitivity to cephalosporins, neonates, renal disease
Do not confuse:
amoxicillin/amoxapine
Amoxil/Amoxapine
Amoxil/amoxicillin
Trimox/Diamox
Trimox/Tylox
Wymox/Tylox

Pharmacokinetics:
PO: Peak 2 hr, duration 6-8 hr; half-life 1-1⅓ hr, metabolized in liver, excreted in urine, crosses placenta, enters breast milk

Interactions:
• Increased amoxicillin level: probenecid
• Decreased effectiveness of oral contraceptives
• Increased anticoagulant action: warfarin
 Delayed or reduced absorption: khat; separate by 2 hr
Lab test interferences:
False positive: Urine glucose, urine protein, direct Coombs' test

NURSING CONSIDERATIONS
Assess:
• I&O ratio; report hematuria, oliguria, since penicillin in high doses is nephrotoxic
• Any patient with a compromised renal system, since drug is excreted slowly in poor renal system function; toxicity may occur rapidly
• Liver function studies: AST, ALT
• Blood studies: WBC, RBC, Hgb and Hct, bleeding time
• Renal studies: urinalysis, protein, blood, BUN, creatinine
• Culture, sensitivity before drug therapy; drug may be given as soon as culture is taken
• Bowel pattern before, during treatment; diarrhea, cramping, blood in stools, report to prescriber, pseudomembranous colitis may occur
• Skin eruptions after administration of penicillin to 1 wk after discontinuing drug
• Respiratory status: rate, character, wheezing, tightness in the chest
• Anaphylaxis: rash, itching, dyspnea, facial/laryngeal edema
Administer:
PO
• Shake suspension well before each dose, may be used alone or mixed in drinks, use immediately
• Give around the clock, caps may be emptied and mixed with liquids if needed

---

 = Nursing alert   = Herb-drug interaction   = Do not crush

Perform/provide:
• Adrenaline, suction, tracheostomy set, endotracheal intubation equipment on unit
• Adequate intake of fluids (2 L) during diarrhea episodes
• Scratch test to assess allergy after securing order from prescriber; usually done when penicillin is only drug of choice
• Storage in tight container; after reconstituting, oral suspension refrigerated for 14 days
Evaluate:
• Therapeutic response: absence of infection; prevention of endocarditis, resolution of ulcer symptoms
Teach patient/family:
• That caps may be opened and contents taken with fluids; chewable form is available
• To take as prescribed, not to double dose
• All aspects of drug therapy: need to complete entire course of medication to ensure organism death (10-14 days); culture may be taken after completed course of medication
◆ To report sore throat, fever, fatigue, diarrhea (may indicate superinfection or agranulocytopenia)
• That drug must be taken in equal intervals around the clock to maintain blood levels; take on empty stomach with a full glass of water
• To wear or carry a Medic Alert ID if allergic to penicillins
Treatment of anaphylaxis: Withdraw drug, maintain airway, administer epinephrine, aminophylline, O_2, IV corticosteroids

amoxicillin/clavulanate potassium (R) A
(a-mox-i-sill'in)
Augmentin, Augmentin ES, Clavulin*
Func. class.: Broad-spectrum antiinfective
Chem. class.: Aminopenicillin β-lactamase inhibitor

Action: Interferes with cell wall replication of susceptible organisms; the cell wall, rendered osmotically unstable, swells and bursts from osmotic pressure; combination increases spectrum of activity against β-lactamase–resistant organisms
Uses: Sinus infections, pneumonia, otitis media, skin infection, UTI; effective for strains of *Escherichia coli, Proteus mirabilis, Haemophilus influenzae, Streptococcus faecalis, Streptococcus pneumoniae,* and some β-lactamase–producing organisms
Dosage and routes:
• *Adult:* **PO** 250-500 mg q8h or 500-875 mg q12h depending on severity of infection
Renal disease
• CrCl 10-30 ml/min dose q12h; CrCl <10 ml/min dose q24h
• *Child ≤40 kg:* **PO** 20-40 mg/kg/day in divided doses q8h or 25-45 mg/kg/day in divided doses q12h
Available forms: Tabs 250, 500, 875 mg/125 mg clavulanate; chew tabs 125, 200, 250, 400 mg; powder for oral susp 125, 200, 250, 400 mg/5 ml
Side effects/adverse reactions:
HEMA: Anemia, ***bone marrow depression, granulocytopenia, leukopenia, eosinophilia,*** thrombocytopenic purpura
GI: Nausea, diarrhea, vomiting, in-

creased AST, ALT, abdominal pain, glossitis, colitis, black tongue, *pseudomembranous colitis*

GU: Oliguria, proteinuria, hematuria, *vaginitis, moniliasis,* **glomerulonephritis**

CNS: Headache, fever, *seizures*

META: Hyperkalemia, hypokalemia, alkalosis, hypernatremia

INTEG: Rash, urticaria

SYST: **Anaphylaxis, respiratory distress, serum sickness**

Contraindications: Hypersensitivity to penicillins

Precautions: Pregnancy (B), lactation, hypersensitivity to cephalosporins; neonates, renal disease

Pharmacokinetics:

PO: Peak 2 hr, duration 6-8 hr; half-life 1-1⅓ hr, metabolized in liver, excreted in urine, crosses placenta, excreted in breast milk, removed by hemodialysis

Interactions:

• Increased amoxicillin levels: probenecid

• Decreased action of: oral contraceptives

• Increased anticoagulant effect: warfarin

🖊 Delayed/reduced absorption: khat; separate by 2 hr

Lab test interferences:

False positive: Urine glucose, urine protein, direct Coombs' test

NURSING CONSIDERATIONS
Assess:

• I&O ratio; report hematuria, oliguria since penicillin in high doses is nephrotoxic

• Any patient with a compromised renal system since drug is excreted slowly in poor renal system function; toxicity may occur

• Liver function studies: AST, ALT

• Blood studies: WBC, RBC, Hgb and Hct, bleeding time

• Renal studies: urinalysis, protein, blood, BUN, creatinine

• Culture, sensitivity before drug therapy; drug may be given as soon as culture is taken

• Bowel pattern before, during treatment; diarrhea, cramping, blood in stools, report to prescriber, pseudomembranous colitis may occur

• Skin eruptions after administration of penicillin to 1 wk after discontinuing drug

• Respiratory status: rate, character, wheezing, tightness in chest

• Anaphylaxis: rash, itching, dyspnea, facial/laryngeal edema

Administer:
PO

◆ Only as directed, 2 (250 mg tab) not equivalent to 1 (500 mg tab) due to strength of clavulanate

• Shake suspension well before each dose, may be used alone or mixed in drinks, use immediately

• Give around the clock

Perform/provide:

• Adrenaline, suction, tracheostomy set, endotracheal intubation equipment on unit

• Adequate intake of fluids (2 L) during diarrhea episodes

• Scratch test to assess allergy after securing order from prescriber; usually done when penicillin is only drug of choice

• Storage refrigerated for 10 days

Evaluate:

• Therapeutic response: absence of infection

Teach patient/family:

• To take as prescribed, not to double dose

• All aspects of drug therapy: need to complete entire course of medication to ensure organism death (10-14 days); culture may be taken after completed course of medication

◆ To report sore throat, fever, fatigue (may indicate superinfection or agranulocytosis)

◆= Nursing alert   🖊= Herb-drug interaction   ⊘= Do not crush

• That drug must be taken in equal intervals around the clock to maintain blood levels

• To wear or carry a Medic Alert ID if allergic to penicillins

• To notify prescriber of diarrhea, cramping, blood in stools; pseudomembranous colitis may occur

• To use alternative contraceptive measures, if using oral contraceptives

Treatment of hypersensitivity: Withdraw drug, maintain airway, administer epinephrine, aminophylline, O_2, IV corticosteroids for anaphylaxis

---

amphetamine (℞)
(am-fet′a-meen)
amphetamine sulfate
Func. class.: Cerebral stimulant
Chem. class.: Amphetamine

Controlled Substance Schedule II
Action: Increases release of norepinephrine, dopamine in cerebral cortex to reticular activating system
Uses: Narcolepsy, exogenous obesity, attention deficit disorder
Dosage and routes:
Narcolepsy
• *Adult:* **PO** 5-60 mg qd in divided doses
• *Child >12 yr:* **PO** 10 mg qd increasing by 10 mg/day at weekly intervals
• *Child 6-12 yr:* **PO** 5 mg qd increasing by 5 mg/wk, max 60 mg/day
Attention deficit disorder
• *Child >6 yr:* **PO** 5 mg qd-bid increasing by 5 mg/day at weekly intervals
• *Child 3-6 yr:* **PO** 2.5 mg qd increasing by 2.5 mg/day at weekly intervals

Obesity
• *Adult:* **PO** 5-30 mg in divided doses 30-60 min before meals
Available forms: Tabs 5, 10 mg
Side effects/adverse reactions:
CNS: Hyperactivity, insomnia, restlessness, talkativeness, dizziness, headache, chills, stimulation, dysphoria, irritability, aggressiveness, tremor, dependence, addiction
GI: Nausea, vomiting, anorexia, dry mouth, diarrhea, constipation, weight loss, metallic taste, cramps
GU: Impotence, change in libido
CV: Palpitations, tachycardia, hypertension, dysrhythmias, decreased heart rate
INTEG: Urticaria
Contraindications: Hypersensitivity to sympathomimetic amines, hyperthyroidism, hypertension, glaucoma, severe arteriosclerosis, drug abuse, cardiovascular disease, anxiety, lactation
Precautions: Gilles de la Tourette's disorder, lactation, child <3 yr, pregnancy (C)
Pharmacokinetics:
PO: Onset 30 min, peak 1-3 hr, duration 4-20 hr, metabolized by liver, excreted by kidneys, crosses placenta, breast milk, half-life 10-30 hr
Interactions:
• Hypertensive crisis: MAOIs or within 14 days of MAOIs
• Increased effect of amphetamine: acetazolamide, antacids, caffeine
• Decreased antidiabetic requirement: insulin, oral antidiabetics
• Altered CNS effect: phenothiazines, haloperidol, tricyclics
• Decreased effect of amphetamine: urinary acidifiers (ascorbic acid, ammonium chloride)
🖋 May decrease amphetamine effect: kava
Lab test interferences:
Increase: Plasma corticosteroids
Interfere: Urinary steroid

NURSING CONSIDERATIONS
Assess:
• VS, B/P, since this drug may reverse antihypertensives; check patients with cardiac disease more often
• CBC, urinalysis, in diabetes: blood sugar, urine sugar; insulin changes may be required since eating will decrease
• Height; growth rate in children may be decreased
• Mental status: mood, sensorium, affect, stimulation, insomnia; aggressiveness may occur
• Physical dependency; should not be used for extended time; dose should be discontinued gradually
 Withdrawal symptoms: headache, nausea, vomiting, muscle pain, weakness
• Drug tolerance will develop after long-term use; dosage should not be increased if tolerance develops
Administer:
PO
• At least 6 hr before hs to avoid sleeplessness
• For obesity only if patient is on weight-reduction program that includes dietary changes, exercise; patient will develop tolerance, and weight loss won't occur without additional methods; give 30-60 min before meals
• Gum, hard candy, frequent sips of water for dry mouth
Evaluate:
• Therapeutic response: decreased activity in attention deficit disorder; absence of sleeping during day in narcolepsy; decrease in weight
Teach patient/family:
• Not to double dose; if dose is missed, take up to 6 hr before hs; that prescription cannot be refilled
• To decrease caffeine consumption (coffee, tea, cola, chocolate), which may increase irritability, stimulation
• To avoid OTC preparations unless approved by prescriber; to avoid alcohol ingestion
• To taper off drug over several weeks, or depression, increased sleeping, lethargy may occur
• To avoid hazardous activities until patient is stabilized on medication
• To get needed rest; patients will feel more tired at end of day
• That seizure threshold is decreased in patients with seizure disorders
Treatment of overdose: Administer fluids, hemodialysis, peritoneal dialysis, antihypertensives for increased B/P; ammonium Cl for increased excretion

---

amphotericin B deoxycholate
(am-foe-ter′i-sin)
Fungizone
amphotericin B lipid based
Abelcet, Amphotec, AmBisome
Func. class: Antifungal
Chem. class.: Amphoteric polyene

Action: Increases cell membrane permeability in susceptible organisms by binding sterols; decreases potassium, sodium, and nutrients in cell
Uses: Histoplasmosis, blastomycosis, coccidioidomycosis, cryptococcosis, aspergillosis, phycomycosis, candidiasis, sporotrichosis causing severe meningitis, septicemia, skin infections, cryptococcal meningitis in HIV-infected patients
Investigational uses: Candiduria (bladder irrigation)

 = Nursing alert   🌿 = Herb-drug interaction   🚫 = Do not crush

Dosage and routes:
Deoxycholate
• *Adult:* IV Give test dose of 1 mg; then 0.25 mg/kg, increase qd slowly to 0.5 mg/kg, may give 1 mg/kg/day or 1.5 mg/kg qid, alternate-day dosing may be used
• *Child:* IV 0.25 mg/kg infused initially, increase by 0.25 mg/kg qod to max of 1 mg/kg/day
• *Adult/child:* **TOP** apply 2-4 × daily
• *Adult/child:* **PO** 1 ml qid
Amphotec
• *Adult/child:* IV 3-4 mg/kg/day, max 6 mg/kg/day
Abelcet
• *Adult/child:* IV 5 mg/kg/day as a 1 mg/ml inf given 2.5 mg/kg/hr
AmBisome
Fungal infections
• *Adult/child:* IV 3-5 mg/kg q24h
Visceral leishmaniasis 3-4 mg/kg q24h days 1-5, decrease dose
Available forms: Amphotericin deoxycholate inj 50 mg vial; oral susp 100 mg/ml, cream, ointment, lotion 3%; *amphotericin B cholesteryl* powder for inj 50 mg/20 ml, 100 mg/50 ml; *amphotericin B lipid complex* susp for inj 100 mg/20 ml vial; amphotericin B liposome powder for inj 50 mg vial

Side effects/adverse reactions:
EENT: Tinnitus, deafness, diplopia, blurred vision
INTEG: Burning, irritation, pain, necrosis at injection site with extravasation, flushing, dermatitis, skin rash (topical route)
CNS: Headache, fever, chills, peripheral nerve pain, paresthesias, peripheral neuropathy, **convulsions,** dizziness
GU: Hypokalemia, azotemia, hyposthenuria, **renal tubular acidosis,** nephrocalcinosis, **permanent renal impairment, anuria, oliguria**

GI: Nausea, vomiting, anorexia, diarrhea, cramps, **hemorrhagic gastroenteritis, acute liver failure**
MS: **Arthralgia, myalgia,** generalized pain, weakness, weight loss
HEMA: Normochromic, normocytic anemia, **thrombocytopenia, agranulocytosis, leukopenia, eosinophilia,** hypokalemia, hyponatremia, hypomagnesemia

Contraindications: Hypersensitivity, severe bone marrow depression
Precautions: Renal disease, pregnancy (B), lactation
Pharmacokinetics:
IV: Peak 1-2 hr, initial half-life 24 hr, metabolized in liver, excreted in urine (metabolites), breast milk, highly bound to plasma proteins; penetrates poorly CSF, bronchial secretions, aqueous humor, muscle, bone

Interactions:
• Increased nephrotoxicity: other nephrotoxic antibiotics (aminoglycosides, cisplatin, vancomycin, cyclosporine, polymyxin B)
• Increased hypokalemia: corticosteroids, digitalis, skeletal muscle relaxants, thiazides
• Increased possibility of nephrotoxicity: gossypol

NURSING CONSIDERATIONS
Assess:
• VS q15-30min during first infusion; note changes in pulse, B/P
• I&O ratio; watch for decreasing urinary output, change in specific gravity; discontinue drug to prevent permanent damage to renal tubules
• Blood studies: CBC, K, Na, Ca, Mg q2wk, BUN, creatinine weekly
• Weight weekly; if weight increases over 2 lb/wk, edema is present; renal damage should be considered
◆ For renal toxicity: increasing BUN, serum creatinine; if BUN is >40 mg/dl or if serum creatinine >3

mg/dl, drug may be discontinued or dosage reduced

⬥ For hepatotoxicity: increasing AST, ALT, alk phosphatase, bilirubin

• For allergic reaction: dermatitis, rash; drug should be discontinued, antihistamines (mild reaction) or epinephrine (severe reaction) administered

• For hypokalemia: anorexia, drowsiness, weakness, decreased reflexes, dizziness, increased urinary output, increased thirst, paresthesias

• For ototoxicity: tinnitus (ringing, roaring in ears) vertigo, loss of hearing (rare)

Administer:

• Do not confuse three different types

IV

• Drug only after C&S confirms organism, drug needed to treat condition; make sure drug is used in life-threatening infections

Deoxycholate

• After diluting 50 mg/10 ml sterile water (no preservatives) (5 mg-1 ml), shake, dilute with 500 ml of D_5W to concentration of 0.1 mg/ml; infuse over 2-6 hr

• Test dose of 1 mg/20 ml D_5W; give over 10-30 min

Intermittent IV inf

• IV using in-line filter (mean pore diameter >1 micron) using distal veins; check for extravasation, necrosis q8h; use an infusion pump; administer over 6 hr; rapid infusion may result in circulation collapse

Additive compatibilities: Heparin, hydrocortisone, sodium bicarbonate

Syringe compatibilities: Heparin

Y-site compatibilities: Aldesleukin, diltiazem, doxorubicin liposome, famotidine, remifentanil, tacrolimus, teniposide, thiotepa, zidovudine

Solution compatibilities: D_5W

IV

• Reconstitute 50 mg vial/10 ml, 100 mg vial/20 ml sterile water for inj (5 mg/5 ml); swirl or shake gently until dissolved, further dilute with D_5W (0.6 mg/ml); wear gloves while preparing

• Test dose 10 ml of final solution (1.6-8.3 mg) over ½ hr, observe for next ½ hr for reactions

• Give 1 mg/kg/hr using infusion pump, do not give rapidly, may increase infusion, if tolerated

• Additive compatibility: Heparin

Cholesteryl

Liposomal complex

IV

• Reconstitute with 12 ml sterile water/50 ml vial (4 mg/ml), shake, use 5 micron filter, dilute in D_5W (1-2 mg/ml), give over 2 hr

Lipid complex

IV

• Shake vial until dissolved, withdraw dose using 18G needle, replace needle from syringe with drug using 5 micron filter needle (use needle for 4 vials or less), empty contents in IV of D_5W (1 mg/ml), give at 2.5 mg/kg/hr, use infusion pump

Perform/provide:

• Acetaminophen and diphenhydramine 30 min prior to inf to reduce fever, chills, headache

• Storage protected from moisture and light; diluted solution is stable for 24 hr at room temperature

Evaluate:

• Therapeutic response: decreased fever, malaise, rash, negative C&S for infecting organism

Teach patient/family:

• That long-term therapy may be needed to clear infection (2 wk-3 mo depending on type of infection)

• To notify prescriber of bleeding, bruising, or soft tissue swelling

---

⬥ = Nursing alert   ▰ = Herb-drug interaction   🚫 = Do not crush

ampicillin (R)
(am-pi-sill'in)
Ampicin*, Apo-Ampi*,
Marcillin, NovoAmpicillin*,
Nu- Ampi*, Omnipen,
Penbriten*, Polycillin,
Principen, Totacillin
Func. class.: Broad-spectrum
antiinfective
Chem. class.: Aminopenicillin

Action: Interferes with cell wall replication of susceptible organisms; the cell wall, rendered osmotically unstable, swells, bursts from osmotic pressure

Uses: Effective for gram-positive cocci *(Staphylococcus aureus, Streptococcus pyogenes, Streptococcus faecalis, Streptococcus pneumoniae),* gram-negative cocci *(Neisseria gonorrhoeae, Neisseria meningitidis),* gram-negative bacilli *(Haemophilus influenzae, Proteus mirabilis, Salmonella, Shigella, Listeria monocytogenes),* gram-positive bacilli

Investigational uses: High-risk patients having C-section

Dosage and routes:
Systemic infections
• *Adult and child ≥40 kg (88 lbs):* **PO** 1-2 g qd in divided doses q6h; **IV/IM** 2-8 g qd in divided doses q4-6h
• *Child <40 kg:* **PO** 25-100 mg/kg/day in divided doses q6h; **IV/IM** 25-50 mg/kg/day in divided doses q8h

Renal disease
• CrCl 10-30 ml/min dose q8-12h; CrCl 30-50 ml/min q6-8hr; <10 ml/min dose q12h

Meningitis
• *Adult:* **IV** 8-14 g/day in divided doses q3-4h

• *Child:* **IV** 100-200 mg/kg/day in divided doses q3-4h

Gonorrhea
• *Adult and child ≥ 45 kg (99 lbs):* **PO** 3.5 g given with 1 g probenecid as a single dose; **IM/IV** 500 mg q6h (≥40 kg); **IM/IV** 50 mg/kg/day in divided doses q6-8h (<40 kg)

Available forms: Powder for inj 125, 250, 500 mg, 1, 2, 10 g; IV inj 500 mg, 1, 2 g; caps 250, 500 mg; powder for oral susp 125, 250, 500 mg/5 ml

Side effects/adverse reactions:
INTEG: Rash, urticaria
HEMA: Anemia, increased bleeding time, ***bone marrow depression, granulocytopenia***
*GI: Nausea, vomiting, diarrhea, **pseudomembranous colitis***
GU: Oliguria, proteinuria, hematuria, vaginitis, moniliasis, ***glomerulonephritis***
CNS: Lethargy, hallucinations, anxiety, depression, twitching, ***coma, seizures***
MISC: ***Anaphylaxis, serum sickness***

Contraindications: Hypersensitivity to penicillins

Precautions: Pregnancy (B), lactation; hypersensitivity to cephalosporins; neonates, renal disease

Do not confuse:
Omnipen/imipenem

Pharmacokinetics:
PO: Peak 2 hr, duration 6-8 hr
IV: Peak 5 min
IM: Peak 1 hr
Half-life 50-110 min; metabolized in liver; excreted in urine, bile, breast milk; crosses placenta, removed by dialysis

Interactions:
• Increased ampicillin concentrations: probenecid
• Decreased effectiveness of oral contraceptives

• Increased ampicillin-induced skin rash: allopurinol

 Delayed/reduced absorption: khat; separate by 2 hr

Lab test interferences:

False positive: Urine glucose, urine protein

NURSING CONSIDERATIONS

Assess:

• I&O ratio; report hematuria, oliguria, since penicillin in high doses is nephrotoxic

◆ Any patient with compromised renal system, since drug is excreted slowly in poor renal system function; toxicity may occur

• Liver function studies: AST, ALT

• Blood studies: WBC, RBC, Hgb and Hct, bleeding time

• Renal studies: urinalysis, protein, blood, BUN, creatinine

• Culture, sensitivity before drug therapy; drug may be taken as soon as culture is taken

• Bowel pattern before, during treatment

• Skin eruptions after administration of penicillin to 1 wk after discontinuing drug

• Respiratory status: rate, character, wheezing, tightness in chest

• Anaphylaxis: rash, itching, dyspnea, facial swelling; stop drug, notify prescriber, have emergency equipment available

Administer:

PO

• On empty stomach for best absorption (1-2 hr ac or 2-3 hr pc)

• Shake suspension well before each dose

IM

• Reconstitute by adding 0.9-1.2 ml/ 125 mg vial; 0.9-1.9 ml/250 mg vial; 1.2-1.8 ml/500 mg vial; 2.4-7.4 ml/ 1 g vial; 6.8 ml/2 g vial

IV

• After diluting with sterile H_2O 0.9-1.2 ml/125 mg drug, administer over 3-5 min (up to 500 mg), 10-15 min (>500 mg) by direct IV; may be diluted in 50 ml or more of D_5W, D_5 0.45% NaCl to a concentration of 30 mg/ml or less; IV sol is stable for 1 hr; give at prescribed rate

Additive compatibilities: Clindamycin, erythromycin, floxacillin, furosemide

Syringe compatibilities: Chloramphenicol, heparin, procaine

Y-site compatibilities: Acyclovir, allopurinol, amifostine, aztreonam, cyclophosphamide, doxorubicin liposome, enalaprilat, esmolol, famotidine, filgrastim, fludarabine, foscarnet, granisetron, heparin, insulin (regular), labetalol, magnesium sulfate, melphalan, meperidine, morphine, multivitamins, ofloxacin, perphenazine, phytonadione, potassium chloride, propofol, remifentanil, tacrolimus, teniposide, theophylline, thiotepa, tolazoline, vit B/C

Perform/provide:

• Adrenaline, suction, tracheostomy set, endotracheal intubation equipment on unit

• Adequate intake of fluids (2 L) during diarrhea episodes

• Scratch test to assess allergy after securing order from prescriber; usually done when penicillin is only drug of choice

• Storage in tight container; after reconstituting, oral suspension refrigerated for 2 wk or stored at room temperature for 1 wk

Evaluate:

• Therapeutic response: absence of temp, draining wounds, other symptoms of infections

Teach patient/family:

• That tabs may be crushed; caps may be opened and mixed with water

• To take oral ampicillin on empty stomach with full glass of water

• All aspects of drug therapy: need

 ◆ = Nursing alert   = Herb-drug interaction   ⊘ = Do not crush

to complete entire course of medication to ensure organism death (10-14 days); culture may be taken after completed course of medication

◆ To report sore throat, fever, fatigue, diarrhea (may indicate superinfection); report rash or other signs of allergy

• That drug must be taken in equal intervals around the clock to maintain blood levels

• To wear or carry a Medic Alert ID if allergic to penicillins

Treatment of anaphylaxis: Withdraw drug, maintain airway, administer epinephrine, aminophylline, O_2, IV corticosteroids

---

ampicillin, sulbactam (℞)

Unasyn

Func. class.: Broad-spectrum antiinfective

Chem. class.: Aminopenicillin with β-lactamase inhibitor

Action: Interferes with cell wall replication of susceptible organisms; the cell wall, rendered osmotically unstable, swells, bursts from osmotic pressure; combination extends spectrum of activity by β-lactamase inhibition

Uses: Skin infections, intraabdominal infections, pneumonia (*Staphylococcus aureus, Escherichia coli, Klebsiella, Proteus mirabilis, Bacteroides fragilis, Haemophilus influenzae, Enterobacter, Acinetobacter calcoaceticus*), intraabdominal infections (*Enterobacter, Klebsiella, Bacteroides, E. coli*), gynecologic infections (*E. coli, Bacteroides*), meningitis, septicemia

Dosage and routes:

• *Adult/child ≥40 kg:* **IM/IV** 1 g ampicillin, 0.5 g sulbactam to 2 g ampicillin and 1 g sulbactam q6h, not to exceed 4 g/day sulbactam

• *Child ≤40 kg:* **IV** 100-200 mg/kg/day (ampicillin component) divided q6h, max 8 g/day

Renal disease

• CrCl 15-29 ml/min dose q12h; CrCl 5-14 ml/min dose q24h

Available forms: Powder for inj 1.5 g (1 g ampicillin, 0.5 g sulbactam), 3 g (2 g ampicillin, 1 g sulbactam), 10 g (10 g ampicillin, 5 g sulbactam)

Side effects/adverse reactions:

HEMA: Anemia, increased bleeding time, **bone marrow depression, granulocytopenia**

GI: Nausea, vomiting, diarrhea, increased AST, ALT, abdominal pain, glossitis, colitis, **pseudomembranous colitis**

GU: Oliguria, proteinuria, hematuria, *vaginitis, moniliasis,* **glomerulonephritis,** dysuria

CNS: Lethargy, hallucinations, anxiety, depression, twitching, **coma, convulsions**

MISC: Anaphylaxis

Contraindications: Hypersensitivity to penicillins ampicillin or sulbactam

Precautions: Pregnancy (B), lactation, hypersensitivity to cephalosporins, neonates, renal disease

Pharmacokinetics:

IV: Peak 5 min; half-life 50-110 min; little metabolized in liver, 75% to 85% of both drugs excreted in urine, diffuses to breast milk, crosses placenta

Interactions:

• Decreased oral contraceptive effect

• Increased ampicillin level: probenecid

• Ampicillin-induced skin rash: allopurinol

🖋 Delayed/reduced absorption: khat; separate by 2 hr

Lab test interferences:

False positive: Urine glucose, urine protein

NURSING CONSIDERATIONS
Assess:

• Bowel pattern before, during treatment

• Respiratory status: rate, character, wheezing, tightness in chest

• I&O ratio; report hematuria, oliguria, since penicillin in high doses is nephrotoxic

◆ Any patient with compromised renal system, since drug is excreted slowly in poor renal system function; toxicity may occur rapidly

• Liver function studies: AST, ALT if on long-term therapy

• Blood studies: WBC, RBC, Hct, Hgb, bleeding time

• Renal studies: urinalysis, protein, blood, BUN, creatinine

• C&S before drug therapy; drug may be given as soon as culture is taken

• Skin eruptions after administration of ampicillin to 1 wk after discontinuing drug

• Allergies before initiation of treatment; reaction of each medication; report allergies on chart in bright red

Administer:

IM

• Reconstitute by adding 3.2 ml sterile water/1.5 g vial; 6.4 ml/3 g vial, give deep in large muscle

IV

• After diluting 1.5 g/3.2 ml sterile H_2O for inj or 3 g/6.4 ml (250 mg ampicillin/125 mg sulbactam); allow to stand until foaming stops; may give over 15 min as direct IV; dilute further in 50 ml or more of D_5W, NaCl, administer within 1 hr after reconstitution; give as an intermittent inf over 15-30 min

Additive compatibilities: Aztreonam

Y-site compatibilities: Amifostine, aztreonam, cefepime, enalaprilat, famotidine, filgrastim, fluconazole, fludarabine, gallium, granisetron, heparin, insulin (regular), meperidine, morphine, paclitaxel, remifentanil, tacrolimus, teniposide, theophylline, thiotepa

Perform/provide:

• Adrenaline, suction, tracheostomy set, endotracheal intubation equipment on unit for possible anaphylaxis

• Adequate intake of fluids (2 L) during diarrhea episodes

• Scratch test to assess allergy after securing order from prescriber; usually done when penicillin is only drug choice

• Storage in tight container, out of light

Evaluate:

• Therapeutic response: absence of fever, draining wounds, negative C&S

Teach patient/family:

• To report sore throat, fever, fatigue, persistent diarrhea (may indicate superinfection)

• To wear or carry Medic Alert ID if allergic to penicillin products

Treatment of anaphylaxis: Withdraw drug, maintain airway, administer epinephrine, aminophylline, O_2, IV corticosteroids

---

amprenavir (R)
(am-pren′ah-veer)
Agenerase
Func. class.: Antiretroviral
Chem. class.: Protease inhibitor

Action: Inhibits human immunodeficiency virus (HIV) protease, which prevents maturation of the infectious virus

Uses: HIV in combination with other antiretroviral agents

◆ = Nursing alert   🖉 = Herb-drug interaction   ⊘ = Do not crush

Research note: One study has documented an increased hypersensitivity to amprenavir in the HIV type 1 virus[2]

Dosage and routes:
• *Adult:* **PO** (cap) 1200 mg bid
• *Child 13-16 yr:* **PO** (cap) 1200 mg bid
• *Child 4-12 yr or wt <50 kg:* **PO** Caps: 20 mg/kg qd or 15 mg/kg tid, max 2400 mg; sol: 22.5 mg/kg bid or 17 mg/kg tid qd, max 2800 mg
Hepatic dose
• *Adult:* **PO** (child—Pugh score 5-8) 450 mg bid in combination; (child—Pugh score 9-12) 300 mg bid in combination
Available forms: Caps 50, 150 mg; oral sol 15 mg/ml
Side effects/adverse reactions:
GI: Diarrhea, abdominal pain, nausea, ***hepatotoxicity***
CNS: Paresthesia, headache
INTEG: Rash, ***Stevens-Johnson syndrome***
HEMA: ***Acute hemolytic anemia***
ENDO: New-onset diabetes, hyperglycemia, exacerbation of preexisting diabetes mellitus, hypertriglyceridemia
Contraindications: Hypersensitivity
Precautions: Liver disease, pregnancy (C), lactation, children, hemophilia, sulfonamide sensitivity, elderly
Pharmacokinetics: Rapidly absorbed, peak 1-2 hr, 90% protein bound, metabolized in liver, excreted unchanged in urine/feces (minimal), half-life 7-10½ hr
Interactions:
• Do not use with: loratadine, midazolam, triazolam, ergots, rifampin, lovastatin, bepridil
◆ Serious life-threatening interactions: amiodarone, lidocaine, quinidine, tricyclics

• Increased amprenavir levels: ketoconazole, ritonavir, cimetidine, itraconazole, indinavir, clarithromycin, erythromycin
• Decreased amprenavir levels: rifamycins, antacids, carbamazepine, phenobarbital, phenytoin
• Drug/food: decreased bioavailability after high-fat meal
⧸ Decreased amprenavir levels: St. John's wort
Lab test interferences: CPK, glucose (low)
NURSING CONSIDERATIONS
Assess:
◆For renal or hepatic failure, pregnancy, or those receiving disulfiram, metronidazole; oral solution contains propylene glycol in greater quantities
• Signs of infection, anemia
• Liver function studies: ALT, AST
• Bowel pattern before, during treatment; if severe abdominal pain with bleeding occurs, drug should be discontinued; monitor hydration
• Skin eruptions, rash, urticaria, itching
• Allergies before treatment, reaction of each medication; place allergies on chart
Teach patient/family:
• To take as prescribed with or without food, avoid high-fat foods; if dose is missed, take as soon as remembered up to 1 hr before next dose; do not double dose, do not share with others
• That drug must be taken in equal intervals around the clock to maintain blood levels for duration of therapy
• To use a nonhormonal method of contraception during treatment, use condoms
• To notify prescriber if diarrhea, nausea, vomiting, rash occurs

---

• That drug does not cure AIDs or prevent transmission to others, only controls symptoms
• That caps and sol are not interchangeable on a mg/mg basis

RARELY USED

amyl nitrite (℞)
(am'il nye'trite)
amyl nitrite, Amyl Nitrite Aspirols, Amyl Nitrite Vaporole

Func. class.: Coronary vasodilator

Uses: Acute angina pectoris, cyanide poisoning
Dosage and routes:
Angina
• *Adult:* **INH** 0.18-0.3 ml as needed, 1-6 inhalations from 1 cap, may repeat in 3-5 min
Cyanide poisoning
• *Adult:* **INH** 0.3 ml ampule inhaled 15 sec until preparation of sodium nitrite infusion is ready
Investigational uses: Cardiac murmur diagnosis
Contraindications: Hypersensitivity to nitrites, severe anemia, increased intracranial pressure, hypertension, pregnancy (X)

---

anagrelide (℞)
(a-na'gre-lide)
Agrylin

Func. class.: Antiplatelet
Chem. class.: Imidazo-quinazolinone

Action: Reduces platelet count and prevents early platelet shape changes in response to aggregating agents thus inhibiting platelet aggregation
Uses: Essential thrombocythemia, polycythemia vera, chronic myelogenous leukemia
Dosage and routes:
• *Adult:* **PO** 0.5 mg qid or 1 mg bid, may be adjusted after 1 wk, max 10 mg/day or 2.5 mg single dose
Available forms: Caps 0.5, 1.0 mg
Side effects/adverse reactions:
MS: Asthenia, back pain
RESP: Dyspnea
GU: Dysuria
GI: Diarrhea, abdominal pain, nausea, flatulence, vomiting, anorexia, constipation, pancreatitis
CV: Postural hypotension, tachycardia, palpitations, *CHF, MI, cardiomyopathy, cardiomegaly, complete heart block, atrial fibrillation,* dysrhythmia, *chest pain*
CNS: Headache, dizziness, *seizures, paresthesia, CVA*
INTEG: Rash
HEMA: Anemia, thrombocytopenia, ecchymosis, lymphadenoma
Contraindications: Hypersensitivity, hypotension
Precautions: Pregnancy (C), lactation, child <16 yr, cardiac, renal, hepatic disease
Pharmacokinetics:
PO: Peak 1 hr, duration >24 hr: metabolized in liver: excreted in feces/urine
Interactions:
• Decreased absorption: sucralfate
• Drug/food: decreased bioavailability
NURSING CONSIDERATIONS
Assess:
• Platelet counts q2day × 1 wk, and qwk thereafter, response should begin after 1-2 wk; Hgb, WBC
• B/P, pulse during treatment until stable; take B/P lying, standing; orthostatic hypotension is common
• Cardiac status: chest pain, what aggravates or ameliorates condition
Administer:
• On an empty stomach: 1 hr before

⬥ = Nursing alert   🍃 = Herb-drug interaction   🚫 = Do not crush

meals or 2 hr after; give with 8 oz water for better absorption

Perform/provide:
• Storage at room temperature

Evaluate:
• Therapeutic response: decreased platelet count

Teach patient/family:
• That medication is not a cure: may have to be taken continuously in evenly spaced doses only as directed
• That it is necessary to quit smoking to prevent excessive vasoconstriction
• To avoid hazardous activities until stabilized on medication; dizziness may occur
• To rise slowly from sitting or lying to prevent orthostatic hypotension
• Not to use alcohol or OTC medications unless approved by prescriber
• To report cardiac reactions, increased bruising, bleeding
• To use contraception (female, child-bearing age)

---

anakinra
See appendix a—selected new drugs

---

anastrozole
(an-a-stroh′zole)
Arimidex
Func. class.: Antineoplastic
Chem. class.: Aromatase inhibitor

Action: Lowers serum estradiol concentrations; many breast cancers have strong estrogen receptors
Uses: Advanced breast carcinoma not responsive to other therapy in estrogen-receptor–positive patients (usually postmenopausal)

Dosage and routes:
• *Adult:* **PO** 1 mg qd
Available forms: Tabs 1 mg

Side effects/adverse reactions:
*HEMA: **Leukopenia***
GI: Nausea, vomiting, altered taste (anorexia), diarrhea, constipation, abdominal pain, dry mouth
GU: Vaginal bleeding, vaginal dryness, pelvic pain, pruritus vulvae, UTI
INTEG: Rash, alopecia
CV: Chest pain, hypertension, thrombophlebitis, edema
CNS: Hot flashes, headache, lightheadedness, depression, dizziness, confusion, insomnia, anxiety
RESP: Cough, sinusitis, dyspnea
MS: Bone pain, myalgia, asthenia

Contraindications: Hypersensitivity, pregnancy (D)
Precautions: Leukopenia, thrombocytopenia, lactation, children, elderly, liver disease, renal disease

Pharmacokinetics:
PO: Peak 4-7 hr, half-life 50 hr, excreted in feces, urine

Lab test interferences:
Increase: GGT, AST, ALT, alk phosphatase, cholesterol, LDL

NURSING CONSIDERATIONS
Assess:
• For side effects during treatment
Administer:
PO
• Give with food
Perform/provide:
• Storage in light-resistant container at room temperature
Evaluate:
• Therapeutic response: decreased tumor size, spread of malignancy
Teach patient/family:
• To report any complaints, side effects to prescriber
• That vaginal bleeding, pruritus, hot

flashes are reversible after discontinuing treatment
• To report vaginal bleeding immediately
• That tumor flare—increase in size of tumor, increased bone pain—may occur and will subside rapidly; may take analgesics for pain
• That hair may be lost during treatment; a wig or hairpiece may make patient feel better; new hair may be different in color, texture

---

anistreplase (R)
(ah-nis′tre-place)
anisoylated plasminogen, APSAC, Eminase

Func. class.: Thrombolytic enzyme
Chem. class.: Anisoylated plasminogen streptokinase activator complex

Action: Promotes thrombolysis by promoting conversion of plasminogen to plasmin
Uses: Acute MI for lysis of coronary artery thrombi
Dosage and routes:
• *Adult:* **IV INJ** 30 U over 2-5 min as soon as possible after onset of symptoms
Available forms: Powder, lyophilized 30 U/vial
Side effects/adverse reactions:
HEMA: Decreased Hct; *GI, GU, intracranial, retroperitoneal,* surface bleeding; *thrombocytopenia*
INTEG: Rash, urticaria, phlebitis at inj site, itching, flushing
CNS: Headache, fever, sweating, agitation, dizziness, paresthesia, tremor, vertigo, *intracranial hemorrhage*
GI: Nausea, vomiting
RESP: Altered respirations, dyspnea, *bronchospasm, lung edema*
MS: Low back pain, arthralgia

CV: Hypotension, *dysrhythmias,* conduction disorders
SYST: Anaphylaxis (rare)
Contraindications: Hypersensitivity, active internal bleeding, intraspinal or intracranial surgery, neoplasms of CNS, severe hypertension, cerebral embolism/thrombosis/hemorrhage, hypersensitivity to this drug or streptokinase
Precautions: Arterial emboli from left side of heart, pregnancy (C), ulcerative colitis/enteritis, renal disease, hepatic disease, hypocoagulation, COPD, subacute bacterial endocarditis, rheumatic valvular disease, intraarterial diagnostic procedure or surgery (10 days), recent major surgery, lactation
Pharmacokinetics: Half-life 105 min
Interactions:
• Increased bleeding potential: aspirin, other NSAIDs, abciximab, eptifibatide, tirofiban, clopidogrel, ticlopidine, some cephalosporins, plicamycin, valproic acid, anticoagulants, dipyridamole
 Increased risk of bleeding: bromelain
Lab test interferences:
Increase: PT, APTT, TT
Decrease: Fibrinogen, plasminogen

NURSING CONSIDERATIONS
Assess:
• VS, B/P, pulse, respirations, neurologic signs, temp at least q4h, temp >104° F (40° C) or indicators of internal bleeding, cardiac rhythm after intracoronary administration; monitor ECG, treat bradycardia, ventricular changes; assess neurologic status, neurologic change may indicate intracranial bleeding; ECG continuously, cardiac enzymes, radionuclide, myocardial scanning/coronary angiography

---

 = Nursing alert   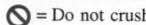 = Herb-drug interaction   🚫 = Do not crush

• Hypersensitivity: fever, rash, itching, chills, facial swelling dyspnea; notify prescriber immediately, stop drug, keep resusciatative equipment nearby; mild reaction may be treated with antihistamines

◆ Bleeding during first hr of treatment (hematuria, hematemesis, bleeding from mucous membranes, epistaxis, ecchymosis), continue to monitor for 24 hr after treatment
• Blood studies (Hct, platelets, PTT, PT, TT, APTT) before starting therapy; PT or APTT must be less than 2 × control before starting therapy; TT or PT q3-4h during treatment

Administer:
IV, direct
• Reconstitute single-dose vial/5 ml sterile water for injection (not bacteriostatic water), and roll (not shake) to enhance reconstitution; give over 2-5 min by direct IV, give within ½ hr of reconstitution or discard, do not add other meds to vial or syringe; give within 6 hr of thrombi identification for best results
• Cryoprecipitate or fresh frozen plasma if bleeding occurs
• Heparin therapy after thrombolytic therapy is discontinued, TT or APTT less than 2 × control (about 3-4 hr)
• About 10% of patients have high streptococcal antibody titers, requiring increased loading doses

Perform/provide:
• Bed rest during entire course of treatment; handle patient as little as possible during therapy
• Storage of powder in refrigerator; use within 30 min after reconstitution
• Avoid invasive procedures: inj, rectal temperature
• Treat fever with acetaminophen
• Pressure of 30 sec to minor bleeding sites, 30 min to sites of arterial puncture followed by

dressing; inform prescriber if hemostasis not attained; apply pressure dressing
Evaluate:
• Therapeutic response: absence of thrombi formation in MI, improved ventricular function

antihemophilic factor VIII (AHF) (℞)

(an-tee-hee-moe-fill'ik)
antihemophilic factor,
Alphanate, Bioclate, Helixate FS, Hemofil M, Humate-P, Hyate C, Koate-DVI, Kogenate, Kogenate FS, Monoclate-P, Recombinate, ReFacto
Func. class.: Hemostatic
Chem. class.: Factor VIII

Action: Necessary for clotting; activates factor X in conjunction with activated factor IX; transforms prothrombin to thrombin
Uses: Hemophilia A, patients with acquired circulating factor VIII inhibitors, factor VIII deficiency
Dosage and routes:
Massive hemorrhage
• *Adult and child:* IV 40-50 U/kg, then 20-25 U/kg q8-12h
Overt bleeding
• *Adult and child:* IV 15-25 U/kg, then 8-15 U/kg q8-12h × 4 days
Hemorrhage near vital organs
• *Adult and child:* IV 15 U/kg, then 8 U/kg q8h × 2 days, then 4 U/kg q8h × 2 days
Minor hemorrhage
• *Adult and child:* IV 8-10 U/kg/ q24h × 2-3 days or 8 U/kg q12h × 2 days, then q24h × 2 days
Joint bleeding
• *Adult and child:* IV 5-10 U/kg q8-12h × 1-2 days
Available forms: Inj 250, 500, 1000,

1500 U/vial (number of units noted on label)

Side effects/adverse reactions:
GI: Nausea, vomiting, abdominal cramps, constipation, diarrhea, anorexia, jaundice, ***viral hepatitis***
INTEG: Rash, flushing, *urticaria,* stinging at injection site
CNS: Headache, *lethargy, chills, fever, flushing*
*HEMA: **Thrombosis, hemolysis, risk of hepatitis B, HIV***
*CV: **Hypotension,*** tachycardia
*RESP: **Bronchospasm,*** rhinitis, dyspnea, nosebleeds
*MISC: **Anaphylaxis***

Contraindications: Hypersensitivity; mouse, hamster, bovine protein
Precautions: Neonates/infants, hepatic disease; blood types A, B, AB; pregnancy (C), factor VIII inhibitor
Pharmacokinetics:
IV: Half-life 4 hr, terminal 15 hr
Interactions:
• Do not admix with other drugs
• Increased bleeding: salicylates, NSAIDs

NURSING CONSIDERATIONS
Assess:
• Blood studies (coagulation factors assay by % normal: 5% prevents spontaneous hemorrhage, 30%-50% for surgery, 80%-100% for severe hemorrhage)
• I&O, urine color; notify prescriber if urine becomes orange, red
• Pulse: discontinue infusion if significant increase
• Hct, Coombs' test with blood types A, B, AB
• Test for factor VIII inhibitors before starting treatment, may require concomitant antiinhibitor coagulant complex therapy
• Allergy: fever, rash, itching, jaundice; give diphenhydramine HCl (Benadryl), continue therapy if reaction is mild

• Blood group of patient, donors (if applicable; most factor VIII not from specific blood group donors)
⬥ Bleeding: ankles, knees, elbows, other joints

Administer:
IV
• After rotating gently to mix
• Using plastic syringe to reconstitute, and administer; adheres to glass; use another needle as a vent when reconstituting
• After dilution with warm NS, D_5W, LR, give within 3 hr

IV infusion
• Give at ≤2 ml/min if concentration exceeds 34 U/ml or over 3 min if concentration is less than 34 U/ml

Perform/provide:
• Storage in refrigerator; do not freeze; after reconstitution, do not refrigerate; give within 3 hr

Evaluate:
• Therapeutic response: absence of bleeding

Teach patient/family:
• To report any signs of bleeding: gums, under skin, urine, stools, emesis; review methods to prevent bleeding
• To avoid salicylates, NSAIDs (increase bleeding tendencies)
• To prepare, administer factor VIII concentrates at first sign of danger
• To advise health professionals of treatment for hemophilia
• The signs of viral hepatitis, AIDS
• That immunization for hepatitis B may be given first
• To report hives, urticaria, chest tightness, hypotension; may be monoclonal antibody-derived factor VIII
• To be checked q2-3mo for HIV screen
• To carry ID describing disease process

⬥ = Nursing alert　　🌿 = Herb-drug interaction　　🚫 = Do not crush

antithrombin III, human (℞)

(an'tee-throm-bin)
ATnativ, Thrombate III

Func. class.: Antithrombin

Chem. class.: Pooled human plasma

Action: Inactivates thrombin and the activated forms of factors IX, X, XI, XII, resulting in inhibition of coagulation

Uses: Hereditary antithrombin III deficiency in connection with surgical or obstetric procedures or for thromboembolism

Dosage and routes: Dosage is individualized; after first dose, antithrombin III level should increase to about 120% of normal; thereafter maintain at levels >80%; this is usually achieved by administering maintenance doses q24h

Available forms: Lyophilized powder, 50 ml infusion bottles containing 500 IU antithrombin III with 10 ml sterile water for injection

Side effects/adverse reactions:

*SYST: **Bleeding,*** surface bleeding, ***anaphylaxis,*** vasodilatory effects

CNS: Dizziness, chills, severe lightheadedness

GI: Nausea, cramps, bowel fullness

RESP: Shortness of breath

Precautions: Pregnancy (B), lactation, children

Pharmacokinetics: Unknown

Interactions:

• Increased anticoagulant effect: heparin, aspirin

• Do not administer with other drugs in syringe or solutions

NURSING CONSIDERATIONS

Assess:

• AT-III levels bid until stabilized, then qd before dose

• VS, B/P, pulse, respirations, neurologic signs, temp at least q4h, temp 104° F (40° C) or indicators of internal bleeding, cardiac rhythm

◆ For child born of parents with hereditary AT-III deficiency, obtain AT-III levels immediately after birth

◆ For neurologic changes that may indicate intracranial bleeding

◆ Retroperitoneal bleeding: back pain, leg weakness, diminished pulses

Administer:

• Heparin after fibrinogen level is over 100 mg/dl; heparin infusion to increase PTT to 1.5-2 × baseline for 3-7 days

IV

• After reconstituting 500 IU/10 ml of NS or D_5W; do not shake; rotate to dissolve; allow to warm to room temperature; use within 3 hr of reconstitution; give 50 IU or less/min; do not exceed 100 IU/min using 0.22 or 0.45 microfilter

Perform/provide:

• Bed rest during entire course of treatment

• Avoidance of venous or arterial puncture, inj, rectal temp

• Treatment of fever with acetaminophen

Evaluate:

• Therapeutic response: absence of thrombi formation

Teach patient/family:

• About drug use and expected results; to report adverse reactions; bleeding, bruising

antithymocyte

See lymphocyte immune globulin

ardeparin (R)

(are-de-pear'in)
Normiflo

Func. class.: Anticoagulant
Chem. class.: Low-molecular-weight heparin

Action: Prevents conversion of fibrinogen to fibrin and prothrombin to thrombin by enhancing inhibitory effects of antithrombin III

Uses: Prevention of deep vein thrombosis after knee replacement surgery

Dosage and routes:
• *Adult:* SC 50 anti–factor Xa U/kg q12h beginning the evening of the day of knee replacement surgery or the following AM continued until patient is fully ambulatory or 2 wk, whichever is first

Available forms: Inj 5000, 10,000 anti–factor Xa U/0.5 ml

Side effects/adverse reactions:
CNS: **Intracranial bleeding,** fever, dizziness, headache
SYST: Hypersensitivity, **hemorrhage, anaphylaxis** possible
HEMA: **Thrombocytopenia,** anemia
INTEG: Pruritus, superficial wound infection, ecchymosis, rash
CV: Chest pain
GI: Nausea, vomiting
RESP: Dyspnea

Contraindications: Hypersensitivity to this drug, pork products, heparin, or other anticoagulants; hemophilia, leukemia with bleeding, thrombocytopenic purpura, cerebrovascular hemorrhage, cerebral aneurysm, severe hypertension, other severe cardiac disease

Precautions: Elderly, pregnancy (C), hepatic disease, severe renal disease, blood dyscrasias, subacute bacterial endocarditis, lactation, child, recent childbirth, peptic ulcer disease, pericarditis, pericardial effusion, recent lumbar puncture, vasculitis, other diseases where bleeding is possible

Pharmacokinetics: Unknown

Interactions:
• Increased risk of bleeding: aspiration, oral anticoagulants, platelet inhibitors, NSAIDs

🌿 May increase risk of bleeding: bromelain, cinchona bark

NURSING CONSIDERATIONS
Assess:
• For blood studies (Hct, occult blood in stools, CBC, platelets, urinalysis) during treatment since bleeding can occur
◆ For bleeding gums, petechiae, ecchymosis, black tarry stools, hematuria, epistaxis, decrease in Hct, B/P; may indicate bleeding, possible hemorrhage; notify prescriber immediately, drug should be discontinued, protamine should be = to dose of drug given; 1 mg protamine = 100 anti–factor Xa U of drug
• For hypersensitivity: fever, skin rash, urticaria; notify prescriber immediately

Administer:
• By SC only; have patient sit or lie down; SC inj may be around the navel in a U-shape, upper outer side of thigh or upper outer quadrangle of the buttocks; rotate inj sites
• Changing needles is not recommended

Evaluate:
• Therapeutic response: absence of deep-vein thrombosis

Teach patient/family:
• To avoid OTC preparations that may cause serious drug interactions unless directed by prescriber; may contain aspirin; other anticoagulants, NSAIDs
• To use soft-bristle toothbrush to avoid bleeding gums, avoid contact

---

◆ = Nursing alert   🌿 = Herb-drug interaction   🚫 = Do not crush

sports, use electric razor, avoid IM injection

• To report any signs of bleeding: gums, under skin, urine, stools; unusual bruising, hematoma at inj site

Treatment of overdose: Protamine sulfate 1% given IV

---

argatroban (℞)

(are-ga-troe'ban)

Acova

Func. class.: Anticoagulant

Chem. class.: Thrombin inhibitor

Action: Direct inhibitor of thrombin that is derived from L-arginine; it reversibly binds to the thrombin active site

Uses: Thrombosis, prophylaxis or treatment

Dosage and routes:

• *Adult:* IV: 2 µg/kg/min (1 mg/ml) give at 6 ml/hr for 50 kg of weight, at 8 ml/hr for 70 kg of weight, at 11 ml/hr for 90 kg of weight, at 13 ml/hr for 110 kg of weight, at 16 ml/hr for 130 kg of weight

Available forms: Inj 100 mg/ml

Side effects/adverse reactions:

*CV: **Atrial fibrillation, ventricular tachycardia***

*SYST: **Sepsis***

CNS: Fever

GI: Nausea, vomiting, abdominal pain, diarrhea, GI bleeding

*GU: **Hematuria,** abnormal kidney function, UTI*

*HEMA: **Hemorrhage, thrombocytopenia***

RESP: Pneumonia, dyspnea

Contraindications: Hypersensitivity, overt major bleeding

Precautions: Intracranial bleeding, renal function impairment, lactation, children, hepatic disease, pregnancy (B)

Pharmacokinetics: Metabolized in the liver, half-life 39-51 mins, excreted in feces

Interactions:

• Increased risk of bleeding: other anticoagulants

• Increased action of argatroban thrombolytics

NURSING CONSIDERATIONS

Assess:

• Obtain baseline in aPTT before treatment; do not start treatment if aPTT ratio ≥2.5, then aPTT 4 hr after initiation of treatment and at least qd thereafter, if aPTT above target, stop inf for 2 hr, then restart at 50%, take aPTT in 4 hr; if below target, increase inf rate by 20%, take aPTT in 4 hr, do not exceed inf rate of 0.21 mg/kg/hr without checking for coagulation abnormalities

• aPTT, which should be 1.5-3 × control

⬥ Bleeding gums, petechiae, ecchymosis, black tarry stools, hematuria/epistaxis, B/P, vaginal bleeding and possible hemorrhage

• Fever, skin rash, urticaria

Administer:

• Avoiding all IM injections that may cause bleeding

IV INF

• Dilute in 0.9% NaCl, D₅, LR to a final conc 1 mg/ml. Dilute each 2.5 ml vial 100-fold by mixing with 250 ml of diluent, mix by repeated inversion of the diluent bag for 1 min; may be slightly hazy

• Dosage adjustment may be made after review of aPTT, not to exceed 10 µg/kg/min

Evaluate:

• Therapeutic response: absence or decrease of thrombosis

Teach patient/family:

• To use soft-bristle toothbrush to avoid bleeding gums, avoid contact sports, use electric razor, avoid IM injection

---

• To report any signs of bleeding: gums, under skin, urine, stools

arsenic trioxide (℞)

Trisenox

Func. class.: Antineoplastic-miscellaneous

Action: Not understood, causes morphological changes and DNA fragmentation

Uses: Acute promyelocytic leukemia

Dosage and routes:

Induction

• *Adult:* **IV** 0.15 mg/kg/day until bone marrow remission, max 60 doses

Consolidation treatment

Wait 3-6 wk after completion of induction

• *Adult:* **IV** 0.15 mg/kg/day × 25 doses over a period of up to 5 wk

• *Available forms:* Inj 1 mg/ml

Side effects/adverse reactions:

META: Increased ALT/AST, hyperkalemia, hypokalemia, hypomagnesemia, hyperglycemia

GU: Vaginal hemorrhage, renal failure, incontinence

HEMA: Leukocytosis, anemia, thrombocytopenia, neutropenia, DIC

CV: Hypotension, hypertension, prolonged QT interval, other ECG changes, chest pain, *tachycardia,* torsades de pointes

GI: Abdominal pain, constipation, diarrhea, dyspepsia, fecal incontinence, GI hemorrhage, dry mouth, *nausea, vomiting, anorexia*

CNS: Anxiety, confusion, insomnia, headache, paresthesia, depression, dizziness, tremor, seizures, agitation, coma, weakness

RESP: **Pleural effusion,** dyspnea, cough, epistaxis, hypoxia, sinusitis, wheezing, rales, tachypnea

MISC: Weight gain or decrease, fatigue, severe edema, rigors, herpes simplex/zoster

Contraindications: Hypersensitivity, pregnancy (D)

Precautions: Elderly, lactation, children

Pharmacokinetics: Metabolized in the liver, stored in the liver, kidney, heart, lung, hair, nails, excreted in urine

NURSING CONSIDERATIONS

Assess:

◆ For APL differentiation syndrome: fever, dyspnea, pulmonary infiltrates, pleural or pericardial effusions, weight gain; this condition can be fatal; give high-dose steroids

• For ECG changes: QT interval prolongation, complete AV block; obtain baseline ECG prior to drug therapy

• Electrolytes: potassium, calcium, magnesium, creatine

Administer:

IV

• Dilute with 100-250 ml D₅ or 0.9% NaCl immediately after withdrawing from ampule, give over 1-2 hr may give over 4 hr if reactions occur

Evaluate:

Therapeutic response: decrease in malignant cells

Teach patient/family:

• To report planned or suspected pregnancy

• That fertility impairment has not been studied

Treatment of overdose:

• Dimercaprol 3 mg/kg IM q4hr, then 250 mg penicillamine PO, max 4 ×/day (≤1 g/day)

◆ = Nursing alert   ● = Herb-drug interaction   Ⓝ = Do not crush ml; inj SC, IM, IV 100, 250, 500 mg/ml

A

ascorbic acid (vit C) (OTC, ℞)

(a-skor'bic)

ascorbic acid, Apo-C*, Ascorbicap, Cebid, Cecon, Cecore-500, Cemill, Cenolate, Cetane, Cevalin, Cevi-Bid, Ce-Vi-Sol, C-Span, Flavorcee, Mega-C/A Plus, Ortho/CS, Sunkist

Func. class.: Vit C—water-soluble vitamin

Action: Needed for wound healing, collagen synthesis, antioxidant, carbohydrate metabolism

Uses: Vit C deficiency, scurvy, delayed wound and bone healing, chronic disease, urine acidification, before gastrectomy

Investigational uses: Acidification of urine, common cold prevention

Dosage and routes:

Scurvy

• *Adult:* **PO/SC/IM/IV** 100 mg-500 mg qd × 2 wk, then 50 mg or more qd

• *Child:* **PO/SC/IM/IV** 100-300 mg qd × 2 wk, then 35 mg or more qd

Wound healing/chronic disease/fracture

• *Adult:* **SC/IM/IV/PO** 200-500 mg qd

• *Child:* **SC/IM/IV/PO** 100-200 mg added doses

Urine acidification

• *Adult:* 4-12 g qd in divided doses

• *Child:* 500 mg q6-8h

Available forms: Tabs 25, 50, 100, 250, 500, 1000, 1500 mg; tabs effervescent 1000 mg; tabs chewable 100, 250, 500 mg; tabs timed release 500, 750, 1000, 1500 mg; caps timed release 500 mg; crys 4 g/tsp; powd 4 g/tsp; liq 35 mg/0.6 ml; sol 100 mg/ml; syr 20 mg/ml, 500 mg/5

Side effects/adverse reactions:

INTEG: Inflammation at inj site

CNS: Headache, insomnia, dizziness, fatigue, flushing

GI: Nausea, vomiting, diarrhea, anorexia, heartburn, cramps

GU: Polyuria, urine acidification, oxalate or urate renal stones, dysuria

HEMA: ***Hemolytic anemia in patients with G6PD***

Contraindications: None significant

Precautions: Gout, pregnancy (C); diabetes, renal calculi (large doses)

Pharmacokinetics:

PO, INJ: Readily absorbed PO, metabolized in liver, unused amounts excreted in urine (unchanged) and metabolites, crosses placenta, breast milk

Interactions:

• Decreased effects of heparin, warfarin (large doses)

Lab test interferences:

False positive: Negatives in glucose tests

False negative: Occult blood

NURSING CONSIDERATIONS

Assess:

• I&O ratio

• Ascorbic acid levels throughout treatment if continued deficiency is suspected

• Nutritional status: citrus fruits, vegetables

• Injection sites for inflammation

Administer:

IV, direct

• Undiluted by direct IV 100 mg over at least 1 min, rapid inf may cause fainting

Intermittent IV inf

• Diluted with D_5W, D_5NaCl, NS, LR, Ringer's, sodium lactate and given over 15 min

---

* = Canada only   Side effects: *italics* = common; **bold italics** = life-threatening

Additive compatibilities: Amikacin, calcium chloride, calcium gluceptate, calcium gluconate, cephalothin, chloramphenicol, chlorpromazine, colistimethate, cyanocobalamin, diphenhydramine, heparin, kanamycin, methicillin, methyldopate, penicillin G potassium, polymyxin B, prednisolone, procaine, prochlorperazine, promethazine, verapamil

Syringe compatibilities: Metoclopramide

Y-site compatibilities: Warfarin

Evaluate:

• Therapeutic response: absence of anorexia, irritability, pallor, joint pain, hyperkeratosis, petechiae, poor wound healing

Teach patient/family:

🚫 Do not break, crush, or chew ext rel tab or caps

• That caps may be opened and contents mixed with jelly

• The necessary foods in diet, such as citrus fruits

• That smoking decreases vit C levels, not to exceed prescribed dose; increases will be excreted in urine, except time release

---

asparaginase (℞)

(a-spare′a-gi-nase)
Elspar, Kidrolase*

Func. class.: Antineoplastic
Chem. class.: Escherichia coli enzyme

Action: Indirectly inhibits protein synthesis in tumor cells; without amino acid, DNA, RNA synthesis is halted; asparagine, protein synthesis is halted; G_1 phase of cell cycle specific; a nonvesicant

Uses: Acute lymphocytic leukemia in combination with other antineoplastics

Dosage and routes:
In combination
• *Adult and child:* **IV** 1000 IU/kg/day × 10 days given over 30 min; **IM** 6000 IU/m²/day
Sole induction
• *Adult and child:* **IV** 200 IU/kg/day × 28 days
Desensitization
• *Adult and child:* Test dose adult/child ID 2 IU **IV/IU** then double dose q10 min, until total dose is administered or reaction occurs
Available forms: Inj 10,000 IU with mannitol

Side effects/adverse reactions:
SYST: **Anaphylaxis**
HEMA: **Thrombocytopenia, leukopenia, myelosuppression, anemia, decreased clotting factors (V, VII, VIII, IX), decreased fibrinogen**
GI: Nausea, vomiting, anorexia, diarrhea, weight loss, cramps, stomatitis, **hepatotoxicity, pancreatitis**
GU: Urinary retention, **renal failure,** glycosuria, polyuria, azotemia, uric acid neuropathy, proteinuria
INTEG: **Rash,** urticaria, chills, fever, perspiration
ENDO: Hyperglycemia
RESP: **Fibrosis, pulmonary infiltrate**
CV: Chest pain
CNS: Neuritis, dizziness, headache, **coma,** depression, fatigue, confusion, hallucinations, lethargy, drowsiness, agitation, Parkinson-like syndrome, **seizures**

Contraindications: Hypersensitivity, infants, pregnancy (C), lactation, pancreatitis

Precautions: Renal disease, hepatic disease

Pharmacokinetics: Half-life 4-9 hr, terminal 1.4-1.8 hr

Interactions:
• Decreased action of methotrexate
• Increased toxicity: vincristine, prednisone

◆ = Nursing alert   ⦸ = Herb-drug interaction   🚫 = Do not crush

• May decrease response to live virus vaccines

Lab test interferences:

Decrease: Thyroid function tests

NURSING CONSIDERATIONS

Assess:

• For signs and symptoms of pancreatitis (nausea, vomiting, severe abdominal pain), anaphylaxis (bronchospasm, dyspnea), cyanosis; more toxic in adults than children

• CBC, differential, platelet count weekly; withhold drug if WBC is <4000 or platelet count is <75,000; notify prescriber of these results

• Pulmonary function tests, chest x-ray studies before, during therapy; chest x-ray film should be obtained q2wk during treatment

• Renal function studies: BUN, serum uric acid, ammonia urine CrCl, electrolytes before, during therapy

• I&O ratio; report fall in urine output of 30 ml/hr

• Monitor temp q4h; may indicate beginning infection

• Liver function tests before, during therapy (bilirubin, AST, ALT, LDH) as needed or monthly

• RBC, Hct, Hgb, since these may be decreased

• Serum, urine glucose levels

• Bleeding: hematuria, guaiac, bruising or petechiae, mucosa or orifices q8h

➔ Dyspnea, rales, nonproductive cough, chest pain, tachypnea, fatigue, increased pulse, pallor, lethargy, swelling around eyes or lips; anaphylaxis may occur; risk of hypersensitivity increases with repeated dose

• Jaundice of skin and sclera, dark urine, clay-colored stools, itchy skin, abdominal pain, fever, diarrhea

• Local irritation, pain, burning, discoloration at injection site

• Symptoms indicating severe allergic reaction: rash, pruritus, urticaria, purpuric skin lesions, itching, flushing, dyspnea

Frequency of stools, characteristics: cramping, acidosis; signs of dehydration: rapid respirations, poor skin turgor, decreased urine output, dry skin, restlessness, weakness

Administer:

IM

• Reconstitute with 2 ml NaCl/10,000 U/vial, refrigerate, use within 8 hr; discard sooner if sol becomes cloudy

IV, direct

• After intradermal skin testing and desensitization, give 0.1 ml (2 IU) intradermally after reconstituting with 5 ml sterile H_2O or 0.9% NaCl for injection; then add 0.1 ml of reconstituted drug to 9.9 ml diluent (20 IU/ml); observe for 1 hr, check for wheal

• Allopurinol or sodium bicarbonate to reduce uric acid levels, alkalinization of urine

Intermittent IV inf

• Using 21G, 23G, 25G needle; administer by slow IV infusion via Y-tube or 3-way stopcock of flowing D_5W or NS infusion over 30 min after diluting 10,000 IU/5 ml of sterile H_2O or 0.9% NaCl (no preservatives) (2000 IU/ml); use of filter may be necessary if fibers are present

Y-site compatibilities: Methotrexate, sodium bicarbonate

Perform/provide:

• Deep-breathing exercises with patient 3-4 ×/day; place in semi-Fowler's position

• Increase fluid intake to 2-3 L/day to prevent urate deposits, calculi formation

• Diet low in purines: absence of organ meats (kidney, liver), dried beans, peas to maintain alkaline urine

• Rinsing of mouth 3-4 ×/day with water, club soda

• Brushing of teeth 2-3 ×/day with soft brush or cotton-tipped applicators for stomatitis; use unwaxed dental floss
• Warm compresses at injection site for inflammation
• Nutritious diet with iron, vitamin supplements
• HOB raised to facilitate breathing
Evaluate:
• Therapeutic response: decreased exacerbations in ALL
Teach patient/family:
• To report any complaints or side effects to nurse or prescriber
• To report any changes in breathing or coughing
Treatment of anaphylaxis:
Administer epinephrine, diphenhydramine, IV corticosteroids, O_2

---

aspirin (OTC)
(as'pir-in)

acetylsalicylic acid, Acuprin, Apo-ASA*, Apo-Asen*, Arthrinol*, Arthrisin*, Artria S.R., A.S.A., Aspergum, Aspirin*, Aspir-Low, Aspirtab, Astrin*, Bayer Aspirin, Coryphen*, Easprin, Ecotrin, 8-Hour Bayer Timed Release, Empirin, Entrophen*, Halfprin, Norwich Extra-Strength, Novasen*, PMS-ASA*, Sloprin, St. Joseph Children's, Supasa*, Therapy Bayer, ZORprin
Func. class.: Nonnarcotic analgesic, nonsteroidal antiinflammatory, antipyretic, antiplatelet
Chem. class.: Salicylate

Action: Blocks pain impulses in CNS, inhibition of prostaglandin synthesis; antipyretic action results from vasodilation of peripheral vessels; decreases platelet aggregation
Uses: Mild to moderate pain or fever including rheumatoid arthritis, osteoarthritis, thromboembolic disorders; transient ischemic attacks, rheumatic fever, postmyocardial infarction, prophylaxis of MI, ischemic stroke, angina
Investigational uses: Prevention of cataracts (long-term use), prevention of pregnancy loss in women with clotting disorders
Dosage and routes:
Arthritis
• *Adult:* **PO** 2.6-5.2 g/day in divided doses q4-6h
• *Child:* **PO** 90-130 mg/kg/day in divided doses q4-6h
Pain/fever
• *Adult:* **PO/RECT** 325-650 mg q4h prn, not to exceed 4 g/day
• *Child:* **PO/RECT** 40-100 mg/kg/day in divided doses q4-6h prn
Kawasaki disease
• *Child:* **PO** 80-120 mg/kg/day in 4 divided doses, maintenance 3-8 mg/kg/day as a single dose × 8 wk
Thromboembolic disorders
• *Adult:* **PO** 325-650 mg/day or bid
Transient ischemic attacks
• *Adult:* **PO** 650 mg qid or 325 mg qid
MI, stroke prophylaxis
• *Adult:* **PO** 81-650 mg/day
Available forms: Tabs 81, 162.5, 325, 500, 650, 975 mg; chewable tabs 80, 81 mg; supp 60, 120, 125, 130, 150, 160, 195, 200, 300, 320, 325, 600, 640, 650 mg, 1.2 g; cream; gum 227 mg; dispersible tabs 325, 500 mg, tabs del rel, enteric coated 80, 165, 300, 325, 500, 600, 650, 975 mg; ext rel tab 325, 650, 800 mg, del rel caps 325, 500 mg
Side effects/adverse reactions:
*HEMA: **Thrombocytopenia, agranulocytosis, leukopenia, neutropenia, hemolytic anemia,*** increased pro-time, APTT, bleeding time
CNS: Stimulation, drowsiness, dizziness, confusion, ***convulsion,*** head-

---

◆ = Nursing alert   **🖊** = Herb-drug interaction   **⊘** = Do not crush

ache, flushing, hallucinations, *coma*
*GI: Nausea, vomiting, **GI bleeding,***
diarrhea, heartburn, anorexia, *hepatitis*
INTEG: Rash, urticaria, bruising
EENT: Tinnitus, hearing loss
CV: Rapid pulse, pulmonary edema
RESP: Wheezing, hyperpnea
ENDO: Hypoglycemia, hyponatremia, hypokalemia
*SYST: **Reye's syndrome (children)***
Contraindications: Hypersensitivity to salicylates, tartrazine (FDC yellow dye #5), GI bleeding, bleeding disorders, children <12 yr, children with flulike symptoms, pregnancy (D) 3rd trimester, lactation, vit K deficiency, peptic ulcer
Precautions: Anemia, hepatic disease, renal disease, Hodgkin's disease, pre/postoperatively, gastritis, asthmatic patients with nasal polyps or aspirin sensitivity, pregnancy (C)
Pharmacokinetics: Well absorbed PO; enteric metabolized by liver, inactive metabolites excreted by kidneys, crosses placenta, excreted in breast milk; half-life 1-3½ hr, up to 30 hr in large dose; rectal products may be erratic
PO: Onset 15-30 min, peak 1-2 hr, duration 4-6 hr
REC: Onset slow, duration 4-6 hr
Interactions:
• Decreased effects of aspirin: antacids (high doses), steroids, urinary alkalizers, corticosteroids
• Increased bleeding: alcohol, heparin, plicamycin, cefamandole
• Increased effects of warfarin, insulin, methotrexate, thrombolytic agents, penicillins, phenytoin, valproic acid, oral hypoglycemics, sulfonamides
• Increased salicylate levels: urinary acidifiers, ammonium chloride, nizatidine

• Decreased effects of probenecid, spironolactone, sulfinpyrazone, sulfonylamides, NSAIDs, beta blockers
• Gastric ulcer: steroids, antiinflammatories, NSAIDs
🌿 Increased risk of bleeding: horse chestnut, kelpware
Lab test interferences:
Increase: Coagulation studies, liver function studies, serum uric acid, amylase, CO_2, urinary protein
Decrease: Serum K, PBI, cholesterol
Interference: Urine catecholamines, pregnancy test, urine glucose tests (Clinistix, Tes-Tape)
NURSING CONSIDERATIONS
Assess:
• Liver function studies: AST, ALT, bilirubin, creatinine if patient is on long-term therapy
• Renal function studies: BUN, urine creatinine if patient is on long-term therapy
• Blood studies: CBC, Hct, Hgb, pro-time if patient is on long-term therapy
• I&O ratio; decreasing output may indicate renal failure (long-term therapy)
◆ Hepatotoxicity: dark urine, clay-colored stools, yellowing of skin, sclera, itching, abdominal pain, fever, diarrhea if patient is on long-term therapy
• Allergic reactions: rash, urticaria; if these occur, drug may have to be discontinued
• Renal dysfunction: decreased urine output
• Ototoxicity: tinnitus, ringing, roaring in ears; audiometric testing needed before, after long-term therapy
• Visual changes: blurring, halos; corneal, retinal damage
• Edema in feet, ankles, legs

• Drug history; many drug interactions
• Pain: location, duration, type, intensity, prior to dose and 1 hr after
• Musculoskeletal status: ROM prior to dose
• Fever; length of time and related symptoms

Administer:

PO

• Crushed or whole; chewable tablets may be chewed

🚫 Do not crush enteric product
• With food or milk to decrease gastric symptoms; give 30 min before or 2 hr after meals

Evaluate:

• Therapeutic response: decreased pain, inflammation, fever

Teach patient/family:

• To report any symptoms of hepatotoxicity, renal toxicity, visual changes, ototoxicity, allergic reactions, bleeding (long-term therapy)
• To take with 8 oz H_2O and sit upright for ½ hr after dose
• Not to exceed recommended dosage; acute poisoning may result
• To read label on other OTC drugs; many contain aspirin
• That the therapeutic response takes 2 wk (arthritis); give ½ hr before planned exercise
• To report tinnitus, confusion, diarrhea, sweating, hyperventilation
• To avoid alcohol ingestion; GI bleeding may occur
• That patients who have allergies may develop allergic reactions
• To avoid buffered or effervescent products
• To discard tabs if vinegar-like smell is detected
• That medication is not to be given to children or teens with flulike symptoms or chickenpox; Reye's syndrome may develop

Treatment of overdose: Lavage, activated charcoal, monitor electrolytes, VS

---

atenolol (℞)

(a-ten'oh-lole)

Apo-Atenol*, atenolol*, Novo-Atenol*, Tenormin

Func. class.: Antihypertensive, antianginal

Chem. class.: β-Blocker, β-1, β-2-blocker (high doses)

Action: Competitively blocks stimulation of β-adrenergic receptor within vascular smooth muscle; produces negative chronotropic activity, negative inotropic activity (decreases rate of SA node discharge, increases recovery time), slows conduction of AV node, decreases heart rate, decreases O_2 consumption in myocardium; also decreases renin-aldosterone-angiotensin system at high doses, inhibits β-2 receptors in bronchial system at higher doses

Uses: Mild to moderate hypertension, prophylaxis of angina pectoris; suspected or known myocardial infarction (IV use)

Investigational uses: Dysrhythmia, mitral valve prolapse, pheochromocytoma, hypertrophic cardiomyopathy, vascular headaches, thyrotoxicosis, tremors, alcohol withdrawal

Dosage and routes:

• *Adult:* IV 5 mg, repeat in 10 min if initial dose is well tolerated, then start **PO** dose 10 min after last **IV** dose
• *Adult:* PO 50 mg qd, increasing q1-2wk to 100 mg qd; may increase to 200 mg qd for angina
• *Elderly:* PO 25 mg/day initially

Renal disease

• CrCl 15-35 ml/min, max 50 mg/day; CrCl <15 ml/min max dose 50

⬥= Nursing alert　　🌿= Herb-drug interaction　　🚫= Do not crush

mg qod; hemodialysis 25-50 mg after dialysis

Available forms: Tabs 25, 50, 100 mg; inj 5 mg/10 ml

Side effects/adverse reactions:

*CV: **Profound hypotension, bradycardia, CHF,** cold extremities, postural hypotension, 2nd- or 3rd-degree heart block*

CNS: Insomnia, fatigue, dizziness, mental changes, memory loss, hallucinations, depression, lethargy, drowsiness, strange dreams, catatonia

GI: Nausea, diarrhea, vomiting, ***mesenteric arterial thrombosis, ischemic colitis***

INTEG: Rash, fever, alopecia

*HEMA: **Agranulocytosis, thrombocytopenia, purpura***

EENT: Sore throat, dry burning eyes

GU: Impotence

ENDO: Increased hypoglycemic response to insulin

*RESP: **Bronchospasm,** dyspnea, wheezing*

Contraindications: Hypersensitivity to β-blockers, cardiogenic shock, 2nd- or 3rd-degree heart block, sinus bradycardia, cardiac failure, pregnancy (D)

Precautions: Major surgery, lactation, diabetes mellitus, renal disease, thyroid disease, CHF, COPD, asthma, well-compensated heart failure

Do not confuse:

atenolol/albuterol

Tenormin/thiamine

Pharmacokinetics:

PO: Peak 2-4 hr; half-life 6-7 hr, excreted unchanged in urine, protein binding 5%-15%

Interactions:

• Increased hypotension, bradycardia: reserpine, hydralazine, methyldopa, prazosin, anticholinergics, digoxin, diltiazem, verapamil, cardiac glycosides, antihypertensives

• Increased hypoglycemic effect: insulin, oral antidiabetics

• Mutual inhibition: sympathomimetics (cough, cold preparations)

Lab test interferences:

Interference: Glucose/insulin tolerance tests

NURSING CONSIDERATIONS

Assess:

• I&O, weight daily

• B/P, pulse q4h; note rate, rhythm, quality

• Apical/radial pulse before administration; notify prescriber of any significant changes (<50 bpm)

• Baselines in renal, liver function tests before therapy begins

• Edema in feet, legs daily

• Skin turgor, dryness of mucous membranes for hydration status

Administer:

PO

• Drug ac, hs, tablet may be crushed or swallowed whole

• Reduced dosage in renal dysfunction

IV, direct

• Undiluted over 5 min

IV infusion

• Diluted in 10-50 ml of D_5W, D_5/NaCl, or NS and give as an infusion at prescribed rate

Y-site compatibilities: Meperidine, meropenem, morphine

Perform/provide:

• Storage protected from light, moisture; place in cool environment

Evaluate:

• Therapeutic response: decreased B/P after 1-2 wk

Teach patient/family:

◆ Not to discontinue drug abruptly, taper over 2 wk

• Not to use OTC products unless directed by prescriber

• To report bradycardia, dizziness, confusion, fever

• To take pulse at home; advise when to notify prescriber

- To limit alcohol, smoking, sodium intake
- To comply with weight control, dietary adjustments, modified exercise program
- To carry Medic Alert ID to identify drug that you are taking, allergies
- To avoid hazardous activities if dizziness is present
- That drug may mask symptoms of hypoglycemia in diabetic patients
- To use contraception while taking this drug

Treatment of overdose: Lavage, IV atropine for bradycardia, IV theophylline for bronchospasm, digitalis, O_2, diuretic for cardiac failure, hemodialysis

---

atorvastatin (Rx)

(at-or'va-sta-tin)
Lipitor
Func. class.: Antilipidemic
Chem. class.: HMG-CoA reductase inhibitor

Action: Inhibits HMG-CoA reductase enzyme, which reduces cholesterol synthesis

Uses: As an adjunct in primary hypercholesterolemia (types Ia, Ib), dysbetalipoproteinemia, elevated triglyceride levels

Dosage and routes:
- *Adult:* PO 10 mg qd, usual range 10-80, dosage adjustments may be made in 2-4 wk intervals

Available forms: Tabs 10, 20, 40 mg

Side effects/adverse reactions:
INTEG: Rash, pruritus, alopecia
GI: Dyspepsia, flatus, *liver dysfunction,* pancreatitis
EENT: Lens opacities
MS: Myalgia
CNS: Headache

Contraindications: Hypersensitivity, pregnancy (X), lactation, active liver disease

Precautions: Past liver disease, alcoholism, severe acute infections, trauma, hypotension, uncontrolled seizure disorders, severe metabolic disorders, electrolyte imbalance

Pharmacokinetics: Metabolized in liver, highly protein bound, excreted primarily in urine, half-life 14 hr; protein binding 98%

Interactions:
- Possible rhabdomyolysis: azole antifungals, cyclosporine, erythromycin, niacin, gemfibrozil, clofibrate
- Increased serum level of digoxin
- Increased levels of oral contraceptives
- Increased levels of atorvastatin: erythromycin, itraconazole
- Increased effects of warfarin

NURSING CONSIDERATIONS

Assess:
- Diet, obtain diet history including fat, cholesterol in diet
- Cholesterol levels periodically during treatment
- Liver function studies q1-2mo during the first 1½ yr of treatment; AST, ALT, liver function tests may be increased
- Renal studies in patients with compromised renal system: BUN, I&O ratio, creatinine
- Ophthalmic exam, 1 mo after treatment begins, annually; lens opacities may occur

◆ For muscle pain, tenderness, obtain CPK if these occur, drug may need to be discontinued

Administer:

PO
- Total daily dose any time of day

Perform/provide:
- Storage in cool environment in tight container protected from light

---

◆ = Nursing alert   = Herb-drug interaction   🚫 = Do not crush

Evaluate:
• Therapeutic response: decrease in cholesterol to desired level after 8 wk

Teach patient/family:
• That blood work and eye exam will be necessary during treatment
• To report blurred vision, severe GI symptoms, headache, muscle pain, weakness
• That previously prescribed regimen will continue: low-cholesterol diet, exercise program, smoking cessation
• Not to take drug if pregnant
• To stay out of the sun, or use sunscreen to prevent photosensitivity (rare)

---

atovaquone (℞)
(a-toe'va-kwon')
Mepron
Func. class.: Antiprotozoal
Chem. class.: Aromatic diamide derivative, analog of ubiquinone

---

Action: Interferes with DNA/RNA synthesis in protozoa
Uses: *Pneumocystis carinii* infections in patients intolerant of trimethoprim-sulfamethoxazole
Dosage and routes:
• *Adult and adolescents 13-16 yr:* **PO** 750 mg with food bid for 21 days
Available forms: 750 mg/5 ml, susp
Side effects/adverse reactions:
CV: Hypotension
HEMA: Anemia, *leukopenia,* neutropenia
INTEG: Pruritus, urticaria, *rash*, oral monilia
GI: Nausea, vomiting, diarrhea, anorexia, increased AST and ALT, acute pancreatitis, constipation, abdominal pain

CNS: Dizziness, headache, anxiety, insomnia
META: Hyperkalemia, hypoglycemia, hyponatremia
Contraindications: Hypersensitivity or history of developing life-threatening allergic reactions to any component of the formulation
Precautions: Blood dyscrasias, hepatic disease, diabetes mellitus, pregnancy (C), lactation, children, elderly
Do not confuse:
Mepron (U.S.)/Mepron (meprobamate in Australia)
Pharmacokinetics: Excreted unchanged in feces (94%), highly protein bound (99%)
Interactions:
• Use caution when administering concurrently with other highly plasma protein-bound drugs with narrow therapeutic indices
• Decreased effect of atovaquone: rifampin, rifabutin
NURSING CONSIDERATIONS
Assess:
• Signs of infection, anemia
• Bowel pattern before, during treatment
• Respiratory status: rate, character, wheezing, dyspnea
• Allergies before treatment, reaction of each medication
Administer:
PO
• With high-fat food because of increased absorption of the drug and higher plasma concentrations
Evaluate:
• Therapeutic response: decreased temp, ability to breathe
Teach patient/family:
• To take with food to increase plasma concentrations

RARELY USED

atracurium (℞)

(a-tra-kyoor'ee-um)

Tracrium

Func. class.: Neuromuscular blocker (nondepolarizing)

Uses: Facilitation of endotracheal intubation, skeletal muscle relaxation during mechanical ventilation, surgery, or general anesthesia

Dosage and routes:

• *Adult and child >2 yr:* **IV BOL** 0.3-0.5 mg/kg, then 0.08-0.10 mg/kg 20-45 min after first dose if needed for prolonged procedures

• *Child, 1 mo-2 yr:* **IV BOL** 0.3-0.4 mg/kg

Contraindications: Hypersensitivity

atropine (℞)

(a'troe-peen)

Atro-Pen

Func. class.: Antidysrhythmic, anticholinergic parasympatholytic, antimuscarinic

Chem. class.: Belladonna alkaloid

Action: Blocks acetylcholine at parasympathetic neuroeffector sites; increases cardiac output, heart rate by blocking vagal stimulation in heart; dries secretions by blocking vagus

Uses: Bradycardia <40-50 bpm, bradydysrhythmia, reversal of anticholinesterase agents, insecticide poisoning, blocking cardiac vagal reflexes, decreasing secretions before surgery, antispasmodic with GU, biliary surgery, bronchodilator

Dosage and routes:

Bradycardia/bradydysrhythmia

• *Adult:* **IV BOL** 0.5-1 mg given q3-5min, not to exceed 2 mg

• *Child:* **IV BOL** 0.01-0.03 mg/kg up to 0.4 mg or 0.3 mg/m²; may repeat q4-6h; min dose 0.1 mg to avoid paradoxical reaction

Organophosphate poisoning

• *Adult and child:* **IM/IV** 2 mg qh until muscarinic symptoms disappear, may need 6 mg qh

Presurgery

• *Adult:* **SC/IM/IV** 0.4-0.6 mg before anesthesia

• *Child:* **SC** 0.1-0.4 mg 30 min before surgery

Available forms: Inj 0.05, 0.1, 0.3, 0.4, 0.5, 0.8, 1 mg/ml; 2 mg/0.7 ml auto injector; tabs 0.4 mg

Side effects/adverse reactions:

GU: Retention, hesitancy, impotence, dysuria

CNS: Headache, dizziness, involuntary movement, confusion, psychosis, anxiety, coma, flushing, drowsiness, insomnia, weakness; delirium (elderly)

GI: Dry mouth, nausea, vomiting, abdominal pain, anorexia, constipation, *paralytic ileus,* abdominal distention, altered taste

CV: Hypotension, paradoxical bradycardia, angina, PVCs, hypertension, *tachycardia,* ectopic ventricular beats

INTEG: Rash, urticaria, contact dermatitis, dry skin, flushing

EENT: Blurred vision, photophobia, glaucoma, eye pain, pupil dilation, nasal congestion

MISC: Suppression of lactation, decreased sweating

Contraindications: Hypersensitivity to belladonna alkaloids, angle-closure glaucoma, GI obstructions, myasthenia gravis, thyrotoxicosis, ulcerative colitis, prostatic hypertrophy, tachycardia/tachydysrhyth-

◆ = Nursing alert   ∥ = Herb-drug interaction   ⊘ = Do not crush

mias, asthma, acute hemorrhage, hepatic disease, myocardial ischemia
Precautions: Pregnancy (C), renal disease, lactation, CHF, tachydysrhythmia, hyperthyroidism, COPD, hepatic disease, child <6 yr, hypertension, elderly, intraabdominal infection, Down syndrome, spastic paralysis, gastric ulcer
Pharmacokinetics: Well absorbed PO, IM, SC; half-life 13-40 hr, excreted by kidneys unchanged (70%-90% in 24 hr); metabolized in liver, 40%-50% crosses placenta, excreted in breast milk
IV: Peak 2-4 min, duration 4-6 hr
IM/SC: Onset 15-50 min; peak 30 min, duration 4-6 hr
PO: Onset ½ hr; peak ½-1 hr; duration 4-6 hr
Interactions:
• Decreased effect of atropine: antacids
• Mucosal lesions: potassium chloride tab
• Decreased absorption: ketoconazole, levodopa
• Increased anticholinergic effects, tricylics, amantadine, antiparkinson agents
🖉 Possible increased action of atropine: chronic use/abuse of cascara sagrada bark, buckthorn bark/berry, rhubarb root, senna leaf/fruits, aloe
NURSING CONSIDERATIONS
Assess:
• I&O ratio; check for urinary retention, daily output
• ECG for ectopic ventricular beats, PVC, tachycardia, in cardiac patients
• For bowel sounds; check for constipation
• Respiratory status: rate, rhythm, cyanosis, wheezing, dyspnea, engorged neck veins

• Increased intraocular pressure: eye pain, nausea, vomiting, blurred vision, increased tearing
• Cardiac rate: rhythm, character, B/P continuously
• Allergic reaction: rash, urticaria
Administer:
PO
• Increased bulk, water in diet if constipation occurs
• ½ hr ac
IM
• Atropine flush may occur in children and is not harmful
IV
• Undiluted or diluted with 10 ml sterile H_2O, give at 0.6 mg/min, give through Y-tube or 3-way stopcock; do not add to IV sol; may cause paradoxical bradycardia lasting 2 min
Additive compatibilities: Dobutamine, furosemide, meropenem, netilmicin, sodium bicarbonate, verapamil
Syringe compatibilities: Benzquinamide, butorphanol, chlorpromazine, cimetidine, dimenhydrinate, diphenhydramine, droperidol, fentanyl, glycopyrrolate, heparin, hydromorphone, hydroxyzine, meperidine, metoclopramide, midazolam, milrinone, morphine, nalbuphine, pentazocine, perphenazine, prochlorperazine, promazine, promethazine, propiomazine, ranitidine, scopolamine, sufentanil
Y-site compatibilities: Amrinone, etomidate, famotidine, heparin, hydrocortisone, meropenem, nafcillin, potassium chloride, sufentanil, vit B/C
Perform/provide:
• Sugarless hard candy, gum, frequent rinsing of mouth for dryness
Evaluate:
• Therapeutic response: decreased dysrhythmias, increased heart rate,

secretions; GI, GU spasms; bronchodilation

Teach patient/family:

• To report blurred vision, chest pain, allergic reactions, constipation, urinary retention

• Not to perform strenuous activity in high temperatures; heat stroke may result

• To take as prescribed; not to skip doses

• Not to operate machinery if drowsiness occurs

• Not to take OTC products without approval of prescriber

Treatment of overdose: O_2, artificial ventilation, ECG; administer dopamine for circulatory depression; administer diazepam or thiopental for convulsions; assess need for antidysrhythmics

---

RARELY USED

auranofin (℞)

(au-rane'oh-fin)

Ridaura

Func. class.: Antiinflammatory

Uses: Rheumatoid arthritis; not for first-line therapy

Investigational uses: SLE, psoriatic arthritis, pemphigus

Dosage and routes:

• *Adult:* **PO** 6 mg qd or 3 mg bid; may increase to 9 mg/day after 3 mo

Contraindications: Hypersensitivity to gold, necrotizing enterocolitis, bone marrow aplasia, child <6 yr, lactation, pulmonary fibrosis, exfoliative dermatitis, blood dyscrasias, recent radiation therapy, renal/hepatic disease, marked hypertension, uncontrolled CHF

Do not confuse:

Ridaura/Cardura

RARELY USED

aurothioglucose/gold sodium thiomalate (℞)

(aur-oh-thye-oh-gloo'kose)

Solganal/Aurolate

Func. class.: Antiinflammatory

Uses: Rheumatoid arthritis, psoriatic arthritis

Dosage and routes:

• *Adult:* **IM** 10 mg, then 25 mg qwk × 2-3 wk, then 50 mg/wk until total of 1 g is administered, then 25-50 mg q3-4wk if there is improvement without toxicity (aurothioglucose) total of 800 mg-1 g

• *Adult:* **IM** 10 mg, then 25 mg after 1 wk, then 50 mg qwk for total of 14-20 doses, then 50 mg q2wk × 4, then 50 mg q3wk × 4, then 50 mg qmo for maintenance (gold sodium thiomalate)

• *Child 6-12 yr:* **IM** 1 mg/kg/wk × 20 wk, or ¼ of adult dose (aurothioglucose)

• *Child:* **IM** 1 mg/kg/wk × 20 wk, then q3-4wk if improvement without toxicity (gold sodium thiomalate) not to exceed 2.5 mg

Contraindications: Hypersensitivity to gold, SLE, uncontrolled diabetes mellitus, marked hypertension, recent radiation therapy, CHF, lactation, renal disease, liver disease

---

◆ = Nursing alert   ⧪ = Herb-drug interaction   ⃠ = Do not crush

azathioprine (R)
(ay-za-thye'oh-preen)
Imuran
Func. class.: Immunosuppressant
Chem. class.: Purine analog

Action: Produces immunosuppression by inhibiting purine synthesis in cells

Uses: Renal transplants to prevent graft rejection, refractory rheumatoid arthritis, refractory ITP, glomerulonephritis, nephrotic syndrome, bone marrow transplant

Investigational uses: Myasthenia gravis, chronic ulcerative colitis, Crohn's disease, Behçet's disease

Dosage and routes:

Prevention of rejection
• *Adult and child:* **PO, IV** 3-5 mg/kg/day, then maintenance (PO) of at least 1-2 mg/kg/day

Refractory rheumatoid arthritis
• *Adult:* **PO** 1/mg/kg/day, may increase dose after 2 mo by 0.5 mg/kg/day, not to exceed 2.5 mg/kg/day

Renal disease
• CrCl 10-50 ml/min 75% of dose; CrCl <10 ml/min 50% of dose

Available forms: Tabs 50 mg; inj 100 mg

Side effects/adverse reactions:

GI: Nausea, vomiting, stomatitis, esophagitis, *pancreatitis, hepatotoxicity, jaundice*

HEMA: **Leukopenia, thrombocytopenia, anemia, pancytopenia**

INTEG: Rash, alopecia

MS: Arthralgia, muscle wasting

Contraindications: Hypersensitivity, pregnancy (D), lactation

Precautions: Severe renal disease, severe hepatic disease, elderly

Do not confuse:
Imuran/Imferon

Pharmacokinetics: Metabolized in liver, excreted in urine (active metabolite), crosses placenta

Lab test interferences:

Interfere: CBC, diff count

Decrease: Uric acid

Increase: LFTs

Interactions:
• Leukopenia: ACE inhibitors; co-trimoxazole, myelopoiesis
• Decreased immune response: vaccines
• Decreased action of warfarin: warfarin
• Increased action of azathioprine: allopurinol
• Do not admix with other drugs

NURSING CONSIDERATIONS

Assess:
• For infection: increased temp, WBC; sputum, urine
• For rheumatoid arthritis, pain, mobility, ROM
• I&O, weight qd, report decreasing urine output; toxicity may occur
• Blood studies: Hgb, WBC, platelets during treatment monthly; if leukocytes are <3000/mm^3 or platelets <100,000/mm^3, drug should be discontinued

◆Hepatotoxicity: dark urine, jaundice, itching, light-colored stools, increased LFTs; drug should be discontinued; liver function studies: alk phosphatase, AST, ALT, bilirubin

Administer:
• All medications PO if possible, avoiding IM injections, since bleeding may occur

PO
• With meals to reduce GI upset

IV
• Prepare in biologic cabinet using gown, gloves, mask
• After diluting 100 mg/10 ml of sterile H_2O for inj; rotate to dissolve; may further dilute with 50 ml or more saline or glucose in saline, give over ½-1 hr

• For several days before transplant surgery

Solution compatibilities: D_5W, NaCl 0.9%, NaCl 0.45%

Evaluate:

• Therapeutic response: absence of graft rejection, immunosuppression in autoimmune disorders

Teach patient/family:

• To take as prescribed, do not miss doses, if dose is missed on qd regimen, skip dose; if on multiple dosing/day, take as soon as remembered

• That therapeutic response may take 3-4 mo in rheumatoid arthritis; to continue with prescribed exercise, rest, other medications

• To report fever, rash, severe diarrhea, chills, sore throat, fatigue, since serious infections may occur

• To use contraceptive measures during treatment, for 12 wk after ending therapy; to avoid vaccinations

• To avoid crowds to reduce risk of infection

• To use soft-bristled toothbrush to prevent bleeding

• That treatment is ongoing to prevent transplant rejection

---

azithromycin (R)

(ay-zi-thro-my′sin)

Zithromax

Func. class.: Antiinfective

Chem. class.: Macrolide (azalide)

Action: Binds to 50S ribosomal subunits of susceptible bacteria and suppresses protein synthesis; much greater spectrum of activity than erythromycin

Uses: Mild to moderate infections of the upper respiratory tract, lower respiratory tract, uncomplicated skin and skin structure infections caused by *Moraxella catarrhalis, Streptococcus pneumoniae, Streptococcus pyogenes, Staphylococcus aureus, Streptococcus agalactiae, Mycoplasma pneumoniae, Haemophilus influenzae, Clostridium, Legionella pneumophila;* nongonococcal urethritis or cervicitis due to *Chlamydia trachomatis;* in children: acute otitis media (*H. influenzae, M. catarrhalis, S. pneumoniae*) PO; acute pharyngitis/tonsillitis (group A streptococcal) PO; acute skin/soft tissue infections (PO); community-acquired pneumonia *(Citrobacter pneumoniae, H. influenzae, M. pneumoniae, S. pneumoniae)* PO; pharyngitis/tonsillitis *(S. pyogenes);* prophylaxis of disseminated *Mycobacterium avium* complex (MAC)

Investigational uses: Bacterial endocarditis prevention

Dosage and routes:

• *Adult:* **PO** 500 mg on day 1, then 250 mg qd on days 2-5 for a total dose of 1.5 g; may give a one-time dose of 1 g for chlamydial infections; 1200 mg qwk for MAC prophylaxis IV 500 mg qd ≥2 days, then 500 mg qd to complete 7-10 day therapy for community-acquired pneumonia; 500 mg qd × 3 days (upper/lower respiratory infections)

• *Adult:* **IV** 500 mg qd × 2 days, then 250 mg qd to complete 7 day therapy for pelvic inflammatory disease (PID)

• *Child ≥2 yr:* 12 mg/kg qd for 5 days

• *Child <6 mo:* 10 mg/kg on day 1, then 5 mg/kg qd days 2-5

Lower respiratory tract infections, acute skin/soft tissue infections, acute pharyngitis/tonsillitis, acute otitis media

• *Child, 3-day regimen:* **PO** 10 mg/kg qd × 3 days

Prevention of acute otitis media

Child: **PO** 10 mg/kg q wk × 6 mo

◆ = Nursing alert   ✐ = Herb-drug interaction   ⊘ = Do not crush

Available forms: Tabs 250, 600 mg; powder for inj 500 mg; powder for oral susp 1 g/packet; susp 100, 200 mg/5 ml

Side effects/adverse reactions:

INTEG: Rash, urticaria, pruritus, photosensitivity

CV: Palpitations, chest pain

CNS: Dizziness, headache, vertigo, somnolence

GI: Nausea, vomiting, diarrhea, **hepatotoxicity,** abdominal pain, stomatitis, heartburn, dyspepsia, flatulence, melena, ***cholestatic jaundice***

GU: Vaginitis, moniliasis, nephritis

Contraindications: Hypersensitivity to azithromycin, erythromycin, or any macrolide

Precautions: Pregnancy (B), lactation; hepatic, renal, cardiac disease; elderly, <6 mo for otitis media, <2 yr for pharyngitis, tonsillitis

Do not confuse:

Zithromax/Zinacef

Pharmacokinetics: Peak 2-4 hr, duration 24 hr, half-life 11-57 hr, excreted in bile, feces, urine primarily as unchanged drug

Interactions:

• Toxicity; ergotamine

• Increased effects of oral anticoagulants, digoxin, theophylline, methylprednisolone, cyclosporine, bromocriptine, disopyramide, triazolam, carbamazepine, phenytoin

• Decreased clearance of: triazolam

◆ Dysrhythmias: astemizole, pimozide; fatal reaction

• Decreased absorption of azithromycin: aluminum, magnesium antacids

Lab interferences:

Increase: CPK, ALT, AST, bilirubin, BUN, creatinine, alk phosphatase

NURSING CONSIDERATIONS

Assess:

• I&O ratio; report hematuria, oliguria in renal disease

• Liver function studies: AST, ALT; CBC with differential

• Renal studies: urinalysis, protein, blood

• C&S before drug therapy; drug may be taken as soon as culture is taken; C&S may be repeated after treatment

• For superinfection: sore throat, mouth, tongue; fever, fatigue, diarrhea, anogenital pruritus

• Bowel pattern before, during treatment

• Respiratory status: rate, character, wheezing, tightness in chest; discontinue drug if these occur

Administer:

PO

• Susp 1 hr ac or 2 hr pc. Reconstitute 1 g packet for susp with 60 ml water, mix, rinse glass with more water and have patient drink to consume all medication

IV

• Reconstitute 500 mg of drug/4.8 ml sterile water for inj (100 mg/ml); shake, dilute with ≥250 ml 0.9% NaCl, 0.45% NaCl, or LR to 1-2 mg/ml

• Give 500 mg/hr or more, never give IM or as a bolus

Perform/provide:

• Storage at room temperature

Evaluate:

• Therapeutic response: C&S negative for infection; decreased signs of infection

Teach patient/family:

◆ To report sore throat, fever, fatigue, severe diarrhea, anal, genital itching (may indicate superinfection)

• Not to take aluminum/magnesiumcontaining antacids simultaneously with this drug (PO)

◆ To notify nurse of diarrhea stools, dark urine, pale stools, yellow discoloration of eyes or skin, severe abdominal pain

• To complete dosage regimen

Treatment of hypersensitivity: Withdraw drug, maintain airway, administer epinephrine, aminophylline, O₂, IV corticosteroids

---

aztreonam (℞)

(az-tree'oh nam)
Azactam
Func. class.: Miscellaneous antibiotic
Chem. class.: Monobactam

Action: Inhibits organisms by inhibiting bacterial cell wall synthesis, which causes death of organism (bactericidal)

Uses: Urinary tract infection; septicemia; skin, muscle, bone infection, lower respiratory tract, intraabdominal infections; and other infections caused by gram-negative organisms

Investigational uses: May be used instead of spectinomycin for acute uncomplicated gonorrhea in patients with penicillin-resistant gonococci

Dosage and routes:

Urinary tract infections
• *Adult:* **IV/IM** 500 mg-1 g q8-12h

Systemic infections
• *Adult:* **IV/IM** 1-2 g q8-12h
• *Child:* **IV/IM** 90-120 mg/kg/day divided q6-8h

Severe systemic infections
• *Adult:* **IV/IM** 2 g q6-8h; do not exceed 8 g/day

Continue treatment for 48 hr after negative culture or until patient is asymptomatic

Available forms: Powder for inj 500 mg, 1, 2 g

Side effects/adverse reactions:

HEMA: Anemia, increased bleeding time, ***bone marrow depression, granulocytopenia***

GI: Nausea, vomiting, diarrhea, increased AST, ALT, abdominal pain, glossitis, colitis, ***pseudomembranous colitis***

CNS: Lethargy, hallucinations, anxiety, depression, twitching, ***coma, convulsions,*** malaise, fever (pediatric)

EENT: Tinnitus, diplopia, nasal congestion

GU: Vaginal candidiasis, vaginitis, breast tenderness, increased BUN, creatinine

INTEG: Rash (pediatric)

Contraindications: Hypersensitivity to this drug, penicillins, cephalosporins

Precautions: Pregnancy (B), lactation, children, impaired renal, hepatic function, elderly

Pharmacokinetics:

IV: Peak immediate, trough 8 hr
IM: Peak 1 hr

Half-life: 1.7 hr; half-life prolonged in renal disease; protein binding 56%; metabolized by liver; excreted in urine 60%-70%; small amounts appear in breast milk, placenta

Interactions:

• Synergistic effect: other antiinfectives, β-lactamase antibiotics, aminoglycosides

• Antagonist effect: Cefoxitin, imipenem

• Increased aztreonam level: Probenecid

• Incompatible with nafcillin, metronidazole, cephradine

Lab test interferences:

Interfere: Urine glucose using Clinitest/Benedict's reagent

False positive: Coombs' test

◆ = Nursing alert   🖉 = Herb-drug interaction   🚫 = Do not crush

Increase: ALT, AST, alk phosphatase, PT, PTT

NURSING CONSIDERATIONS

Assess:

• Signs of bruising, bleeding, anemia

• Bowel pattern before, during treatment

• I&O ratio; report hematuria, oliguria, since this drug in high doses is nephrotoxic

◆ Any patient with compromised renal system, since drug is excreted slowly in poor renal system function; toxicity may occur rapidly

• Liver function studies: AST, ALT

• Blood studies: WBC, RBC, Hgb, Hct, bleeding time

• Renal studies: urinalysis, protein, blood, serum creatinine, BUN

• Skin eruptions after administration of drug to 1 wk after discontinuing drug

• Allergies before initiation of treatment, reaction of medication; highlight allergies on chart

• Give drug after C&S completed

Administer:

IM

• Dilute each g with at least 3 ml of 0.9% NaCl; give into large muscle

IV, direct

• After diluting with 6-10 ml sterile H_2O/15-30 ml drug; give over 3-5 min

IV inf

• After diluting with 3 ml or more sterile H_2O/1 g drug; then dilute with 50-100 ml of D_5W, 0.9% NaCl, LR, D_5, D_{10} solution; give over ½-1 hr, by Y-tube or 3-way stopcock; flush tubing before and after administration

Additive compatibilities: Ampicillin/sulbactam, cefazolin, ciprofloxacin, clindamycin, gentamicin, tobramycin

Syringe compatibilities: Clindamycin

Y-site compatibilities: Allopurinol, amifostine, amikacin, aminophylline, ampicillin, ampicillin/sulbactam, bleomycin, bumetanide, buprenorphine, butorphanol, calcium gluconate, carboplatin, carmustine, cefazolin, cefepime, cefonicid, cefoperazone, cefotaxime, cefotetan, cefoxitin, ceftazidime, ceftizoxime, ceftriaxone, cefuroxime, cimetidine, ciprofloxacin, cisatracurium, cisplatin, clindamycin, cyclophosphamide, cytarabine, dacarbazine, dactinomycin, dexamethasone, diltiazem, diphenhydramine, dobutamine, dopamine, doxorubicin, doxorubicin liposome, doxycycline, droperidol, enalaprilat, etoposide, famotidine, filgrastim, floxuridine, fluconazole, fludarabine, fluorouracil, foscarnet, furosemide, gallium, gentamicin, granisetron, haloperidol, heparin, hydrocortisone, hydromorphone, hydroxyzine, idarubicin, ifosfamide, imipenem-cilastatin, insulin (regular), leucovorin, magnesium sulfate, mannitol, mechlorethamine, melphalan, meperidine, mesna, methotrexate, methylprednisolone, metoclopramide, mezlocillin, minocycline, morphine, nalbuphine, netilmicin, ondansetron, piperacillin, piperacillin/tazobactam, plicamycin, potassium chloride, promethazine, propofol, ranitidine, remifentanil, sargramostim, sodium bicarbonate, teniposide, theophylline, thiotepa, ticarcillin, ticarcillin/clavulanate, tobramycin, trimethoprim-sulfamethoxazole, vinblastine, vincristine, vinorelbine, zidovudine

Perform/provide:

• Adequate fluid intake (2 L) during diarrhea episodes

• Storage in refrigerator for 1 wk; room temperature ≤48 hr, discard if precipitate forms

Evaluate:
• Therapeutic response: absence of fever, purulent drainage, redness, inflammation, temp
Teach patient/family:
• That culture may be taken after completed course of medication
• To report sore throat, fever, fatigue (may indicate superinfection)

RARELY USED

bacitracin (℞)
(bass-i-tray′sin)
BACI-IM, Baciquent, Bacitin*
Func. class.: Antiinfective, misc.

Uses:
Staphylococcal pneumonia, empyema
Dosage and routes:
• *Infant >2.5 kg:* **IM** 1000 U/kg/day in divided doses q8-12h
• *Infant ≤2.5 kg:* **IM** 900 U/kg/day in divided doses q8-12h
Contraindications: Hypersensitivity, severe renal disease (IM use)

---

baclofen (℞)
(bak′loe-fen)
Lioresal, Lioresal Intrathecal
Func. class.: Skeletal muscle relaxant, central acting
Chem. class.: GABA chlorophenyl derivative

Action: Inhibits synaptic responses in CNS by decreasing GABA, which decreases neurotransmitter function; decreases frequency, severity of muscle spasms
Uses: Spasticity in spinal cord injury, multiple sclerosis
Investigational uses: Pain in trigeminal neuralgia, hiccoughs
Dosage and routes:
• *Adult:* **PO** 5 mg tid × 3 days, then

10 mg tid × 3 days, then 15 mg tid × 3 days, then 20 mg tid × 3 days, then titrated to response, not to exceed 80 mg/day. **IT:** Use implantable intrathecal **INF** pump; use screening trial of 3 separate **BOL** doses if needed (50 μg/ml, 75 μg/1.5 ml, 100 μg/2 ml). Initial: double screening dose that produced result and give over 24 hr: increase by 10%-30% q24h only. Maintenance: 1200-1500 μg/day; **PO** 5-10 mg tid, taper before discontinuing drug
• *Child >2 yr:* **PO** 10-15 mg/kg/day divided q8h titrate to max 40 mg/day
• *Child ≥8 yr:* as above, max 60 mg/day
• *Child:* **IT** 25-1200 μg/day infusion, titrated to response in screening phase
Available forms: Tabs 10, 20 mg; intrathecal inj 10 mg/20 ml (500 μg/ml), 10 mg/5 ml (2000 μg/ml)
Side effects/adverse reactions:
CNS: Dizziness, weakness, fatigue, drowsiness, headache, *disorientation,* insomnia, paresthesias, tremors, **seizures**
EENT: Nasal congestion, blurred vision, mydriasis, tinnitus
CV: Hypotension, chest pain, palpitations, edema
GI: Nausea, constipation, *vomiting,* increased AST, alk phosphatase, abdominal pain, dry mouth, anorexia
GU: Urinary frequency
INTEG: Rash, pruritus
Contraindications: Hypersensitivity
Precautions: Peptic ulcer disease, renal disease, hepatic disease, stroke, seizure disorder, diabetes mellitus, pregnancy (C), lactation, elderly
Do not confuse:
Lioresal/Lotensin
Pharmacokinetics:
PO: Peak 2-3 hr, duration >8 hr, half-life 2½-4 hr, partially metab-

---

⬦ = Nursing alert   🍃 = Herb-drug interaction   🚫 = Do not crush olized in liver, excreted in urine (unchanged)

INTRATHECAL: CSF levels with plasma levels 100 times oral route; onset ½-1 hr, peak 4 hr, duration 4-8 hr

Interactions:

• Increased CNS depression: alcohol, tricyclics, opiates, barbiturates, sedatives, hypnotics, MAOIs

🌢 May increase CNS depression: kava

Lab test interferences:

Increase: AST, alk phosphatase, blood glucose

NURSING CONSIDERATIONS
Assess:

• B/P, weight, blood sugar, and hepatic function periodically

◆ For increased seizure activity in epilepsy patient; this drug decreases seizure threshold

• I&O ratio; check for urinary frequency

• EEG in epileptic patients; poor seizure control has occurred in patients taking this drug

• Allergic reactions: rash, fever, respiratory distress

• Severe weakness, numbness in extremities

• Tolerance: increased need for medication, more frequent requests for medication, increased pain

• CNS depression: dizziness, drowsiness, psychiatric symptoms

Administer:
PO

• With meals for GI symptoms
IT

• Dosage, as individual titration is required

• Do not use IT inj IV, IM, SC, epidural

Additive compatibilities: Morphine

Perform/provide:

• Storage in tight container at room temperature

• Assistance with ambulation if dizziness or drowsiness occurs

Evaluate:

• Therapeutic response: decreased pain, spasticity

Teach patient/family:

• Not to discontinue medication quickly; hallucinations, spasticity, tachycardia will occur; drug should be tapered off over 1-2 wk

• Not to take with alcohol, other CNS depressants

• To avoid hazardous activities if drowsiness or dizziness occurs

• To avoid using OTC medication: cough preparations, antihistamines, unless directed by prescriber

Treatment of overdose: Induce emesis of conscious patient, lavage, dialysis

---

balsalazide (R)

(ball-sal′a-zide)
Colazal
Func. class.: Antiinflammatory
Chem. class.: Salicylate derivative

Action: Delivered intact to the colon, bioconverted to 4-aminobenzoyl-β-alanine

Uses: Active, mild to moderate ulcerative colitis

Dosage and routes:

• *Adult:* **PO** 750 mg tid × 8 wk, may take up to 12 wk

Available forms: Tabs 750 mg

Side effects/adverse reactions:

EENT: Dry eyes, rhinitis, sinusitis, watery eyes, blurred vision

*SYST: **Anaphylaxis***

GI: Nausea, vomiting, abdominal pain, diarrhea, rectal bleeding, flatulence, dyspepsia, dry mouth, constipation

CNS: Headache, insomnia, fatigue, fever, dizziness

MS: Arthralgia, back pain, myalgia

Contraindications: Hypersensitivity to salicylates

Precautions: Pregnancy (B), child <14 yr, lactation; pyloric stenosis

Pharmacokinetics:

PO: Low and variably absorbed, peak 1½ hr, excreted in urine as metabolites, plasma protein binding 99%

Lab test interferences:

False positive: Urinary glucose test

NURSING CONSIDERATIONS

Assess:

• Kidney function studies: BUN, creatinine, urinalysis (long-term therapy)

• Allergic reaction: rash, dermatitis, urticaria, pruritus, dyspnea, bronchospasm

Administer:

• With food in evenly divided doses

• With resuscitative equipment available; severe allergic reactions may occur

• Total daily dose evenly spaced to minimize GI intolerance

Perform/provide:

• Storage in tight, light-resistant container at room temperature

Evaluate:

• Therapeutic response: absence of fever, mucus in stools, resolution of symptoms of ulcerative colitis

---

basiliximab (Rx)

(bas-ih-liks'ih-mab)

Simulect

Func. class.: Immunosuppressive

Chem. class.: Murine/human monoclonal antibody (Interleukin-2) receptor antagonist

Action: Binds to and blocks the IL-2 receptor, which is selectively expressed on the surface of activated T-lymphocytes; impairs the immune system to antigenic challenges

Uses: Acute allograft rejection in renal transplant patients when used with cyclosporine and corticosteroids

Dosage and routes:

• *Adult:* **IV** 20 mg × 2 doses; 1st dose within 2 hr before transplant surgery; 2nd dose given 4 days after transplantation

• *Child 2-15 yr:* **IV** 12 mg/m^2 × 2 doses; 1st dose within 2 hr before transplant surgery; 2nd dose given 4 days after transplantation

Available forms: Powder for inj 20 mg

Side effects/adverse reactions:

INTEG: Acne

CNS: Pyrexia, chills, tremors, headache, insomnia, weakness

META: Acidosis, hypercholesterolemia, hyperuricemia, hyperkalemia, hypocalcemia, hypokalemia, hypophosphatemia

RESP: Dyspnea, wheezing, **pulmonary edema,** cough

CV: Chest pain, angina, **cardiac failure,** hypotension, *hypertension, edema*

MS: Arthralgia, myalgia

GI: Vomiting, nausea, diarrhea, constipation, abdominal pain, **GI bleeding,** gingival hyperplasia, stomatitis

MISC: Infection, moniliasis

Contraindications: Hypersensitivity

Precautions: Pregnancy (B), infections, elderly, lactation, children

Pharmacokinetics:

Peak ½ hr (adults) terminal half-life 7 days (adult), 9½ days (children)

NURSING CONSIDERATIONS

Assess:

• For infection: increased temp, WBC, sputum, urine

• Blood studies: Hgb, WBC, plate-

◆ = Nursing alert   ⫽ = Herb-drug interaction   ⊘ = Do not crush

lets during treatment qmo; if leukocytes are <3000/mm^3, drug should be discontinued
• Liver function studies: alk phosphatase, AST, ALT, bilirubin
• Hepatotoxicity: dark urine, jaundice, itching, light-colored stools; drug should be discontinued
Administer:
• All medications PO if possible; avoid IM injection, since infection may occur
IV
• After adding 5 ml sterile water for inj, shake gently to dissolve, reconstitute to a vol of 50 ml with 0.9% NaCl or D$_5$, gently invert bag, do not shake, give over ½ hr, do not admix
Evaluate:
• Therapeutic response: absence of graft rejection
Teach patient/family:
• To report fever, chills, sore throat, fatigue, since serious infection may occur
• To avoid crowds, persons with known upper respiratory infections
• To use contraception during treatment

---

beclomethasone (℞)

(be-kloe-meth'a-sone)
Beclodisk*, Becloforte Inhaler*, Beclovent, Beclovent Rotocaps*, Qvar, Vanceril
Func. class.: Corticosteroid, synthetic
Chem. class.: Glucocorticoid

Action: Prevents inflammation by depression of migration of polymorphonuclear leukocytes, fibroblasts, reversal of increased capillary permeability and lysosomal stabilization; does not suppress hypothalamus and pituitary function

Uses: Chronic asthma, rhinitis
Dosage and routes:
• *Adult:* **INH** 2-4 puffs tid-qid, not to exceed 20 inhalations/day (42 μg/actuation); 2 puffs bid, max 10 INH/day (84 μg/actuation)
• *Child: 6-12 yr:* **INH** 1-2 puffs tid-qid, not to exceed 10 inhalations/day (42 μg/actuations); 2 puffs bid, max 5 INH/day (84 μg/actuations)
Available forms: Aerosol 42, 50, 84, 250 μg/actuation; INH cap 100, 200 μg
Side effects/adverse reactions:
CNS: Headache
EENT: Hoarseness, candidal infections of oral cavity, sore throat
GI: Dry mouth, dyspepsia
*MISC: **Angioedema, adrenal insufficiency,** facial edema*
*RESP: **Bronchospasm,** wheezing, cough*
Contraindications: Hypersensitivity, status asthmaticus (primary treatment), nonasthmatic bronchial disease; bacterial, fungal, viral infections of mouth, throat, lungs; children <12 yr
Precautions: Nasal disease/surgery, pregnancy (C), lactation
Pharmacokinetics:
INH: Onset 10 min, excreted in feces, urine (metabolites), half-life 2.8 hr, crosses placenta, metabolized in lungs, liver (by CYP3A), GI system
NURSING CONSIDERATIONS
Assess:
• For fungal infection in mucous membranes
• Adrenal function periodically for HPA axis suppression during prolonged therapy, monitor growth/development
Administer:
• INH with water to decrease possibility of fungal infections
• Titrated dose, use lowest effective dose

Perform/provide:
• Gum, rinsing of mouth for dry mouth

Evaluate:
• Therapeutic response: decreased dyspnea, wheezing, dry rales on auscultation

Teach patient/family:
• To carry or wear ID as steroid user
• To gargle/rinse mouth after each use to prevent oral fungal infections
• That in times of stress, systemic corticosteroids may be needed to prevent adrenal insufficiency; do not discontinue oral drug abruptly, taper slowly
• To notify prescriber if therapeutic response decreases; dosage adjustment may be needed
• Proper administration technique
• To wash inhaler with warm water and dry after each use
• All aspects of drug usage, including cushingoid symptoms
• The symptoms of adrenal insufficiency: nausea, anorexia, fatigue, dizziness, dyspnea, weakness, joint pain, depression

---

benazepril (℞)
(ben-aze'uh-pril)
Lotensin

Func. class.: Antihypertensive
Chem. class.: Angiotensin-converting enzyme (ACE) inhibitor

Action: Selectively suppresses renin-angiotensin-aldosterone system; inhibits ACE, preventing conversion of angiotensin I to angiotensin II

Uses: Hypertension, alone or in combination with thiazide diuretics

Dosage and routes:
• *Adult:* **PO** 10 mg qd initially, then 20-40 mg/day divided bid or qd (without a diuretic); 5 mg **PO** qd (with a diuretic)
• *Renal dose:* CrCl <30 ml/min 5 mg **PO** qd, max 40 mg/day
• *Geriatric:* **PO** 5-10 mg/day initially

Available forms: Tabs 5, 10, (20,) 40 mg

Side effects/adverse reactions:
CV: Hypotension, postural hypotension, syncope, palpitations, angina
GU: Increased BUN, creatinine, decreased libido, impotence, urinary tract infection
HEMA: **Neutropenia, agranulocytosis**
INTEG: Rash, flushing, sweating
RESP: Cough, asthma, bronchitis, dyspnea, sinusitis
META: Hyperkalemia, hyponatremia
GI: Nausea, constipation, vomiting, gastritis, melena
CNS: Anxiety, hypertonia, insomnia, paresthesia, headache, dizziness, fatigue
MS: Arthralgia, arthritis, myalgia
MISC: **Angioedema**

Contraindications: Hypersensitivity to ACE inhibitors, pregnancy (D) 2nd/3rd trimester, lactation, children

Precautions: Impaired renal, liver function, dialysis patients, hypovolemia, blood dyscrasias, CHF, COPD, asthma, elderly, bilateral renal artery stenosis, pregnancy (C) 1st trimester

Do not confuse:
Lotensin/Lioresal
Lotensin/Loniten

Pharmacokinetics:
PO: Peak ½-1 hr, serum protein binding 97%, half-life 10-11 hr, metabolized by liver (metabolites), excreted in urine

Interactions:
• Increased hypotension, phenothi-

◆ = Nursing alert   ✒ = Herb-drug interaction   ⊘ = Do not crush

azines, nitrates, acute alcohol ingestion: diuretics, other antihypertensives

• Increased hyperkalemia: potassium-sparing diuretics, potassium supplements

• Increased serum levels of lithium, digoxin

Lab test interferences:

Increase: AST, ALT, alk phosphatase, bilirubin, uric acid, blood glucose

Drug/food: Decreased perindopril to perindoprilat conversion

False positive: ANA titer

NURSING CONSIDERATIONS

Assess:

• Blood studies: neutrophils, decreased platelets; WBC with diff baseline and q3mo, if neutrophils <1000/mm³ discontinue treatment

• B/P at peak/trough level of drug, orthostatic hypotension, syncope when used with diuretic

• Renal studies: protein, BUN, creatinine; increased levels may indicate nephrotic syndrome; monitor urine for protein, increased LFTs, uric acid and glucose may be increased

• Potassium levels, although hyperkalemia rarely occurs

• Allergic reactions: rash, fever, pruritus, urticaria; drug should be discontinued if antihistamines fail to help

• Renal symptoms: polyuria, oliguria, frequency, dysuria

• Edema in feet, legs qd, weight qd in CHF

Perform/provide:

• Storage in tight container at 86° F (30° C) or less

Evaluate:

• Therapeutic response: decrease in B/P

Teach patient/family:

• Not to discontinue drug abruptly

• Not to use OTC products (cough, cold, allergy) unless directed by prescriber; do not use salt substitutes containing potassium without consulting prescriber

• The importance of complying with dosage schedule, even if feeling better

• To notify prescriber of pregnancy, drug will need to be discontinued

• To rise slowly to sitting or standing position to minimize orthostatic hypotension

• To notify prescriber of mouth sores, sore throat, fever, swelling of hands or feet, irregular heartbeat, chest pain

• To report excessive perspiration, dehydration, vomiting, diarrhea; may lead to fall in B/P

• That drug may cause dizziness, fainting, light-headedness; may occur during first few days of therapy

• That drug may cause skin rash or impaired perspiration

• How to take B/P, and normal readings for age group

Treatment of overdose: 0.9% NaCl IV INF, hemodialysis

RARELY USED

benzonatate (℞)

(ben-zoe′na-tate)
Tessalon Perles
Func. class.: Antitussive, nonnarcotic

Uses: Nonproductive cough

Dosage and routes:

• *Adult and child:* **PO** 100 mg tid, not to exceed 600 mg/day; *Child <10 yr:* **PO** 8 mg/kg in 3-6 divided doses

Contraindications: Hypersensitivity

RARELY USED

benzoyl peroxide (OTC)
(ben'zoe-ill per-ox'ide)
Func. class.: Antiacne medication

Uses: Mild to moderate acne
Dosage and routes:
• *Adult and child:* **TOP** apply to affected area qd or bid
Contraindications: Hypersensitivity to benzoic acid derivatives

---

RARELY USED

benzquinamide (℞)
(benz-kwin'a-mide)
Emete-Con
Func. class.: Antiemetic

Uses: To inhibit nausea, vomiting associated with anesthetic, surgery
Dosage and routes:
• *Adult:* **IM** 50 mg or 0.5-1 mg/kg, may be repeated in 1 hr, then q3-4h prn; **IV** 25 mg or 0.2-0.4 mg/kg as a one-time dose
Contraindications: Hypersensitivity, hypertension

---

benztropine (℞)
(benz'troe-peen)
Apo-Benztropin*,
benztropine mesylate,
Cogentin
Func. class.: Cholinergic blocker, antiparkinson agent
Chem. class.: Tertiary amine

Action: Blockade of central acetylcholine receptors
Uses: Parkinson symptoms, EPS associated with neuroleptic drugs, acute dystonic reactions

Dosage and routes:
Drug-induced EPS
• *Adult:* **IM/IV** 1-4 mg qd-bid; give **PO** dose as soon as possible; **PO** 1-2 mg bid/tid, increase by 0.5 mg q5-6 days
• *Child:* **IM/IV** 0.02-0.05 mg/kg/dose 1-2 ×/day
• *Geriatric:* **PO** 0.5 mg qd-bid, increase by 0.5 mg q5-6d
Parkinson symptoms
• *Adult:* **PO** 1-2 mg/day in 1-2 divided doses, increase 0.5 mg q5-6d titrated to patient response, max 6 mg qd
Acute dystonic reactions
• *Adult:* **IM/IV** 1-2 mg, may increase to 1-2 mg bid (PO)
Available forms: Tabs 0.5, 1, 2 mg; inj 1 mg/ml
Side effects/adverse reactions:
MS: Muscular weakness, cramping
INTEG: Rash, urticaria, dermatoses
MISC: Increased temperature, flushing, decreased sweating, hyperthermia, heat stroke, numbness of fingers
CNS: Anxiety, restlessness, irritability, delusions, hallucinations, headache, sedation, depression, incoherence, dizziness, memory loss; confusion, delirium (elderly)
EENT: Blurred vision, photophobia, dilated pupils, difficulty swallowing, dry eyes, mydriasis, increased intraocular tension, angle-closure glaucoma
CV: Palpitations, tachycardia, hypotension, bradycardia
GI: Dryness of mouth, constipation, nausea, vomiting, abdominal distress, *paralytic ileus,* epigastric distress
GU: Hesitancy, retention, dysuria
Contraindications: Hypersensitivity, narrow-angle glaucoma, myasthenia gravis, GI/GU obstruction, child <3 yr, peptic ulcer, megacolon, prostate hypertrophy

---

◆ = Nursing alert   ∅ = Herb-drug interaction   ⊘ = Do not crush

Precautions: Pregnancy (C), elderly, lactation, tachycardia, liver, kidney disease, drug abuse history, dysrhythmias, hypotension, hypertension, psychiatric patients, children

Pharmacokinetics:

IM/IV: Onset 15 min, duration 6-10 hr
PO: Onset 1 hr, duration 6-10 hr

Interactions:

• Increased anticholinergic effect: antihistamines, phenothiazines, tricyclics, disopyramide, quinidine

• Decreased absorption: antidiarrheals

NURSING CONSIDERATIONS
Assess:

• I&O ratio; commonly causes decreased urinary output; urinary hesitancy, retention; palpate bladder if retention occurs

• Parkinsonism, EPS: shuffling gait, muscle rigidity, involuntary movements, loss of balance

• Constipation; increase fluids, bulk, exercise if this occurs

• Mental status: affect, mood, CNS depression, worsening of mental symptoms during early therapy

• Use caution in hot weather; drug may increase susceptibility to stroke by decreasing sweating

• For benztropine "buzz" or "high," patients may imitate EPS

Administer:
PO

• With or after meals to prevent GI upset; may give with fluids other than water

• At hs to avoid daytime drowsiness in patient with parkinsonism

IM

• Use for dystonic reactions only

IV

• Undiluted IV (1 mg = 1 ml) give 1 mg/1 min; keep in bed for at least 1 hr after dose

Syringe compatibilities: Chlorpromazine, fluphenazine, metoclopramide, perphenazine, thiothixene

Y-site compatibilities: Fluconazole, tacrolimus

Perform/provide:

• Storage at room temperature

• Hard candy, gum, frequent drinks, to relieve dry mouth

Evaluate:

• Therapeutic response: absence of involuntary movements

Teach patient/family:

• That tabs may be crushed and mixed with food

• Not to discontinue this drug abruptly; to taper off over 1 wk, or withdrawal symptoms may occur (EPS, tremors, insomia, tachycardia, restlessness)

• To avoid driving, other hazardous activities; drowsiness may occur

• To avoid OTC medication: cough, cold preparations with alcohol, antihistamines unless directed by prescriber

• To change positions slowly to prevent orthostatic hypotension

• To use good oral hygiene, frequent sips of water, sugarless gum for dry mouth

---

bepridil (℞)

(be'pri-dil)
Bepadin, Vascor
Func. class.: Calcium channel blocker, antianginal

Action: Inhibits calcium ion influx across cell membrane during cardiac depolarization; produces relaxation of coronary vascular smooth muscle, dilates coronary arteries, decreases SA/AV node conduction, dilates peripheral arteries

Uses: Chronic stable angina, used alone or in combination with propranolol

---

Dosage and routes:
Angina
• *Adult:* **PO** 200 mg qd, after 10 days may increase dose if needed, max dose 400 mg/day
Available forms: Tabs, film-coated, 200, 300, 400 mg

Side effects/adverse reactions:
*CV: **Dysrhythmia**,* edema, ***CHF***, bradycardia, hypotension, palpitations, AV block, ***torsades de pointes***
GI: Nausea, vomiting, diarrhea, gastric upset, constipation, increased liver function studies
GU: Nocturia, polyuria
CNS: Headache, fatigue, drowsiness, dizziness, anxiety, depression, weakness, insomnia, confusion, light-headedness, nervousness
*HEMA: **Agranulocytosis***

Contraindications: Sick sinus syndrome, 2nd- or 3rd-degree heart block, Wolff-Parkinson-White syndrome, hypotension less than 90 mm Hg systolic, cardiogenic shock, history of serious ventricular dysrhythmias

Precautions: CHF, hypotension, hepatic injury, pregnancy (C), lactation, children, renal disease, idiopathic hypertropic subaortic stenosis (IHSS), concomitant β-blocker therapy

Do not confuse:
bepridil/Prepidil

Pharmacokinetics: Onset 1 hr, peak 2-3 hr, duration 24 hr, 99% plasma protein bound, half-life 42 hr; completely metabolized in the liver and excreted in urine and feces

Interactions:
• Increased prolongation of QT, depression of AV node: cardiac glycosides, antidysrhythmics
• Increased hypotension: fentanyl
• Increased levels of digoxin
🌿 Increased antianginal effect: cat's claw, chicory

🌿 Increased hypotensive effects: grapefruit juice

Lab test interferences:
Increase: Liver function tests, aminotransferase, CPK, LDH

NURSING CONSIDERATIONS
Assess:
• Cardiac status: B/P, pulse, respiration, ECG intervals (PR, QRS, QT), dysrhythmias; may increase QT interval, altered T wave
• I&O ratios, weight qd, monitor for CHF: weight gain, jugular vein distention, edema, rales/crackles, dyspnea, restlessness

Administer:
PO
• Before meals, hs; adjust no more frequently than q10 days; may give with food/fluids to decrease GI upset

Evaluate:
• Therapeutic response: decreased anginal pain, increased activity tolerance

Teach patient/family:
• How to take pulse before taking drug; record or graph should be kept; use demonstration, return demonstration
• To avoid hazardous activities until stabilized on drug, dizziness no longer a problem
• To limit caffeine consumption
🚫 Not to break, crush, or chew tabs
• To avoid OTC drugs unless directed by a prescriber
• The importance of compliance with all areas of medical regimen: diet, exercise, stress reduction, drug therapy
• To notify prescriber of swelling, weight gain, dyspnea, irregular heart beat
• To maintain good oral hygiene to prevent gingival hyperplasia

◆ = Nursing alert   🌿 = Herb-drug interaction   🚫 = Do not crush

Treatment of overdose: Defibrillation, atropine for AV block, vasopressor for hypotension

---

RARELY USED

beractant (R)

(ber-ak'tant)
Survanta
Func. class.: Natural lung surfactant

Uses: Prevention and treatment (rescue) of respiratory distress syndrome in premature infants
Dosage and routes:
• **INTRATRACHEAL INSTILL:** 4 doses can be administered in the 1st 48 hrs of life; give doses no more frequently than q6h; each dose is 100 mg of phospholipids/kg birth weight (4 ml/kg)

---

betamethasone (R)

(bay-ta-meth'a-sone)
Betnelan*, Betnesol*,
Celestone, Selestoject*
Func. class.: Corticosteroid, synthetic, long-acting

Action: Decreases inflammation by suppressing migration of polymorphonuclear leukocytes, fibroblasts, reversal of increased capillary permeability and lysosomal stabilization
Uses: Immunosuppression, severe inflammation, prevention of neonatal respiratory distress syndrome (by administration to mother)
Dosage and routes:
• *Adult:* **PO** 0.6-7.2 mg qd; **IM/IV** 0.6-7.2 mg qd in joint or soft tissue (sodium phosphate)
• *Child:* **PO** 17.5 µg/kg/day in 3 divided doses; **IM** 17.5 µg/kg/day in 3 divided doses every 3rd day or

5.8-8.75 µg/kg/day as a single dose (adrenal insufficiency)
• *Child:* **PO** 62.5-250 µg/kg/day in 3 divided doses; **IM** 20.8-125 µg/kg/day of the base q12-24h (other uses)
Available forms: Betamethasone: tabs 500; 600 µg, tabs, effervescent 500 µg*, syr 600 µg/5 ml; ext rel tab 1 mg; sol for inj (phosphate) 3 mg/ml; susp for inj (phosphate/acetate) 6 mg/ml
Side effects/adverse reactions:
INTEG: Acne, poor wound healing, ecchymosis, bruising, petechiae
CNS: Depression, flushing, sweating, headache, ecchymosis, bruising, mood changes
*CV: Hypertension, **circulatory collapse, thrombophlebitis, embolism,** tachycardia, **necrotizing angiitis, CHF***
*HEMA: **Thrombocytopenia***
MS: Fractures, osteoporosis, weakness
*GI: Diarrhea, nausea, abdominal distention, **GI hemorrhage,** increased appetite, **pancreatitis***
EENT: Fungal infections, increased intraocular pressure, blurred vision
Contraindications: Psychosis, hypersensitivity, idiopathic thrombocytopenia, acute glomerulonephritis, amebiasis, fungal infections, nonasthmatic bronchial disease, child <2 yr, AIDS, TB
Precautions: Pregnancy (C), lactation, diabetes mellitus, glaucoma, osteoporosis, seizure disorders, ulcerative colitis, CHF, myasthenia gravis, renal disease, esophagitis, peptic ulcer
Pharmacokinetics:
PO: Onset 1-2 hr, peak 1 hr, duration 3 days
IM/IV: Onset 10 min, peak 4-8 hr, duration 1-1½ days
Metabolized in liver, excreted in urine as steroids, crosses placenta

---

Interactions:

• Decreased action of betamethasone: barbiturates, rifampin, phenytoin

• Decreased effects of anticoagulants, antidiabetics, insulin, isoniazid, toxoids, vaccines, salicylates

• GI bleeding: NSAIDs, alcohol, salicylates, indomethacin

🍃 Potassium deficiency: chronic use/abuse of cascara sagrada bark, buckthorn bark/berry, rhubarb root, senna leaf/fruits, aloe

🍃 Increased action/side effects: squill, lily of the valley, pheasant's eye

Lab test interferences:

Increase: Cholesterol, sodium, blood glucose, uric acid, calcium, urine glucose

Decrease: Calcium, potassium, T_4, T_3, thyroid ^{131}I uptake test, urine 17-OHCS, 17-KS, PBI

False negative: Skin allergy tests

NURSING CONSIDERATIONS

Assess:

• Potassium, blood sugar, urine glucose while on long-term therapy; hypokalemia and hyperglycemia

• Weight daily; notify prescriber of weekly gain >5 lb

• B/P q4h, pulse; notify prescriber if chest pain occurs

• I&O ratio; be alert for decreasing urinary output and increasing edema

• Plasma cortisol levels during long-term therapy (normal level: 138-635 nmol/L SI units when drawn at 8 AM)

Administer:

PO

• With food or milk to decrease GI symptoms

IM

• Inject deeply in large muscle mass, rotate sites, avoid deltoid, use 21G needle

• In one dose in AM to prevent adrenal suppression, avoid SC administration; may damage tissue

IV

• Only sodium phosphate product; give >1 min; may be given by IV INF in compatible sol

• After shaking suspension (parenteral)

• Titrated dose; use lowest effective dose

Y-site compatibilities: Heparin, hydrocortisone, potassium chloride, vit B/C

Perform/provide:

• Assistance with ambulation in patient with bone tissue disease to prevent fractures

Evaluate:

• Therapeutic response: ease of respirations, decreased inflammation

• Infection: increased temperature, WBC even after withdrawal of medication; drug masks infection symptoms

• Potassium depletion: paresthesias, fatigue, nausea, vomiting, depression, polyuria, dysrhythmias, weakness

• Edema, hypertension, cardiac symptoms

• Mental status: affect, mood, behavioral changes, aggression

Teach patient/family:

• That ID as steroid user should be carried

• To notify prescriber if therapeutic response decreases; dosage adjustment may be needed

◆ Not to discontinue abruptly; adrenal crisis can result

• To avoid OTC products: salicylates, alcohol in cough products, cold preparations unless directed by prescriber

• All aspects of drug usage including cushingoid symptoms

• The symptoms of adrenal insufficiency: nausea, anorexia, fatigue,

◆ = Nursing alert   🍃 = Herb-drug interaction   🚫 = Do not crush

dizziness, dyspnea, weakness, joint pain

bethanechol (R)

(be-than'e-kole)
bethanechol chloride,
Duvoid, Urebeth, Urecholine
Func. class.: Cholinergic agonist

Chem. class.: Synthetic choline ester

Action: Stimulates muscarinic Ach receptors directly; mimics effects of parasympathetic nervous system stimulation; stimulates gastric motility, stimulates micturition; increases lower esophageal sphincter pressure

Uses: Urinary retention (postoperative, postpartum), neurogenic atony of bladder with retention

Dosage and routes:
• *Adult:* **PO** 25-50 mg bid-qid; **SC** 5 mg tid-qid prn
• *Child:* **PO** 0.6 mg/kg/day divided in 3-4 doses/day; SC 0.06 mg/kg tid or 0.15 mg/kg qid
Test dose
• *Adult:* SC 2.5 mg repeated 15-30 min intervals × 4 doses to determine effective dose
Available forms: Tabs 5, 10, 25, 50 mg; inj 5 mg/ml

Side effects/adverse reactions:
INTEG: Rash, urticaria, flushing, increased sweating
CNS: Dizziness
GI: Nausea, bloody diarrhea, belching, vomiting, cramps, fecal incontinence
CV: Hypotension, bradycardia, orthostatic hypotension, reflex tachycardia, **cardiac arrest, circulatory collapse**
GU: Urgency

*RESP: **Acute asthma, dyspnea, bronchoconstriction***
EENT: Miosis, increased salivation, lacrimation, blurred vision
Contraindications: Hypersensitivity, severe bradycardia, asthma, severe hypotension, hyperthyroidism, peptic ulcer, parkinsonism, seizure disorders, CAD, COPD, coronary occlusion, mechanical obstruction, peritonitis, recent urinary or GI surgery
Precautions: Hypertension, pregnancy (C), lactation, child <8 yr
Pharmacokinetics:
PO: Onset 30-90 min, duration 1-6 hr
SC: Onset 5-15 min, duration 2 hr, excreted by kidneys
Interactions:
• Increased action or toxicity: cholinergic agonists, anticholinesterase agents
• Severe hypotension: ganglionic blockers
Lab test interferences:
Increase: AST, lipase/amylase, bilirubin, BSP

NURSING CONSIDERATIONS
Assess:
• B/P, pulse; observe after parenteral dose for 1 hr
• I&O ratio; check for urinary retention or urge incontinence
• Bradycardia, hypotension, bronchospasm, headache, dizziness, convulsions, respiratory depression; drug should be discontinued if toxicity occurs
Administer:
• To avoid nausea and vomiting, take on an empty stomach
SC
◆ Parenteral dose by SC route; use of IM, IV may result in cardiac arrest
◆ Only with atropine sulfate available for cholinergic crisis
• Only after all other cholinergics have been discontinued

• Increased doses if tolerance occurs

Perform/provide:
• Storage at room temperature
• Bedpan/urinal if given for urinary retention
• Use of rectal tube if ordered, to increase passage of gas when used for abdominal distention

Evaluate:
• Therapeutic response: absence of urinary retention, abdominal distention

Teach patient/family:
• To take drug exactly as prescribed; 1 hr ac or 2 hr pc
• To make position changes slowly; orthostatic hypotension may occur

Treatment of overdose: Administer atropine 0.6-1.2 mg IV or IM (adult)

---

bexarotene (R)
Targretin
Func. class.: Retinoid, 2nd generation

Action: Selectively binds and activates retinoid X receptors (RXRs) that are partially responsible for cellular proliferation and differentiation. Inhibits some tumor cells

Uses: Cutaneous T-cell lymphoma

Investigational uses: Breast cancer

Research note: Bexarotene has been proven effective and safe for refractory advanced-stage cutaneous T-cell lymphoma[3]

Dosage and routes:
• *Adult:* **PO** 300 mg/day/m^2, may increase to 400 mg/day with proper monitoring

Available forms: Cap 75 mg

Side effects/adverse reactions:
CNS: Headache, fatigue, lethargy
GI: Nausea, abdominal pain, diarrhea, **acute pancreatitis**
INTEG: Rash, asthenia, dry skin

HEMA: **Leukopenia, neutropenia,** anemia
SYST: Infection, hypothyroidism

Contraindications: Hypersensitivity to retinoids, pregnancy (X)

Precautions: Lactation, sunburn, hepatic, renal disease, children

Pharmacokinetics: Unknown

Interactions:
• Increased bexarotene levels: azole antiinfectives, grapefruit juice
• Decreased bexarotene levels: barbiturates, rifampins, phenytoin
• Limit intake of vit A ≤15,000 IU/day
• Decreased action of: tamoxifen, oral contraceptives
• Increased action of: antidiabetics

NURSING CONSIDERATIONS

Assess:
• Area of body involved, what helps or aggravates condition; cysts, dryness, itching
• Cholesterol, HDL, triglycerides may be elevated
• CBC for leukopenia, neutropenia, anemia

Administer:
• With food

Perform/provide:
• Storage at room temperature

Evaluate:
• Therapeutic response: decrease in size and number of lesions

Teach patient/family:
• To watch for hypoglycemia in diabetic patients on insulin
• To limit vit A intake to ≤15,000 IU/day to avoid toxicity
• To avoid sunlight, sunlamps, or use protective clothing, sunscreen
• To avoid pregnancy while taking this drug and ≥1 mo after discontinuing therapy

---

⬥ = Nursing alert   🖋 = Herb-drug interaction   🚫 = Do not crush

bicalutamide (℞)

(bye-kal-u′ta-mide)
Casodex
Func. class.: Antineoplastic hormone

Chem. class.: Nonsteroidal antiandrogen

Action: Binds to cytosol androgen in target tissue, which competitively inhibits the action to androgens
Uses: Prostate cancer in combination with luteinizing hormone–releasing hormone (LHRH) analog
Dosage and routes:
• *Adult:* **PO** 50 mg qd with LHRH
Available forms: Tabs 50 mg
Side effects/adverse reactions:
GI: Diarrhea, constipation, nausea, vomiting, increased liver enzymes, anorexia, dry mouth, melena, abdominal pain
CV: Hot flashes, hypertension, chest pain, ***CHF,*** edema
CNS: Dizziness, paresthesia, insomnia, anxiety, neuropathy, headache
INTEG: Rash, sweating, dry skin, pruritus, alopecia
GU: Nocturia, hematuria, UTI, impotence, gynecomastia, urinary incontinence, frequency, dysuria, retention, urgency, breast tenderness, decreased libido, *hot flashes*
MISC: Infection, anemia, dyspnea, bone pain, headache, asthenia, *back pain,* flulike symptoms
Contraindications: Hypersensitivity, pregnancy (X)
Precautions: Renal, hepatic disease, elderly, lactation
Pharmacokinetics: Well absorbed, metabolized by liver, excreted in urine, feces; half-life 5.8 days
Interactions:
• May displace anticoagulants from their binding sites

Lab test interferences:
Increase: AST, ALT, bilirubin, BUN, creatinine
Decrease: Hgb, WBC
NURSING CONSIDERATIONS
Assess:
• For diarrhea, constipation, nausea, vomiting
• For hot flashes, gynecomastia (assure patient that these are common side effects)
• Prostate specific antigen (PSA), liver function studies
Administer:
PO
• At same time each day, either AM or PM, with/without food
• With LHRH treatment; start at same time for both drugs
Evaluate:
• Therapeutic response: decreased tumor size, decreased spread of malignancy
Teach patient/family:
• To recognize, report signs of anemia, hepatoxicity, renal toxicity
• That hair may be lost, but is reversible after therapy is completed
• Not to use other products, unless approved by prescriber
• To report severe diarrhea
• To use contraception while taking this drug

biperiden (℞)

(bye-per′i-den)
Akineton
Func. class.: Cholinergic blocker

Action: Centrally acting competitive anticholinergic
Uses: Parkinson symptoms, EPS secondary to neuroleptic drug therapy
Dosage and routes:
Extrapyramidal symptoms
• *Adult:* **PO** 2 mg qd-tid; **IM/IV** 2

mg q30min, if needed, not to exceed 8 mg/24 hr
• *Child:* **IM** 40 μg/kg or 1.2 mg/m², may repeat q½h

Parkinson symptoms
• *Adult:* **PO** 2 mg tid-qid; max 16 mg/24 hr

Available forms: Tabs 2 mg; inj 5 mg/ml (lactate)

Side effects/adverse reactions:
CNS: Confusion, anxiety, restlessness, irritability, delusions, hallucinations, headache, sedation, depression, incoherence, dizziness, euphoria, tremors, memory loss
EENT: Blurred vision, photophobia, dilated pupils, difficulty swallowing, mydriasis, increased intraocular tension, angle-closure glaucoma
CV: Palpitations, tachycardia, postural hypotension, bradycardia
GI: Dryness of mouth, constipation, nausea, vomiting, abdominal distress, ***paralytic ileus***
GU: Hesitancy, retention, dysuria
INTEG: Rash, urticaria, dermatoses
MISC: Increased temp, flushing, decreased sweating, hyperthermia, ***heat stroke,*** numbness of fingers, weakness, cramping

Contraindications: Hypersensitivity, narrow-angle glaucoma, myasthenia gravis, GI/GU obstruction, megacolon, stenosing peptic ulcers, prostatic hypertrophy

Precautions: Pregnancy (C), elderly, lactation, tachycardia, dysrhythmias, liver or kidney disease, drug abuse, hypotension, hypertension, psychiatric patients, children <8 yr

Pharmacokinetics:
IM/IV: Onset 15 min, duration 6-10 hr
PO: Onset 1 hr, duration 6-10 hr

Interactions:
• Increased schizophrenic symptoms: haloperidol

• Increased anticholinergic effect: antihistamines, phenothiazines, amantadine, tricyclics, quinidine
• Decreased biperiden absorption: antacids, antidiarrheals
• Increased sedation: alcohol

NURSING CONSIDERATIONS
Assess:
• I&O ratio; retention commonly causes decreased urinary output
• Parkinsonism, EPS: shuffling gait, muscle rigidity, involuntary movements
• Patient response if anticholinergics are given
• Urinary hesitancy, retention; palpate bladder if retention occurs
• Constipation; increase fluids, bulk, exercise if this occurs
• For tolerance over long-term therapy; dose may have to be increased or changed
• Mental status: affect, mood, CNS depression, worsening of mental symptoms during early therapy

Administer:
PO
• With or after meals to prevent GI upset; may give with fluids other than water
• At hs to avoid daytime drowsiness in patients with parkinsonism
IM/IV
• With patient recumbent to prevent postural hypotension, give undiluted 2 mg or less over 1 min or more

Perform/provide:
• Storage at room temperature
• Hard candy, gum, frequent drinks to relieve dry mouth

Evaluate:
• Therapeutic response: absence of involuntary movements

Teach patient/family:
• To use caution in hot weather; drug may increase susceptibility to heat stroke, decreases sweating

---

◆ = Nursing alert   ⫽ = Herb-drug interaction   ⊘ = Do not crush

• Not to discontinue this drug abruptly; to taper off over 1 wk
• To avoid driving, other hazardous activities; drowsiness may occur
• To avoid OTC medication: cough, cold preparations with alcohol, antihistamines unless directed by prescriber

---

bisacodyl (℞, OTC)

(bis-a-koe′dill)
Bisac-Evac, Bisaco-Lax, Bisacolax*, Bisc-Evac, Bisco-Lax, Carter's Little Pills, Dacodyl, Deficol, Dulcagen, Dulcolax, Fleet Bisacodyl, Fleet Laxative, Laxit*, Therelax
Func. class.: Laxative, stimulant
Chem. class.: Diphenylmethane

Action: Acts directly on intestine by increasing motor activity; thought to irritate colonic intramural plexus

Uses: Short-term treatment of constipation, bowel or rectal preparation for surgery, examination

Dosage and routes:
• *Adult ≥12 yr:* **PO** 5-15 mg in PM or AM; may use up to 30 mg for bowel or rectal preparation; **RECT** 10 mg, single dose
• *Child >3 yr:* **PO** 5-10 mg as a single dose; **RECT** 10 mg as a single dose
• *Child <2 yr:* **RECT** 5 mg as a single dose

Available forms: Enteric-coated tabs 5 mg; supp 5, 10 mg; rect sol 10 mg/37 ml; enema 0.33 mg/ml, 10 mg/5 ml; powder for rectal sol/ 1.5 mg bisacodyl/2.5 g tannic acid

Side effects/adverse reactions:
CNS: Muscle weakness
GI: Nausea, vomiting, anorexia, cramps, diarrhea, rectal burning (suppositories)
META: Protein-losing enteropathy, alkalosis, hypokalemia, **tetany,** electrolyte, fluid imbalances

Contraindications: Hypersensitivity, rectal fissures, abdominal pain, nausea, vomiting, appendicitis, acute surgical abdomen, ulcerated hemorrhoids, acute hepatitis, fecal impaction, intestinal/biliary tract obstruction

Precautions: Pregnancy (C), lactation

Pharmacokinetics:
PO: Onset 6-10 hr
RECT: Onset 15-60 min
Metabolized by liver; excreted in urine, bile, feces, breast milk

Interactions:
• Gastric irritation: antacids, milk, H₂-blockers
⌀ Increased action/side effects: lily of the valley, pheasant's eye, squill

NURSING CONSIDERATIONS
Assess:
• Blood, urine electrolytes if drug is used often by patient
• I&O ratio to identify fluid loss
• Cause of constipation; identify whether fluids, bulk, or exercise missing from lifestyle
• Cramping, rectal bleeding, nausea, vomiting; if these symptoms occur, drug should be discontinued

Administer:
PO
• Alone only with water for better absorption; do not take within 1 hr of other drugs or within 1 hr of antacids, milk, or cimetidine
• In AM or PM

Evaluate:
• Therapeutic response: decrease in constipation

Teach patient/family:
🚫 To swallow tabs whole; do not break, crush, or chew tabs

• Not to use laxatives for long-term therapy; bowel tone will be lost
• That normal bowel movements do not always occur daily
• Not to use in presence of abdominal pain, nausea, vomiting
• To notify prescriber if constipation is unrelieved or if symptoms of electrolyte imbalance occur: muscle cramps, pain, weakness, dizziness

---

bismuth subsalicylate (OTC)

(bis'muth sub-sal-iss'uh-late)
Bismatrol, Bismatrol Extra Strength, Bismed, Pepto-Bismol, Pepto-Bismol Maximum Strength, Pink Bismuth, PMS-Bismuth Subsalicylate

Func. class.: Antidiarrheal
Chem. class.: Salicylate

Action: Inhibits prostaglandin synthesis responsible for GI hypermotility; stimulates absorption of fluid and electrolytes

Uses: Diarrhea (cause undetermined), prevention of diarrhea when traveling; may be included to treat *Helicobacter pylori*

Dosage and routes:
Antidiarrheal
• *Adult:* **PO** 524 mg q½h or 1048 mg q1h, max 4.2 mg/24 hr
• *Child 9-12 yr:* **PO** 262 mg q½-1hr, max 2.1 mg/24 hr
• *Child 6-9 yr:* **PO** 174.6 mg q½-1hr, max 1.4 mg/24 hr
• *Child 3-6 yr:* **PO** 88 mg q½-1hr, max 704 mg/24 hr

Available forms: Tabs 262 mg; chewable tabs 262, 300 mg; susp 262 mg/15 ml, 524 mg/15 ml

Side effects/adverse reactions:
HEMA: Increased bleeding time
GI: Increased fecal impaction (high doses), dark stools
CNS: Confusion, twitching
EENT: Hearing loss, tinnitus, metallic taste, blue gums, black tongue (chew tabs)

Contraindications: Child <3 yr, history of GI bleeding, renal disease
Precautions: Anticoagulant therapy, immobility
Pharmacokinetics:
PO: Onset 1 hr, peak 2 hr, duration 4 hr
Interactions:
• Possible salicylate toxicity: salicylates
• Increased effects of oral anticoagulants, oral antidiabetics
• Decreased absorption of: tetracycline
🌿 Increased absorption of bismuth: sarsaparilla root
Lab test interferences:
Interference: Radiographic studies of GI system

NURSING CONSIDERATIONS
Assess:
• Electrolytes (K, Na, Cl) if diarrhea is severe or continues long term; assess skin turgor
• Bowel pattern before drug therapy, after treatment
Administer:
PO
• Increased fluids to rehydrate the patient
• Shake liquid before using
Evaluate:
• Therapeutic response: decreased diarrhea or absence of diarrhea when traveling
Teach patient/family:
• To chew or dissolve in mouth; do not swallow whole; shake liquid before using
• To avoid other salicylates unless directed by prescriber; not to give to children, possibility of Reye's syndrome

---

◆ = Nursing alert   🌿 = Herb-drug interaction   ⊘ = Do not crush

• That stools may turn black; tongue may darken; impaction may occur in debilitated patients

• To stop use if symptoms do not improve within 2 days or become worse, or if diarrhea is accompanied by high fever

---

bisoprolol (℞)

(bis-oh'pro-lole)
Zebeta
Func. class.: Antihypertensive
Chem. class.: β₁-Blocker

Action: Preferentially and competitively blocks stimulation of β_1-adrenergic receptors within cardiac muscle (decreases rate of SA node discharge, increases recovery time), slows conduction of AV node, decreases heart rate, which decreases O_2 consumption in myocardium; decreases renin-aldosterone-angiotensin system; inhibits β_2-receptors in bronchial and vascular smooth muscle at high doses

Uses: Mild to moderate hypertension

Investigational uses: Angina pectoris, supraventricular tachycardia

Dosage and routes:

• *Adult:* **PO** 5 mg qd; may increase if necessary to 20 mg qd

Renal/hepatic dose: 2.5 mg **PO,** titrate upward

Available forms: Tabs 5, 10 mg

Side effects/adverse reactions:

MS: Joint pain, arthralgia

MISC: Facial swelling, weight gain, decreased exercise tolerance

CV: Ventricular dysrhythmias, profound hypotension, bradycardia, CHF, cold extremities, postural hypotension, *2nd- or 3rd-degree heart block*

CNS: Vertigo, headache, insomnia, fatigue, dizziness, mental changes, memory loss, hallucinations, depression, lethargy, drowsiness, strange dreams, catatonia, peripheral neuropathy

GI: Nausea, diarrhea, vomiting, *mesenteric arterial thrombosis,* ischemic colitis, flatulence, gastritis, gastric pain

INTEG: Rash, fever, alopecia, pruritus, sweating

HEMA: Agranulocytosis, thrombocytopenia, purpura, eosinophilia

EENT: Sore throat; dry, burning eyes

GU: Impotence, decreased libido

ENDO: Increased hypoglycemic response to insulin

RESP: Bronchospasm, dyspnea, wheezing, cough, nasal stuffiness

Contraindications: Hypersensitivity to β-blockers, cardiogenic shock, heart block (2nd, 3rd degree), sinus bradycardia, CHF, cardiac failure

Precautions: Major surgery, pregnancy (C), lactation, children, diabetes mellitus, renal or hepatic disease, thyroid disease, COPD, asthma, well-compensated heart failure, aortic or mitral valve disease, peripheral vascular disease, myasthenia gravis

Do not confuse:

Zebeta/Diabeta

Pharmacokinetics:

PO: Peak 2-4 hr; half-life 9-12 hr, 50% excreted unchanged in urine, protein binding 30%; metabolized in liver to inactive metabolites

Interactions:

• Decreased antihypertensive effect: NSAIDs

• Hypotension: reserpine, guanethidine

• Myocardial depression: calcium channel blockers

Lab test interferences:

Increase: AST and ALT

Interference: Glucose/insulin tolerance tests

NURSING CONSIDERATIONS
Assess:
• B/P during beginning treatment, periodically thereafter; pulse q4h: note rate, rhythm, quality
• Apical/radial pulse before administration; notify prescriber of any significant changes (pulse <50 bpm)
• Baselines in renal, liver function tests before therapy begins
• I&O, weight qd, watch for CHF: increased weight, jugular vein distention, dyspnea, rales, crackles
• Edema in feet, legs daily
• Skin turgor, dryness of mucous membranes for hydration status, especially elderly

Administer:
PO
• Drug ac, hs, tablet may be crushed or swallowed whole, may give without regard to meals
• Reduced dosage in renal and hepatic dysfunction

Perform/provide:
• Storage protected from light, moisture; place in cool environment

Evaluate:
• Therapeutic response: decreased B/P after 1-2 wk

Teach patient/family:
• Not to discontinue drug abruptly, may cause precipitate angina, evaluate noncompliance
• Not to use OTC products containing α-adrenergic stimulants (such as nasal decongestants, OTC cold preparations) unless directed by prescriber
• To report bradycardia, dizziness, confusion, depression, fever, cold extremities
• To take pulse at home; advise when to notify prescriber
• To avoid alcohol, smoking, sodium intake
• To comply with weight control, dietary adjustments, modified exercise program

• To carry Medic Alert ID to identify drug taking, allergies
• To avoid hazardous activities if dizziness is present
◆ To report symptoms of CHF: difficulty breathing, especially on exertion or when lying down, night cough, swelling of extremities

Treatment of overdose: Lavage, IV atropine for bradycardia, IV theophylline for bronchospasm; digitalis, O_2, diuretic for cardiac failure; hemodialysis, IV glucose for hypoglycemia; IV diazepam (or phenytoin) for seizures

---

RARELY USED

bitolterol (℞)
(bye-tole'ter-ole)
Tornalate
Func. class.: Bronchodilator, adrenergic β_2-agonist

Uses: Asthma, bronchospasm
Dosage and routes:
Inhaler
• *Adult and child >12 yr:* **INH** 2 puffs, wait 1-3 min before 3rd puff if needed, not to exceed 3 **INH** q6h or 2 **INH** q4h
Nebulization
• *Adult and child >12 yr:* **INH** 0.5 ml (1 mg) tid by intermittent flow or 1.25 mg tid by continuous flow, max 8 mg (intermittent), 14 mg (continuous)

Contraindications: Hypersensitivity to sympathomimetics

◆ = Nursing alert   ▨ = Herb-drug interaction   ⊘ = Do not crush

bivalirudin (R)

(bye-val-i-rue′din)

Angiomax

Func. class.: Anticoagulant

Chem. class.: Thrombin inhibitor

Action: Direct inhibitor of thrombin that is highly specific

Uses: Unstable angina in patients undergoing percutaneous transluminal coronary angioplasty (PTCA)

Dosage and routes:

• *Adult:* **IV BOL** 1 mg/kg, then **IV INF** 2.5 mg/kg/hr for 4 hr; another **IV INF** may be used at 0.2 mg/kg/hr for ≤20 hr; this drug is intended to be used with aspirin (325 mg qd) adjusted to body weight

Available forms: Inj, lyophilized 250 mg

Side effects/adverse reactions:

CV: Hypo/hypertension, bradycardia

CNS: Headache, insomnia, anxiety, nervousness, fever

GI: Nausea, vomiting, abdominal pain, dyspepsia

*HEMA: **Hemorrhage***

MS: Back pain

MISC: Pain at inj site, pelvic pain, urinary retention

Contraindications: Hypersensitivity, active bleeding

Precautions: Renal function impairment, lactation, children, hepatic disease, pregnancy (B)

Pharmacokinetics: Excreted in urine, half-life 25 min

Interactions:

• Increased risk of bleeding: anticoagulants, thrombolytics

NURSING CONSIDERATIONS

Assess:

➡ Fall in B/P or Hct, that may indicate hemorrhage

• Fever, skin rash, urticaria

Administer:

• To each 250 mg vial add 5 ml of sterile water for inj, swirl until dissolved, further dilute reconstituted vial with 50 ml of D_5W or 0.9% NaCl (5 mg/ml); the dose is adjusted to body weight

• Reduced dose in renal impairment

Evaluate

• Therapeutic response: anticoagulation in PTCA

Teach patient/family:

• Reason for drug and expected results

bleomycin (R)

(blee-oh-mye′sin)

Blenoxane

Func. class.: Antineoplastic, antibiotic

Chem. class.: Glycopeptide

Action: Inhibits synthesis of DNA, RNA, protein; derived from *Streptomyces verticillus;* replication is decreased by binding to DNA, which causes strand splitting; phase specific in the G_2 and M phases; a nonvesicant

Uses: Cancer of head, neck, penis, cervix, vulva of squamous cell origin, Hodgkin's disease, lymphosarcoma, reticulum cell sarcoma, testicular carcinoma, malignant pleural effusion

Dosage and routes:

• *Adult and child:* **SC/IV/IM** 0.25-0.5 U/kg 1-2 times/wk or 10-20 U/m², then 1 U/day or 5 U/wk; may also be given by **CONT INF**; do not exceed total dose, 400 U in lifetime

Malignant pleural effusion

• *Adult:* 60 U as a single bolus intrapleural inj; 0.9% NaCl given through a thoracostomy tube following drainage of excess pleural

---

Side effects: *italics* = common; ***bold italics*** = life-threatening

fluid and complete lung expansion, remove after 4 hr

Available forms: Powder for inj, 15 U/vial

Side effects/adverse reactions:

*SYST: **Anaphylaxis,** radiation recall, Raynaud's phenomenon*

GI: Nausea, vomiting, anorexia, stomatitis, weight loss, ulceration of mouth, lips

INTEG: Rash, hyperkeratosis, nail changes, alopecia, fever and chills, pruritus, acne, stria, peeling

*RESP: **Fibrosis,** pneumonitis, wheezing, **pulmonary toxicity***

CNS: Fever, chills, pain at tumor site, headache, confusion

IDIOSYNCRATIC REACTION: Hypotension, confusion, fever, chills, wheezing

Contraindications: Hypersensitivity, pregnancy (D)

Precautions: Renal, hepatic, respiratory disease

Pharmacokinetics: Half-life 2 hr; when CrCl >35 ml/min, half-life is increased in lower clearance; metabolized in liver, 50% excreted in urine (unchanged)

Interactions:

• Increased toxicity: other antineoplastics, radiation therapy, general anesthesia

Lab test interferences:

Increase: Uric acid

• Decreased serum phenytoin levels: phenytoin

NURSING CONSIDERATIONS

Assess:

• IM test dose in lymphoma

• Pulmonary function tests: chest x-ray film before and during therapy; should be obtained q2wk during treatment

• Temp q4h; fever may indicate beginning infection

• Serum creatinine

• Dyspnea, rales, unproductive cough, chest pain, tachypnea, fatigue, increased pulse, pallor, lethargy

• Effects of alopecia and skin color on body image; discuss feelings about body changes

• Buccal cavity q8h for dryness, sores, ulceration, white patches, oral pain, bleeding, dysphagia

• Local irritation, pain, burning, discoloration at injection site

◆ Symptoms indicating anaphylaxis: rash, pruritus, urticaria, purpuric skin lesions, itching, flushing, wheezing, hypotension; have emergency equipment available

Administer:

• Antiemetic 30-60 min before giving drug to prevent vomiting, continue antiemetics 6-10 hr after treatment

• Topical or systemic analgesics for pain of stomatitis as ordered; antihistamines and antipyretics for fever and chills

IM/SC

• After reconstituting 15 U/1-5 ml sterile H_2O, D_5W, 0.9% NaCl, or bacteriostatic water for inj, rotate inj sites; do not use products containing benzyl alcohol when giving to neonates

Direct IV

• After reconstituting 15 U or less/5 ml or more of D_5W or 0.9% NaCl; after further diluting with 50-100 ml D_5W or 0.9% NaCl, give 15 U or less/10 min through Y-tube or 3-way stopcock

• In lymphoma, two test doses 2-5 U before initial dose; monitor for anaphylaxis

Intrapleural

• 60 U/50-100 ml of 0.9% NaCl, administered by MD through thoracotomy tube

Additive compatibilities: Amikacin, cephapirin, dexamethasone, di-

---

◆ = Nursing alert   ✍ = Herb-drug interaction   🚫 = Do not crush phenhydramine, fluorouracil, gentamicin, heparin, hydrocortisone, phenytoin, streptomycin, tobramycin, vinblastine, vincristine

Solution compatibilities: 0.9% NaCl

Syringe compatibilities: Cisplatin, cyclophosphamide, doxorubicin, droperidol, fluorouracil, furosemide, heparin, leucovorin, methotrexate, metoclopramide, mitomycin, vinblastine, vincristine

Y-site compatibilities: Allopurinol, amifostine, aztreonam, cefepime, cisplatin, cyclophosphamide, doxorubicin, doxorubicin liposome, droperidol, filgrastim, fludarabine, fluorouracil, granisetron, heparin, leucovorin, melphalan, methotrexate, metoclopramide, mitomycin, ondansetron, paclitaxel, piperacillin/tazobactam, sargramostim, teniposide, thiotepa, vinblastine, vincristine, vinorelbine

Perform/provide:
• Storage for 2 wk after reconstituting at refrigerated or 24 hr at room temperature; discard unused portions
• Deep-breathing exercises with patient tid-qid; place in semi-Fowler's position
• Liquid diet: carbonated beverage; gelatin may be added if patient is not nauseated or vomiting
• Rinsing of mouth tid-qid with water, club soda; brushing of teeth with baking soda bid-tid with soft brush or cotton-tipped applicators for stomatitis; use unwaxed dental floss
• HOB raised to facilitate breathing

Evaluate:
• Therapeutic response: decrease in size of tumor

Teach patient/family:
• To report any complaints, side effects to nurse or prescriber
• To report any changes in breathing, coughing, fever
• That hair may be lost during treatment, and wig or hairpiece may make patient feel better; that new hair may be different in color, texture
• To avoid foods with citric acid, hot or rough texture
• To report any bleeding, white spots, ulcerations in mouth; to examine mouth qd and report symptoms
• To use contraception during treatment
• Not to receive vaccines during treatment

---

bosentan
See appendix a—selected new drugs

---

bretylium (℞)
(bre-til'ee-um)
Bretylate*, bretylium tosylate, Bretylol
Func. class.: Antidysrhythmic (Class III)
Chem. class.: Quaternary ammonium compound

Action: After a transient release of norepinephrine, inhibits further release by postganglionic nerve endings; prolongs duration of action potential and effective refractory period

Uses: Life-threatening ventricular tachycardia, cardioversion, ventricular fibrillation; for short-term use only

Dosage and routes:
Severe ventricular fibrillation
• *Adult:* **IV BOL** 5 mg/kg, over 15-30 sec; increase to 10 mg/kg repeated q15min, up to 30 mg/kg; **IV INF** 1-2 mg/min or give 5-10 mg/kg over 10 min q6h (maintenance)

Ventricular tachycardia
• *Adult:* **IV INF** 500 mg diluted in 50 ml D_5W or NS, infuse over 10-30 min, may repeat in 1 hr, maintain with 1-2 mg/min or 5-10 mg/kg over 10-30 min q6h; **IM** 5-10 mg/kg undiluted; repeat in 1-2 hr if needed; maintain with same dose q6-8h
• *Child:* 2-5 mg/kg/dose

Renal disease
• CrCl 10-50 ml/min 25%-50% dose; CrCl <10 ml/min avoid use

Available forms: Inj 50 mg/ml; 1, 2, 4 mg/ml prefilled syringes

Side effects/adverse reactions:
CNS: Syncope, dizziness, confusion, psychosis, anxiety
GI: Nausea, vomiting
CV: Hypotension, postural hypotension, bradycardia, angina, PVCs, substernal pressure, transient hypertension, precipitation of angina
*RESP: **Respiratory depression***

Contraindications: Hypersensitivity, digitalis toxicity, aortic stenosis, pulmonary hypertension

Precautions: Renal disease, pregnancy (C), lactation, children

Pharmacokinetics: Well absorbed by IM/IV routes
IV: Onset 5 min, duration 6-24 hr
IM: Onset ½-2 hr, duration 6-24 hr
Half-life 4-17 hr, excreted unchanged by kidneys (70%-80% in 24 hr), not metabolized

Interactions:
• Increased or decreased effects of bretylium: quinidine, procainamide, propranolol, other antidysrhythmics
• Hypotension: antihypertensives
• Increased effects of: sympathomimetics
🖊 Increased action of bretylium: chronic use/abuse of cascara sagrada bark, aloe, buckthorn bark/berry, rhubarb root, senna leaf/fruits

NURSING CONSIDERATIONS
Assess:
• ECG continuously to determine drug effectiveness, PVCs, other dysrhythmias
• IV INF rate to avoid causing nausea, vomiting
• For dehydration or hypovolemia
• B/P continuously for hypotension, hypertension; orthostatic hypotension; keep supine until hypotension subsides
• I&O ratio
• If systolic B/P <75 mm Hg, notify prescriber
• For rebound hypertension after 1-2 hr
• Cardiac status: rate, rhythm, character, continuously
Administer:
IM
• Inj, rotate sites, inject <5 ml in any one site to prevent tissue necrosis, may repeat 1-2 hr
IV, direct
• Undiluted over 15-30 sec (ventricular fibrillation); may repeat in 15-30 min, not to exceed 30 mg/kg/24 hr
Intermittent IV inf
• Dilute 500 mg of drug/50 ml or more D_5W, 0.9% NaCl, D_5/0.45%, D_5/0.9% NaCl, D_5/LR, give over 15-30 min
Continuous IV inf
• Dilute further; give at 1-2 mg diluted drug/min via infusion pump
• Reduced dosage slowly with ECG monitoring, discontinue over 3-5 days, maintain on oral dysrhythmic
Additive compatibilities: Aminophylline, atracurium, calcium chloride, calcium gluconate, digoxin, dopamine, esmolol, insulin (regular), lidocaine, potassium chloride, quinadine, verapamil
Y-site compatibilities: Amiodarone, amrinone, cisatracurium, diltiazem,

---

◆ = Nursing alert   🖊 = Herb-drug interaction   🚫 = Do not crush

dobutamine, famotidine, isoproterenol, ranitidine, remifentanil
Perform/provide:
• Place patient in supine position unless otherwise ordered; assist with ambulation
• Have suction equipment available
Evaluate:
• Therapeutic response: absence of ventricular tachycardia, fibrillation
Teach patient/family:
• To make position changes slowly; orthostatic hypotension may occur
Treatment of overdose: O$_2$, artificial ventilation, ECG; administer dopamine for circulatory depression; administer diazepam or thiopental for convulsions

---

bromocriptine (℞)

(broe-moe-krip'teen)
Alti-Bromocriptine*, Apo-Bromocriptine*, Parlodel
Func. class.: Dopamine receptor agonist, antiparkinson agent
Chem. class.: Ergot alkaloid derivative

Action: Inhibits prolactin release by activating postsynaptic dopamine receptors; activation of striatal dopamine receptors may be reason for improvement in Parkinson's disease

Uses: Parkinson's disease, amenorrhea/galactorrhea caused by hyperprolactinemia, acromegaly

Investigational uses: Pituitary adenomas, neuroleptic malignant syndrome

Dosage and routes:

Hyperprolactinemia
• *Adult:* PO 1.25-2.5 mg with meals; may increase by 2.5 mg q3-7d, usual 5-7.5 mg

Acromegaly
• *Adult:* PO 1.25-2.5 mg × 3 days

hs; may increase by 1.25-2.5 mg q3-7d; usual range 20-30 mg/day, max 100 mg/day

Parkinson's disease
• *Adult:* PO 1.25 mg bid with meals, may increase q2-4wk by 2.5 mg/day, not to exceed 100 mg qd

Pituitary adenoma
• *Adult:* PO 1.25 mg bid-tid, may increase over several weeks

Neuroleptic malignant syndrome
• *Adult:* PO 5 mg qd, max 20 mg/day

Available forms: Caps 5 mg; tabs 2.5 mg

Side effects/adverse reactions:
EENT: Blurred vision, diplopia, burning eyes, nasal congestion
CNS: Headache, depression, restlessness, anxiety, nervousness, confusion, *convulsions,* hallucinations, dizziness, fatigue, drowsiness, abnormal involuntary movements, psychosis
GU: Frequency, retention, incontinence, diuresis
GI: Nausea, vomiting, anorexia, cramps, constipation, diarrhea, dry mouth, GI hemorrhage
INTEG: Rash on face, arms, alopecia; coolness, pallor of fingers, toes
CV: Orthostatic hypotension, decreased B/P, palpitation, extra systole, *shock,* dysrhythmias, bradycardia, *MI*

Contraindications: Hypersensitivity to ergot, severe ischemic disease, severe peripheral vascular disease

Precautions: Lactation, hepatic disease, renal disease, children, pituitary tumors, pregnancy (B)

Do not confuse:
Parlodel/pindolol

Pharmacokinetics:
PO: Peak 1-3 hr, duration 4-8 hr, 90%-96% protein bound, half-life 3 hr, metabolized by liver (inactive

---

metabolites), 85%-98% of dose excreted in feces

Interactions:

• Decreased action of bromocriptine: phenothiazines, oral contraceptives, progestins, estrogens, haloperidol, loxapine, methyldopa, metoclopramide, MAOIs, reserpine

• Increased action of antihypertensives, levodopa

• Disulfiram-like reaction: alcohol

⫽ Decreased effect of bromocriptine: chaste tree fruit

Lab test interferences:

Increase: Growth hormone, AST, ALT, CK, BUN, uric acid, alk phosphatase

NURSING CONSIDERATIONS
Assess:

• B/P; establish baseline, compare with other reading; this drug decreases B/P

• Parkinson's symptoms: pill-rolling, shuffling gait, restlessness, tremors, before and during treatment

• For resolution of symptoms of neuroleptic malignant syndrome: decreased temp, seizures, sweating, pulse

• Change in size of soft tissue volume, in acromegaly

Administer:

PO

• With meal to prevent GI symptoms

• At hs so dizziness, orthostatic hypotension do not occur

Perform/provide:

• Storage at room temperature in tight container

Evaluate:

• Therapeutic response (Parkinson's disease): decreased dyskinesia, decreased slow movements, decreased drooling

Teach patient/family:

• That tabs may be crushed and mixed with food

• To change position slowly to prevent orthostatic hypotension

• To use contraceptives during treatment with this drug; pregnancy may occur; to use methods other than oral contraceptives

• That therapeutic effect for Parkinson's disease may take 2 mo: galactorrhea, amenorrhea

• To avoid hazardous activity if dizziness occurs

• To report symptoms of MI immediately

---

brompheniramine (℞)

(brome-fen-ir′a-meen)
Bromfenac, brompheniramine, Chlorphed, Dehist, Dimetane, Dimetane Extentabs, Dimetapp Allergy Liqui-Gels, Nasahist-B

Func. class.: Antihistamine

Chem. class.: Alkylamine, H_1-receptor antagonist

Action: Acts on blood vessels, GI, respiratory system by competing with histamine for H_1-receptor site; decreases allergic response by blocking histamine

Uses: Allergy symptoms, rhinitis

Dosage and routes:

• *Adult and child >12 yr:* **PO** 4-8 mg tid-qid, not to exceed 36 mg/day; time rel 8-12 mg bid-tid, not to exceed 36 mg/day; **IM/IV/SC** 10 mg q6-12h, not to exceed 40 mg/day

• *Child 6-12 yr:* **PO** 2 mg tid-qid, not to exceed 12 mg/day; **IM/IV/SC** 0.125 mg/kg

• *Child 2-6 yr:* 1 mg q4-6h, max 6 mg/day

Available forms: Tabs 4 mg; elix 2 mg/5 ml; inj 10 mg/ml; caps 4 mg

Side effects/adverse reactions:

CNS: Dizziness, drowsiness, poor coordination, fatigue, anxiety, euphoria, confusion, paresthesia, neuritis

CV: Hypotension, palpitations, tachycardia

RESP: Increased thick secretions, wheezing, chest tightness

*HEMA: **Thrombocytopenia, agranulocytosis, hemolytic anemia***

GI: Nausea, vomiting, anorexia, constipation, diarrhea

INTEG: Photosensitivity

GU: Retention, dysuria, frequency, impotence

EENT: Blurred vision, dilated pupils, tinnitus, nasal stuffiness, dry nose, throat, mouth

Contraindications: Hypersensitivity to H$_1$-receptor antagonists, acute asthma attack, lower respiratory tract disease, child <2 yr

Precautions: Increased intraocular pressure, renal disease, cardiac disease, hypertension, bronchial asthma, seizure disorder, stenosed peptic ulcers, hyperthyroidism, prostatic hypertrophy, bladder neck obstruction, pregnancy (C), lactation

Pharmacokinetics:

PO: Peak 2-5 hr, duration to 48 hr; metabolized in liver, excreted by kidneys, excreted in breast milk, half-life 12-34 hr

Interactions:

• Increased CNS depression: barbiturates, opiates, hypnotics, tricyclics, alcohol

• Increased anticholinergic effect: MAOIs

• Incompatible with aminophylline, insulins, pentobarbital

🍃 Increased CNS depression: kava

🍃 Increased anticholinergic effect: henbane leaf

Lab test interferences:

Interfere: Skin allergy tests

NURSING CONSIDERATIONS

Assess:

• Be alert for urinary retention, frequency, dysuria; drug should be discontinued if these occur

• CBC during long-term therapy

• Blood dyscrasias: thrombocytopenia, agranulocytosis (rare) during long-term therapy

• Respiratory status: rate, rhythm, increase in bronchial secretions, wheezing, chest tightness

Administer:

PO

• With meals if GI symptoms occur; absorption may slightly decrease

IV, direct

• Undiluted or diluted with 10 ml 0.9% NaCl, given over 1 min or more

IV inf

• Dilute in D$_5$W, 0.9% NaCl given at prescribed rate

Perform/provide:

• Hard candy, gum, frequent rinsing of mouth for dryness

• Storage in tight container at room temperature

Evaluate:

• Therapeutic response: absence of running or congested nose or rashes

Teach patient/family:

🚫 Not to break, crush, or chew sustained release forms

• All aspects of drug use; to notify prescriber if confusion/sedation/hypotension occurs

• To avoid driving, other hazardous activities if drowsiness occurs

• To avoid use of alcohol, other CNS depressants while taking drug

Treatment of overdose: Administer ipecac syrup or lavage, diazepam, vasopressors, barbiturates (short-acting)

budesonide (Ŗ)

(byoo-des'oh-nide)
Entocort EC, Pulmicort
Func. class.: Glucocorticoid
Chem. class.: Nonhalogenated

Action: Prevents inflammation by depression of migration of polymorphonuclear leukocytes, fibroblasts, reversal of increased capillary permeability and lysosomal stabilization; does not suppress hypothalamus and pituitary function

Uses: Rhinitis, asthma; Crohn's disease

Dosage and routes:
• *Adult and child ≥6 yr:* **INH** 400-600 µg/day

Available forms: Dry powder for INH 200 µg/metered dose (turbuhaler); inh susp 0.25 mg/2 ml, 0.5 mg/2 ml

Side effects/adverse reactions:
CNS: Headache, insomnia, hypertonia, syncope
EENT: Sinusitis, pharyngitis, rhinitis, oral candidiasis
GI: Dry mouth, dyspepsia, nausea, vomiting, abdominal pain, oral candidiasis
MISC: Ecchymosis, fever, *hypersensitivity,* flulike symptoms
MS: Back pain, myalgias, fractures
RESP: Nasal irritation, cough, nasal bleeding, *respiratory infections, bronchospasm*

Contraindications: Hypersensitivity, status asthmaticus

Precautions: Pregnancy (C), lactation, children, TB, fungal, bacterial, systemic viral infections, ocular herpes simplex, nasal septal ulcers

Pharmacokinetics: Unknown

Interactions:
• Decreased budesonide metabolism: ketoconazole

NURSING CONSIDERATIONS
Assess:
• Respiratory status: rate, rhythm, increase in bronchial secretions, wheezing, chest tightness; provide fluids to 2 L/day to decrease thickness of secretions; check for oral candidiasis
• For bronchospasm, stop treatment and give bronchodilator
• With viral infections, corticosteroid use can mask infections
• For increased intraocular pressure, discontinue use if increase occurs

Administer:
Inhalation
• Use scissors to open pouch
• Use Turbuhaler upright to load, prime when using first time, turn grip to the right, then left to click in place; to provide dose turn to right, then to the left, click in place. Place mouthpiece between lips, inhale forcefully, do not exhale through Turbuhaler, rinse after use

Perform/provide:
• Storage at 59°-86° F (15°-30° C); keep away from heat, open flame

Evaluate:
• Therapeutic response: absence of asthma, rhinitis

Teach patient/family:
• To notify prescriber of pharyngitis, nasal bleeding
• Not to exceed recommended dose; adrenal suppression may occur
• To carry medical ID identifying steroid use
• To read and follow package directions
• To prevent exposure to infections, especially viral

◆ = Nursing alert   🍃 = Herb-drug interaction   ⊘ = Do not crush

bumetanide (R̸)

(byoo-met′a-nide)
Bumex
Func. class.: Loop diuretic,
antihypertensive
Chem. class.: Sulfonamide de-
rivative

Action: Acts on ascending loop of
Henle by inhibiting reabsorption of
chloride, sodium
Uses: Edema in CHF, liver disease,
renal disease (nephrotic syndrome),
pulmonary edema, ascites (nephrotic
syndrome), hypertension, anasarca
Investigational uses: May be used
alone or as adjunct with antihypertensives such as spironolactone, triamterene
Dosage and routes:
• *Adult:* **PO** 0.5-2.0 mg qd; may
give 2nd or 3rd dose at 4-5 hr intervals, not to exceed 10 mg/day;
may be given on alternate days or
intermittently; **IV/IM** 0.5-1.0 mg;
may give 2nd or 3rd dose at 2-3 hr
intervals, not to exceed 10 mg/day
• *Child:* **PO/IM/IV** 0.02-0.1 mg/kg
q12h, max 10 mg/day
Available forms: Tabs 0.5, 1, 2 mg;
inj 0.25 mg/ml
Side effects/adverse reactions:
GU: Polyuria, **renal failure,** glycosuria
*ELECT: Hypokalemia, hypochlor-
emic alkalosis, hypomagnesemia,
hyperuricemia, hypocalcemia, hyponatremia*
CNS: Headache, fatigue, weakness,
vertigo
GI: Nausea, diarrhea, dry mouth,
vomiting, anorexia, cramps, upset
stomach, abdominal pain, ***acute pancreatitis, jaundice***
EENT: **Loss of hearing,** ear pain,
tinnitus, blurred vision
INTEG: Rash, pruritus, purpura,

Stevens-Johnson syndrome, sweat-
ing, photosensitivity
MS: Muscular cramps, arthritis, stiff-
ness, tenderness
ENDO: Hyperglycemia
HEMA: ***Thrombocytopenia***
CV: ***Chest pain,*** hypotension, ***cir-
culatory collapse,*** ECG changes, de-
hydration
Contraindications: Hypersensitiv-
ity to sulfonamides, anuria, hepatic
coma
Precautions: Dehydration, ascites,
severe renal disease, pregnancy (C),
hepatic cirrhosis, lactation
Do not confuse:
Bumex/Buprenex
Pharmacokinetics:
PO: Onset ½-1 hr, peak 1-2 hr, du-
ration 4 hr
IM: Onset 40 min, duration 4 hr
IV: Onset 5 min, peak 15-30 min,
duration 2-3 hr, excreted by kid-
neys, crosses placenta, excreted in
breast milk
Interactions:
• Decreased diuretic effect: indo-
methacin, NSAIDs, probenecid
• Ototoxicity: aminoglycosides
• Increased toxicity: lithium, digitalis
• Increased diuresis, electrolyte loss:
metolazone
• Hypokalemia: potassium-wasting
drugs, corticosteroids
• Decreased effects of antidiabetics
NURSING CONSIDERATIONS
Assess:
• Hearing with high IV doses
• Weight, I&O daily to determine
fluid loss; if urinary output decreases
or azotemia occurs, drug should
be discontinued; the safest dosage
schedule is on alternate days
• B/P lying, standing; postural hy-
potension may occur
• Electrolytes: K, Na, Cl; include
BUN, blood sugar, CBC, serum cre-
atinine, blood pH, ABGs, uric acid,
Ca, Mg

• Blood glucose if patient is diabetic; blood uric acid levels in those with gout
• Improvement in edema of feet, legs, sacral area daily if medication is being used in CHF
• Signs of metabolic alkalosis: drowsiness, restlessness
• Signs of hypokalemia: postural hypotension, malaise, fatigue, tachycardia, leg cramps, weakness
• Rashes, temp elevation qd
• Confusion, especially in elderly; take safety precautions if needed
• For digitalis toxicity in patients taking digitalis products; lithium toxicity in those taking lithium

Administer:
• In AM to avoid interference with sleep if using drug as a diuretic
• Potassium replacement if potassium is less than 3.0

PO
• With food if nausea occurs; absorption may be decreased slightly

IV, direct
• Direct IV undiluted over at least 2 min through Y-tube or 3-way stopcock or heplock

Intermittent IV
• Dilute in LR, D₅W, 0.9% NaCl (rarely given by this method), give over 12 hr in renal disease

Additive compatibilities: Floxacillin, furosemide

Syringe compatibilities: Doxapram

Y-site compatibilities: Allopurinol, amifostine, aztreonam, cefepime, cisatracurium, cladribine, diltiazem, filgrastim, granisetron, lorazepam, melphalan, meperidine, morphine, piperacillin/tazobactam, propofol, remifentanil, teniposide, thiotepa, vinorelbine

Evaluate:
• Therapeutic response: decreased edema, B/P

Teach patient/family:
• To increase fluid intake to 2-3

L/day unless contraindicated, to take K supplement, to rise slowly from lying or sitting position
• To recognize adverse reactions: muscle cramps, weakness, nausea, dizziness
• To take with food or milk for GI symptoms
• To take early in day to prevent nocturia
• To use sunscreen to prevent photosensitivity

Treatment of overdose: Lavage if taken orally; monitor electrolytes; administer dextrose in saline; monitor hydration, CV, renal status

---

buprenorphine (℞)
(byoo-pre-nor'feen)
Buprenex
Func. class.: Opioid analgesic
Chem. class.: Thebaine derivative

Controlled Substance Schedule V
Action: Depresses pain impulse transmission at the spinal cord level by interacting with opioid receptors
Uses: Moderate to severe pain
Dosage and routes:
• *Adult:* **IM/IV** 0.3 mg q6h prn, reduce dosage in elderly, may repeat after ½ hr; epidural 60-180 µg over 48 hr
• *Child 2-12 yr:* **IM/IV** 2-6 µg/kg q4-6h
• *Geriatric:* **PO** 0.15 mg q6h prn
Available forms: Inj 0.3 mg/ml (1 ml vials)
Side effects/adverse reactions:
*CNS: Drowsiness, dizziness, confusion, headache, sedation, euphoria, **increased intracranial pressure,** amnesia*
GI: Nausea, vomiting, anorexia, constipation, cramps, dry mouth

---

GU: Increased urinary output, dysuria, urinary retention

INTEG: Rash, urticaria, bruising, flushing, diaphoresis, pruritus

EENT: Tinnitus, blurred vision, *miosis,* diplopia

CV: Palpitations, bradycardia, change in B/P, tachycardia

*RESP: **Respiratory depression,*** dyspnea, hypo-, hyperventilation

Contraindications: Hypersensitivity, addiction (narcotic)

Precautions: Addictive personality, pregnancy (C), lactation, increased intracranial pressure, MI (acute), severe heart disease, respiratory depression, hepatic disease, renal disease

Do not confuse:
Buprenex/Bumex

Pharmacokinetics:

IM: Onset 10-30 min, peak ½ hr, duration 3-4 hr

IV: Onset 1 min, peak 5 min, duration 2-5 hr

Metabolized by liver; excreted by kidneys/feces; crosses placenta; excreted in breast milk; half-life 2½-3½ hr; 96% bound to plasma proteins

Interactions:

• Effects may be increased with other CNS depressants: alcohol, opioids, sedative/hypnotics, antipsychotics, skeletal muscle relaxants, MAOIs

🖉 Increased CNS depression: kava

NURSING CONSIDERATIONS

Assess:

• I&O ratio; check for decreasing output; may indicate urinary retention

• CNS changes, dizziness, drowsiness, hallucinations, euphoria, LOC, pupil reaction; withdrawal in narcotic-dependent persons; if dependence occurs, within 2 wk of discontinuing drug withdrawal symptoms will occur

• Allergic reactions: rash, urticaria

• Respiratory dysfunction: respiratory depression, character, rate, rhythm; notify prescriber if respirations are <12/min

• Need for pain medication, tolerance; location, intensity, severity

Administer:

IM

• In deep muscle mass

IV, direct

• Undiluted over 3-5 min (0.3 mg over 2 min), titrate to patient response

• With antiemetic if nausea, vomiting occur

• When pain is beginning to return; determine dosage interval by patient response

Additive compatibilities: Atropine, bupivacaine, diphenhydramine, droperidol, glycopyrrolate, haloperidol, hydroxyzine, promethazine, scopolamine

Syringe compatibilities: Midazolam

Y-site compatibilities: Allopurinol, amifostine, aztreonam, cefepime, cisatracurium, cladribine, filgrastim, granisetron, melphalan, piperacillin/tazobactam, propofol, remifentanil, teniposide, thiotepa, vinorelbine

Perform/provide:

• Assistance with ambulation if needed

Evaluate:

• Therapeutic response: decrease in pain, absence of grimacing

Teach patient/family:

• To report any symptoms of CNS changes, allergic reactions

• That tolerance may result when used for extended periods

• To avoid hazardous activities

---

bupropion (℞)

(byoo-proe′pee-on)
Wellbutrin, Wellbutrin SR,
Zyban
Func. class.: Misc. antidepressant, smoking deterrent
Chem. class.: Aminoketone

Action: Inhibits reuptake of dopamine, serotonin, norepinephrine
Uses: Depression (Wellbutrin), smoking cessation (Zyban)
Dosage and routes:
Depression
• *Adult:* **PO** 100 mg bid initially, then increase after 3 days to 100 mg tid if needed; may increase after 1 mo to 150 mg tid
• *Geriatric:* **PO** 50-100 mg/day, may increase by 50-100 mg q3-4 day
Smoking cessation
• *Adult:* **PO** 150 mg bid, begin with 150 mg qd × 3 days, then 300 mg/day; continue for 7-12 wk
Available forms: Tabs 75, 100 mg; tab sust rel 50, 100, (Zyban) 150 mg
Side effects/adverse reactions:
CNS: Headache, agitation, confusion, seizures, delusions, *insomnia,* sedation, tremors
CV: Dysrhythmias, hypertension, palpitations, tachycardia, hypotension, *complete AV block*
GI: Nausea, vomiting, dry mouth, increased appetite, constipation
GU: Impotence, urinary frequency, retention
INTEG: Rash, pruritus, sweating
EENT: Blurred vision, auditory disturbance
Contraindications: Hypersensitivity, eating disorders
Precautions: Renal and hepatic disease, recent MI, cranial trauma, pregnancy (B), lactation, children <18 yr, elderly, seizure disorder

Pharmacokinetics: Onset 2-4 wk, half-life 14 hr; metabolized by liver, steady state 1½-5 wk
Interactions:
• Increased adverse reactions, seizures: levodopa, MAOIs, phenothiazines, antidepressants, benzodiazepines, alcohol, theophylline, systemic steroids
• Increased bupropion toxicity: ritonavir
• Decreased bupropion effect: carbamazepine, phenobarbital, phenytoin
• Increased bupropion level: cimetidine
 Increased CNS depression: kava
 May increase anticholinergic effect: belladonna leaf/root
NURSING CONSIDERATIONS
Assess:
• For increased risk of seizures; if patient has excessively used CNS depressants and OTC stimulants, dosage of bupropion should not be exceeded
• For smoking cessation after 7-12 wk; if progress has not been made, drug should be discontinued
• Mental status: mood, sensorium, affect, suicidal tendencies, increase in psychiatric symptoms
Administer:
PO
🚫 Do not crush, break, chew sust rel tab
• Increased fluids, bulk in diet if constipation occurs
• With food or milk for GI symptoms
• Gum, hard candy, or frequent sips of water for dry mouth
Perform/provide:
• Assistance with ambulation during beginning therapy, since sedation occurs
• Safety measures, primarily in elderly

 = Nursing alert   = Herb-drug interaction   🚫 = Do not crush

Evaluate:
• Therapeutic response: decreased depression, ability to function in daily activities, ability to sleep throughout the night, smoking cessation

Teach patient/family:
• That therapeutic effects may take 2-4 wk; not to increase dose without prescriber's approval; that treatment for smoking cessation lasts 7-12 wk
• To use caution in driving, other activities requiring alertness; sedation, blurred vision may occur
• To avoid alcohol ingestion, other CNS depressants
• Not to use with nicotine patches unless directed by prescriber, may increase B/P
• That risk of seizures is increased when dose is exceeded, or if patient has seizure disorder
• To notify prescriber, if pregnancy is suspected or planned

Treatment of overdose: ECG monitoring; induce emesis, lavage, activated charcoal; administer anticonvulsant

---

buspirone (℞)
(byoo-spye'rone)
BuSpar
Func. class.: Antianxiety, sedative
Chem. class.: Azaspirodecanedione

Action: Acts by inhibiting the action of serotonin (5-HT); has shown little potential for abuse, a good choice in substance abuse
Uses: Management and short-term relief of anxiety disorders
Dosage and routes:
• *Adult:* **PO** 5 mg tid; may increase by 5 mg/day q2-3d, not to exceed 60 mg/day

Available forms: Tabs 5, 10, 15 mg
Side effects/adverse reactions:
CNS: Dizziness, headache, depression, stimulation, insomnia, nervousness, light-headedness, numbness, paresthesia, incoordination, tremors, excitement, involuntary movements, confusion, akathisia
GI: Nausea, dry mouth, diarrhea, constipation, flatulence, increased appetite, rectal bleeding
CV: Tachycardia, palpitations, hypotension, hypertension, ***CVA, CHF, MI***
EENT: Sore throat, tinnitus, blurred vision, nasal congestion; red, itching eyes; change in taste, smell
GU: Frequency, hesitancy, menstrual irregularity, change in libido
MS: Pain, weakness, muscle cramps, spasms
RESP: Hyperventilation, chest congestion, shortness of breath
INTEG: Rash, edema, pruritus, alopecia, dry skin
MISC: Sweating, fatigue, weight gain, fever
Contraindications: Hypersensitivity, child
Precautions: Pregnancy (B), lactation, elderly, impaired hepatic/renal function
Pharmacokinetics: Half-life 2-3 hr rapidly absorbed, metabolized by liver, excreted in feces
Interactions:
• Decreased buspirone effects: rifampin
• Increased B/P: MAOIs; do not use together
• Increased CNS depression: psychotropic drugs, alcohol (avoid use)
🌿 Increased CNS depression: kava
🌿 Increased peak concentration of buspirone: grapefruit juice

---

Side effects: *italics* = common; ***bold italics*** = life-threatening

NURSING CONSIDERATIONS
Assess:
- B/P (lying, standing), pulse; if systolic B/P drops 20 mm Hg, hold drug, notify prescriber
- CNS reactions, since some reactions may be unpredictable
- Mental status: mood, sensorium, affect, sleeping pattern, drowsiness, dizziness

Administer:
PO
- With food or milk for GI symptoms
- Crushed if patient unable to swallow medication whole
- Sugarless gum, hard candy, frequent sips of water for dry mouth

Perform/provide:
- Assistance with ambulation during beginning therapy; drowsiness, dizziness occur
- Safety measures if drowsiness occurs
- Check to see PO medication swallowed

Evaluate:
- Therapeutic response: decreased anxiety, restlessness, sleeplessness

Teach patient/family:
- That drug may be taken with food
- To avoid OTC preparations unless approved by prescriber
- To avoid activities requiring alertness, since drowsiness may occur
- To avoid alcohol ingestion, other psychotropic medications, unless directed by prescriber
- Not to discontinue medication abruptly after long-term use
- To rise slowly because fainting may occur, especially elderly
- That drowsiness may worsen at beginning of treatment
- That 1-2 wk of therapy may be required before therapeutic effects occur

Treatment of overdose: Gastric lavage, VS, supportive care

busulfan (Rx)
(byoo-sul'fan)
Myleran

Func. class.: Antineoplastic alkylating agent

Chem. class.: Nitrosurea

Action: Changes essential cellular ions to covalent bonding with resultant alkylation; this interferes with normal biologic function of DNA; activity is not phase specific; action is due to myelosuppression

Uses: Chronic myelocytic leukemia

Dosage and routes:
- *Adult:* **PO** 4-8 mg/day initially until WBC levels fall to 10,000/mm^3, then drug is stopped until WBC levels raise over 50,000/mm^3, then 1-3 mg/day; **IV** 0.8 mg/kg q6h × 4 days, given with cyclophosphamide
- *Child:* **PO** 0.06-0.12 mg/kg or 1.8-4.6 mg/m^2 day; dose is titrated to maintain WBC levels at 20,000/mm^3

Available forms: Tabs 2 mg; sol for inj 6 mg/ml

Side effects/adverse reactions:
PO
GI: Anorexia, constipation, diarrhea, dry mouth, nausea, vomiting
*RESP: **Alveolar hemorrhage,** atelectasis, cough, hemoptysis, hypoxia, pleural effusion, pneumonia, sinusitis*
CV: Hypotension, thrombosis, chest pain, tachycardia, atrial fibrillation, heart block, pericardial effusion
IV
*CNS: **Cerebral hemorrhage, coma, seizures,** anxiety, depression, dizziness, headache, encephalopathy, weakness, mental changes*
EENT: Pharyngitis, epistaxis
*HEMA: **Thrombocytopenia, leukopenia, pancytopenia, severe bone marrow depression***

GI: Nausea, vomiting, *diarrhea, weight loss*

GU: Impotence, sterility, amenorrhea, gynecomastia, ***renal toxicity,*** hyperuremia, adrenal insufficiency–like syndrome

INTEG: Dermatitis, hyperpigmentation, alopecia

RESP: ***Irreversible pulmonary fibrosis,*** pneumonitis

OTHER: ***Chromosomal aberrations***

Contraindications: Radiation, chemotherapy, lactation, pregnancy (3rd trimester) (D), blastic phase of chronic myelocytic leukemia, hypersensitivity

Precautions: Childbearing age women and men, leukopenia, thrombocytopenia, anemia, hepatotoxicity, renal toxicity

Pharmacokinetics: Well absorbed orally; excreted in urine; crosses placenta; excreted in breast milk, half-life 2.5 hr

Interactions:

• Increased toxicity: other antineoplastics or radiation

• Increased risk of bleeding: anticoagulants, aspirin

NURSING CONSIDERATIONS

Assess:

• CBC, differential, platelet count weekly; withhold drug if WBC is $<15,000/mm^3$ or platelet count is $<150,000/mm^3$; notify prescriber of results; institute thrombocytopenia precautions

• Pulmonary function tests, chest x-ray films before, during therapy; chest film should be obtained q2wk during treatment; pulmonary fibrosis may occur up to 10 yr after treatment with busulfan

• Renal function studies: BUN, serum uric acid, urine CrCl before, during therapy

• I&O ratio; report fall in urine output <30 ml/hr

• Monitor for cold, fever, sore throat (may indicate beginning infection)

• For decreased hyperuricemia

• Bleeding: hematuria, guaiac, bruising or petechiae, mucosa or orifices q8h, no rectal temps

• Dyspnea, rales, nonproductive cough, chest pain, tachypnea

• Food preferences; list likes, dislikes

• Edema in feet, joint, stomach pain, shaking

• Inflammation of mucosa, breaks in skin; use viscous xylocaine for oral pain

Administer:

PO

• Give at same time qd, on empty stomach

IV

• Prepared in biologic cabinet, using gloves, gown, mask; dilute with 10 times volume of drug with D_5W or 0.9% NaCl, (0.5 mg/ml). When withdrawing drug, use needle with 5 micron filter provided, remove amount needed, remove filter and inject drug into diluent; always add drug to diluent, not vice versa; stable for 8 hr room temperature (using D_5W) or 12 hr refrigerated

• Give antiemetics before IV route, on schedule

• Give phenytoin prior to IV route, to prevent seizures (using 0.9% NaCl) give by central venous catheter over 2 hr q6h × 4 days, use infusion pump, do not admix

Perform/provide:

• Comprehensive oral hygiene

• Strict medical asepsis, protective isolation if WBC levels are low

• Deep breathing exercises with patient tid-qid; place in semi-Fowler's position for pulmonary reactions

• Increase fluid intake to 2-3 L/day to prevent urate deposits, calculi formation

• Diet low in purines: organ meats (kidney, liver), dried beans, peas to maintain alkaline urine
• Storage in tight container

Evaluate:
• Therapeutic response: decreased exacerbations of chronic myelocytic leukemia

Teach patient/family:
• About protective isolation precautions
• To avoid use of products containing aspirin or ibuprofen, razors, commercial mouthwash
• To report signs of anemia (fatigue, headache, irritability, faintness, shortness of breath)
• To report symptoms of bleeding (hematuria, tarry stools)
• That impotence or amenorrhea can occur, are reversible after discontinuing treatment
• To report any changes in breathing or coughing even several months after treatment

---

butorphanol (R̟)
(byoo-tor′fa-nole)
Stadol, Stadol NS
Func. class.: Opioid analgesic

Controlled Substance Schedule IV
Action: Depresses pain impulse transmission at the spinal cord level by interacting with opioid receptors
Uses: Moderate to severe pain
Investigational uses: Migraine headache, pain
Dosage and routes:
• *Adult:* **IM** 1-4 mg q3-4h prn; **IV** 0.5-2 mg q3-4h prn; **INTRANA-SAL,** 1 spray in one nostril q3-4h; may give another dose 1-1½ hr later; repeat if needed q3-4h
Geriatric: ½ adult dose at 2× the interval

Renal disease
• CrCl 10-50 ml/min 75% dose; CrCl <10 ml/min 50% dose
Available forms: Inj 1, 2 mg/ml; nasal spray 10 mg/ml
Side effects/adverse reactions:
CNS: Drowsiness, dizziness, confusion, headache, sedation, euphoria, weakness, hallucinations
GI: Nausea, vomiting, anorexia, constipation, cramps
GU: Increased urinary output, dysuria, urinary retention
INTEG: Rash, urticaria, bruising, flushing, diaphoresis, pruritus
EENT: Tinnitus, blurred vision, miosis, diplopia
CV: Palpitations, bradycardia, change in B/P
*RESP: **Respiratory depression,** pulmonary hypertension*
Contraindications: Hypersensitivity, addiction (narcotic), CHF, myocardial infarction
Precautions: Addictive personality, pregnancy (C), lactation, increased intracranial pressure, respiratory depression, hepatic disease, renal disease, child <18 yr
Do not confuse:
Stadol/Haldol
Pharmacokinetics:
IM: Onset 10-30 min, peak ½ hr, duration 3-4 hr
IV: Onset 1 min, peak 5 min, duration 2-4 hr
INTRANASAL: Onset within 15 min, peak 1-2 hr, duration 4-5 hr
Metabolized by liver; excreted by kidneys; crosses placenta; excreted in breast milk; half-life 2½-3½ hr
Interactions:
• Increased CNS effects: alcohol, opioids, sedative/hypnotics, antipsychotics, skeletal muscle relaxants
◆ Severe, fatal reactions: MAOIs
✿ Increased CNS depression: kava

◆ = Nursing alert   ✿ = Herb-drug interaction   ⊘ = Do not crush

NURSING CONSIDERATIONS
Assess:
• For decreasing output; may indicate urinary retention

◆ For withdrawal symptoms in opioid-dependent patients: pulmonary embolus, vascular occlusion, abscesses, ulcerations

• CNS changes: dizziness, drowsiness, hallucinations, euphoria, LOC, pupil reaction

• Allergic reactions: rash, urticaria

• Respiratory dysfunction: respiratory depression, character, rate, rhythm; notify prescriber if respirations are <10/min

• Need for pain medication, physical dependence

Administer:
• With antiemetic if nausea, vomiting occur

• When pain is beginning to return; determine dosage interval by patient response

IM
• Deeply in large muscle mass

IV
• Undiluted at a rate of <2 mg/>3-5 min, titrate to patient response

Syringe compatibilities: Atropine, chlorpromazine, cimetidine, diphenhydramine, droperidol, fentanyl, hydroxyzine, meperidine, methotrimerprazine, metoclopramide, midazolam, morphine, pentazocine, perphenazine, prochlorperazine, promethazine, scopolamine, thiethylperazine

Y-site compatibilities: Allopurinol, amifostine, aztreonam, cefepime, cisatracurium, cladribine, doxorubicin liposome, enalaprilat, esmolol, filgrastim, fludarabine, granisetron, labetalol, melphalan, paclitaxel, piperacillin/tazobactam, propofol, remifentanil, sargramostim, tenoposide, thiotepa, vinorelbine

Perform/provide:
• Storage in light-resistant container at room temperature

• Assistance with ambulation

• Safety measures: night-light, call bell within easy reach, especially elderly

Evaluate:
• Therapeutic response: decrease in pain

Teach patient/family:
• To report any symptoms of CNS changes, allergic reactions

• That physical dependency may result when used for extended periods

• That withdrawal symptoms may occur: nausea, vomiting, cramps, fever, faintness, anorexia

Treatment of overdose: Naloxone HCl (Narcan) 0.2-0.8 mg IV, O$_2$, IV fluids, vasopressors

---

RARELY USED

cabergoline (℞)
(ka-bear′joe-leen)
Dostinex
Func. class.: Dopamine receptor/agonist

Uses: Reduced prolactin/secretion in postpartum lactation

Dosage and routes:
Hyperprolactinemic indications
• *Adult:* **PO** 0.25 mg 2×/wk, may increase by 0.25 mg 2×/wk at 4 wk intervals, max 1 mg 2×/wk; maintenance therapy may be needed for 6 mo

Contraindications: Hypersensitivity, uncontrolled hypertension

---

calcifediol (R)
(kal-si-fe-dye'ole)
Calderol
Func. class.: Vit D analog, 25-hydroxyvitamin D₃
Chem. class.: Sterol

Action: Increases intestinal absorption of calcium for bones; increases renal tubular absorption of phosphate; increases mobilization of calcium from bones, bone resorption

Uses: Metabolic bone disease with chronic renal failure, osteopenia, osteomalacia, hypocalcemia

Dosage and routes:
• *Adult:* **PO** 300-350 μg qwk divided into qd or qod doses; may increase q4wk
• *Supplement Elderly:* **PO** 20 μg qd
Available forms: Caps 20, 50 μg

Side effects/adverse reactions:
EENT: Tinnitus, conjunctivitis, photophobia, rhinorrhea
CNS: Drowsiness, headache, vertigo, fever, lethargy
GI: Nausea, diarrhea, vomiting, jaundice, anorexia, dry mouth, constipation, cramps, metallic taste, thirst
MS: Myalgia, arthralgia, decreased bone development, weakness
GU: Polyuria, hypercalciuria, hyperphosphatemia, hematuria
CV: Dysrhythmias

Contraindications: Hypersensitivity, hyperphosphatemia, hypercalcemia, vit D toxicity

Precautions: Pregnancy (C), renal calculi, lactation, CV disease, elderly

Pharmacokinetics: Absorbed by the small intestine; stored in liver and fat deposits, activated in kidneys, excreted in bile and feces; peak 4 hr, duration 15-20 days; half-life 12-22 days

Interactions:
• Decreased absorption of calcifediol: cholestyramine, colestipol, mineral oil, fat-soluble vitamins
• Hypercalcemia: thiazide diuretics, calcium supplements
• Cardiac dysrhythmias: cardiac glycosides
• Decreased effect of this drug: corticosteroids
• Hypermagnesemia: magnesium antacids
• Increased metabolism of vit D: phenytoin
• Toxicity: other vit D products

Lab test interferences:
False increase: Cholesterol
Interfere: Alk phosphatase, electrolytes

NURSING CONSIDERATIONS
Assess:
• BUN, urinary calcium, AST, ALT, cholesterol, creatinine, uric acid, chloride, magnesium, electrolytes, urine pH, phosphate; may increase; calcium should be kept at 9-10 mg/dl, vit D 50-135 IU/dl, phosphate 70 mg/dl
• Alk phosphatase; may be decreased
• For increased blood level, since toxic reactions may occur rapidly
• For dry mouth, metallic taste, polyuria, bone pain, muscle weakness, headache, fatigue, tinnitus, change in LOC, irregular pulse, dysrhythmias, increased respirations, anorexia, nausea, vomiting, cramps, diarrhea, constipation; may indicate hypercalcemia
• Renal status: decreased urinary output (oliguria, anuria), edema in extremities, weight gain 5 lb, periorbital edema
• Nutritional status, diet for sources of vit D (milk, some seafood), calcium (dairy products, dark

◆ = Nursing alert   ◖ = Herb-drug interaction   ⊘ = Do not crush green vegetables), phosphates (dairy products)

Administer:

PO

• May be taken without regard to food

🚫 Do not break, crush, or chew caps

• May be increased q4wk depending on blood level

Perform/provide:

• Storage in tight, light-resistant container at room temperature

• Restriction of sodium, potassium if required; ensure adequate calcium intake

• Restriction of fluids if required for chronic renal failure

Evaluate:

• Therapeutic response: calcium levels 9-10 mg/dl, decreasing symptoms of bone disease

Teach patient/family:

• The symptoms of hypercalcemia

• About foods rich in calcium

• To advise prescriber of all other medications, supplements taken

---

calcitonin (human) (℞)

(kal-sih-toh′nin)

Cibacalcin

calcitonin (salmon) (℞)

Calcimir, Miacalcin, Miacalcin Nasal Spray, Osteocalcin, Salmonine

Func. class.: Parathyroid agents (calcium regulator)

Chem. class.: Polypeptide hormone

Action: Decreases bone resorption, blood calcium levels; increases deposits of calcium in bones; opposes parathyroid hormone

Uses: Paget's disease, postmenopausal osteoporosis, hypercalcemia

Dosage and routes:

Human

Paget's disease

• *Adult:* SC 0.5 mg/day initially; may require 0.5 mg bid × 6 mo, then decrease until symptoms reappear

Salmon

Postmenopausal osteoporosis

• *Adult:* SC/IM 100 IU/day; NASAL 200 IU (1 spray) qd alternating nostrils qd, activate pump before 1st dose

Paget's disease

• *Adult:* SC/IM 100 IU qd, maintenance 50-100 IU qd or qod

Hypercalcemia

• *Adult:* SC/IM 4 IU/kg q12h, increase to 8 IU/kg q6h if response is unsatisfactory

Available forms: Human: **INJ** (SC) 500 mg vial; *salmon:* **INJ** 100 IU, 200 IU/ml, **NASAL** spray 200 IU/actuation

Side effects/adverse reactions:

INTEG: Rash, flushing, pruritus of earlobes, edema of feet, reaction at inj site

CNS: Headache, tetany, chills, weakness, dizziness, fever

GU: Diuresis, nocturia, urine sediment, frequency

GI: Nausea, diarrhea, vomiting, anorexia, abdominal pain, salty taste, epigastric pain

MS: Swelling, tingling of hands

CV: Chest pressure

EENT: Nasal congestion, eye pain

RESP: Dyspnea

SYST: **Anaphylaxis**

Contraindications: Hypersensitivity

Precautions: Renal disease, children, lactation, osteogenic sarcoma, pregnancy (C), pernicious anemia

Pharmacokinetics:

IM/SC: Onset 15 min, peak 4 hr, duration 8-24 hr; metabolized by kidneys, excreted as inactive metabolites via kidneys

---

NURSING CONSIDERATIONS
Assess:
- GI symptoms, polyuria, flushing, head swelling, tingling, headache; may indicate hypercalcemia
- Nutritional status; diet for sources of vit D (milk, some seafood), calcium (dairy products, dark green vegetables), phosphates
- BUN, creatinine, uric acid, chloride, electrolytes, urine pH, urinary calcium, magnesium, phosphate, urinalysis (calcium should be kept at 9-10 mg/dl, vit D 50-135 IU/dl), alk phosphatase baseline, q3-6mo
- Increased drug level, since toxic reactions occur rapidly; have calcium chloride on hand if calcium level drops too low; check for tetany
- Urine for sediment

Administer:
Human
SC
- By SC route only; rotate injection sites; use within 6 hr of reconstitution; give hs to minimize nausea, vomiting

Salmon
IM
- After test dose of 10 IU/ml, 0.1 ml intradermally; watch 15 min; give only with epinephrine and emergency meds available
- IM injection slowly in deep muscle mass; rotate sites

Perform/provide:
- Storage at <77° F (25° C); protect from light

Evaluate:
- Therapeutic response: calcium levels 9-10 mg/dl, decreasing symptoms of Paget's disease

Teach patient/family:
- The method of injection if patient will be responsible for self-medication
- To report difficulty swallowing or any change in side effects to prescriber immediately

Nasal
- To use alternating nostrils for nasal spray

---

calcitriol (℞)
(kal-sih-try'ole)
Calcijex, Rocaltrol (1,25-dihydroxycholecalciferol), vitamin D₃
Func. class.: Parathyroid agent (calcium regulator)
Chem. class.: Vit D hormone

Action: Increases intestinal absorption of calcium, provides calcium for bones, increases renal tubular resorption of phosphate
Uses: Hypocalcemia in chronic renal disease, hypoparathyroidism pseudohypoparathyroidism
Dosage and routes:
- *Adult:* **IV** 0.5 µg tid, initially; may increase by 0.25-0.5 µg/dose q2-4wk; 0.5-3 µg tid maintenance

Predialysis
- *Adult:* **PO** 0.25 µg/day, max 0.5 µg/day
- *Child:* **PO** 0.25 µg/day, max 0.5 µg/day
- *Child <3 yr:* **PO** 10-15 µg/kg/day

Hypocalcemia during chronic dialysis
- *Adult:* **PO** 0.5-3 µg/day
- *Child:* **PO** 0.25-2 µg/day

Renal osteodystrophy
- *Adult:* **PO** 0.25 µg qod-3 µg/day
- *Child:* **PO** 0.014-0.041 µg/kg/day

Hypoparathyroidism
- *Adult:* **PO** 0.25-2.7 µg/day
- *Child:* **PO** 0.04-0.08 µg/kg/day

Available forms: Caps 0.25, 0.5 µg; inj 1 µg, 2 µg/ml
Side effects/adverse reactions:
CNS: Drowsiness, headache, vertigo, fever, lethargy
GI: Nausea, diarrhea, vomiting, jaundice, anorexia, dry mouth, constipation, cramps, metallic taste

---

◆ = Nursing alert   ◢ = Herb-drug interaction   ⊘ = Do not crush

MS: Myalgia, arthralgia, decreased bone development, weakness

GU: Polyuria, hypercalciuria, hyperphosphatemia, hematuria, thirst

EENT: Blurred vision, photophobia

CV: Palpitations

Contraindications: Hypersensitivity, hyperphosphatemia, hypercalcemia, vit D toxicity

Precautions: Pregnancy (C), renal calculi, lactation, CV disease

Do not confuse:
calcitriol/Calciferol

Pharmacokinetics:

PO: Absorbed readily from GI tract, peak 10-12 hr, duration 3-5 days, half-life 3-6 hr

Interactions:

• Decreased absorption of calcitriol: cholestyramine, mineral oil, fat-soluble vitamins

• Hypercalcemia: thiazide diuretics, calcium supplements

• Cardiac dysrhythmias: cardiac glycosides, verapamil

• Hypermagnesemia: magnesium antacids

• Increased metabolism of vit D: phenytoin

• Toxicity: other vit D products

• Drug/food: large amounts of high-calcium foods may cause hypercalcemia

Lab test interferences:

False increase: Cholesterol

Interfere: Alk phosphatase, electrolytes

NURSING CONSIDERATIONS

Assess:

• BUN, urinary calcium, AST, ALT, cholesterol, creatinine, albumin, uric acid, chloride, magnesium, electrolytes, urine pH, phosphate; may increase calcium, should be kept at 9-10 mg/dl, vit D 50-135 IU/dl, phosphate 70 mg/dl

• Alk phosphatase; may be decreased

• For increased drug level, since toxic reactions may occur rapidly

• For dry mouth, metallic taste, polyuria, bone pain, muscle weakness, headache, fatigue, change in LOC, dysrhythmias, increased respirations, anorexia, nausea, vomiting, cramps, diarrhea, constipation; may indicate hypercalcemia

• Renal status: decreased urinary output (oliguria, anuria), edema in extremities, weight gain 5-7 lb, periorbital edema

• Nutritional status, diet for sources of vit D (milk, some seafood); calcium (dairy products, dark green vegetables), phosphates (dairy products) must be avoided

Administer:

PO

• Give without regard to meals

IV

• Give by direct IV over 1 min

Perform/provide:

• Storage protected from light, heat, moisture

• Restriction of sodium, potassium if required

• Restriction of fluids if required for chronic renal failure

Evaluate:

• Therapeutic response: calcium 9-10 mg/dl, decreasing symptoms of hypocalcemia, hypoparathyroidism

Teach patient/family:

• The symptoms of hypercalcemia

• About foods rich in calcium

• To avoid products with sodium: cured meats, dairy products, cold cuts, olives, beets, pickles, soups, meat tenderizers in chronic renal failure

• To avoid products with potassium: oranges, bananas, dried fruit, peas, dark green leafy vegetables, milk, melons, beans in chronic renal failure

• To avoid OTC products containing calcium, potassium, or sodium in chronic renal failure

• To avoid all preparations containing vit D

• To monitor weight weekly

🚫 Not to break, crush, or chew caps

---

calcium carbonate
(PO-OTC, IV-℞)

Alka-Mints, Amitone, Apo-Cal*, BioCal, Calcarb, Calci-Chew, Calci-Mix, Calcilac, Calcite*, Calglycine*, Cal-Plus, Calsan*, Caltrate 600, Caltrate Jr., Chooz, Dicarbosil, Equilet, Gencalc, Liquid-Cal, Liquid-Cal-600, Maalox Antacid Caplets, Mallamint, Mylanta Lozenges*, Nephro-Calci, Nu-Cal*, Os-Cal 500, Oysco 500, Oystercal 500, Oyst-Cal 500, Rolaids Calcium Rich, Titralac, Tums, Tums E-X Extra Strength

Func. class.: Antacid, calcium supplement

Chem. class.: Calcium product

Action: Neutralizes gastric acidity

Uses: Antacid, calcium supplement; not suitable for chronic therapy

Dosage and routes:

Antacid

• *Adult:* **PO** 350 mg-1.5 g or 2 pieces of gum 1 hr pc and hs

Osteoporosis

• *Adult:* **PO** 1-2 g bid-tid

Available forms: Chewable tabs 350, 420, 500, 750, 850, 1000, 1250 mg; tabs 500, 600, 650, 1000, 1250 mg; gum 500 mg; susp 1250 mg/5 ml; lozenges 600 mg

Side effects/adverse reactions:

GI: Constipation, anorexia, nausea,

vomiting, flatulence, diarrhea, rebound hyperacidity, eructation

Contraindications: Hypersensitivity, hypercalcemia, hyperparathyroidism, bone tumors

Precautions: Elderly, fluid restriction, decreased GI motility, GI obstruction, dehydration, renal disease, pregnancy (C), lactation

Pharmacokinetics: ⅓ of dose absorbed by small intestine, onset 20 min, duration 20-180 min, excreted in feces and urine, crosses placenta

Interactions:

• Increased plasma levels of quinidine, amphetamines

• Decreased levels of salicylates, calcium channel blockers, ketoconazole, tetracyclines, iron salts

🌿 Increased action/side effects: lily of the valley, pheasant's eye, squill

NURSING CONSIDERATIONS

Assess:

• Ca^+ (serum, urine), Ca^+ should be 8.5-10.5 mg/dl, urine Ca^+ should be 150 mg/day, monitor weekly

◆ Milk-alkali syndrome: nausea, vomiting, disorientation, headache

• Constipation; increase bulk in the diet if needed

• Hypercalcemia: headache, nausea, vomiting, confusion

Administer:

PO

• As antacid 1 hr pc and hs

• As supplement 1½ hr pc and hs

• Only with regular tablets or capsules; do not give with enteric-coated tablets

• Laxatives or stool softeners if constipation occurs

Evaluate:

• Therapeutic response: absence of pain, decreased acidity

Teach patient/family:

• To increase fluids to 2 L unless contraindicated, to add bulk to diet for constipation, notify prescriber of constipation

---

◆ = Nursing alert   🌿 = Herb-drug interaction   🚫 = Do not crush

- Not to switch antacids unless directed by prescriber, not to use as antacid for >2 wk without approval by prescriber
- That therapeutic dose recommendations are figured as elemental calcium

calcium chloride
calcium gluceptate
calcium gluconate
calcium lactate (℞)
Func. class.: Electrolyte replacement—calcium product

Action: Cation needed for maintenance of nervous, muscular, skeletal function, enzyme reactions, normal cardiac contractility, coagulation of blood; affects secretory activity of endocrine, exocrine glands

Uses: Prevention and treatment of hypocalcemia, hypermagnesemia, hypoparathyroidism, neonatal tetany, cardiac toxicity caused by hyperkalemia, lead colic, hyperphosphatemia, vit D deficiency

Dosage and routes:

Calcium chloride
- *Adult:* **IV** 500 mg-1 g q1-3d as indicated by serum calcium levels, give at <1 ml/min; **IV** 200-800 mg injected in ventricle of heart
- *Child:* **IV** 25 mg/kg over several min

Calcium gluconate
- *Adult:* **PO** 0.5-2 g bid-qid; **IV** 0.5-2 g at 0.5 ml/min (10% solution)
- *Child:* **PO/IV** 500 mg/kg/day in divided doses

Calcium lactate
- *Adult:* **PO** 325 mg-1.3 g tid with meals
- *Child:* **PO** 500 mg/kg/day in divided doses

Available forms: Many; check product listings

Side effects/adverse reactions:
INTEG: Pain, burning at IV site, severe venous thrombosis, necrosis, extravasation
HYPERCALCEMIA: Drowsiness, lethargy, muscle weakness, headache, constipation, ***coma,*** anorexia, nausea, vomiting, polyuria, thirst
CV: Shortened QT, heart block, hypotension, bradycardia, ***dysrhythmias; cardiac arrest (IV)***
GI: Vomiting, nausea, constipation
Contraindications: Hypercalcemia, digitalis toxicity, ventricular fibrillation, renal calculi
Precautions: Pregnancy (C), lactation, children, renal disease, respiratory disease, cor pulmonale, digitalized patient, respiratory failure
Pharmacokinetics: Crosses placenta, enters breast milk, excreted via urine and feces; half-life unknown
PO: Onset, peak, duration unknown; absorption (PO) from GI tract
IV: Onset immediate, duration ½-2 hr
Interactions:
- Increased dysrhythmias: digitalis glycosides
- Increased action/side effects: lily of the valley, pheasant's eye, squill
Lab test interferences:
Increase: 11-OHCS
False decrease: Magnesium
Decrease: 17-OHCS
NURSING CONSIDERATIONS
Assess:
- ECG for decreased QT and T wave inversion: hypercalcemia, drug should be reduced or discontinued, consider cardiac monitoring
- Calcium levels during treatment (8.5-11.5 g/dl is normal level)
- Cardiac status: rate, rhythm, CVP, (PWP, PAWP if monitored directly)

Administer:
PO
• With or following meals to enhance absorption
IM
• IM injection may cause severe burning, necrosis, tissue sloughing; warm sol to body temp before administering (only gluconate/gluceptate)
IV
• Undiluted or diluted with equal amounts of NS to a 5% sol for inj, give 0.5-1 ml/min
• Through small-bore needle into large vein; if extravasation occurs, necrosis will result (IV)

Calcium chloride
Additive compatibilities: Amikacin, ascorbic acid, bretylium, cephapirin, chloramphenicol, dopamine, hydrocortisone, isoproterenol, lidocaine, methicillin, norepinephrine, penicillin G potassium, penicillin G sodium, pentobarbital, phenobarbital, sodium bicarbonate, verapamil, vit B/C

Syringe compatibilities: Milrinone

Y-site compatibilities: Amrinone, dobutamine, epinephrine, esmolol, morphine, paclitaxel

Calcium gluceptate
Additive compatibilities: Ascorbic acid injection, isoproterenol, lidocaine, norepinephrine, phytonadione, sodium bicarbonate

Calcium gluconate
Additive compatibilities: Amikacin, aminophylline, ascorbic acid injection, bretylium, cephapirin, chloramphenicol, cisatracurium, corticotropin, dimenhydrinate, doxorubicin liposome, erythromycin, furosemide, heparin, hydrocortisone, lidocaine, magnesium sulfate, methicillin, norepinephrine, penicillin G potassium, penicillin G sodium, phenobarbital, potassium chloride,

remifentanil, tobramycin, vancomycin, verapamil, vit B/C

Syringe compatibilities: Aldesleukin, allopurinol, amifostine, aztreonam, cefazolin, cefepime, ciprofloxacin, cladribine, dobutamine, enalaprilat, epinephrine, famotidine, filgrastim, granisetron, heparin/hydrocortisone, labetalol, melphalan, midazolam, netilmicin, piperacillin/tazobactam, potassium chloride, prochlorperazine, propofol, sargramostim, tacrolimus, teniposide, thiotepa, tolazoline, vinorelbine, vit B/C

Perform/provide:
• Seizure precautions: padded side rails, decreased stimuli (noise, light); place airway suction equipment, padded mouth gag if Ca levels are low
• Store at room temperature

Evaluate:
• Therapeutic response: decreased twitching, paresthesias, muscle spasms, absence of tremors, convulsions, dysrhythmias, dyspnea, laryngospasm, negative Chvostek's sign, negative Trousseau's sign

Teach patient/family:
• To remain recumbent ½ hr after IV dose
• To add foods high in vit D
• To add calcium-rich foods to diet: dairy products, shellfish, dark green leafy vegetables; decrease oxalate-rich and zinc-rich foods: nuts, legumes, chocolate, spinach, soy
• To prevent injuries, avoid immobilization

◆ = Nursing alert   ∅ = Herb-drug interaction   ⊘ = Do not crush

calcium polycarbophil (OTC)

(pol-ee-kar′boe-fil)
Equalactin, Fiberall, FiberCon, Fiber-Lax, Mitrolan
Func. class.: Laxative
Chem. class.: Bulk-forming

Action: Attracts water, expands in intestine to increase peristalsis; also absorbs excess water in stool; decreases diarrhea

Uses: Constipation, irritable bowel syndrome (diarrhea), acute, nonspecific diarrhea

Dosage and routes:
• *Adult:* **PO** 1 g qd-qid prn, not to exceed 6 g/24 hr
• *Child 6-12 yr:* **PO** 500 mg bid prn, not to exceed 3 g/24 hr
• *Child 3-6 yr:* **PO** 500 mg bid prn, not to exceed 1.5 g/24 hr
Available forms: Chew tabs 500, 1000 mg; tabs 500 mg

Side effects/adverse reactions:
GI: **Obstruction**, abdominal distention, flatus, laxative dependence

Contraindications: Hypersensitivity, GI obstruction

Precautions: Pregnancy (C), lactation

Pharmacokinetics:
PO: Onset 12-24 min, peak 1-3 days

Interactions:
🖊 Increased action/side effects: lily of the valley, pheasant's eye, squill

NURSING CONSIDERATIONS
Assess:
• Cause of constipation; identify whether fluids, bulk, or exercise is missing from lifestyle
• Cramping, rectal bleeding, nausea, vomiting; if these symptoms occur, drug should be discontinued

Administer:
PO
• Alone for better absorption; do not take within 1 hr of other drugs
• In morning or evening (oral dose)
Evaluate:
• Therapeutic response: decreased constipation
Teach patient/family:
• Not to use laxatives for long-term therapy; laxative dependence will result
• That normal bowel movements do not always occur daily
• Not to use in presence of abdominal pain, nausea, vomiting
• To notify prescriber if constipation is unrelieved or if symptoms of electrolyte imbalance occur: muscle cramps, pain, weakness, dizziness
• To chew thoroughly (chew tab) and follow with 6-8 oz water

calfactant (℞)

(cal-fak′tant)
Infasurf
Func. class.: Natural lung surfactant extract

Action: Replenishes surfactant and restores surface activity to the lungs in premature infants

Uses: Prevention and treatment (rescue) of respiratory distress syndrome in premature infants

Dosage and routes:
• Newborn: **INTRATRACHEAL INSTILL:** 3 ml/kg of birth wt, given as 2 doses of 1.5 ml/kg, repeat doses of 3 ml/kg of birth wt until up to 3 doses 12 hr apart have been given
Available forms: Susp 35 mg phospholipids/ml in 0.9% NaCl with 0.65 mg proteins in single-use vials containing 6 ml susp

Side effects/adverse reactions:
Concurrent illnesses that have occurred during treatment are in bold
*RESP: **Pulmonary air leaks, pulmonary interstitial emphysema, apnea, pulmonary hemorrhage***
*SYST: **Patent ductus arteriosus, intracranial hemorrhage, severe intracranial hemorrhage, necrotizing enterocolitis, posttreatment sepsis, posttreatment infection**,* bradycardia, oxygen desaturation, pallor, vasoconstriction, hypotension, hypertension

Precautions: Bradycardia, rales, infections

Pharmacokinetics: Becomes lung associated within hours of administration

NURSING CONSIDERATIONS
Assess:
• Respiratory rate, rhythm, character, chest expansion, color, transcutaneous saturation, ABGs
• Endotracheal tube placement before dosing; for apnea after endotracheal administration
• Reflux of drug into the endotracheal tube during administration; stop drug if this occurs, and if needed, increase peak inspiratory pressure on the ventilator by 4-5 cm H_2O until tube is cleared
• Infant for repeat dosing using radiographic confirmation of RDS; repeat doses should be given as above; ventilator settings for repeat doses FIo_2 were decreased by 0.2 or amount to prevent cyanosis; ventilator rate of 30/min; inspiratory time <1 sec; if infant's pretreatment rate was >30, it was left unchanged during dosing; resume usual ventilator management after dosing

Administer:
• After suctioning
• By endotracheal administration only by persons trained in neonatal intubation and ventilation
• After using a No. 5 Fr end-hole catheter inserted into the endotracheal tube with the tip protruding just beyond the end of the endotracheal tube; shorten the catheter before insertion; do not insert the drug into the mainstem bronchus
• Divide doses and administer with infant in different positions
• Determine dosing by weight of infant; slowly withdraw contents into plastic syringe through 20G needle; do not filter or shake; attach premeasured No. 5 Fr catheter to syringe; fill with drug and discard excess through catheter so only dose to be given remains in syringe
• For prevention dosing, stabilize, weigh, and intubate infant; give drug within 15 min of birth if possible; position infant and inject first dose through catheter over 2-3 sec; remove catheter and manually ventilate with O_2 to prevent cyanosis (60 bpm) and sufficient positive pressure to promote adequate air exchange and chest wall excursion
• For rescue dosing, give dosing as soon as infant is placed on ventilator after birth; immediately before administering dose, change ventilator settings to 60/min, inspiratory time 0.5 sec, FIo_2 1; position infant and inject first dose through catheter over 2-3 sec; remove catheter; return to mechanical ventilator
• Ventilate infant for >30 sec or until stable after prevention or rescue strategy; reposition for next dose; same procedure for subsequent dosing; do not suction for at least 1 hr after dosing unless airway obstruction is evident; resume ventilator therapy after dosing

Perform/provide:
• Reduction in peak ventilator inspiratory pressures immediately if chest expansion improves substantially after dose

• Reduction in FIo$_2$ in small, repeated steps when infant becomes pink and transcutaneous oxygen saturation is in excess of 95%; oxygen saturation should remain between 90% and 95%
• Suctioning of all infants before administration to prevent mucus plugging; if endotracheal tube obstruction is suspected, remove obstruction and replace tube immediately
• Storage in refrigerator; protect from light; warm to room temperature for >20 min or warm in hand >8 min before giving; do not use artificial warming methods; enter a vial only once; unopened, unused vials that have been warmed to room temperature may be rerefrigerated within 8 hr of warming; do not warm and return to refrigerator more than once

Evaluate:
• Therapeutic response: significant improvement in respiratory status

---

candesartan (R)

(can-deh-sar′tan)
Atacand
Func. class.: Antihypertensive
Chem. class.: Angiotensin II receptor (type AT$_1$)

Action: Blocks the vasoconstrictor and aldosterone-secreting effects of angiotensin II; selectively blocks the binding of angiotensin II to the AT$_1$ receptor found in tissues
Uses: Hypertension, alone or in combination

Dosage and routes:
• *Adult:* **PO,** single agent 16 mg qd initially in patients who are not volume depleted, range 8-32 mg/day; with diuretic, or volume depletion

2-32 mg/day as single dose or divided bid
Available forms: Tabs 4, 8, 16, 32 mg
Side effects/adverse reactions:
CNS: Dizziness, fatigue, headache
GI: Diarrhea, nausea, abdominal pain, vomiting
MS: Arthralgia, pain
RESP: Cough, upper respiratory infection
*SYST: **Angioedema***
CV: Chest pain, peripheral edema
EENT: Sinusitis, rhinitis, pharyngitis

Contraindications: Hypersensitivity, pregnancy (D) 2nd and 3rd trimesters
Precautions: Hypersensitivity to ACE inhibitors; pregnancy (C) 1st trimester, lactation; children; elderly
Pharmacokinetics: Extensively metabolized, excreted in urine and feces

NURSING CONSIDERATIONS
Assess:
• For pregnancy, this drug can cause fetal death when given in pregnancy
• Response and adverse reactions especially in renal disease
• For severe hypotension, place supine, give 0.9% NaCl IV for volume depletion
• B/P, pulse q4h; note rate, rhythm, quality; electrolytes: K, Na, Cl; baselines in renal, liver function tests before therapy begins
• Skin turgor, dryness of mucous membranes for hydration status; for angioedema: facial swelling, dyspnea
Administer:
• Without regard to meals
Evaluate:
• Therapeutic response: decreased B/P
Teach patient/family:
• To comply with dosage schedule, even if feeling better

• To notify prescriber of mouth sores, fever, swelling of hands or feet, irregular heartbeat, chest pain
• That excessive perspiration, dehydration, vomiting, diarrhea may lead to fall in blood pressure; to consult prescriber if these occur
• That drug may cause dizziness, fainting; light-headedness may occur
• To rise slowly to sitting or standing position to minimize orthostatic hypotension
• To notify prescriber immediately if pregnant; not to use during lactation
• To avoid all OTC medications, unless approved by prescriber
• To inform all health-care providers of medication use
• To use proper technique for obtaining B/P and acceptable parameters

---

capecitabine (℞)

(cap-eh-sit'ah-bean)

Xeloda

Func. class.: Antineoplastic, antimetabolite

Chem. class.: Fluoropyrimidine carbamate

Action: Competes with physiologic substrate of DNA synthesis, thus interfering with cell replication in the S phase of cell cycle (before mitosis); drug is converted to 5-FU

Uses: Metastatic breast, colorectal cancer

Dosage and routes:
• *Adult:* **PO** 2500 mg/m^2/day in 2 divided doses q12h at end of meal × 2 wk, then 1 wk rest period; given in 3 wk cycles

Available forms: Tabs 150, 500 mg

Side effects/adverse reactions:

HEMA: **Neutropenia, lymphopenia,** **thrombocytopenia, myelosuppression,** anemia

GI: Nausea, vomiting, anorexia, diarrhea, stomatitis, abdominal pain, constipation, anorexia, dyspepsia, *intestinal obstruction*

OTHER: Hyperbilirubinemia, eye irritation, pyrexia, edema, myalgia, limb pain, *pyrexia,* dehydration

INTEG: **Hand and foot syndrome, dermatitis,** nail disorder

CNS: Dizziness, headache, *paresthesia, fatigue,* insomnia

Contraindications: Hypersensitivity to 5-FU, infants, pregnancy (D), severe renal impairment (CrCl <30 ml/min)

Precautions: Renal disease, hepatic disease, lactation, children, elderly

Pharmacokinetics: Readily absorbed, peak 1½ hr; food decreases absorption; extensively metabolized in the liver; elimination half-life 45 min

Interactions:
• Increased toxicity: leucovorin
• Increased capecitabine levels: antacids
• Increased risk of bleeding: warfarin

NURSING CONSIDERATIONS

Assess:
• CBC (RBC, Hct, Hgb), differential, platelet count weekly; withhold drug if WBC is <4000/mm^3, platelet count is <75,000/mm^3, or RBC, Hct, Hgb low; notify prescriber of these results
• Renal function studies: BUN, serum uric acid, urine creatinine clearance, electrolytes before and during therapy
• Monitor temp q4h; fever may indicate beginning infection; no rectal temps
• Liver function tests before and during therapy: bilirubin, ALT, AST, alk phosphatase, as needed or monthly

---

◆ = Nursing alert   ⫙ = Herb-drug interaction   ⊘ = Do not crush

- Bleeding: hematuria, heme-positive stools, bruising or pete-chiae, mucosa or orifices q8h
- Dyspnea, rales, unproductive cough, chest pain, tachypnea, fatigue, increased pulse, pallor, lethargy; personality changes, with high doses
- Edema in feet, joint pain, stomach pain, shaking
- For hand and foot syndrome: paresthesia, tingling, painful/painless swelling, blistering, erythema with severe pain of hands or feet
- For toxicity: severe diarrhea, nausea, vomiting, stomatitis
- Buccal cavity q8h for dryness, sores or ulceration, white patches, oral pain, bleeding, dysphagia
- GI symptoms: frequency of stools, cramping, if severe diarrhea occurs, fluid and electrolytes may need to be given

Administer:
- Antiemetic 30-60 min before giving drug and prn

Perform/provide:
- Rinsing of mouth tid-qid with water, club soda; brushing of teeth bid-tid with soft brush or cotton-tipped applicators for stomatitis; use un-waxed dental floss

Evaluate:
- Therapeutic response: decreased tumor size, spread of malignancy

Teach patient/family:
- To avoid foods with citric acid, hot or rough texture if stomatitis is present
- To avoid pregnancy while on this drug; to avoid using while lactating
- Not to double dose, if dose is missed
- ◆ To immediately report severe diarrhea, vomiting, stomatitis, fever over 100° F (37.8° C), hand and foot syndrome, anorexia
- To report signs of infection: increased temp, sore throat, flulike symptoms
- To report signs of anemia: fatigue, headache, faintness, shortness of breath, irritability
- To report bleeding; to avoid use of razors, commercial mouthwash

---

captopril (℞)
(kap'toe-pril)
Capoten, Novo-Captoril*
Func. class.: Antihypertensive
Chem. class.: Angiotensin-con-verting enzyme inhibitor (ACE)

Action: Selectively suppresses renin-angiotensin-aldosterone system; inhibits ACE; preventing conversion of angiotensin I to angiotensin II
Uses: Hypertension, CHF, left ventricular dysfunction after MI, diabetic nephropathy
Dosage and routes:
Malignant hypertension
- *Adult:* **PO** 25 mg increasing q2h until desired response, not to exceed 450 mg/day
Hypertension
- *Adult:* **PO** initial dose: 25 mg bid-tid; may increase to 50 mg bid-tid at 1-2 wk intervals; usual range: 25-150 mg bid-tid; max 450 mg
- *Child:* **PO** 0.3-0.5 mg/kg/dose, titrate up to 6 mg/kg/day in 2-4 divided doses
- *Neonate:* **PO** 10 µg (0.01 mg)/kg bid-tid, may increase as needed
CHF
- *Adult:* **PO** 12.5 mg bid-tid; may increase to 50 mg bid-tid; after 14 days, may increase to 150 mg tid if needed
LVD after MI
- *Adult:* **PO** 50 mg tid, may begin treatment 3 days after MI; give 6.25 mg as a single dose, then 12.5 mg

tid, increase to 25 mg tid for several days, then to 50 mg tid

Diabetic nephropathy
• *Adult:* **PO** 25 mg tid

Renal dose
• *Adult:* **PO** 6.25-12.5 mg bid-tid
• *Child:* **PO** 150 μg (0.15)/kg tid

Available forms: Tabs 12.5, 25, 50, 100 mg

Side effects/adverse reactions:

CV: Hypotension, postural hypotension, *tachycardia,* angina

GU: Impotence, dysuria, nocturia, proteinuria, **nephrotic syndrome, acute reversible renal failure,** polyuria, oliguria, urinary frequency

HEMA: **Neutropenia, agranulocytosis, pancytopenia, thrombocytopenia,** anemia

INT: Rash, *angioedema*

RESP: **Bronchospasm,** *dyspnea, cough*

GI: Loss of taste, increased LFTs

CNS: Fever, chills

MISC: **Angioedema,** hyperkalemia

Contraindications: Hypersensitivity, lactation, heart block, children, potassium-sparing diuretics, bilateral renal artery stenosis

Precautions: Dialysis patients, hypovolemia, leukemia, scleroderma, SLE, blood dyscrasias, CHF, diabetes mellitus, renal disease, thyroid disease, COPD, asthma, pregnancy (C)

Pharmacokinetics:

PO: Peak 1 hr; duration 6-12 hr; half-life 6-7 hr; metabolized by liver (metabolites), excreted in urine; crosses placenta; excreted in breast milk

Interactions:

• Increased hypotension: diuretics, other antihypertensives, phenothiazines, nitrates, acute alcohol ingestion
• Decreased captopril effect: antacids, NSAIDs
• Possible toxicity: lithium, digoxin
• Hypoglycemia: insulin, oral antidiabetics
• Do not use with potassium-sparing diuretics, sympathomimetics, potassium supplements
• Drug/food: decreased perindopril to perindoprilat conversion

Lab test interferences:

False positive: Urine acetone, ANA titer

NURSING CONSIDERATIONS

Assess:

• Blood studies: decreased platelets; WBC with diff baseline and periodically q3mo, if neutrophils <1000/mm^3, discontinue treatment
• B/P, pulse rates baseline, frequently
• Renal studies: protein, BUN, creatinine; watch for increased levels that may indicate nephrotic syndrome
• Baselines in renal, liver function tests before therapy begins and periodically, increased LFTs, uric acid and glucose may be increased
• Edema in feet, legs daily, weight daily in CHF
• Allergic reaction: rash, fever, pruritus, urticaria; drug should be discontinued if antihistamines fail to help
• Symptoms of CHF: edema, dyspnea, wet rales, B/P

Administer:

• 1 hr ac or 1½ hr pc

Perform/provide:

• Storage in tight container at 86° F (30° C) or less

Evaluate:

• Therapeutic response: decrease in B/P in hypertension, edema, moist rales (CHF)

Teach patient/family:

• That tabs may be crushed and mixed with food; to take 1 hr before meals or 1½ hr pc; not to discontinue drug abruptly

---

◆ = Nursing alert   🍃 = Herb-drug interaction   🚫 = Do not crush

- Not to use OTC products (cough, cold, or allergy) unless directed by prescriber
- To avoid sunlight or wear sunscreen if in sunlight; photosensitivity may occur
- To comply with dosage schedule, even if feeling better
- To rise slowly to sitting or standing position to minimize orthostatic hypotension
- To notify prescriber of mouth sores, sore throat, fever, swelling of hands or feet, irregular heartbeat, chest pain, signs of angioedema
- That excessive perspiration, dehydration, vomiting; diarrhea may lead to fall in blood pressure; consult prescriber if these occur
- That dizziness, fainting, lightheadedness may occur during first few days of therapy
- That skin rash or impaired perspiration may occur
- How to take B/P and when to notify prescriber
- To report if pregnancy is suspected or planned

Treatment of overdose: 0.9% NaCl IV/INF; hemodialysis

---

carbamazepine (℞)

(kar-ba-maz′e-peen)
Apo-Carbamazepine*,
Atretol, Carbatrol, Epitol,
Novo-Carbamaz*, Tegretol,
Tegretol CR*, Tegretol-XR
Func. class.: Anticonvulsant
Chem. class.: Iminostilbene derivative

Action: Inhibits nerve impulses by limiting influx of sodium ions across cell membrane in motor cortex

Uses: Tonic-clonic, complex-partial, mixed seizures; trigeminal neuralgia, diabetic neuropathy

Investigational uses: Diabetes insipidus, bipolar disorder, neurogenic pain, schizophrenia, psychotic behavior with dementia, rectal administration

Dosage and routes:
Seizures
- *Adult and child >12 yr:* **PO** 200 mg bid, may be increased by 200 mg/day in divided doses q6-8h; maintenance 800-1200 mg/day maximum 1200 mg/day; adjustment is needed to minimum dose to control seizures; ext rel give bid; rectal administration of oral susp 200 mg/10 ml or 6 mg/kg as a single dose
- *Child 6-12 yr:* **PO** tabs 100 mg bid or susp 50 mg qid; may increase by 100 mg qwk; ext rel tabs qd-bid
- *Child <6 yr:* **PO** 10-20 mg/kg/day in 2-3 divided doses, may increase by 100 mg/day qwk

Trigeminal neuralgia
- *Adult:* **PO** 100 mg bid with meals; may increase 100 mg q12h until pain subsides, not to exceed 1.2 g/day; maintenance is 200-400 mg bid

Available forms: Tabs, chewable 100, 200 mg; tabs 200 mg; ext-rel tabs 100, 200, 400 mg; oral susp 100 mg/5 ml

Side effects/adverse reactions:
*HEMA: **Thrombocytopenia, agranulocytosis, leukocytosis, neutropenia, aplastic anemia, eosinophilia,*** increased PT
ENDO: SIADH (elderly)
CNS: Drowsiness, dizziness, confusion, fatigue, ***paralysis,*** headache, hallucinations, ***worsening of seizures***
GI: Nausea, constipation, diarrhea, anorexia, vomiting, abdominal pain, stomatitis, glossitis, increased liver enzymes, ***hepatitis***
*INTEG: Rash, **Stevens-Johnson syndrome,*** urticaria

EENT: Tinnitus, dry mouth, blurred vision, diplopia, nystagmus, conjunctivitis

CV: **Hypertension, CHF, dysrhythmias, AV block,** hypotension, aggravation of cardiac artery disease

RESP: Pulmonary hypersensitivity (fever, dyspnea, pneumonitis)

GU: Frequency, retention, albuminuria, glycosuria, impotence, increased BUN

Contraindications: Hypersensitivity to carbamazepine or tricyclics, bone marrow depression, concomitant use of MAOIs

Precautions: Glaucoma, hepatic disease, renal disease, cardiac disease, psychosis, pregnancy (C), lactation, child <6 yr

Do not confuse:

Tegretol/Toradol

Pharmacokinetics:

PO: Onset slow, peak 4-8 hr; metabolized by liver; excreted in urine, feces; crosses placenta, blood-brain barrier; excreted in breast milk; half-life 14-16 hr

Interactions:

• CNS toxicity: lithium

• Increased carbamazepine levels: cimetidine, clarithromycin, danazol, diltiazem, erythromycin, fluoxetine, fluvoxamine, isoniazid, propoxyphene, valproic acid, verapamil

• Decreased effects of benzodiazepines, doxycycline, felbamate, haloperidol, oral contraceptives, phenobarbital, phenytoin, primidone, theophylline, thyroid hormones, warfarin

• Increased effects of desmopressin, lithium, lypressin, vasopressin

◆ Fatal reaction: MAOIs

🖊 Increased peak concentration of carbamazepine: grapefruit juice

🖊 Decreased carbamazepine metabolism, increased levels: quinine

NURSING CONSIDERATIONS

Assess:

• Renal studies: urinalysis, BUN, urine creatinine q3mo

◆ Blood studies: RBC, Hct, Hgb, reticulocyte counts qwk for 4 wk then qmo; if myelosuppression occurs, drug should be discontinued

• Hepatic studies: ALT, AST, bilirubin

• Drug levels during initial treatment or when changing dose; should remain at 4-12 µg/ml; anorexia may indicate increased blood levels

• Description of seizures: frequency, duration, aura

• Mental status: mood, sensorium, affect, behavioral changes; if mental status changes, notify prescriber

• Eye problems: need for ophthalmic examinations before, during, after treatment (slit lamp, fundoscopy, tonometry)

• Allergic reaction: purpura, red, raised rash; if these occur, drug should be discontinued

◆ Blood dyscrasias: fever, sore throat, bruising, rash, jaundice

◆ Toxicity: bone marrow depression, nausea, vomiting, ataxia, diplopia, cardiovascular collapse, Stevens-Johnson syndrome

Administer:

PO

• With food, milk to decrease GI symptoms

🚫 Do not crush, break, or chew ext rel product

• Chewable tabs; tell patient to chew tab, not swallow it whole

• Shake oral susp before use

• Mix an equal amount of water, D_5W, 0.9% NaCl when giving by NG tube, flush tube with 100 ml of above sol

Perform/provide:

• Storage at room temperature

• Hard candy, gum, frequent rinsing for dry mouth

◆ = Nursing alert   🖊 = Herb-drug interaction   🚫 = Do not crush

• Assistance with ambulation during early part of treatment; dizziness occurs
Evaluate:
• Therapeutic response: decreased seizure activity, document on patient's chart
Teach patient/family:
• To carry Medic Alert ID stating patient's name, drugs taken, condition, prescriber's name, phone number
• To avoid driving, other activities that require alertness usually the first 3 days of treatment
• Not to discontinue medication quickly after long-term use
• That urine may turn pink to brown
Treatment of overdose: Lavage, VS

---

carbidopa-levodopa (℞)

(kar-bi-doe'pa) (lee-voe-doe'pa)
carbidopa/levodopa,
Sinemet, Sinemet CR
Func. class.: Antiparkinson agent
Chem. class.: Catecholamine

Action: Decarboxylation of levodopa to periphery is inhibited by carbidopa; more levodopa is made available for transport to brain and conversion to dopamine in the brain
Uses: Parkinson's disease, parkinsonism resulting from carbon monoxide, chronic manganese intoxication, cerebral arteriosclerosis, restless leg syndrome
Dosage and routes:
Beginning therapy for those not taking levodopa
• *Adult:* **PO** 10 mg carbidopa/100 mg levodopa tid-qid or 25 mg carbidopa/100 mg levodopa tid, may increase qd to desired response

For those not taking levodopa ER
50 mg carbidopa/200 mg levodopa bid
For those taking levodopa ER
Begin treatment with 10% more levodopa/day given q4-8h, may increase or decrease dose q3d
For those taking levodopa <1.5 g/day
• *Adult:* **PO** 25 mg carbidopa/100 mg levodopa tid-qid, may increase qd to desired response
For those taking levodopa >1.5 g/day
• *Adult:* **PO** 25 mg carbidopa/250 mg levodopa tid-qid, may increase qd to desired response
Available forms: Tabs 10/100, 25/100, 25 mg carbidopa/250 mg levodopa; ext rel tab: 25 mg/100 mg, 50 mg/200 mg carbidopa/levodopa (Sinemet CR)
Side effects/adverse reactions:
HEMA: **Hemolytic anemia, leukopenia, agranulocytosis**
CNS: Involuntary choreiform movements, hand tremors, fatigue, headache, anxiety, twitching, numbness, weakness, confusion, agitation, insomnia, nightmares, psychosis, hallucination, hypomania, severe depression, dizziness
GI: Nausea, vomiting, anorexia, abdominal distress, dry mouth, flatulence, dysphagia, bitter taste, diarrhea, constipation
INTEG: Rash, sweating, alopecia
CV: Orthostatic hypotension, tachycardia, hypertension, palpitation
EENT: Blurred vision, diplopia, dilated pupils
MISC: Urinary retention, incontinence, weight change, dark urine
Contraindications: Hypersensitivity, narrow-angle glaucoma, malignant melanoma, history of malignant melanoma or undiagnosed skin lesions resembling melanoma

---

Precautions: Renal disease, wide-angle glaucoma, cardiac disease, hepatic disease, respiratory disease, MI with dysrhythmias, convulsions, peptic ulcer, pregnancy (C), lactation

Pharmacokinetics:

PO: Peak 1-3 hr, excreted in urine (metabolites)

Interactions:
• Hypertensive crisis: MAOIs
• Decreased effects of levodopa: anticholinergics, hydantoins, papaverine, pyridoxine, benzodiazepines
• Increased effects of levodopa: antacids, metoclopramide
• Drug/food: increased pyridoxine will decrease levodopa effect
• Decreased absorption of levodopa: protein
🍃 Decreased action, increased EPS: Indian snakeroot
🍃 Increased Parkinson symptoms: kava

Lab test interferences:
False positive: Urine ketones, Coombs' test
False negative: Urine glucose
False increase: Uric acid, urine protein
Decrease: VMA, BUN, creatinine

NURSING CONSIDERATIONS

Assess:
• B/P, respiration; orthostatic B/P
• Mental status: affect, mood, behavioral changes, depression, complete suicide assessment
• Muscle twitching, blepharospasm that may indicate toxicity
• Renal, liver, hematopoietic tests, also for diabetes, acromegaly if on long-term therapy

Administer:

PO
• Drug until NPO before surgery
• Adjust dosage to response
• With meals if GI symptoms occur; limit protein taken with drug

• Only after MAOIs have been discontinued for 2 wk; if previously on levodopa, discontinue for at least 8 hr before change to carbidopa-levodopa

Perform/provide:
• Assistance with ambulation during beginning therapy

Evaluate:
• Therapeutic response: decrease in akathisia, improved mood

Teach patient/family:
🚫 Not to crush or chew cont rel tabs; may be broken in half
• To change positions slowly to prevent orthostatic hypotension
• To report side effects: twitching, eye spasms; indicate overdose
• To use drug exactly as prescribed; if discontinued abruptly, parkinsonian crisis may occur; prescriber may recommend drug-free holidays
• That urine, sweat may darken
• To use physical activities to maintain mobility, lessen spasms
• That improvement may not occur for 3-4 mo

---

carboplatin (℞)

(kar-boe-pla'-tin)
Paraplatin, Paraplatin-AQ*

Func. class.: Antineoplastic alkylating agent

Chem. class.: Platinum coordination compound

Action: Produces interstrand DNA cross-links and, to a lesser extent, DNA-protein cross-links; activity is not cell cycle phase specific

Uses: Initial treatment of advanced ovarian cancer in combination with other agents; palliative treatment of ovarian carcinoma recurrent after treatment with other antineoplastic agents

---

◆ = Nursing alert   🍃 = Herb-drug interaction   🚫 = Do not crush

Dosage and routes (single agent):
• *Adult:* IV INF initially 300 mg/m^2 given with cyclophosphamide, q4-6wk; refractory tumors 360 mg/m^2 single dose, may repeat q4wk, as needed

Renal dose
CrCl 41-59 ml/min 250 mg/m^2, CrCl 16-40 ml/min 200 mg/m^2

Available forms: Inj 50, 150, 450 mg/vial

Side effects/adverse reactions:
EENT: Tinnitus, hearing loss, *vestibular toxicity,* visual changes
HEMA: ***Thrombocytopenia, leukopenia, pancytopenia, neutropenia,*** anemia, bleeding
CV: Cardiac abnormalities
GI: Severe nausea, vomiting, diarrhea, weight loss, mucositis, anorexia, constipation, taste change
GU: **Renal tubular damage,** renal insufficiency, impotence, sterility, amenorrhea, gynecomastia
INTEG: Alopecia, dermatitis, rash, erythema, pruritus, urticaria
CNS: **Convulsions, central neurotoxicity,** peripheral neuropathy, dizziness, confusion
META: Hypomagnesemia, hypocalcemia, hypokalemia, hyponatremia, hyperuremia
SYST: **Anaphylaxis**

Contraindications: Hypersensitivity to this drug, platinum products, mannitol; severe bone marrow depression, significant bleeding, pregnancy (D)

Precautions: Radiation therapy within 1 mo, chemotherapy within 1 mo, lactation, liver disease

Do not confuse:
carboplatin/cisplatin

Pharmacokinetics: Initial half-life 1-2 hr, postdistribution half-life 2 ½-6 hr, not bound to plasma proteins, excreted by the kidneys

Interactions:
• Increased nephrotoxicity or ototoxicity: aminoglycosides
• Increased risk of bleeding: aspirin
• Increased toxicity: radiation, bone marrow suppressants
• Increased myelosuppression: myelosuppressives
• Decreased phenytoin levels: phenytoin

Lab test interferences:
Increase: AST, BUN, alk phosphatase, bilirubin, creatinine

NURSING CONSIDERATIONS
Assess:
• CBC, differential, platelet count weekly; withhold drug if neutrophil count is <2000/mm^3 or platelet count is <100,000/mm^3; notify prescriber of results
• Renal function studies: BUN, creatinine, serum uric acid, urine CrCL before and during therapy; I&O ratio; report fall in urine output to <30 ml/hr
• Monitor temp q4h (may indicate beginning of infection)
• Liver function tests before and during therapy (bilirubin, AST, ALT, LDH) as needed or monthly; jaundice of skin, sclera, dark urine, clay-colored stools, itchy skin, abdominal pain, fever, diarrhea
• For anaphylaxis: hypotension, rash, pruritus, wheezing, tachycardia; notify prescriber after discontinuing drug, resuscitation equipment should be available
• Bleeding; hematuria, stool guaiac, bruising or petechiae, mucosa or orifices q8h
• Dyspnea, rales, unproductive cough, chest pain, tachypnea
• Effects of alopecia on body image; discuss feelings about body changes
• Edema in feet, joint pain, stomach pain, shaking

Administer:
• Antiemetic 30-60 min before giving drug and prn for vomiting
IV
• After diluting 10 mg/ml of sterile water for inj, D₅W, NS (10 mg/ml); then further dilute with the same sol 1-4 mg/ml; give over 15 min or more (INT INF)
• IV INF over 5-6 hr; do not use needles or IV administration sets containing aluminum; may cause precipitate or loss of potency
• Diuretic (furosemide 40 mg IV) after infusion
Additive compatibilities: Cisplatin, etoposide, floxuridine, ifosfamide, ifosfamide/etoposide, paclitaxel
Solution compatibilities: D₅/0.2% NaCl, D₅/0.45% NaCl, D₅/0.9% NaCl, 0.9% NaCl, D₅W, sterile water for inj
Y-site compatibilities: Allopurinol, amifostine, aztreonam, cefepime, cladribine, doxorubicin liposome, filgrastim, fludarabine, granisetron, melphalan, ondansetron, paclitaxel, piperacillin/tazobactam, propofol, sargramostim, teniposide, thiotepa, vinorelbine
Perform/provide:
• Storage protected from light at room temperature; reconstituted sol stable for 8 hr at room temperature
Evaluate:
• Therapeutic response: decreasing size of tumor, spread of malignancy
Teach patient/family:
• That impotence or amenorrhea can occur; reversible after treatment is discontinued, to notify prescriber if pregnancy is suspected
• Not to breastfeed during treatment
• To avoid OTC drugs with aspirin
• To notify prescriber of fever, fatigue, sore throat, and bleeding, bruising

• That hair may be lost during treatment; a wig or hairpiece may make patient feel better; new hair may be different in color, texture

carboprost (℞)
(kar′boe-prost)
Hemabate, Prostin/15M*
Func. class.: Oxytocic, abortifacient
Chem. class.: Prostaglandin

Action: Stimulates uterine contractions, causing complete abortion in approximately 16 hr
Uses: Abortion at 13-20 wk gestation, postpartum hemorrhage caused by uterine atony not controlled by other methods
Dosage and routes:
To induce abortion
• *Adult:* **IM** 250 μg, then 250 μg q1½- 3½ h, may increase to 500 μg if no response, not to exceed 12 mg total dose
Postpartum hemorrhage
• *Adult:* **IM** 250 μg, repeat at 15-90 min intervals; max total dosage 2 mg
Available forms: Inj 250 μg/ml
Side effects/adverse reactions:
CNS: Fever, chills, headache
GI: Nausea, vomiting, diarrhea
Contraindications: Hypersensitivity, severe hepatic disease, severe renal disease, PID, respiratory disease, cardiac disease
Precautions: Asthma, anemia, jaundice, diabetes mellitus, convulsive disorders, past uterine surgery, pregnancy (C)
Pharmacokinetics: Onset 15 min, peak 2 hr; metabolized in lungs, liver; excreted in urine (metabolites)
Interactions:
• Increased action: other oxytocics
🖋 Hypertension: ephedra

➡ = Nursing alert 🖋 = Herb-drug interaction 🚫 = Do not crush

C

NURSING CONSIDERATIONS
Assess:
• B/P, pulse; watch for change that may indicate hemorrhage
• Respiratory rate, rhythm, depth; notify prescriber of abnormalities
• For length, duration of contraction; notify prescriber of contractions lasting over 1 min or absence of contractions
• For incomplete abortion, pregnancy must be terminated by another method; drug is teratogenic

Administer:
• In deep muscle mass; rotate injection sites if additional doses are given

Evaluate:
• Therapeutic response: expulsion of fetus, control of bleeding

Teach patient/family:
• To report increased blood loss, abdominal cramps, increased temp, foul-smelling lochia

---

carisoprodol (R)

(kar-eye-soe-proe'dole)
carisoprodol, Soma, Vanadom

Func. class.: Skeletal muscle relaxant, central acting

Chem. class.: Meprobamate congener

Action: Depresses CNS by blocking interneuronal activity in descending reticular formation, spinal cord, producing sedation

Uses: Relieving pain, stiffness in musculoskeletal disorders

Dosage and routes:
• *Adult and child >12 yr:* **PO** 350 mg tid and hs
• *Child 6-12 yr:* **PO** 6.25 mg/kg qid

Available forms: Tabs 350 mg

Side effects/adverse reactions:
CNS: Dizziness, weakness, drowsi-ness, headache, tremor, depression, insomnia, ataxia, irritability
EENT: Diplopia, temporary loss of vision
HEMA: Eosinophilia
RESP: Asthmatic attacks
CV: Postural hypotension, tachycardia
GI: Nausea, vomiting, hiccups, epigastric discomfort
INTEG: Rash, pruritus, fever, facial flushing, ***erythema multiforme***
*SYST: **Angioedema, anaphylaxis***

Contraindications: Hypersensitivity, child <12 yr, intermittent porphyria

Precautions: Renal disease, hepatic disease, addictive personality, pregnancy (C), elderly, lactation

Pharmacokinetics:
PO: Onset ½ hr, peak 4 hr, duration 4-6 hr; metabolized by liver; excreted in urine; crosses placenta; excreted in breast milk (large amounts); half-life 8 hr

Interactions:
• Increased CNS depression: alcohol, tricyclics, narcotics, barbiturates, sedatives, hypnotics
🖊 May increase CNS depression: kava

NURSING CONSIDERATIONS
Assess:
• Pain, stiffness, mobility, activities of daily living baseline and throughout treatment
• ECG in epileptic patients; poor seizure control has occurred with patients taking this drug
• Idiosyncratic reaction, anaphylaxis within a few min or hr of 1st to 4th dose
• Allergic reactions: rash, fever, respiratory distress
• Severe weakness, numbness in extremities
• CNS depression: dizziness, drowsiness, psychiatric symptoms

---

Administer:
PO
• With meals for GI symptoms
Perform/provide:
• Storage in tight container at room temperature
• Assistance with ambulation if dizziness, drowsiness occurs, especially elderly
Evaluate:
• Therapeutic response: decreased pain, spasticity
Teach patient/family:
• Not to take with alcohol, other CNS depressants
• To avoid hazardous activities if drowsiness, dizziness occur
• To avoid using OTC medication: cough preparations, antihistamines, unless directed by prescriber
Treatment of overdose: Induce emesis of conscious patient, lavage, dialysis

---

carmustine (R)

(kar-mus'teen)
BiCNU, BCNU, Gliadel
Func. class.: Antineoplastic alkylating agent
Chem. class.: Nitrosourea

Action: Alkylates DNA, RNA; is able to inhibit enzymes that allow synthesis of amino acids in proteins; activity is not cell cycle phase specific

Uses: Brain tumors such as glioblastoma, medulloblastoma, astrocytoma; multiple myeloma, Hodgkin's disease, other lymphomas; GI, breast, bronchogenic, renal carcinomas, other lymphomas

Dosage and routes:
• *Adult:* IV 75-100 mg/m² over 1-2 hr × 2 days or 150-200 mg/m² × 1 dose q6-8wk or 40 mg/m²/day × 5 days q6wk; if WBC is 3000-3999/mm³ give 50% of dose; if WBC is 2000-2999/mm³ and platelets are 25,000-75,000/mm³ give 25% of dose; withhold dose if WBC is <2000/mm³ and platelets are <25,000/mm³
• *Adult:* **INTRACAVITARY** wafer: 8 inserted into resection cavity
Available forms: Powder for inj 100 mg; wafer 7.7 mg (intracavitary)

Side effects/adverse reactions:
HEMA: **Thrombocytopenia, leukopenia, myelosuppression, anemia**
GI: Nausea, vomiting, anorexia, stomatitis, **hepatotoxicity**
GU: Azotemia, **renal failure**
INTEG: Burning, hyperpigmentation at injection site
RESP: **Fibrosis, pulmonary infiltrate**

Contraindications: Hypersensitivity, leukopenia, thrombocytopenia
Precautions: Pregnancy (D), lactation
Pharmacokinetics: Degraded within 15 min; crosses blood-brain barrier; 70% excreted in urine within 96 hr; 10% excreted as CO_2; fate of 20% is unknown

Interactions:
• Increased toxicity: other antineoplastics, radiation, cimetidine
• Risk of bleeding: aspirin, anticoagulants
• Myelosuppression: myelosuppressive agents

NURSING CONSIDERATIONS
Assess:
• CBC, differential, platelet count weekly; withhold drug if WBC is <4000 or platelet count is <100,000; notify prescriber of results
• Liver function tests: AST, ALT, bilirubin
• Pulmonary function tests, chest x-ray films before, during therapy; chest film should be obtained q2wk during treatment

---

- Renal function studies: BUN, serum uric acid, urine CrCl before, during therapy; I&O ratio; report fall in urine output of 30 ml/hr
- Monitor for cold, cough, fever (may indicate beginning infection)
- Bleeding: hematuria, guaiac, bruising, petechiae, mucosa, orifices q8h
- Dyspnea, rales, unproductive cough, chest pain, tachypnea

Administer:
- Blood transfusions or RBC colony-stimulating factors to counter anemia
- Antiemetic 30-60 min before giving drug to prevent vomiting
- All medications PO, if possible, avoid IM inj if platelets are <100,000/mm^3

Wafer
- Foil pouches may be kept at room temperature for 6 hr if unopened
- 🚫 If wafers are broken in several pieces, they should not be used

IV
- After diluting 100 mg drug/3 ml ethyl alcohol (provided); then further dilute 27 ml sterile H$_2$O for inj; then dilute with 100-500 ml 0.9% NaCl or D$_5$W, give over 1 hr or more, reduce rate if discomfort is felt; use only glass containers

Y-site compatibilities: Amifostine, aztreonam, cefepime, filgrastim, fludarabine, granisetron, melphalan, ondansetron, piperacillin/tazobactam, sargramostim, teniposide, thiotepa, vinorelbine

Perform/provide:
- Storage of reconstituted sol in refrigerator for 24 hr, or room temperature for 8 hr
- Rinsing of mouth tid-qid with water or club soda; use of sponge brush for stomatitis
- Warm compresses at injection site for inflammation; reduce flow rate if patient complains of burning at infusion site

Evaluate:
- Therapeutic response: decreasing size of tumor, spread of malignancy

Teach patient/family:
- To report any changes in breathing or coughing
- To avoid foods with citric acid, hot or rough texture if stomatitis is present; to report any bleeding, white spots, ulceration in mouth to prescriber; tell patient to examine mouth qd
- To avoid use of aspirin, ibuprofen, razors, commercial mouthwash
- To report signs of anemia (fatigue, irritability, shortness of breath, faintness); to report signs of infection (sore throat, fever)
- To use contraception during treatment
- Not to receive vaccines during treatment

carteolol (℞)
(kar-tee'oh-lole)
Cartrol
Func. class.: Antihypertensive
Chem. class.: Nonselective β-blocker

Action: Produces fall in B/P without reflex tachycardia or significant reduction in heart rate through mixture of α-blocking, β-blocking effects and intrinsic sympathomimetic activity; elevated plasma renins are reduced

Uses: Mild to moderate hypertension, ophthalmic, intraocular, open-angle glaucoma

Dosage and routes:
- *Adult:* **PO** 2.5 mg qd initially, may gradually increase to desired response, max 10 mg/day (see ophthalmics, Appendix C)

Renal disease
• CrCl >60 ml/min give dose q24h;
CrCl 20-60 ml/min give dose q48h;
CrCl <20 ml/min give dose q72h
Available forms: Tabs 2.5, 5 mg
Side effects/adverse reactions:
CV: Orthostatic hypotension, *bradycardia, CHF, chest pain, ventricular dysrhythmias, AV block, peripheral vascular insufficiency,* palpitations
CNS: Dizziness, mental changes, drowsiness, fatigue, headache, catatonia, depression, anxiety, nightmares, paresthesia, lethargy, insomnia, decreased concentration
GI: Nausea, vomiting, diarrhea, dry mouth, flatulence, constipation, anorexia
INTEG: Rash, alopecia, urticaria, pruritus, fever
HEMA: Agranulocytosis, thrombocytopenic purpura (rare)
EENT: Tinnitus, visual changes, sore throat, double vision, dry, burning eyes
GU: Impotence, dysuria, ejaculatory failure, urinary retention
RESP: Bronchospasm, dyspnea, wheezing, nasal stuffiness, pharyngitis
MS: Joint pain, arthralgia, muscle cramps, pain
OTHER: Facial swelling, decreased exercise tolerance, weight change, Raynaud's disease, lupus-like syndrome
Contraindications: Hypersensitivity to β-blockers, cardiogenic shock, heart block (2nd or 3rd degree), sinus bradycardia, bronchial asthma
Precautions: Major surgery, pregnancy (C), lactation, CHF, diabetes mellitus, renal disease, thyroid disease, COPD, well-compensated heart failure, nonallergic bronchospasm
Do not confuse:
Ocupress/Ocufen

Pharmacokinetics:
PO: Onset 1-2 hr, peak 2-4 hr, duration 8-12 hr, half-life 6-8 hr; metabolized by liver (metabolites inactive); excreted in urine, bile; crosses placenta; excreted in breast milk
Interactions:
• Decreased carteolol effect: thyroid agents
• Increased myocardial depression: phenytoin (IV), verapamil
• Increased hypertension: MAOIs, amphetamines
• Decreased CV effect: dopamine, dobutamine
• Decreased antihypertensive effect: NSAIDs
• Increased hypotension: other antihypertensives, clonidine, nitrates, general anesthetics, alcohol (large amts)
• Increased hypoglycemic effect: insulin, oral antidiabetics
• Decreased bronchodilating effects of theophylline, β-agonists
NURSING CONSIDERATIONS
Assess:
• I&O, weight daily; edema in feet, legs daily, jugular vein distention, dyspnea, rales, crackles
• B/P, pulse q4h; note rate, rhythm, quality; apical/radial pulse before administration; notify prescriber of any significant changes
• Baselines in renal, liver function tests before therapy begins
• Skin turgor, dryness of mucous membranes for hydration status
• Blood glucose in those taking insulin/oral antidiabetics
Administer:
PO
• Drug ac, hs; tablet may be crushed or swallowed whole
Perform/provide:
• Storage in dry area at room temperature; do not freeze

◆ = Nursing alert   ✦ = Herb-drug interaction   ⊘ = Do not crush

Evaluate:
• Therapeutic response: decreased B/P after 1-2 wk

Teach patient/family:
• Not to discontinue drug abruptly; taper over 2 wk or may precipitate angina
• Not to use OTC products containing α-adrenergic stimulants (nasal decongestants, OTC cold preparations) unless directed by prescriber
• To report bradycardia, dizziness, confusion, depression, fever
• To take pulse, B/P at home, advise when to notify prescriber
• To avoid alcohol, smoking, sodium intake
• To comply with weight control, dietary adjustments, modified exercise program
• To carry Medic Alert ID to identify drug being taken, allergies
• To avoid hazardous activities if dizziness is present
• To report symptoms of CHF: difficulty breathing, especially on exertion or when lying down, night cough, swelling of extremities
• To take medication hs to minimize orthostatic hypotension

Treatment of overdose: Lavage, IV atropine for bradycardia, IV theophylline for bronchospasm, digitalis, O₂, diuretic for cardiac failure; administer vasopressor (norepinephrine) for hypotension, isoproterenol for heart block

---

carvedilol (℞)

(kar-ved′i-lole)
Coreg
Func. class.: Antihypertensive, α/β-adrenergic blocker

Action: A mixture of nonselective α/β-adrenergic blocking activity; decreases cardiac output, exercise-induced tachycardia, reflex orthostatic tachycardia; causes vasodilation, reduction in peripheral vascular resistance

Uses: Essential hypertension alone or in combination with other antihypertensives, CHF

Investigational uses: Angina pectoris, idiopathic cardiomyopathy

Dosage and routes:

Essential hypertension
• *Adult:* **PO** 6.25 mg bid × 7-14 days; if tolerated well, then increase to 12.5 mg bid × 7-14 days; if tolerated well, may be increased (if needed) to 25 mg bid; not to exceed 50 mg qd

Congestive heart failure
• *Adult:* **PO** 3.125 mg bid × 2 wk; if tolerated well, give 6.25 mg bid × 2 wk, then double q2wk to max dose, 25 mg bid <85 kg or 50 mg bid >85 kg

Angina pectoris
• *Adult:* **PO** 25-50 mg bid

Idiopathic cardiomyopathy
• *Adult:* **PO** 6.25-25 mg bid

Available forms: Tabs 3.125, 6.25, 12.5, 25 mg

Side effects/adverse reactions:

CNS: Dizziness, fatigue, weakness, somnolence, insomnia, ataxia, hyperesthesia, paresthesia, vertigo, depression

GI: Diarrhea, abdominal pain, increased alk phosphatase, ALT/AST

*CV: **Bradycardia,** postural hypotension,* dependent edema, peripheral edema, ***AV block,*** extrasystoles, hypertension, hypotension, palpitations, peripheral ischemia, ***CHF, pulmonary edema***

GU: Decreased libido, *impotence*

RESP: Rhinitis, pharyngitis, dyspnea

MISC: Fatigue, injury, back pain, UTI, viral infection, hypertriglyceridemia, ***thrombocytopenia,*** *hyperglycemia*

Side effects: *italics* = common; ***bold italics*** = life-threatening

Contraindications: Hypersensitivity, bronchial asthma, class IV decompensated cardiac failure, 2nd- or 3rd-degree heart block, cardiogenic shock, severe bradycardia, pulmonary edema

Precautions: Cardiac failure, hepatic injury, peripheral vascular disease, anesthesia, major surgery, diabetes mellitus, thyrotoxicosis, elderly, pregnancy (C), lactation, children, emphysema, chronic bronchitis, renal disease

Pharmacokinetics: Readily and extensively absorbed PO, >98% protein binding, extensively metabolized by liver, excreted through bile into feces, terminal half-life 7-10 hr with increases in elderly, hepatic disease

Interactions:
• Increased hypoglycemia: antidiabetic agents
• Decreased heart rate, B/P: clonidine
• Increased concentrations of digoxin
• Increased toxicity of carvedilol: cimetidine, other antihypertensives, nitrates, acute alcohol ingestion
• Decreased levels of carvedilol: rifampin, NSAIDs, thyroid med
• Conduction disturbances: calcium channel blockers
• Bradycardia, hypotension: MAOIs, reserpine

NURSING CONSIDERATIONS
Assess:
◆Renal studies, including protein, BUN, creatinine; watch for increased levels that may indicate nephrotic syndrome; obtain baselines in renal, liver function studies before beginning treatment
• Liver function studies, jaundice; if LFTs are elevated, drug should be discontinued
• I&O, weight daily
• B/P during beginning treatment, periodically thereafter; pulse q4h, note rate, rhythm, quality; apical/radial pulse before administration; notify prescriber of significant changes
• Edema in feet, legs daily, fluid overload: dyspnea, weight gain, jugular vein distention, fatigue, rales, crackles

Administer:
PO
• Drug ac, hs; tablets may be crushed or swallowed whole
• Reduced dosage in renal dysfunction; may give with food

Evaluate:
• Therapeutic response: decreased B/P in hypertension

Teach patient/family:
• To comply with dosage schedule, even if feeling better, that improvement may take several wk
• To rise slowly to sitting or standing position to minimize orthostatic hypotension
• To report bradycardia, dizziness, confusion, depression, fever, weight gain, SOB, cold extremities, rash, sore throat, bleeding, or bruising
• To take pulse, B/P at home; advise when to notify prescriber
• Not to discontinue drug abruptly, taper over 1-2 wk
• To avoid hazardous activities until stabilized on medication; dizziness may occur
• To avoid all OTC medications unless approved by prescriber
• To carry ID with drug name, prescriber at all times
• To inform all health care providers of drugs taken

cascara sagrada/ cascara sagrada aromatic fluid extract/ cascara sagrada fluid extract (OTC)

(kas-kar′a)

Func. class.: Laxative
Chem. class.: Anthraquinone

Action: Direct chemical irritation in colon; increases propulsion of stool

Uses: Constipation; bowel or rectal preparation for surgery or examination

Dosage and routes:
• *Adult:* PO 325 mg hs; **FLUID** 1 ml qd; **AROMATIC FLUID** 5 ml qd
• *Child 2-12 yr:* **PO/FLUID/ AROMATIC FLUID** ½ adult dose
• *Child <2 yr:* **PO/FLUID/AR-OMATIC FLUID** ¼ adult dose
Available forms: Tabs 325 mg; fluid extract 1 g/ml; aromatic fluid extract 1 g/ml

Side effects/adverse reactions:
GI: Nausea, vomiting, anorexia, cramps, diarrhea
META: Hypocalcemia, enteropathy, alkalosis, hypokalemia, *tetany*

Contraindications: Hypersensitivity, GI bleeding, obstruction, CHF, lactation, abdominal pain, nausea/vomiting, appendicitis, acute surgical abdomen, alcoholics (aromatic form)

Precautions: Pregnancy (C)

Pharmacokinetics:
PO: Peak 6-12 hr; metabolized by liver; excreted in urine, feces, breast milk

Interactions:
• Decreased absorption of these drugs: antibiotics, digitalis, nitrofurantoin, salicylates, tetracyclines, oral anticoagulants

🍃 Increased action/side effects: lily of the valley, pheasant's eye, squill

NURSING CONSIDERATIONS

Assess:
• Monitor blood, urine electrolytes if drug is used often by patient; check I&O ratio to identify fluid loss
• Cause of constipation; identify whether fluids, bulk, or exercise missing from lifestyle
• Cramping, rectal bleeding, nausea, vomiting; if these symptoms occur, drug should be discontinued

Administer:
• Alone for better absorption; do not take within 1 hr of other drugs or within 1 hr of antacids, milk
• In morning or evening (oral dose)

Evaluate:
• Therapeutic response: decrease in constipation

Teach patient/family:
🚫 To swallow tabs whole; do not break, crush, or chew
• Not to use laxatives for long-term therapy; bowel tone will be lost
• That normal bowel movements do not always occur daily
• Not to use in presence of abdominal pain, nausea, vomiting
• To notify prescriber if constipation unrelieved or of symptoms of electrolyte imbalance: muscle cramps, pain, weakness, dizziness

cefaclor
See cephalosporins—2nd generation

cefadroxil
cefazolin
See cephalosporins—1st generation

cefdinir
See cephalosporins—3rd generation

cefditoren
See appendix a—selected new drugs

cefepime
cefixime
See cephalosporins—3rd generation

cefamandole
cefmetazole
cefonicid
See cephalosporins—2nd generation

cefoperazone
cefotaxime
See cephalosporins—3rd generation

cefotetan
cefoxitin
See cephalosporins—2nd generation

cefpodoxime
See cephalosporins—3rd generation

cefprozil
See cephalosporins—2nd generation

ceftazidime
ceftibuten
ceftizoxime
ceftriaxone
See cephalosporins—3rd generation

cefuroxime
See cephalosporins—2nd generation

celecoxib (℞)
(sel-eh-cox′ib)
Celebrex
Func. class.: Nonsteroidal antiinflammatory
Chem. class.: COX-2 inhibitor

Action: Inhibits prostaglandin synthesis by decreasing enzyme needed for biosynthesis; analgesic, antiinflammatory, antipyretic properties
Uses: Acute, chronic rheumatoid arthritis, osteoarthritis, familial adenomatous polyposis (FAP)
Investigational uses: Colorectal polyps
Dosage and routes:
Osteoarthritis
• *Adult:* **PO** 200 mg/day as a single dose or 100 mg bid
Rheumatoid arthritis
• *Adult:* **PO** 100-200 mg bid
Familial adenomatous polyposis (FAP)
• *Adult:* **PO** 400 mg bid
Colorectal polyps
• *Adult:* **PO** 400 mg bid × 6 mo
Available forms: Caps 100, 200 mg
Side effects/adverse reactions:
CNS: Fatigue, anxiety, depression, nervousness, paresthesia, dizziness, insomnia
*CV: **Tachycardia,** angina, **MI,** palpitations, dysrhythmias, hypertension, fluid retention*
EENT: Tinnitus, hearing loss, blurred vision, glaucoma, cataract, conjunctivitis, eye pain
GI: Nausea, anorexia, vomiting, constipation, dry mouth, diverticulitis, gastritis, gastroenteritis, hemorrhoids, hiatal hernia, stomatitis, **GI bleeding**
*GU: **Nephrotoxicity:** dysuria, **hematuria, oliguria, azotemia,** cystis, UTI*
*HEMA: **Blood dyscrasias,** epistaxis, bruising, anemia*
INTEG: Purpura, rash, pruritus, sweating, erythema, petechiae, photosensitivity, alopecia
RESP: Pharyngitis, shortness of breath, pneumonia, coughing
Contraindications: Hypersensitivity to aspirin, iodides, other NSAIDs, sulfonamides, 3rd trimester of pregnancy, asthma triad, asthma

◆ = Nursing alert ✦ = Herb-drug interaction ⊘ = Do not crush

Precautions: Pregnancy 1st/2nd trimester (C), 3rd trimester (D), lactation, bleeding, GI, cardiac, renal, hepatic, disorders, hypersensitivity to other antiinflammatory agents, glucocorticoids, anticoagulants, geriatrics, hypertension, severe dehydration, children <18 yr

Do not confuse:
Celebrex/Celexa

Pharmacokinetics: Well absorbed, crosses placenta, bound to plasma proteins, metabolized in liver, excreted by kidneys, peak 3 hr

Interactions:
• Increased effect of: anticoagulants
• Decreased effect of: aspirin, ACE inhibitors, thiazide, diuretics, furosemide
• Increased adverse reactions: glucocorticoids, NSAIDs, aspirin
• Increased toxicity: lithium, antineoplastics
• Increased celecoxib blood level: fluconazole

NURSING CONSIDERATIONS
Assess:
• For pain of rheumatoid arthritis, osteoarthritis; check ROM, inflammation of joints, characteristics of pain
• FAP clients for decreasing number of polyps
• Blood counts during therapy; watch for decreasing platelets; if low, therapy may need to be discontinued, restarted after hematologic recovery
◆ For blood dyscrasias (thrombocytopenia): bruising, fatigue, bleeding, poor healing

Administer:
PO
• With food or milk to decrease gastric symptoms, do not increase dose
🚫 Do not crush, dissolve, or chew caps

Evaluate:
• Therapeutic response: decreased pain, inflammation in arthritic conditions; decreased number of polyps

Teach patient/family:
• To check with prescriber to determine when drug should be discontinued prior to surgery
• That drug must be continued for prescribed time to be effective; to avoid other NSAIDs, aspirin, sulfonamides
• To notify prescriber if pregnancy is planned or suspected
• To notify prescriber of GI symptoms: black, tarry stools; cramping or rash; edema of extremities, weight gain
• To report bleeding, bruising, fatigue, malaise since blood dyscrasias do occur
🚫 To take with a full glass of water to enhance absorption; do not crush, break, or chew

cephalexin
See cephalosporins—1st generation

CEPHALOSPORINS—1ST GENERATION

cefadroxil (℞)
(sef-a-drox'ill)
cefadroxil, Duricef, Ultracef
cefazolin (℞)
(sef-a'zoe-lin)
Ancef, cefazolin, Kefzol
cephalexin (℞)
(sef-a-lex'in)
Apo-Cephalex*, Cefanex, C-Lexin, cephalexin, Keflex, Keftab, Novo-Lexin*, Nu-Cephalex*
cephalothin (℞)
(sef-a-loe'thin)
cephalothin, Keflin
cephapirin (℞)
(sef-a-pye'rin)
Cefadyl, cephapirin
cephradine (℞)
(sef'ra-deen)
cephradine, Velosef
Func. class.: Antiinfective
Chem. class.: Cephalosporin
(1st generation)

Action: Inhibits bacterial cell wall synthesis, rendering cell wall osmotically unstable, leading to cell death by binding to cell wall membrane

Uses:

cefadroxil: Gram-negative bacilli: *Escherichia coli, Proteus mirabilis, Klebsiella* (UTI only); gram-positive organisms: *Streptococcus pneumoniae, Streptococcus pyogenes, Staphylococcus aureus;* upper, lower respiratory tract, urinary tract, skin infections, otitis media; tonsillitis; and UTIs

cefazolin: Gram-negative bacilli: *Haemophilus influenzae, Escherichia coli, Proteus mirabilis, Klebsiella;* gram-positive organisms: *Staphylococcus aureus;* upper, lower respiratory tract, urinary tract, skin infections, bone, joint, biliary, genital infections, endocarditis, surgical prophylaxis, septicemia

cephalexin: Gram-negative bacilli: *Haemophilus influenzae, Escherichia coli, Proteus mirabilis, Klebsiella;* gram-positive organisms: *Streptococcus pneumoniae, Streptococcus pyogenes, Staphylococcus aureus;* upper, lower respiratory tract, urinary tract, skin, bone infections, otitis media

cephalothin: Gram-negative bacilli: *Haemophilus influenzae, Escherichia coli, Proteus mirabilis, Klebsiella, Salmonella, Shigella;* gram-positive organisms: *Streptococcus pneumoniae, Streptococcus pyogenes, Staphylococcus aureus;* upper, lower respiratory tract, skin infections, bone infections, endocarditis, septicemia, bacterial peritonitis

cephapirin: Gram-negative bacilli: *Haemophilus influenzae, Escherichia coli, Proteus mirabilis, Klebsiella;* gram-positive organisms: *Streptococcus pneumoniae, Streptococcus viridans, Staphylococcus aureus;* lower respiratory tract, skin infections, endocarditis, bacterial peritonitis

cephradine: Gram-negative bacilli: *Haemophilus influenzae, Escherichia coli, Proteus mirabilis, Klebsiella;* gram-positive organisms: *Streptococcus pneumoniae, Streptococcus pyogenes, Staphylococcus aureus;* serious respiratory tract, skin infections, urinary tract infections, otitis media

Dosage and routes:

cefadroxil
• *Adult:* **PO** 1-2 g qd or q12h in divided doses, give a loading dose of 1 g initially
• *Child:* **PO** 30/kg/day in divided doses bid

◆ = Nursing alert   ✐ = Herb-drug interaction   ⊘ = Do not crush

Renal dose: CrCl 25-50 ml/min 1 g, then 500 mg q12h; CrCl 10-24 ml/min 500 mg q24h; CrCl <10 ml/min 500 mg q36h

Available forms: Caps 500 mg; tabs 1 g; oral susp 125, 250, 500 mg/5 ml

cefazolin
Life-threatening infections
• *Adult:* **IM/IV** 1-2 g q6h
• *Child >1 mo:* **IM/IV** 100 mg/kg in 3-4 divided doses
Mild/moderate infections
• *Adult:* **IM/IV** 250 mg-1 g q8h
• *Child >1 mo:* **IM/IV** 25-50 mg/kg in 3-4 equal doses

Renal dose: CrCl 35-54 ml/min: 250-1000 mg q12h; CrCl 10-34 ml/min: 50% of dose q12h; CrCl <10 ml/min: 50% of dose q18-24h

Available forms: Inj 500 mg, 1 g; infusion 500 mg, 1 g/50 ml vial

cephalexin
Moderate infections
• *Adult:* **PO** 250-500 mg q6h
• *Child:* **PO** 25-50 mg/kg/day in 4 equal doses
Moderate skin infections
• *Adult:* **PO** 500 mg q12h
Endocarditis prophylaxis
• 2 g 1 hr before procedure
Severe infections
• *Adult:* **PO** 500 mg-1 g q6h
• *Child:* **PO** 50-100 mg/kg/day in 4 equal doses

Renal dose: CrCl <40 ml/min give q8-12h; CrCl 5-10 ml/min give q12h; CrCl <5 ml/min give q24h

Available forms: Caps 250, 500 mg; tabs 250, 500 mg, 1 g; oral susp 125, 250 mg/5ml

cephalothin
Renal dose: CrCl 26-50 ml/min 1.5 g q6h; CrCl 10-25 ml/min 1 g q6h; CrCl <10 ml/min 500 mg q6h
Moderate infections
• *Adult:* **IM/IV** 500 mg-1 g q4-6h
• *Child:* **IM/IV** 14-27 mg/kg q4h or 20-40 mg/kg q6h

Uncomplicated gonorrhea
• *Adult:* **IM** 2 g as a single dose
Severe infections
• *Adult:* **IM/IV** 1-2 g q4h
• *Child:* **IM/IV** 80-160 mg/kg/day in divided doses q4h

Available forms: Powder for inj 1, 2, 20 g

cephapirin
• *Adult:* **IM/IV** 500 mg-1 g q4-6h
• *Child:* **IM/IV** 40-80 mg/kg/day in divided doses q6h or 10-20 mg/kg q6h

Renal dose: CrCl <10 ml/min give q12h

Available forms: Powder for inj 500 mg, 1, 2, 20 g; IV only 1, 2, 4 g

cephradine
• *Adult:* **PO** 250 mg-1 g q6-12h
• *Child >1 yr:* **PO** 6-12 mg/kg q6h

Renal dose: CrCl >20 ml/min 500 mg q6h; CrCl 5-20 ml/min 250 mg q6h

Available forms: Caps 250, 500 mg; oral susp 125, 250 mg/5ml

Side effects/adverse reactions:
CNS: Headache, dizziness, weakness, paresthesia, fever, chills
GI: Nausea, vomiting, *diarrhea, anorexia,* pain, glossitis, bleeding; increased AST, ALT, bilirubin, LDH, alk phosphatase; abdominal pain, ***pseudomembranous colitis***
GU: Proteinuria, vaginitis, pruritus, candidiasis, increased BUN, ***nephrotoxicity, renal failure***
HEMA: ***Leukopenia, thrombocytopenia, agranulocytosis,*** anemia, ***neutropenia, lymphocytosis, eosinophilia, pancytopenia, hemolytic anemia***
INTEG: Rash, urticaria, dermatitis, ***anaphylaxis***
RESP: Dyspnea
Contraindications: Hypersensitivity to cephalosporins, infants <1 mo
Precautions: Hypersensitivity to penicillins, pregnancy (B), lactation, renal disease

Do not confuse:
cephalexin/cefaclor
cephapirin/cephradine
Kefzol/Cefzil
Pharmacokinetics:

cefadroxil: Peak 1-1½ hr, duration 12-24 hr, half-life 1-2 hr; 20% bound by plasma proteins; crosses placenta; excreted in breast milk

cefazolin
IM: Peak ½-2 hr, duration 6-12 hr, half-life 1½-2¼ hr
IV: Peak 10 min, duration 6-12 hr; eliminated unchanged in urine; 70%-86% protein bound

cephalexin: Peak 1 hr, duration 6-12 hr, half-life 30-72 min; 5%-15% bound by plasma proteins; 90%-100% eliminated unchanged in urine; crosses placenta; excreted in breast milk

cephalothin
IV: Peak 15 min
IM: Peak 30 min
Half-life ½-1 hr, 65%-80% bound by plasma proteins, 50%-75% eliminated unchanged in urine in 8 hr; crosses placenta, excreted in breast milk, deacetylated in kidneys, liver

cephapirin
IV: Peak 5 min, duration 4-6 hr
IM: Peak 30 min, duration 4-6 hr
Half-life 21-47 min; 44%-50% bound by plasma proteins; 40%-70% eliminated unchanged in urine; crosses placenta; excreted in breast milk; metabolized in liver

cephradine: Peak 1 hr, duration 6-12 hr, half-life 0.75-1.5 hr; 20% bound by plasma proteins; 80%-90% eliminated unchanged in urine; crosses placenta; excreted in breast milk

Interactions:
• Increased toxicity: aminoglycosides, loop diuretics, probenecid
Lab test interferences:
False increase: Creatinine (serum urine), urinary 17-KS

False positive: Urinary protein, direct Coombs' test, urine glucose
Interference: Cross-matching
NURSING CONSIDERATIONS
Assess:
• Sensitivity to penicillin and other cephalosporins
◆ Nephrotoxicity: increased BUN, creatinine
• I&O daily
• Blood studies: AST, ALT, CBC, Hct, bilirubin, LDH, alk phosphatase, Coombs' test monthly if patient is on long-term therapy
• Electrolytes: K, Na, Cl monthly if patient is on long-term therapy
• Bowel pattern qd; if severe diarrhea occurs, drug should be discontinued; may indicate pseudomembranous colitis
• Urine output: if decreasing, notify prescriber; may indicate nephrotoxicity
◆ Anaphylaxis: rash, urticaria, pruritus, chills, fever, joint pain; angioedema; may occur few days after therapy begins
• Bleeding: ecchymosis, bleeding gums, hematuria, stool guaiac daily
◆ Overgrowth of infection: perineal itching, fever, malaise, redness, pain, swelling, drainage, rash, diarrhea, change in cough, sputum
Administer:
cefadroxil
• For 10-14 days to ensure organism death, prevent superinfection
• With food if needed for GI symptoms
• Shake susp, refrigerate, discard after 2 wk
• After C&S completed
cefazolin
• IV; check for irritation, extravasation often; dilute in 10 ml sterile H$_2$O for inj and run over 3-5 min; may be further diluted with 50-100 ml of NS, D$_5$W sol and run over ½-1 hr by Y-tube or 3-way stopcock

◆ = Nursing alert   ∥ = Herb-drug interaction   ⊘ = Do not crush

• For 10-14 days to ensure organism death, prevent superinfection
• After C&S completed

Additive compatibilities: Aztreonam, clindamycin, famotidine, fluconazole, metronidazole, verapamil

Syringe compatibilities: Heparin, vit B

Y-site compatibilities: Acyclovir, allopurinol, amifostine, atracurium, aztreonam, calcium gluconate, cyclophosphamide, diltiazem, doxorubicin liposome, enalaprilat, esmolol, famotidine, filgrastim, fluconazole, fludarabine, foscarnet, heparin, hydromorphone, insulin (regular), labetalol, lidocaine, magnesium sulfate, melphalan, meperidine, midazolam, morphine, multivitamins, ondansetron, perphenazine, pancuronium, remifentanil, sargramostim, tacrolimus, teniposide, theophylline, thiotepa, vecuronium, vit B/C, warfarin

cephalexin
• Shake susp, refrigerate, discard after 2 wk
• For 10-14 days to ensure organism death, prevent superinfection
• With food if needed for GI symptoms
• After C&S

cephalothin
• Clear solution; do not give cloudy sol
• IV after diluting 1 g or less/10 ml or more of sterile H_2O for inj; give over 3-5 min; may be further diluted with 50 ml D_5W, NS by Y-tube or 3-way stopcock; run over 15-30 min; discontinue primary IV during administration; may also be given by continuous infusion
• Store 96 hr refrigerated, 24 hr room temperature
• IM after reconstituting with 4 ml sterile H_2O for inj/1 g vial
• For 10-14 days to ensure organism death, prevent superinfection

• After C&S
• Insert IM in deep muscle mass, massage

Additive compatibilities: Ascorbic acid, chloramphenicol, clindamycin, fluorouracil, hydrocortisone, isoproterenol, magnesium sulfate, metaraminol, methicillin, methotrexate, potassium chloride, prednisolone, procaine, sodium bicarbonate, vit B/C

Syringe compatibilities: Cimetidine

Y-site compatibilities: Cyclophosphamide, famotidine, heparin, hydromorphone, magnesium sulfate, meperidine, morphine, multivitamins, perphenazine, potassium chloride, vit B/C

cephapirin
• IV after diluting 1 g or less/10 ml or more NS, D_5W, or bacteriostatic H_2O for inj; give 1 g or less/5 min or more; may be further diluted in 50-100 ml of D_5W, NS; run over 15 min; discontinue primary IV during administration; may also be given by continuous infusion, store refrigerated 96 hr, room temperature 24 hr
• For 10-14 days to ensure organism death, prevent superinfection
• After C&S

Additive compatibilities: Bleomycin, calcium chloride, calcium gluconate, chloramphenicol, diphenhydramine, ergonovine, heparin, hydrocortisone, metaraminol, oxacillin, penicillin G potassium, pentobarbital, phenobarbital, phytonadione, potassium chloride, sodium bicarbonate, succinylcholine, verapamil, vit B, warfarin

Y-site compatibilities: Acyclovir, cyclophosphamide, famotidine, heparin, hydrocortisone, hydromorphone, magnesium sulfate, meperidine, morphine, multivitamins, perphenazine, potassium chloride, vit B/C

cephradine
• Shake suspension well before each dose
• For 10-14 days to ensure organism death, prevent superinfection
• With food if needed for GI symptoms
• After C&S

Evaluate:
• Therapeutic response: decreased symptoms of infection, negative C&S

Teach patient/family:
• Not to drink alcohol or use meds with alcohol: reaction may occur
• To use yogurt or buttermilk to maintain intestinal flora, decrease diarrhea
• To take all medication prescribed for length of time ordered
◆ To report sore throat, bruising, bleeding, joint pain (may indicate blood dyscrasias [rare])

Treatment of anaphylaxis: Epinephrine, antihistamines; resuscitate if needed

---

CEPHALOSPORINS—2ND GENERATION

cefaclor (℞)
(sef'a-klor)
Ceclor

cefamandole (℞)
(sef-a-man'dole)
Mandol

cefmetazole (℞)
(sef-met'a-zole)
Zefazone

cefonicid (℞)
(se-fon'i-sid)
Monocid

cefotetan (℞)
(sef'oh-tee-tan)
Cefotan

cefoxitin (℞)
(se-fox'i-tin)
Mefoxin

cefprozil (℞)
(sef-proe'zill)
Cefzil

cefuroxime (℞)
(sef-yoor-ox'eem)
Ceftin, Kefurox, Zinacef

loracarbef (℞)
(lor-a-kar'beff)
Lorabid

Func. class.: Antiinfective
Chem. class.: Cephalosporin (2nd generation)

Action: Inhibits bacterial cell wall synthesis, rendering cell wall osmotically unstable, leading to cell death by binding to cell wall membrane

Uses:

cefaclor: Gram-negative bacilli: *Haemophilus influenzae, Escherichia coli, Proteus mirabilis, Klebsiella;* gram-positive organisms: *Streptococcus pneumoniae, Strep-*

◆ = Nursing alert   🌿 = Herb-drug interaction   🚫 = Do not crush

tococcus pyogenes, *Staphylococcus aureus;* respiratory tract, urinary tract, skin, bone, joint infections, otitis media

cefamandole: Gram-negative bacilli: *Haemophilus influenzae, Escherichia coli, Proteus mirabilis, Klebsiella;* gram-positive organisms: *Streptococcus pneumoniae, Streptococcus pyogenes, Staphylococcus aureus;* upper, lower respiratory tract, urinary tract, skin infections, peritonitis, septicemia, surgical prophylaxis

cefmetazole: Gram-negative bacilli: *Haemophilus influenzae, Escherichia coli, Proteus, Klebsiella, Bacteroides fragilis;* gram-positive organisms: *Streptococcus pneumoniae, Streptococcus pyogenes, Staphylococcus aureus;* anaerobes, including *Clostridium;* infections of lower respiratory tract, urinary tract, skin, bone, intraabdominal infections

cefonicid: Gram-negative bacilli: *Haemophilus influenzae, Escherichia coli, Proteus mirabilis, Klebsiella;* gram-positive organisms: *Streptococcus pneumoniae, Streptococcus pyogenes, Staphylococcus aureus;* lower respiratory tract, urinary tract, skin infections, otitis media, peritonitis, septicemia

cefotetan: Gram-negative organisms: *Haemophilus influenzae, Escherichia coli, Escherichia aerogenes, Proteus mirabilis, Klebsiella, Citrobacter, Enterobacter, Salmonella, Shigella, Acinetobacter, Bacteroides fragilis, Neisseria, Serratia;* gram-positive organisms: *Streptococcus pneumoniae, Streptococcus pyogenes, Staphylococcus aureus;* upper, lower, serious respiratory tract, urinary tract, skin, bone, joint, gynecologic, gonococcal, intraabdominal infections

cefoxitin: Gram-negative bacilli: *Haemophilus influenzae, Escherichia coli, Proteus, Klebsiella, Bacteroides fragilis, Neisseria gonorrhoeae;* gram-positive organisms: *Streptococcus pneumoniae, Streptococcus pyogenes, Staphylococcus aureus;* anaerobes including *Clostridium,* lower respiratory tract, urinary tract, skin, bone, gynecologic, gonococcal infections, septicemia, peritonitis

cefprozil: Pharyngitis/tonsillitis, otitis media, secondary bacterial infection of acute bronchitis, and acute bacterial exacerbation of chronic bronchitis and uncomplicated skin and skin structure infections; acute sinusitis

cefuroxime: Gram-negative bacilli: *Haemophilus influenzae, Escherichia coli, Neisseria, Proteus mirabilis, Klebsiella;* gram-positive organisms: *Streptococcus pneumoniae, Streptococcus pyogenes, Staphylococcus aureus;* serious lower respiratory tract, urinary tract, skin, bone, joint, gonococcal infections, septicemia, meningitis

loracarbef: Gram-negative bacilli: *Haemophilus influenzae, Escherichia coli, Proteus mirabilis, Klebsiella;* gram-positive organisms: *Streptococcus pneumoniae, Streptococcus pyogenes, Staphylococcus aureus;* upper and lower respiratory tract, urinary tract, skin infections, otitis media, pharyngitis, tonsillitis

Dosage and routes:

cefaclor

• *Adult:* **PO** 250-500 mg q8h, not to exceed 4 g/day or 375-500 mg (ext rel) q12h × 7-10 days

• *Child >1 mo:* **PO** 20-40 mg/kg qd in divided doses q8h, or total daily dose may be divided and given q12h, not to exceed 1 g/day

Acute bacterial exacerbations of chronic bronchitis or acute bronchitis

• *Adult:* 500 mg/12 hr × 1 wk (ext rel)

Pharyngitis/tonsillitis

• *Adult:* 375 mg/12 hr × 10 days (ext rel)

Available forms: Caps 250, 500 mg; oral susp 125, 187, 250, 375 mg/5 ml; tabs, ext rel 375, 500 mg

cefamandole

• *Adult:* **IM/IV** 500 mg-1 g q4-8h; may give up to 2 g q4h for severe infections

• *Child >1 mo:* **IM/IV** 8.3-16.7 mg/kg q4h, not to exceed adult dose

• Dosage reduction indicated in renal impairment (CrCl <50 ml/min)

Available forms: Inj 1, 2, 10 g

cefmetazole

Renal dose: CrCl <50 ml/min 1-2 g q12h; CrCl 10-29 ml/min 1-2 g q24h; CrCl <10 ml/min 1-2 g q48h

• *Adult:* **IV** 2 g divided q6-12h × 5-14 days

Available forms: Powder for inj 1, 2 g/vial

cefonicid

Life-threatening infections

• *Adult:* **IM/IV BOL** or **INF** 0.5-2 g/24 hr; divide in two doses if giving 2 g

• Dosage reduction indicated in renal impairment

Available forms: Inj 500 mg, 1, 10 g

cefotetan

Renal dose: CrCl 10-30 ml/min give q24h; CrCl <10 ml/min give q48h

• *Adult:* **IV/IM** 1-2 g q12h × 5-10 days

Perioperative prophylaxis

• *Adult:* **IV** 1-2 g ½-1 hr before surgery

Available forms: Inj 1, 2, 10 g

cefoxitin

Renal dose: CrCl <50 ml/min give q8-12h; CrCl 10-29 ml/min give q24h; CrCl <10 ml/min give q24-48h

• *Adult:* **IM/IV** 1-2 g q6-8h

• Dosage reduction indicated in renal impairment (CrCl <50 ml/min)

Uncomplicated gonorrhea: 2 g IM as single dose with 1 g **PO** probenecid at same time

Severe infections

• *Adult:* **IM/IV** 2 g q4h

• *Child ≥3 mo:* **IM/IV** 80-160 mg/kg/day divided q4-6h; max 12 g/day

Available forms: Powder for inj 1, 2, 10 g

cefprozil

Renal dose: CrCl <30 ml/min 50% of dose

Upper respiratory infections

• *Adult:* **PO** 500 mg q24h × 10 days

Otitis media

• *Child 6 mo-12 yr:* **PO** 15 mg/kg q12h × 10 days

Lower respiratory infections

• *Adult:* **PO** 500 mg q12h × 10 days

Skin/skin structure infections

• *Adult:* **PO** 250-500 mg q12h × 10 days

Available forms: Tabs 250, 500 mg; susp 125, 250 mg/5 ml

cefuroxime

• *Adult and child:* **PO** 250 mg q12h; may increase to 500 mg q12h in serious infections

• *Adult:* **IM/IV** 750 mg-1.5 g q8h for 5-10 days

Urinary tract infections

• *Adult:* **PO** 125 mg q12h; may increase to 250 mg q12h if needed

Otitis media

• *Child <2 yr:* **PO** 125 mg bid

• *Child >2 yr:* **PO** 250 mg bid

Surgical prophylaxis

• *Adult:* **IV** 1.5 g ½-1 hr preop

Severe infections

• *Adult:* **IM/IV** 1.5 g q6h; may give up to 3 g q8h for bacterial meningitis

• *Child >3 mo:* **IM/IV** 50-100 mg/kg/day; may give up to 200-240 mg/kg/day **IV** in divided doses for bacterial meningitis (not recommended)

• Dosage reduction indicated in se-

---

vere renal impairment (CrCl <20 ml/min)

Uncomplicated gonorrhea

• *Adult:* 1.5 g **IM** as single dose with oral probenecid in 2 separate sites

Available forms: Tabs 125, 250, 500 mg; inj 150, 750 mg, 1.5, 7.5 g; inj 750 mg; 1.5 g powder; susp 125, 250 mg/5 ml

loracarbef

Renal dose: CrCl 10-49 ml/min 50% of dose; CrCl <10 ml/min q3-5 days

• *Adult and child >13:* **PO** 200-400 mg q12h

• *Child <12 yr:* **PO** 15-30 mg/kg/day in 2 divided doses q12h

Available forms: Caps 200, 400 mg; 100, 200 mg/5 ml oral susp

Side effects/adverse reactions:

CNS: Dizziness, headache, fatigue, paresthesia, fever, chills, confusion

GI: Diarrhea, nausea, vomiting, anorexia, dysgeusia, glossitis, bleeding; increased AST, ALT, bilirubin, LDH, alk phosphatase; abdominal pain, loose stools, flatulence, heartburn, stomach cramps, colitis, jaundice

INTEG: Rash, urticaria, dermatitis, *Stevens-Johnson syndrome*

GU: Vaginitis, pruritus, candidiasis, increased BUN, *nephrotoxicity, renal failure,* pyuria, dysuria, reversible interstitial nephritis

HEMA: Leukopenia, thrombocytopenia, agranulocytosis, anemia, *neutropenia, lymphocytosis, eosinophilia, pancytopenia, hemolytic anemia, leukocytosis, granulocytopenia*

RESP: Dyspnea

SYST: Anaphylaxis, serum sickness

Contraindications: Hypersensitivity to cephalosporins or related antibiotics, seizures

Precautions: Pregnancy (B), lactation, children, renal disease

Do not confuse:
cefaclor/cephalexin
Cefotan/Ceftin
cefprozil/Cafazolin
cefprozil/cefuroxime
Cefzil/Ceftin
Cefzil/Kefzol

Pharmacokinetics:

cefaclor:

PO: Peak ½-1 hr, ext rel peak 1½-2½ hr, half-life 36-54 min; 25% bound by plasma proteins; 60%-85% eliminated unchanged in urine in 8 hr; crosses placenta; excreted in breast milk (low concentrations)

cefamandole: Peak 1-1½ hr, half-life ½-1 hr; 60%-75% bound by plasma proteins; crosses placenta; excreted in breast milk; poor penetration into CSF

cefmetazole

IM: Peak 30-45 min; 68% bound by plasma proteins, excreted by kidneys; half-life 1-3 hr

cefonicid

IV: Onset 5 min

IM: Peak 1 hr

Half-life 4½ hr; excreted in breast milk (small amounts); 98% protein bound; poor penetration in CSF

cefotetan

IV/IM: Peak 1½-3 hr; half-life 3-5 hr, 70%-90% bound by plasma proteins, 50%-80% eliminated unchanged in urine, crosses placenta, excreted in breast milk

cefoxitin

IV: Peak 3 min

IM: Peak 15-60 min

Half-life 1 hr, 55%-75% bound by plasma proteins, 90%-100% eliminated unchanged in urine; crosses placenta, blood-brain barrier; eliminated in breast milk, not metabolized

cefprozil

PO: Peak 6-10 hr; plasma protein binding 99%; elimination half-life

25 hr; extensively metabolized to an active metabolite

cefuroxime: 65% excreted unchanged in urine, half-life 1-2 hr in normal renal function

loracarbef

PO: Peak 1 hr, half-life 1 hr; excreted in urine as unchanged drug

Interactions:

• Increased effect/toxicity: aminoglycosides, furosemide, probenecid

• Disulfiram-like reaction: alcohol

• Antagonist effect: chloramphenicol, do not use together

Lab test interferences:

False increase: Creatinine (serum urine), urinary 17-KS

False positive: Urinary protein, direct Coombs' test, urine glucose testing (Clinitest)

Interference: Cross-matching

NURSING CONSIDERATIONS

Assess:

⬧ Nephrotoxicity: increased BUN, creatinine

• I&O ratio

• Blood studies: AST, ALT, CBC, Hct, bilirubin, LDH, alk phosphatase, Coombs' test qmo if patient is on long-term therapy

• Electrolytes: K, Na, Cl qmo if patient is on long-term therapy

• Bowel pattern qd; if severe diarrhea occurs, drug should be discontinued; may indicate pseudomembranous colitis

• Urine output; if decreasing, notify prescriber (may indicate nephrotoxicity)

⬧ Anaphylaxis: rash, flushing, urticaria, pruritus, dyspnea

• Bleeding: ecchymosis, bleeding gums, hematuria, stool guaiac daily

⬧ Overgrowth of infection: perineal itching, fever, malaise, redness, pain, swelling, drainage, rash, diarrhea, change in cough, sputum

Administer:

cefaclor

• Shake susp, refrigerate, discard after 2 wk

• For 10-14 days to ensure organism death, prevent superinfection

• With food if needed for GI symptoms

• After C&S completed

🚫 Do not break, crush, or chew ext rel tabs

cefamandole

• IV; check often for irritation, extravasation; dilute 1 g or less of drug/10 ml or more normal saline or sterile H_2O for inj; run over 3-5 min; may be further diluted with 100 ml of compatible sol and run over 15-30 min via Y-tube or 3-way stopcock; may also be diluted in 1 L compatible sol, run over prescribed rate

• For 10-14 days to ensure organism death, prevent superinfection

• After C&S completed

Additive compatibilities: Clindamycin, floxacillin, furosemide, metronidazole, verapamil

Syringe compatibilities: Heparin

Y-site compatibilities: Acyclovir, cyclophosphamide, hydromorphone, magnesium sulfate, meperidine, morphine, perphenazine

cefmetazole

• For 10-14 days to ensure organism death, prevent superinfection

• After C&S completed

Solution compatibilities: D_5W, 0.9% NaCl

Additive compatibilities: Clindamycin, famotidine, KCl

• IV after diluting 3.7 or 10 ml sterile H_2O for inj, 2 g/7 or 15 ml, shake, let stand until clear, run over 3-5 min; may be further diluted in 50-100 ml of D_5W, NS, LR to 1-20 mg/ml and run over ½-1 hr by Y-tube or 3-way stopcock

---

⬧ = Nursing alert   ▰ = Herb-drug interaction   🚫 = Do not crush

C

cefonicid
• IV direct dilute 0.5 g/2 ml or 1 g/2.5 ml sterile H_2O for inj and give by Y-tube or 3-way stopcock over 3-5 min
• IV INT INF may be further diluted in 50-100 ml D_5W, NS and given over 30 min; slight yellowing of sol does not affect potency
• IV; check for irritation, extravasation often
Additive compatibilities: Clindamycin
Y-site compatibilities: Acyclovir, amifostine, aztreonam, teniposide, thiotepa

cefotetan
• IV direct after diluting 1 g/10 ml sterile H_2O for inj and give over 3-5 min; may be diluted further with 50-100 ml of normal saline or D_5W, shake; run over ½-1 hr by Y-tube or 3-way stopcock; discontinue primary inf during administration
• May be stored 96 hr refrigerated or 24 hr room temperature
Y-site compatibilities: Allopurinol, amifostine, aztreonam, diltiazem, famotidine, filgrastim, fluconazole, fludarabine, heparin, insulin (regular), melphalan, meperidine, morphine, paclitaxel, remifentanil, sargramostim, tacrolimus, teniposide, theophylline, thiotepa

cefoxitin
• IV after diluting 1 g or less/10 ml or more D_5W, NS and give over 3-5 min; may be diluted further with 50-100 ml of normal saline or D_5W; run over ½-1 hr by Y-tube or 3-way stopcock; discontinue primary inf during administration; by cont inf at prescribed rate; may store 96 hr refrigerated or 24 hr room temperature
• For 10-14 days to ensure organism death, prevent superinfection
• After C&S completed

Additive compatibilities: Amikacin, cimetidine, clindamycin, gentamicin, kanamycin, multivitamins, sodium bicarbonate, tobramycin, verapamil, vit B/C
Syringe compatibilities: Heparin, insulin
Y-site compatibilities: Acyclovir, amifostine, amphotericin B cholesteryl sulfate complex, aztreonam, cyclophosphamide, diltiazem, doxorubicin liposome, famotidine, fluconazole, foscarnet, hydromorphone, magnesium sulfate, meperidine, morphine, ondansetron, perphenazine, remifentanil, teniposide, thiotepa

cefprozil
• For 10-14 days to ensure organism death, prevent superinfection
• After C&S
• Refrigerate/shake susp prior to use

cefuroxime
• For 10-14 days to ensure organism death, prevent superinfection
• With food if needed for GI symptoms
• After C&S

Additive compatibilities: Clindamycin, floxacillin, furosemide, metronidazole, netilmicin
Y-site compatibilities: Acyclovir, allopurinol, amifostine, atracurium, aztreonam, cyclophosphamide, diltiazem, famotidine, fludarabine, foscarnet, hydromorphone, melphalan, meperidine, morphine, ondansetron, pancuronium, perphenazine, remifentanil, sargramostim, tacrolimus, teniposide, thiotepa, vecuronium

loracarbef
• Oral susp should be shaken before giving; store for 2 wk at room temperature, discard after 2 wk
• 1 hr before or 2 hr after a meal
• After C&S is completed
• For 7 days to ensure organism death, prevent superinfection

---

Evaluate:
• Therapeutic response: negative C&S
Teach patient/family:
• If diabetic, to use blood glucose testing
• Not to drink alcohol or take meds with alcohol or reaction may occur
• To complete full course of drug therapy, to report persistent diarrhea
• To take on an empty stomach 1 hr before or 2 hr after a meal
🚫 Not to break, crush, or chew caps
• To notify prescriber if breastfeeding or of any side effects
Treatment of anaphylaxis: Epinephrine, antihistamines; resuscitate if needed

CEPHALOSPORINS—3RD GENERATION

cefdinir (℞)
(sef'dih-ner)
Omnicef
cefepime (℞)
(sef'e-peem)
Maxipime
cefixime (℞)
(sef-icks'ime)
Suprax
cefoperazone (℞)
(sef-oh-per'a-zone)
Cefobid
cefotaxime (℞)
(sef-oh-taks'eem)
Claforan
cefpodoxime (℞)
(sef-poe-docks'eem)
Vantin
ceftazidime (℞)
(sef'tay-zi-deem)
Ceptaz, Fortaz, Magnacef*, Pentacef, Tazicef, Tazidime
ceftibuten (℞)
(sef-ti-byoo'tin)
Cedax
ceftizoxime (℞)
(sef-ti-zox'eem)
Cefizox
ceftriaxone (℞)
(sef-try-ax'one)
Rocephin
moxalactam (℞)
(mox'a-lak-tam)
Moxam
Func. class.: Broad-spectrum antibiotic
Chem. class.: Cephalosporin (3rd generation)

Action: Inhibits bacterial cell wall synthesis, rendering cell wall osmotically unstable, leading to cell death

⬥ = Nursing alert   🌿 = Herb-drug interaction   🚫 = Do not crush

Uses:

cefdinir: Gram-negative bacilli: *Haemophilus influenzae, Haemophilus parainfluenzae, Moraxella catarrhalis;* gram-positive organisms: *Streptococcus pneumoniae, Streptococcus pyogenes, Staphylococcus aureus;* acute exacerbations of chronic bronchitis

cefepime: Gram-negative bacilli: *Escherichia coli, Proteus, Klebsiella;* gram-positive organisms: *Streptococcus pneumoniae, Streptococcus pyogenes, Staphylococcus aureus;* lower respiratory tract, urinary tract, skin, bone infections

cefixime: Uncomplicated UTI *(Escherichia coli, Proteus mirabilis),* pharyngitis and tonsillitis *(Streptococcus pyogenes),* otitis media *(Haemophilus influenzae), Moraxella catarrhalis,* acute bronchitis, and acute exacerbations of chronic bronchitis *(Streptococcus pneumoniae, H. influenzae)*

cefoperazone: Gram-negative bacilli: *Haemophilus influenzae, Escherichia coli, Proteus mirabilis, Klebsiella, Enterobacter, Serratia, Citrobacter, Providencia, Proteus aeruginosa;* lower respiratory tract, urinary tract, skin, bone infections, bacterial septicemia, peritonitis, PID

cefotaxime: Gram-negative organisms: *Haemophilus influenzae, Escherichia coli, Neisseria gonorrhoeae, Neisseria meningitidis, Proteus mirabilis, Klebsiella, Citrobacter, Serratia, Salmonella, Shigella;* gram-positive organisms: *Streptococcus pneumoniae, Streptococcus pyogenes, Staphylococcus aureus;* serious lower respiratory tract, urinary tract, skin, bone, gonococcal infections; bacteremia, septicemia, meningitis

cefpodoxime: Gram-negative bacilli: *Neisseria gonorrhoeae, Haemophilus influenzae, Escherichia coli, Proteus mirabilis, Klebsiella;* gram-positive organisms: *Streptococcus pneumoniae, Streptococcus pyogenes, Staphylococcus aureus;* upper and lower respiratory tract, urinary tract, skin infections; otitis media, sexually transmitted diseases

ceftazidime: Gram-negative organisms: *Haemophilus influenzae, Escherichia coli, Escherichia aerogenes, Proteus aeruginosa, Proteus mirabilis, Klebsiella, Citrobacter, Enterobacter, Salmonella, Shigella, Acinetobacter, Bacteroides fragilis, Neisseria, Serratia;* gram-positive organisms: *Streptococcus pneumoniae, Streptococcus pyogenes, Staphylococcus aureus;* serious upper/lower respiratory tract, urinary tract, skin, gynecologic, bone, joint, intraabdominal infections; septicemia, meningitis

ceftibuten: Pharyngitis/tonsillitis, otitis media, secondary bacterial infection of acute bronchitis

ceftizoxime: Gram-negative bacilli: *Haemophilus influenzae, Escherichia coli, Escherichia aerogenes, Proteus mirabilis, Klebsiella, Enterobacter;* gram-positive organisms: *Streptococcus pneumoniae, Streptococcus pyogenes, Staphylococcus aureus;* serious lower respiratory tract, urinary tract, skin, intraabdominal infections, septicemia, meningitis, bone and joint infections, PID caused by *Neisseria gonorrhoeae*

ceftriaxone: Gram-negative bacilli: *Haemophilus influenzae, Escherichia coli, Escherichia aerogenes, Proteus mirabilis, Klebsiella, Citrobacter, Enterobacter, Salmonella, Shigella, Acinetobacter, Bacteroides fragilis, Neisseria, Serratia;* gram-positive organisms: *Streptococcus pneumoniae, Streptococcus pyogenes, Staphylococcus aureus;* serious lower respiratory tract, urinary tract, skin, gonococcal, intraabdominal infections, septicemia, meningitis, bone, joint infections

moxalactam: Gram-negative bacilli: *Haemophilus influenzae, Escherichia coli, Proteus mirabilis, Klebsiella, Citrobacter, Salmonella, Shigella, Serratia;* gram-positive organisms: *Streptococcus pneumoniae, Streptococcus pyogenes, Staphylococcus aureus;* serious lower respiratory tract, urinary tract, skin, bone infections; septicemia, meningitis, intraabdominal infections

Dosage and routes:
cefdinir
Uncomplicated skin and skin structure infections/community-acquired pneumonia
• *Adult and child ≥13 yr:* **PO** 300 mg q12h × 10 days
• *Child 6 mo-12 yr:* **PO** 7 mg/kg q12h or 14 mg/kg q24h × 10 days, max 60 mg qd
Acute exacerbations of chronic bronchitis/acute maxillary sinusitis
• *Adult and child ≥13 yr:* **PO** 300 mg q12h or 600 mg q24h × 10 days or 300 mg bid × 5 days in some infections
Pharyngitis/tonsillitis
• *Adult and child ≥13 yr:* **PO** 300 mg q12h or 600 mg q24h × 10 days
• *Child 6 mo-12 yr:* **PO** 7 mg/kg q12h × 5-10 days or 14 mg/kg q24h × 10 days
Renal dose
• CrCl <30 ml/min 300 mg qd (adult); 7 mg/kg qd (child)
cefepime
Urinary tract infections (mild to moderate)
• *Adult:* **IV/IM** 0.5-1 g q12h × 7-10 days
Urinary tract infections (severe)
• *Adult:* **IV** 2 g q12h × 10 days
Pneumonia (moderate to severe)
• *Adult:* **IV** 1-2 g q12h × 10 days

• Dosage reduction indicated in renal impairment (CrCl <50 ml/min)
Uncomplicated gonorrhea
• **IM** 2 g as a single dose with 1 g **PO** probenecid at the same time
Available forms: Powder for inj 500 mg, 1, 2 g
cefixime
Renal dose: CrCl 21-60 ml/min give 75% of dose; CrCl <20 ml/min give 50% of dose
• *Adult:* **PO** 400 mg qd as a single dose or 200 mg q12h
• *Child >50 kg or >12 yr:* **PO** use adult dosage
• *Child <50 kg or <12 yr:* **PO** 8 mg/kg/day as a single dose or 4 mg/kg q12h
Available forms: Tabs 200, 400 mg; powder for oral susp 100 mg/5 ml
cefoperazone
Hepatic dose: give 50% of dose
Mild/Moderate infections
• *Adult:* **IM/IV** 1-2 g q12h
Severe infections
• *Adult:* **IM/IV** 6-12 g/day divided in 2-4 equal doses
Available forms: Inj 1, 2 g
cefotaxime
• *Adult:* **IM/IV** 1-2 g q12h as a single dose
• *Child 1 mo-12 yr:* **IM/IV** 50-180 mg/kg/day divided q6h
Severe infections
• *Adult:* **IM/IV** 2 g q4h, not to exceed 12 g/day
• *Child 1 mo-12 yr:* **IM/IV** 50 mg/kg q6h
Uncomplicated gonorrhea
• *Adult:* **IM** 1 g
Dosage reduction indicated for severe renal impairment (CrCl <30 ml/min)
Available forms: Powder for inj 1, 2, 10 g; frozen inj 20, 40 mg/ml
cefpodoxime
• Reduce dose in renal disease
• *Adult >13 yr:* Pneumonia: 200 mg q12h for 14 days; *uncomplicated*

gonorrhea: 200 mg single dose; *skin and skin structure:* 400 mg q12h for 7-14 days; *pharyngitis and tonsillitis:* 100 mg q12h for 10 days; *uncomplicated UTI:* 100 mg q12h for 7 days; dosing interval increased in presence of severe renal impairment

• *Child 5 mo-12 yr: acute otitis media:* 5 mg/kg q12h for 10 days; *pharyngitis/tonsillitis:* 5 mg/kg q12h (max 100 mg/dose or 200 mg/day) × 5-10 days

Available forms: Tabs 100, 200 mg/granules for susp 50, 100 mg/5 ml

ceftazidime
Renal dose: CrCl <50 ml/min give q12h; CrCl 10-30 ml/min give q24h; CrCl <10 ml/min give q48h

• *Adult:* **IV/IM** 1-2 g q8-12h × 5-10 days

• *Child:* **IV** 30-50 mg/kg q8h not to exceed 6 g/day

• *Neonate:* **IV** 30-50 mg/kg q12h

Available forms: Inj 500 mg, 1, 2, 6 g

ceftibuten
Renal dose: CrCl <50 ml/min give 200 mg q24h; CrCl 5-20 ml/min give 100 mg q24h

• *Adult:* **PO** 400 mg qd × 10 days

• *Child 6 mo-12 yr:* **PO** 9 mg/kg qd × 10 days

Available forms: Caps 400 mg; 90, 180 mg/5 ml

ceftizoxime
Renal dose: CrCl <80 ml/min give 500-1500 mg q8h; CrCl 10-49 ml/min give 250-1000 mg q12h

• *Adult:* **IM/IV** 1-2 g q8-12h, may give up to 4 g q8h in life-threatening infections

• *Child <6 mo:* **IM/IV** 50 mg/kg q6-8h

PID
• *Adult:* **IV** 2 g q8h, may increase to 4 g q8h in severe infections

Available forms: Powder for inj 500 mg, 1, 2, 10 g; premixed 1 g, 2 g/50 ml

ceftriaxone
• *Adult:* **IM/IV** 1-2 g qd, max 2 g q12h

• *Child:* **IM/IV** 50-75 mg/kg/day in equal doses q12h

Uncomplicated gonorrhea
• *Adult:* 250 mg **IM** as single dose

• Reduce dosage in severe renal impairment (CrCl <10 ml/min)

Meningitis
• *Adult and child:* **IM/IV** 100 mg/kg/day in equal doses q12h, max 4 g/day

Surgical prophylaxis
• *Adult:* **IV** 1 g ½-2 hr preop

Available forms: Inj 500 mg, 1, 2, 10 g

moxalactam
• *Adult:* **IM/IV** 2-4 g q8-12h

Mild infections
• *Adult:* **IM/IV** 250-500 mg q8-12h

Severe infections
• *Adult:* **IM/IV** 2-6 g q8h

• *Child:* **IM/IV** 50 mg/kg q6-8h

• Dosage reduction indicated even for mild renal impairment (CrCl <80 ml/min)

Available forms: Powder for inj 1, 2, 10 g

Side effects/adverse reactions:

CNS: Headache, dizziness, weakness, paresthesia, fever, chills, seizures

GI: Nausea, vomiting, diarrhea, anorexia, pain, glossitis, ***bleeding;*** increased AST, ALT, bilirubin, LDH, alk phosphatase; abdominal pain, ***pseudomembranous colitis***

*GU: **Proteinuria,*** vaginitis, pruritus, candidiasis, increased BUN, ***nephrotoxicity, renal failure***

*HEMA: **Leukopenia, thrombocytopenia, agranulocytosis,*** anemia, ***neutropenia, lymphocytosis, eosinophilia, pancytopenia, hemolytic anemia***

INTEG: Rash, urticaria, dermatitis

RESP: Dyspnea

*SYST: **Anaphylaxis,*** serum sickness

Contraindications: Hypersensitivity to cephalosporins, infants <1 mo
Precautions: Hypersensitivity to penicillins, pregnancy (B), lactation, renal disease, children
Do not confuse:
Vantin/Ventolin
ceftazidime/ceftizoxime
Pharmacokinetics:
cefdinir
Unchanged in urine; crosses placenta, blood-brain barrier; eliminated in breast milk; not metabolized
cefepime
Peak 79 min, half-life 2 hr, 20% bound by plasma proteins, 90% excreted unchanged in urine; crosses placenta, blood-brain barrier; excreted in breast milk; not metabolized
cefixime
PO: Peak 1-2 hr, half-life 3-4 hr, 65% bound by plasma proteins, 50% eliminated unchanged in urine; crosses placenta; excreted in breast milk
cefoperazone
IV: Onset 5 min, peak 5-20 min, duration 6-8 hr
IM: Peak 1-2 hr, duration 6-8 hr
Half-life 2 hr; 70%-75% is eliminated unchanged in bile; 20%-30% unchanged in urine; excreted in breast milk (small amounts)
cefotaxime
IV: Onset 5 min
IM: Onset 30 min
Half-life 1 hr; 35%-65% is bound by plasma proteins; 40%-65% is eliminated unchanged in urine in 24 hr; 25% metabolized to active metabolites; excreted in breast milk (small amounts)
cefpodoxime
Half-life 2-3 hr; 25% bound by plasma proteins; 30% eliminated unchanged in urine in 8 hr; crosses placenta; excreted in breast milk

ceftazidime
IV/IM: Peak 1 hr, half-life ½-1 hr, 90% bound by plasma proteins, 80% eliminated unchanged in urine, crosses placenta, excreted in breast milk
ceftibuten
PO: Peak 6-10 hr; plasma protein binding 99%; elimination half-life 25 hr; extensively metabolized to an active metabolite
ceftizoxime
IV: Onset 5 min
IM: Peak 1 hr
Half-life 5-8 hr; 90% bound by plasma proteins; 36%-60% eliminated unchanged in urine; crosses placenta; excreted in breast milk
ceftriaxone
IV: Onset 5 min
IM: Peak 1 hr
Half-life 5-8 hr, 90% bound by plasma proteins, 35%-60% eliminated unchanged in urine; crosses placenta; excreted in breast milk
moxalactam
IV: Peak 5 min
IM: Peak ½-2 hr
Half-life 1½-2½ hr, 25% bound by plasma proteins; 60%-97% eliminated unchanged in urine in 24 hr; crosses placenta, blood-brain barrier; excreted in breast milk; not metabolized
Interactions:
• Increased toxicity: aminoglycosides, furosemide, probenecid
Lab test interferences:
False increase: Urinary 17-KS
False positive: Urinary protein, direct Coombs' test, urine glucose
Interference: Cross-matching
NURSING CONSIDERATIONS
Assess:
• Sensitivity to penicillin, other cephalosporins
◆Nephrotoxicity: increased BUN, creatinine

◆ = Nursing alert   ∥ = Herb-drug interaction   ⊘ = Do not crush

• Blood studies: AST, ALT, CBC, Hct, bilirubin, LDH, alk phosphatase, Coombs' test monthly if patient is on long-term therapy

• Electrolytes: K, Na, Cl monthly if patient is on long-term therapy

• Bowel pattern qd; if severe diarrhea occurs, drug should be discontinued; may indicate pseudomembranous colitis

• IV site for extravasation, phlebitis; change site q72h

◆ Urine output: if decreasing, notify prescriber; may indicate nephrotoxicity

◆ Anaphylaxis: rash, urticaria, pruritus, chills, fever, joint pain, angioedema; may occur few days after therapy begins

• Bleeding: ecchymosis, bleeding gums, hematuria, stool guaiac

◆ Overgrowth of infection: perineal itching, fever, malaise, redness, pain, swelling, drainage, rash, diarrhea, change in cough, sputum

Administer:

cefdinir

• Oral susp after adding 39 ml water to the 60 ml bottle; 65 ml water to the 120 ml bottle; discard unused portion after 10 days

• After C&S completed

cefepime

• IV after diluting in 50-100 ml or more D_5, NS and give over 30 min

• For 7-10 days to ensure organism death, prevent superinfection

Solution compatibilities: 0.9% NaCl, D_5, D_5W, 0.5%, 10% lidocaine, bacteriostatic water for inj with parabens/benzyl alcohol

Y-site compatibilities: Doxorubicin liposome

cefixime

• For 10-14 days to ensure organism death, prevent superinfection

cefoperazone

• IV after diluting 1 g/ml sterile H_2O for inj, or 0.9% NaCl; shake, give

over 3-5 min; each g may be further diluted with 20-40 ml D_5W, NS given over 30 min or as a cont inf over 6-24 hr to a concentration no greater than 25 mg/ml

• IM for concentration >250 mg/ml, dilute in sterile water, then lidocaine, inject deeply

• For 10-14 days to ensure organism death, prevent superinfection

Additive compatibilities: Cimetidine, clindamycin, furosemide

Syringe compatibilities: Heparin

Y-site compatibilities: Acyclovir, allopurinol, aztreonam, cyclophosphamide, enalaprilat, esmolol, famotidine, foscarnet, fludarabine, hydromorphone, magnesium sulfate, melphalan, morphine, teniposide, thiotepa

cefotaxime

• IV after diluting 1 g/10 ml D_5W, NS, sterile H_2O for inj and give over 3-5 min by Y-tube or 3-way stopcock; may be diluted further with 50-100 ml of normal saline or D_5W; run over ½-1 hr; discontinue primary inf during administration; or may be diluted in larger vol of sol and given as a cont inf over 6-24 hr

• For 10-14 days to ensure organism death, prevent superinfection

Additive compatibilities: Clindamycin, metronidazole, verapamil

Syringe compatibilities: Heparin, ofloxacin

Y-site compatibilities: Acyclovir, amifostine, aztreonam, cyclophosphamide, diltiazem, famotidine, fludarabine, hydromorphone, lorazepam, magnesium sulfate, melphalan, meperidine, midazolam, morphine, ondansetron, perphenazine, sargramostim, teniposide, thiotepa, tolazoline, vinorelbine

cefpodoxime

• For 10-14 days to ensure organism death, prevent superinfection

• With food to enhance absorption

Y-site compatibilities: Famotidine, fluconazole, fludarabine, insulin (regular), meperidine, morphine, sargramostim

ceftazidime

• IV after diluting 1 g/10 ml sterile H_2O for inj, shake, invert needle, push plunger, insert needle through stopper and keep in sol, expel bubbles and give over 3-5 min; may be diluted further with 50-100 ml of normal saline or D_5W; run over ½-1 hr, give through Y-tube or 3-way stopcock, discontinue primary inf during administration; store for 96 hr refrigerated, 24 hr room temperature

• For 5-10 days to ensure organism death, prevent superinfection

Syringe compatibilities: Hydromorphone

Additive compatibilities: Ciprofloxacin, clindamycin, fluconazole, metronidazole, ofloxacin

Y-site compatibilities: Acyclovir, allopurinol, amifostine, aztreonam, ciprofloxacin, diltiazem, enalaprilat, esmolol, famotidine, filgrastim, fludarabine, foscarnet, granisetron, heparin, hydromorphone, labetalol, meperidine, melphalan, morphine, ondansetron, paclitaxel, ranitidine, remifentanil, tacrolimus, teniposide, theophylline, thiotepa, vinorelbine, zidovudine

ceftibuten

• For 10 days to ensure organism death, prevent superinfection

ceftizoxime

• IV after diluting 1 g/10 ml sterile water, shake and give over 3-5 min; may be diluted further with 50-100 ml NS or D_5W give through Y-tube or 3-way stopcock; run over ½-1 hr

• For 10-14 days to ensure organism death, prevent superinfection

Additive compatibilities: Clindamycin

Y-site compatibilities: Acyclovir, allopurinol, amphotericin B cholesteryl sulfate complex, aztreonam, doxorubicin liposome, enalaprilat, esmolol, famotidine, fludarabine, foscarnet, hydromorphone, labetalol, melphalan, meperidine, morphine, ondansetron, remifentanil, sargramostim, teniposide, vinorelbine

ceftriaxone

• For 10-14 days to ensure organism death, prevent superinfection

• IV after diluting 250 mg/2.4 ml D_5W, H_2O for inj, 0.9% NaCl; may be further diluted with 50-100 ml NS, D_5W, $D_{10}W$, shake; run over ½-1 hr

Additive compatibilities: Amino acids or sodium bicarbonate, metronidazole

Y-site compatibilities: Acyclovir, allopurinol, aztreonam, cisatracurium, diltiazem, doxorubicin liposome, fludarabine, foscarnet, heparin, melphalan, meperidine, methotrexate, morphine, paclitaxel, remifentanil, sargramostim, tacrolimus, teniposide, theophylline, vinorelbine, warfarin, zidovudine

moxalactam

• For 10-14 days to ensure organism death, prevent superinfection

• IV after diluting 1 g/10 ml sterile H_2O, D_5, 0.9% NaCl; give through Y-tube over 3-5 min; may be further diluted 1 g/20 ml in D_5, 0.9% NaCl, give over ½ hr; may be added to 500-1000 ml, give over 6-24 hr

• Vit K for bleeding (10 mg/wk)

Additive compatibilities: Metronidazole, ranitidine, verapamil

Syringe compatibilities: Heparin

Y-site compatibilities: Cyclophosphamide, hydromorphone, magnesium sulfate, meperidine, morphine, perphenazine

Evaluate:

• Therapeutic response: decreased symptoms of infection; negative C&S

◆ = Nursing alert   🖋 = Herb-drug interaction   ⊘ = Do not crush

Teach patient/family:
• If diabetic, to check blood glucose
• To report sore throat, bruising, bleeding, joint pain; may indicate blood dyscrasias (rare)
• To report persistent diarrhea
Treatment of anaphylaxis: Epinephrine, antihistamines; resuscitate if needed

cephalothin
cephapirin
cephradine

See cephalosporins—1st generation

cetirizine (℞)

(se-teer'i-zeen)
Zyrtec
Func. class.: Antihistamine (2nd generation, peripherally selective)
Chem. class.: Piperazine, H_1-histamine antagonist

Action: Acts on blood vessels, GI, respiratory system by competing with histamine for H_1-receptor site; decreases allergic response by blocking pharmacologic effects of histamine; minimal anticholinergic action
Uses: Rhinitis, allergy symptoms
Dosage and routes:
• *Adult and child ≥6 yr:* **PO** 5-10 mg qd
• *Child 2-6:* **PO** 2.5 mg qd, may increase to 5 mg qd or 2.5 mg bid
• *Geriatric:* **PO** 5 mg qd, may increase to 10 mg/day
Renal/hepatic dose: CrCl 11-31 ml/min 5 mg qd
Available forms: Tabs 5, 10 mg; syrup 5 mg/5 ml
Side effects/adverse reactions:
RESP: Thickening of bronchial secretions, dry nose, throat

GI: Dry mouth
CNS: Headache, stimulation, *drowsiness,* sedation, *fatigue,* confusion, blurred vision, tinnitus, restlessness, tremors, paradoxical excitation in children or elderly
INTEG: Rash, eczema, photosensitivity, urticaria
Contraindications: Hypersensitivity to this drug or hydroxyzine, newborn or premature infants, lactation, severe hepatic disease
Precautions: Pregnancy (B), elderly, children, respiratory disease, narrow-angle glaucoma, prostatic hypertrophy, bladder neck obstruction, asthma, elderly
Pharmacokinetics:
Onset ½ hr, peak 1-2 hr, duration 24 hr, protein binding 93%, half-life 8.3 hr, decreased in children, increased in hepatic/renal disease
Interactions:
• Increased CNS depression: alcohol, other CNS depressants
• Increased anticholinergic/sedative effect: MAOIs
• Drug/food: food decreases absorption by 1.7 hr
⚕ Increased CNS depression: kava
Lab test interferences:
False negative: Skin allergy tests
NURSING CONSIDERATIONS
Assess:
• Allergy symptoms: pruritus, urticaria, watering eyes, baseline and during treatment
• Respiratory status: rate, rhythm, increase in bronchial secretions, wheezing, chest tightness
Administer:
• Without regard to meals
Perform/provide:
• Hard candy, gum, frequent rinsing of mouth for dryness
• Storage in tight, light-resistant container

Evaluate:
• Therapeutic response: absence of running or congested nose or rashes
Teach patient/family:
• All aspects of drug use; to notify prescriber if confusion, sedation, hypotension occur
• To avoid driving, other hazardous activity if drowsiness occurs
• To avoid alcohol, other CNS depressants
• That drug is not recommended during lactation
• To avoid exposure to sunlight; burns may occur
Treatment of overdose: Administer ipecac syrup or lavage, diazepam, vasopressors, barbiturates (short-acting)

---

cetrorelix (R)
(set-roe-ree'lix)
Cetrotide
Func. class.: Gonadotropin-releasing hormone antagonist
Chem. class.: Synthetic decapeptide

Action: Inhibitor of pituitary gonadotropin secretion; initially increases LH and FSH, induces a rapid suppression of gonadotropin secretion
Uses: For inhibition of premature LH surges in women undergoing controlled ovarian hyperstimulation
Dosage and routes:
Single-dose regimen
• *Adult:* SC 3 mg when serum estradiol level is at appropriate stimulation response, usually on stimulation day 7; if hCG has not been given withiin 4 days after inj of 3 mg cetrorelix, give 0.25 mg qd until day of hCG administration
Multiple-dose regimen
• *Adult:* SC 0.25 mg is given on stimulation day 5 (either morning or evening) or 6 (morning) and continued qd until day hCG is given
Available forms: Inj 0.25, 3 mg
Side effects/adverse reactions:
CNS: Headache
ENDO: Ovarian hyperstimulation syndrome, abdominal pain (gyn)
GI: Nausea
INTEG: Pain on injection; local site reactions
SYST: **Fetal death**
Contraindications: Hypersensitivity, pregnancy (X), latex allergy, lactation
Pharmacokinetics: Excreted in feces/urine, half-life depends on dosage, metabolized to metabolites, protein binding 86%
NURSING CONSIDERATIONS
Assess:
• For suspected pregnancy, drug should not be used
• For latex allergy, drug should not be used
• For ALT, AST, GGT, alk phosphatase
Administer:
• SC using abdomen, around navel or upper thigh, swab inj area with disinfectant, clean a 2 in circle and allow to dry, pinch up area between thumb and finger, insert needle 45-90° to surface; if positioned correctly, no blood will be drawn back into syringe, reposition needle without removing it
• Do not administer if patient is pregnant
Perform/provide:
• Protection from light
Evaluate:
• Therapeutic response: pregnancy
Teach patient/family:
• To report abdominal pain, vaginal bleeding
• To teach self-administration technique if needed

◆ = Nursing alert   ✐ = Herb-drug interaction   ⊘ = Do not crush

chloral hydrate (℞)

(klor-al hye'drate)
Aquachloral, chloral hydrate,
Novo-Chlorhydrate*,
PMS-chloral hydrate*

Func. class.: Sedative/hypnotic
Chem. class.: Chloral derivative

Controlled Substance Schedule IV
(USA), Schedule F (Canada)
Action: Reduction product trichloroethanol produces mild cerebral depression, which causes sleep
Uses: Sedation, short-term treatment of insomnia
Dosage and routes:
Sedation
• *Adult:* **PO/RECT** 250 mg tid pc
• *Child:* **PO** 25-50 mg/kg tid, not to exceed 500 mg tid
Insomnia
• *Adult:* **PO/RECT** 500 mg-1 g ½ hr before hs
• *Child:* **PO/RECT** 50-75 mg/kg (one dose)
Procedure sedation
• *Child:* **PO/RECT** 25-50 mg/kg, not to exceed 100 mg/kg or 2 g
Renal disease
• CrCl <50 ml/min avoid use
Available forms: Caps 250, 500, 650 mg; syr 250, 500 mg/5 ml; supp 325, 500 mg
Side effects/adverse reactions:
HEMA: Eosinophilia, leukopenia
CNS: Drowsiness, dizziness, stimulation, nightmares, ataxia, hangover (rare), light-headedness, headache, paranoia
GI: Nausea, vomiting, flatulence, diarrhea, unpleasant taste, ***gastric necrosis***
INTEG: Rash, urticaria, ***angioedema,*** fever, purpura, eczema
CV: Hypotension, ***dysrhythmias***
RESP: Depression

Contraindications: Hypersensitivity to this drug or triclofos, severe renal disease, severe hepatic disease, GI disorders (oral forms), gastritis
Precautions: Severe cardiac disease, depression, suicidal individuals, asthma, intermittent porphyria, pregnancy (C), lactation, elderly
Pharmacokinetics:
PO: Onset 30 min-1 hr, duration 4-8 hr
RECT: Onset slow, duration 4-8 hr; metabolized by liver; excreted by kidneys (inactive metabolite) and feces; crosses placenta; excreted in breast milk; metabolite is highly protein bound
Interactions:
• Increased action: oral anticoagulants, furosemide
• Increased action of both drugs: alcohol, CNS depressants
⚠ Increased CNS depression: kava
Lab test interferences:
Interference: Urine catecholamines, urinary 17-OHCS
NURSING CONSIDERATIONS
Assess:
• Mental status: mood, sensorium, affect, memory (long-, short-term)
• Physical dependency: more frequent requests for medication, tremors, anxiety, pinpoint pupils
• Respiratory dysfunction: respiratory depression, character, rate, rhythm; hold drug if respirations <10/min or if pupils dilated (rare)
• History of substance abuse, cardiac disease, gastritis
Administer:
• ½-1 hr before hs for sleeplessness
🚫 On empty stomach with full glass of water or juice for best absorption and to decrease corrosion (do not break, crush, or chew); after meals to decrease GI symptoms if using for sedation

Perform/provide:

• Assistance with ambulation after receiving dose, especially elderly

• Safety measure: night-light, call bell within easy reach

• Check to see PO medication swallowed

• Check dose of syrup carefully, fatal overdoses have occurred

• Storage in dark container, suppositories in refrigerator

Evaluate:

• Therapeutic response: ability to sleep at night, decreased amount of early morning awakening if taking drug for insomnia

Teach patient/family:

• To avoid driving, other activities requiring alertness

• To avoid alcohol ingestion, CNS depressants; serious CNS depression may result

• Not to discontinue medication quickly after long-term use; drug should be tapered over 1-2 wk

• That effects may take 2 nights for benefits to be noticed

🚫 Not to break, crush, or chew caps

• Alternative measures to improve sleep (reading, exercise several hours before hs, warm bath, warm milk, TV, self-hypnosis, deep breathing)

Treatment of overdose: Lavage, activated charcoal; monitor electrolytes, vital signs

---

chlorambucil (℞)

(klor-am′byoo-sil)
Leukeran
Func. class.: Antineoplastic alkylating agent
Chem. class.: Nitrogen mustard

Action: Alkylates DNA, RNA; inhibits enzymes that allow synthesis of amino acids in proteins; activity is not cell cycle phase specific

Uses: Chronic lymphocytic leukemia, Hodgkin's disease, other lymphomas, macroglobulinemia, nephrotic syndrome, breast carcinoma, choreocarcinoma, ovarian carcinoma

Dosage and routes:

• *Adult:* **PO** 0.1-0.2 mg/kg/day for 3-6 wk initially, then 2-6 mg/day; maintenance 0.2 mg/kg for 2-4 wk; course may be repeated at 2-4 wk intervals, or 0.4 mg/kg (12 mg/m^2) 2 × /wk, may increase by 0.1 mg/kg (3 mg/m^2) q2wk, adjust as needed

• *Geriatric:* **PO** initially ≤2-4 mg/day

• *Child:* **PO** 0.1-0.2 mg/kg/day (4.5 mg/m^2/day) in divided doses or 4.5 mg/m^2/day as 1 dose or in divided doses

Available forms: Tabs 2 mg

Side effects/adverse reactions:

CNS: **Convulsions**

HEMA: **Thrombocytopenia, leukopenia, pancytopenia** (prolonged use), **permanent bone marrow depression**

GI: Nausea, vomiting, diarrhea, weight loss, **hepatotoxicity,** *jaundice*

GU: Hyperuremia

INTEG: Alopecia (rare), dermatitis, rash, **Stevens-Johnson syndrome**

RESP: **Fibrosis, pneumonitis**

Contraindications: Radiation therapy within 1 mo, chemotherapy within 1 mo, thrombocytopenia, smallpox vaccination, pregnancy (D), lactation

Precautions: *Pneumococcus* vaccination

Do not confuse:

Leukeran/leucovorin
Leukeran/Leukine

Pharmacokinetics: Well absorbed orally; metabolized in liver; excreted in urine; half-life 2 hr

Interactions:

• Increased toxicity: other antineoplastics, radiation

◆ = Nursing alert   ⫮ = Herb-drug interaction   🚫 = Do not crush

• Increased risk of bleeding: anticoagulants, salicylates

NURSING CONSIDERATIONS

Assess:

• Bleeding: hematuria, guaiac, bruising or petechiae, mucosa or orifices q8h

• Jaundice of skin, sclera, dark urine, clay-colored stools, itchy skin, abdominal pain, fever, diarrhea

• Dyspnea, rales, unproductive cough, chest pain, tachypnea

• Effects of alopecia on body image; discuss feelings about body changes (rare)

• CBC, differential, platelet count weekly; withhold drug if WBC is <2000 or granulocyte count is <1000/mm³; notify prescriber of results

• Pulmonary function tests, chest x-ray films before, during therapy; chest film should be obtained q2wk during treatment

• Renal function studies: BUN, serum uric acid, urine CrCl before, during therapy; I&O ratio; report urine output of <30 ml/hr

• Monitor temp q4h (may indicate beginning infection)

• Liver function tests before, during therapy (bilirubin, AST, ALT, LDH) as needed or monthly

Administer:

PO

• All drugs PO if possible, avoid IM inj when platelets <150,000/mm³

• Antacid before oral agent; give drug 2 hr after evening meal, before bedtime or 1 hr before breakfast

• Antiemetic 30-60 min before giving drug to prevent vomiting

• Allopurinol to maintain uric acid levels, alkalinization of urine; increase fluid intake to 2-3 L/day to prevent urate deposits, calculi formation

Perform/provide:

• Storage in tight container

Evaluate:

• Therapeutic response: decreased size of tumor, spread of malignancy

Teach patient/family:

• To report signs of infection: increased temperature, sore throat, flu-like symptoms

• To report signs of anemia: fatigue, headache, faintness, shortness of breath, irritability

• To report bleeding; avoid use of razors, commercial mouthwash

• To avoid use of aspirin products, ibuprofen

• To avoid vaccinations during treatment

• To use contraception during and several months after completion of therapy, may cause irreversible gonadal suppression

• To report any changes in breathing or coughing

• To drink 2-3 L of fluid qd unless contraindicated

---

chloramphenicol (℞)

(klor-am-fen′i-kole)

chloramphenicol,
Chloromycetin,
Pentamycetin*

Func. class.: Antiinfective, misc

Chem. class.: Dichloroacetic acid derivative

Action: Binds to 50S ribosomal subunit, which interferes with or inhibits protein synthesis

Uses: Infections caused by *Haemophilus influenzae, Salmonella typhi, Rickettsia, Neisseria,* mycoplasma; not to be used if less toxic drugs can be used

Dosage and routes:

• *Adult and child:* **PO/IV** 50-75 mg/kg/day in divided doses q6h, 100 mg/kg/day (for meningitis only) max 4 g/day

---

Side effects: *italics* = common; ***bold italics*** = life-threatening

• *Premature infants and neonates:*
IV/PO 25 mg/kg/day in divided doses q12-24h
Available forms: Inj 1 g; caps 250 mg
Side effects/adverse reactions:
HEMA: **Anemia, thrombocytopenia, aplastic anemia, granulocytopenia, leukopenia** (rare)
EENT: Optic neuritis, blindness
GI: *Nausea, vomiting, diarrhea,* abdominal pain, xerostomia, glossitis, colitis, pruritus ani
INTEG: Itching, urticaria, contact dermatitis, rash
CV: **Gray syndrome in newborns: failure to feed, pallor, cyanosis, abdominal distention, irregular respiration, vasomotor collapse**
CNS: Headache, *depression,* confusion, peripheral neuritis
Contraindications: Hypersensitivity, severe renal disease, severe hepatic disease, minor infections
Precautions: Hepatic disease, renal disease, infants, children, bone marrow depression (drug-induced), pregnancy (C), lactation
Pharmacokinetics:
PO/IV: Peak 1-2 hr, duration 8 hr, half-life 1½-4 hr; conjugated in liver; excreted in urine (up to 15% as free drug, up to 80% in neonates), excreted in breast milk, feces; crosses placenta
Interactions:
• Increased action of: barbiturates, anticoagulants, hydantoins, iron products, antidiabetics
• Decreased action of: vit B_{12}, folic acid, penicillins, rifampin
NURSING CONSIDERATIONS
Assess:
• Signs of infection, anemia
◆ Any patient with compromised renal system; drug is excreted slowly in poor renal system function; toxicity may occur rapidly
• Liver studies: AST, ALT

• Blood studies: WBC, RBC, Hct, Hgb, platelets, serum iron, reticulocytes; drug should be discontinued if bone marrow is depressed
• Renal studies: urinalysis, protein, blood, BUN, creatinine
• C&S before drug therapy; may be given as soon as culture is taken
• Drug level in impaired hepatic, renal systems; peak 15-20 mg/ml 3 hr after dose, trough 5-10 mg/ml prior to next dose
• Bowel pattern before, during treatment
• Skin eruptions, itching, dermatitis after administration
• Allergies before treatment, reaction of each medication
◆ Neonates for beginning Gray syndrome: cyanosis, abdominal distention, irregular respiration, failure to feed; drug should be discontinued immediately
Administer:
• Oral form on empty stomach with full glass of water
• IM route not recommended
IV
• After diluting 1 g/10 ml of sterile H_2O for inj or D_5W (10% sol); give >1 min; may be further diluted in 50-100 ml of D_5W; give through Y-tube, 3-way stopcock, or additive inf set; run over ½-1 hr
Additive compatibilities: Amikacin, aminophylline, ascorbic acid, calcium chloride or gluconate, cephalothin, cephapirin, colistimethate, corticotropin, cyanocobalamin, dimenhydrinate, dopamine, ephedrine, heparin, hydrocortisone, kanamycin, lidocaine, magnesium sulfate, metaraminol, methicillin, methyldopate, methylprednisolone, metronidazole, nafcillin, oxacillin, oxytocin, penicillin G potassium, penicillin G sodium, pentobarbital, phenylephrine, phytonadione, plasma protein fraction, potassium

---

◆ = Nursing alert   🖊 = Herb-drug interaction   ⊘ = Do not crush

chloride, promazine, ranitidine, sodium bicarbonate, thiopental, verapamil, vit B/C

Syringe compatibilities: Ampicillin, cloxacillin, heparin, methicillin, penicillin G sodium

Y-site compatibilities: Acyclovir, cyclophosphamide, enalaprilat, esmolol, foscarnet, hydromorphone, labetalol, magnesium sulfate, meperidine, morphine, perphenazine, tacrolimus

Perform/provide:

• Storage of capsules in tight container at room temperature, reconstituted sol at room temperature 30 days

Evaluate:

• Therapeutic response: decreased symptoms of infection

Teach patient/family:

• All aspects of drug therapy: the need to complete entire course to ensure organism death (10-14 days); culture may be taken after complete course of medication

🚫 Not to break, crush, or chew caps

• To report sore throat, fever, fatigue, unusual bleeding, bruising; could indicate bone marrow depression (may occur weeks or months after termination of drug)

• That drug must be taken in equal intervals around clock to maintain blood levels

Treatment of hypersensitivity:
Withdraw drug, maintain airway, administer epinephrine, aminophylline, O_2, IV corticosteroids

chlordiazepoxide (℞)

(klor-dye-az-e-pox'ide)
Apo-Chlordiazepoxide*, chlordiazepoxide HCl*, Libritabs, Librium, Novopoxide*

Func. class.: Antianxiety
Chem. class.: Benzodiazepine

Controlled Substance Schedule IV
Action: Potentiates the actions of GABA, especially in the limbic system, reticular formation
Uses: Short-term management of anxiety, acute alcohol withdrawal, preoperatively for relaxation
Dosage and routes:
Mild anxiety
• *Adult:* **PO** 5-10 mg tid-qid
• *Child >6 yr:* **PO** 5 mg bid-qid, not to exceed 10 mg bid-tid
Severe anxiety
• *Adult:* **PO** 20-25 mg tid-qid
Preoperatively
• *Adult:* **PO** 5-10 mg tid-qid on day before surgery; **IM** 50-100 mg 1 hr before surgery
Alcohol withdrawal
• *Adult:* **PO/IM/IV** 50-100 mg, not to exceed 300 mg/day
Available forms: Caps 5, 10, 25 mg; tabs 5, 10, 25 mg; inj 100 mg ampule
Side effects/adverse reactions:
CNS: Dizziness, drowsiness, confusion, headache, anxiety, tremors, stimulation, fatigue, depression, insomnia, hallucinations
GI: Constipation, dry mouth, nausea, vomiting, anorexia, diarrhea
INTEG: Rash, dermatitis, itching
*CV: Orthostatic hypotension, **ECG changes, tachycardia,*** hypotension
EENT: Blurred vision, tinnitus, mydriasis
Contraindications: Hypersensitivity to benzodiazepines, narrow-angle glaucoma, psychosis, pregnancy (D), lactation, child <6 yr

* = Canada only   Side effects: *italics* = common; ***bold italics*** = life-threatening

Precautions: Elderly, debilitated, hepatic disease, renal disease
Do not confuse:
Librium/Librax
Pharmacokinetics:
PO: Onset 30 min, peak ½ hr, duration 4-6 hr; metabolized by liver, excreted by kidneys; crosses placenta, excreted in breast milk; half-life 5-30 hr (increased in elderly)
Interactions:
• Increased CNS depression: CNS depressants, alcohol
• Increased chlordiazepoxide: cimetidine, disulfiram, fluoxetine, isoniazid, ketoconazole, metoprolol, oral contraceptives, propranolol, valproic acid
• Decreased action of: levodopa
• Decreased action of chlordiazepoxide: barbiturates, rifamycins
⧄ Increased CNS depression: kava
Lab test interferences:
False increase: 17-OHCS
False positive: Pregnancy test (some methods)

NURSING CONSIDERATIONS
Assess:
• B/P (lying, standing), pulse; if systolic B/P drops 20 mm Hg, hold drug, notify prescriber
• Blood studies: CBC during long-term therapy; blood dyscrasias have occurred rarely
• Hepatic studies: AST, ALT, bilirubin, creatinine, LDH, alk phosphatase during long-term therapy
• I&O; may indicate renal dysfunction
• For ataxia, oversedation in elderly, debilitated patients
• Mental status: mood, sensorium, affect, sleeping pattern, drowsiness, dizziness
• Physical dependency, withdrawal symptoms: headache, nausea, vomiting, muscle pain, weakness after long-term use

• Suicidal tendencies, paradoxic reactions such as excitement, stimulation, acute rage
• For pregnancy; drug should be avoided during pregnancy
Administer:
PO
• With food or milk for GI symptoms
• Crushed if patient is unable to swallow medication whole
IM
• Add 2 ml diluent to powder, rotate until clear, use immediately
• Preferred route is IM
IV
• 5 ml NS/100 mg powder; agitate ampule gently; give through Y-tube or 3-way stopcock; give 100 mg or less ≥1 min; do not use IM diluent for IV use
• Keep powder from light; refrigerate, mix when ready to use
Solution compatibilities: D_5W, 0.9% NaCl
Y-site compatibilities: Heparin, hydrocortisone, potassium chloride, vit B/C
Perform/provide:
• Assistance with ambulation during beginning therapy, since drowsiness/dizziness occurs
• Check to see PO medication has been swallowed if patient is depressed, suicidal
• Sugarless gum, hard candy, frequent sips of water for dry mouth
Evaluate:
• Therapeutic response: decreased anxiety, restlessness, sleeplessness
Teach patient/family:
• That drug may be taken with food
• Not to use drug for everyday stress or use longer than 4 mo, unless directed by prescriber
• Not to take more than prescribed amount; may be habit forming
• To avoid OTC preparations unless approved by prescriber

◆ = Nursing alert   ⧄ = Herb-drug interaction   ⊗ = Do not crush

- To avoid driving, activities that require alertness; drowsiness may occur
- To avoid alcohol ingestion, other psychotropic medications, unless directed by prescriber
- Not to discontinue medication abruptly after long-term use; may precipitate seizures
- To rise slowly or fainting may occur, especially elderly
- That drowsiness may be worse at beginning of treatment
- To notify prescriber if pregnancy is suspected or planned

Treatment of overdose: Lavage, VS, supportive care, give flumazenil

---

chloroquine (℞)

(klor'oh-kwin)
Aralen HCl, Aralen Phosphate, chloroquine phosphate
Func. class.: Antimalarial
Chem. class.: Synthetic 4-aminoquinoline derivative

Action: Inhibits parasite replications, transcription of DNA to RNA by forming complexes with DNA of parasite

Uses: Malaria of *Plasmodium vivax, P. malariae, P. ovale, P. falciparum* (some strains), amebiasis

Dosage and routes:

Malaria suppression
- *Adult and child:* PO 5 mg base/kg/wk on same day of week, not to exceed 300 mg base; treatment should begin 1-2 wk before exposure and for 8 wk after; if treatment begins after exposure, 600 mg base for adult and 10 mg base/kg for children in 2 divided doses 6 hr apart

Extraintestinal amebiasis
- *Adult:* IM 160-200 mg base qd × 10-12 days or PO (HCl) 600 mg base qd × 2 days, then 300 mg base qd × 2-3 wk (phosphate)
- *Child:* IM/PO 10 mg/kg qd (HCl) × 2-3 wk, not to exceed 300 mg/day

Available forms: Tabs 250 mg (150 mg base), 500 mg (300 mg base) phosphate; inj 50 mg (40 mg base)/ml HCl

Side effects/adverse reactions:

CV: Hypotension, ***heart block, asystole with syncope,*** ECG changes
INTEG: Pruritus, pigmentary changes, skin eruptions, lichen planus–like eruptions, eczema, ***exfoliative dermatitis***
CNS: Headache, stimulation, fatigue, ***convulsion,*** psychosis
EENT: Blurred vision, corneal changes, retinal changes, difficulty focusing, tinnitus, vertigo, deafness, photophobia, corneal edema
GI: Nausea, vomiting, anorexia, diarrhea, cramps
*HEMA: **Thrombocytopenia, agranulocytosis, hemolytic anemia, leukopenia***

Contraindications: Hypersensitivity, retinal field changes

Precautions: Pregnancy (C), children, blood dyscrasias, severe GI disease, neurologic disease, alcoholism, hepatic disease, G6PD deficiency, psoriasis, eczema, lactation, porphyria

Pharmacokinetics: Metabolized in liver; excreted in urine, feces, breast milk; crosses placenta
PO: Peak 1-3 hr, half-life 3-5 days
IM: Peak 30 min

Interactions:
- Decreased action of chloroquine: magnesium, aluminum compounds, kaolin
- Reduced oral clearance and metabolism of chloroquine: cimetidine

NURSING CONSIDERATIONS

Assess:
- Ophthalmic test if long-term treatment or dosage >150 mg/day

---

• Liver studies qwk: AST, ALT, bilirubin
• Blood studies: CBC, since blood dyscrasias occur
• ECG during therapy; watch for depression of T waves, widening of QRS complex
• Allergic reactions: pruritus, rash, urticaria
• Blood dyscrasias: malaise, fever, bruising, bleeding (rare)
• For ototoxicity (tinnitus, vertigo, change in hearing); audiometric testing should be done before, after treatment
◆ For toxicity: blurring vision; difficulty focusing; headache; dizziness; decreased knee, ankle reflexes, seizures, CV collapse; drug should be discontinued immediately
Administer:
• IM after aspirating to avoid injection into blood system, which may cause hypotension, asystole, heart block; rotate injection sites
PO
• Before or after meals at same time each day to maintain drug level
Additive compatibilities: Promethazine
Perform/provide:
• Storage in tight, light-resistant container at room temperature; keep injection in cool environment
Evaluate:
• Therapeutic response: decreased symptoms of infection
Teach patient/family:
• To use sunglasses in bright sunlight to decrease photophobia
• That urine may turn rust or brown color
• To report hearing, visual problems, fever, fatigue, bruising, bleeding, which may indicate blood dyscrasias
Treatment of overdose: Induce vomiting, gastric lavage, administer barbiturate (ultrashort-acting), va-

sopressor; tracheostomy may be necessary

---

chlorothiazide (℞)
(klor-oh-thye'a-zide)
Diuril
Func. class.: Diuretic
Chem. class.: Thiazide; sulfonamide derivative

Action: Acts on distal tubule and thick ascending limb of the loop of Henle by increasing excretion of water, sodium, chloride, potassium, magnesium
Uses: Edema, hypertension, diuresis
Dosage and routes:
Edema, hypertension
• *Adult:* **PO/IV** 500 mg-2 g qd may divide bid
Diuresis
• *Adult:* **IV** 250 mg q6-12h
• *Child >6 mo:* **PO** 10-20 mg/kg/day may divide bid
• *Child <6 mo:* **PO** up to 40 mg/kg/day in 2 doses
Available forms: Tabs 250, 500 mg; inj 500 mg; oral susp 250 mg/5 ml
Side effects/adverse reactions:
CNS: Paresthesia, anxiety, depression, headache, *dizziness, fatigue, weakness,* insomnia
CV: Irregular pulse, orthostatic hypotension, palpitations, volume depletion
EENT: Blurred vision
ELECT: Hypokalemia, hypercalcemia, hyponatremia, hypochloremia, hypophosphatemia, hypomagnesemia
GI: Nausea, vomiting, anorexia, constipation, diarrhea, cramps, pancreatitis, GI irritation, ***hepatitis***
GU: Urinary frequency, polyuria, ***uremia,*** glucosuria, hematuria
*HEMA: **Aplastic anemia, hemolytic***

◆ = Nursing alert   ✂ = Herb-drug interaction   🚫 = Do not crush *anemia, leukopenia, agranulocytosis, thrombocytopenia, neutropenia*

INTEG: Rash, urticaria, purpura, photosensitivity, fever, alopecia

META: Hyperglycemia, *hyperuricemia,* increased creatinine, BUN

Contraindications: Hypersensitivity to thiazides or sulfonamides, hepatic coma, anuria, renal decompensation, pregnancy (B), lactation

Precautions: Hypokalemia, renal disease, hepatic disease, gout, COPD, SLE, diabetes mellitus, elderly, hyperlipidemia

Do not confuse:
chlorothiazide/chlorpromazine, chlorthalidone, chlorpropamide

Pharmacokinetics: Not well absorbed PO

PO: Onset 2 hr, peak 4 hr, duration 6-12 hr; crosses placenta, excreted in breast milk, excreted unchanged by kidneys; half-life 2 hr

Interactions:

• Increased toxicity: lithium, nondepolarizing skeletal muscle relaxants, digitalis, allopurinol

• Increased hypotension: other antihypertensives, alcohol, nitrates

• Decreased absorption of thiazides: cholestyramine, colestipol

• Decreased diuretic action: NSAIDs

• Hypokalemia: ticarcillin, glucocorticoids, amphotericin, mezlocillin, piperacillin

🖉 Hypokalemia: chronic use/abuse cascara sagrada bark, aloe, buckthorn bark/berry, licorice root, senna pod/leaf

Lab test interferences:
False negative: Phentolamine and tyramine tests
Interference: Urine steroid tests
Increase: BSP retention, Ca, amylase, parathyroid test
Decrease: PBI, PSP

NURSING CONSIDERATIONS
Assess:

• Weight, I&O daily to determine fluid loss; effect of drug may be decreased if used qd

• Rate, depth, rhythm of respirations; effect of exertion

• B/P lying, standing; postural hypotension may occur, especially in elderly

• Electrolytes: K, Na, Cl; include BUN, blood glucose, CBC, serum creatinine, blood pH, ABGs, uric acid, Ca, Mg

• Glucose in urine if patient is diabetic

• Signs of metabolic alkalosis: drowsiness, restlessness

• Rashes, temp elevation qd

• Confusion, especially in elderly; take safety precautions if needed

Administer:

• In AM to avoid interference with sleep if using drug as a diuretic

• K replacement if K less than 3 mg/dl

• With food if nausea occurs; absorption may be decreased slightly; tablets may be crushed

• After shaking suspension

IV

• After diluting 0.5 g/18 ml or more of sterile water for inj; may be diluted further with 0.9% NaCl, D_5W, check for extravasation; give over 5 min (0.5 g/5 min)

Additive compatibilities: Cimetidine, lidocaine, nafcillin, ranitidine, sodium bicarbonate

Evaluate:

• Therapeutic response: improvement in edema of feet, legs, sacral area daily if medication is being used for CHF; decreased B/P; increased urinary output

Teach patient/family:

• To rise slowly from lying or sitting position; orthostatic hypotension may occur

• To notify prescriber of muscle weakness, cramps, nausea, dizziness

• That drug may be taken with food or milk; to take at same time each day; not to double dose; dehydration may occur

• That blood sugar may be increased in diabetics

• To take early in day to avoid nocturia

• To use sunscreen; use protective clothing to prevent photosensitivity

• To weigh weekly and notify prescriber of change of >3 lb

• To eat diet high in K if recommended by prescriber; teach high potassium foods

• Not to take OTC medications without consulting prescriber

Treatment of overdose: Lavage if taken orally; monitor electrolytes; administer dextrose in saline; monitor hydration, CV, renal status

---

chlorpheniramine
(OTC, ℞)

(klor-fen-ir′a-meen)
Aller-Chlor, Chlo-Amine, Chlorate, chlorpheniramine maleate, Chlor-Trimeton, Chlor-Tripolon*, GenAllerate, Novo-Pheniram*, Pedia Care Allergy Formula, Phenetron, Teldrin

Func. class.: Antihistamine (1st generation, nonselective)

Chem. class.: Alkylamine, H_1-receptor antagonist

Action: Acts on blood vessels, GI system, respiratory system, by competing with histamine for H_1-receptor site; decreases allergic response by blocking histamine

Uses: Allergy symptoms, rhinitis

Dosage and routes:

• *Adult and child ≥12 yr:* **PO** 2-4 mg tid-qid, not to exceed 24 mg/day; **TIME-REL** 8-12 mg bid-tid, not to exceed 24 mg/day; **IM/IV/SC** 5-40 mg/day, max 40 mg/day

• *Child 6-12 yr:* **PO** 2 mg q4-6h, not to exceed 12 mg/day; **SUS REL** 8 mg hs or qd, **SUS REL** not recommended for child <6 yr; **SC** 87.5 µg/kg or 2.5 mg/m^2 q6h

• *Child 2-5 yr:* **PO** 1 mg q4-6h, not to exceed 4 mg/day

Available forms: Tabs, chewable 2 mg; tabs 4, 8, 12 mg; tabs, time-rel 8, 12 mg; caps, time-rel 8, 12 mg; syr 1 mg/5 ml, 2 mg/5 ml, 2.5 mg/5 ml; inj 10, 100 mg/ml

Side effects/adverse reactions:

CNS: Dizziness, drowsiness, poor coordination, fatigue, anxiety, euphoria, confusion, paresthesia, neuritis

RESP: Increased thick secretions, wheezing, chest tightness

HEMA: **Thrombocytopenia, agranulocytosis, hemolytic anemia**

GI: Nausea, anorexia, diarrhea

INTEG: Photosensitivity

GU: Retention, dysuria, urinary frequency

EENT: Blurred vision, dilated pupils, tinnitus, nasal stuffiness, dry nose, throat, mouth

Contraindications: Hypersensitivity to H_1-receptor antagonists, acute asthma attack, lower respiratory tract disease, stenosed peptic ulcers, bladder neck obstruction

Precautions: Increased intraocular pressure, renal disease, cardiac disease, hypertension, bronchial asthma, seizure disorder, hyperthyroidism, prostatic hypertrophy, pregnancy (B), lactation, elderly

Do not confuse:

Teldrin/Tedral

Pharmacokinetics:

PO: Onset ½ hr, duration 4-12 hr; *PO-ER:* Duration 8-24 hr; *SC/IM/*

◆ = Nursing alert　　　🖋 = Herb-drug interaction　　　🚫 = Do not crush

IV: duration 4-12 hr; detoxified in liver; excreted by kidneys (metabolites/free drug); half-life 12-15 hr

Interactions:

• Increased CNS depression: barbiturates, opiates, hypnotics, tricyclics, alcohol

• Increased effect of chlorpheniramine: MAOIs

• Increased anticholinergic action: atropine, phenothiazines, quinidine, haloperidol

⚕ Increased CNS depression: kava

⚕ Increased anticholinergic effect: henbane leaf

Lab test interferences:

False negative: Skin allergy tests

NURSING CONSIDERATIONS

Assess:

• Be alert for urinary retention, frequency, dysuria; drug should be discontinued

• Respiratory status: rate, rhythm, increase in bronchial secretions, wheezing, chest tightness

Administer:

PO

• With meals for GI symptoms; absorption may slightly decrease

IV

• Undiluted at ≥10 mg/1 min

• The 100 mg/ml form is not to be used IV; for IM/SC use

Perform/provide:

• Hard candy, gum, frequent rinsing of mouth for dryness

• Storage in tight container at room temperature

Evaluate:

• Therapeutic response: absence of running, congested nose, rashes

Teach patient/family:

🚫 Not to break, crush, or chew sustained-release forms

• All aspects of drug use; to notify prescriber of confusion/sedation/hypotension, difficulty voiding

• To avoid driving, other hazardous activity if drowsiness occurs, especially elderly

• To avoid concurrent use of alcohol, other CNS depressants

Treatment of overdose: Administer ipecac syrup or lavage, diazepam, vasopressors, barbiturates (short-acting)

---

chlorpromazine (℞)

(klor-proe'ma-zeen)
Chlorpromanyl*, chlorpromazine HCl, Largactil*, Novo-Chlorpromazine*, Thorazine, Thor-Prom

Func. class.: Antipsychotic/neuroleptic/antiemetic

Chem. class.: Phenothiazine-aliphatic

Action: Depresses cerebral cortex, hypothalamus, limbic system, which control activity aggression; blocks neurotransmission produced by dopamine at synapse; exhibits a strong α-adrenergic, anticholinergic blocking action; mechanism for antipsychotic effects is unclear

Uses: Psychotic disorders, mania, schizophrenia, anxiety, intractable hiccups in adults, nausea, vomiting; preoperatively for relaxation; acute intermittent porphyria, behavioral problems in children, nonpsychotic, demented patients, Tourette's syndrome

Investigational uses: Vascular headache

Dosage and routes:

Psychosis

• *Adult:* **PO** 10-50 mg q1-4h initially, then increase up to 2 g/day if necessary; **IM** 10-50 mg q1-4h

• *Geriatric:* Use lowest effective dose

Side effects: *italics* = common; ***bold italics*** = life-threatening

• *Child:* **PO** 0.5 mg/kg q4-6h; **IM** 0.5 mg/kg q6-8h; **RECT** 1 mg/kg q6-8h

Nausea and vomiting

• *Adult:* **PO** 10-25 mg q4-6h prn; **IM** 25-50 mg q3h prn; **RECT** 50-100 mg q6-8h prn, not to exceed 400 mg/day; **IV** 25-50 mg qd-qid

• *Child ≥ 6 mo:* **PO** 0.55 mg/kg q4-6h; **IM** q6-8h; **RECT** 1.1 mg/kg q6-8h; max **IM** ≤ 5 yr or ≤ 22.7 kg 40 mg; max **IM** 5-10 yr or 22.7-45.5 kg, 75 mg

Intractable hiccups

• *Adult:* **PO** 25-50 mg tid-qid; **IM** 25-50 mg (only if PO dose does not work); **IV** 25-50 mg in 500-1000 ml **NS** (only for severe hiccups)

Available forms: Tabs 10, 25, 50, 100, 200 mg; sus-rel caps 30, 75, 150, 200, 300 mg; syr 10, 25, 100 mg/5 ml; conc 30, 40, 100 mg/ml; supp 25, 100 mg; inj 25 mg/ml

Side effects/adverse reactions:

CV: Orthostatic hypotension, hypertension, ***cardiac arrest,*** ECG changes, ***tachycardia***

EENT: Blurred vision, glaucoma, dry eyes

GI: Dry mouth, nausea, vomiting, anorexia, constipation, diarrhea, jaundice, weight gain

GU: Urinary retention, enuresis, impotence, amenorrhea, gynecomastia, breast engorgement

HEMA: Anemia, ***leukopenia, leukocytosis, agranulocytosis***

INTEG: Rash, photosensitivity, dermatitis

*RESP: **Laryngospasm,*** dyspnea, ***respiratory depression***

CNS: EPS: pseudoparkinsonism, akathisia, dystonia, tardive dyskinesia, seizures, *headache,* ***neuroleptic malignant syndrome***

Contraindications: Hypersensitivity, circulatory collapse, liver damage, cerebral arteriosclerosis, coronary disease, severe hypertension/ hypotension, blood dyscrasias, coma, child <6 mo, brain damage, bone marrow depression, alcohol/ barbiturate withdrawal, narrow-angle glaucoma

Precautions: Pregnancy (C), lactation, seizure disorders, hypertension, hepatic disease, cardiac disease, elderly, prostatic enlargement

Do not confuse:

chlorpromazine/chlorpropamide
chlorpromazine/prochlorperazine

Pharmacokinetics:

PO: Absorption variable, widely distributed; onset erratic 30-60 min, duration 4-6 hr

PO-ER: Onset 30-60 min, peak unknown, duration 10-12 hr

REC: Onset erratic, duration 3 hr

IM: Well absorbed; peak 15-20 min, duration 4-8 hr

IV: Onset 5 min, peak 10 min, duration unknown

Metabolized by liver, excreted in urine (metabolites), crosses placenta, enters breast milk; 95% bound to plasma proteins; elimination half-life 10-30 hr

Interactions:

• Lowered seizure threshold: anticonvulsants

• Oversedation: other CNS depressants, alcohol, barbiturate anesthetics, antihistamines, sedatives/hypnotics, antidepressants

• Toxicity: epinephrine

• Decreased absorption: aluminum hydroxide, magnesium hydroxide antacids

• Decreased antiparkinson activity: levodopa, bromocriptine

• Decreased serum chlorpromazine: lithium, barbiturates

• Decreased anticoagulant effect: warfarin

• Increased effects of both drugs: β-adrenergic blockers, alcohol

• Increased anticholinergic effects:

◆ = Nursing alert   ⫻ = Herb-drug interaction   ⊘ = Do not crush

anticholinergics, antidepressants, antiparkinsonian agents
• Agranulocystosis: antithyroid agents
• Increased valproic acid level
🖋 Increased CNS depression: kava
🖋 Increased anticholinergic effect: henbane leaf

Lab test interferences:

Increase: Liver function tests, cardiac enzymes, cholesterol, blood glucose, prolactin, bilirubin, PBI, cholinesterase, ^{131}I, alk phosphatase, leukocytes, granulocytes, platelets
Decrease: Hormones (blood and urine)
False positive: Pregnancy tests, PKU
False negative: Urinary steroids, 17-OHCS

NURSING CONSIDERATIONS
Assess:
• Mental status: orientation, mood, behavior, presence and type of hallucinations before initial administration and monthly
• Any potentially reversible causes of behavior problems in the elderly before and during therapy
• Swallowing of PO medication; check for hoarding or giving of medication to other patients
• I&O ratio; palpate bladder if low urinary output occurs, especially in elderly
• Bilirubin, CBC, liver function studies, ocular exam; agranulocytosis may occur, monthly
• Urinalysis recommended before, during prolonged therapy
• Affect, orientation, LOC, reflexes, gait, coordination, sleep pattern disturbances
• B/P sitting, standing, lying; take pulse and respirations q4h during initial treatment; establish baseline before starting treatment; report drops of 30 mm Hg; obtain baseline ECG, Q-wave and T-wave changes

• Dizziness, faintness, palpitations, tachycardia on rising
◆ For neuroleptic malignant syndrome: hyperpyrexia, muscle rigidity, increased CPK, altered mental status, for acute dystonia (check chewing, swallowing, eyes, pin rolling)
• EPS including akathisia (inability to sit still, no pattern to movements), tardive dyskinesia (bizarre movements of the jaw, mouth, tongue, extremities), pseudoparkinsonism (rigidity, tremors, pill rolling, shuffling gait)
• Skin turgor daily
• Constipation, urinary retention daily; increase bulk, H_2O in diet

Administer:
• IM, inject in deep muscle mass, do not give SC
• Rectal after placing in refrigerator for ½ hr if too soft to insert
• Antiparkinsonian agent for EPS
PO
• With full glass of water, milk; or with food to decrease GI upset
• Drug in liquid form mixed in glass of juice or cola if hoarding is suspected
• Periodically attempt dosage reduction in behavioral problems
IV
• After diluting 1 mg/1 ml with NS, give 1 mg or less/2 min or more; may be further diluted in 500-1000 ml of NS

Additive compatibilities: Ascorbic acid, ethacrynate, netilmicin, theophylline, vit B/C
Syringe compatibilities: Atropine, benztropine, butorphanol, diphenhydramine, doxapram, droperidol, fentanyl, glycopyrrolate, hydromorphone, hydroxyzine, meperidine, metoclopramide, midazolam, morphine, pentazocine, perphenazine, prochlorperazine, promazine, promethazine, scopolamine

Y-site compatibilities: Amsacrine, cisatracurium, cisplatin, cladribine, cyclophosphamide, cytarabine, doxorubicin, doxorubicin liposome, famotidine, filgrastim, fluconazole, granisetron, heparin, hydrocortisone, ondansetron, potassium chloride, propofol, teniposide, thiotepa, vinorelbine, vit B/C

Perform/provide:

• Supervised ambulation until stabilized on medication; do not involve in strenuous exercise program because fainting is possible; patient should not stand still for long periods

• Increased fluids to prevent constipation

• Candy, gum, sips of water for dry mouth

• Storage in tight, light-resistant container, oral sol in amber bottle

Evaluate:

• Therapeutic response: decrease in emotional excitement, hallucinations, delusions, paranoia, reorganization of patterns of thought, speech, increase in target behaviors

Teach patient/family:

• To use good oral hygiene; frequent rinsing of mouth, sugarless gum for dry mouth

• To avoid hazardous activities until drug response is determined

🚫 Not to break, crush, or chew time-rel caps

• That orthostatic hypotension occurs often and to rise gradually from sitting or lying position

• To remain lying down for at least 30 min after IM injection

• To avoid hot tubs, hot showers, tub baths, since hypotension may occur; that in hot weather, heat stroke may occur; take extra precautions to stay cool

• To avoid abrupt withdrawal of this drug or EPS may result; drug should be withdrawn slowly

• To avoid OTC preparations (cough, hay fever, cold) unless approved by prescriber, since serious drug interactions may occur; avoid use with alcohol, CNS depressants; increased drowsiness may occur

• To use a sunscreen and sunglasses to prevent burns

• To take antacids 2 hr before or after this drug

• To report sore throat, malaise, fever, bleeding, mouth sores; CBC should be drawn and drug discontinued

• Contraceptive measures

• That urine may turn pink or red

Treatment of overdose: Lavage if orally ingested; provide airway; *do not induce vomiting or use epinephrine*

RARELY USED

chlorpropamide (℞)

(klor-proe′pa-mide)

Chloronase*, Chlorpropamide, Diabinese, Novopropamide*

Functional class.: Antidiabetic

Uses: Stable adult-onset diabetes mellitus (type II) NIDDM

Dosage and routes:

• *Adult:* **PO** 100-250 mg qd, initially, then 100-500 mg maintenance according to response; not to exceed 750 mg/day

Contraindications: Hypersensitivity to sulfonylureas, juvenile or brittle diabetes, pregnancy (D), lactation, renal failure

---

🔽 = Nursing alert   🔹 = Herb-drug interaction   🚫 = Do not crush

C

chlorthalidone (℞)

(klor-thal'i-done)
Apo-Chlorthalidone*, chlorthalidone, Hygroton, Thalitone, Uridon*

Func. class.: Diuretic
Chem. class.: Thiazide-like phthalimidine derivative

Action: Acts on distal tubule and thick ascending limb of the loop of Henle by increasing excretion of water, sodium, chloride, potassium, magnesium, bicarbonate, possible arteriolar dilation

Uses: Edema, hypertension, diuresis, edema in CHF, nephrotic syndrome

Dosage and routes:
• *Adult:* PO 25-200 mg/day or 100 mg every other day
• *Geriatric:* PO 12.5 mg qd, initially
• *Child:* PO 2 mg/kg or 60 mg/m^2 3 ×/wk

Available forms: Tabs 25, 50, 100 mg

Side effects/adverse reactions:
GU: Urinary frequency, polyuria, **uremia,** glucosuria, impotence
CNS: Paresthesia, headache, *dizziness, fatigue, weakness*
GI: Nausea, vomiting, anorexia, constipation, diarrhea, cramps, pancreatitis, GI irritation, **hepatitis**
EENT: Blurred vision
INTEG: Rash, urticaria, purpura, photosensitivity, fever
META: Hyperglycemia, hyperuremia, increased creatinine, BUN, gout
*HEMA: **Aplastic anemia, hemolytic anemia, leukopenia, agranulocytosis, thrombocytopenia, neutropenia***
CV: Irregular pulse, orthostatic hypotension, palpitations, volume depletion

ELECT: Hypokalemia, hypomagnesemia, hypercalcemia, hyponatremia, hypochloremia

Contraindications: Hypersensitivity to thiazides or sulfonamides, anuria, renal decompensation, lactation

Precautions: Hypokalemia, renal disease, pregnancy (B), hepatic disease, gout, diabetes mellitus, elderly, hyperlipidemia

Do not confuse:
Uridon/Vicodin
Hygroton/Regroton

Pharmacokinetics:
PO: Onset 2 hr, peak 6 hr, duration 24-72 hr; excreted unchanged by kidneys; crosses placenta; enters breast milk; half-life 40 hr

Interactions:
• Increased toxicity of: lithium, nondepolarizing skeletal muscle relaxants, allopurinol
• Decreased absorption of thiazides: cholestyramine, colestipol
• Hyperglycemia, hypotension: diazoxide
• Increased hypotensive effect: alcohol
• Hypokalemia: glucocorticoids, amphotericin B
⧪ Potassium deficiency: chronic use/abuse of aloe, buckthorn bark/berry, cascara sagrada bark, licorice root, senna pod/leaf

Lab test interferences:
Increase: BSP retention, Ca, cholesterol, triglycerides, amylase
Decrease: PBI, PSP, parathyroid test

NURSING CONSIDERATIONS
Assess:
• Weight, I&O daily to determine fluid loss; effect of drug may be decreased if used qd
• Rate, depth, rhythm of respiration, effect of exertion, B/P lying, standing; postural hypotension may occur

---

* = Canada only   Side effects: *italics* = common; **bold italics** = life-threatening

• Electrolytes: K, Mg, Na, Cl; include BUN, blood sugar, CBC, serum creatinine, blood pH, ABGs, uric acid, Ca
• Blood glucose levels if patient is diabetic
• Signs of metabolic alkalosis: drowsiness, restlessness
• Signs of hypokalemia: postural hypotension, malaise, fatigue, tachycardia, leg cramps, weakness
• Rashes, temp elevation qd
• Confusion, especially in elderly; take safety precautions if needed

Administer:
• In AM to avoid interference with sleep if using drug as a diuretic
• K replacement if K less than 3 mg/dl
• With food if nausea occurs; absorption may be decreased slightly

Evaluate:
• Therapeutic response: improvement in edema of feet, legs, sacral area daily if medication used in CHF

Teach patient/family:
• To rise slowly from lying or sitting position
• To notify prescriber of muscle weakness, cramps, nausea, dizziness
• That drug may be taken with food or milk
• That blood sugar may be increased in diabetics
• To use sunscreen to protect against photosensitivity
• To take early in day to avoid nocturia

Treatment of overdose: Lavage if taken orally, monitor electrolytes, administer dextrose in NS, monitor hydration, CV, renal status

chlorzoxazone (R)
(klor-zox′a-zone)
EZE-DS, chlorzoxazone, Paraflex, Parafon Forte DSC, Relaxazone, Remular, Remular-S, Strifon Forte DSC
Func. class.: Skeletal muscle relaxant, central acting
Chem. class.: Benzoxazole derivative

Action: Inhibits multisynaptic reflex arcs causing skeletal muscle relaxation

Uses: Relieving pain, spasm in musculoskeletal conditions

Dosage and routes:
• *Adult:* **PO** 250-750 mg tid-qid
• *Child:* **PO** 20 mg/kg/day in divided doses bid-tid

Available forms: Tabs 250, 500 mg

Side effects/adverse reactions:
GU: Urine discoloration
HEMA: **Granulocytopenia, anemia**
CNS: Dizziness, drowsiness, headache, insomnia, stimulation, malaise
GI: Nausea, vomiting, anorexia, diarrhea, constipation, **GI bleeding**
INTEG: Rash, pruritus, petechiae, ecchymoses, **angioedema**
SYST: **Anaphylaxis, angioedema**

Contraindications: Hypersensitivity, impaired hepatic function

Precautions: Pregnancy (unknown), lactation, hepatic disease, elderly

Pharmacokinetics:
PO: Onset 1 hr, peak 1-2 hr, duration 3-4 hr, half-life 1 hr; metabolized in liver; excreted in urine (metabolites)

Interactions:
• Increased CNS depression: alcohol, tricyclics, opiates, barbiturates, sedatives, hypnotics
🖋 May increase CNS depression: kava

◆ = Nursing alert 🖋 = Herb-drug interaction 🚫 = Do not crush

NURSING CONSIDERATIONS
Assess:
• Blood studies: CBC, WBC, differential for blood dyscrasias if on long-term therapy
• Allergic reactions: rash, fever, respiratory distress
• CNS depression: dizziness, drowsiness, psychiatric symptoms
Administer:
• With meals for GI symptoms
Perform/provide:
• Storage in tight container at room temperature
Evaluate:
• Therapeutic response: decreased pain, spasticity
Teach patient/family:
• Not to discontinue abruptly; insomnia, nausea, headache, spasticity, tachycardia will occur; drug should be tapered over 1-2 wk
• Not to take with alcohol, other CNS depressants; take with food
• To avoid hazardous activities if drowsiness, dizziness occurs
• To avoid using OTC medication: cough preparations, antihistamines, unless directed by prescriber
• That urine may be orange or purple
Treatment of overdose: Gastric lavage or induce emesis, then administer activated charcoal; use other supportive treatment as necessary; monitor cardiac function

---

cholestyramine (R)
(koe-less-tir'a-meen)
LoCHOLEST, LoCHOLEST
Light, Prevalite, Questran,
Questran Light
Func. class.: Antilipemic
Chem. class.: Bile acid sequestrant

Action: Absorbs, combines with bile acids to form insoluble complex that is excreted through feces; loss of bile acids lowers cholesterol levels
Uses: Primary hypercholesterolemia, pruritus associated with biliary obstruction, diarrhea caused by excess bile acid, xanthomas
Dosage and routes:
• *Adult:* **PO** 4 g ac, and hs, not to exceed 32 g/day
• *Child:* **PO** 240 mg/kg/day in 3 divided doses with food or drink, max 8 g/day
Available forms: Pwd 9 g/4 g cholestyramine
Side effects/adverse reactions:
CNS: Headache, dizziness, drowsiness, vertigo, tinnitus
MS: Muscle, joint pain
GI: Constipation, abdominal pain, nausea, fecal impaction, hemorrhoids, flatulence, vomiting, steatorrhea, peptic ulcer
INTEG: Rash, irritation of perianal area, tongue, skin
*HEMA: **Bleeding,** decreased protime
META: Decreased vit A, D, K, red cell folate content; ***hyperchloremic acidosis***
Contraindications: Hypersensitivity, biliary obstruction
Precautions: Pregnancy (C), lactation, children
Pharmacokinetics:
PO: Excreted in feces, maximum effect in 2 wk
Interactions:
• Decreased absorption of: warfarin, thiazides, cardiac glycosides; acetaminophen, beta-blockers, corticosteroids, iron, thyroid hormones, fat-soluble vitamins
Lab test interferences:
Interfere: cholecystography
NURSING CONSIDERATIONS
Assess:
• Cardiac glycoside level, if both drugs are being administered
• For signs of vit A, D, K deficiency

• Fasting LDL, HDL, total cholesterol, triglyceride levels, electrolytes if on extended therapy
• Bowel pattern daily; increase bulk, H₂O in diet for constipation

Administer:
• Drug ac, hs; give all other medications 1 hr before cholestyramine or 4 hr after cholestyramine to avoid poor absorption
• Drug mixed with applesauce or stirred into beverage (2-6 oz), let stand for 2 min; do not take dry, avoid inhaling powder
• Supplemental doses of vit A, D, K, if levels are low

Evaluate:
• Therapeutic response: decreased cholesterol level (hyperlipidemia); diarrhea, pruritus (excess bile acids)

Teach patient/family:
◆ The symptoms of hypoprothrombinemia: bleeding mucous membranes, dark tarry stools, hematuria, petechiae; report immediately
• The importance of compliance
• That risk factors should be decreased: high-fat diet, smoking, alcohol consumption, absence of exercise

---

choline salicylate (℞)
(koe′leen sa-liss′ih-late)
Arthropan, choline/magnesium salicylates CMT, Tricosal, Trilisate
Func. class.: Nonnarcotic analgesic
Chem. class.: Salicylate

Action: Blocks pain impulses in CNS that occur in response to inhibition of prostaglandin synthesis; antipyretic action results from inhibition of hypothalamic heat-regulating center to produce vasodilation to allow heat dissipation

Uses: Mild to moderate pain or fever including arthritis, juvenile rheumatoid arthritis

Dosage and routes:
Choline salicylate
• *Adult and child >12 yr:* **PO** 870-1740 mg qid; max 6 ×/day
Pain/fever
• *Adult:* **PO** 435-870 mg q3-4h prn
Choline/magnesium salicylates
• *Adult:* **PO** 2-3 g salicylate/day divided bid-tid
• *Child >37 kg:* **PO** 2.2 g of salicylate/day divided bid
• *Child <37 kg:* **PO** 50 mg of salicylate/kg/day divided bid

Available forms: Choline salicylate liq 870 mg/5 ml; choline/magnesium salicylate tabs 500, 750, 1000 mg; liq 500 mg/5 ml

Side effects/adverse reactions:
*HEMA: **Thrombocytopenia, agranulocytosis, leukopenia, neutropenia, hemolytic anemia,*** increased pro-time
CNS: Stimulation, drowsiness, dizziness, confusion, ***convulsion,*** headache, flushing, hallucinations, ***coma***
GI: Nausea, vomiting, GI bleeding, diarrhea, heartburn, anorexia, ***hepatitis, hepatotoxicity***
INTEG: Rash, urticaria, bruising, sweating
EENT: Tinnitus, hearing loss
CV: Rapid pulse, pulmonary edema
RESP: Wheezing, hyperpnea, hyperventilation
ENDO: Hypoglycemia, hyponatremia, hypokalemia

Contraindications: Hypersensitivity to salicylates, GI bleeding, bleeding disorders, children <3 yr, vit K deficiency, children with flulike symptoms

Precautions: Anemia, hepatic disease, renal disease, Hodgkin's disease, pregnancy (C), lactation

---

◆ = Nursing alert   ∥ = Herb-drug interaction   ⊘ = Do not crush

C

Pharmacokinetics:
Absorbed via GI tract, onset 15-30 min; metabolized by liver; crosses placenta; excreted in breast milk, by kidneys, half-life 2-3 hr, large doses 15-30 hr

Interactions:
• Decreased effects of aspirin: antacids (high doses), steroids, urinary alkalizers, corticosteroids
• Increased bleeding: alcohol, heparin, plicamycin, cefamandole
• Increased effects of warfarin, insulin, methotrexate, thrombolytic agents, penicillins, phenytoin, valproic acid, oral hypoglycemics, sulfonamides
• Increased salicylate levels: urinary acidifiers, ammonium chloride, nizatidine
• Decreased effects of probenecid, spironolactone, sulfinpyrazone, sulfonylamides, NSAIDs, β-blockers
• Gastric ulcer: steroids, antiinflammatories, NSAIDs

⚕ Increased risk of bleeding: horse chestnut, kelpware

Lab test interferences:
Increase: Coagulation studies, liver function studies, serum uric acid, amylase, CO_2, urinary protein
Decrease: Serum K, PBI, cholesterol
Interference: Urine catecholamines, pregnancy test

NURSING CONSIDERATIONS
Assess:
• Pain: location, intensity, character baseline and 1-2 hr after dose
• Liver function studies: AST, ALT, bilirubin, creatinine (long-term therapy)
• Renal function studies: BUN, urine creatinine (long-term therapy)
• Blood studies: CBC, Hct, Hgb, PT (long-term therapy)
• I&O ratio; decreasing output may indicate renal failure (long-term therapy)

◆ Hepatotoxicity: dark urine; clay-colored stools; yellowing of skin, sclera; itching; abdominal pain; fever; diarrhea (long-term therapy)
• Allergic reactions: rash, urticaria; drug may have to be discontinued
• Renal dysfunction: decreased urine output
• Ototoxicity: tinnitus, ringing, roaring in ears; audiometric testing needed before, after long-term therapy
• Visual changes: blurring, halos, corneal, retinal damage
• Edema in feet, ankles, legs
• Drug history; many interactions

Administer:
• Mixed with fruit juice, carbonated beverage, water

Evaluate:
• Therapeutic response: decreased pain, fever, stiffness of joints

Teach patient/family:
• To report any symptoms of hepatotoxicity, renal toxicity, visual changes, ototoxicity, allergic reactions, bleeding (long-term therapy)
• Not to exceed recommended dosage; acute poisoning may result
• To read label on other OTC drugs; many contain aspirin
• That therapeutic response takes 2 wk (arthritis)
• To avoid alcohol ingestion; GI bleeding may occur
• That if anticoagulants are given with this drug, this drug should be decreased 2 wk before surgery

Treatment of overdose: Lavage, activated charcoal, monitor electrolytes, VS

choriogonadotropin (℞)

(chore-i-oh-gon'a-doe-troe-pin)
Ovidrel
Func. class.: Ovulation stimulant

Action: hCG is an analog of LH and binds to LH/hCG receptor
Uses: Final follicular maturation ovulation induction
Dosage and routes:
Infertile women undergoing OI
• *Adult:* SC 250 µg following last dose of FS agent
Infertile women undergoing ART
• *Adult:* SC 250 µg 1 day following last dose of FS agent
Available forms: Powder for inj, lyophilized 285 µg r-hCG
Side effects/adverse reactions:
CV: Vasomotor flushing, phlebitis, *deep-vein thrombosis*
CNS: Headache, depression, restlessness, anxiety, nervousness, fatigue, insomnia, dizziness, flushing, lability
GI: Nausea, vomiting, abdominal pain, bloating, diarrhea
INTEG: Rash
GU: Polyuria, urinary frequency, birth defects, spontaneous abortions, multiple ovulation, breast pain, oliguria, abnormal uterine bleeding
Contraindications: Hypersensitivity, pregnancy (X), hepatic disease, undiagnosed uterine bleeding, uncontrolled thyroid or adrenal dysfunction, intracranial lesion, ovarian cysts
Precautions: Hypertension, depression, convulsions, diabetes mellitus
Pharmacokinetics: Half-life 29 hr
Lab test interferences:
Increase: FSH/LH, ALT

NURSING CONSIDERATIONS
Administer:
• After reconstituting with 1 ml sterile water for inj, discard unused portion, store vial at room temperature, protect from light
Evaluate
• Therapeutic response: fertility
Teach patient/family:
• That multiple births are common
• To notify prescriber immediately if low abdominal pain occurs; may indicate ovarian cyst, cyst rupture
• The method for taking, recording basal body temp to determine whether ovulation has occurred
• If ovulation can be determined (there is a slight decrease in temp, then a sharp increase for ovulation), to attempt coitus 3 days before and qod until after ovulation
• If pregnancy is suspected, to notify prescriber immediately

cidofovir (℞)

(si-doh-foh'veer)
Vistide
Func. class.: Antiviral
Chem. class.: Nucleotide analog

Action: Suppresses cytomegalovirus (CMV) replication by selective inhibition of viral DNA synthesis
Uses: CMV retinitis in patients with HIV, used with probenecid
Dosage and routes:
• Dilute in 100 ml 0.9% saline sol before administration; probenecid must be given PO 2 g 3 hr prior to the cidofovir infusion and 1 g at 2 and 8 hr after ending the cidofovir infusion; give 1 L of 0.9% saline sol IV with each INF of cidofovir, give saline INF over 1-2 hr period immediately prior to cidofovir; patient should be given a 2nd L if the patient can tolerate the fluid load (2nd

L given at time of cidofovir or immediately afterward and should be given over a 1-3 hr period)

Renal dose
• CrCl <50 ml/min reduce dose

Induction
• *Adult:* **IV INF** initially, 5 mg/kg given over 1 hr at a constant rate qwk × 2 consecutive wk; then **IV INF** 5 mg/kg given over 1 hr q2wk

Available forms: Inj 75 mg/ml

Side effects/adverse reactions:

*CNS: Fever, chills, **coma,** confusion, abnormal thought, dizziness, bizarre dreams, headache, psychosis, tremors, somnolence, paresthesia, amnesia, anxiety, insomnia, **seizures***

CV: Dysrhythmias, hypertension/hypotension

EENT: Retinal detachment in CMV retinitis

GI: Abnormal LFTs, *nausea, vomiting, anorexia, diarrhea,* abdominal pain, **hemorrhage**

GU: **Hematuria,** increased creatinine, BUN, **nephrotoxicity**

HEMA: **Granulocytopenia, thrombocytopenia, irreversible neutropenia, anemia, eosinophilia**

INTEG: Rash, alopecia, pruritus, acne, urticaria, pain at inj site, phlebitis

RESP: Dyspnea

Contraindications: Hypersensitivity to this drug or probenecid, sulfa drugs

Precautions: Preexisting cytopenias, renal function impairment, pregnancy (C), lactation, children <6 mo, elderly, platelet count <25,000/mm^3

Pharmacokinetics: Unknown

Interactions:
• Nephrotoxicity: amphotericin B, foscarnet, aminoglycosides, pentamidine IV, NSAIDs

NURSING CONSIDERATIONS

Assess:
• Culture before treatment is initiated; cultures of blood, urine, and throat may all be taken; CMV is not confirmed by this method; the diagnosis is made by an ophth exam
• Kidney, liver function, increased hemopoietic studies and BUN; serum creatinine, AST, ALT, creatinine, creatinine clearance, A-G ratio, baseline and drip treatment, blood counts should be done q2wk; watch for decreasing granulocytes, Hgb; if low, therapy may have to be discontinued and restarted after hematologic recovery; blood transfusions may be required
• For GI symptoms: severe nausea, vomiting, diarrhea; severe symptoms may necessitate discontinuing drug
• Electrolytes and minerals: calcium, phosphorus, magnesium, sodium, potassium; watch closely for tetany during first administration
• For symptoms of blood dyscrasias (anemia, granulocytopenia); bruising, fatigue, bleeding, poor healing
• Allergic reactions: flushing, rash, urticaria, pruritus
• For leukopenia, neutropenia, thrombocytopenia: WBCs, platelets q2d during 2×/day dosing and qwk thereafter; check for leukopenias, with qd WBC count in patients with prior leukopenia, with other nucleoside analogs, or for whom leukopenia counts are <1000 cells/mm^3 at start of treatment
• Monitor serum creatinine or creatinine clearance at least q2wk; give only to those with creatinine levels ≤1.5 mg/dl, CrCl >55 ml/min, urine protein <100 mg/dl

Administer:

IV
• Mix under strict aseptic conditions using gloves, gown, and mask,

and using precautions for antineoplastic

• After diluting in 100 ml 0.9% NaCl

• Slowly; do not give by bolus IV, SC inj

• Use diluted sol within 12 hr, do not refrigerate or freeze; do not use sol with particulate matter or discoloration

Evaluate:

• Therapeutic response: decreased symptoms of CMV

Teach patient/family:

• To notify prescriber if sore throat, swollen lymph nodes, malaise, fever occur; may indicate other infections

• To report perioral tingling, numbness in extremities, and paresthesias

• That serious drug interactions may occur if OTC products are ingested; check first with prescriber

• That drug is not a cure, but will control symptoms

• That regular ophthalmic exams must be continued

• That major toxicities may necessitate discontinuing drug

• To use contraception during treatment and that infertility may occur; men should use barrier contraception for 90 days after treatment

Treatment of overdose: Discontinue drug; use hemodialysis, and increase hydration

---

cilostazol (℞)

(sih-los′tah-zol)

Pletal

Func. class.: Platelet aggregation inhibitor

Chem. class.: Quinolinone derivative

Action: Inhibits cellular phosphodiesterase; reversibly inhibits platelet aggregation induced by throm-bin, ADP, collagen, arachidonic acid, epinephrine, and sheer stress

Uses: Intermittent claudication

Research note: One study has documented improved glucose tolerance and insulin resistance in rats[4]

Dosage and routes:

• *Adult:* **PO** 100 mg bid taken ≥30 min ac or 2 hr pc breakfast and dinner or 50 mg bid if using drugs that inhibit CYP3A4 and CYP2C19; 12 wk of treatment may be needed for beneficial effect

Available forms: Tabs 50, 100 mg

Side effects/adverse reactions:

CNS: Dizziness, headache

CV: Palpitations, tachycardia, nodal dysrhythmia, postural hypotension

GI: Nausea, vomiting, *diarrhea,* GI discomfort, colitis, cholelithiasis, ulcer, esophagitis, gastritis, anorexia, *flatulence, dyspepsia*

*HEMA: **Bleeding (epistaxis, hematuria, retinal hemorrhage, GI bleeding), thrombocytopenia,** anemia, polycythemia*

INTEG: Rash, urticaria, dry skin

GU: Cystitis, frequency, vaginitis, ***vaginal hemorrhage***

EENT: Blindness, diplopia, ear pain, tinnitus, retinal hemorrhage

MISC: Back pain, headache, infection, myalgia, peripheral edema, chills, fever, malaise, diabetes mellitus

RESP: Cough, pharyngitis, rhinitis, asthma, pneumonia

Contraindications: Hypersensitivity, CHF

Precautions: Past liver disease, renal disease, elderly, pregnancy (C), lactation, children, increased bleeding risk, low platelet count, platelet dysfunction, active bleeding

Pharmacokinetics: 95%-98% protein binding, metabolism-hepatic extensively by cytochrome P450 enzymes, excreted urine (74%), feces (20%), half-life 11-13 hr

---

◆ = Nursing alert   ✔ = Herb-drug interaction   ⃠ = Do not crush

Interactions:
• Possible increased bleeding tendencies: anticoagulants
• Increased cilostazol levels: diltiazem, erythromycin, omeprazole; exercise caution when coadministering with fluvoxamine, fluoxetine, nefazodone, ketoconazole, itraconazole, fluconazole and reduce dose to 50 mg bid
• Drug/food: do not use with grapefruit juice

NURSING CONSIDERATIONS
Assess:
• For underlying CV disease since CV risk is great
• For CV lesions with repeated oral administration
• For congestive heart failure
• Blood studies: CBC; CBC q2 wk, Hct, Hgb, PT

Administer:
• Give bid 1 hr ac or 2 hr pc; do not give with grapefruit juice

Evaluate:
• Therapeutic response: improved walking distance and duration, decreased pain

Teach patient/family:
• To report any unusual bleeding to prescriber
• To report side effects such as diarrhea, skin rashes, subcutaneous bleeding
• That effects may take 2-4 wk, treatment of up to 12 wk may be required for necessary effect
• About potential risk for patients with chf
• To take 1 hr ac or 2 hr pc
• That reading the patient package insert is necessary

cimetidine (OTC, ℞)
(sye-met′i-deen)
Apo-Cimetidine*, cimetidine, Novo-Cimetidine*, Peptol*, Tagamet, Tagamet HB
Func. class.: H_2-histamine receptor antagonist
Chem. class.: Imidazole derivative

Action: Inhibits histamine at H_2-receptor site in the gastric parietal cells, which inhibits gastric acid secretion

Uses: Short-term treatment of duodenal and gastric ulcers and maintenance; management of GERD and Zollinger-Ellison syndrome

Investigational uses: Prevention of aspiration pneumonitis, stress ulcers, upper GI bleeding, herpes infection, hirsutism, cutaneous/nongenital warts, weight loss

Dosage and routes:
Treatment of active ulcers
• *Adult:* **PO** 300 mg qid with meals, hs × 8 wk or 400 mg bid, 800 mg hs; after 8 wk give hs dose only; **IV BOL** 300 mg/20 ml 0.9% NaCl over 1-2 min q6h; **IV INF** 300 mg/50 ml D_5W over 15-20 min; **IM** 300 mg q6h, not to exceed 2400 mg/day
• *Child:* **PO** 20-40 mg/kg/day; **IM/IV** 5-10 mg/kg q6-8h

Prophylaxis of duodenal ulcer
• *Adult and child >16 yr:* 400 mg hs

GERD
• *Adult:* **PO** 800-1600 mg/day in divided doses

Hypersecretory conditions (Zollinger-Ellison syndrome)
• *Adult:* **PO/IM/IV** 300-600 mg q6h; may increase to 12 g/day if needed

Upper GI bleeding prophylaxis
• *Adult:* **IV** 50 mg/hr; lowered in renal disease

Aspiration pneumonitis prophylaxis
• *Adult:* **IM/IV** 300 mg **IM** 1 hr before anesthesia, then 300 mg **IV** q4h until patient is alert, max 2400 mg/day

Hirsutism
• *Adult:* **PO** 300 mg qid × 5 days or 1600 mg qd up to 6 mo

Warts
• *Adult:* **PO** 400-800 mg tid × 12 wk or 30-40 mg/kg/day given tid × 3 mo

Weight loss
• *Adult:* **PO** 200-400 mg tid × 8-12 wk

Renal disease
• CrCl 20-40 ml/min 300 mg q8h; CrCl <20 ml/min 300 mg q12h

Available forms: Tabs 100, 200, 300, 400, 800 mg; liq 200, 300 mg/5 ml; inj 300 mg/2 ml, 300 mg/50 ml 0.9% NaCl

Side effects/adverse reactions:
CNS: Confusion, headache, depression, dizziness, anxiety, weakness, psychosis, tremors, *convulsions*
CV: Bradycardia, tachycardia, *dysrhythmias*
GI: Diarrhea, abdominal cramps, *paralytic ileus, jaundice*
GU: Gynecomastia, galactorrhea, impotence, increase in BUN, creatinine
HEMA: Agranulocytosis, thrombocytopenia, neutropenia, aplastic anemia, increase in PT
INTEG: Urticaria, rash, alopecia, sweating, flushing, *exfoliative dermatitis*

Contraindications: Hypersensitivity

Precautions: Pregnancy (B), lactation, child <16 yr, organic brain syndrome, hepatic disease, renal disease, elderly

Pharmacokinetics: Well absorbed (PO, IM)

IM/IV: Onset 10 min, peak ½ hr, duration 4-5 hr
PO: Peak 1-1½ hr, half-life 1½-2 hr; 30%-40% metabolized by liver, excreted in urine unchanged, crosses placenta, enters breast milk

Interactions:
• Increased toxicity due to CYP450 pathway: benzodiazepines, β-blockers, calcium channel blockers, carbamazepine, chloroquine, lidocaine, metronidazole, moricizine, phenytoin, quinidine, quinine, sulfonylureas, theophylline, tricyclics, valproic acid, warfarin
• Decreased absorption of cimetidine: antacids, sucralfate
• Decreased absorption: ketoconazole

Lab test interferences:
Increase: Alk phosphatase, AST, creatinine, prolactin
False positive: Gastroccult, hemoccult
False negative: Skin tests

NURSING CONSIDERATIONS
Assess:
• Gastric pH (5 or more should be maintained), also epigastric pain and duration, intensity; aggravating, ameliorating factors
• I&O ratio, BUN, creatinine, CBC with differential periodically

Administer:
• With meals for prolonged drug effect; antacids 1 hr before or 1 hr after cimetidine

IV
• After diluting 300 mg/20 ml of 0.9% NaCl for inj; give ≥5 min; may be diluted 300 mg/50 ml of D_5W; run over 15-20 min; or total daily dose (900 mg) diluted in 100-1000 ml D_5W given over 24 hr

Additive compatibilities: Acetazolamide, amikacin, aminophylline, atracurium, cefoperazone, cefoxitin, chlorothiazide, clindamycin, colistimethate, dexamethasone, di-

---

◆ = Nursing alert   ∥ = Herb-drug interaction   ⊘ = Do not crush

goxin, epinephrine, erythromycin, ethacrynate, floxacillin, flumazenil, furosemide, gentamicin, insulin (regular), isoproterenol, lidocaine, lincomycin, meropenem, metaraminol, methylprednisolone, norepinephrine, nitroprusside, penicillin G potassium, phytonadione, polymyxin B, potassium chloride, protamine, quinidine, tacrolimus, vancomycin, verapamil, vit B/C

Syringe compatibilities: Atropine, butorphanol, cephalothin, diazepam, diphenhydramine, doxapram, droperidol, fentanyl, glycopyrrolate, heparin, hydromorphone, hydroxyzine, lorazepam, meperidine, midazolam, morphine, nafcillin, nalbuphine, penicillin G sodium, pentazocine, perphenazine, prochlorperazine, promazine, promethazine, scopolamine

Y-site compatibilities: Acyclovir, amifostine, aminophylline, amrinone, atracurium, aztreonam, cisatracurium, cisplatin, cladribine, cyclophosphamide, cytarabine, diltiazem, doxorubicin, doxorubicin liposome, enalaprilat, esmolol, filgrastim, fluconazole, fludarabine, foscarnet, gallium, granisetron, haloperidol, heparin, hetastarch, idarubicin, labetalol, melphalan, meropenem, methotrexate, midazolam, ondansetron, paclitaxel, pancuronium, piperacillin/tazobactam, propofol, remifentanil, sargramostim, tacrolimus, teniposide, theophylline, thiotepa, tolazoline, vecuronium, vinorelbine, zidovudine

Perform/provide:
• Storage of diluted sol at room temperature up to 48 hr

Evaluate:
• Therapeutic response: decreased pain in abdomen; healing of ulcers, absence of gastroesophageal reflux, gastric pH 5

Teach patient/family:
• That gynecomastia, impotence may occur, are reversible
• To avoid driving, other hazardous activities until patient is stabilized on this medication; drowsiness or dizziness may occur
• To avoid black pepper, caffeine, alcohol, harsh spices, extremes in temperature of food
• To avoid OTC preparations: aspirin, cough, cold preparations; condition may worsen
• That smoking decreases the effectiveness of the drug
• That drug must be taken exactly as prescribed and continued for prescribed time to be effective; doses not to be doubled
• To report bruising, fatigue, malaise; blood dyscrasias may occur
• To report to prescriber diarrhea, black tarry stools, sore throat, rash

ciprofloxacin (℞)
(sip-ro-floks'a-sin)
Cipro, Cipro IV
Func. class.: Broad-spectrum antiinfective
Chem. class.: Fluoroquinolone

Action: Interferes with conversion of intermediate DNA fragments into high-molecular-weight DNA in bacteria; DNA gyrase inhibitor

Uses: Infection caused by susceptible *Escherichia coli, Enterobacter cloacae, Proteus mirabilis, Klebsiella pneumoniae, Proteus vulgaris, Citrobacter freundii, Serratia marcescens, Proteus aeruginosa, Staphylococcus aureus, Staphylococcus epidermidis, Enterobacter, Campylobacter jejuni, Salmonella;* chronic bacterial prostatitis, acute sinusitis, postexposure inhalation anthrax

Dosage and routes:
Uncomplicated urinary tract infections
• *Adult:* **PO** 250 mg q12h; **IV** 200 mg q12h
Complicated/severe urinary tract infections
• *Adult:* **PO** 500 mg q12h; **IV** 400 mg q12h
Respiratory, bone, skin, joint infections
• *Adult:* **PO** 500-750 mg q12h; **IV** 400 mg q12h
Renal disease
• CrCl <50 ml/min **PO** 250-500 mg q12h; CrCl 5-29 ml/min **PO** 250-500 mg q18h; **IV** 200-400 mg q18-24h
Available forms: Tabs 250, 500, 750 mg; inj 200 mg/20 ml, 400 mg/40 ml, 200 mg/100 ml D$_5$, 400 mg/200 ml D$_5$; oral susp 250, 500 mg/5 ml
Side effects/adverse reactions:
CNS: Headache, dizziness, fatigue, insomnia, depression, *restlessness, seizures,* confusion
GI: Nausea, diarrhea, increased ALT, AST, dry mouth, flatulence, heartburn, *vomiting,* oral candidiasis, dysphagia, *pseudomembranous colitis*
INTEG: Rash, pruritus, urticaria, photosensitivity, flushing, fever, chills
MS: Tremor, arthralgia, tendon rupture
*MISC: **Anaphylaxis, Stevens-Johnson syndrome***
Contraindications: Hypersensitivity to quinolones
Precautions: Pregnancy (C), lactation, children, renal disease, epilepsy
Pharmacokinetics:
PO: Peak 1 hr, half-life 3-4 hr; excreted in urine as active drug, metabolites
Interactions:
• Decreased absorption of cipro-

flaxin: antacids containing magnesium, aluminum; zinc, iron, sucralfate, enteral feedings, calcium
• Nephrotoxicity: cyclosporine
• Increased serum levels of ciprofloxacin: probenecid; monitor for toxicity
• Increased levels of: theophylline, warfarin, monitor blood levels
🖋 Possible toxicity: yerba maté
• Drug/food: increased effect of: caffeine; decreased absorption: dairy products, food

NURSING CONSIDERATIONS
Assess:
• CNS symptoms: headache, dizziness, fatigue, insomnia, depression
• Kidney, liver function studies: BUN, creatinine, AST, ALT
• I&O ratio, urine pH <5.5 is ideal
◆ Anaphylaxis: fever, flushing, rash, urticaria, pruritus
Administer:
• 2 hr before or 2 hr after antacids, zinc, iron, calcium
IV
• Over 1 hr as an INF, comes in premixed plastic INF container or diluted 20 or 40 ml vial to a final conc of 0.5-2 mg/ml of NS or D$_5$W; give through Y-tube or 3-way stopcock
• After clean-catch urine for C&S
Additive compatibilities: Amikacin, aztreonam, ceftazidime, cyclosporine, gentamicin, metronidazole, netilmicin, piperacillin, potassium acetate, potassium chloride, potassium phosphates, prednisolone, promethazine, propofol, ranitidine, Ringer's, sodium chloride, tobramycin, vit B/C
Y-site compatibilities: Amifostine, amino acids, aztreonam, calcium gluconate, ceftazidime, cisatracurium, digoxin, diltiazem, diphenhydramine, dobutamine, dopamine, doxorubicin liposome, gallium, gentamicin, granisetron, hydroxyzine,

◆ = Nursing alert   🖋 = Herb-drug interaction   🚫 = Do not crush

lidocaine, lorazepam, metoclopramide, midazolam, midodrine, piperacillin, potassium acetate, potassium chloride, potassium phosphates, prednisolone, promethazine, propofol, ranitidine, remifentanil, Ringer's, sodium chloride, tacrolimus, teniposide, thiotepa, tobramycin, verapamil

Perform/provide:
• Limited intake of alkaline foods, drugs: milk, dairy products, alkaline antacids, sodium bicarbonate

Evaluate:
• Therapeutic response: decreased pain, frequency, urgency, C&S; absence of infection

Teach patient/family:
• Not to take any products containing magnesium or calcium (such as antacids), iron, or aluminum with this drug or within 2 hr of drug
• That photosensitivity may occur; patient should avoid sunlight or use sunscreen to prevent burns
• That fluids must be increased to 3 L/day to avoid crystallization in kidneys
• If dizziness occurs, to ambulate, perform activities with assistance
• To complete full course of drug therapy, not to double or miss doses
• To contact prescriber if adverse reaction occurs or if inflammation or pain in tendon occurs
• To use frequent rinsing of mouth, sugarless candy or gum for dry mouth
• Not to use theophylline with this product, will cause toxicity, contact prescriber if taking theophylline

cisplatin (℞)

(sis′pla-tin)
Platinol*, Platinol-AQ
Func. class.: Antineoplastic alkylating agent
Chem. class.: Inorganic heavy metal

Action: Alkylates DNA, RNA; inhibits enzymes that allow synthesis of amino acids in proteins; activity is not cell cycle phase specific

Uses: Advanced bladder cancer, adjunctive in metastatic testicular cancer, adjunctive in metastatic ovarian cancer, head, neck cancer, esophagus, prostate, lung and cervical cancer, lymphoma

Dosage and routes:
Dosage protocols may vary
Testicular cancer
• *Adult:* **IV** 20 mg/m^2 qd × 5 days, repeat q3wk for 3 cycles or more, depending on response
Bladder cancer
• *Adult:* **IV** 50-70 mg/m^2 q3-4wk
Metastatic ovarian cancer
• *Adult:* **IV** 100 mg/m^2 q4wk or 50 mg/m^2 q3wk with cyclophosphamide; mix with 2 L NaCl and 37.5 g mannitol over 6 hr
Available forms: Inj 0.5*, 1 mg/ml; powder for inj 10, 50 mg vials

Side effects/adverse reactions:
EENT: Tinnitus, hearing loss, vestibular toxicity
*HEMA: **Thrombocytopenia, leukopenia, pancytopenia***
CV: Cardiac abnormalities
GI: Severe nausea, vomiting, diarrhea, weight loss
*GU: **Renal tubular damage,** renal insufficiency, impotence, sterility, amenorrhea, gynecomastia, hyperuremia*
*INTEG: **Alopecia,** dermatitis*

CNS: **Seizures,** peripheral neuropathy
RESP: **Fibrosis**
META: Hypomagnesemia, hypocalcemia, hypokalemia, hypophosphatemia
SYST: **Anaphylaxis**

Contraindications: Radiation therapy or chemotherapy within 1 mo, thrombocytopenia, smallpox vaccination, pregnancy (D)

Precautions: Pneumococcus vaccination, lactation

Do not confuse:
cisplatin/carboplatin

Pharmacokinetics: Absorption complete, metabolized in liver, excreted in urine; half-life 30-100 hr, accumulates in body tissues for several months, enters breast milk

Interactions:
• Risk of bleeding: aspirin, NSAIDs, alcohol
• Ototoxicity: bumetanide, ethacrynic acid, furosemide
• Decreased antibody response: live virus vaccines
• Increased myelosuppression: myelosuppressive agents, radiation
• Increased nephrotoxicity: aminoglycosides, loop diuretics
• Decreased effects of: phenytoin

Lab test interferences:
Positive: Coombs' test
Increase: Uric acid, BUN, creatinine
Decrease: Creatinine clearance, calcium, phosphate, potassium, magnesium

NURSING CONSIDERATIONS
Assess:
For bone marrow depression
• CBC, differential, platelet count weekly; withhold drug if WBC is <4000 or platelet count is <100,000; notify prescriber of results
• Renal function studies: BUN, creatinine, serum uric acid, urine CrCl before, electrolytes during therapy;

dose should not be given if BUN <25 mg/dl; creatinine <1.5 mg/dl; I&O ratio; report fall in urine output of <30 ml/hr
• For anaphylaxis: wheezing, tachycardia, facial swelling, fainting; discontinue drug and report to prescriber; resuscitation equipment should be nearby
• Monitor temp q4h (may indicate beginning infection)
• Liver function tests before, during therapy (bilirubin, AST, ALT, LDH) as needed or monthly
• Bleeding: hematuria, guaiac, bruising or petechiae, mucosa or orifices q8h; obtain prescription for viscous lidocaine (Xylocaine)
• Effects of alopecia on body image; discuss feelings about body changes
• Jaundice of skin, sclera; dark urine; clay-colored stools; itchy skin; abdominal pain; fever; diarrhea
• Edema in feet, joint pain, stomach pain, shaking

Administer:
IV
• Do not use aluminum equipment during any preparation or administration, will form precipitate; do not refrigerate unopened powder or solution, protect from sunlight
• Prepare in biologic cabinet using gown, gloves, mask, do not allow drug to come in contact with skin, use soap and water if contact occurs
• For intermittent inf, dilute 10 mg/10 ml or 50 mg/50 ml sterile H$_2$O for inj; withdraw prescribed dose, dilute ½ dose with 1000 ml D$_5$ 0.2 NaCl or D$_5$ 0.45 NaCl with 37.5 g mannitol; IV INF is given over 3-4 hr; use a 0.45 µm filter; total dose 2 L over 6-8 hr; check site for irritation, phlebitis
• For continuous inf give over 24 hr × 5 days

◆ = Nursing alert   ▮ = Herb-drug interaction   🚫 = Do not crush

• Hydrate patient with 0.9% NaCl over 8-12 hr before treatment
• Epinephrine, antihistamines, corticosteroids for hypersensitivity reaction
• Antiemetic 30-60 min before giving drug and prn
• Allopurinol to maintain uric acid levels, alkalinization of urine
• Diuretic (furosemide 40 mg IV) or mannitol after infusion

Additive compatibilities: Carboplatin, cyclophosphamide with etoposide, etoposide, etoposide with floxuridine, floxuridine, floxuridine with leucovorin, hydroxyzine, ifosfamide, ifosfamide with etoposide, leucovorin, magnesium sulfate, mannitol, ondansetron

Solution compatibilities: D_5/0.225% NaCl, D_5/0.45% NaCl, D_5/0.9% NaCl, D_5/0.45% NaCl with mannitol 1.875%, D_5/0.33% NaCl with KCl 20 mEq and mannitol 1.875%, 0.9% NaCl, 0.45% NaCl, 0.3% NaCl, 0.225% NaCl

Syringe compatibilities: Bleomycin, cyclophosphamide, doxapram, doxorubicin, droperidol, fluorouracil, furosemide, heparin, leucovorin, methotrexate, metoclopramide, mitomycin, vinblastine, vincristine

Y-site compatibilities: Allopurinol, aztreonam, bleomycin, chlorpromazine, cimetidine, cladribine, cyclophosphamide, dexamethasone, diphenhydramine, doxorubicin, doxorubicin liposome, droperidol, famotidine, filgrastim, fludarabine, fluorouracil, furosemide, ganciclovir, granisetron, heparin, hydromorphone, leucovorin, lorazepam, melphalan, methotrexate, methylprednisolone, metoclopramide, mitomycin, morphine, ondansetron, paclitaxel, prochlorperazine, promethazine, propofol, ranitidine, sargramostim, teniposide, vinblastine, vincristine, vinorelbine

Perform/provide:
• Comprehensive oral hygiene
• All medications PO, if possible, avoid IM inj when platelets <100,000/mm³
• Increase fluid intake to 2-3 L/day to prevent urate deposits, calculi formation; elimination of drug

Evaluate:
• Therapeutic response: decreased tumor size, spread of malignancy

Teach patient/family:
• To report signs of infection: increased temp, sore throat, flulike symptoms
• To report signs of anemia: fatigue, headache, faintness, shortness of breath, irritability
• To report bleeding: avoid use of razors, commercial mouthwash
• To avoid aspirin, ibuprofen, NSAIDs, alcohol; may cause GI bleeding
• To report any complaints or side effects to nurse or prescriber
• That impotence or amenorrhea can occur; reversible after discontinuing treatment
• To report any changes in breathing, coughing
• That hair may be lost during treatment; a wig or hairpiece may make patient feel better; new hair may be different in color, texture
• To report numbness, tingling in face or extremities, poor hearing or joint pain, swelling
• Not to receive vaccines during treatment
• To use contraception during treatment and 4 mo after; this drug may cause infertility

---

citalopram (℞)

(sigh-tal'oh-pram)
Celexa
Func. class.: Antidepressant
Chem. class.: Selective serotonin reuptake inhibitor (SSRI)

Action: Inhibits CNS neuron uptake of serotonin but not of norepinephrine

Uses:
Major depressive disorder

Investigational uses: Fibromyalgia, premenstrual disorders

Dosage and routes:
• *Adult:* **PO** 20 mg qd AM or PM, may increase if needed to 40 mg/day after 1 wk; maintenance: after 6-8 wk of initial treatment, continue for 24 wk (32 wk total), reevaluate long-term usefulness (max 60 mg/day)
• *Geriatric:* **PO** 20 mg qd initially, may increase to 40 mg/day
Fibromyalgia
• *Adult:* **PO** 20 mg qd × 4 wk; increase dose to 40 mg qd × 4 wk
Hepatic dose
• *Adult:* **PO** 20 mg/day, may increase to 40 mg/day if no response
Available forms: Tabs 20, 40 mg

Side effects/adverse reactions:
*CNS: Headache, nervousness, insomnia, drowsiness, anxiety, tremor, dizziness, fatigue, sedation, poor concentration, abnormal dreams, agitation, **convulsions,** apathy, euphoria, hallucinations, delusions, psychosis, **suicidal attempts***
GI: Nausea, diarrhea, dry mouth, anorexia, dyspepsia, constipation, cramps, vomiting, taste changes, flatulence, decreased appetite
INTEG: Sweating, rash, pruritus, acne, alopecia, urticaria
RESP: Infection, pharyngitis, nasal congestion, sinus headache, sinusitis, cough, dyspnea, bronchitis, asthma, hyperventilation, pneumonia
*CV: Hot flashes, palpitations, angina pectoris, **hemorrhage,** hypertension, tachycardia, 1st-degree AV block, bradycardia, MI, thrombophlebitis*
MS: Pain, arthritis, twitching
GU: Dysmenorrhea, decreased libido, urinary frequency, UTI, amenorrhea, cystitis, impotence, urine retention
EENT: Visual changes, ear/eye pain, photophobia, tinnitus
SYST: Asthenia, viral infection, fever, allergy, chills

Contraindications: Hypersensitivity

Precautions: Pregnancy (B), lactation, children, elderly

Pharmacokinetics:
PO: Metabolized in liver; excreted in urine; steady state 28-35 days; peak 2-4 hr; half-life 35 hr

Interactions:
• Increased effect of tricyclics, use cautiously
• Increased CNS effects: CNS depressants
 Fatal reactions: do not use with MAOIs
• Increased citalopram levels: macrolides, azole antifungals
• Increased plasma levels of: β-blockers
• Decreased citalopram levels; carbamazepine
• Increased serotonergic effects: lithium
 Avoid use with St. John's wort; fatal reaction may occur

Lab test interferences:
• *Increase:* Serum bilirubin, blood glucose, alk phosphatase
• *Decrease:* VMA, 5-HIAA
• *False increase:* Urinary catecholamines

 = Nursing alert   = Herb-drug interaction   ⃠ = Do not crush

NURSING CONSIDERATIONS
Assess:

• Mental status: mood, sensorium, affect, suicidal tendencies, increase in psychiatric symptoms, depression, panic

• B/P (lying/standing), pulse q4h; if systolic B/P drops 20 mm Hg, hold drug, notify prescriber; take vital signs q4h in patients with cardiovascular disease

• Weight qwk; appetite may decrease or increase with drug

• ECG for flattening of T wave, bundle branch, AV block, dysrhythmias in cardiac patients

• Alcohol consumption; if alcohol is consumed, hold dose until AM
Administer:

• With food or milk for GI symptoms

• Crushed if patient is unable to swallow medication whole

• Dosages hs if oversedation occurs during the day; may take entire dose hs
Perform/provide:

• Storage at room temperature; do not freeze

• Assistance with ambulation during therapy, since drowsiness, dizziness occur

• Safety measures primarily in elderly

• Check to see if PO medication swallowed

• Gum, hard candy, frequent sips of water for dry mouth
Evaluate:

• Therapeutic response: decreased depression
Teach patient/family:

• That therapeutic effect may take 2-3 wk

• To use caution in driving, other activities requiring alertness because of drowsiness, dizziness, blurred vision

• To avoid alcohol ingestion, other CNS depressants

• To notify prescriber if pregnant or plan to become pregnant or breastfeed

---

RARELY USED

cladribine (CdA) (℞)
(kla′dri-been)
Leustatin
Func. class.: Antineoplastic antiinfective

Uses: Treatment of active hairy cell leukemia; may be useful in chronic lymphocytic leukemia, non-Hodgkin's lymphomas, acute myeloid leukemia, autoimmune hemolytic anemia
Dosage and routes:

• *Adult:* **IV** 0.09 mg/kg diluted with 0.9% NaCl qs to 100 ml; pass through 0.22 µm microfilter, given for 1 wk
Contraindications: Hypersensitivity, lactation

---

clarithromycin (℞)
(klare-ith′row-my-sin)
Biaxin, Biaxin XL
Func. class.: Antiinfective
Chem. class.: Macrolide

Action: Binds to 50S ribosomal subunits of susceptible bacteria and suppresses protein synthesis
Uses: Mild to moderate infections of the upper respiratory tract, lower respiratory tract, uncomplicated skin and skin structure infections caused by *Streptococcus pneumoniae, Mycoplasma pneumoniae, Legionella pneumophila, Moraxella catarrhalis, Neisseria gonorrhoeae, Corynebacterium diphtheriae, Listeria*

Side effects: *italics* = common; **bold italics** = life-threatening

monocytogenes, Haemophilus influenzae, Streptococcus pyogenes, Staphlococcus aureus, Mycobacterium avium (MAC) complex infection in AIDS patients, *Mycobacterium intracellulare, Helicobacter pylori* in combination with omeprazole

Dosage and routes:

• *Adult:* **PO** 250-500 mg q12h for 7-14 days; 500 mg q12h continues for *M. avium* complex (MAC)

• *Child:* **PO** 15 mg/kg/day (max 1000 mg) divided q12h × 10 days

H. pylori *infection*

• *Adult:* **PO** 500 mg qd plus omeprazole 2 × 20 mg q AM (day 1-14), then omeprazole 20 mg q AM (days 15-28)

Acute maxillary sinusitis/acute bacterial bronchitis

• *Adult:* **PO** 500 mg q12h × 10 days

Available forms: Tabs 250, 500 mg; granules for oral susp 125 mg/5 ml, 250 mg/5 ml; ext rel tab

Side effects/adverse reactions:

INTEG: Rash, urticaria, pruritus, *Stevens-Johnson syndrome*

CV: Ventricular dysrhythmias

HEMA: Leukopenia, thrombocytopenia, increased INR

GI: Nausea, vomiting, diarrhea, hepatotoxicity, abdominal pain, stomatitis, heartburn, anorexia, *abnormal taste, pseudomembranous colitis*

GU: Vaginitis, moniliasis

MISC: Headache

Contraindications: Hypersensitivity to this drug or macrolide antibiotics

Precautions: Pregnancy (C), lactation, hepatic, renal disease, elderly

Pharmacokinetics: Peak 2 hr, duration 12 hr, half-life 4-6 hr; metabolized by liver; excreted in bile, feces

Interactions:

• Dysrhythmias: cisapride, pimozide

• Increased clarithromycin levels: fluconazole

• Increased effects of oral anticoagulants, digoxin, theophylline, carbamazepine

• Decreased action: zidovudine

Lab test interferences:

Increase: 17-OHCS/17-KS, AST, ALT, BUN, creatinine, LDH, total bilirubin

Decrease: Folate assay, WBC

NURSING CONSIDERATIONS

Assess:

• LFTs, renal studies; report hematuria, oliguria

• C&S before drug therapy; drug may be given as soon as culture is taken; C&S may be repeated after treatment

• Bowel pattern before, during treatment

• Skin eruptions, itching

• Respiratory status: rate, character, wheezing, tightness in chest; discontinue drug

• Allergies before treatment, reaction of each medication

Administer:

• Adequate intake of fluids (2 L) during diarrhea episodes

• q12h to maintain serum level

Perform/provide:

• Storage at room temperature

Evaluate:

• Therapeutic response: C&S negative for infection

Teach patient/family:

• To take with full glass H_2O; may give with food to decrease GI symptoms

🚫 Not to crush tabs

🔶 To report sore throat, fever, fatigue; may indicate superinfection

🔶 To notify nurse of diarrhea, dark urine, pale stools, yellow discoloration of eyes or skin, severe abdominal pain

• To take at evenly spaced intervals; complete dosage regimen

---

🔶 = Nursing alert   🌿 = Herb-drug interaction   🚫 = Do not crush

• To notify prescriber if pregnancy is suspected or planned

Treatment of hypersensitivity: Withdraw drug, maintain airway, administer epinephrine, aminophylline, O_2, IV corticosteroids

clindamycin HCl (℞)
(klin-da-my′sin)
Cleocin HCl
clindamycin palmitate (℞)
Cleocin Pediatric, Dalacin C Palmitate
clindamycin phosphate (℞)
Cleocin Phosphate, Dalacin C, Dalacin C Phosphate

Func. class.: Antiinfective, misc.

Chem. class.: Lincomycin derivative

Action: Binds to 50S subunit of bacterial ribosomes, suppresses protein synthesis

Uses: Infections caused by staphylococci, streptococci, *Rickettsia, Fusobacterium, Actinomyces, Peptococcus, Bacteroides, Pneumocystis carinii*

Dosage and routes:
• *Adult:* **PO** 150-450 mg q6h, max 1.8 g/day; **IM/IV** 1.2-1.8 g/day in 2-4 divided doses, not to exceed 4800 mg/day
• *Child >1 mo:* **PO** 8-25 mg/kg/day in divided doses q6-8h; **IM/IV** 20-40 mg/kg/day in divided doses q6-8h (3-4 equal doses)
• *Child <1 mo:* 15-20 mg/kg/day divided q6-8h
• *PID: Adult:* **IV** 600 mg qid plus gentamicin or 900 mg q8h
Bacterial endocarditis prophylaxis
• *Adult:* 600 mg 1 hr prior to procedure

Available forms:
Phosphate: inj 150, 300, 600 mg base/4 ml; 900 mg base/ml; inj INF in D_5 300 mg, 600 mg, 900 mg; HCl: caps 75, 150, 300 mg; palmitate: oral sol 75 mg/ml

Side effects/adverse reactions:
*HEMA: **Leukopenia, eosinophilia, agranulocytosis, thrombocytopenia, polyarthritis***
*GI: Nausea, vomiting, abdominal pain, diarrhea, **pseudomembranous colitis,** anorexia, weight loss, increased AST, ALT, bilirubin, alk phosphatase; jaundice*
GU: Vaginitis, urinary frequency
EENT: Rash, urticaria, pruritus, erythema, pain, abscess at injection site

Contraindications: Hypersensitivity to this drug or lincomycin, tartrazine dye; ulcerative colitis/enteritis

Precautions: Renal disease, liver disease, GI disease, elderly, pregnancy (B), lactation, tartrazine sensitivity

Pharmacokinetics:
PO: Peak 45 min, duration 6 hr
IM: Peak 3 hr, duration 8-12 hr; half-life 2½ hr; metabolized in liver; excreted in urine, bile, feces as inactive metabolites; crosses placenta; excreted in breast milk

Interactions:
• Decreased absorption: kaolin
• May block clindamycin effect: erythromycin
• Increased neuromuscular blockade: neuromuscular blockers

Lab test interferences:
Increase: Alk phosphatase, bilirubin, CPK, AST, ALT

NURSING CONSIDERATIONS
Assess:
• Liver studies: AST, ALT if on long-term therapy
• Blood studies: WBC, RBC, Hct, Hgb, platelets, serum iron, reticu-

locytes; drug should be discontinued if bone marrow depression occurs

• C&S before drug therapy; drug may be given as soon as culture is taken

• B/P, pulse in patient receiving drug parenterally

• Bowel pattern before, during treatment; if severe diarrhea occurs, drug should be discontinued; may indicate pseudomembranous colitis

• Skin eruptions, itching, dermatitis after administration

• Respiratory status: rate, character, wheezing, tightness in chest

• Allergies before treatment, reaction of each medication

Administer:

• IM deep injection; rotate sites

• Orally with at least 8 oz H_2O

IV

• By infusion only; do not administer bolus dose; dilute 300 mg or less/50 ml or more of D_5W, NS; may be further diluted in greater amounts of D_5W, NS and given as a cont inf in acute PID; give first dose 10 mg/min over ½ hr, then 0.75 mg/min; increased rates may be used to keep serum blood levels higher; run >10 min; no more than 1200 mg in a single 1-hr inf

Additive compatibilities: Amikacin, ampicillin, aztreonam, cefamandole, cefazolin, cefepime, cefonicid, cefoperazone, cefotaxime, cefoxitin, ceftazidime, ceftizoxime, cefuroxime, cephalothin, cimetidine, fluconazole, heparin, hydrocortisone, kanamycin, methylprednisolone, metoclopramide, metronidazole, netilmicin, ofloxacin, penicillin G, piperacillin, potassium chloride, sodium bicarbonate, tobramycin, verapamil, vit B/C

Syringe compatibilities: Amikacin, aztreonam, gentamicin, heparin

Y-site compatibilities: Amifostine, amiodarone, amphotericin B cholesteryl, amsacrine, aztreonam, cefpirome, cisatracurium, cyclophosphamide, diltiazem, doxorubicin liposome, enalaprilat, esmolol, fludarabine, foscarnet, granisetron, heparin, hydromorphone, labetalol, magnesium sulfate, melphalan, meperidine, midazolam, morphine, multivitamins, ondansetron, perphenazine, piperacillin/tazobactam, propofol, remifentanil, sargramostim, tacrolimus, teniposide, theophylline, thiotepa, vinorelbine, vit B/C, zidovudine

Perform/provide:

• Storage at room temperature (caps) up to 2 wk (reconstituted)

• Epinephrine, suction, tracheostomy set, endotracheal intubation equipment on unit

• Adequate intake of fluids (2 L) during diarrhea episodes

Evaluate:

• Therapeutic response: decreased temp, negative C&S

Teach patient/family:

• To take oral drug with full glass H_2O; may give with food to reduce GI symptoms; antiperistaltic drugs may worsen diarrhea

• All aspects of drug therapy: need to complete entire course of medication to ensure organism death (10-14 days); culture may be taken after medication course completed

◆ To report sore throat, fever, fatigue; may indicate superinfection

🚫 Not to break, crush, or chew caps

• That drug must be taken in equal intervals around clock to maintain blood levels

• To notify nurse or prescriber of diarrhea

◆ = Nursing alert   ∥ = Herb-drug interaction   🚫 = Do not crush

C

Treatment of hypersensitivity:
Withdraw drug; maintain airway; administer epinephrine, aminophylline, O_2, IV corticosteroids

---

RARELY USED

clofazimine (℞)

(kloe-fa′zi-meen)
Lamprene
Func. class.: Leprostatic

Uses: Lepromatous leprosy, dapsone-resistant leprosy, lepromatous leprosy complicated by erythema nodosum leprosum
Dosage and routes:
Erythema nodosum leprosum
• *Adult:* **PO:** 100-200 mg qd × 3 mo, then taper dosage to 100 mg when disease is controlled; do not exceed 200 mg/day
Dapsone-resistant leprosy
• *Adult:* **PO:** 100 mg/day in combination with at least one other antileprosy drug × 3 yr, then 100 mg qd clofazimine (only)
Contraindications: Hypersensitivity to this drug

---

clomiphene (℞)

(kloe′mi-feen)
Clomid, clomiphene citrate, Milophene, Serophene
Func. class.: Ovulation stimulant
Chem. class.: Nonsteroidal antiestrogenic

Action: Increases LH, FSH release from the pituitary, which increases maturation of ovarian follicle, ovulation, development of corpus luteum
Uses: Female infertility (ovulatory failure)

Dosage and routes:
• *Adult:* **PO** 50-100 mg qd × 5 days or 50-100 mg qd beginning on day 5 of cycle; may be repeated until conception occurs or 3 cycles of therapy have been completed
Available forms: Tabs 50 mg
Side effects/adverse reactions:
CV: Vasomotor flushing, phlebitis, **deep-vein thrombosis**
EENT: Blurred vision, diplopia, photophobia
CNS: Headache, depression, restlessness, anxiety, nervousness, fatigue, insomnia, dizziness, flushing
GI: Nausea, vomiting, constipation, abdominal pain, bloating
INTEG: Rash, dermatitis, urticaria, alopecia
GU: Polyuria, urinary frequency, birth defects, spontaneous abortions, multiple ovulation, breast pain, oliguria, abnormal uterine bleeding
Contraindications: Hypersensitivity, pregnancy (X), hepatic disease, undiagnosed uterine bleeding, uncontrolled thyroid or adrenal dysfunction, intracranial lesion, ovarian cysts
Precautions: Hypertension, depression, convulsions, diabetes mellitus
Do not confuse:
clomiphene/clomipramine
Pharmacokinetics: Metabolized in liver, excreted in feces
Lab test interferences:
Increase: FSH/LH, BSP, thyroxine, TBG
NURSING CONSIDERATIONS
Administer:
• After discontinuing estrogen therapy
• At same time qd to maintain drug level
Evaluate:
• Therapeutic response: fertility
Teach patient/family:
• That multiple births are common
• To notify prescriber immediately

if low abdominal pain occurs; may indicate ovarian cyst, cyst rupture
• To notify prescriber of photophobia, blurred vision, diplopia
• That if dose is missed, to double at next time; if more than one dose is missed, to call prescriber
• That response usually occurs 4-10 days after last day of treatment
• The method for taking, recording basal body temp to determine whether ovulation has occurred
• If ovulation can be determined (there is a slight decrease in temp, then a sharp increase for ovulation), to attempt coitus 3 days before and qod until after ovulation
• If pregnancy is suspected, to notify prescriber immediately

---

clomipramine (R)

(kloe-mip′ra-meen)
Anafranil
Func. class.: Antidepressant, tricyclic
Chem. class.: Tertiary amine

Action: Potentiates serotonin and norepinephrine; also increases dopamine metabolism; moderate anticholinergic effect

Uses: Obsessive-compulsive disorder, depression, dysphoria, phobias, anxiety, agoraphobia

Dosage and routes:
Obsessive-compulsive disorder
• *Adult:* PO 25 mg hs and increase gradually over 4 wk to 75-300 mg/day in divided doses
• *Child 10-18 yr:* PO 25-50 mg/day gradually increased; or 3 mg/kg/day, whichever is smaller, not to exceed 200 mg/day
Depression
• *Adult:* PO 50-150 mg/day in a single or divided dose

Anxiety/agoraphobia
• *Adult:* PO 25-75 mg/day
Available forms: Caps 10, 25, 50, 75 mg

Side effects/adverse reactions:
*HEMA: **Agranulocytosis, neutropenia, pancytopenia***
CV: Hypotension, tachycardia, ***cardiac arrest***
*CNS: Dizziness, tremors, mania, **seizures,** aggressiveness, EPS*
ENDO: Galactorrhea, hyperprolactinemia
META: Hyponatremia
GI: Constipation, dry mouth, nausea, dyspepsia
GU: Delayed ejaculation, anorgasmia, urinary retention
INTEG: Diaphoresis, photosensitivity

Contraindications: Hypersensitivity, immediate post-MI
Precautions: Seizures, suicidal patients, elderly, pregnancy (C), lactation, cardiac disease
Do not confuse:
clomipramine/clomiphene
clomipramine/desipramine
Pharmacokinetics: Onset ≥2 wk, peak 2-6 hr; extensively bound to tissue and plasma proteins; demethylated in liver; active metabolites excreted in urine; half-life: 19-37 hr; steady state 1-2 wk
Interactions:
• Decreased clomipramine levels: barbiturates, carbamazepine, phenytoin
• Increased clomipramine levels: cimetidine, fluoxetine, fluvoxamine, sertraline; do not use together
• Increased hypertensive effect: clonidine, epinephrine, norepinephrine
• Increased CNS depression: alcohol, CNS depressants
• Hypertensive crisis, convulsions, hypertensive episode: MAOIs
✎ Increased CNS depression: kava

🖉 Increased anticholinergic effect: belladonna leaf/root, henbane leaf

🖉 Increased action of clomipramine: scopolia root

Lab test interferences:

Increase: Prolactin, TBG

Decrease: Serum thyroid hormone

NURSING CONSIDERATIONS
Assess:

• B/P (lying, standing), pulse q4h; if systolic B/P drops 20 mm Hg, withhold drug, notify prescriber; take vital signs q4h in patients with cardiovascular disease

• ECG for flattening of T wave, QTc prolongation, bundle branch block, AV block, dysrhythmias in cardiac patients

• Blood studies: CBC, leukocytes, differential, cardiac enzymes if patient is receiving long-term therapy

• Hepatic studies: AST, ALT, bilirubin

• Mental status: mood, sensorium, affect, suicidal tendencies; increase in psychiatric symptoms: depression, panic, frequency of obsessive-compulsive behaviors

• Urinary retention, constipation; constipation more likely in children

• Withdrawal symptoms: headache, nausea, vomiting, muscle pain, weakness; not usual unless drug discontinued abruptly

• Alcohol consumption; if alcohol consumed, withhold dose until AM

Administer:

• Increased fluids, bulk in diet for constipation, especially elderly

• With food or milk for GI symptoms

Perform/provide:

• Storage in tight container at room temperature; do not freeze

• Assistance with ambulation during beginning therapy, since drowsiness/dizziness occurs

• Safety measures, primarily in elderly

• Checking to see PO medication swallowed

• Gum, hard candy, or frequent sips of water for dry mouth

Evaluate:

• Therapeutic response: decreased anxiety, depression

Teach patient/family:

🚫 Not to break, crush, or chew caps

• That the effects may take 2-3 wk

• To use caution in driving, other activities requiring alertness because of drowsiness, dizziness, blurred vision

• To avoid alcohol ingestion, other CNS depressants

• Not to discontinue medication quickly after long-term use; may cause nausea, headache, malaise

• To wear sunscreen, protective clothing to prevent photosensitivity

Treatment of overdose: ECG monitoring; induce emesis; lavage, activated charcoal; anticonvulsant

---

clonazepam (℞)

(kloe-na'zi-pam)
Klonopin, Rivotril*,
Syn-Clonazepam*

Func. class.: Anticonvulsant
Chem. class.: Benzodiazepine derivative

Controlled Substance Schedule IV

Action: Inhibits spike, wave formation in absence seizures (petit mal), decreases amplitude, frequency, duration, spread of discharge in minor motor seizures

Uses: Absence, atypical absence, akinetic, myoclonic seizures, Lennox-Gastaut syndrome

Investigational uses: Parkinsonian dysarthrosis, acute manic episodes, adjunction schizophrenia, neuralgias, multifocal tic disorders, restless leg syndrome, rectal administration

Dosage and routes:
• *Adult:* **PO** not to exceed 1.5 mg/day in 3 divided doses; may be increased 0.5-1 mg q3d until desired response, not to exceed 20 mg/day; rectal 0.02 mg/kg
• *Child <10 yr or <30 kg:* **PO** 0.01-0.03 mg/kg/day in divided doses q8h, not to exceed 0.05 mg/kg/day; may be increased 0.25-0.5 mg q3d until desired response, not to exceed 0.1-0.2 mg/kg/day; rectal 0.05-0.1 mg/kg

Available forms: Tabs 0.5, 1, 2 mg; oral susp; IV sol

Side effects/adverse reactions:
HEMA: **Thrombocytopenia, leukocytosis, eosinophilia**
CNS: Drowsiness, dizziness, confusion, behavioral changes, tremors, insomnia, headache, suicidal tendencies, slurred speech
GI: Nausea, constipation, polyphagia, anorexia, xerostomia, diarrhea, gastritis, sore gums
INTEG: Rash, alopecia, hirsutism
EENT: Increased salivation, nystagmus, diplopia, abnormal eye movements
RESP: **Respiratory depression,** dyspnea, congestion
CV: Palpitations, bradycardia
GU: Dysuria, enuresis, nocturia, retention

Contraindications: Hypersensitivity to benzodiazepines, acute narrow-angle glaucoma
Precautions: Open-angle glaucoma, chronic respiratory disease, lactation, renal, hepatic disease, elderly, pregnancy (C)
Do not confuse:
Klonopin/clonidine
Pharmacokinetics:
PO: Peak 1-2 hr; metabolized by liver; excreted in urine; half-life 18-50 hr

Interactions:
• Increased CNS depression: alcohol, barbiturates, opiates, antidepressants, other anticonvulsants, general anesthetics, hypnotics, sedatives
• Decreased clonazepam effect: carbamazepine, phenobarbital, phenytoin
🌿 Increased CNS depression: kava
Lab test interferences:
Increase: AST, alk phosphatase
NURSING CONSIDERATIONS
Assess:
• Blood level: ther level 20-80 ng/ml
• Renal studies: urinalysis, BUN, urine creatinine
• Blood studies: RBC, Hct, Hgb, reticulocyte counts qwk for 4 wk, then qmo
• Hepatic studies: ALT, AST, bilirubin, creatinine
• Drug levels during initial treatment (therapeutic 20-80 ng/ml)
• Signs of physical withdrawal if medication suddenly discontinued
• Mental status: mood, sensorium, affect, oversedation, behavioral changes; if mental status changes, notify prescriber
• Eye problems: need for ophthalmic exam before, during, after treatment (slit lamp, fundoscopy, tonometry)
• Allergic reaction: red, raised rash; drug should be discontinued
◆ Blood dyscrasias: fever, sore throat, bruising, rash, jaundice
• Toxicity: bone marrow depression, nausea, vomiting, ataxia, diplopia, cardiovascular collapse
Administer:
• With food, milk for GI symptoms Oral suspension
• May use rectally (1 mg/ml of clonazepam with 1 ml of water); use plastic tube (volume 2.2-3.3 ml)

◆ = Nursing alert　　🌿 = Herb-drug interaction　　🚫 = Do not crush

IV solution
• May use rectally 1 ml syringe inserted 3 cm into rectum
Perform/provide:
• Storage at room temperature
• Assistance with ambulation during early part of treatment; dizziness occurs, especially elderly
Evaluate:
• Therapeutic response: decreased seizure activity, document on patient's chart
Teach patient/family:
• To carry ID card or Medic Alert bracelet stating name, drugs taken, condition, prescriber's name, phone number
• To avoid driving, other activities that require alertness
• To avoid alcohol ingestion, CNS depressants; increased sedation may occur
• Not to discontinue medication quickly after long-term use; taper off over several wk
Treatment of overdose: Lavage, activated charcoal, monitor electrolytes, VS, administer vasopressors

---

clonidine (℞)

(klon'i-deen)

Catapres, Catapres-TTS, clonidine HCl, Dixarit*, Duraclon

Func. class.: Antihypertensive, centrally acting analgesic

Chem. class.: Central α-adrenergic agonist

Action: Inhibits sympathetic vasomotor center in CNS, which reduces impulses in sympathetic nervous system; blood pressure, pulse rate, cardiac output decrease, prevents pain signal transmission in CNS by α-adrenergic receptor stimulation of the spinal cord

Uses: Mild to moderate hypertension, used alone or in combination; severe pain in cancer patients

Investigational uses: Opioid withdrawal, prevention of vascular headaches, treatment of menopausal symptoms, dysmenorrhea, attention deficit hyperactivity disorder

Dosage and routes:

Hypertension
• *Adult:* **PO/TRANS** 0.1 mg bid, then increase by 0.1-0.2 mg/day until desired response; range 0.2-0.8 mg/day in divided doses
• *Geriatric:* **PO** 0.1 mg hs, may increase gradually
• *Child:* 5-10 µg/kg/day in divided doses q8-12h, max 0.9 mg/day

Opioid withdrawal
• *Adult:* **PO** 0.3-1.2 mg/day; may decrease by 50% × 3 days then decrease by 0.1-0.2 mg/day or discontinue

Severe pain
• *Adult:* **CONT EPIDURAL INF** 30 µg/hr
• *Child:* **CONT EPIDURAL INF** 0.5 µg/kg/hr, then titrate to response

ADHD
• *Child:* 0.05 mg/day titrate up to max 0.4 mg/day

Menopausal symptoms
• *Adult:* **TD** 0.1 mg patch q1wk; **PO** 0.05-0.4 mg bid

Available forms: Tabs 0.025*, 0.1, 0.2, 0.3 mg; TRANS 2.5, 5, 7.5 mg delivering 0.1, 0.2, 0.3 mg/24 hr, respectively; inj 100, 500 µg/ml

Side effects/adverse reactions:

CNS: Drowsiness, sedation, headache, fatigue, nightmares, insomnia, mental changes, anxiety, depression, hallucinations, delirium

*CV: Orthostatic hypotension, palpitations, **CHF,*** ECG abnormalities

EENT: Taste change, parotid pain

ENDO: Hyperglycemia

GI: Nausea, vomiting, malaise, constipation, *dry mouth*

GU: Impotence, dysuria, nocturia, gynecomastia

INTEG: Rash, alopecia, facial pallor, pruritus, hives, edema, burning papules, excoriation (transdermal patches)

MS: Muscle, joint pain; leg cramps

MISC: Withdrawal symptoms

Contraindications: Hypersensitivity; (epidural) bleeding disorders, anticoagulants

Precautions: MI (recent), diabetes mellitus, chronic renal failure, Raynaud's disease, thyroid disease, depression, COPD, child <12 yr (transdermal), asthma, pregnancy (C), lactation, elderly, noncompliant patients

Do not confuse:

clonidine/Klonopin

Catapres/Cataflam

Pharmacokinetics: Absorbed well

PO: Onset ½ to 1 hr, peak 2-4 hr, duration 8-12 hr; half-life 12-21 hr

TD: Onset 3 days, duration 1 wk; metabolized by liver (metabolites), excreted in urine (30% unchanged, inactive metabolites), feces; crosses blood-brain barrier, excreted in breast milk

Interactions:

• Increased CNS depression: opiates, sedatives, hypnotics, anesthetics, alcohol

• Decreased hypotensive effects: tricyclics, MAOIs, appetite suppressants, amphetamines

• Increased hypotensive effects: diuretics, other antihypertensive nitrates

• Increased bradycardia: β-blockers, cardiac glycosides

• AV block: verapamil

• Decreased effect of: levodopa

Lab test interferences:

Increase: Blood glucose

Decrease: VMA, urinary catecholamines, aldosterone

NURSING CONSIDERATIONS

Assess:

• Blood studies: neutrophils, decreased platelets

• Renal studies: protein, BUN, creatinine; increased levels may indicate nephrotic syndrome

• Baselines in renal, liver function tests before therapy begins; K levels, although hyperkalemia rare

• B/P, pulse if used for hypertension, report significant changes

• For opiate withdrawal including fever, diarrhea, nausea, vomiting, cramps, insomnia, shivering, dilated pupils

• Pain: location, intensity, character; alleviating, aggravating factors, baseline and frequently

• Edema in feet, legs daily; monitor I&O; check for falling output

• Allergic reaction: rash, fever, pruritus, urticaria; drug should be discontinued if antihistamines fail to help

• Allergic reaction from patches: rash, urticaria, angioedema; should not continue to use

• Symptoms of CHF: edema, dyspnea, wet rales, B/P

• Renal symptoms: polyuria, oliguria, frequency

Administer:

• PO: give last dose at hs

• Transdermal patch qwk; apply to site without hair; best absorption over chest or upper arm; rotate sites with each application; clean site before application; apply firmly, especially around edges

Perform/provide:

• Storage of patches in cool environment, tablets in tight container

Evaluate:

• Therapeutic response: decrease in B/P in hypertension, decrease in withdrawal symptoms (opioid), decrease in pain

---

◆ = Nursing alert   ⫸ = Herb-drug interaction   ⊘ = Do not crush

Teach patient/family:
• To avoid hazardous activities, since drug may cause drowsiness
• To administer 1 hr before meals (PO)
• To notify all health care providers of medication use
• Not to discontinue drug abruptly or withdrawal symptoms may occur: anxiety, increased B/P, headache, insomnia, increased pulse, tremors, nausea, sweating
• Not to use OTC (cough, cold, or allergy) products unless directed by prescriber
• To comply with dosage schedule even if feeling better
• To rise slowly to sitting or standing position to minimize orthostatic hypotension, especially elderly
• To notify prescriber of mouth sores, sore throat, fever, swelling of hands, feet, irregular heartbeat, chest pain, signs of angioedema
• About excessive perspiration, dehydration, vomiting; diarrhea may lead to fall in blood pressure; consult prescriber if these occur
• That drug may cause dizziness, fainting; light-headedness may occur during first few days of therapy
• That drug may cause dry mouth; use hard candy, saliva product, or frequent rinsing of mouth
• That compliance is necessary; not to skip or stop drug unless directed by prescriber
• That drug may cause skin rash or impaired perspiration
• To use patch; patch comes in two parts: drug patch and overlay to keep patch in place
• That response may take 2-3 days if drug is given transdermally; instruct on administration of patch
Treatment of overdose: Supportive treatment; administer tolazoline, atropine, dopamine prn

clopidogrel (Rx)

(klo-pid'oh-grel)
Plavix
Func. class.: Platelet aggregation inhibitor
Chem. class.: Thienopyridine derivative

Action: Inhibits first and second phases of ADP-induced effects in platelet aggregation
Uses: Reducing the risk of stroke, MI in high-risk patients
Investigational uses: Loading dose
Dosage and routes:
• *Adult:* **PO** 75 mg qd with or without food
Loading dose
• *Adult:* **PO** 150-600 mg then 75-150 mg qd
Available forms: Tabs 75 mg
Side effects/adverse reactions:
INTEG: Rash, pruritus
GI: Nausea, vomiting, diarrhea, GI discomfort, *GI bleeding*
HEMA: Epistaxis, purpura, *bleeding, neutropenia*
CV: Edema, hypertension
CNS: Headache, dizziness
MS: Arthralgia, back pain
RESP: Upper respiratory tract infection, dyspnea, rhinitis, bronchitis, cough
MISC: UTI, depression, hypercholesterolemia, chest pain, fatigue, *intracranial hemorrhage*
Contraindications: Hypersensitivity, active bleeding
Precautions: Past liver disease, pregnancy (B), lactation, children, increased bleeding risk, neutropenia, agranulocytosis
Pharmacokinetics: Rapidly absorbed, peak 1-3 hr, metabolized by liver, excreted in urine, feces
Interactions:
• Increased bleeding tendencies: an-

---

ticoagulants, aspirin, NSAIDs, abciximab, eptifibatide, tirofiban, thrombolytics, ticlopidine

• May increase the action of: some NSAIDs, phenytoin, tolbutamide, tamoxifen, torsemide, fluvastatin, warfarin

NURSING CONSIDERATIONS

Assess:

• For symptoms of stroke, MI during treatment

• Liver function studies: AST, ALT, bilirubin, creatinine (long-term therapy)

• Blood studies: CBC, Hct, Hgb, PT, cholesterol (long-term therapy)

Administer:

• With food to decrease gastric symptoms

Evaluate:

• Therapeutic response: absence of stroke, MI

Teach patient/family:

• That blood work will be necessary during treatment

• To report any unusual bruising, bleeding to prescriber

• To take with food or just after eating to minimize GI discomfort

• To report side effects such as diarrhea, skin rashes, subcutaneous bleeding

---

clorazepate (℞)

(klor-az′e-pate)

Apo-Clorazepate*, clorazepate, Gen-XENE, Novo-Clopate*, Tranxene, Tranxene-SD

Func. class.: Antianxiety, anticonvulsant, sedative/hypnotic

Chem. class.: Benzodiazepine

Controlled Substance Schedule IV
Action: Potentiates the actions of GABA, especially in limbic system, reticular formation

Uses: Anxiety, acute alcohol withdrawal, adjunct in seizure disorders

Dosage and routes:

Anxiety

• *Adult:* **PO** 15-60 mg/day

• *Geriatric:* **PO** 7.5 mg qd-bid

Alcohol withdrawal

• *Adult:* **PO** 30 mg then 30-60 mg in divided doses; day 2, 45-90 mg in divided doses; day 3, 22.5-45 mg in divided doses; day 4, 15-30 mg in divided doses; then reduce daily dose to 7.5-15 mg

Seizure disorders

• *Adult and child >12 yr:* **PO** 7.5 mg tid; may increase by 7.5 mg/wk or less, not to exceed 90 mg/day

• *Child 9-12 yr:* **PO** 7.5 mg bid; may increase by 7.5 mg/wk or less, not to exceed 60 mg/day

Available forms: Caps 3.75, 7.5, 15 mg; tabs 3.75, 7.5, 15 mg

Side effects/adverse reactions:

CNS: Dizziness, drowsiness, confusion, headache, anxiety, tremors, stimulation, fatigue, depression, insomnia, hallucinations, lethargy

GI: Constipation, dry mouth, nausea, vomiting, anorexia, diarrhea

INTEG: Rash, dermatitis, itching

*CV: Orthostatic hypotension, **ECG changes, tachycardia,*** hypotension

EENT: Blurred vision, tinnitus, mydriasis

Contraindications: Hypersensitivity to benzodiazepines, narrow-angle glaucoma, psychosis, pregnancy (D), lactation, child <9 yr

Precautions: Elderly, debilitated, hepatic disease, renal disease

Pharmacokinetics:

PO: Onset 1 hr, peak 1-2 hr, duration up to 24 hr; metabolized by liver, excreted by kidneys; crosses placenta, breast milk; half-life 30-100 hr

---

◆ = Nursing alert   ∥ = Herb-drug interaction   ⊘ = Do not crush

Interactions:
• Increased effects of clorazepate: CNS depressants, alcohol, valproic acid, antidepressants, MAOIs, cimetidine, oral contraceptives, disulfiram, fluoxetine, isoniazid, ketoconazole, propoxyphene, some β-blockers
• Decreased action of clorazepate: rifampin, barbiturates
⧸ Increased CNS depression: kava

Lab test interferences:
Increase: AST, ALT
Decrease: Hct

NURSING CONSIDERATIONS
Assess:
• B/P (lying, standing), pulse; if systolic B/P drops 20 mm Hg, hold drug, notify prescriber
• Blood studies: CBC during long-term therapy; blood dyscrasias have occurred rarely
• Hepatic studies: AST, ALT, bilirubin, creatinine, LDH, alk phosphatase
• I&O; may indicate renal dysfunction
• Mental status: mood, sensorium, affect, sleeping pattern, drowsiness, dizziness; for delirium, tremors, hallucination in alcohol withdrawal
• Physical dependency, withdrawal symptoms: headache, nausea, vomiting, muscle pain, weakness after long-term use
• Suicidal tendencies, anxiety level
• Seizures: location, duration, intensity

Administer:
• With food, milk for GI symptoms
• Crushed if patient cannot swallow whole (tab only)

Perform/provide:
• Assistance with ambulation during beginning therapy because of drowsiness/dizziness, especially elderly
• Safety measures, including side rails
• Check to see PO medication has been swallowed
• Sugarless gum, hard candy, frequent sips of water for dry mouth

Evaluate:
• Therapeutic response: decreased anxiety, restlessness, insomnia

Teach patient/family:
• That drug may be taken with food
• That drug is not to be used for everyday stress or used longer than 4 mo unless directed by prescriber; not to take more than prescribed amount; may be habit forming
🚫 Not to break, crush, or chew caps
• To avoid OTC preparations unless approved by prescriber
• To avoid driving, activities that require alertness; drowsiness may occur, especially in elderly
• To avoid alcohol ingestion, other psychotropic medications, unless directed by prescriber
• Not to discontinue medication abruptly after long-term use
• To rise slowly because fainting may occur
• That drowsiness may worsen at beginning of treatment

Treatment of overdose: Lavage, VS, supportive care, flumazenil

cloxacillin (℞)
(klox-a-sill′in)
Apo-Cloxi*, cloxacillin
Cloxapen, Novo-Cloxin*,
Nu-Clox*, Orbenin*
Func. class.: Broad-spectrum antiinfective
Chem. class.: Penicillinase-resistant penicillin

Action: Interferes with cell wall replication of susceptible organisms;

the cell wall, rendered osmotically unstable, swells, bursts from osmotic pressure, resists the penicillinase action that inactivates penicillin

Uses: Gram-positive cocci *(Staphylococcus aureus, Streptococcus pyogenes, Streptococcus pneumoniae)*, penicillinase-producing staphylococci

Dosage and routes:
• *Adult:* **PO** 1-4 g/day in divided doses q6h
• *Child:* **PO** 50-100 mg/kg in divided doses q6h, max 4 g/day

Available forms: Caps 250, 500 mg; oral sol 125 mg/5 ml

Side effects/adverse reactions:

HEMA: Anemia, increased bleeding time, ***bone marrow depression, granulocytopenia***

GI: Nausea, vomiting, diarrhea, increased AST, ALT, abdominal pain, glossitis, colitis, ***pseudomembranous colitis***

GU: Oliguria, proteinuria, hematuria, *vaginitis, moniliasis,* ***glomerulonephritis***

CNS: Lethargy, hallucinations, anxiety, depression, twitching, ***coma, seizures***

SYST: ***Anaphylaxis, serum sickness***

Contraindications: Hypersensitivity to penicillins; neonates, severe renal, hepatic disease

Precautions: Pregnancy (B), lactation, hypersensitivity to cephalosporins

Pharmacokinetics:

PO: Peak 1 hr, duration 6 hr; half-life 30-60 min; metabolized in liver; excreted in urine, bile, breast milk; crosses placenta, poor penetration in CSF

Interactions:
• Increased cloxacillin concentrations: probenecid
• Increased action of anticoagulants

• Food/drug: citric juices/food decreases absorption of cloxacillin

🍃 Delayed/reduced absorption: khat

Lab test interferences:

False positive: Urine glucose, urine protein

Decrease: Uric acid

NURSING CONSIDERATIONS
Assess:

◆ Anaphylaxis: pruritus, rash, dyspnea, laryngeal edema; have emergency equipment available; skin eruptions after administration of penicillin to 1 wk after discontinuing drug

• For infection: temp, draining wounds, WBC, sputum, urine, stool before and during treatment

• I&O ratio; report hematuria, oliguria, since penicillin in high doses is nephrotoxic

◆ Any patient with compromised renal system, since drug is excreted slowly in poor renal system function; toxicity may occur rapidly

• Liver studies: AST, ALT
• Blood studies: WBC, RBC, H&H, bleeding time
• Renal studies: urinalysis, protein, blood
• C&S before drug therapy; drug may be taken as soon as culture is taken
• Bowel pattern before, during treatment

Administer:
• After C&S completed
• Shake suspension well before each dose

Perform/provide:
• Adrenaline, suction, tracheostomy set, endotracheal intubation equipment on unit
• Adequate intake of fluids (2 L) during diarrhea episodes
• Scratch test to assess allergy after

◆ = Nursing alert   🍃 = Herb-drug interaction   🚫 = Do not crush

securing order from prescriber; usually done when penicillin is only drug of choice

• Storage in tight container; after reconstituting, store in refrigerator for 2 wk, room temperature 3 days

Evaluate:
• Therapeutic response: absence of fever, draining wounds

Teach patient/family:

🚫 Not to break, crush, or chew caps

• All aspects of drug therapy, including need to complete entire course of medication to ensure organism death (10-14 days); culture may be taken after course of medication completed

• To report sore throat, fever, fatigue (may indicate superinfection)

• To wear or carry a Medic Alert ID if allergic to penicillins

• To notify prescriber of diarrhea, fever

• To take on an empty stomach with a full glass of water

Treatment of overdose: Withdraw drug; maintain airway; administer epinephrine, aminophylline, O₂, IV corticosteroids for anaphylaxis

---

clozapine (℞)
(kloz′a-peen)
clozapine, Clozaril
Func. class.: Antipsychotic
Chem. class.: Tricyclic dibenzodiazepine derivative

Action: Interferes with dopamine receptor binding with lack of extrapyramidal symptoms; also acts as an adrenergic, cholinergic, histaminergic, serotonergic antagonist

Uses: Management of psychotic symptoms in schizophrenic patients for whom other antipsychotics have failed

Dosage and routes:
• *Adult:* **PO** 25 mg qd or bid; may increase by 25-50 mg/day; normal range 300-450 mg/day after 2 wk; do not increase dose more than 2 × per wk; do not exceed 900 mg/day; use lowest dose to control symptoms

Available forms: Tabs 25, 100 mg

Side effects/adverse reactions:
*CNS: **Neuroleptic malignant syndrome**, sedation, salivation, dizziness, headache, tremors, sleep problems, akinesia, fever, **seizures**, sweating, akathisia, confusion, fatigue, insomnia, depression, slurred speech, anxiety*
GI: Drooling or excessive salivation, constipation, nausea, abdominal discomfort, vomiting, diarrhea, anorexia
MS: Weakness; pain in back, neck, legs; spasm
CV: Tachycardia, hypotension, hypertension, chest pain, ECG changes
GU: Urinary abnormalities, incontinence, ejaculation dysfunction, frequency, urgency, retention, dysuria
RESP: Dyspnea, nasal congestion, throat discomfort
*HEMA: **Leukopenia, neutropenia, agranulocytosis, eosinophilia, thrombocytopenia***

Contraindications: Hypersensitivity, myeloproliferative disorders, severe granulocytopenia, CNS depression, coma

Precautions: Pregnancy (B); lactation; children <16; hepatic, renal, cardiac disease; seizures; prostatic enlargement; elderly, narrow-angle glaucoma

Do not confuse:
Clozaril/Clinoril

Pharmacokinetics: Steady state 2.5 hr; 95% protein bound; completely metabolized by liver; excreted in urine and feces (metabolites); half-life 8-12 hr

---

Interactions:
• Decreased effect of: phenytoin
• Increased anticholinergic effects: anticholinergics
• Increased hypotension: antihypertensives, nitrates, large quantities of alcohol
• Increased CNS depression: CNS depressants, psychoactives, alcohol
• Increased bone marrow suppression: antineoplastics, other drugs suppressing bone marrow
• Increased plasma concentrations: warfarin, digoxin, other highly protein-bound drugs
• Drug/food: decreased clozapine level: caffeine

*Increased CNS depression: kava, St. John's wort

Lab test interferences:
Increase: LFTs, cardiac enzymes, cholesterol, blood glucose, bilirubin, PBI, cholinesterase, ^{131}I
False positive: Pregnancy tests, PKU
False negative: Urinary steroids, 17-OHCS

NURSING CONSIDERATIONS
Assess:
• Swallowing of PO medication; check for hoarding or giving of medication to other patients
• I&O ratio; obtain baseline before treatment begins; palpate bladder if low urinary output occurs
• Bilirubin, CBC, liver function studies monthly; discontinue treatment if WBC <3000/mm^3 or ANC <1500/mm^3 test qwk; may resume when normal; if WBC <2000/mm^3 or ANC <1000/mm^3 discontinue
• Urinalysis is recommended before, during prolonged therapy
• Affect, orientation, LOC, reflexes, gait, coordination, sleep pattern disturbances
• B/P standing and lying; take pulse and respirations q4h during initial treatment; establish baseline before starting treatment; report drops of 30 mm Hg
• Dizziness, faintness, palpitations, tachycardia on rising
• EPS including akathisia (inability to sit still, no pattern to movements), tardive dyskinesia (bizarre movements of the jaw, mouth, tongue, extremities), pseudoparkinsonism (rigidity, tremors, pill rolling, shuffling gait)
• For neuroleptic malignant syndrome: tachycardia, seizures, fever, dyspnea, diaphoresis, increased or decreased B/P, notify prescriber immediately
• Skin turgor daily
• Constipation, urinary retention daily; if these occur, increase bulk, water in diet, especially elderly

Perform/provide:
• Decreased sensory input by dimming lights, avoiding loud noises
• Supervised ambulation until stabilized on medication; do not involve in strenuous exercise program because fainting is possible; patient should not stand still for long periods
• Increased fluids to prevent constipation
• Storage in tight, light-resistant container

Evaluate:
• Therapeutic response: decrease in emotional excitement, hallucinations, delusions, paranoia, reorganization of patterns of thought, speech

Teach patient/family:
• About symptoms of agranulocytosis and need for blood tests qwk for 6 mo, then q2wk; report flulike symptoms
• That orthostatic hypotension often occurs, and to rise gradually from sitting or lying position

⬦ = Nursing alert   〼 = Herb-drug interaction   🚫 = Do not crush

• To avoid hot tubs, hot showers, tub baths; hypotension may occur

• To avoid abrupt withdrawal of this drug because EPS may result; drug should be withdrawn slowly

• To avoid OTC preparations (cough, hay fever, cold) unless approved by prescriber, since serious drug interactions may occur; avoid use with alcohol or CNS depressants, increased drowsiness may occur

• About compliance with drug regimen

• About EPS and necessity for meticulous oral hygiene, since oral candidiasis may occur

• To report sore throat, malaise, fever, bleeding, mouth sores; if these occur, CBC should be drawn and drug discontinued

• That heat stroke may occur in hot weather; take extra precautions to stay cool

• To avoid driving, other hazardous activities; seizures may occur

• To notify prescriber if pregnant or if pregnancy is intended

Treatment of overdose: Lavage, activated charcoal; provide an airway; do not induce vomiting

---

coagulation factor VIIa, recombinant (℞)

NovoSeven

Func. class.: Antihemophilic

Action: Promotes hemostasis by activating the intrinsic pathway of coagulation

Uses: Bleeding in hemophilia A or B, with inhibitors to factor VIII or IX

Research note: One study concluded that a high-fat meal does not activate blood coagulation factor VII[5]

Dosage and routes:

• *Adult:* **IV BOL** 90 µg/kg q2h until hemostasis occurs, or until therapy is deemed to be inadequate; posthemostatic doses q3-6h may be required

Available forms: Lyophilized powder, 1.2 mg/vial (1200 µg/vial), 4.8 mg/vial (4800 µg/vial) recombinant human coagulation factor VIIa (rFVIIa)

Side effects/adverse reactions:

CNS: Fever, headache

SYST: ***Hemorrhage NOS, hemarthrosis, fibrinogen plasma decreased,*** hypertension, bradycardia, ***DIC, coagulation disorder, thrombosis***

INTEG: Pain, redness at inj site, pruritus, purpura, rash

Contraindications: Hypersensitivity to this product or mouse, hamster, or bovine products

Precautions: Pregnancy (B), lactation, children

Pharmacokinetics: Half-life 2.3 hr

Interactions:

• Do not use with activated prothrombin complex concentrates or prothrombin complex concentrate

NURSING CONSIDERATIONS

Assess:

• VS, B/P, pulse, respirations, neurologic signs, temp at least q4h, temp 104° F (40° C) or indicators of internal bleeding, cardiac rhythm

• PT, aPTT, plasma FVII clotting

• For thrombosis, dose should be reduced or stopped

Administer:

IV

• Bring to room temperature; for 1.2 mg vial/2.2 ml sterile water for inj; 4.8 mg vial/8.5 ml sterile water for inj • Remove caps from stop, cleanse stopper with alcohol, allow to dry, draw back plunger of sterile syringe and allow air into syringe, insert needle of syringe into sterile water

for inj, inject the air and withdraw amount required, insert syringe needle with diluent into drug vial, aim to side so liquid runs down vial wall, gently swirl until dissolved, use within 3 hr, give by bol over 3-5 min
• Do not admix, keep refrigerated until ready to use, avoid sunlight
Evaluate:
• Therapeutic response: hemostasis

---

codeine (℞)

(koe′deen)
Paveral*
Func. class.: Opiate analgesic, antitussive
Chem. class.: Opiate, phenanthrene derivative

Controlled Substance Schedule II, III, IV, V (depends on route)
Action: Depresses pain impulse transmission at the spinal cord level by interacting with opioid receptors, decreases cough reflex, GI motility
Uses: Moderate to severe pain, nonproductive cough
Investigational uses: Diarrhea
Dosage and routes:
Pain
• *Adult:* **PO** 15-60 mg q4h prn; **IM/SC** 15-60 mg q4h prn
• *Child:* **PO** 3 mg/kg/day in divided doses q4h prn
Cough
• *Adult:* **PO** 10-20 mg q4-6h, not to exceed 120 mg/day
• *Child:* **PO** 1-1.5 mg/kg/day in 4 divided doses, not to exceed 60 mg/day
Diarrhea
• *Adult:* **PO** 30 mg; may repeat qid prn
Renal disease
• CrCl 10-50 ml/min 75% of dose; CrCl <10 ml/min 50% of dose

Available forms: Inj 30, 60 mg/ml; tabs 15, 30, 60 mg; oral sol 10 mg/5 ml, 15 mg/5 ml
Side effects/adverse reactions:
CNS: Drowsiness, sedation, dizziness, agitation, dependency, lethargy, restlessness, euphoria, *seizures*
GI: Nausea, vomiting, anorexia, constipation
RESP: **Respiratory depression, respiratory paralysis**
CV: Bradycardia, palpitations, orthostatic hypotension, tachycardia, *circulatory collapse*
GU: Urinary retention
INTEG: Flushing, rash, urticaria, pruritus
SYST: **Anaphylaxis**
Contraindications: Hypersensitivity to opiates, respiratory depression, increased intracranial pressure, seizure disorders, severe respiratory disorders
Precautions: Elderly, cardiac dysrhythmias, pregnancy (C), lactation
Do not confuse:
codeine/Lodine
Pharmacokinetics: Onset 10-30 min, peak ½-1 hr, duration 4-6 hr; metabolized by liver; excreted by kidneys, in breast milk; crosses placenta; half-life 3 hr
Interactions:
• Increased CNS depression: alcohol, opiates, sedative/hypnotics, antipsychotics, skeletal muscle relaxants
• Increased toxicity: MAOIs, use cautiously
🍃 Increased CNS depression: kava
NURSING CONSIDERATIONS
Assess:
• I&O ratio; check for decreasing output; may indicate urinary retention, especially elderly
• GI function: nausea, vomiting, constipation
• By using pain-scoring method

⬥ = Nursing alert   🍃 = Herb-drug interaction   🚫 = Do not crush

- For productive cough
- Cough: type, duration, ability to raise secretion
- CNS changes, dizziness, drowsiness, hallucinations, euphoria, LOC, pupil reaction
- Allergic reactions: rash, urticaria
- Respiratory dysfunction: respiratory depression, character, rate, rhythm; notify prescriber if respirations are <10/min, shallow
- Need for pain medication, tolerance

Administer:

IV

- Give slowly by direct inj
- With antiemetic for nausea, vomiting
- When pain is beginning to return; determine dosage interval by patient response

Syringe compatibilities: Glycopyrrolate, hydroxyzine

Y-site compatibilities: Cefmetazole

Perform/provide:

- Storage in light-resistant container at room temperature
- Assistance with ambulation if needed
- Safety measures: top side rails, night-light, call bell

Evaluate:

- Therapeutic response: decrease in pain, absence of grimacing, decreased cough; decreased diarrhea

Teach patient/family:

- To report any symptoms of CNS changes, allergic reactions
- That physical dependency may result after extended periods
- To change position slowly; orthostatic hypotension may occur
- To avoid hazardous activities if drowsiness, dizziness occurs
- To avoid alcohol, other CNS depressants unless directed by prescriber

colchicine (R)

(kol'chi-seen)

Func. class.: Antigout agent
Chem. class.: Colchicum autumnale alkaloid

Action: Inhibits microtubule formation of lactic acid in leukocytes, which decreases phagocytosis and inflammation in joints

Uses: Gout, gouty arthritis (prevention, treatment); to arrest progression of neurologic disability in multiple sclerosis

Investigational uses: Hepatic cirrhosis, familial Mediterranean fever, pericarditis

Dosage and routes:

Prevention

- *Adult:* **PO** 0.5-1.8 mg qd depending on severity; **IV** 0.5-1 mg 1-2 × day

Treatment

- *Adult:* **PO** 0.5-1.2 mg, then 0.5-1.2 mg q1h, until pain decreases or side effects occur; **IV** 2 mg, then 0.5 mg q6h until response, max 4 mg total

Pericarditis

- *Adult:* **PO** 0.5-3 mg qd × 3 days, then 1 mg qd up to 1 yr

Available forms: Tabs 0.5, 0.6 mg; inj 1 mg/2 ml

Side effects/adverse reactions:

MISC: Myopathy, alopecia, reversible azoospermia, peripheral neuritis

GU: Hematuria, *oliguria, renal damage*

HEMA: Agranulocytosis, thrombocytopenia, aplastic anemia, pancytopenia

GI: Nausea, vomiting, anorexia, malaise, metallic taste, cramps, peptic ulcer, diarrhea

INTEG: Chills, dermatitis, pruritus, purpura, erythema

Contraindications: Hypersensitivity; serious GI, renal, hepatic, cardiac disorders; pregnancy (D) IV
Precautions: Blood dyscrasias, pregnancy (C) PO, hepatic disease, elderly, lactation, children
Pharmacokinetics:
PO: Peak ½-2 hr, half-life 20 min; deacetylates in liver; excreted in feces (metabolites/active drug)
Interactions:
• Increased GI effects: NSAIDs
• Increased bone marrow depression: radiation, bone marrow depressants, cyclosporine
• Decreased action of vit B_{12}, may cause reversible malabsorption
• Increased colchicine effect: erythromycin
• Increased blood dyscrasias: phenylbutazone
• Decreased colchicine effect: loop diuretics
Lab test interferences:
Increase: Alk phosphatase, AST, ALT
False positive: RBC, Hgb
NURSING CONSIDERATIONS
Assess:
• I&O ratio; observe for decrease in urinary output
• CBC, platelets, reticulocytes before, during therapy (q3mo)
• Coombs' test for Coombs' negative hemolytic anemia
• For toxicity: weakness, abdominal pain, nausea, vomiting, diarrhea
Administer:
PO
• On empty stomach only, to facilitate absorption
IV
• Do not give IM or SC
• Give over 2-5 min
• Wait ≥1 wk after giving a full course of IV colchicine before giving subsequent doses

Evaluate:
• Therapeutic response: decreased stone formation on x-ray, decreased pain in kidney region, absence of hematuria, decreased pain in joints
Teach patient/family:
• To increase fluid intake to 3-4 L/day
• To avoid alcohol, OTC preparations that contain alcohol; skin rashes have occurred
• To report any pain, redness, or hard area, usually in legs
• The importance of complying with medical regimen; the possibility of bone marrow depression occurring
Treatment of overdose: D/C medication, may need opioids to treat diarrhea

---

colesevelam (℞)
(coal-see-vel′am)
Welchol
Func. class.: Antilipemic
Chem. class.: Bile acid sequestrant

Action: Absorbs, combines with bile acids to form insoluble complex that is excreted through feces; loss of bile acids lowers cholesterol levels
Uses: Elevated LDL cholesterol, alone or in combination with HMG-CoA reductase inhibitor
Dosage and routes:
• *Adult:* **PO** Monotherapy: 3 625-mg tabs bid with meals or 6 tabs qd with a meal; may increase to 7 tabs if needed
• Combination therapy: 3 tabs bid with meals or 6 tabs qd with a meal given with an HMG-CoA reductase inhibitor
Available forms: Tabs 625 mg
Side effects/adverse reactions:
CNS: Headache, dizziness, drowsiness, vertigo, tinnitus

◆ = Nursing alert　　🌿 = Herb-drug interaction　　⊘ = Do not crush

MS: Muscle, joint pain

GI: Constipation, abdominal pain, nausea, fecal impaction, hemorrhoids, flatulence, vomiting, steatorrhea, peptic ulcer

INTEG: Rash, irritation of perianal area, tongue, skin

HEMA: Decreased vit A, D, K, red cell folate content; ***hyperchloremic acidosis, bleeding,*** decreased protime

Contraindications: Hypersensitivity, biliary obstruction

Precautions: Pregnancy (C), lactation, children

Pharmacokinetics:

PO: Excreted in feces, maximum effect in 2 wk

Interactions:

• Decreased absorption of phenylbutazone, warfarin, thiazides, digitalis, penicillin G, tetracyclines, cephalexin, phenobarbital, folic acid, corticosteroids, iron, thyroid, clindamycin, trimethoprim, chenodiol, fat-soluble vitamins

Lab test interferences:

Increase: Liver function studies, Cl, PO_4

NURSING CONSIDERATIONS

Assess:

• Cardiac glycoside level, if both drugs are being administered

• For signs of vit A, D, K deficiency

• Fasting LDL, HDL, total cholesterol, triglyceride levels, electrolytes if on extended therapy

• Bowel pattern daily; increase bulk, H_2O in diet for constipation

Administer:

• Drug ac, hs; give all other medications 1 hr before colesevelam or 4 hr after colesevelam to avoid poor absorption

• Supplemental doses of vit A, D, K, if levels are low

Evaluate:

• Therapeutic response: decreased cholesterol level (hyperlipidemia); diarrhea, pruritus (excess bile acids)

Teach patient/family:

◆The symptoms of hypoprothrombinemia: bleeding mucous membranes, dark tarry stools, hematuria, petechiae; report immediately

• The importance of compliance; toxicity may result if doses missed

• That risk factors should be decreased: high-fat diet, smoking, alcohol consumption, absence of exercise

• Not to discontinue suddenly

---

colestipol (℞)

(koe-les´ti-pole)

Colestid

Func. class.: Antilipemic

Chem. class.: Bile acid sequestrant

Action: Absorbs, combines with bile acids to form insoluble complex excreted through feces; loss of bile acids lowers cholesterol levels

Uses: Primary hypercholesterolemia, xanthomas, digitalis toxicity, pruritus due to biliary obstruction, diarrhea due to bile acids

Dosage and routes:

• *Adult:* **PO** tabs 2 g qd-bid, may increase q1mo, max 16 g/day; granules: 5 g qd-bid, may increase q1mo, max 30 g/day

Available forms: Granules 300 g, 500 g bottles, 5 g packets; tabs 1 g

Side effects/adverse reactions:

GI: Constipation, abdominal pain, nausea, fecal impaction, hemorrhoids, flatulence, vomiting, steatorrhea, peptic ulcer

INTEG: Rash, irritation of perianal area, tongue, skin

*HEMA: **Bleeding, decreased PT***

META: Decreased vit A, D, K, red folate content; ***hyperchloremic acidosis***

Contraindications: Hypersensitivity, biliary obstruction

Precautions: Pregnancy (B), lactation, children, bleeding disorders

Pharmacokinetics:

PO: Onset 24-48 hr, peak/duration 30 days, excreted in feces

Interactions:

• May reduce action of: thiazides, digitalis, warfarin, penicillin G, folic acid, phenylbutazone, tetracycline, corticosteroids, iron, thyroid agents, clindamycin, trimethoprim, chenodiol, fat-soluble vitamins, cephalexin, phenobarbital

• Antagonize colestipol: oral antidiabetics

Lab test interferences:

Increase: Liver function studies, chloride, PO_4

NURSING CONSIDERATIONS
Assess:

• Cardiac glycoside levels, if both drugs are being administered

• For signs of vit A, D, K deficiency

• Serum cholesterol, triglyceride levels, electrolytes (extended therapy)

• Bowel pattern daily; increase bulk, water in diet if constipation develops

Administer:

• Drug ac, hs; give all other medications 1 hr before colestipol or 4 hr after colestipol to avoid poor absorption

• Drug mixed in applesauce or stirred into beverage (2-6 oz); do not take dry; let stand for 2 min

🚫 Tabs should be swallowed whole; do not break, crush, or chew

• Supplemental doses of vit A, D, K if levels are low

Evaluate:

• Therapeutic response: decreased triglycerides, diarrhea, pruritus (excess bile acids)

Teach patient/family:

◆ The symptoms of hypoprothrombinemia: bleeding mucous membranes; dark, tarry stools; hematuria, petechiae; report immediately

• That compliance is needed; not to miss or double doses

• That risk factors should be decreased: high-fat diet, smoking, alcohol consumption, absence of exercise

---

RARELY USED

colfosceril (℞)

(kole-foss′er-ill)

Exosurf Neonatal

Func. class.: Synthetic lung surfactant

Uses: Treatment of respiratory distress syndrome (RDS) in premature infants

Dosage and routes:

Prophylactic treatment: *Endotracheally:* 5 ml/kg as soon as possible after birth and repeat doses 12 and 24 hr later to infants remaining on mechanical ventilation

Rescue treatment: *Endotracheally:* Administer in two 2.5 ml/kg doses; give initial dose after treatment of RDS, then second dose in 12 hr

---

RARELY USED

corticotropin (ACTH) (℞)

(kor-ti-koe-troe′pin)

ACTH, Acthar, corticotropin, H.P. Acthar Gel

Func. class.: Pituitary hormone

Uses: Testing adrenocortical function, treatment of adrenal insufficiency caused by administration of

---

◆ = Nursing alert   🌿 = Herb-drug interaction   🚫 = Do not crush

corticosteroids (long term), multiple sclerosis, infantile spasms

Dosage and routes:

Testing of adrenocortical function

• *Adult:* **IM/SC** up to 80 U in divided doses; **IV** 10-25 U in 500 ml D$_5$W given over 8 hr

Inflammation

• *Adult:* **SC/IM** 40 U in 4 divided doses (aqueous) or 40 U q12-24h (gel/repository form)

Infantile spasms

• *Infant:* **IM Gel** 20 U/day × 2 wks, increase if needed

Contraindications: Hypersensitivity, scleroderma, osteoporosis, CHF, peptic ulcer disease, hypertension, systemic fungal infections, smallpox vaccination, recent surgery, ocular herpes simplex, primary adrenocortical insufficiency/hyperfunction

---

cortisone (℞)

(kor'ti-sone)

Cortone*, Cortone Acetate

Func. class.: Corticosteroid, synthetic

Chem. class.: Glucocorticoid, short-acting

Action: Decreases inflammation by suppression of migration of polymorphonuclear leukocytes, fibroblasts, reversal of increased capillary permeability and lysosomal stabilization

Uses: Inflammation, severe allergy, adrenal insufficiency, collagen disorders, respiratory, dermatologic disorders

Dosage and routes:

• *Adult:* **PO/IM** 25-300 mg qd or q2d, titrated to response

• *Child:* **PO** 2.5-10 mg/kg/day; **IM** 1-5 mg/kg/day

Available forms: Tabs 5, 10, 25 mg; inj 50 mg/ml

Side effects/adverse reactions:

INTEG: Acne, poor wound healing, ecchymosis, bruising, petechiae

CNS: Depression, flushing, sweating, headache, mood changes

*CV: Hypertension, **circulatory collapse, thrombophlebitis, embolism,*** tachycardia, ***necrotizing angiitis, CHF,*** edema

*HEMA: **Thrombocytopenia***

MS: Fractures, osteoporosis, weakness

*GI: Diarrhea, nausea, abdominal distention, **GI hemorrhage,*** increased appetite, ***pancreatitis***

EENT: Fungal infections, increased intraocular pressure, blurred vision

Contraindications: Psychosis, hypersensitivity, idiopathic thrombocytopenia, acute glomerulonephritis, amebiasis, fungal infections, nonasthmatic bronchial disease, pregnancy (D), child <2 yr, AIDS, TB

Precautions: Pregnancy (C), lactation, diabetes mellitus, glaucoma, osteoporosis, seizure disorders, ulcerative colitis, CHF, myasthenia gravis, renal disease, esophagitis, peptic ulcer

Pharmacokinetics:

PO: Peak 2 hr, duration 1½ days

IM: Peak 20-48 hr, duration 1½ days

Interactions:

• Decreased action of cortisone: barbiturates, rifampin, phenytoin, rifampin, theophylline

• Increased GI symptoms: salicylates, indomethacin, NSAIDs

• Decreased effects of anticoagulants, antidiabetics, toxoids, vaccines, salicylates

• Increased side effects: alcohol, salicylates, indomethacin, potassium-wasting diuretics

• Increased action of cortisone: salicylates, estrogens, indomethacin, oral contraceptives, ketoconazole, macrolide antiinfectives

🌿 Potassium deficiency: chronic use/abuse cascara sagrada bark, aloe, buckthorn bark/berry, rhubarb root, senna leaf/fruits

Lab test interferences:

Increase: Cholesterol, Na, blood glucose, uric acid, Ca, urine glucose

Decrease: Ca, K, T_4, T_3, thyroid ^{131}I uptake test, urine 17-OHCS, 17-KS, PBI skin allergy tests

NURSING CONSIDERATIONS
Assess:

• K, blood sugar, urine glucose while on long-term therapy; hypokalemia and hyperglycemia

• Weight daily; notify prescriber of weekly gain >5 lb

• B/P q4h, pulse; notify prescriber if chest pain occurs

• I&O ratio; be alert for decreasing urinary output and increasing edema

• Plasma cortisol levels during long-term therapy (normal level: 138-635 nmol/L SI units if drawn at 8 AM)

• Infection: fever, WBC even after withdrawal of medication; drug masks infection

• K depletion: paresthesias, fatigue, nausea, vomiting, depression, polyuria, dysrhythmias, weakness

• Edema, hypertension, cardiac symptoms

• Mental status: affect, mood, behavioral changes, aggression

Administer:

• After shaking suspension (parenteral)

• Titrated dose; use lowest effective dose

• IM inj deeply in large mass; rotate sites; avoid deltoid; use a 21G needle

• In one dose in AM to prevent adrenal suppression; avoid SC administration; tissue may be damaged; never administer by IV route

• With food or milk to decrease GI symptoms

Perform/provide:

• Assistance with ambulation in patient with bone tissue disease to prevent fractures

Evaluate:

• Therapeutic response: ease of respirations, decreased inflammation

Teach patient/family:

• That medical ID as steroid user should be carried at all times

• To notify prescriber if therapeutic response decreases; dosage adjustment may be needed

◆ Not to discontinue abruptly or adrenal crisis can result

• To avoid OTC products: salicylates, alcohol in cough products, cold preparations unless directed by prescriber

• All aspects of drug usage, including cushingoid symptoms

• The symptoms of adrenal insufficiency: nausea, anorexia, fatigue, dizziness, dyspnea, weakness, joint pain

---

RARELY USED

cosyntropin (℞)
(koe-sin-troe'pin)
Cortrosyn, Synacthen*, Tetracosactrin
Func. class.: Pituitary hormone

Uses: Testing adrenocortical function

Dosage and routes:

• *Adult and child >2 yr:* **IM/IV** 0.25-1 mg between blood sampling;

Child <2 yr: **IM/IV** 0.125 mg

Contraindications: Hypersensitivity

◆ = Nursing alert   🌿 = Herb-drug interaction   🚫 = Do not crush

cromolyn (OTC, ℞)

(kroe'moe-lin)

Intal, Nasalcrom, Rynacrom*

Func. class.: Antiasthmatic

Chem. class.: Mast cell stabilizer

Action: Stabilizes the membrane of the sensitized mast cell, preventing release of chemical mediators after an antigen-IgE interaction

Uses: Allergic rhinitis, severe perennial bronchial asthma, prevention of exercise-induced bronchospasm, acute bronchospasm induced by environmental pollutants, mastocytosis

Dosage and routes:

Allergic rhinitis

• *Adult and child >6 yr:* **NASAL SOL** 1 spray in each nostril tid-qid, not to exceed 6 doses/day

Bronchospasm

• *Adult and child >6 yr:* **INH** 20 mg <1 hr before exercise

Bronchial asthma

• *Adult and child >6 yr:* **INH** 20 mg qid; **NEB** 20 mg qid by nebulization

Systemic mastocytosis

• *Adult and child >12 yr:* **PO** 200 mg qid ac and hs

• *Child 2-12 yr:* **PO** 100 mg qid ½ ac and hs

Available forms: Nasal sol 5.2 mg/metered spray (40 mg/ml); caps for inh, 20 mg; neb sol 20 mg/2 ml; aerosol 800 μg/actuation

Side effects/adverse reactions:

EENT: Throat irritation, cough, nasal congestion, burning eyes, nasal stinging, sneezing

CNS: *Headache, dizziness,* neuritis

GU: Urinary frequency, dysuria

GI: Nausea, vomiting, anorexia, dry mouth, bitter taste

INTEG: Rash, urticaria, angioedema

MS: Joint pain/swelling

Contraindications: Hypersensitivity to this drug or lactose, status asthmaticus

Precautions: Pregnancy (B), lactation, renal disease, hepatic disease, safety not established; child <5 yr (aerosol); <2 yr (nebulizer); <6 yr (nasal sol)

Pharmacokinetics: Excreted unchanged in feces; half-life 80 min

NURSING CONSIDERATIONS

Assess:

• Eosinophil count during treatment

• Respiratory status: rate, rhythm, characteristics, cough, wheezing, dyspnea

Administer:

• For oral dose, dissolve powder in caps mixed with hot water; further dilute in cold water

• By inhalation/nebulizer only

Perform/provide:

• Gargle, sip of water to decrease irritation in throat

Evaluate:

• Therapeutic response: decrease in asthmatic symptoms; congested, runny nose

Teach patient/family:

• To clear mucus before using

• Proper inhalation technique: exhale; using inhaler, inhale deeply with head tipped back to open airway; remove; hold breath; exhale; repeat until all of drug is inhaled, use demonstration; return demonstration

• That therapeutic effect may take up to 4 wk

• Not to swallow capsule

• That drug is preventive only, not restorative

RARELY USED

crotamiton (℞)
(kroe-tam'i-ton)
Func. class.: Scabicide

Uses: Scabies, pruritus
Dosage and routes:
Scabies:
• *Adult and child:* **CREAM** wash area with soap, water; remove visible crusts, apply cream, apply another coat in 24 hr, remove with soap, water in 48 hr
Pruritus: Massage into affected area, repeat as necessary
Contraindications: Hypersensitivity, skin inflammation, abrasions, breaks in skin, mucous membranes

---

cyanocobalamin (vit B₁₂)
(OTC, ℞)
(sye-an-oh-koe-bal'a-min)
Alphamin, Anacobin*, Bedoz*, Cobex, Cobolin-M, Crystamine, Crysti-1000, Cyanabin*, Cyanoject, Cyomin, Ener-B, Hydrobexan, Hydro Cobex, Hydro-Crysti-12
hydroxocobalamin
hydroxycobal, la-12, nascobal, neuroforte-r, rubesol-1000, rubramin pc, shovite, vibal la, vibral, vitamin B₁₂

Func. class.: Vit B₁₂, water-soluble vitamin

Action: Needed for adequate nerve functioning, protein and carbohydrate metabolism, normal growth, RBC development, cell reproduction

Uses: Vit B₁₂ deficiency, pernicious anemia, vit B₁₂ malabsorption syndrome, Schilling test, increased requirements with pregnancy, thyrotoxicosis, hemolytic anemia, hemorrhage, renal and hepatic disease
Dosage and routes:
Cyanocobalamin
• *Adult:* **PO** up to 1000 μg/day **SC/IM** 30-100 μg/day × 1 wk, then 100-200 μg/mo
Schilling test
• *Adult and child:* **IM** 1000 μg in one dose
• *Child:* **PO** up to 1000 μg/day **SC/IM** 30-50 μg/day × 2 wk, then 100 μg/mo; nasal 500 μg qwk
Hydroxocobalamin
• *Adult:* **SC/IM** 30-50 μg/day × 5-10 days, then 100-200 μg/mo
• *Child:* **SC/IM** 30-50 μg/day × 5-10 days, then 100 μg/mo
Available forms: Cyanocobalamin: tabs 25, 50, 100, 250, 500, 1000, 5000 μg; ext rel tabs: 100, 200, 500, 1000 μg; lozenges: 100, 250, 500 μg; nasal jel 500 μg/spray; inj 100, 1000 μg/ml; hydroxocobalamin: inj 1000 μg/ml
Side effects/adverse reactions:
CNS: Flushing, optic nerve atrophy
GI: Diarrhea
CV: CHF, peripheral vascular thrombosis, *pulmonary edema*
INTEG: Itching, rash, pain at inj site
META: Hypokalemia
SYST: Anaphylactic shock
Contraindications: Hypersensitivity, optic nerve atrophy
Precautions: Pregnancy (A), lactation, children
Pharmacokinetics: Gastric intrinsic factor must be present for absorption to occur; stored in liver, kidneys, stomach; 50%-90% excreted in urine; crosses placenta, excreted in breast milk

---

◆ = Nursing alert   🌿 = Herb-drug interaction   ⊘ = Do not crush

Interactions:
• Decreased absorption: aminoglycosides, anticonvulsants, colchicine, chloramphenicol, aminosalicylic acid, K preparation, cimetidine
• Increased absorption: prednisone

Lab test interferences:

False positive: Intrinsic factor

NURSING CONSIDERATIONS

Assess:

• For vit B_{12} deficiency: red, beefy tongue, psychosis, pallor, neuropathy
• GI function: diarrhea, constipation
• K levels during beginning treatment in megaloblastic anemia; q6mo in pernicious anemia; folic acid, plasma vit B_{12} (after 1 wk), reticulocyte counts
• Nutritional status: egg yolks, fish, organ meats, dairy products, clams, oysters: good sources of vit B_{12}
• For pulmonary edema, worsening of CHF in cardiac patients

Administer:

PO

• With fruit juice to disguise taste; immediately after mixing
• With meals if possible for better absorption

Nasal

• Avoid use within 1 hr of hot fluids/food

IM

• By IM inj for pernicious anemia for life unless contraindicated

IV

• IV route not recommended but may be admixed in TPN solution

Additive compatibilities: Ascorbic acid, chloramphenicol, metaraminol, vit B/C

Solution compatibilities: Dextrose/Ringer's or lactated Ringer's combinations, dextrose/saline combinations, D_5W, $D_{10}W$, 0.45% NaCl, Ringer's or lactated Ringer's sol

Y-site compatibilities: Heparin, hydrocortisone, potassium chloride, vit B/C

Perform/provide:

• Protection from light and heat

Evaluate:

• Therapeutic response: decreased anorexia, dyspnea on exertion, palpitations, paresthesias, psychosis, visual disturbances

Teach patient/family:

• That treatment must continue for life for pernicious anemia
• To eat well-balanced diet
• To avoid contact with persons with infection; infections common

Treatment of overdose: Discontinue drug

---

cyclobenzaprine (℞)

(sye-kloe-ben'za-preen)
cyclobenzaprine HCl,
cycloflex, Flexeril

Func. class.: Skeletal muscle relaxant, central acting

Chem. class.: Tricyclic amine salt

Action: Unknown; may be related to antidepressant effects

Uses: Adjunct for relief of muscle spasm and pain in musculoskeletal conditions

Dosage and routes:

Muscloskeletal disorders

• *Adult:* **PO** 10 mg tid × 1 wk, not to exceed 60 mg/day × 3 wk
• *Child:* 20-40 mg/kg/day in 2-4 divided doses

Fibromyalgia

• *Adult:* **PO** 10-40 mg hs

Available forms: Tabs 10 mg

Side effects/adverse reactions:

CNS: Dizziness, weakness, drowsiness, headache, tremor, depression, insomnia, confusion, paresthesia

---

EENT: Diplopia, temporary loss of vision

CV: Postural hypotension, tachycardia, ***dysrhythmias***

GI: Nausea, vomiting, hiccups, dry mouth, constipation

INTEG: Rash, pruritus, fever, facial flushing, sweating

GU: Urinary retention, frequency, change in libido

Contraindications: Acute recovery phase of myocardial infarction, dysrhythmias, heart block, CHF, hypersensitivity, child <12 yr, intermittent porphyria, thyroid disease

Precautions: Renal disease, hepatic disease, addictive personality, pregnancy (B), lactation, elderly

Do not confuse:

cyclobenzaprine/cyproheptadine

Pharmacokinetics:

PO: Onset 1 hr, peak 3-8 hr, duration 12-24 hr, half-life 1-3 days; metabolized by liver; excreted in urine; crosses placenta; excreted in breast milk

Interactions:

• Increased CNS depression: alcohol, tricyclics, opiates, barbiturates, sedatives, hypnotics

• Do not use within 14 days of MAOI

🍃 Increased CNS depression: kava

NURSING CONSIDERATIONS

Assess:

• For pain: location, duration, mobility, stiffness, baseline and periodically

• Blood studies: CBC, WBC, differential for blood dyscrasias

• Liver function studies: AST, ALT, alk phosphatase; hepatitis may occur

• ECG in epileptic patients; poor seizure control has occurred

• Allergic reactions: rash, fever, respiratory distress

• Severe weakness, numbness in extremities

• Psychologic dependency: increased need for medication, more frequent requests for medication, increased pain

• CNS depression: dizziness, drowsiness, psychiatric symptoms

Administer:

• With meals for GI symptoms

Perform/provide:

• Storage in tight container at room temperature

• Assistance with ambulation if dizziness, drowsiness occur, especially elderly

Evaluate:

• Therapeutic response: decreased pain, spasticity; muscle spasms of acute, painful musculoskeletal conditions generally short term; long-term therapy seldom warranted

Teach patient/family:

• Not to discontinue medication abruptly; insomnia, nausea, headache, spasticity, tachycardia will occur; drug should be tapered off over 1-2 wk

• Not to take with alcohol, other CNS depressants

• To avoid hazardous activities if drowsiness/dizziness occurs

• To avoid using OTC medication: cough preparations, antihistamines, unless directed by prescriber

• To use gum, frequent sips of water for dry mouth

Treatment of overdose: Empty stomach with emesis, gastric lavage, then administer activated charcoal; use anticonvulsants if indicated; monitor cardiac function

---

◆ = Nursing alert   🍃 = Herb-drug interaction   🚫 = Do not crush

cyclophosphamide (℞)

(sye-kloe-foss'fa-mide)
Cytoxan, Neosar,
Procytox*

Func. class.: Antineoplastic alkylating agent

Chem. class.: Nitrogen mustard

Action: Alkylates DNA, RNA; inhibits enzymes that allow synthesis of amino acids in proteins; is also responsible for cross-linking DNA strands; activity is not cell cycle phase specific

Uses: Hodgkin's disease; lymphomas; leukemia; cancer of female reproductive tract, breast; lung, prostate; multiple myeloma; neuroblastoma; retinoblastoma; Ewing's sarcoma

Dosage and routes:
• *Adult:* PO initially 1-5 mg/kg over 2-5 days, maintenance is 1-5 mg/kg; **IV** initially 40-50 mg/kg in divided doses over 2-5 days, maintenance 10-15 mg/kg q7-10d, or 3-5 mg/kg q3d
• *Child:* **PO/IV** 2-8 mg/kg or 60-250 mg/m^2 in divided doses for 6 or more days; maintenance 10-15 mg/kg q7-10d or 30 mg/kg q3-4wk; dose should be reduced by half when bone marrow depression occurs

Renal disease
• CrCl 25-50 ml/min 50% of dose; CrCl <25 ml/min avoid use

Available forms: Inj 100, 200, 500, 750 mg, 1, 2 g; tabs 25, 50 mg

Side effects/adverse reactions:
CV: **Cardiotoxicity** (high doses)
HEMA: **Thrombocytopenia, leukopenia, pancytopenia; myelosuppression**
GI: *Nausea, vomiting, diarrhea, weight loss,* colitis, **hepatotoxicity**
GU: **Hemorrhagic cystitis,** *hematuria, neoplasms, amenorrhea, azoospermia, sterility, ovarian fibrosis*
INTEG: *Alopecia,* dermatitis
RESP: **Fibrosis**
ENDO: Syndrome of inappropriate antidiuretic hormone (SIADH), gonadal suppression
CNS: Headache, dizziness
META: Hyperuricemia
MISC: Secondary neoplasms

Contraindications: Lactation, pregnancy (D)

Precautions: Radiation therapy

Do not confuse:
cyclophosphamide/cyclosporine
Cytoxan/Cytosar
Cytoxan/Cytotec

Pharmacokinetics: Metabolized by liver; excreted in urine; half-life 4-6½ hr; 50% bound to plasma proteins

Interactions:
• Increased toxicity of cyclophosphamide: barbiturates
• Potentiation of neuromuscular blockade: succinylcholine
• Increased bone marrow depression: allopurinol, thiazides
• Increased hypoglycemia: insulin
• Decreased digoxin levels: digoxin
• Decreased cyclophosphamide effect: chloramphenicol, corticosteroids
• Decreased antibody response: live virus vaccines
• Increased action of: warfarin

Lab test interferences:
Increase: Uric acid
False positive: Pap smear
False negative: PPD, mumps, trichophytin, *Candida*
Decrease: Pseudocholinesterase

NURSING CONSIDERATIONS
Assess:
• For hemorrhagic cystitis; renal function studies: BUN, serum uric acid, urine CrCl before, during therapy; I&O ratio; report fall in urine output of <30 ml/hr

• CBC, differential, platelet count baseline, weekly; withhold drug if WBC is <2500 or platelet count is <75,000; notify prescriber of results
• Pulmonary function tests, chest x-ray films before, during therapy; chest film should be obtained q2wk during treatment
• Monitor temp q4h (may indicate beginning infection)
• Liver function tests before, during therapy (bilirubin, AST, ALT, LDH) as needed or monthly
• Bleeding: hematuria, guaiac, bruising or petechiae, mucosa or orifices q8h
• Dyspnea, rales, unproductive cough, chest pain, tachypnea
• Effects of alopecia on body image, discuss feelings about body changes
• Jaundice of skin, sclera; dark urine; clay-colored stools; itchy skin; abdominal pain; fever; diarrhea
• Buccal cavity q8h for dryness, sores or ulceration, white patches, oral pain, bleeding, dysphagia; obtain prescription for viscous lidocaine (Xylocaine)

◆ Symptoms indicating severe allergic reaction: rash, pruritus, urticaria, purpuric skin lesions, itching, flushing

Administer:
• In AM so drug can be eliminated before hs
• Fluids IV or PO before chemotherapy to hydrate patient
• Antacid before oral agent, give after evening meal, before bedtime
• Antiemetic 30-60 min before giving drug and prn
• Allopurinol or sodium bicarbonate to maintain uric acid levels, alkalinization of urine

IV
• IV after diluting 100 mg/5 ml of sterile H_2O or bacteriostatic H_2O; shake; let stand until clear; may be further diluted in up to 250 ml D_5 or NS; give 100 mg or less/min through 3-way stopcock of glucose or saline inf
• Using 21, 23, 25G needle; check site for irritation, phlebitis

Additive compatibilities: Cisplatin with etoposide, fluorouracil, hydroxyzine, methotrexate, methotrexate/fluorouracil, mitoxantrone, ondansetron

Solution compatibilities: Amino acids 4.25%/D_{25}, D_5/0.9% NaCl, D_5W, 0.9% NaCl

Syringe compatibilities: Bleomycin, cisplatin, doxapram, doxorubicin, droperidol, fluorouracil, furosemide, heparin, leucovorin, methotrexate, metoclopramide, mitomycin, vinblastine, vincristine

Y-site compatibilities: Allopurinol, amifostine, amikacin, ampicillin, azlocillin, aztreonam, bleomycin, cefamandole, cefazolin, cefepime, cefoperazone, cefotaxime, cefoxitin, cefuroxime, cephalothin, cephapirin, chloramphenicol, chlorpromazine, cimetidine, cisplatin, cladribine, clindamycin, dexamethasone, diphenhydramine, doxorubicin, doxorubicin liposome, doxycycline, droperidol, erythromycin, famotidine, filgrastim, fludarabine, fluorouracil, furosemide, gallium, ganciclovir, gentamicin, granisetron, heparin, hydromorphone, idarubicin, kanamycin, leucovorin, lorazepam, melphalan, methotrexate, methylprednisolone, metoclopramide, metronidazole, mezlocillin, minocycline, mitomycin, morphine, moxalactam, nafcillin, ondansetron, oxacillin, paclitaxel, penicillin G potassium, piperacillin, piperacillin/tazobactam, prochlorperazine, promethazine, propofol, ranitidine, sargramostim, sodium bicarbonate, teniposide, thiotepa, ticarcillin, ticarcillin-clavulanate, tobramycin,

◆ = Nursing alert   ⚫ = Herb-drug interaction   🚫 = Do not crush trimethoprim - sulfamethoxazole, vancomycin, vinblastine, vincristine, vinorelbine

Perform/provide:
• Storage in tight container at room temperature
• Strict medical asepsis, protective isolation if WBC levels are low
• Increase fluid intake to 2-3 L/day to prevent urate deposits, calculi formation, reduce incidence of hemorrhagic cystitis
• Diet low in purines: organ meats (kidney, liver), dried beans, peas to maintain alkaline urine
• Rinsing of mouth tid-qid with water, club soda; brushing of teeth bid-tid with soft brush or cotton-tipped applicators for stomatitis; use unwaxed dental floss
• Warm compresses at injection site for inflammation

Evaluate:
• Therapeutic response: decreased tumor size, spread of malignancy

Teach patient/family:
• About protective isolation
• That amenorrhea can occur; reversible after stopping treatment
• To report any changes in breathing or coughing
• That hair may be lost during treatment; a wig or hairpiece may make patient feel better; new hair may be different in color, texture
• To avoid foods with citric acid, hot or rough texture
• To report any bleeding, white spots, ulcerations in mouth to prescriber; tell patient to examine mouth qd
• To report signs of infection: increased temperature, sore throat, flu-like symptoms
• To report signs of anemia: fatigue, headache, faintness, shortness of breath, irritability
• To report bleeding: avoid use of razors, commercial mouthwash

• To avoid use of aspirin products, ibuprofen
• To avoid vaccinations during therapy

---

cyclosporine (Ŗ)
(sye′kloe-spor-een)
Neoral, Sandimmune, SangCya

Func. class.: Immunosuppressant

Chem. class.: Fungus-derived peptide

Action: Produces immunosuppression by inhibiting lymphocytes (T)
Uses: Organ transplants (liver, kidney, heart) to prevent rejection, rheumatoid arthritis, psoriasis
Investigational uses: Recalcitrant ulcerative colitis
Dosage and routes:
Prevention of transplant rejection
• *Adult and child:* **PO** 15 mg/kg several hr before surgery, daily for 2 wk, reduce dosage by 2.5 mg/kg/wk to 5-10 mg/kg/day; **IV** 5-6 mg/kg several hr before surgery, daily, switch to PO form as soon as possible
Rheumatoid arthritis
• *Adult:* **PO** 2.5 mg/kg/day divided bid, may increase 0.5-0.75 mg/kg/day after 8-12 wk, max 4 mg/kg/day
Psoriasis
• *Adult:* **PO** 2.5 mg/kg/day divided bid, × 4 wk, then increase by 0.5 mg/kg/day q2wk, max 4 mg/kg/day
Available forms: Microemulsion oral sol (Neoral) 100 mg/ml; microemulsion soft gel cap (Neoral) 25, 100 mg; soft gel caps 25, 100 mg; oral sol 100 mg/ml; inj 50 mg/ml

---

Side effects/adverse reactions:
GI: Nausea, vomiting, diarrhea, *oral Candida, gum hyperplasia, **hepatotoxicity**,* pancreatitis
INTEG: Rash, acne, *hirsutism*
*CNS: Tremors, headache, **seizures***
*GU: **Albuminuria, hematuria, proteinuria, renal failure***
META: Hyperkalemia, hypomagnesemia, hyperlipidemia, hyperuricemia
MISC: Gingival hyperplasia, infection
Do not confuse:
cyclosporine/Cycloserine
cyclosporine/cyclophosphamide
Contraindications: Hypersensitivity
Precautions: Severe renal disease, severe hepatic disease, pregnancy (C)
Do not confuse:
cyclosporine/Cycloserine
cyclosporine/cyclophosphamide
Pharmacokinetics: Peak 4 hr, highly protein bound, half-life (biphasic) 1.2 hr, 25 hr; metabolized in liver; excreted in feces; crosses placenta; excreted in breast milk
Interactions:
• Increased levels of: digoxin, etoposide
• Increased action, toxicity of cyclosporine: amiodarone, amphotericin B, androgens, azole antifungals, calcium channel blockers, carvedilol, cimetidine, colchicine, corticosteroids, foscarnet, imipenem-cilastatin, ketoconazole, macrolides, metoclopramide, oral contraceptives, NSAIDs, melphalan, fluconazole
• Decreased action of cyclosporine: carbamazepine, phenobarbital, phenytoin, rifamycins, sulfamethoxazole/trimethoprim
• Decreased antibody reaction: live virus vaccines
• Do not use with tacrolimus

• Drug/food: Slowed metabolism of drug: grapefruit juice
• Decreased absorption of neoral products
NURSING CONSIDERATIONS
Assess:
• Renal studies: BUN, creatinine at least monthly during treatment, 3 mo after treatment
• Liver function studies: alk phosphatase, AST, ALT, bilirubin
• Drug blood level during treatment
• Hepatotoxicity: dark urine, jaundice, itching, light-colored stools; drug should be discontinued
• For nephrotoxicity: 6 wk post op, acute tubular necrosis, CyA trough level >200 ng/ml, gradual rise in Cr (0.15 mg/dl/day), Cr plateau <25% above baseline, intracapsular pressure <40 mm Hg
Administer:
PO
• Use pipette provided to draw up oral sol; may mix with milk or juice, wipe pipette, do not wash
• For several days before transplant surgery
• With corticosteroids
• With meals for GI upset or in chocolate milk
• With oral antifungal for *Candida* infections
• Microemulsion products (Neoral) and other products are not interchangeable
IV
• After diluting each 50 mg/20-100 ml of 0.9% NaCl or D_5W; run over 2-6 hr, may give as a continuous inf over 24 hr; use an infusion pump, glass inf bottles only
Additive compatibilities: Ciprofloxacin
Solution compatibilities: D_5W, NaCl 0.9%
Y-site compatibilities: Cefmetazole, propofol, sargramostim

♦ = Nursing alert　　🍃 = Herb-drug interaction　　🚫 = Do not crush

Evaluate:
• Therapeutic response: absence of rejection
Teach patient/family:
• To report fever, chills, sore throat, fatigue, since serious infections may occur; tremors, bleeding gums, increased B/P
• To use contraceptive measures during treatment, for 12 wk after ending therapy
🚫 Not to break, crush, or chew caps

---

cyproheptadine (Rx)
(si-proe-hep′ta-deen)
cyproheptadine HCl,
Periactin, PMS-
Cyproheptadine*
Func. class.: Antihistamine, H_1-receptor antagonist
Chem. class.: Piperidine

Action: Acts on blood vessels, GI, respiratory system by competing with histamine for H_1-receptor site; decreases allergic response by blocking histamine
Uses: Allergy symptoms, rhinitis, pruritus, cold, urticaria
Investigational uses: Appetite stimulant, management of vascular headache, nightmares, posttraumatic stress disorder
Dosage and routes:
• *Adult:* PO 4 mg tid-qid, not to exceed 0.5 mg/kg/day
• *Child 7-14 yr:* PO 4 mg bid-tid, not to exceed 16 mg/day
• *Child 2-6 yr:* PO 2 mg bid-tid, not to exceed 12 mg/day
Nightmares, posttraumatic stress disorder
• *Adult:* PO 4-12 mg qhs, max 32 mg
Available forms: Tabs 4 mg; syr 2 mg/5 ml

Side effects/adverse reactions:
HEMA: **Hemolytic anemia, leukopenia, thrombocytosis, agranulocytosis**
SYST: **Anaphylactic shock**
CNS: Dizziness, drowsiness, poor coordination, fatigue, anxiety, euphoria, confusion, paresthesia, neuritis
CV: Hypotension, palpitations, tachycardia
RESP: Increased thick secretions, wheezing, chest tightness
GI: Constipation, dry mouth, nausea, vomiting, anorexia, diarrhea, weight gain
INTEG: Rash, urticaria, photosensitivity
GU: Retention, dysuria, frequency, increased appetite
EENT: Blurred vision, dilated pupils; tinnitus; nasal stuffiness; dry nose, throat, mouth
Contraindications: Hypersensitivity to H_1-receptor antagonist, acute asthma attack, lower respiratory tract disease
Precautions: Increased intraocular pressure, renal disease, cardiac disease, hypertension, bronchial asthma, seizure disorder, stenosed peptic ulcers, hyperthyroidism, prostatic hypertrophy, bladder neck obstruction, pregnancy (B), lactation, elderly
Do not confuse:
cyproheptadine/cyclobenzaprine
Pharmacokinetics:
PO: Duration 4-6 hr; metabolized in liver; excreted by kidneys; excreted in breast milk
Interactions:
• Increased CNS depression: barbiturates, opiates, hypnotics, tricyclics, alcohol
• Increased effect of cyproheptadine: MAOIs
🌿 Increased CNS depression: kava
🌿 Increased anticholinergic effect: henbane leaf

Lab test interferences:
False negative: Skin allergy tests
NURSING CONSIDERATIONS
Assess:
• I&O ratio; be alert for urinary retention, frequency, dysuria; drug should be discontinued
• CBC during long-term therapy
• Respiratory status: rate, rhythm, increase in bronchial secretions, wheezing, chest tightness
• Cardiac status: palpitations, increased pulse, hypotension
Administer:
• With meals for GI symptoms; absorption may slightly decrease
Perform/provide:
• Hard candy, gum, frequent rinsing of mouth for dryness
• Storage in airtight container at room temperature
Evaluate:
• Therapeutic response: absence of running or congested nose, rashes
Teach patient/family:
• All aspects of drug use; to notify prescriber of confusion, sedation, hypotension
• That this drug decreases anticoagulant (oral) effect
• To avoid driving, other hazardous activity if drowsiness occurs, especially elderly
• To avoid concurrent use of alcohol, other CNS depressants
Treatment of overdose: Ipecac syrup or lavage, diazepam, vasopressors, barbiturates (short-acting)

cytarabine (℞)
(sye-tare′a-been)
Ara-C, Cytosar*, Cytosar-U, cytosine arabinoside, DepoCyt
Func. class.: Antineoplastic, antimetabolite
Chem. class.: Pyrimidine nucleoside

Action: Competes with physiologic substrate of DNA synthesis, thus interfering with cell replication in the S phase of the cell cycle (before mitosis)

Uses: Acute myelocytic leukemia, acute lymphocytic leukemia, chronic myelocytic leukemia, lymphomatous meningitis (IT), and in combination for non-Hodgkin's lymphomas in children

Dosage and routes:
Acute myelocytic leukemia
• *Adult:* **IV INF** 200 mg/m^2/day × 5 days q2wk as single agent or 2-6 mg/kg/day (100-200 mg/m^2/day) as single dose or 2-3 divided doses for 5-10 days until remission, used in combination; maintenance 70-200 mg/m^2/day for 2-5 days qmo; **SC** maintenance 1 mg/kg q1-2×/wk
Lymphomatous meningitis
Liposomal (DepoCyt): Adult **IT:** 50 mg q14d × 2 doses (wk 1, 3) then 50 mg q14d × 3 doses (wk 5, 7, 9) followed by 1 dose wk 13; then 50 mg q28d × 4 doses (wk 17, 21, 25, 29); if neurotoxicity occurs, reduce dose to 25 mg, if it persists, discontinue use
In combination
• *Child:* **IV INF** 100 mg/m^2/day × 5-10 days
Available forms: Powder for inj 100, 500 mg, 1, 2 g; liposomal for intrathecal use 10 mg/ml

Side effects/adverse reactions:
HEMA: Thrombophlebitis, bleeding,
thrombocytopenia, leukopenia, my-
elosuppression, anemia
META: Hyperuricemia
GI: Nausea, vomiting, anorexia, di-
*arrhea, stomatitis, **hepatotoxicity,***
abdominal pain, hematemesis, ***GI***
hemorrhage
EENT: Sore throat, conjunctivitis
GU: Urinary retention, ***renal fail-***
ure, hyperuricemia
INTEG: Rash, fever, freckling, cellulitis
*RESP: **Pneumonia,*** dyspnea, ***pul-***
monary edema (high doses)
CV: Chest pain, ***cardiopathy***
CNS: Neuritis, dizziness, headache,
personality changes, ataxia, mechan-
ical dysphasia, ***coma; chemical***
arachnoiditis (IT)
*SYST: **Anaphylaxis***
CYTARABINE SYNDROME: *Fever,*
myalgia, bone pain, chest pain, *rash,*
conjunctivitis, malaise (6-12 hr after administration)
Contraindications: Hypersensitivity, infants, pregnancy (D)
Precautions: Renal disease, hepatic
disease, lactation
Do not confuse:
Cytosar/Cytoxan
Cytosar/Cytovene
Pharmacokinetics:
INTRATHECAL: Half-life 100-236 hr;
metabolized in liver; excreted in
urine (primarily inactive metabolite); crosses blood-brain barrier,
placenta
IV/SC: Distribution half-life 10 min,
elimination half-life 1-3 hr
Interactions:
• Increased toxicity, bone marrow
depression: radiation or other anti-
neoplastics
• Decreased effects of oral digoxin

NURSING CONSIDERATIONS
Assess:
• CBC (RBC, Hct, Hgb), differential, platelet count weekly; withhold
drug if WBC is <1000/mm^3, platelet count is <50,000/mm^3, or RBC,
Hct, Hgb low; notify prescriber of
these results
• Renal function studies: BUN, serum uric acid, urine CrCl, electrolytes before and during therapy
• I&O ratio; report fall in urine output to <30 ml/hr
• Monitor temp q4h; fever may indicate beginning infection; no rectal
temps
• Liver function tests before and during therapy: bilirubin, ALT, AST,
alk phosphatase, as needed or
monthly; check for jaundice of skin,
sclera; dark urine; clay-colored
stools; pruritus; abdominal pain; fever; diarrhea
• Blood uric acid during therapy
◆ For anaphylaxis: rash, pruritus,
facial swelling, dyspnea; resuscitation equipment should be nearby
◆Chemical arachnoiditis (IT): headache, nausea, vomiting, fever; neck
ridigity pain, meningism, CSF pleo-
cytosis; may be decreased by dexamethasone
• Cytarabine syndrome 6-12hr after
inf: fever, myalgia, bone pain, chest
pain, rash, conjunctivitis, malaise;
corticosteroids may be ordered
• Bleeding: hematuria, heme-positive stools, bruising or petechiae,
mucosa or orifices q8h
◆ Dyspnea, rales, unproductive
cough, chest pain, tachypnea, fatigue, increased pulse, pallor, lethargy; personality changes, with high
doses; pulmonary edema may be fatal (rare)
• Buccal cavity q8h for dryness,
sores or ulceration, white patches,
oral pain, bleeding, dysphagia

• Local irritation, pain, burning, discoloration at injection site
• GI symptoms: frequency of stools, cramping, antispasmodic may be used
• Acidosis, signs of dehydration: rapid respirations, poor skin turgor, decreased urine output, dry skin, restlessness, weakness

Administer:
• Antiemetic 30-60 min before giving drug and prn
• Allopurinol to maintain uric acid levels and alkalinization of the urine
• Topical or systemic analgesics for pain

IT
• Liposomal: withdraw drug immediately before use; use within 4 hr, do not save unused portions, or use in-line filter; give directly into CSF by intraventricular reservoir or by direct inj into lumbar site
• Give slowly over 1-5 min, follow with lumbar puncture, instruct patient to lie flat, give dexamethasone 4 mg bid PO or IV × 5 days beginning on day of liposomal inj

IV
• After diluting 100 mg/5 ml of sterile H_2O for inj; given by direct IV over 1-3 min through free-flowing tubing (IV); may be further diluted in 50-100 ml NS or D_5W, given over 30 min to 24 hr depending on dose; also may be given by continuous inf

Additive compatibilities: Corticotropin, daunorubicin with etoposide, etoposide, hydroxyzine, lincomycin, mitoxantrone, ondansetron, potassium chloride, prednisolone, sodium bicarbonate, vincristine
Solution compatibilities: Amino acids, D_5/LR, D_5/0.2% NaCl, D_5/0.9% NaCl, D_{10}/0.9% NaCl, D_5W, invert sugar 10% in electrolyte #1, Ringer's LR, 0.9% NaCl, sodium lactate ⅙ mol/L, TPN #57
Syringe compatibilities: Metoclopramide
Y-site compatibilities: Amifostine, amsacrine, aztreonam, cefepime, chlorpromazine, cimetidine, cladribine, dexamethasone, diphenhydramine, doxorubicin liposome, droperidol, famitodine, filgrastim, fludarabine, gentamicin, granisetron, heparin, hydrocortisone, hydromorphone, idarubicin, lorazepam, melphalan, methotrexate, methylprednisolone, metoclopramide, morphine, ondansetron, paclitaxel, piperacillin/tazobactam, prochlorperazine, promethazine, propofol, ranitidine, sargramostim, sodium bicarbonate, teniposide, thiotepa, vinorelbine

Perform/provide:
• Strict medical asepsis and protective isolation if WBC levels are low
• Increase fluid intake to 2-3 L/day to prevent urate deposits and calculi formation, unless contraindicated
• Diet low in purines: absence of organ meats (kidney, liver), dried beans, peas to prevent increased urate deposits
• Rinsing of mouth tid-qid with water, club soda; brushing of teeth bid-tid with soft brush or cotton-tipped applicators for stomatitis; use unwaxed dental floss

Evaluate:
• Therapeutic response: decreased tumor size, spread of malignancy

Teach patient/family:
• To report any coughing, chest pain, changes in breathing; may indicate beginning pneumonia, pulmonary edema
• To avoid foods with citric acid, hot or rough texture if stomatitis is present, use sponge brush and rinse with water after each meal; to report stomatitis: any bleeding, white spots,

---

⬥ = Nursing alert   ▮ = Herb-drug interaction   ⊘ = Do not crush

ulcerations in mouth; tell patient to examine mouth qd, report any symptoms
• To report signs of infection: increased temp, sore throat, flulike symptoms; avoid crowds, persons with infections
• To report signs of anemia: fatigue, headache, faintness, shortness of breath, irritability
• To report bleeding; avoid use of razors, commercial mouthwash, salicylates, NSAIDs
• To use thrombocytopenia precautions
• To take fluids to 3 L/day to prevent renal damage
• To use contraception during treatment and 4 mo thereafter
• To avoid receiving vaccines during treatment
• To continue using dexamethasone with IT administration, that fever, headache, nausea, vomiting are likely to occur

dacarbazine (℞)

(da-kar′ba-zeen)
dacarbazine, DTIC*, DTIC-Dome

Func. class.: Antineoplastic alkylating agent

Chem. class.: Cytotoxic triazine

Action: Alkylates DNA, RNA; inhibits enzymes that allow synthesis of amino acids in proteins; also responsible for cross-linking DNA strands; activity is not cell cycle phase specific

Uses: Hodgkin's disease, sarcomas, neuroblastoma, malignant melanoma

Dosage and routes:
Malignant melanoma
• *Adult:* **IV** 2-4.5 mg/kg or 250

mg/m² qd × 5 days; repeat q3wk depending on response
Hodgkin's disease
• *Adult:* IV 150 mg/m² qd × 5 days with other agents, repeat q4wk; or 375 mg/m² on day 1 when given in combination, repeat q15d
• *Available forms:* Inj 100, 200 mg
Side effects/adverse reactions:
HEMA: ***Thrombocytopenia, leukopenia,*** anemia
GI: Nausea, anorexia, vomiting, ***hepatotoxicity*** (rare)
CNS: Facial paresthesia, flushing, fever, malaise
INTEG: Alopecia, dermatitis, pain at injection site
SYST: ***Anaphylaxis***
Contraindications: Lactation
Precautions: Radiation therapy, pregnancy (1st trimester) (C)
Pharmacokinetics: Metabolized by liver; excreted in urine; half-life 35 min, terminal 5 hr, 5% protein bound
Interactions:
• Decreased effectiveness of dacarbazine: phenytoin, phenobarbital
• Toxicity: bone marrow suppressants
• Bleeding: salicylates, anticoagulants
NURSING CONSIDERATIONS
Assess:
• CBC, differential, platelet count weekly; withhold drug if WBC <4000 or platelet count <75,000; notify prescriber of results
• Monitor temp q4h (may indicate beginning infection)
• Liver function tests before, during therapy (bilirubin, AST, ALT, LDH) as needed or monthly
• Bleeding: hematuria, guaiac, bruising or petechiae, mucosa or orifices q8h
• Effects of alopecia on body image, discuss feelings about body changes

• Jaundice of skin, sclera; dark urine; clay-colored stools; itchy skin; abdominal pain; fever; diarrhea
• Inflammation of mucosa, breaks in skin
Administer:
• Antiemetic 30-60 min before giving drug to prevent vomiting
• Antibiotics for prophylaxis of infection
IV
• After diluting 100 mg/9.9 ml of sterile H_2O for inj (10 mg/ml), give by direct IV over 1 min through Y-tube or 3-way stopcock; may be further diluted in 50-250 ml D_5W or NS for inj, given as an inf over ½ hr
• Watch for extravasation; give Na thiosulfate 10% 4 ml plus sterile H_2O 5 ml, 3-5 ml SC if needed
Additive compatibilities: Bleomycin, carmustine, cyclophosphamide, cytarabine, dactinomycin, doxorubicin, fluorouracil, mercaptopurine, methotrexate, ondansetron, vinblastine
Additive incompatibilities: Hydrocortisone sodium succinate, cysteine
Y-site compatibilities: Amifostine, aztreonam, filgrastim, fludarabine, granisetron, melphalan, ondansetron, paclitaxel, sargramostim, teniposide, thiotepa, vinorelbine
Perform/provide:
• Storage in light-resistant container, dry area
• Strict medical asepsis, protective isolation if WBC levels are low
• Increase fluid intake to 2-3 L/day to prevent urate deposits, calculi formation
• Warm compresses at infusion site for inflammation
Evaluate:
• Therapeutic response: decreased tumor size, spread of malignancy
Teach patient/family:
• That patient should avoid prolonged exposure to sun

• That hair may be lost during treatment; a wig or hairpiece may make the patient feel better; new hair may be different in color, texture
• To report signs of infection: fever, sore throat, flulike symptoms
• To report signs of anemia: fatigue, headache, faintness, shortness of breath, irritability
• To report bleeding; avoid use of razors, commercial mouthwash
• To avoid use of aspirin products or ibuprofen
• To use contraceptives during and for several months after therapy

---

daclizumab (Ŗ)
(dah-kliz′uh-mab)
Zenapax
Func. class.: Immunosuppressive
Chem. class.: Humanized IgG1 monoclonal antibody

Action: Binds to the IL-2 (interleukin-2) receptor antagonist
Uses: Acute allograft rejection in renal transplant patients
Dosage and routes:
• *Adult:* IV 1 mg/kg as part of a regimen that includes cyclosporine and corticosteroids, mix calculated vol with 50 ml of 0.9% NaCl and give via peripheral/central vein over 15 min
Available forms: Inj 25 mg/ml
Side effects/adverse reactions:
CNS: Chills, tremors, headache, prickly sensation
*RESP: Dyspnea, wheezing, **pulmonary edema,*** coughing, atelectasis, congestion, hypoxia
GI: Vomiting, nausea, diarrhea, constipation, abdominal pain, pyrosis
CV: Hypertension, ***tachycardia, thrombosis,*** bleeding
GU: Oliguria, dysuria, ***renal tubu-***

⬥ = Nursing alert   ▰ = Herb-drug interaction   ⊘ = Do not crush

lar necrosis, renal damage, ***hydro-nephrosis***
INTEG: Impaired wound healing
Contraindications: Hypersensitivity
Precautions: Pregnancy (C), child <2 yr, lactation, elderly
NURSING CONSIDERATIONS
Assess:
• Blood studies: Hgb, WBC, platelets during treatment qmo; if leukocytes are <3000/mm³, drug should be discontinued
• Liver function studies: alk phosphatase, AST, ALT, bilirubin
• Hepatotoxicity: dark urine, jaundice, itching, light-colored stools; drug should be discontinued
• For anaphylaxis, have corticosteroids, epinephrine available
Administer:
• All other medications PO if possible
• Avoid IM injection, since infection may occur
• Protect undiluted sol from direct light; should be used with drugs for immunosuppression
Solution compatibilities: 0.9% NaCl
Evaluate:
• Therapeutic response: absence of graft rejection
Teach patient/family:
• To report fever, chills, sore throat, fatigue, since serious infection may occur
• To use contraception (women) before, during, and for 4 mo after treatment
• To avoid vaccinations during treatment
• To increase fluid intake during treatment

dactinomycin (℞)
(dak-ti-noe-mye'sin)
Cosmegen
Func. class.: Antineoplastic, antibiotic

Action: Inhibits DNA, RNA, protein synthesis; derived from *Streptomyces parvullus;* replication is decreased by binding to DNA, which causes strand splitting; cell cycle nonspecific; a vesicant
Uses: Sarcomas, melanomas, trophoblastic tumors in women, testicular cancer, Wilms' tumor, rhabdomyosarcoma
Dosage and routes:
• *Adult:* IV 500 µg/m²/day × 5 days; stop drug for 2-4 wk; then repeat cycle
• *Child:* IV 15 µg/kg/day × 5 days, not to exceed 500 µg/day; stop drug until bone marrow recovery, then repeat cycle
Available forms: Inj 0.5 mg/vial
Side effects/adverse reactions:
HEMA: ***Thrombocytopenia, leukopenia, aplastic anemia***
GI: Nausea, vomiting, anorexia, stomatitis, ***hepatotoxicity,*** *abdominal pain, diarrhea*
INTEG: Rash, alopecia, pain at injection site, folliculitis, acne, desquamation, ***extravasation***
EENT: Chelitis, dysphagia, esophagitis
CNS: Malaise, fatigue, lethargy, fever
MS: Myalgia
Contraindications: Hypersensitivity, herpes infection, child <6 mo
Precautions: Renal disease, hepatic disease, pregnancy (C), lactation, bone marrow depression
Pharmacokinetics: Half-life 36 hr; IV onset 2-5 min; concentrates in kidneys, liver, spleen; does not cross

blood-brain barrier; excreted in feces and urine

Interactions:
• Increased toxicity: other antineoplastics, radiation

Lab test interferences:
Increase: Uric acid

NURSING CONSIDERATIONS
Assess:
• CBC, differential, platelet count weekly; withhold drug if WBC is <4000/mm^3 or platelet count is <75,000/mm^3; notify prescriber
• Renal function studies: BUN, serum uric acid, urine CrCl, electrolytes before, during therapy
• I&O ratio; report fall in urine output to <30 ml/hr
• Monitor temp q4h; fever may indicate beginning infection
• Liver function tests before, during therapy: bilirubin, AST, ALT, alk phosphatase, as needed or monthly; check for jaundice of skin, sclera; dark urine; clay-colored stools; itchy skin; abdominal pain; fever; diarrhea
• Bleeding: hematuria, guaiac stools, bruising, petechiae, mucosa or orifices q8h
• Food preferences; list likes, dislikes
• Effects of alopecia on body image; discuss feelings about body changes
• Inflammation of mucosa, breaks in skin
• Buccal cavity q8h for dryness, sores, ulceration, white patches, oral pain, bleeding, dysphagia
⬧ Symptoms indicating severe allergic reaction: rash, pruritus, urticaria, purpuric skin lesions, itching, flushing
• GI symptoms: frequency of stools, cramping, nausea, vomiting, anorexia
• Acidosis, signs of dehydration: rapid respirations, poor skin turgor, decreased urine output, dry skin, restlessness, weakness, sunken eyeball in children

Administer:
• Antiemetic 30-60 min before giving drug to prevent vomiting
IV
• After diluting 0.5 mg/1.1 ml of sterile H_2O for inj without preservative; use 2.2 ml (0.25 mg/ml), give by direct IV at 0.5 mg or less/min through Y-tube or 3-way stopcock if inf in progress; may be further diluted if required in 50 ml D_5W or NS for infusion; run over 10-15 min; change needles between reconstitution and direct IV administration
• Hydrocortisone, sodium thiosulfate to infiltration area, and ice compress after stopping infusion

Y-site compatibilities: Allopurinol, amifostine, aztreonam, cefepime, fludarabine, granisetron, melphalan, ondansetron, sargramostim, teniposide, thiotepa, vinorelbine

Perform/provide:
• Strict hand-washing technique, gloves and protective covering
• Liquid diet: carbonated beverages; gelatin may be added if patient is not nauseated or vomiting
• Rinsing of mouth tid-qid with water, club soda; brushing of teeth bid-qid with soft brush or cotton-tipped applicators for stomatitis; use unwaxed dental floss to prevent injury
• Storage in cool, dark environment; do not expose to bright light or freeze

Evaluate:
• Therapeutic response: decreased tumor size, spread of malignancy

Teach patient/family:
• That contraception is needed during treatment and for 4-6 mo after discontinuing therapy
• To avoid vaccinations without order by prescriber
• That hair may be lost during treatment after 1-2 wk and that wig or

---

⬧ = Nursing alert   ⫽ = Herb-drug interaction   ⊘ = Do not crush

hairpiece may make patient feel better; that new hair may be different in color, texture
• To avoid foods with citric acid, hot or rough texture when stomatitis is present
• To report any bleeding, white spots, ulcerations in mouth to prescriber; tell patient to examine mouth qd
• To avoid crowds, persons with known infection when granulocyte count is low
• To increase fluids to 3 L/day

dalteparin (Ŗ)
(dahl'ta-pear-in)
Fragmin
Func. class.: Anticoagulant
Chem. class.: Low molecular weight heparin
Action: Prevents conversion of fibrinogen to fibrin and prothrombin to thrombin by enhancing inhibitory effects of antithrombin III
Uses: Unstable angina/non-Q-wave MI; prevention of deep vein thrombosis in abdominal surgery patients
Investigational uses: Systemic anticoagulation in venous/arterial thromboembolic complications
Dosage and routes:
Hip replacement surgery
• *Adult:* SC 2500 IU 2 hr prior to surgery and 2nd dose in the evening the day of surgery, then 5000 IU SC 1st postop day and qd 5-10 days
Unstable angina/non-Q-wave MI
• *Adult:* SC 120 IU/kg, do not exceed 10,000 IU q12h with concurrent aspirin, continue until stable
Systemic anticoagulation
• *Adult:* SC 200 IU/kg qd or 100 IU/kg bid
DVT, prophylaxis
• *Adult:* SC 2500 IU qd, 1-2 hr prior to abdominal surgery and repeat qd

× 5-10 days; in high-risk patients 5000 IU may be used
Available forms: Prefilled syringes, 2500, 5000 IU/0.2 ml; 10,000 IU multidose vials
Side effects/adverse reactions:
CNS: ***Intracranial bleeding***
SYST: Hypersensitivity, ***hemorrhage, anaphylaxis*** possible
HEMA: ***Thrombocytopenia***
INTEG: Pruritus, superficial wound infection
Contraindications: Hypersensitivity to this drug, heparin, or other anticoagulants; hemophilia, leukemia with bleeding, thrombocytopenic purpura, cerebrovascular hemorrhage, cerebral aneurysm, severe hypertension, other severe cardiac disease
Precautions: Elderly, pregnancy (B), hepatic disease, severe renal disease, blood dyscrasias, subacute bacterial endocarditis, acute nephritis, lactation, children, recent childbirth, peptic ulcer disease, pericarditis, pericardial effusion, recent lumbar puncture, vasculitis, other diseases where bleeding is possible
Pharmacokinetics: 87% absorbed, excreted by kidneys, half-life 2 hr, peak 4 hr, onset and duration unknown
Interactions:
• Increased risk of bleeding: aspirin, oral anticoagulants, platelet inhibitors
⬆ Possible increased risk of bleeding: bromelain, cinchona bark
NURSING CONSIDERATIONS
Assess:
• For blood studies (Hct, CBC, platelets, occult blood in stools) during treatment since bleeding can occur
◆ For bleeding gums, petechiae, ecchymosis, black tarry stools, hematuria, epistaxis, decrease in Hct,

B/P; may indicate bleeding, possible hemorrhage; notify prescriber immediately, drug should be discontinued

• For hypersensitivity: fever, skin rash, urticaria; notify prescriber immediately

• For needed dosage change q1-2wk; dose may need to be decreased if bleeding occurs

Administer:
• Do not give IM or IV drug route; approved is SC only; do not mix with other inj or sol

• By SC only; have patient sit or lie down; SC inj may be 2 in from umbilicus in a U-shape, upper outer side of thigh or upper outer quadrangle of the buttocks; rotate inj sites

• Changing needles is not recommended

Evaluate:
• Therapeutic response: absence of deep-vein thrombosis

Teach patient/family:
• To avoid OTC preparations that contain aspirin; other anticoagulants, serious drug interaction may occur

• To use soft-bristle toothbrush to avoid bleeding gums, avoid contact sports, use electric razor, avoid IM injection

• To report any signs of bleeding: gums, under skin, urine, stools; unusual bruising

• To take missed dose as soon as possible, but not if almost time for next dose

Treatment of overdose: Protamine sulfate 1% given IV; 1 mg protamine/100 anti-Xa IU of dalteparin given

danaparoid (℞)
(dan-a-pair'oid)
Orgaran
Func. class.: Anticoagulant
Chem. class.: Low molecular weight heparin

Action: Prevents conversion of fibrinogen to fibrin and prothrombin to thrombin by enhancing inhibitory effects of antithrombin III

Uses: Prevention of vein thrombosis in hemodialysis, stroke, elective surgery for malignancy or total hip replacement, hip fracture surgery

Dosage and routes:
Prevention of venous thrombosis
• *Adult:* SC 750 anti–factor-Xa units bid × 7-10 days, begin 1-4 hr presurgery and restart 2 hr after surgery
Hemodialysis
• *Adult:* SC 2400-4800 anti-Xa units given predialysis
Available forms: Inj 750 anti-Xa units/0.6 ml

Side effects/adverse reactions:
SYST: Hypersensitivity, ***hemorrhage***
HEMA: ***Thrombocytopenia***
INTEG: Rash, pruritus, inj site pain
CV: ***Hemorrhage,*** peripheral edema
CNS: Insomnia, headache
GI: Nausea, vomiting, constipation
MS: Asthenia

Contraindications: Hypersensitivity to this drug, sulfites, pork; hemophilia, leukemia with bleeding, thrombocytopenia, purpura, cerebrovascular hemorrhage, cerebral aneurysm, severe hypertension, other severe cardiac disease

Precautions: Hypersensitivity to heparin, elderly, pregnancy (B), hepatic disease, severe renal disease, blood dyscrasias, subacute bacterial endocarditis, acute nephritis, lactation, children, recent childbirth, pep-

◆ = Nursing alert   ∥ = Herb-drug interaction   ⊘ = Do not crush

tic ulcer disease, pericarditis, pericardial effusion, recent lumbar puncture, vasculitis, other diseases where bleeding is possible

Pharmacokinetics: 100% absorbed, excreted by kidneys, half-life 24 hr, peak 4 hr

Interactions:

• Increased risk of bleeding: aspirin, oral anticoagulants, platelet inhibitors, NSAIDs, penicillin, dextran

🌿 Increased risk of bleeding: bromelain, cinchona bark

NURSING CONSIDERATIONS
Assess:

• For blood studies (Hct, CBC, occult blood in stools) during treatment since bleeding can occur; aPTT, ACT, anti–factor-Xa test, platelets

• For bleeding gums, petechiae, ecchymosis, black tarry stools, hematuria, epistaxis, decrease in Hct, B/P; may indicate bleeding, possible hemorrhage; notify prescriber immediately, drug should be discontinued

• For hypersensitivity: fever, skin, rash, urticaria; notify prescriber immediately

• For needed dosage change q1-2wk; dose may need to be decreased if bleeding occurs

Administer:

• By SC, have patient sit or lie down; SC inj may be around the navel in a U-shape, upper outer side of thigh or upper outer quadrangle of the buttocks; rotate inj sites

• Changing needles is not recommended

Evaluate:

• Therapeutic response: absence of deep-vein thrombosis

Teach patient/family:

• To avoid OTC preparations that may cause serious drug interactions unless directed by prescriber;

may contain aspirin, other anticoagulants

• To use soft-bristle toothbrush to avoid bleeding gums, avoid contact sports, use electric razor, avoid IM injection

• To report any signs of bleeding: gums, under skin, urine, stools; unusual bruising

Treatment of overdose: Protamine sulfate 1% given IV; 1 mg protamine/100 anti–factors-Xa IU of danaparoid given

---

danazol (℞)
(da′na-zole)
Cyclomen*, danazol, Danocrine
Func. class.: Androgen, anabolic steroid
Chem. class.: α-Ethinyl testosterone derivative

Action: Atrophy of endometrial tissue; decreases FSH, LH, which are controlled by pituitary; this leads to amenorrhea/anovulation

Uses: Endometriosis, prevention of hereditary angioedema, fibrocystic breast disease

Dosage and routes:
Endometriosis
• *Adult:* **PO** 100-500 mg bid uninterrupted for 3-9 mo
Fibrocystic breast disease
• *Adult:* **PO** 100-400 mg qd in 2 divided doses × 2-6 mo
Hereditary angioedema prevention
• *Adult:* **PO** 200 mg bid-tid until desired response, then decrease dose to 100 mg at 1-3 mo intervals
Available forms: Caps 50, 100, 200 mg
Side effects/adverse reactions:
INTEG: Rash, *acneiform lesions,* oily hair, skin, flushing, sweating, acne

vulgaris, alopecia, *hirsutism,* pruritus
CNS: Dizziness, headache, fatigue, tremors, paresthesias, flushing, sweating, anxiety, *lability,* insomnia, carpal tunnel syndrome
MS: Cramps, spasms, joint swelling
CV: Increased B/P
GU: Hematuria, *amenorrhea,* atrophic vaginitis, decreased libido, *decreased breast size,* clitoral hypertrophy, testicular atrophy
GI: Nausea, vomiting, constipation, *weight gain,* **cholestatic jaundice**
EENT: Conjunctival edema, nasal congestion, voice weakness
ENDO: Abnormal GTT
Contraindications: Severe renal, severe cardiac, severe hepatic disease, hypersensitivity, genital bleeding (abnormal), pregnancy (X), children
Precautions: Migraine headaches, seizure disorders
Do not confuse:
danazol/Dantrium
Interactions:
• Increased action: anticoagulants, oral antidiabetics, insulin, corticosteroids
• Nephrotoxicity: cyclosporine
Lab test interferences:
Increase: Cholesterol
Decrease: Cholesterol, T_4, T_3, thyroid ^{131}I uptake test, 17-KS, PBI
Interference: GTT
NURSING CONSIDERATIONS
Assess:
• For pain before and alter treatment in endometriosis, fibrocystic breast disease; tenderness, nodules in fibrocystic breast disease
• K, blood, urine glucose while on long-term therapy; LFTs, periodically, semen volume, sperm count, motility in hereditary angioedema
• Weight daily; notify prescriber if

weekly weight gain is >5 lb; drug should be decreased or discontinued
• I&O ratio; be alert for decreasing urinary output, increasing edema
• Edema, hypertension, cardiac symptoms, jaundice
• Mental status: affect, mood, behavioral changes, aggression, sleep disorders, depression, anxiety, lability
• Signs of virilization: deepening of voice, decreased libido, facial hair that may not be reversible
• Hypercalcemia: GI symptoms, polydipsia, polyuria, increased calcium levels above 11 mg/dl, loss of muscle tone
Administer:
• Start treatment during menstruation in endometriosis, fibrocystic breast disease
• With food or milk to decrease GI symptoms (i.e., nausea, vomiting, anorexia, dyspepsia)
Perform/provide:
• Storage in airtight container at room temperature; do not freeze
Evaluate:
• Therapeutic response: decreased pain in endometriosis; decreased size, pain in fibrocystic breast disease
Teach patient/family:
🚫 Not to break, crush, or chew caps
• To notify prescriber if therapeutic response decreases
• Not to discontinue medication abruptly; to taper over several wk
• To report menstrual irregularities; that amenorrhea usually occurs but menstruation resumes 2-3 mo after termination of therapy without medical intervention
• About routine breast self-exam and to report any increase in nodule size

• That drug should induce anovulation; reversible within 60-90 days after drug is discontinued and treatment will need to be resumed

• That endometriosis tends to recur after drug is discontinued

• To use nonhormonal contraception

• That virilization may occur, to notify prescriber

• To use sunscreen or stay out of the sun to prevent burns

---

dantrolene (R)

(dan′troe-leen)

Dantrium

Func. class.: Skeletal muscle relaxant, direct acting

Chem. class.: Hydantoin

Action: Interferes with intracellular release of calcium from the sarcoplasmic reticulum necessary to initiate contraction; slows catabolism in malignant hyperthermia

Uses: Spasticity in multiple sclerosis, stroke, spinal cord injury, cerebral palsy, malignant hyperthermia

Dosage and routes:

Spasticity

• *Adult:* PO 25 mg/day; may increase by 25-100 mg bid-qid, not to exceed 400 mg/day × 1 wk

• *Child:* PO 1 mg/kg/day given in divided doses bid-tid; dosage may increase gradually, not to exceed 100 mg qid

Prevention of malignant hyperthermia

• *Adult and child:* PO 4-8 mg/kg/day in 3-4 divided doses × 1-2 days prior to procedures, give last dose 4 hr preop; IV 2.5 mg/kg prior to anesthesia

Malignant hyperthermia

• *Adult and child:* IV 1 mg/kg, may repeat to total dose of 10 mg/kg; PO 4-8 mg/kg/day in 4 divided doses × 3 days to prevent further hyperthermia; post-crisis follow-up 4-8 mg/kg/day for 1-3 days

Available forms: Caps 25, 50, 100 mg; powder for inj 20 mg/vial

Side effects/adverse reactions:

CNS: Dizziness, weakness, fatigue, drowsiness, headache, disorientation, insomnia, paresthesias, tremors, **seizures**

EENT: Nasal congestion, blurred vision, mydriasis

HEMA: Eosinophilia

CV: Hypotension, chest pain, palpitations

GI: Hepatic injury, nausea, constipation, vomiting, increased AST, alk phosphatase, abdominal pain, dry mouth, anorexia, hepatitis, dyspepsia

GU: Urinary frequency, nocturia, impotence, crystalluria

INTEG: Rash, pruritus, photosensitivity

Contraindications: Hypersensitivity, compromised pulmonary function, active hepatic disease, impaired myocardial function

Precautions: Peptic ulcer disease, renal disease, hepatic disease, stroke, seizure disorder, diabetes mellitus, pregnancy (C), lactation, elderly

Do not confuse:

Dantrium/danazol

Pharmacokinetics:

PO: Peak 5 hr; highly protein bound; half-life 8 hr; metabolized in liver; excreted in urine (metabolites)

Interactions:

• Dysrhythmias: verapamil

• Increased CNS depression: alcohol, tricyclics, opiates, barbiturates, sedatives, hypnotics, antihistamines

• Hepatotoxicity: estrogens, other hepatotoxics

• Considered incompatible in sol or syringe; compatibility unknown

---

NURSING CONSIDERATIONS
Assess:
• For increased seizure activity, ECG in epilepsy patient; poor seizure control has occurred
• I&O ratio; check for urinary retention, frequency, hesitancy, especially elderly
• Hepatic function by frequent determination of AST, ALT, bilirubin, alk phosphatase, GGTP; renal function studies, BUN, creatinine, CBC
• Allergic reactions: rash, fever, respiratory distress
• Severe weakness, numbness in extremities; prescriber should be notified and drug discontinued
• Tolerance: increased need for medication, more frequent requests for medication, increased pain
• CNS depression: dizziness, drowsiness, insomnia, psychiatric symptoms
◆ Signs of hepatotoxicity: jaundice, yellow sclera, pain in abdomen, nausea, fever; prescriber should be notified, drug should be discontinued

Administer:
PO
• With meals for GI symptoms, caps may be opened and mixed with food/liquid
IV
• IV after diluting 20 mg/60 ml sterile H_2O for inj without bacteriostatic agent (333 µg/ml); shake until clear; give by rapid IV push through Y-tube or 3-way stopcock; follow by prescribed doses immediately; may also give by intermittent inf over 1 hr prior to anesthesia

Perform/provide:
• Storage in tight container at room temperature; protect diluted sol from light, use within 6 hr
• Gum, frequent sips of water for dry mouth
• Assistance with ambulation if dizziness/drowsiness occurs

Evaluate:
• Therapeutic response: decreased pain, spasticity

Teach patient/family:
• Not to discontinue medication quickly; hallucinations, spasticity, tachycardia will occur; drug should be tapered off over 1-2 wk; notify prescriber of abdominal pain, jaundiced sclera, clay-colored stools, change in color of urine
• Not to take with alcohol, other CNS depressants
• That if improvement does not occur within 6 wk, prescriber may discontinue
• To avoid hazardous activities if drowsiness, dizziness occurs
• To avoid using OTC medication: cough preparations, antihistamines, unless directed by prescriber
Ⓝ Not to break, crush, or chew caps
• To use sunscreen or stay out of the sun to prevent burns

Treatment of overdose: Induce emesis of conscious patient; lavage, dialysis

---

RARELY USED

dapsone (DDS) (℞)
(dap'sone)
Avlosulfon*, Dapsone
Func. class.: Leprostatic

Uses: Hansen's disease, PCP (*Pneumocystis carinii* pneumonia), malaria, dermatitis herpetiformis

Dosage and routes:
Hansen's disease
• *Adult:* **PO** 100 mg qd with rifampin 600 mg qd × 6 mo, then dapsone alone for 3-10 yr
• *Child:* **PO** 1-2 mg/kg/day

◆ = Nursing alert   🖋 = Herb-drug interaction   Ⓝ = Do not crush

D

PCP

• *Adult:* **PO** 50-100 mg/day usually given with trimethoprim 20 mg/kg/day in 4 divided doses for 3 wk
• *Child:* **PO** 2 mg/kg/day

Contraindications: Hypersensitivity to sulfones, severe anemia

---

darbepoetin alfa
See appendix a—selected new drugs

---

daunorubicin (℞)
(daw-noe-roo′bi-sin)
Cerubidine

daunorubicin citrate liposome
DaunoXome
Func. class.: Antineoplastic, antiinfective

Chem. class.: Anthracycline glycoside

Action: Inhibits DNA synthesis, primarily; derived from *Streptomyces coerulorubidus;* replication is decreased by binding to DNA, which causes strand splitting; cell cycle specific (S phase); a vesicant

Uses: Myelogenous, monocytic leukemia, acute nonlymphocytic leukemia, Ewing's sarcoma, Wilms' tumor, neuroblastoma, rhabdomyosarcoma; daunorubicin citrate liposome: advanced Kaposi's sarcoma in HIV

Dosage and routes:
Use decreased dose for those >60 yr of age
Daunorubicin
Single agent
• *Adult:* **IV** 60 mg/m²/day × 3-5 days q4wk
In combination
• *Adult:* **IV** 45 mg/m²/day × 3 days, then 2 days of subsequent courses in combination
• *Child:* **IV** 25-60 mg/m² depending on cycle
Daunorubicin citrate liposome
• *Adult:* **IV** 40 mg/m² q2wk
Renal dose
• *Adult:* **IV** serum Cr >3 mg/dl reduce dose by 50%
Hepatic dose
• *Adult:* **IV** serum bilirubin 1.2-3 mg/dl reduce dose by 25%; bilirubin >3 mg/dl reduce dose by 50%

Available forms: Inj 20 mg pwd/vial, sol for inj 5 mg/ml; liposome: dispersion for inj 2 mg/ml

Side effects/adverse reactions:
Daunorubicin
HEMA: **Thrombocytopenia, leukopenia, anemia**
GI: *Nausea, vomiting, anorexia, mucositis,* **hepatotoxicity**
GU: Impotence, sterility, amenorrhea, gynecomastia, hyperuricemia
INTEG: *Rash,* **extravasation,** dermatitis, reversible alopecia, cellulitis, thrombophlebitis at injection site
CV: **Dysrhythmias, CHF, pericarditis, myocarditis,** peripheral edema
CNS: Fever, chills
SYST: **Anaphylaxis**
Daunorubicin citrate liposome
CV: Chest pain, edema
GI: Cramps, diarrhea, constipation, stomatitis
INTEG: Sweating, pruritus
MS: Arthralgia, back pain
CNS: Fatigue, headache, depression, insomnia, dizziness, malaise, neuropathy

Contraindications: Hypersensitivity, pregnancy (D), lactation, systemic infections, cardiac disease

Precautions: Renal, hepatic disease; gout; bone marrow depression

Pharmacokinetics: Half-life 18½ hr, liposome 55½ hr; metabolized by liver; crosses placenta; excreted in breast milk, urine, bile

---

Do not confuse:

daunorubicin/doxorubicin

Interactions:

• Increased risk of bleeding: NSAIDs, salicylates

• Increased toxicity: other antineoplastics, radiation, cyclophosphamide

• Decreased antibody reaction: live virus vaccines

Lab test interferences:

Increase: Uric acid

NURSING CONSIDERATIONS

Assess:

• CBC, differential, platelet count weekly, leukocyte nadir within 2 wk after administration, recovery within 3 wk; do not administer if absolute granulocyte count is <750/mm³ (liposome)

• Blood, urine uric acid levels baseline and during therapy

• Renal function studies: BUN, urine CrCl, electrolytes baseline, before each dose

• I&O ratio; report fall in urine output to <30 ml/hr

• Monitor temp q4h; fever may indicate beginning infection

• Liver function tests baseline, before each dose: bilirubin, AST, ALT, alk phosphatase; check for jaundice of skin, sclera; dark urine; clay-colored stools; itchy skin; abdominal pain; fever; diarrhea

• Chest x-ray, echocardiography, radionuclide angiography, ECG; watch for ST-T wave changes, low QRS and T, possible dysrhythmias (sinus tachycardia, heart block, PVCs); watch for CHF (jugular vein distention, weight gain, edema, rales or crackles), may occur after 2-6 mo of treatment

• Bleeding: hematuria, guaiac stools, bruising or petechiae, mucosa or orifices q8h

• Effects of alopecia on body image; discuss feelings about body changes

• Buccal cavity q8h for dryness, sores or ulceration, white patches, oral pain, bleeding, dysphagia

• Local irritation, pain, burning at injection site

• GI symptoms: frequency of stools, cramping

• Acidosis, signs of dehydration: rapid respirations, poor skin turgor, decreased urine output, dry skin, restlessness, weakness

Administer:

• Antiemetic 30-60 min before giving drug and 6-10 hr after treatment to prevent vomiting

• Allopurinol or sodium bicarbonate to reduce uric acid levels, alkalinization of urine

IV (Cerubidine)

• After diluting 20 mg/4 ml sterile H₂O for inj (5 mg/ml), rotate, further dilute in 10-15 ml 0.9% NaCl; give over 3-5 min by direct IV through Y-tube or 3-way stopcock of inf of D₅ or 0.9% NaCl; or dilute in 50 ml 0.9% NaCl and give over 10-15 min; or dilute in 100 ml and give over 30 min

• Hydrocortisone for extravasation; apply ice compress after stopping infusion

Additive compatibilities: Cytarabine/etoposide, hydrocortisone; not recommended for admixing

Solution compatibilities: D₃.₃/0.3% NaCl, D₅W, Normosol R, Ringer's, 0.9% NaCl

Y-site compatibilities: Amifostine, filgrastim, granisetron, melphalan, methotrexate, ondansetron, sodium bicarbonate, teniposide, thiotepa, vinorelbine

IV (DaunoXome)

• Dilute with D₅W to (1 mg/ml) give over 60 min, do not use in-line

---

◆ = Nursing alert   ∥ = Herb-drug interaction   ⊘ = Do not crush

filter, reconstituted sol may be stored ≤6 hr refrigerated; do not admix
Perform/provide:
• Increased fluid intake to 2-3 L/day to prevent urate and calculi formation
• Diet low in purines: absence of organ meats (kidney, liver), dried beans, peas to reduce uric acid level
• Rinsing of mouth tid-qid with water, club soda; brushing of teeth bid-qid with soft brush or cotton-tipped applicators for stomatitis; use unwaxed dental floss
Evaluate:
• Therapeutic response: decreased tumor size, spread of malignancy
Teach patient/family:
• To report signs of infection, bleeding, bruising, shortness of breath, swelling, change in heart rate
• That hair may be lost during treatment and wig or hairpiece may make patient feel better; tell patient that new hair may be different in color, texture
• To avoid pregnancy while on this drug, and 4 mo thereafter
• To avoid foods with citric acid, hot or rough texture
• To report any bleeding, white spots, ulcerations in mouth; tell patient to examine mouth qd
• That urine and other body fluids may be red-orange for 48 hr
• To avoid vaccines while taking this drug
• To avoid crowds, those with known infections
• To avoid alcohol, aspirin, NSAIDs

RARELY USED

deferoxamine (℞)
(de-fer-ox′a-meen)
Desferal
Func. class.: Heavy metal antagonist

Uses: Acute, chronic iron intoxication, hemochromatosis, hemosiderosis
Dosage and routes:
Acute iron toxicity
• *Adult and child:* **IM/IV** 1 g, then 500 mg q4h × 2 doses, then 500 mg q4-12h × 2 doses, not to exceed 15 mg/kg/hr or 6 g/24 hr
Chronic iron toxicity
• *Adult and child:* **IM** 500 mg-1 g/day plus **IV INF** 2 g given by separate line with each blood transfusion, not to exceed 15 mg/kg/hr or 6 g/24 hr; **SC** 1-2 g over 8-24 hr by SC infusion pump
Contraindications: Hypersensitivity, anuria, severe renal disease, child <3 yr
Do not confuse:
deferoxamine/cefuroxime

delavirdine (℞)
(de-la-veer′deen)
Rescriptor
Func. class.: Nonnucleoside reverse transcriptase inhibitor (NNRTI)

Action: Binds directly to reverse transcriptase and blocks RNA, DNA causing a disruption of the enzyme's site
Uses: HIV-1 in combination with zidovudine or didanosine
Dosage and routes:
• *Adult and child ≥ 16 yr:* 400 mg tid
Available forms: Tabs 100 mg

Side effects: *italics* = common; ***bold italics*** = life-threatening

Side effects/adverse reactions:
CNS: Headache, fatigue
GI: Diarrhea, abdominal pain, nausea, anorexia, vomiting, dyspepsia, ***hepatotoxicity***
GU: ***Nephrotoxicity***
HEMA: ***Neutropenia, leukopenia, thrombocytopenia, anemia, granulocytopenia***
INTEG: Rash
MS: Pain myalgia

Contraindications: Hypersensitivity to this drug or atevirdine

Precautions: Liver disease, pregnancy (C), lactation, children, renal disease, myleosuppression

Pharmocokinetics:
Highly protein bound, half-life 6 hr, peak 1 hr, duration 8 hr, extensively metabolized

Interactions:
• Increased levels of: alprazolam, clarithromycin, dapsone, ergots, felodipine, midazolam, nifedipine, indinavir, amprenavir, saquinavir
• Decreased delavirdine levels: antacids, anticonvulsants, rifamycins, protease inhibitors
• Decreased action of: oral contraceptives
• Increased delavirdine levels: fluoxetine, ketoconazole
• Increased levels of both drugs: quinidine, warfarin, clarithromycin
◆ Serious life-threatening adverse reaction: amphetamines, ergots, benzodiazipines, calcium channel blockers, sedative/hypnotics, antidysrhythmics, sildenafil, pimozide, cisapride

NURSING CONSIDERATIONS
Assess:
• For signs of infection, anemia
• Liver studies: ALT, AST; renal studies
• C&S before drug therapy; drug may be taken as soon as culture is taken; repeat C&S after treatment; determine the presence of other sexually transmitted disease
• Bowel pattern before, during treatment; if severe abdominal pain with bleeding occurs, drug should be discontinued; monitor hydration
• For skin eruptions; rash, urticaria, itching
• For allergies before treatment, reaction to each medication; place allergies on chart
• Plasma delavirdine concentrations (trough 10 micromolar)
• CBC, blood chemistry, plasma HIV RNA, absolute CD4+/CD8+/ cell counts/%, serum β-2 microglobulin, serum ICD+24 antigen levels
• For signs of delavirdine toxicity: severe nausea/vomiting, maculopapular rash

Administer:
• Dispersion by adding 4 tab/3-4 oz water, let stand, stir, swallow, rinse glass, swallow

Evaluate:
• Therapeutic response: increased CD4 cell count, decreased viral load, improvement in symptoms of HIV

Teach patient/family:
• To take as prescribed; if dose is missed, take as soon as remembered up to 1 hr before next dose; do not double dose
• That tabs may be dissolved in ½ cup of water, stir, when dissolved, drink right away, rinse cup with water, and drink that to get all medication
• To make sure health care provider knows of all the medications being taken
• That if severe rash, mouth sores, swelling, aching muscles/joints, or eye redness occur, stop taking and notify health care provider
• Not to breastfeed if taking this drug

◆ = Nursing alert   /// = Herb-drug interaction   ⊘ = Do not crush

RARELY USED

demeclocycline (R)
(dem-e-kloe-sye'kleen)
Declomycin
Func. class.: Antiinfective
Chem. class.: Tetracycline

Uses: Uncommon gram-positive/gram-negative bacteria, protozoa, *Rickettsia, Mycoplasma, Haemophilus ducreyi, Yersinia pestis, Campylobacter fetus, Chlamydia trachomatis,* psittacosis, granuloma inguinale

Dosage and routes:
• *Adult:* **PO** 150 mg q6h or 300 mg q12h
• *Child >8 yr:* **PO** 6-12 mg/kg/day in divided doses q6-12h
Gonorrhea
• *Adult:* **PO** 600 mg, then 300 mg q12h × 4 days, total 3 g
Contraindications: Hypersensitivity to tetracyclines, children <8 yr, pregnancy (D)

denileukin diftitox (R)
(den-ih-loo'kin dif'tih-tox)
Ontak
Func. class.: Antineoplastic—misc.

Action: A recombinant DNA-derived cytotoxic protein; inhibits cellular protein synthesis
Uses: Cutaneous T-cell lymphoma that expresses CD25 component of the IL-2 receptor
Research note: Research has concluded that denileukin is effective for cutaneous T-cell lymphoma[6]
Dosage and routes:
• *Adult:* **IV** 9-18 μg/kg/day given for 5 days q21 days, given over ≥15 min

Available forms: Sol for inj, frozen 150 μg/ml
Side effects/adverse reactions:
CNS: Dizziness, paresthesia, nervousness, confusion, insomnia
CV: Hypotension, vasodilation, tachycardia, thrombosis, hypertension, dysrhythmias
GI: Nausea, anorexia, vomiting, diarrhea, constipation, dyspepsia, dysphagia
GU: Hematuria, albuminuria, pyuria, creatinine increase
*HEMA: **Thrombocytopenia, leukopenia,** anemia*
INTEG: Rash, pruritus, sweating
META: Hypoalbuminemia, edema, hypocalcemia, weight decrease, dehydration, hypokalemia
MISC: Fever, chills, asthenia, infection, pain, headache, chest pain, flu-like symptoms
MS: Myalgia, arthralgia
RESP: Dyspnea, cough, pharyngitis, rhinitis
Contraindications: Hypersensitivity to denileukin, diphtheria toxin, IL-2
Precautions: Radiation therapy, pregnancy (C), lactation, elderly, children
Pharmacokinetics: Concentrates in liver/kidneys; metabolized by proteolytic degradation
Interactions:
• Increased bone marrow depression: radiation, other antineoplastics
• Decreased antibody reaction: live vaccines
NURSING CONSIDERATIONS
Assess:
• CBC, differential, platelet count weekly; withhold drug if WBC <4000/mm^3 or platelet count <75,000/mm^3; notify prescriber of results
• Monitor temp q4h (may indicate beginning infection)

• Liver function tests before, during therapy (bilirubin, AST, ALT, LDH) as needed or monthly

• Bleeding: hematuria, guaiac, bruising or petechiae, mucosa or orifices q8h

• Jaundice of skin, sclera; dark urine; clay-colored stools; itchy skin; abdominal pain; fever; diarrhea

• For vascular leak syndrome after 2wk of treatment, hypotension, edema, hypoalbuminemia; monitor weight, B/P, serum albumin, edema

• Obtain CD25 expression on skin biopsy samples

Administer:

• Antiemetic 30-60 min before giving drug to prevent vomiting

• Antibiotics for prophylaxis of infection

IV

• Prepare and hold sol in plastic syringes or soft plastic IV bags only

• Draw calculated dose from vial, inject into empty IV infusion bag, for each 1 ml of drug removed from vial, no more than 9 ml of sterile saline without preservative should be added to IV bag; infuse over ≥15 min; do not give by bolus; do not admix with other drugs; do not use a filter

• Use within 6 hr, discard unused portions

Perform/provide:

• Storage in light-resistant container, dry area

• Warm compresses at infusion site for inflammation

Evaluate:

• Therapeutic response: decreased tumor size, spread of malignancy

Teach patient/family:

• To report signs of infection: fever, sore throat, flulike symptoms

• To report signs of anemia: fatigue, headache, faintness, shortness of breath, irritability

• To report bleeding; avoid use of razors, commercial mouthwash

• To avoid use of aspirin products or ibuprofen

RARELY USED

desipramine
(dess-ip'ra-meen)
desipramine HCl, Norpramin, Pertofrane
Func. class.: Antidepressant, tricyclic

Uses: Depression
Dosage and routes:

• *Adult:* **PO** 75-150 mg/day in divided doses; may increase to 300 mg/day or may give daily dose hs

• *Adolescent and elderly:* **PO** 25-50 mg/day, may increase to 100 mg/day

Contraindications: Hypersensitivity to tricyclics, recovery phase of myocardial infarction, narrow-angle glaucoma, convulsive disorders, prostatic hypertrophy, child <12 yr

---

desloratadine
See appendix a—selected new drugs

---

desmopressin (℞)
(des-moe-press'in)
DDAVP, Stimate
Func. class.: Pituitary hormone
Chem. class.: Synthetic antidiuretic hormone

Action: Promotes reabsorption of water by action on renal tubular epithelium; causes smooth muscle constriction, increase in plasma factor VIII levels, which increases platelet aggregation resulting in vasopressor effect, similar to vasopressin

---

◆ = Nursing alert   ∥ = Herb-drug interaction   ⊘ = Do not crush

Uses: Hemophilia A, von Willebrand's disease type 1, nonnephrogenic diabetes insipidus, symptoms of polyuria/polydipsia caused by pituitary dysfunction, nocturnal enuresis

Dosage and routes:

Primary nocturnal enuresis

• *Adult and child ≥6 yr:* **INTRANASAL** 20 µg (10 µg in each nostril) hs, may increase to 40 µg; **PO** 0.2 mg hs, may be increased to max 0.6 mg hs

Diabetes insipidus

• *Adult:* **INTRANASAL** 0.1-0.4 ml qd in divided doses (1-4 sprays with pump); **IV/SC** 0.5-1 ml qd in divided doses

• *Child 3 mo to 12 yr:* **INTRANASAL** 0.05-0.3 ml qd in divided doses

Hemophilia/von Willebrand's disease

• *Adult and child >3 mo:* **IV** 0.3 µg/kg in NaCl over 15-30 min; may repeat if needed

Antihemorrhagic

• *Adult and child >3 mo:* **IV** 0.3 µg/kg

• *Adult and child <50 kg:* **INTRANASAL** 1 spray in one nostril

• *Adult and child >50 kg:* 1 spray each nostril

Available forms: Inj 4, 15 µg/ml, Rhihal Tube del 2.5 mg/vial (0.1 mg/ml); tabs 0.1, 0.2 mg; nasal spray pump 10 µg/spray (0.1 mg/ml); nasal sol 1.5 mg/ml (150 µg/dose)

Side effects/adverse reactions:

EENT: Nasal irritation, congestion, rhinitis

CNS: Drowsiness, headache, lethargy, flushing

GU: Vulval pain

GI: Nausea, heartburn, cramps

CV: Increased B/P

*SYST: **Anaphylaxis (IV)***

Contraindications: Hypersensitivity, nephrogenic diabetes insipidus

Precautions: Pregnancy (B), CAD, lactation, hypertension

Pharmacokinetics:

NASAL: Onset 1 hr, peak 1-4 hr, duration 8-20 hr, half-life 8 min, 76 min (terminal)

PO: Onset 1 hr, peak 4-7 hr

IV: Onset 1 min, peak ½ hr, duration more than 3 hr

Interactions:

• Increased antidiuretic action: carbamazepine, chlorpropamide, clofibrate

• Decreased antidiuretic action: lithium, alcohol, demeclocycline, heparin, large doses of epinephrine

NURSING CONSIDERATIONS

Assess:

• Pulse, B/P when giving IV or SC

• I&O ratio, weight daily; check for edema in extremities; if water retention is severe, diuretic may be prescribed

• Water intoxication: lethargy, behavioral changes, disorientation, neuromuscular excitability

• Intranasal use: nausea, congestion, cramps, headache; usually decreased with decreased dose

◆ For severe allergic reaction including anaphylaxis (IV route)

• For nasal mucosa changes: congestion, edema, discharge, scarring (nasal route)

• Urine vol/osmolality and plasma osmolality (diabetes insipidus)

• Factor VIII coagulant activity before using for hemostasis

Administer:

• Undiluted over 1 min in diabetes insipidus

• Diluted, one single dose/50 ml of 0.9% NaCl (adult and child >10 kg), a single dose/10 ml as an IV INF over 15-30 min in von Willebrand's disease or hemophilia A

Perform/provide:

• Storage in refrigerator or cool environment

Evaluate:
• Therapeutic response: absence of severe thirst, decreased urine output, osmolality

Teach patient/family:
• The proper technique for nasal instillation: to insert tube into nostril to instill drug
• To avoid OTC products: cough, hay fever products, since these preparations may contain epinephrine, decrease drug response; do not use with alcohol
• To wear Medic Alert ID specifying therapy
• That if dose is missed, take when remembered up to 1 hr before next dose; do not double dose

---

dexamethasone (℞)
(dex-ah-meth′a-sone)
Decadron, Deronil*
Dexasone*, Dexon, Hexadrol, Mymethasone
dexamethasone acetate (℞)
Dalalone DP, Dalalone LA, Decadron-LA, Decaject-LA, Dexacen LA-8, Dexasone-LA, Dexone LA, Solurex-LA
dexamethasone sodium phosphate (℞)
Dalalone, Decadron Phosphate, Decaject, Dexacen-4, Dexone, Hexadrol Phosphate, Solurex
Func. class.: Corticosteroid
Chem. class.: Glucocorticoid, long-acting

Action: Decreases inflammation by suppression of migration of polymorphonuclear leukocytes, fibroblasts, reversal of increased capillary permeability and lysosomal stabilization

Uses: Inflammation, allergies, neoplasms, cerebral edema, septic shock, collagen disorders

Dosage and routes:
Inflammation
• *Adult:* **PO** 0.75-9 mg/day or phosphate **IM** 0.5-9 mg/day; or acetate **IM** 4-16 mg q1-3wk
• *Child:* **PO** 0.08-0.3 mg/kg/day in divided doses q6-12h

Shock (Phosphate)
• *Adult:* **IV** single dose 1-6 mg/kg or **IV** 40 mg q2-6h as needed up to 72h

Cerebral edema
• *Adult: (Phosphate)* **IV** 10 mg, then 4-6 mg **IM** q6h × 2-4 days, then taper over 1 wk
• *Child:* **PO** 0.2 mg/kg/day in divided doses

Adrenocortical insufficiency
• *Child:* 23.3 µg/kg/day in 3 divided doses

Supression test
• *Adult:* **PO** 1 mg at 11 PM or 0.5 mg q6h × 48 hr

Available forms: dexamethasone: Tabs 0.25, 0.5, 0.75, 1, 1.5, 2, 4, 6 mg; elix 0.5 mg/5 ml; oral sol 0.5 mg/5 ml, 1 mg/1 ml; inj acetate 8, 16 mg/ml; inj phosphate 4, 10, 20, 24 mg/ml

Side effects/adverse reactions:
INTEG: Acne, poor wound healing, ecchymosis, petechiae
CNS: Depression, *flushing, sweating,* headache, mood changes, euphoria, psychosis, *seizures*
CV: Hypertension, *circulatory collapse, thrombophlebitis, embolism,* tachycardia, edema
HEMA: ***Thrombocytopenia***
MS: Fractures, osteoporosis, weakness
GI: Diarrhea, nausea, abdominal distention, **GI hemorrhage,** *increased appetite,* **pancreatitis**

◆ = Nursing alert   🌿 = Herb-drug interaction   🚫 = Do not crush

EENT: Fungal infections, increased intraocular pressure, blurred vision
ENDO: HPA suppression
META: Hypokalemia
Contraindications: Psychosis, hypersensitivity, idiopathic thrombocytopenia, acute glomerulonephritis, amebiasis, fungal infections, nonasthmatic bronchial disease, child <2 yr, AIDS, TB
Precautions: Pregnancy (C), lactation, diabetes mellitus, glaucoma, osteoporosis, seizure disorders, ulcerative colitis, CHF, myasthenia gravis, renal disease, peptic ulcer, esophagitis
Do not confuse:
Decadron/Percodan
Pharmacokinetics:
PO: Onset 1 hr, peak 1-2 hr, duration 2½ days
IM: (acetate) Peak 8 hr, duration 6 days
Half-life 3-4½ hr
Interactions:
• Decreased action of dexamethasone: cholestyramine, colestipol, barbiturates, rifampin, ephedrine, phenytoin, theophylline, antacids
• Decreased effects of anticoagulants, anticonvulsants, antidiabetics, ambenonium, neostigmine, isoniazid, toxoids, vaccines, anticholinesterases, salicylates, somatrem
• Increased side effects: alcohol, salicylates, indomethacin, amphotericin B, digitalis, cyclosporine, diuretics
• Increased action of dexamethasone: salicylates, estrogens, indomethacin, oral contraceptives, ketoconazole, macrolide antiinfectives
🖊 Potassium deficiency: aloe, buckthorn bark/berry, cascara sagrada bark, ephedra, senna pod/leaf
Lab test interferences:
Increase: Cholesterol, Na, blood glucose, uric acid, Ca, urine glucose
Decrease: Ca, K, T₄, T₃, thyroid ^{131}I uptake test, urine 17-OHCS, 17-KS, PBI skin allergy tests

NURSING CONSIDERATIONS
Assess:
• K, blood sugar, urine glucose while on long-term therapy; hypokalemia and hyperglycemia
• Weight daily; notify prescriber of weekly gain >5 lb
• B/P q4h, pulse; notify prescriber of chest pain
• I&O ratio; be alert for decreasing urinary output, increasing edema
• Plasma cortisol levels during long-term therapy (normal: 138-635 nmol/L SI units when drawn at 8 AM)
• Infection: fever, WBC even after withdrawal of medication; drug masks infection
• Potassium depletion: paresthesias, fatigue, nausea, vomiting, depression, polyuria, dysrhythmias, weakness
• Edema, hypertension, cardiac symptoms
• Mental status: affect, mood, behavioral changes, aggression
Administer:
• Titrated dose; use lowest effective dose
• IM inj deeply in large muscle mass; rotate sites; avoid deltoid; use 21G needle
• In one dose in AM to prevent adrenal suppression; avoid SC administration, may damage tissue
• With food or milk to decrease GI symptoms
IV
• Undiluted direct over 1 min or less or diluted with 0.9% NaCl or D₅W and give as an IV INF at prescribed rate
• After shaking suspension (parenteral); do not give suspension IV
Dexamethasone sodium phosphate
Additive compatibilities: Aminophylline, bleomycin, cimetidine,

floxacillin, furosemide, granisetron, lidocaine, meropenem, mitomycin, nafcillin, netilmicin, ondansetron, prochlorperazine, ranitidine, verapamil

Syringe compatibilities: Granisetron, metoclopramide, ranitidine, sufentanil

Y-site compatibilities: Acyclovir, allopurinol, amifostine, amikacin, amphotericin B cholesteryl, amsacrine, aztreonam, cefepime, cefpirome, cisatracurium, cisplatin, cladribine, cyclophosphamide, cytarabine, doxorubicin, doxorubicin liposome, famotidine, filgrastim, fluconazole, fludarabine, foscarnet, granisetron, heparin, lorazepam, melphalan, meperidine, meropenem, morphine, ondansetron, paclitaxel, piperacillin/tazobactam, potassium chloride, propofol, remifentanil, sargramostim, sodium bicarbonate, sufentanil, tacrolimus, teniposide, theophylline, thiotepa, vinorelbine, vit B/C, zidovudine

Perform/provide:
• Assistance with ambulation in patient with bone tissue disease to prevent fractures

Evaluate:
• Therapeutic response: ease of respirations, decreased inflammation

Teach patient/family:
• That ID as steroid user should be carried
• To notify prescriber if therapeutic response decreases; dosage adjustment may be needed
◆ Not to discontinue abruptly or adrenal crisis can result
• Symptoms of adrenal insufficiency: nausea, anorexia, fatigue, dizziness, dyspnea, weakness, joint pain
• To avoid OTC products: salicylates, alcohol in cough products, cold preparations unless directed by prescriber

• To teach patient all aspects of drug usage, including cushingoid symptoms; to notify health-care provider of infection

---

dexmedetomidine
Precedex
Func. class.: Sedative, α_2 adrenoceptor agonist

Action: Produces α_2 activity seen at low and moderate doses, also α_1 at high doses

Uses: Sedation in mechanically ventilated, intubated patients ICU

Research note: One study has concluded that more research is needed before wider applications of this drug can be pursued[7]

Dosage and routes:
• *Adult:* **IV** loading dose of 1 µg/kg over 10 min then 0.2-0.7 µg/kg/hr, do not use for more than 24 hr
Available forms: Inj 100 µg/ml

Side effects/adverse reactions:
GI: Nausea, thirst
GU: Oliguria
CV: Bradycardia, hypotension, hypertension, *atrial fibrillation, infarction*
RESP: Pulmonary edema, pleural effusion, hypoxia
HEMA: Leukocytosis, anemia

Contraindications: Hypersensitivity

Precautions: Elderly, respiratory depression, severe respiratory disorders, cardiac dysrhythmias, pregnancy (C), lactation, children, renal disease

Pharmacokinetics: Rapid distribution, excreted in urine; metabolized in liver

Interactions:
• Increased CNS depression: alcohol, opioids, sedative/hypnotics, antipsychotics, skeletal muscle relaxants, inhalational anesthetics

---

◆ = Nursing alert   🌿 = Herb-drug interaction   🚫 = Do not crush

NURSING CONSIDERATIONS
Assess:
- Injection site: phlebitis, burning, stinging
- ECG for changes: atrial fibrillation
- CNS changes: movement, jerking, tremors, dizziness, LOC, pupil reaction
- Respiratory dysfunction: respiratory depression, character, rate, rhythm; notify prescriber if respirations are <10/min

Administer:
IV
- After diluting with D_5W 0.9% NaCl, withdraw 2 ml of drug and add to 48 ml of 0.9% NaCl to a total of 50 ml, shake to mix well
- Only with resuscitative equipment available
- Only by qualified persons trained in ICU sedation

Solution compatibilities: LR, D_5W, 0.9% NaCl, 20% mannitol

Additive compatibilities: Thiopental, etomidate, vecuronium, pancuronium, succinylcholine, atracurium, mivacurium, glycopyrrolate, phenylephrine, atropine, midazolam, morphine, fentanyl

Perform/provide:
- Safety measures: side rails, nightlight, call bell within easy reach

Evaluate:
- Therapeutic response: induction of anesthesia

---

dexmethylphenidate
See appendix a—selected new drugs

---

dextran 40 (℞)
(deks′tran)
Dextran 40, Gentran 40, LMD 10%, Rheomacrodex
Func. class.: Plasma volume expander
Chem. class.: Low molecular weight polysaccharide

Action: Similar to human albumin, which expands plasma volume by drawing fluid from interstitial space to intravascular space

Uses: Expand plasma volume, prophylaxis of embolism, thrombosis

Dosage and routes:
Shock
- *Adult:* **IV INF** 500 ml over 15-30 min, total dose in 24 hr not to exceed 20 ml/kg; subsequent doses given slowly; if given >24 hr, not to exceed 10 ml/kg/day; not to exceed therapy >5 days

Thrombosis/embolism
- *Adult:* **IV INF** 500-1000 ml, then 500 ml/day × 3 days, then 500 ml q2-3 days × 2 wk if needed

Available forms: 10% dextran 40/D_5W, 10% dextran 40/0.9% NaCl

Side effects/adverse reactions:
HEMA: Decreased hematocrit, platelet function; ***increased bleeding/coagulation times***
INTEG: Rash, urticaria, pruritus, ***angioedema,*** chills, fever, flushing
RESP: Wheezing, dyspnea, ***bronchospasm, pulmonary edema***
CV: Hypotension, ***cardiac arrest***
GU: ***Osmotic nephrosis, renal failure, stasis,*** hyponatremia
GI: Nausea, vomiting, increased AST, ALT
SYST: ***Anaphylaxis***
Contraindications: Hypersensitiv-

---

ity, renal failure, CHF (severe), extreme dehydration

Precautions: Active hemorrhage, pregnancy (C)

Pharmacokinetics:

IV: Expands blood vol 1-2 × amount infused; excreted in urine and feces

Interactions:

• Incompatible with chlortetracycline, phytonadione, promethazine

Lab test interferences:

False increase: Blood glucose, urinary protein, bilirubin, total protein

Interference: Rh test, blood typing/crossmatching

NURSING CONSIDERATIONS

Assess:

• VS q5min × 30 min; Hgb/Hct, if falling by 30%, notify prescriber

• CVP during infusion (5-10 cm H_2O—normal range)

• Urine output q1h; watch for increase in urinary output (common); if output does not increase, decrease or discontinue infusion

• I&O ratio and specific gravity, urine osmolarity; if specific gravity is very low, renal clearance is low; drug should be discontinued

• Allergy: rash, urticaria, pruritus, wheezing, dyspnea, bronchospasm, drug should be discontinued immediately

◆ Circulatory overload: increased pulse, respirations, SOB, wheezing, chest tightness, chest pain

• Dehydration after infusion: decreased output, decreased specific gravity of urine, increased temp, poor skin turgor, increased specific gravity, dry skin

Administer:

IV

• After prescribed dilution; may give inital 500 mg at 15-30 min; distribute remainder of daily dose over 8-24 hr

• After crossmatch is drawn, if blood is to be given also

• D_5W sol in heart failure patients as ordered

Additive compatibilities: Cloxacillin

Y-site compatibilities: Enalaprilat, famotidine

Perform/provide:

• Storage at constant temperature (15°-30° C [59°-86° F]); discard unused portions, protect from freezing

Evaluate:

• Therapeutic response: increased plasma volume

---

dextran 70/75 (R)

(deks'tran)

Dextran 75, Gentran 70, Gentran 75, Macrodex

Func. class.: Plasma volume expander

Chem. class.: High molecular weight polysaccharide

Action: Similar to human albumin, which expands plasma volume by drawing fluid from interstitial spaces to intravascular space

Uses: Expand plasma volume in hypovolemic shock or impending shock

Dosage and routes:

• *Adult:* **IV INF** 500-1000 ml not to exceed 20-40 ml/min, not to exceed 10 ml/kg/24 hr if therapy >24 hr

Available forms: 70/75 dextran in 0.9% NaCl, D_5%

Side effects/adverse reactions:

HEMA: Decreased hematocrit, platelet function; *increased bleeding/coagulation times*

INTEG: Rash, urticaria, pruritus, *angioedema*, chills, fever, flushing

RESP: Wheezing, dyspnea, *bronchospasm, pulmonary edema*

◆ = Nursing alert　　🌿 = Herb-drug interaction　　🚫 = Do not crush

CV: Hypotension, ***cardiac arrest***

GU: ***Osmotic nephrosis, renal failure, stasis,*** hypernatremia

GI: Nausea, vomiting, increased AST, ALT

SYST: ***Anaphylaxis***

Contraindications: Hypersensitivity, renal failure, CHF (severe), extreme dehydration

Precautions: Active hemorrhage, pregnancy (C)

Pharmacokinetics:

IV: Onset within mins, duration 12 hr, expands blood vol 1-2 × amount infused; excreted in urine, feces

Lab test interferences:

False increase: Blood glucose, urinary protein, bilirubin, total protein

Interference: Rh test, blood typing/crossmatching

NURSING CONSIDERATIONS

Assess:

• VS q5min × 30 min; Hgb/Hct, if falling by 30%, notify prescriber

• CVP during infusion (5-10 cm H_2O—normal range)

• Urine output q1h; watch for increase in urinary output (common); if output does not increase, decrease or discontinue infusion

• I&O ratio and specific gravity, urine osmolarity; if specific gravity is very low, renal clearance is low; drug should be discontinued

• Allergy: rash, urticaria, pruritus, wheezing, dyspnea, bronchospasm; drug should be discontinued immediately

◆ Circulatory overload: increased pulse, respirations, SOB, wheezing, chest tightness, chest pain

• Dehydration after infusion: decreased output, increased temp, poor skin turgor, increased specific gravity, dry skin

Administer:

• After prescribed dilution, may give inital 500 mg at 20-40 ml/min, reduce flow to lowest rate

• After crossmatch is drawn, if blood is to be given also

• D_5W sol in heart failure patients as ordered

D

Perform/provide:

• Storage at constant temperature (<25° C [77° F]); discard unused portions; do not use unless clear

Evaluate:

• Therapeutic response: increased plasma volume

---

dextroamphetamine (℞)

(dex-troe-am-fet′a-meen)
Dexedrine, dextroamphetamine, Dextrostat
Func. class.: Cerebral stimulant
Chem. class.: Amphetamine

Controlled Substance Schedule II

Action: Increases release of norepinephrine, dopamine in cerebral cortex to reticular activating system

Uses: Narcolepsy, attention deficit disorder with hyperactivity (ADHD)

Dosage and routes:

Narcolepsy

• *Adult:* **PO** 5-60 mg qd in divided doses

• *Child >12 yr:* **PO** 10 mg qd increasing by 10 mg/day at weekly intervals

• *Child 6-12 yr:* **PO** 5 mg qd increasing by 5 mg/wk (max 60 mg/day)

ADHD

• *Adult:* **PO** 5-60 mg/day in divided doses

• *Child >6 yr:* **PO** 5 mg qd-bid increasing by 5 mg/day at weekly intervals

Side effects: *italics* = common; ***bold italics*** = life-threatening

• *Child 3-6 yr:* **PO** 2.5 mg qd increasing by 2.5 mg/day at weekly intervals

Available forms: Tabs 5, 10 mg; caps sus rel 5, 10, 15 mg

Side effects/adverse reactions:

CNS: Hyperactivity, insomnia, restlessness, talkativeness, dizziness, headache, chills, stimulation, dysphoria, irritability, aggressiveness, tremor, dependence, addiction

GI: Anorexia, dry mouth, diarrhea, constipation, weight loss, metallic taste

GU: Impotence, change in libido

CV: Palpitations, tachycardia, hypertension, decrease in heart rate, *dysrhythmias*

INTEG: Urticaria

Contraindications: Hypersensitivity to sympathomimetic amines, hyperthyroidism, hypertension, glaucoma, severe arteriosclerosis, drug abuse, cardiovascular disease, anxiety

Precautions: Gilles de la Tourette's disorder, pregnancy (C), lactation, child <3 yr

Pharmacokinetics:

PO: Onset 30 min, peak 1-3 hr, duration 4-20 hr; metabolized by liver; urine excretion pH dependent; crosses placenta, breast milk; half-life 10-30 hr

Interactions:

◆ Hypertensive crisis: MAOIs or within 14 days of MAOIs

• Delayed absorption of: barbiturates, phenytoin

• Increased effect of dextroamphetamine: acetazolamide, antacids, sodium bicarbonate

• Increased CNS effect: haloperidol, tricyclics, phenothiazines

• Decreased effect of dextroamphetamine: ascorbic acid, ammonium chloride

• Decreased effect of: adrenergic blockers, antidiabetics

• Drug/food: increased amine effect: caffeine

NURSING CONSIDERATIONS

Assess:

• VS, B/P; this drug may reverse antihypertensives; check patients with cardiac disease often

• CBC, urinalysis; in diabetes: blood sugar, urine sugar; insulin changes may be required, since eating will decrease

• Height, growth rate in children; growth rate may be decreased

• Mental status: mood, sensorium, affect, stimulation, insomnia, irritability

• Tolerance or dependency: an increased amount may be used to get same effect; will develop after long-term use

• Overdose: pain, fever, dehydration, insomnia, hyperactivity

Administer:

• At least 6 hr before hs to avoid sleeplessness

Perform/provide:

• Gum, hard candy, frequent sips of water for dry mouth

Evaluate:

• Therapeutic response: increased CNS stimulation, decreased drowsiness

Teach patient/family:

🚫 Not to break, crush, or chew sus rel forms

• To decrease caffeine consumption (coffee, tea, cola, chocolate); may increase irritability, stimulation

• To avoid OTC preparations unless approved by prescriber

• To taper drug over several wk; depression, increased sleeping, lethargy

• To avoid alcohol ingestion

• To avoid hazardous activities until stabilized on medication

• To get needed rest; patient will feel more tired at end of day

Treatment of overdose: Adminis-

◆ = Nursing alert   🌿 = Herb-drug interaction   🚫 = Do not crush

ter fluids, hemodialysis or peritoneal dialysis; antihypertensive for increased B/P, ammonium Cl for increased excretion

dextromethorphan
(OTC)

(dex-troe-meth-or′fan)
Balminil DM*, Benylin DM*, Broncho-Grippol-DM*, Children's Hold, Creo-Terpin, Delsym, dextromethorphan, Hold DM, Koffex*, Neo-DM*, Orex DM*, Pertussin, Pertussin ES, Robidex*, Robitussin Cough Calmers, Robitussin Pediatric, Sedatuss*, St. Joseph Cough Suppressant, Scot-Tussin DM, Sucrets Cough Control, Suppress, Vicks Formula 44

Func. class.: Antitussive, nonnarcotic

Chem. class.: Levorphanol derivative

Action: Depresses cough center in medulla by direct effect

Uses: Nonproductive cough

Investigational uses: Neuropathy

Dosage and routes:
• *Adult and child ≥12 yr:* **PO** 10-20 mg q4h, or 30 mg q6-8h, not to exceed 120 mg/day; **SUS-REL LIQ** 60 mg q12h, not to exceed 120 mg/day
• *Child 6-12 yr:* **PO** 5-10 mg q4h; **SUS-REL LIQ** 30 mg bid, not to exceed 60 mg/day
• *Child 2-6 yr:* **PO** 2.5-5 mg q4h, or 7.5 mg q6-8h, not to exceed 30 mg/day

Neuropathy
• *Adult:* **PO** doses vary widely

Available forms: Loz 2.5, 5, 7.5, 15 mg; sol; liq 3.5 mg, 7.5, 15 mg/5 ml, 3.5, 5, 7.5, 10, 15 mg/5 ml; syr 15 mg/15 ml, 10 mg/5 ml; sus action liq equivalent to 30 mg/5 ml; caps 30 mg; ext rel susp 30 mg/5 ml

Side effects/adverse reactions:
CNS: Dizziness, sedation
GI: Nausea

Contraindications: Hypersensitivity, asthma/emphysema, productive cough

Precautions: Nausea/vomiting, fever, persistent headache, pregnancy (C)

Pharmacokinetics:
PO: Onset 15-30 min, duration 3-6 hr
SUS: Duration 12 hr

Interactions:
• Do not give with MAOIs or within 2 wk of MAOIs
• Increased CNS depression: alcohol, antidepressants, antihistamines, opioids, sedative/hypnotics
• Increased adverse reactions: amiodarone, fluoxetine, quinidine

NURSING CONSIDERATIONS
Assess:
• Cough: type, frequency, character, including sputum

Administer:
• Decreased dose to elderly patients; metabolism may be slowed

Perform/provide:
• Increased fluids to liquefy secretions
• Humidification of patient's room

Evaluate:
• Therapeutic response: absence of cough

Teach patient/family:
• To avoid driving, other hazardous activities until patient is stabilized on this medication
• To avoid smoking, smoke-filled rooms, perfumes, dust, environmental pollutants, cleaners that increase cough
• To avoid alcohol, CNS depressants
• To notify prescriber if cough persists over a few days

**dextrose
(D-glucose) (R̶)**
Glucose, Glutose, Insta-
Glucose
Func. class.: Caloric

Action: Needed for adequate utilization of amino acids; decreases protein, nitrogen loss; prevents ketosis
Uses: Increases intake of calories; increases fluids in patients unable to take adequate fluids, calories orally; acute hypoglycemia
Dosage and routes:
• *Adult and child:* **IV** depends on individual requirements
Available forms: Inj 2.5%, 5%, 10%, 20%, 30%, 40%, 50%, 60%, 70%; oral gel 40%; chew tab 5 g
Side effects/adverse reactions:
CNS: Confusion, *loss of consciousness,* dizziness
CV: Hypertension, *CHF, pulmonary edema*
GU: Glycosuria, osmotic diuresis
ENDO: Hyperglycemia, rebound hypoglycemia, hyperosmolar syndrome, hyperglycemic nonketotic syndrome
INTEG: Chills, flushing, warm feeling, rash, urticaria, extravasation necrosis
Contraindications: Hyperglycemia, delirium tremens, hemorrhage (cranial/spinal), CHF
Precautions: Renal, liver, cardiac disease, diabetes mellitus
Interactions:
• Increased fluid retention/electrolyte excretion: coricosteroids
NURSING CONSIDERATIONS
Assess:
• Electrolytes (K, Na, Ca, Cl, Mg), blood glucose, ammonia, phosphate
• Injection site for extravasation: redness along vein, edema at site,

necrosis, pain; hard, tender area; site should be changed immediately
• Monitor temp q4h for increased fever, indicating infection; if infection suspected, infusion is discontinued, tubing, bottle, catheter tip cultured
• Serum glucose in patients receiving hypotonic glucose 50% and over
• Nutritional status: calorie count by dietitian
Administer:
• Only (4%) protein and dextrose (up to 12.5%) via peripheral vein; stronger sol: central IV administration
• May be given undiluted via prepared sol; give 10% sol, 5 ml/15 sec; 10% sol, 1000 ml/3 hr or more; 20% sol, 500 ml/½-1 hr; 50% sol, 10 ml/min; control rate, rapid infusions may cause fluid shifts
• Oral glucose preparations (gel, chew tabs) are to be used in conscious patients only; check serum blood glucose after first dose
• After changing IV catheter, dressing q24h with aseptic technique
Evaluate:
• Therapeutic response: increased weight
Teach patient/family:
• The reason for dextrose infusion
• To review hypoglycemia/hyperglycemia symptoms
• To review blood glucose monitoring procedure

---

dezocine (R̶)
(dez'oh-seen)
Dalgan
Func. class.: Narcotic agonist-antagonist analgesic
Chem. class.: Opioid, synthetic
Action: Depresses pain impulse transmission at the spinal cord level by interacting with opioid receptors

---

⬥ = Nursing alert   ∥ = Herb-drug interaction   ⃠ = Do not crush

Uses: Severe pain
Dosage and routes:
• *Adult:* **IM** 5-20 mg q3-6h, not to exceed 120 mg/day; **IV** 2.5-10 mg q2-4h
Available forms: Inj 5, 10, 15 mg/ml single-dose vials, multiple dose 10 mg/ml
Side effects/adverse reactions:
CV: Hypotension, pulse irregularity, hypertension, chest pain, pallor, edema, thrombophlebitis, bradycardia
CNS: Drowsiness, dizziness, confusion, sedation, anxiety, headache, depression, delirium, sleep disturbances, dependency, euphoria
GI: Nausea, vomiting, anorexia, constipation, cramps, abdominal pain, dry mouth, diarrhea
INTEG: Injection site reactions, pruritus, rash, sweating, chills
RESP: **Respiratory depression,** hiccups
GU: Urinary frequency, hesitancy, retention
EENT: Blurred vision, slurred speech, diplopia, miosis
Contraindications: Hypersensitivity
Precautions: Addictive personality, pregnancy (C), lactation, increased intracranial pressure, respiratory depression, hepatic disease, renal disease, children <18 yr, elderly, biliary surgery, COPD, sulfite sensitivity
Pharmacokinetics:
IM: Onset 30 min, peak 50-90 min, duration 2-4 hr
IV: Onset 10 min, peak 30 min, duration 2-4 hr
Metabolized by liver; excreted by kidneys; may cross placenta
Interactions:
• Incompatibility: not known
• Increased CNS depression: alcohol, narcotics, sedative/hypnotics, antipsychotics, skeletal muscle relaxants, general anesthetics, tranquilizers
NURSING CONSIDERATIONS
Assess:
• I&O ratio; decreasing output may indicate urinary retention
• CNS changes: dizziness, drowsiness, hallucinations, euphoria, LOC, pupil reaction
• Allergic reactions: rash, urticaria
• Respiratory dysfunction: respiratory depression, character, rate, rhythm of respirations; notify prescriber if <10/min, shallow
• Need for pain medication, physical dependence
Administer:
• Undiluted 5 mg or less over 2-3 min
• With antiemetic if nausea, vomiting occur
• When pain is beginning to return; determine dosage interval by patient response
Perform/provide:
• Storage in light-resistant area at room temperature
• Assistance with ambulation
• Safety measures: top side rails, night-light, call bell in easy reach
Evaluate:
• Therapeutic response: decrease in pain
Teach patient/family:
• To report any symptoms of CNS changes, allergic reactions
• That physical dependency may result after extended use
• That withdrawal symptoms may occur: nausea, vomiting, cramps, fever, faintness, anorexia
Treatment of overdose: Naloxone 0.2-0.8 mg IV, O_2, IV fluids, vasopressors

diazepam (℞)

(dye-az'-e-pam)
Apo-Diazepam*, Diastat,
Diazemuls*, diazepam,
Novodiapam*, PMS-
Diazepam*, Valium,
Valrelease, Vivol*
Func. class.: Antianxiety, anti-
convulsant, skeletal muscle re-
laxant, central acting
Chem. class.: Benzodiazepine

Controlled Substance Schedule IV
Action: Potentiates the actions of
GABA, especially in limbic system,
reticular formation; enhances pre-
sympathetic inhibition, inhibits spi-
nal polysynaptic afferent paths
Uses: Anxiety, acute alcohol with-
drawal, adjunct in seizure disor-
ders; preoperatively as a relaxant,
skeletal muscle relaxation; rectally
for acute repetitive seizures
Investigational uses: Panic attacks
Dosage and routes:
Anxiety/convulsive disorders
• *Adult:* **PO** 2-10 mg bid-qid; **EXT
REL** 15-30 mg qd
• *Geriatric:* **PO** 1-2 mg qd-bid, in-
crease slowly as needed
• *Child >6 mo:* **PO** 1-2.5 mg tid-qid
Muscle relaxation
• *Adult:* **PO** 2-10 mg tid-qid or ext
rel 15-30 mg qd; **IV/IM** 5-10 mg
repeat in 2-4 hr
• *Geriatric:* **PO** 2-5 mg bid-qid;
IV/IM 2-5 mg, may repeat in 2-4 hr
Tetanic muscle spasms
• *Child <5 yr:* **IM/IV** 5-10 mg q3-4h
prn
• *Infant >30 days:* **IM/IV** 1-2 mg
q3-4h prn
Status epilepticus
• *Adult:* **IV BOL** 5-20 mg, 2 mg/
min, may repeat q5-10min, not to
exceed 60 mg; may repeat in 30 min
if seizures reappear

• *Child:* **IV BOL** 0.1-0.3 mg/kg
(1 mg/min over 3 min); may repeat
q15min × 2 doses
• *Adult:* **RECT** 0.2 mg/kg, may repeat 4-12 hr later
• *Child 6-11 yr:* **RECT** 0.3 mg/kg,
may repeat 4-12 hr later
• *Child 2-5 yr:* **RECT** 0.5 mg/kg,
may repeat 4-12 hr later
Alcohol withdrawal
• *Adult:* **PO** 10 mg tid-qid in 1st 24
hr, then 5 mg tid-qid; **IV/IM** 10 mg,
then 5-10 mg after 3 hr
Available forms: Tabs 2, 5, 10 mg;
caps ext rel 15 mg; inj emulsified 5
mg/ml; oral sol 5 mg/5 ml; gel, rectal delivery system 2.5, 10, 15, 20
mg, twin packs; sterile emulsion for
inj 5 mg/ml
Side effects/adverse reactions:
HEMA: **Neutropenia**
RESP: **Respiratory depression**
CNS: Dizziness, drowsiness, confusion, headache, anxiety, tremors,
stimulation, fatigue, depression, insomnia, hallucinations
CV: Orthostatic hypotension, **ECG
changes, tachycardia,** hypotension
EENT: Blurred vision, tinnitus, mydriasis
GI: Constipation, dry mouth, nausea, vomiting, anorexia, diarrhea
INTEG: Rash, dermatitis, itching
Contraindications: Hypersensitivity to benzodiazepines, narrow-angle
glaucoma, psychosis, pregnancy (D),
lactation, coma, respiratory depression
Precautions: Elderly, debilitated,
hepatic disease, renal disease, addiction
Do not confuse:
diazepam/Ditropan
Pharmacokinetics:
PO: Rapidly absorbed; onset ½ hr,
duration 2-3 hr
IM: Onset 15-30 min, duration 1-1½
hr; absorption slow and erratic

◆ = Nursing alert   ∥ = Herb-drug interaction   ⊘ = Do not crush

IV: Onset immediate, duration 15 min

Metabolized by liver, excreted by kidneys, crosses placenta, excreted in breast milk, crosses the blood-brain barrier; half-life 20-50 hr, more reliable by mouth

Interactions:

• Increased toxicity: barbiturates, SSRIs, cimetidine, CNS depressants, valproic acid

• Decreased metabolism of diazepam: oral contraceptives, valproic acid, disulfiram, isoniazid, propranolol

• Increased CNS depression: CNS depressants, alcohol

🌿 Increased action of diazepam: kava

Lab test interferences:

Increase: AST/ALT, serum bilirubin

False increase: 17-OHCS

Decrease: RAIU

NURSING CONSIDERATIONS
Assess:

• B/P (lying, standing), pulse; respiratory rate; if systolic B/P drops 20 mm Hg, hold drug, notify prescriber; respirations q5-15min if given IV

• Blood studies: CBC during long-term therapy; blood dyscrasias (rare)

• Degree of anxiety; what precipitates anxiety and whether drug controls symptoms

• For alcohol withdrawal symptoms, including hallucinations (visual, auditory), delirium, irritability, agitation, fine to coarse tremors

• For seizure control and type, duration, intensity of convulsions

• Hepatic studies: AST, ALT, bilirubin, creatinine, LDH, alk phosphatase

• IV site for thrombosis or phlebitis, which may occur rapidly

• Mental status: mood, sensorium, affect, sleeping pattern, drowsiness, dizziness

• Physical dependency, withdrawal symptoms: headache, nausea, vomiting, muscle pain, weakness after long-term use

• Suicidal tendencies

Administer:

• With food or milk for GI symptoms; crushed if patient is unable to swallow medication whole; do not crush ext rel capsules

• Sugarless gum, hard candy, frequent sips of water for dry mouth

• Reduced opioid dose by ⅓ if given concomitantly with diazepam

IV

• Into large vein; give IV 5 mg or less/1 min or total dose over 3 min or more (children, infants); continuous infusion is not recommended

Additive compatibilities: Netilmicin, verapamil

Syringe compatibilities: Cimetidine

Y-site compatibilities: Cefmetazole, dobutamine, nafcillin, quinidine, sufentanil

Sterile emulsion for INJ

• Use IV only, within 6 hr, flush line after use and after 6 hr

Rectal

• Do not use more than 5 ×/mo or for an episode q5d

Perform/provide:

• Assistance with ambulation during beginning therapy, for drowsiness, dizziness, safety measures

• Check to see PO medication has been swallowed

Evaluate:

• Therapeutic response: decreased anxiety, restlessness, insomnia

Teach patient/family:

• That drug may be taken with food

• That drug is not to be used for everyday stress or used longer than 4 mo unless directed by prescriber;

no more than prescribed amount; may be habit forming
• To avoid OTC preparations unless approved by prescriber
• To avoid driving, activities that require alertness; drowsiness may occur
• To avoid alcohol, other psychotropic medications unless directed by prescriber; that smoking may decrease diazepam effect
• Not to discontinue medication abruptly after long-term use
• To rise slowly or fainting may occur, especially in elderly
• That drowsiness may worsen at beginning of treatment
• To avoid use during pregnancy
🚫 Not to break, crush, or chew ext rel caps

Treatment of overdose: Lavage, VS, supportive care, flumazenil

---

diazoxide (R)
(dye-az-ox′ide)
diazoxide parenteral,
Hyperstat IV
Func. class.: Antihypertensive
Chem. class.: Vasodilator

Action: Vasodilates arteriolar smooth muscle by direct relaxation; a reduction in blood pressure with concomitant increases in heart rate, cardiac output; reduces release of insulin from the pancreas
Uses: Hypertensive crisis when urgent decrease of diastolic pressure required; increase blood glucose levels in hyperinsulinism
Dosage and routes:
Hypoglycemia
• *Adult and child:* **PO** 3-8 mg/kg/day in 2-3 divided doses q8-12h
• *Infants and neonates:* **PO** 8-15 mg/kg/day in 2-3 divided doses 8-12h

Hypertension
• *Adult:* **IV BOL** 1-3 mg/kg rapidly up to a max of 150 mg in a single injection; dose may be repeated at 5-15 min intervals until desired response is achieved; give IV in 30 sec or less
• *Child:* **IV BOL** 1-2 mg/kg rapidly; administration same as adult, not to exceed 150 mg
Available forms: Caps 50 mg; oral susp 50 mg/ml; inj 15 mg/ml, 300 mg/20 ml
Side effects/adverse reactions:
CV: **Hypotension,** T-wave changes, angina pectoris, palpitations, *supraventricular tachycardia, edema,* rebound hypertension, *shock, MI*
CNS: **Headache,** sleepiness, euphoria, anxiety, EPS, confusion, tinnitus, blurred vision, dizziness, weakness, *seizures, cerebral ischemia, paralysis*
GI: Nausea, vomiting, dry mouth
INTEG: Rash
HEMA: Decreased hemoglobin, Hct, *thrombocytopenia*
GU: Breast tenderness; increased BUN, fluid, electrolyte imbalances; Na, water retention
ENDO: Hyperglycemia in diabetics, transient hyperglycemia in nondiabetics
Contraindications: Hypersensitivity to thiazides, sulfonamides, hypertension of aortic coarctation or AV shunt, pheochromocytoma, dissecting aortic aneurysm
Precautions: Tachycardia, fluid, electrolyte imbalances, pregnancy (C), lactation, impaired cerebral or cardiac circulation, children
Pharmacokinetics:
IV: Onset 1-2 min, peak 5 min, duration 3-12 hr; *PO:* onset 1 hr, peak 8-12 hr, duration 8 hr, half-life 20-36 hr, excreted slowly in urine, crosses blood-brain barrier, placenta

---

Interactions:
- Severe hypotension: antihypertensives
- Increased hyperuricemic, antihypertensive effects of diazoxide: thiazide diuretics
- Hyperglycemia: sulfonylureas
- Decreased anticonvulsant effect: hydantoins

NURSING CONSIDERATIONS
Assess:
- B/P q5min until stabilized, then q1h × 2 hr, then q4h
- Pulse, jugular venous distention q4h
- Electrolytes, blood studies: K, Na, Cl, CO_2, CBC, serum glucose
- Weight daily, I&O
- Edema in feet, legs daily
- Skin turgor, mucous membranes for hydration status
- Rales, dyspnea, orthopnea
- IV site for extravasation
- Signs of CHF: dyspnea, edema, wet rales
- Postural hypotension, take B/P sitting, standing

Administer:
- Undiluted; give over ½ min or less
- To patient in recumbent position; keep in that position for 1 hr after administration

Syringe compatibilities: Heparin
Perform/provide:
- Storage protected from light

Evaluate:
- Therapeutic response: decreased B/P, primarily diastolic pressure

Treatment of overdose: Dopamine, or norepinephrine for hypotension, Trendelenburg maneuver

diclofenac potassium (℞)
(dye-kloe'fen-ak)
Cataflam, Voltaren Rapide*

diclofenac sodium
Apo-Dilo*, Novo-Difenac*, Nu-Diclo, Voltaren, Voltaren-Sr

Func. class.: Nonsteroidal antiinflammatory, nonopioid analgesic
Chem. class.: Phenylacetic acid

Action: Inhibits prostaglandin synthesis by decreasing enzyme needed for biosynthesis; analgesic, antiinflammatory, antipyretic

Uses: Acute, chronic rheumatoid arthritis, osteoarthritis; ankylosing spondylitis, analgesia, primary dysmenorrhea; ophthalmic: postoperative inflammation after cataract extraction

Dosage and routes:
Osteoarthritis
- *Adult:* **PO** 100-150 mg/day in 2-3 divided doses (potassium)

Rheumatoid arthritis
- *Adult:* **PO** 150-200 mg/day in 2-4 divided doses (potassium); 50 mg tid-qid, then reduce to lowest dose needed (25 mg tid) (sodium)

Ankylosing spondylitis
- *Adult:* **PO** 100-125 mg/day in 4-5 divided doses, give 25 mg qid and 25 mg hs if needed (potassium)

Postcataract surgery
- *Adult:* **OPHTH** 1 gtt of 0.1% sol qid × 2 wk 24 hr post surgery

Analgesia/primary dysmenorrhea
- *Adult:* **PO** 50 mg tid, max 150 mg/day (potassium)

Available forms: Potassium: tabs 50, 75 mg; sodium: tabs delayed rel (enteric-coated) 25, 50, 75 mg; ext rel tabs 75, 100 mg; supp 50, 100 mg

---

Side effects/adverse reactions:
*SYST: **Anaphylaxis***
GI: Nausea, anorexia, vomiting, diarrhea, ***jaundice, cholestatic hepatitis,*** constipation, flatulence, cramps, dry mouth, peptic ulcer, GI bleeding, ***hepatotoxicity***
CNS: Dizziness, headache, drowsiness, fatigue, tremors, confusion, insomnia, anxiety, depression, nervousness, paresthesia, muscle weakness
*CV: **CHF,*** tachycardia, peripheral edema, palpitations, ***dysrhythmias,*** hypotension, hypertension, fluid retention
INTEG: Purpura, rash, pruritus, sweating, erythema, petechiae, photosensitivity, alopecia
*GU: **Nephrotoxicity: dysuria, hematuria, oliguria, azotemia, cystitis, UTI***
*HEMA: **Blood dyscrasias,*** epistaxis, bruising
EENT: Tinnitus, hearing loss, blurred vision, ***laryngeal edema***
RESP: Dyspnea, hemoptysis, pharyngitis, ***bronchospasm,*** rhinitis, shortness of breath
Contraindications: Hypersensitivity to aspirin, iodides, other nonsteroidal antiinflammatory agents, asthma
Precautions: Pregnancy (B) 1st trimester; lactation, children, bleeding disorders, GI disorders, cardiac disorders, hypersensitivity to other antiinflammatory agents, CrCl <30 ml/min
Do not confuse:
Cataflam/Catapres
Pharmacokinetics:
PO: Peak 2-3 hr, elimination half-life 1-2 hr, 90% bound to plasma proteins, metabolized in liver to metabolite, excreted in urine
Interactions:
• Decreased antihypertensive effect: β-blockers, diuretics

• Increased anticoagulant effect: anticoagulants
• Increased toxicity: phenytoin, lithium, cyclosporine, methotrexate
• Increased GI side effects: aspirin, other NSAIDs
• GI toxicity: aspirin
• Hyperkalemia: potassium-sparing diuretics
• Need for dosage adjustment: antidiabetics
NURSING CONSIDERATIONS
Assess:
• For pain: location, character, aggravating, alleviating factors, ROM, before and 1 hr after dose
• Blood counts during therapy; watch for decreasing platelets; if low, therapy may need to be discontinued, restarted after hematologic recovery
• For clients with asthma, aspirin hypersensitivity, nasal polyps; may develop hypersensitivity
• LFTs (may be elevated) and uric acid (may be decreased—serum; increased—urine) periodically; also BUN, creatinine, electrolytes (may be elevated)
◆ Blood dyscrasias (thrombocytopenia): bruising, fatigue, bleeding, poor healing
Evaluate:
• Therapeutic response: decreased inflammation in joints, decreased inflammation after cataract surgery
Teach patient/family:
• That drug must be continued for prescribed time to be effective; to contact prescriber prior to surgery as when to discontinue this drug
• To report bleeding, bruising, fatigue, malaise; blood dyscrasias do occur
🚫 Not to break, crush, or chew enteric products
• To avoid aspirin, alcoholic beverages, NSAIDs, acetaminophen, or

other OTC medications unless approved by prescriber

• To take with food, milk, or antacids to avoid GI upset, to swallow whole

• To use caution when driving; drowsiness, dizziness may occur

• To take with a full glass of water to enhance absorption, remain upright for ½ hr; if dose is missed, take as soon as remembered within 2 hr if taking 1-2 ×/day, do not double doses

• To report hepatotoxicity: flulike symptoms, nausea, vomiting, jaundice, pruritus, lethargy

• To use sunscreen to prevent photosensitivity

---

dicloxacillin (℞)

(dye-klox-a-sill'-in)
dicloxacillin sodium, Dycill, Dynapen, Pathocil
Func. class.: Antiinfective
Chem. class.: Penicillinase-resistant penicillin

Action: Interferes with cell wall replication of susceptible organisms; osmotically unstable cell wall swells, bursts from osmotic pressure

Uses: Effective for gram-positive cocci (*Staphylococcus aureus, Streptococcus pyogenes, S. viridans, S. faecalis, S. bovis, S. pneumoniae*), infections caused by penicillinase-producing *Staphylococcus*

Dosage and routes:

• *Adult/child ≥40 kg:* **PO** 0.5-4 g/day in divided doses q6h, max 4 g/day

• *Child ≤40 kg:* **PO** 12.5-50 mg/kg in divided doses q6h, max 4 g/day

Available forms: Caps 125, 250, 500 mg; powder for oral susp 62.5 mg/5 ml

Side effects/adverse reactions:

HEMA: Anemia, increased bleeding time, **bone marrow depression, granulocytopenia**

GI: Nausea, vomiting, diarrhea, increased AST, ALT, abdominal pain, glossitis, **pseudomembranous colitis**

GU: **Oliguria, proteinuria, hematuria,** *vaginitis, moniliasis,* **glomerulonephritis**

CNS: Lethargy, hallucinations, anxiety, depression, twitching, **coma, convulsions**

SYST: **Anaphylaxis**

Contraindications: Hypersensitivity to penicillins; neonates

Precautions: Hypersensitivity to cephalosporins, pregnancy (B), lactation, severe renal or hepatic disease

Do not confuse:

Pathocil/Bactocil

Pharmacokinetics:

PO: Peak 1 hr, duration 4-6 hr, half-life 30-60 min; metabolized in liver; excreted in urine, bile, breast milk; crosses placenta

Interactions:

• Increased dicloxacillin concentrations: aspirin, probenecid, oral contraceptives

• Increased effect of anticoagulants

• Food/drug: citric juices/food decrease absorption of dicloxacillin

🍃 Delayed/reduced absorption: khat, separate by 2 hr

Lab test interferences:

False positive: Urine glucose, urine protein

NURSING CONSIDERATIONS

Assess:

• I&O ratio; report hematuria, oliguria, since penicillin in high doses is nephrotoxic

◆ Any patient with compromised renal system, since drug is excreted slowly in poor renal system function; toxicity may occur rapidly

---

- Blood studies: WBC, RBC, Hgb, Hct, bleeding time
- Renal studies: urinalysis, protein, blood
- C&S before drug therapy; drug may be given as soon as culture is taken
- WBC and differential, ALT, AST, BUN, creatinine for patients on long-term therapy
- Bowel pattern before, during treatment
- Anaphylaxis: pruritus, rash, dyspnea, laryngeal edema; have emergency equipment available; skin eruptions after administration of penicillin to 1 wk after discontinuing drug
- For infection: temp, draining wounds, WBC, sputum, urine, stool, before, during treatment

Administer:
- Drug after C&S
- On an empty stomach with a full glass of water
- Susp after shaking well before each dose

Perform/provide:
- Adrenalin, suction, tracheostomy set, endotracheal intubation equipment
- Adequate fluid intake (2 L) during diarrhea episodes
- Scratch test to assess allergy after securing order from prescriber; usually done when penicillin is only drug of choice
- Storage in tight container; after reconstituting, store in refrigerator up to 2 wk

Evaluate:
- Therapeutic response: absence of fever, draining wounds

Teach patient/family:
- All aspects of drug therapy, including need to complete course of medication to ensure organism death (10-14 days); culture may be taken after completed course

- To report sore throat, fever, fatigue; may indicate superinfection
- 🚫 Not to break, crush, or chew caps
- To wear or carry Medic Alert ID if allergic to penicillins
- To notify prescriber of diarrhea, fever

Treatment of anaphylaxis: Withdraw drug; maintain airway; administer epinephrine, aminophylline, O_2, IV corticosteroids

---

RARELY USED

dicyclomine (℞)

(dye-sye'kloe-meen)
Antispas, Bentyl, Bentylol*, Byclomine, Dibent, dicyclomine HCL, Dilomine, Di-Spaz, Formulex*, Lomine*, Neoquess, Or-Tyl, Spasmoject
Func. class.: Gastrointestinal anticholinergic

Uses: Treatment of peptic ulcer disease in combination with other drugs; infant colic, urinary incontinence

Dosage and routes:
- *Adult:* **PO** 10-20 mg tid-qid; **IM** 20 mg q4-6h
- *Child >2 yr:* **PO** 10 mg tid-qid
- *Child 6 mo-2 yr:* **PO** 5 mg tid-qid

Contraindications: Hypersensitivity to anticholinergics, narrow-angle glaucoma, GI obstruction, myasthenia gravis, paralytic ileus, GI atony, toxic megacolon

---

◆ = Nursing alert   🌿 = Herb-drug interaction   🚫 = Do not crush

didanosine (℞)

(dye-dan'oh-seen)

ddl, dideoxyinosine, Videx, Videx EC

Func. class.: Antiretroviral

Chem. class.: Nucleoside reverse transcriptase inhibitor

Action: Nucleoside analog incorporating into cellular DNA by viral reverse transcriptase, thereby terminating the cellular DNA chain

Uses: HIV infection in combination with other antiretrovirals

Dosage and routes:

• Reduce dosage CrCl <60 ml/min

• *Adult:* **PO** >60 kg, 200 mg bid tabs, or 250 mg bid buffered pwd; caps, del rel 400 mg qd; <60 kg, 125 mg bid tabs, or 167 mg bid buffered pwd; caps, del rel 250 mg qd

• *Child:* **PO** tabs 90-120 mg/m^2 q12h; buffered pwd packets 112.5-150 mg/m^2 q12h; **PO** (child BSA 1.1-1.4 m^2) tab 100 mg q8-12h; recon pedi pwd 125 mg q8-12h; **PO** (child BSA 0.8-1 m^2) tabs 75 mg q8-12h; recon pedi pwd 94 mg q8-12h; **PO** (child BSA 0.5-0.7 m^2) tabs 50 mg q8-12h; recon pedi pwd 62 mg q8-12h; **PO** (child BSA <0.4 m^2) tabs 25 mg q8-12h; recon pedi pwd 31 mg q8-12h

Available forms: Tabs, buffered, chewable/dispersible 25, 50, 100, 150 mg; pwd for oral sol, buffered 100, 167, 250, 375 mg/packet; pwd for oral sol, pedi 10 mg, 20 mg/ml; caps, del rel 125, 200, 250, 400

Side effects/adverse reactions:

GI: **Pancreatitis,** *diarrhea, nausea,* vomiting, *abdominal pain,* constipation, stomatitis, dyspepsia, liver abnormalities, flatulence, taste perversion, dry mouth, oral thrush, melena, increased ALT, AST, alk phosphatase, amylase, **hepatic failure**

GU: Increased bilirubin, uric acid

CNS: **Peripheral neuropathy, seizures,** confusion, *anxiety,* hypertonia, abnormal thinking, asthenia, *insomnia,* **CNS depression,** pain, dizziness, chills, fever

RESP: Cough, pneumonia, dyspnea, asthma, epistaxis, hypoventilation, sinusitis

INTEG: *Rash, pruritus,* alopecia, ecchymosis, hemorrhage, petechiae, sweating

MS: Myalgia, arthritis, myopathy, muscular atrophy

CV: Hypertension, vasodilation, dysrhythmia, syncope, **CHF,** palpitation

EENT: Ear pain, otitis, photophobia, visual impairment, retinal depigmentation

HEMA: **Leukopenia, granulocytopenia, thrombocytopenia, anemia**

SYST: **Lactic acidosis, anaphylaxis**

Contraindications: Hypersensitivity

Precautions: Renal, hepatic disease, pregnancy (B), lactation, children, sodium-restricted diets, elevated amylase, preexistant peripheral neuropathy, phenylketonuria, hyperuricemia

Pharmacokinetics:

PO: Peak 0.67 hr; del rel 2 hr; elimination half-life 1.62 hr, extensive metabolism is thought to occur; administration within 5 min of food will decrease absorption

Interactions:

• Increased didanosine level: allopurinol

• Decreased absorption: ketoconazole, dapsone

• Increased side effects from: magnesium, aluminum antacids

• Decreased concentrations of fluoroquinolones, other antiretrovirals, itraconazole, tetracyclines

- Drug/food: any food decreases rate of absorption
- Do not use with acidic juices

NURSING CONSIDERATIONS

Assess:

- Peripheral neuropathy: tingling or pain in hands and feet, distal numbness; onset usually occurs 2-6 mo after beginning treatment, may persist if drug is not discontinued

◆Pancreatitis: abdominal pain, nausea, vomiting, elevated liver enzymes; drug should be discontinued, since condition can be fatal

- For anaphylaxis, lactic acidosis
- Children by dilated retinal exam q6mo to rule out retinal depigmentation
- CBC, differential, platelet count qmo; withhold drug if WBC is <4000 or platelet count is <75,000; notify prescriber of results; alk phosphatase, monitor amylase; viral load, CD4 count
- Renal function studies: BUN, serum uric acid, urine CrCl before, during therapy
- Temp q4h, may indicate beginning infection
- Liver function tests before, during therapy (bilirubin, AST, ALT) as needed or qmo

Administer:

- Pediatric powder for oral sol after preparation by pharmacist; dilution is required using purified USP water, then antacid (10 mg/ml), refrigerate, shake before use
- On an empty stomach ≥30 min, ac or 2 hr pc

Perform/provide:

- Cleanup of powdered products; use wet mop or damp sponge
- Storage of tabs, caps in tightly closed bottle at room temperature; store oral sol after dissolving at room temperature ≤4 hr

Evaluate:

- Therapeutic response: absence of infection; symptoms of HIV

Teach patient/family:

- To avoid use with alcohol
- To report numbness/tingling in extremities
- To take on an empty stomach; not to take dapsone at same time as ddI; do not mix powder with fruit juice; chew tab or crush and dissolve in water; drink powder immediately after mixing
- To report signs of infection: increased temp, sore throat, flulike symptoms
- To report signs of anemia: fatigue, headache, faintness, shortness of breath, irritability
- To report bleeding; avoid use of razors, commercial mouthwash
- That hair may be lost during therapy (rare); a wig or hairpiece may make patient feel better

---

RARELY USED

dienestrol (℞)

(dye-en-ess'trole)

DV, Ortho Dienestrol

Func. class.: Estrogen

Uses: Atrophic vaginitis, kraurosis vulvae

Dosage and routes:

- *Adult:* **VAG CREAM** 1-2 applications qd × 2 wk, then ½ dose × 2 wk, then 1 application

Contraindications: Breast cancer, thromboembolic disorders, reproductive cancer, genital bleeding (abnormal, undiagnosed), pregnancy (X), lactation

---

◆ = Nursing alert   🖊 = Herb-drug interaction   🚫 = Do not crush

RARELY USED

diflunisal (R)

(dye-floo'ni-sal)

diflunisal, Dolobid

Func. class.: Nonsteroidal anti-inflammatory/analgesic (non-opioid)

Uses: Mild to moderate pain or fever including arthritis; 3-4 times more potent than aspirin

Dosage and routes:

• *Adult:* **PO** loading dose 1 g; then 500-1000 mg/day in 2 divided doses, q12h, not to exceed 1500 mg/day

• *Geriatric:* ½ adult dose

Contraindications: Hypersensitivity to salicylates, GI bleeding, bleeding disorders, children <12 yr, vit K deficiency

digoxin (R)

(di-jox'in)

digoxin, Lanoxicaps, Lanoxin

Func. class.: Cardiac glycoside, inotropic, antidysrhythmic

Chem. class.: Digitalis preparation

Action: Inhibits the sodium-potassium ATPase, which makes more calcium available for contractile proteins, resulting in increased cardiac output; increases force of contraction (+ inotropic effect); decreases heart rate (chronotropic effect); decreases AV conduction speed

Uses: CHF, atrial fibrillation, atrial flutter, atrial tachycardia, cardiogenic shock, paroxysmal atrial tachycardia, rapid digitalization in these disorders

Dosage and routes:

• *Adult:* **IV** *digitalizing dose* 0.6-1.0 mg given as 50% of the dose initially, additional fractions given at 4-8 hr intervals; **PO digitalizing dose** 0.75-1.25 mg given as 50% of the dose initially, additional fractions given at 4-8 hr intervals; **maintenance** 0.063-0.5 mg/day (tabs), or 0.350-0.5 mg/day (gelatin cap)

• *Child >10 yr:* **IV digitalizing dose** 8-12 μg/kg given as 50% of the dose initially, additional fractions given at 4-8 hr intervals; **PO digitalizing dose** 0.01-0.015 mg/kg given as 50% of the dose initially, additional fractions given at 6-8 hr intervals; **maintenance** 25%-35% of the loading dose qd as a single dose

• *Child 5-10 yr:* **IV digitalizing dose** 0.015-0.03 mg/kg given as 50% of the dose initially, additional fractions given at 4-8 hr intervals; **PO digitalizing dose** 0.02-0.035 mg/kg given as 50% of the dose initially, additional fractions given at 6-8 hr intervals; **maintenance** 25%-35% of the loading dose qd in 2 divided doses

• *Child 2-5 yr:* **IV digitalizing dose** 0.025-0.035 mg/kg given as 50% of the dose initially, additional fractions given at 4-8 hr intervals; **PO digitalizing dose** 0.03-0.04 mg/kg given as 50% of the dose initially, additional fractions given at 6-8 hr intervals; **maintenance** 25%-35% of the loading dose qd in 2 divided doses

• *Child 1-2 yr:* **IV digitalizing dose** 0.03-0.05 mg/kg given as 50% of the dose initially, additional fractions given at 4-8 hr intervals; **PO digitalizing dose** 0.035-0.06 mg/kg given as 50% of the dose initially, additional fractions given at 4-8 hr intervals; **maintenance** 25%-35% of the loading dose qd in 2 divided doses

• *Infants:* **IV digitalizing dose** 0.02-0.03 mg/kg given as 50% of the dose initially, additional fractions given at 4-8 hr intervals; **PO digitalizing dose** 0.025-0.035 mg/kg given as 50% of the dose initially, additional fractions given at 6-8 hr intervals; **maintenance** 25%-35% of the loading dose qd in 2 divided doses

• *Infants, premature:* **IV digitalizing dose** 0.015-0.025 mg/kg given as 50% of the dose initially, additional fractions given at 4-8 hr intervals; **PO digitalizing dose** 0.02-0.03 mg/kg given as 50% of the dose initially, additional fractions given at 6-8 hr intervals; **maintenance** 20%-30% of the loading dose qd in 2 divided doses

Available forms: Caps 0.05, 0.1, 0.2 mg; elix 0.05 mg/ml; tabs 0.125, 0.25, 0.5 mg; inj 0.5*, 0.25 mg/ml; pediatric inj 0.01 mg/ml

Side effects/adverse reactions:

CNS: Headache, drowsiness, apathy, confusion, disorientation, fatigue, depression, hallucinations

*CV: **Dysrhythmias, hypotension,** bradycardia, **AV block***

EENT: Blurred vision, yellow-green halos, photophobia, diplopia

GI: Nausea, vomiting, anorexia, abdominal pain, diarrhea

Contraindications: Hypersensitivity to digitalis, ventricular fibrillation, ventricular tachycardia, carotid sinus syndrome, 2nd- or 3rd-degree heart block

Precautions: Renal disease, acute MI, AV block, severe respiratory disease, hypothyroidism, elderly, pregnancy (C), sinus nodal disease, lactation, hypokalemia

Do not confuse:
Lanoxin/Lasix
Lanoxin/Lomotil
Lanoxin/Xanax

Pharmacokinetics:

PO: Onset ½-2 hr, peak 6-8 hr, duration 3-4 days

IV: Onset 5-30 min, peak 1-5 hr, duration variable

Half-life 1.5 days, excreted in urine

Interactions:

• Decreased digoxin absorption: antacids kaolin/pectin

• Hypercalcemia, hypomagnesemia, digitalis toxicity: thiazides, parenteral Ca

• Hypokalemia, digitalis toxicity: diuretics, amphotericin B, carbenicillin, ticarcillin, corticosteroids

• Decreased digoxin level: thyroid agents, cholestyramine, colestipol, metoclopramide

• Increased digoxin blood levels: propantheline, quinidine, verapamil, amiodarone, anticholinergics, diltiazem, nifedipine

• Increased bradycardia: β-adrenergic blockers, antidysrhythmics

🍀 Increased action: aloe, buckthorn bark/berry, cascara sagrada bark, castor bean oil, May apple root, rhubarb root, senna pod/leaf, yellow dock root, oleander, pheasant's eye, purple foxglove, squill

🍀 Dysrhythmias: ephedra

🍀 Bradycardia: Indian snakeroot

🍀 Cardiac toxicity: hawthorn

🍀 Digoxin toxicity: licorice

🍀 Decreased digoxin absorption: psyllium

🍀 Increased hypokalemia: cocoa seeds, coffee seeds, cola seeds, guarana seeds, horsetail, licorice, yerba maté

Lab test interferences:

Increase: CPK

NURSING CONSIDERATIONS

Assess:

• Apical pulse for 1 min before giving drug; if pulse <60 in adult or <90 in an infant, take again in 1 hr; if <60 in adult, call prescriber; note rate, rhythm, character; monitor ECG continuously during parenteral loading dose

◆ = Nursing alert   🍀 = Herb-drug interaction   🚫 = Do not crush

D

• Electrolytes: K, Na, Cl, Mg, Ca; renal function studies: BUN, creatinine; blood studies: ALT, AST, bilirubin, Hct, Hgb before initiating treatment and periodically thereafter
• I&O ratio, daily weights; monitor turgor, lung sounds, edema
• Monitor drug levels (therapeutic level 0.5-2 ng/ml)
• Cardiac status: apical pulse, character, rate, rhythm

Administer:

PO

• PO with or without food; may crush tabs, mix with food/fluids
• K supplements if ordered for K levels <3, or foods high in K: bananas, orange juice

IV

• Undiluted or 1 ml of drug/4 ml sterile H₂O, D₅, or NS; give >5 min through Y-tube or 3-way stopcock; during digitalization close monitoring is necessary

Additive compatibilities: Bretylium, cimetidine, floxacillin, furosemide, lidocaine, ranitidine, verapamil

Syringe compatibilities: Heparin, milrinone

Y-site compatibilities: Amrinone, cefmetazole, ciprofloxacin, cisatracurium, diltiazem, famotidine, meperidine, meropenem, midazolam, milrinone, morphine, potassium chloride, propofol, remifentanil, tacrolimus, vit B/C

Perform/provide:

• Storage protected from light

Evaluate:

• Therapeutic response: decreased weight, edema, pulse, respiration, rales; increased urine output; serum digoxin level (0.5-2 ng/ml)

Teach patient/family:

• Not to stop drug abruptly; teach all aspects of drug, to take exactly as ordered; how to monitor heart rate
• To avoid OTC medications, since many adverse drug interactions may occur; do not take antacid at same time
• To notify prescriber of loss of appetite, lower stomach pain, diarrhea, weakness, drowsiness, headache, blurred or yellow vision, rash, depression, toxicity
• The toxic symptoms of this drug and when to notify prescriber
• To maintain a sodium-restricted diet as ordered
🚫 Not to break, crush, or chew caps
• To report shortness of breath, difficulty breathing, weight gain, edema, persistent cough

Treatment of overdose: Discontinue drug; give K; monitor ECG; give adrenergic-blocking agent, digoxin immune FAB

---

digoxin immune FAB (ovine) (℞)

(di-jox′in im-myoon′ FAB)

Digibind

Func. class.: Antidote—digoxin specific

Action: Antibody fragments bind to free digoxin or digitoxin to reverse toxicity by not allowing digoxin or digitoxin to bind to sites of action

Uses: Life-threatening digoxin or digitoxin toxicity

Dosage and routes:

Digoxin toxicity

• *Adult:* IV dose (mg) = dose ingested (mg) × serum digoxin conc × 5.6 × wt in kg ÷ 1000; if ingested amount is unknown, give 800 mg IV; if digoxin liquid caps, **IV,** do not multiply ingested dose by 0.8

Available forms: Inj 38 mg/vial (binds 0.5 mg digoxin or digitoxin)
Side effects/adverse reactions:

CV: CHF, ventricular rate increase, *atrial fibrillation,* low cardiac output

RESP: Impaired respiratory function, rapid respiratory rate
META: Hypokalemia
MISC: Anaphylaxis
INTEG: Hypersensitivity, allergic reactions, facial swelling, redness

Contraindications: Mild digoxin toxicity, hypersensitivity

Precautions: Children, lactation, cardiac disease, renal disease, pregnancy (C), allergy to ovine proteins

Pharmacokinetics:

IV: Peaks after completion of infusion, onset 30 min (variable); not known if crosses placenta, breast milk; half-life biphasic—14-20 hr; prolonged in renal disease; excreted by kidneys

Interactions:

• Considered incompatible with all drugs in syringe or sol

Lab test interferences:

Interference: Immunoassay digoxin

NURSING CONSIDERATIONS
Assess:

• Hypokalemia: ST depression, flat T waves, presence of U wave, ventricular dysrhythmia; K levels may decrease rapidly

Administer:

• After diluting 38 mg/4 ml of sterile H_2O for inj 10 mg/ml mix; may be further diluted with normal saline, sol should be clear, colorless

• By bolus if cardiac arrest is imminent or IV over 30 min using a 0.22 μm filter

Perform/provide:

• Storage of reconstituted sol for up to 4 hr in refrigerator

Evaluate:

• Therapeutic response: correction of digoxin toxicity; check digoxin

levels 0.5-2 ng/ml; digitoxin level 9-25 ng/ml

Teach patient/family:

• The purpose of medication; to report fever, chills, itching, swelling, dyspnea

---

dihydroergotamine (℞)
(dye-hye-droe-er-got′a-meen)
D.H.E. 45,
Dihydroergotamine-Sandoz*
Func. class.: α-Adrenergic blocker
Chem. class.: Ergot alkaloid (dihydrogenated)

Action: Constricts smooth muscle in periphery, cranial blood vessels; inhibits norepinephrine uptake

Uses: Vascular headache (migraine or histamine)

Dosage and routes:

• *Adult:* **IM/IV** 1 mg; may repeat q1-2h if needed, not to exceed 3 mg/day or 6 mg/wk

Available forms: Inj 1 mg/ml

Side effects/adverse reactions:

CNS: Numbness in fingers, toes, general weakness
CV: Transient tachycardia, chest pain, bradycardia, increase or decrease in B/P, *gangrene*
GI: Nausea, vomiting
MS: Muscle pain

Contraindications: Hypersensitivity to ergot preparations, occlusion (peripheral vascular), CAD, hepatic disease, pregnancy (X), renal disease, peptic ulcer, hypertension, lactation, children, uremia

Pharmacokinetics:

IM: Onset 15-30 min, peak 2 hr, duration 3-4 hr
IV: Onset 5 min, peak 45 min, duration 3-4 hr; half-life 1.3-4 hr

---

◆ = Nursing alert   ∥ = Herb-drug interaction   ⊘ = Do not crush

Interactions:

• Ergot toxicity symptoms: macrolide antiinfectives

• Increased vasoconstriction: β-blockers

• Incompatible with any drug in syringe or sol

NURSING CONSIDERATIONS

Assess:

• Weight daily, check for peripheral edema in feet, legs

• For stress level, activity, recreation, coping mechanisms

• Neurologic status: LOC, blurring vision, nausea, vomiting, tingling in extremities that precedes headache

• Ingestion of tyramine (pickled products, beer, wine, aged cheese), food additives, preservatives, colorings, artificial sweeteners, chocolate, caffeine; may precipitate these headaches

Administer:

• IV undiluted; give over 3 min

• At beginning of headache; dose must be titrated to patient response

• Only to women who are not pregnant; harm to fetus may occur

Perform/provide:

• Storage in dark area; do not use discolored solutions

• Quiet, calm environment with decreased stimulation for noise, bright light, excessive talking

Evaluate:

• Therapeutic response: decrease in frequency, severity of headache

Teach patient/family:

• Not to use OTC medications; serious drug interactions may occur

• To report side effects: increased vasoconstriction starting with cold extremities, then paresthesia, weakness

• That an increase in headaches may occur when this drug is discontinued after long-term use

◆ To keep drug out of reach of children; death may occur

• Not to use during pregnancy

---

dihydrotachysterol (Ŗ)

(dye-hye-droh-tak-iss′ter-ole)

DHT Intensol*, Hytakerol

Func. class.: Parathyroid agent (calcium regulator)

Chem. class.: Vitamin D analog

Action: Increases intestinal absorption of calcium for bones, increases renal tubular absorption of phosphate; regulates calcium levels by regulating calcitonin, parathyroid hormone

Uses: Renal osteodystrophy, hypoparathyroidism, pseudohypoparathyroidism, familial hypophosphatemia, postoperative tetany

Dosage and routes:

Hypophosphatemia

• *Adult and child:* **PO** 0.5-2 mg qd, maintenance 0.3-1.5 mg qd

Hypoparathyroidism/pseudohypoparathyroidism

• *Adult:* **PO** 0.8-2.4 mg qd × 4 days, maintenance 0.2-2 mg qd regulated by serum Ca levels

• *Child:* **PO** 1-5 mg qd × 1 wk, maintenance 0.2-1 mg qd regulated by serum Ca levels

Renal osteodystrophy

• *Adult:* **PO** 0.1-0.6 mg qd, then 0.2-1 mg/day

Available forms: Tabs 0.125, 0.2, 0.4 mg; caps 0.125 mg; oral sol 0.2, 0.25 mg/5 ml, 0.2 mg/ml* (Intensol)

Side effects/adverse reactions:

EENT: Tinnitus

CNS: Drowsiness, headache, vertigo, fever, lethargy, depression

GI: Nausea, diarrhea, vomiting, jaundice, anorexia, dry mouth, constipation, cramps, metallic taste, thirst

MS: Myalgia, arthralgia, decreased bone development, weakness, ataxia

GU: Polyuria, hypercalciuria, hyperphosphatemia, hematuria, nocturia, renal calculi

*CV: **Dysrhythmias,*** hypertension

Contraindications: Hypersensitivity, renal disease, hyperphosphatemia, hypercalcemia

Precautions: Pregnancy (C), renal calculi, lactation, CV disease

Pharmacokinetics:

PO: Onset 2 wk; readily absorbed from small intestine; metabolized by liver, excreted in feces (active/inactive)

Interactions:

• Decreased absorption of dihydrotachysterol: cholestyramine, colestipol mineral oil

• Hypercalcemia: thiazide diuretics, Ca supplements

• Cardiac dysrhythmias: cardiac glycosides, verapamil

• Decreased effect of dihydrotachysterol: corticosteroids, phenytoin, barbiturates

Lab test interferences:

False increase: Cholesterol

NURSING CONSIDERATIONS
Assess:

• BUN, urinary Ca, AST, ALT, cholesterol, creatinine, alk phosphatase, uric acid, chlorine, magnesium, electrolytes, urine pH, phosphate; may increase calcium, should be kept at 9-10 mg/dl, vit D 50-135 IU/dl, phosphate 70 mg/dl

• Alk phosphatase; may be decreased

• For increased blood level, since toxic reactions may occur rapidly

• For dry mouth, metallic taste, polyuria, bone pain, muscle weakness, headache, fatigue, tinnitus, change in LOC, irregular pulse, dysrhythmias, increased respirations, an-

orexia, nausea, vomiting, cramps, diarrhea, constipation; may indicate hypercalcemia

• Renal status: decreased urinary output (oliguria, anuria), edema in extremities, weight gain >5 lb, periorbital edema

• Nutritional status, diet for sources of vit D (milk, some seafood), Ca (dairy products, dark green vegetables), phosphates (dairy products) must be avoided

Administer:

• PO, may be increased q4wk depending on blood level

Perform/provide:

• Storage in tight, light-resistant containers at room temperature

• Restriction of Na, K if required

• Restriction of fluids if required for chronic renal failure

Evaluate:

• Therapeutic response: prevention of bone deficiencies

Teach patient/family:

• The symptoms of hypercalcemia

• About foods rich in calcium, vit D

🚫 Not to break, crush, or chew caps

---

diltiazem (℞)

(dil-tye'a-zem)

Apo-Diltiaz*, Cardizem, Cardizem CD, Cardizem SR, Dilacor-XR, diltiazem, Tiazac

Func. class.: Calcium channel blocker

Chem. class.: Benzothiazepine

Action: Inhibits calcium ion influx across cell membrane during cardiac depolarization; produces relaxation of coronary vascular smooth muscle, dilates coronary arteries, slows SA/AV node conduction times, dilates peripheral arteries

---

 = Nursing alert   *🌿* = Herb-drug interaction   🚫 = Do not crush

D

Uses: Angina pectoris due to coronary insufficiency, hypertension, vasospasm; parenteral: atrial fibrillation, flutter, paroxysmal supraventricular tachycardia

Dosage and routes:
• *Adult:* PO 30 mg qid, increasing dose gradually to 180-360 mg/day in divided doses or 60-120 mg bid; may increase to 240-360 mg/day
• *Adult:* IV BOL 0.25 mg/kg over 2 min initially, then 0.35 mg/kg may be given after 15 min; if no response, may give **CONT INF** 5-15 mg/hr for up to 24 hr
• *Adult:* PO (Cardizem CD) qd

Available forms: Tabs 30, 60, 90, 120 mg; caps ext rel 120, 180, 240, 300, 360 mg; cap, sus rel 60, 90, 120, 180, 240 mg; inj 5 mg/ml (5, 10 ml)

Side effects/adverse reactions:
CV: Dysrhythmia, edema, CHF, bradycardia, hypotension, palpitations, *heart block*
GI: Nausea, vomiting, diarrhea, gastric upset, *constipation,* increased liver function studies
GU: Nocturia, polyuria, *acute renal failure*
INTEG: Rash, pruritus, flushing, photosensitivity
CNS: Headache, fatigue, drowsiness, dizziness, depression, weakness, insomnia, tremor, paresthesia

Contraindications: Sick sinus syndrome, 2nd- or 3rd-degree heart block, hypotension less than 90 mm Hg systolic, acute MI, pulmonary congestion

Precautions: CHF, hypotension, hepatic injury, pregnancy (C), lactation, children, renal disease

Do not confuse:
Cardizem CD/Cardizem SR
Cardizem/Cardene
Cardizem SR/Cardene SR

Pharmacokinetics: Onset 30-60 min; peak 2-3 hr, immediate rel, 6-11 sus rel; half-life 3½-9 hr; metabolized by liver; excreted in urine (96% as metabolites)

Interactions:
• Increased effects of: β-blockers, digoxin, lithium, carbamazepine, cyclosporine, anesthetics
• Increased effects of diltiazem: cimetidine
🍴 Increased hypotensive effects: grapefruit juice

NURSING CONSIDERATIONS
Assess:
• Cardiac status: B/P, pulse, respiration, ECG and intervals PR, QRS, QT; if systolic B/P <90 mm Hg or HR <60 bpm, hold dose, notify prescriber

Administer:
• Before meals, hs (PO)
IV
• IV undiluted over 2 min or diluted 125 mg/100 ml, 250 mg/250 ml of D_5W, 0.9% NaCl, D_5/0.45% NaCl, give 10 mg/hr, may increase by 5 mg/hr to 15 mg/hr, continue infusion up to 24 hr

Y-site compatibilities: Albumin, amikacin, amphotericin B, aztreonam, bretylium, bumetanide, cefazolin, cefotaxime, cefotetan, cefoxitin, ceftazidime, ceftriaxone, cefuroxime, cimetidine, ciprofloxacin, clindamycin, digoxin, dobutamine, dopamine, doxycycline, epinephrine, erythromycin, esmolol, fentanyl, fluconazole, gentamicin, hetastarch, hydromorphone, imipenem-cilastatin, labetalol, lidocaine, lorazepam, meperidine, metoclopramide, metronidazole, midazolam, milrinone, morphine, multivitamins, nicardipine, nitroglycerin, norepinephrine, oxacillin, penicillin G potassium, pentamidine, piperacillin, potassium chloride, potassium phosphates, ranitidine, sodium nitroprusside, theophylline, ticarcillin, ticarcillin/clavulanate, tobramycin, trimethoprim-sulfamethoxazole, vancomycin, vecuronium

Perform/provide:

• Storage in tight container at room temperature

Evaluate:

• Therapeutic response: decreased anginal pain, decreased B/P

Teach patient/family:

• How to take pulse before taking drug; record or graph should be kept

• To avoid hazardous activities until stabilized on drug, dizziness is no longer a problem

• To limit caffeine consumption

• To avoid OTC drugs unless directed by prescriber

• The importance of complying with all areas of medical regimen: diet, exercise, stress reduction, drug therapy

🚫 Not to break, crush, or chew sus rel caps or tabs

• To report dizziness, shortness of breath, palpitations

• Not to discontinue abruptly

• To take with a full glass of water

Treatment of overdose: Atropine for AV block, vasopressor for hypotension

---

dimenhydrinate
(OTC, ℞)

(dye-men-hye′dri-nate)

Apo-Dimenhydrinate*, Calm-X, Children's Dramamine, dimenhydrinate, Dimetabs, Dinate, Dramamine, Dramanate, Dymenate, Gravol*, Gravol L/A*, Hydrate, Nauseatol*, Novo-Dimenate*, PMS-Dimenhydrinate*, Travamine*, Triptone Caplets

Func. class.: Antiemetic, antihistamine, anticholinergic

Chem. class.: H$_1$-Receptor antagonist, ethanolamine derivative

Action: Vestibular stimulation is decreased

Uses: Motion sickness, nausea, vomiting

Dosage and routes:

• *Adult:* **PO** 50-100 mg q4h; **IM/IV** 50 mg q4h as needed

• *Child:* **IM/PO** 5 mg/kg divided in 4 equal doses

Available forms: Tabs 50 mg; inj 50 mg/ml; elixir 15 mg/5 ml*; chew tabs 50 mg

Side effects/adverse reactions:

CNS: Drowsiness, restlessness, headache, dizziness, insomnia, confusion, nervousness, tingling, vertigo

GI: Nausea, anorexia, vomiting, *constipation*

CV: Hypertension, *hypotension*, palpitation

INTEG: Rash, urticaria, fever, chills, flushing

EENT: Dry mouth, blurred vision, diplopia, nasal congestion, photosensitivity

MISC: Anaphylaxis

➡ = Nursing alert   ⫻ = Herb-drug interaction   🚫 = Do not crush

Contraindications: Hypersensitivity to narcotics, shock

Precautions: Children, cardiac dysrhythmias, elderly, asthma, pregnancy (B), lactation, prostatic hypertrophy, bladder-neck obstruction, narrow-angle glaucoma, stenosing peptic ulcer, pyloroduodenal obstruction

Pharmacokinetics:
IM/PO: Duration 4-6 hr

Interactions:
• Increased effect: alcohol, other CNS depressants

 Increased anticholinergic effect: henbane leaf

Lab test interferences:
False negative: Allergy skin testing

NURSING CONSIDERATIONS
Assess:
• VS, B/P; check patients with cardiac disease more often
• Signs of toxicity of other drugs or masking of symptoms of disease: brain tumor, intestinal obstruction
• Observe for drowsiness, dizziness

Administer:
• IM injection in large muscle mass; aspirate to avoid IV administration
• Tablets may be swallowed whole, chewed, or allowed to dissolve

IV
• After diluting 50 mg/10 ml of NaCl inj; give 50 mg or less over 2 min

Additive compatibilities: Amikacin, calcium gluconate, chloramphenicol, corticotropin, erythromycin, heparin, hydroxyzine, methicillin, norepinephrine, penicillin G potassium, pentobarbital, phenobarbital, potassium chloride, prochlorperazine, vancomycin, vit B/C

Syringe compatibilities: Atropine, diphenhydramine, droperidol, fentanyl, heparin, hydromorphone, meperidine, metoclopramide, morphine, pentazocine, perphenazine, ranitidine, scopolamine

Y-site compatibilities: Acyclovir
• Therapeutic response: absence of nausea, vomiting

Teach patient/family:
• That a false-negative result may occur with skin testing; these procedures should not be scheduled for 4 days after discontinuing use
• To avoid hazardous activities, activities requiring alertness; dizziness may occur; instruct patient to request assistance with ambulation
• To avoid alcohol, other depressants

RARELY USED

dimercaprol (℞)
(dye-mer-cap′role)
BAL in Oil, British
Anti-Lewisite*,
dimercaptopropanol
Func. class.: Heavy metal antagonist
Chem. class.: Chelating agent

Uses: Arsenic, gold, mercury, lead poisoning

Dosage and routes:
Severe gold/arsenic poisoning
• *Adult:* **IM** 3 mg/kg q4h × 2 days then qid × 1 day, then bid × 10 days
Mild gold/arsenic poisoning
• *Adult:* **IM** 2.5 mg/kg qid × 2 days, then bid × 1 day, then qd × 10 days
Acute lead poisoning
• *Adult:* **IM** 4 mg/kg, then q4h with edetate calcium disodium 12.5 mg/kg **IM,** not to exceed 5 mg/kg/dose
Mercury poisoning
• *Adult:* **IM** 5 mg/kg, then 2.5 mg/kg/day or bid × 10 days
Contraindications: Hypersensitivity, anuria, hepatic insufficiency, poisoning of other metals (iron, cad-

---

mium, selenium), severe renal disease, child <3 yr, pregnancy (D)

---

dinoprostone (R)
(dye-noe-prost′one)
Cervidil Vaginal Insert,
Prepidil, Endocervical Gel,
Prostin E Vaginal Suppository
Func. class.: Oxytocic, abortifacient
Chem. class.: Prostaglandin E_2

Action: Stimulates uterine contractions, causing abortion; acts within 30 hr for complete abortion

Uses: Abortion during 2nd trimester, benign hydatidiform mole, expulsion of uterine contents in fetal deaths to 28 wk, missed abortion, to efface and dilate the cervix in pregnancy at term

Dosage and routes:
Abortifacient
• *Adult:* **VAG SUPP** 20 mg, repeat q3-5h until abortion occurs, max dose is 240 mg
Cervical ripening
• *Adult:* **GEL** warm to room temperature, choose correct length shielded catheter (10 or 20 mm), fill catheter by pushing plunger; patient should remain recumbent for 15-30 min; insert one 10 mg insert
Available forms: Vag supp 20 mg; gel 0.5 mg/3 g (prefilled syringe); 10 mg insert
Side effects/adverse reactions:
CNS: Headache, dizziness, chills, fever
CV: Hypotension, *dysrhythmias*
GI: Nausea, vomiting, diarrhea
GU: Vaginitis, vaginal pain, vulvitis, vaginismus
INTEG: Rash, skin color changes
MS: Leg cramps, joint swelling, weakness

EENT: Blurred vision
INSERT: Uterine hyperstimulation, fever, nausea, vomiting, diarrhea, abdominal pain
GEL: Uterine contractile abnormality, GI side effects, back pain, fever
FETAL: Bradycardia (i.e., deceleration)
SUPPOSITORY: Uterine rupture, anaphylaxis

Contraindications: Hypersensitivity, uterine fibrosis, cervical stenosis, pelvic surgery, pelvic inflammatory disease, respiratory disease
Precautions: Hepatic disease, renal disease, cardiac disease, asthma, anemia, jaundice, diabetes mellitus, convulsive disorders, hypertension, hypotension, pregnancy (C)
Do not confuse:
Prepidil/bepridil
Interactions
• Increased effect: other oxytocics
• Decreased oxytocic effect: alcohol
🍃 Hypertension: ephedra
Pharmacokinetics:
SUPP: Onset 10 min, duration 2-3 hr; metabolized in spleen, kidney, lungs; excreted in urine

NURSING CONSIDERATIONS
Assess:
• Dilation, effacement of cervix and uterine contraction, fetal heart tones, check for contractions over 1 min
• For fever that occurs ½ hr after suppository insertion (abortion)
• Respiratory rate, rhythm, depth; notify prescriber of abnormalities, pulse, B/P, temp
• Vaginal discharge: check for itching, irritation; indicates vaginal infection
• For fever, chills: increase fluids or give tepid sponge bath or blanket
Administer:
• By gel: after warming to room temp, remove seal from end of syringe, and remove the protective end cap and insert into plunger stopper

---

◆ = Nursing alert   🍃 = Herb-drug interaction   🚫 = Do not crush

D

assembly; make sure patient is in dorsal position
Antiemetic/antidiarrheal before administration of this drug
Evaluate:
• Therapeutic response: expulsion of fetus
Teach patient/family:
• To remain supine for 10-15 min after insertion of supp 2 hr after insert, 15-30 min after gel
• To report excessive cramping, bleeding, chills, fever
• Some methods of pain, comfort control

---

diphenhydramine
(OTC, ℞)

(dye-fen-hye′dra-meen)
Allerdryl*, AllerMax*, Allermed, Banophen, Benadryl, Benadryl 25, Benadryl Kapseals, Benahist 10, Benahist 50, Ben-Allergin-50, Benoject-10, Benoject-50, Benylin Cough, Bydramine, Compoz, Diphenadryl, Diphen Cough, Diphenhist, diphenhydramine HCl, Dormin, Genahist, Hydramine, Hydramyn, Hydril, Hyrexin-50, Insomnal*, Nidryl, Nighttime Sleep Aid, Nordryl, Nordryl Cough, Nytol, Phendry, Siladryl, Sleep-Eze 3, Sominex 2, Tusstat, Twilite, Uni-Bent Cough, Wehdryl
Func. class.: Antihistamine (1st generation, nonselective)
Chem. class.: Ethanolamine derivative, H_1-receptor antagonist

Action: Acts on blood vessels, GI, respiratory system by competing with histamine for H_1-receptor site; decreases allergic response by blocking histamine

Uses: Allergy symptoms, rhinitis, motion sickness, antiparkinsonism, nighttime sedation, infant colic, nonproductive cough
Dosage and routes:
• *Adult:* **PO** 25-50 mg q4-6h, not to exceed 400 mg/day; **IM/IV** 10-50 mg, not to exceed 400 mg/day
• *Child >12 kg:* **PO/IM/IV** 5 mg/kg/day in 4 divided doses, not to exceed 300 mg/day
Nighttime sleep aid
• *Adult and child ≥12 yr:* **PO** 25-50 mg hs
Antitussive (syrup only)
• *Adult and child ≥12 yr:* 25 mg q4h, max 100 mg/24 hr
• *Child 6-12 yr:* 12.5 mg q4h, max 50 mg/24 hr
• *Child 2-6 yr:* 6.25 mg q4h, max 25 mg/24 hr
Renal disease
• CrCl 10-50 ml/min dose q6-12h; CrCl <10 ml/min dose q12-18h
Available forms: Caps 25, 50 mg; tabs 25, 50 mg; chew tabs 25 mg; elix 12.5 mg/5 ml; syr 12.5 mg/5 ml; inj 10, 50 mg/ml
Side effects/adverse reactions:
CNS: Dizziness, drowsiness, poor coordination, fatigue, anxiety, euphoria, confusion, paresthesia, neuritis, *seizures*
RESP: Increased thick secretions, wheezing, chest tightness
HEMA: Thrombocytopenia, agranulocytosis, hemolytic anemia
GI: Nausea, anorexia, diarrhea
INTEG: Photosensitivity
GU: Retention, dysuria, frequency
EENT: Blurred vision, dilated pupils, tinnitus, nasal stuffiness, dry nose, throat, mouth
MISC: Anaphylaxis
Contraindications: Hypersensitivity to H_1-receptor antagonist, acute asthma attack, lower respiratory tract disease
Precautions: Increased intraocu-

---

lar pressure, renal disease, cardiac disease, hypertension, bronchial asthma, seizure disorder, stenosed peptic ulcers, hyperthyroidism, prostatic hypertrophy, bladder neck obstruction, pregnancy (B), lactation

Do not confuse:
diphenhydramine/dicyclomine

Pharmacokinetics:
PO: Peak 1-3 hr, duration 4-7 hr
IM: Onset ½ hr, peak 1-4 hr, duration 4-7 hr; *IV:* Onset immediate, duration 4-7 hr; metabolized in liver, excreted by kidneys; crosses placenta, excreted in breast milk; half-life 2-7 hr

Interactions:
• Increased CNS depression: barbiturates, opiates, hypnotics, tricyclics, alcohol
• Increased effect of diphenhydramine: MAOIs

💉 Increased anticholinergic effect: henbane leaf

Lab test interferences:
False negatives: Skin allergy tests

NURSING CONSIDERATIONS
Assess:
• Be alert for urinary retention, frequency, dysuria; drug should be discontinued
• CBC during long-term therapy; blood dyscrasias may occur
• Respiratory status: rate, rhythm, increase in bronchial secretions, wheezing, chest tightness

Administer:
• With meals for GI symptoms; absorption may slightly decrease
• Deep IM in large muscle; rotate site
• hs only if using for sleep aid
IV
• Undiluted; give 25 mg/1 min

Additive compatibilities: Amikacin, aminophylline, ascorbic acid, bleomycin, cephapirin, erythromycin, hydrocortisone, lidocaine, methicillin, methyldopa, nafcillin, netilmicin, penicillin G potassium, penicillin G sodium, polymyxin B, vit B/C

Syringe compatibilities: Atropine, butorphanol, chlorpromazine, cimetidine, dimenhydrinate, droperidol, fentanyl, fluphenazine, glycopyrrolate, hydromorphone, hydroxyzine, meperidine, metoclopramide, midazolam, morphine, nalbuphine, pentazocine, perphenazine, prochlorperazine, promazine, promethazine, ranitidine, scopolamine, sufentanil, thiothixene

Y-site compatibilities: Acyclovir, aldesleukin, amifostine, amsacrine, aztreonam, ciprofloxacin, cisatracurium, cisplatin, cladribine, cyclophosphamide, cytarabine, doxorubicin, doxorubicin liposome, famotidine, filgrastim, fluconazole, fludarabine, gallium, granisetron, heparin, hydrocortisone, idarubicin, melphalan, meperidine, meropenem, methotrexate, ondansetron, paclitaxel, piperacillin/tazobactam, potassium chloride, propofol, remifentanil, sargramostim, sufentanil, tacrolimus teniposide, thiotepa, vinorelbine, vit B/C

Perform/provide:
• Hard candy, gum, frequent rinsing of mouth for dryness
• Storage in tight container at room temperature

Evaluate:
• Therapeutic response: absence of running or congested nose or rashes, improved sleep

Teach patient/family:
• All aspects of drug use; to notify prescriber of confusion, sedation, hypotension
• To avoid driving, other hazardous activity if drowsiness occurs
• That photosensitivity may occur
• To avoid concurrent use of alcohol, other CNS depressants

Treatment of overdose: Adminis-

ter ipecac syrup or lavage, diazepam, vasopressors, barbiturates
(short-acting)

---

diphenoxylate/
atropine (R)

(dye-fen-ox'ee-late a'troe-peen)
Logene, Lomanate, Lomotil,
Lonox

Func. class.: Antidiarrheal
Chem. class.: Phenylpiperidine
derivative opiate agonist

**Controlled Substance Schedule
IV (US)**

Action: Inhibits gastric motility by
acting on mucosal receptors responsible for peristalsis

Uses: Acute nonspecific and acute
exacerbations of chronic functional
diarrhea

Dosage and routes:
• *Adult:* **PO** 5 mg qid titrated to
patient response needed, not to exceed 8 tabs/24 hr
• *Child 2-12 yr:* **PO** 0.3-0.4 mg/kg/
day in divided dose
Available forms: Tabs 2.5 mg with
atropine 0.025 mg; liquid 2.5 mg
with atropine 0.025 mg/5 ml
Side effects/adverse reactions:
RESP: **Respiratory depression**
MISC: **Anaphylaxis, angioedema**
CNS: Dizziness, drowsiness, light-
headedness, headache, fatigue, nervousness, insomnia, confusion
GI: Nausea, vomiting, dry mouth,
epigastric distress, constipation,
paralytic ileus
EENT: Burning eyes, blurred vision
Contraindications: Hypersensitivity, pseudomembranous enterocolitis, jaundice, glaucoma, child <2 yr,
severe electrolyte imbalances, diarrhea associated with organisms that
penetrate intestinal mucosa
Precautions: Hepatic disease, renal

disease, ulcerative colitis, pregnancy
(C), lactation, severe liver disease
Do not confuse:
Lomotil/Lamictal
Lomotil/Lanoxin
Lomotil/Lasix
Pharmacokinetics:
PO: Onset 40-60 min, peak 2 hr,
duration 3-4 hr, terminal half-life
12-14 hr; metabolized in liver to
inactive metabolite; excreted in
urine, feces
Interactions:
• Do not use with MAOIs; hyper-
tensive crisis may occur
• Increased action of: alcohol, nar-
cotics, barbiturates, other CNS de-
pressants, anticholinergics
NURSING CONSIDERATIONS
Assess:
• Electrolytes (K, Na, Cl) if on long-
term therapy
• Bowel pattern before; for rebound
constipation after termination of
medication; bowel sounds
• Response after 48 hr; if none, drug
should be discontinued
• Abdominal distention, toxic mega-
colon, which may occur in ulcera-
tive colitis
• Hepatic function if on long-term
therapy
Administer:
• For 48 hr only; if no response,
drug should be discontinued
Evaluate:
• Therapeutic response: decreased
diarrhea
Teach patient/family:
• To avoid OTC products unless directed by prescriber (may contain
alcohol); do not use alcohol or CNS
depressants
• Not to exceed recommended dose
• That drug may be habit forming
• Not to engage in hazardous activities; drowsiness may occur, not to
use for longer than 48 hr for acute
diarrhea

dipyridamole (℞)

(dye-peer-id'a-mole)
Apo-Dipyridamole*, dipyrida-
mole*, Novo-Dipiradol*,
Persantine, Persantine IV
Func. class.: Coronary vasodi-
lator, antiplatelet agent
Chem. class.: Nonnitrate

Action: Inhibits adenosine uptake,
which produces coronary vasodilation; increases oxygen saturation in
coronary tissues, coronary blood
flow; acts on small resistance vessels with little effect on vascular
resistance; may increase development of collateral circulation; decreases platelet aggregation by the
inhibition of phosphodiesterase (an
enzyme)

Uses: Prevention of transient ischemic attacks, inhibition of platelet
adhesion to prevent myocardial reinfarction, thromboembolism, with
warfarin in prosthetic heart valves,
prevention of coronary bypass graft
occlusion with aspirin; possibly effective for long-term therapy of
chronic angina pectoris

Dosage and routes:
TIA
• *Adult:* PO 50 mg tid, 1 hr ac, not
to exceed 400 mg qd
Inhibition of platelet adhesion
• *Adult:* PO 50-75 mg qid in com-
bination with aspirin or warfarin;
IV 570 µg/kg
Available forms: Tabs 25, 50, 75
mg; inj 10 mg/2 ml

Side effects/adverse reactions:
CV: Postural hypotension
*CNS: Headache, dizziness, weak-
ness, fainting, syncope*
*GI: Nausea, vomiting, anorexia, di-
arrhea*
INTEG: Rash, flushing

Contraindications: Hypersensitivity, hypotension
Precautions: Pregnancy (B), lactation
Pharmacokinetics:
PO: Peak 2-2½ hr, duration 6 hr;
therapeutic response may take several months; metabolized in liver;
excreted in bile; undergoes entero-
hepatic recirculation
Interactions:
• Prevention of coronary vasodilation: theophylline
• Increased risk of bleeding:
NSAIDs, cefamandole, cefotetan,
cefoperazone, plicamycin, valproic
acid, sulfinpyrazole, anticoagulants,
thrombolytics

NURSING CONSIDERATIONS
Assess:
• B/P, pulse during treatment until
stable; take B/P lying, standing; or-
thostatic hypotension is common
• Cardiac status: chest pain, what
aggravates or ameliorates condition
Administer:
• IV after diluting each 5 mg/2 ml
or more D₅W, 0.45% NaCl, or 0.9%
NaCl to a total vol of 20-50 ml; give
over 4 min; do not give undiluted
• On an empty stomach: 1 hr before
meals or 2 hr after; give with 8 oz
water for better absorption
Perform/provide:
• Storage at room temperature
Evaluate:
• Therapeutic response: decreased
chest pain (angina), decreased platelet adhesion
Teach patient/family:
• That medication is not cure; may
have to be taken continuously in
evenly spaced doses only as directed
• That it is necessary to quit smoking to prevent excessive vasoconstriction
• To avoid hazardous activities un-

til stabilized on medication; dizziness may occur
• To rise slowly from sitting or lying to prevent orthostatic hypotension
• Not to use alcohol or OTC medications unless approved by prescriber
Treatment of overdose: Administer IV phenylephrine

---

dirithromycin (Rx)
(dye-rith-roe-mye'sin)
Dynabac
Func. class.: Antiinfective
Chem. class.: Macrolide

Action: Binds to 50S ribosomal subunits of susceptible bacteria, suppresses protein synthesis
Uses: Infections of the respiratory tract caused by *Moraxella catarrhalis, Streptococcus* sp., *(S. pneumoniae, S. agalactiae, S. viridans), Legionella pneumophilia, Mycoplasma pneumoniae, Streptococcus pyogenes, Staphylococcus aureus, Bordetella pertussis, Propionibacterium acnes*
Dosage and routes:
• *Adult:* **PO** 500 mg qd, given for 7-14 days depending on infections
Available forms: Tabs, enteric coated 250 mg
Side effects/adverse reactions:
GI: Abdominal pain, nausea, diarrhea, vomiting, dyspepsia, GI disorders, flatulence, abnormal stools, anorexia, constipation, ***pseudomembranous colitis***
CNS: Headache, dizziness, insomnia
HEMA: Increased platelet count, increased eosinophils
RESP: Cough, dyspnea
INTEG: Pruritus, urticaria
Contraindications: Hypersensitivity to this drug or any other macrolide, or erythromycin, bacteremias

Precautions: Pregnancy (C), lactation, children, hepatic, renal disease
Pharmacokinetics: Rapidly absorbed, widely distributed, no hepatic metabolism, excreted in bile, feces (up to 97%), plasma half-life 8 hr, terminal 44 hr
Interactions:
• Absorption of dirithromycin slightly enhanced: antacids, H_2-antagonists
• May alter effect of: theophylline
• Drug/food: increased absorption with food
NURSING CONSIDERATIONS
Assess:
• Report hematuria, oliguria in renal disease
• Liver studies: AST, ALT if on long-term therapy
• Renal studies: Urinalysis, protein, blood if on long-term therapy
• C&S before drug therapy; drug may be given as soon as culture is taken; C&S may be repeated after treatment
• Bowel pattern before, during treatment; pseudomembranous colitis may occur
• Skin eruptions, itching
• Respiratory status: rate, character, wheezing, tightness in chest; discontinue drug
• Allergies before treatment, reaction of each medication; place allergies on chart, notify all people giving drugs
Administer:
• Adequate intake of fluids (2 L) during diarrhea episodes
🚫 Whole; do not break, crush, or chew tablets
• With food or within 1 hr of food at same time each day
Perform/provide:
• Storage at room temperature, in tight container

Evaluate:
• Therapeutic response: C&S negative for infection

Teach patient/family:
• To take with full glass of water; to give with food
• To report sore throat, fever, fatigue; may indicate superinfection
• To notify prescriber of diarrhea stools, dark urine, pale stools, jaundiced eyes or skin, severe abdominal pain
• To take at evenly spaced intervals; complete dosage regimen

Treatment of hypersensitivity:
Withdraw drug, maintain airway, administer epinephrine, aminophylline, O_2, IV corticosteroids

---

disopyramide (R)
(dye-soe-peer'a-mide)
disopyramide, Norpace,
Norpace CR, Rhythmodan
Func. class.: Antidysrhythmic
(Class IA)
Chem. class.: Nonnitrate

Action: Prolongs duration of action potential and effective refractory period; reduces disparity in refractory period between normal and infarcted myocardium; prevents increased myocardial excitability and conduction contractility

Uses: PVCs, ventricular tachycardia, supraventricular tachycardia, atrial flutter, fibrillation

Investigational uses: Supraventricular tachycardia (prevention, treatment)

Dosage and routes:
Renal disease
• CrCl 30-40 ml/min dose q8h; CrCl 15-30 ml/min dose q12h; CrCl <15 ml/min dose q24h
• *Adult:* **PO** 100-200 mg q6h, in renal dysfunction 100 mg q6h; **SUS REL CAPS** 200 mg q12h

• *Child 12-18 yr:* **PO** 6-15 mg/kg/day, in divided doses q6h
• *Child 4-12 yr:* **PO** 10-15 mg/kg/day in divided doses q6h
• *Child 1-4 yr:* **PO** 10-20 mg/kg/day in divided doses q6h
• *Child <1 yr:* **PO** 10-30 mg/kg/day, in divided doses q6h

Available forms: Caps 100, 150 mg (as phosphate); cont rel caps 100, 150 mg; tabs, sus rel 250 mg*

Side effects/adverse reactions:
GU: Urinary retention, hesitancy, impotence
CNS: Headache, dizziness, psychosis, fatigue, depression, paresthesias, anxiety, insomnia
GI: Dry mouth, constipation, nausea, anorexia, flatulence, diarrhea, vomiting
CV: Hypotension, bradycardia, angina, PVCs, tachycardia, increased QRS, QT segments, *cardiac arrest,* edema, weight gain, AV block, *CHF,* syncope, chest pain
META: Hypoglycemia
INTEG: Rash, pruritus, urticaria
MS: Weakness, pain in extremities
EENT: Blurred vision; dry nose, throat, eyes; narrow-angle glaucoma
*HEMA: **Thrombocytopenia, agranulocytosis,** anemia (rare), decreased Hgb, Hct*

Contraindications: Hypersensitivity, 2nd- or 3rd-degree block, cardiogenic shock, CHF (uncompensated), sick sinus syndrome, QT prolongation

Precautions: Pregnancy (C), lactation, diabetes mellitus, renal disease, children, hepatic disease, myasthenia gravis, narrow-angle glaucoma, cardiomyopathy, conduction abnormalities

Pharmacokinetics:
PO: Peak 30 min-3 hr, duration 6-12 hr; half-life 4-10 hr; metabolized in liver; excreted in feces, urine, breast milk; crosses placenta

---

◆ = Nursing alert   ∥ = Herb-drug interaction   ⊘ = Do not crush

Interactions:

• Increased effects of disopyramide: quinidine, procainamide, propranolol, lidocaine, atenolol, other antidysrhythmics, erythromycin

• Increased side effects of disopyramide: anticholinergics

• Decreased effects of disopyramide: phenytoin, rifampin, phenobarbital

🍃 Increased action: aloe, buckthorn bark/berry, cascara sagrada bark, senna pod/leaf

Lab test interferences:

Increase: Liver enzymes, lipids, BUN, creatinine

Decrease: Hgb/Hct, blood glucose

NURSING CONSIDERATIONS

Assess:

• Apical pulse for 1 min; if less than 60, check again in 1 hr; if still less than 60, notify prescriber

• ECG; check for increased QT, widening QRS; drug should be discontinued

• Weight daily; a rapid weight gain should be reported

• For dehydration or hypovolemia, I&O ratio, electrolytes (Na, K, Cl)

• Liver, kidney function studies (AST, ALT, bilirubin, BUN, creatinine) during treatment

• Diabetics for signs of hypoglycemia (rare)

• B/P continuously for hypotension, hypertension

• For rebound hypertension after 1-2 hr

• Constipation: increased bulk in diet, water, stool softeners, or laxatives needed

• Cardiac rate, respiration: rate, rhythm, character

• Urinary hesitancy, frequency, or a change in I&O ratio; check for edema daily; check for toxicity

Administer:

🚫 Do not break, crush, or chew sus rel cap; give 1 hr before or 2 hr after meals

• Sugar-free gum, frequent sips of water for dry mouth

• Reduced dosage slowly with ECG monitoring

Evaluate:

• Therapeutic response: decreased dysrhythmias

Teach patient/family:

• To take drug exactly as prescribed; if dose is missed, take within 3-4 hr of next dose; do not double dose

• To avoid alcohol, or severe hypotension may occur; to avoid OTC drugs, or serious drug interactions may occur

• To make position change slowly during early therapy to prevent orthostatic hypotension

• To avoid hazardous activities if dizziness or blurred vision occurs

• The importance of complying with drug regimen; tell patient that this drug does not cure condition

Treatment of overdose: O_2, artificial ventilation, ECG, dopamine for circulatory depression, diazepam or thiopental for convulsions, gastric lavage

---

RARELY USED

disulfiram (℞)

(dye-sul'fi-ram)
Antabuse, disulfiram
Func. class.: Alcohol deterrent

Uses: Chronic alcoholism (as adjunct)

Dosage and routes:

• *Adult:* **PO** 250-500 mg qd × 1-2 wk, then 125-500 mg qd until fully socially recovered

Contraindications: Hypersensitivity, alcohol intoxication, psychoses, CV disease, pregnancy (X), lactation

dobutamine (℞)

(doe-byoo′ta-meen)
dobutamine, Dobutrex

Func. class.: Adrenergic direct-acting β_1-agonist, cardiac stimulant

Chem. class.: Catecholamine

Action: Causes increased contractility, increased coronary blood flow and heart rate by acting on β_1-receptors in heart; minor α and β_2 effects

Uses: Cardiac decompensation due to organic heart disease or cardiac surgery

Investigational uses: Cardiogenic shock in children

Unlabeled uses: Congenital heart disease in children undergoing cardiac cath

Dosage and routes:
• *Adult:* **IV INF** 2.5-10 µg/kg/min; may increase to 40 µg/kg/min if needed
• *Child:* **IV INF** 5-20 µg/kg/min over 10 min for cardiac cath

Available forms: Inj 12.5 mg/ml

Side effects/adverse reactions:
CNS: Anxiety, headache, dizziness
CV: Palpitations, tachycardia, hypertension, PVCs, angina
GI: Heartburn, nausea, vomiting
MS: Muscle cramps (leg)

Contraindications: Hypersensitivity, idiopathic hypertrophic subaortic stenosis

Precautions: Pregnancy (B), lactation, children, hypertension

Do not confuse:
dobutamine/dopamine
Dobutrex/Diamox

Pharmacokinetics:
IV: Onset 1-2 min, peak 10 min, half-life 2 min; metabolized in liver (inactive metabolites); excreted in urine

Interactions:
• Severe hypertension: guanethidine
• Dysrhythmias: general anesthetics, bretylium
• Decreased action of dobutamine: other β-blockers
• Dysrhythmias: bretylium, general anesthetics
• Increased pressor effect and dysrhythmias: tricyclics, MAOIs, oxytocics

NURSING CONSIDERATIONS
Assess:
• Hypovolemia; if present, correct first; administer cardiac glycoside before dobutamine
• Oxygenation/perfusion deficit (check B/P, chest pain, dizziness, loss of consciousness)
• Heart failure: S_3 gallop, dyspnea, neck vein distention, bibasilar crackles in patients with CHF, cardiomyopathy
• ECG during administration continuously; if B/P increases, drug is decreased; CVP or PWP, cardiac output during infusion
• Serum electrolytes, urine output
⬥ Sulfite sensitivity, which may be life-threatening

Administer:
IV
• Diluting each 250 mg/10 ml of sterile H_2O or D_5W for inj; may be further diluted in 50 ml or more given at prescribed rate; should be gradually increased to desired rate; use a CVP catheter or large peripheral vein, use infusion pump, titrate to patient response
• Change IV site q48h
• Plasma expanders for hypovolemia

Additive compatibilities: Amiodarone, atracurium, atropine, dopamine, enalaprilat, epinephrine, flumazenil, hydralazine, isoproterenol, lidocaine, meperidine, meropenem, metaraminol, morphine,

⬥ = Nursing alert   🖋 = Herb-drug interaction   🚫 = Do not crush

nitroglycerin, norepinephrine, phentolamine, phenylephrine, procainamide, propranolol, ranitidine

Syringe compatibilities: Heparin, ranitidine

Y-site compatibilities: Amifostine, amiodarone, amrinone, atracurium, aztreonam, bretylium, calcium chloride, calcium gluconate, ciprofloxacin, cisatracurium, cladribine, diazepam, diltiazem, dopamine, doxorubicin liposome, enalaprilat, epinephrine, famotidine, fentanyl, fluconazole, granisetron, haloperidol, hydromorphone, insulin (regular), labetalol, lidocaine, lorazepam, magnesium sulfate, meperidine, milrinone, morphine, nicardipine, nitroglycerin, norepinephrine, pancuronium, potassium chloride, propofol, ranitidine, remifentanil, sodium nitroprusside, streptokinase, tacrolimus, theophylline, thiotepa, tolazoline, vecuronium, verapamil, zidovudine

Perform/provide:
• Storage of reconstituted solution for 24 hr if refrigerated

Evaluate:
• Therapeutic response: increased B/P with stabilization, increased urine output

Teach patient/family:
• The reason for drug administration; to report dyspnea, headache, IV site discomfort

Treatment of overdose: Administer a β_1-adrenergic blocker; reduce IV or discontinue, ensure oxygenation/ventilation; for severe tachydysrhythmias (ventricular) give lidocaine or propranolol

---

docusate calcium (OTC)
(dok'yoo-sate cal'see-um)
DC Softgels, Pro-Cal-Sof, Sulfalax Calcium, Surfak
docusate sodium (OTC)
Colace, Correctol Extra Gentle, Dialose, Diocto, Dioeze, Disonate, Di-Sosul, DOK, DOS, D-S-S, Ex-Lax, Modane, Regulax SS, Regulex*, Silace
Func. class.: Laxative, emollient
Chem. class.: Anionic surfactant

Action: Increases water, fat penetration in intestine; allows for easier passage of stool

Uses: To soften stools

Dosage and routes:
• *Adult:* **PO** 50-300 mg qd (sodium) or 240 mg (calcium or potassium) prn; **ENEMA** 5 ml (sodium)
• *Child >12 yr:* **ENEMA** 2 ml (sodium)
• *Child 6-12 yr:* **PO** 40-120 mg qd (sodium)
• *Child 3-6 yr:* **PO** 20-60 mg qd (sodium)
• *Child <3 yr:* **PO** 10-40 mg qd (sodium)

Available forms: Calcium: caps 50, 240 mg; *sodium:* caps 50, 100, 240, 250 mg; tabs 50, 100 mg; syr 20 mg/5 ml 50, 60/15 ml; liq 150 mg/15 ml; oral sol 10, 50 mg/ml; enema 283 mg/3.9 cap

Side effects/adverse reactions:
GI: Nausea, anorexia, cramps, diarrhea
INTEG: Rash
EENT: Bitter taste, throat irritation
Contraindications: Hypersensitivity, obstruction, fecal impaction, nausea/vomiting

Precautions: Pregnancy (C), lactation

Pharmacokinetics: Onset 24-72 hr

Interactions:

• Toxicity: mineral oil

NURSING CONSIDERATIONS
Assess:

• Cause of constipation; identify whether fluids, bulk, or exercise are missing from lifestyle

• Cramping, rectal bleeding, nausea, vomiting; if these symptoms occur, drug should be discontinued

Administer:

• In milk, fruit juice to decrease bitter taste

• In morning or evening (oral dose)

Perform/provide:

• Storage in cool environment; do not freeze

Evaluate:

• Therapeutic response: decrease in constipation

Teach patient/family:

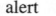 To swallow tabs whole; do not break, crush, or chew

• That normal bowel movements do not always occur daily

• Not to use in presence of abdominal pain, nausea, vomiting

• To notify prescriber if constipation unrelieved or if symptoms of electrolyte imbalance occur: muscle cramps, pain, weakness, dizziness, excessive thirst

• Inform patient that drug may take up to 3 days to soften stools

• Take oral prep with a full glass of water unless on fluid restrictions and increase fluid intake

---

dofetilide (R)

Tikosyn

Func. class.: Antidysrhythmic (Class III)

Action: Blocks cardiac ion channel carrying the rapid component of delayed potassium current, no effect on sodium channels

Uses: Atrial fibrillation, flutter

Research note: One study has concluded that dofetilide can be used in structural heart disease to maintain sinus rhythm[8]

Dosage and routes:

• *Adult:* **PO** 125-500 µg bid depending on CrCl

Renal dose

• CrCl >60 ml/min 500 µg bid; CrCl 40-60 ml/min 250 µg bid; CrCl 20-40 ml/min 125 µg bid; CrCl <20 ml/min do not use

Available forms: Caps 125, 250, 500 µg

Side effects/adverse reactions:

CNS: Syncope, dizziness

GI: Nausea, vomiting, severe diarrhea, anorexia

CV: Hypotension, postural hypotension, bradycardia, angina, PVCs, substernal pressure, transient hypertension, precipitation of angina

Contraindications: Hypersensitivity, digitalis toxicity, aortic stenosis, pulmonary hypertension, children, QT syndromes, severe renal disease

Precautions: Renal disease, pregnancy (C), lactation

Pharmacokinetics: Well absorbed

Interactions:

• Increased hypokalemia: potassium-depleting diuretics

• Do not use with cimetidine, ketoconazole, verapamil, prochlorperazine, trimethoprim-sulfamethizole, amiloride, metformin, megestrol, prochlorperazine, triamterene

NURSING CONSIDERATIONS
Assess:

• ECG continuously to determine drug effectiveness, PVCs, other dysrhythmias; renal function, QTc q3mo; this drug is only available to facilities that have been educated in this administration, patient must be hospitalized

---

◆ = Nursing alert   ✍ = Herb-drug interaction   ⊘ = Do not crush

• B/P continuously for hypotension, hypertension; orthostatic hypotension; keep supine until hypotension subsides
• Cardiac status: rate, rhythm, character, continuously

Administer:
PO
• For 3 days hospitalized

Perform/provide:
• Place patient in supine position unless otherwise ordered; assist with ambulation

Evaluate:
• Therapeutic response: control in atrial fibrillation

Teach patient/family:
• To make position changes slowly; orthostatic hypotension may occur
• Notify prescriber if fast heartbeats with fainting or dizziness occur
• Notify all prescribers of all medications and supplements taken

---

dolasetron (Ŗ)
(do-la′se-tron)
Anzemet
Func. class.: Antiemetic
Chem. class.: 5-HT3 receptor antagonist

Action: Prevents nausea, vomiting by blocking serotonin peripherally, centrally, and in the small intestine
Uses: Prevention of nausea, vomiting associated with cancer chemotherapy, radiotherapy, and prevention of postoperative nausea, vomiting
Investigational uses: Radiotherapy-induced nausea/vomiting
Dosage and routes:
Prevention of nausea/vomiting of cancer chemotherapy
• *Adult and child 2-16 yr:* **IV** 1.8

mg/kg as a single dose, ½ hr prior to chemotherapy
• *Adult:* **PO** 100 mg 1 hr prior to chemotherapy
• *Child 2-16 yr:* **PO** 1.8 mg/kg/hr prior to chemotherapy; max 100 mg
Prevention of postoperative nausea/vomiting
• *Adult:* **IV** 12.5 mg as a single dose, 15 min before cessation of anesthesia; **PO** 100 mg 2 hr before surgery (prevention only)
• *Child 2-16 yr:* **IV** 0.35 mg/kg as a single dose, 15 min before cessation of anesthesia; **PO** 1.2 mg/kg 2 hr before surgery (prevention only)
Available forms: Tabs 50, 100 mg; inj 20 mg/ml (12.5 mg/0.625 ml)
Side effects/adverse reactions:
GI: Diarrhea, constipation, increased AST, ALT, abdominal pain, anorexia
CNS: Headache, dizziness, fatigue, drowsiness
MISC: Rash, ***bronchospasm***
GU: Urinary retention, oliguria
*CV: **Dysrhythmias,*** ECG changes, hypotension, tachycardia, hypertension, bradycardia
Contraindications: Hypersensitivity
Precautions: Pregnancy (B), lactation, children, elderly
Pharmacokinetics: Unknown
Interactions:
• Dysrhythmias: antidysrhythmics
• Increased dolasetron levels: cimetidine
• Decreased dolasetron levels: rifampin
NURSING CONSIDERATIONS
Assess:
• For absence of nausea, vomiting during chemotherapy
• For hypersensitivity reaction: rash, bronchospasm
• For cardiac conduction conditions, electrolyte imbalances, or dysrhythmias

Administer:
• By inj 100 mg/½ min or less or diluted in 50 ml compatible sol; give over 15 min

Perform/provide:
• Storage at room temperature 48 hr after dilution

Evaluate:
• Therapeutic response: absence of nausea, vomiting during cancer chemotherapy

Teach patient/family:
• To report diarrhea, constipation, nausea, vomiting, rash, or changes in respirations
• Not to mix product for oral administration in juice until immediately before administration
• May cause headache, use analgesic

---

donepezil (Ɍ)
(don-ep-ee'zill)
Aricept
Func. class.: Reversible cholinesterase inhibitor

Action: Elevates acetylcholine concentrations (cerebral cortex) by slowing degradation of acetylcholine released in cholinergic neurons; does not alter underlying dementia

Uses: Treatment of mild to moderate dementia in Alzheimer's disease

Dosage and routes:
• *Adult:* PO 5 mg qd hs; may increase to 10 mg qd after 4-6wk
Available forms: Tabs 5, 10 mg

Side effects/adverse reactions:
CNS: Dizziness, *insomnia,* somnolence, *headache,* fatigue, abnormal dreams, syncope, *seizures*
CV: Hypotension or hypertension
GI: Nausea, vomiting, anorexia; *diarrhea*
GU: Urinary frequency, UTI, incontinence
INTEG: Rash, flushing

RESP: Rhinitis, URI, cough, pharyngitis
*CV: **Atrial fibrillation***
MS: Cramps, arthritis

Contraindications: Hypersensitivity to this drug or piperidine derivatives

Precautions: Sick sinus syndrome, history of ulcers, GI bleeding, hepatic disease, bladder obstruction, asthma, pregnancy (C), lactation, children, seizures, asthma, COPD

Pharmacokinetics: Well absorbed PO, metabolized to metabolites, elimination half-life 10 hr single dose, 70 hr multiple dosing

Interactions:
• Decreased activity of anticholinergics
• Synergistic effects: succinylcholine, cholinesterase inhibitors, cholinergic agonists
• Increased gastric acid secretions: NSAIDs
• Decreased donepezil effect: carbamazepine, dexamethasone, phenytoin, phenobarbital, rifampin

NURSING CONSIDERATIONS
Assess:
• B/P: hypotension, hypertension
• Mental status: affect, mood, behavioral changes, depression, complete suicide assessment
• GI status: nausea, vomiting, anorexia, diarrhea
• GU status: urinary frequency, incontinence

Administer:
• Between meals; may be given with meals for GI symptoms
• Dosage adjusted to response no more than q6wk

Perform/provide:
• Assistance with ambulation during beginning therapy; dizziness, ataxia may occur

Evaluate:
• Therapeutic response: decrease in confusion, improved mood

◆ = Nursing alert   ✒ = Herb-drug interaction   ⊘ = Do not crush

Teach patient/family:
• To report side effects: twitching, nausea, vomiting, sweating; indicates overdose
• To use drug exactly as prescribed; at regular intervals, preferably between meals; may be taken with meals for GI upset
• To notify prescriber of nausea, vomiting, diarrhea (dose increase or beginning treatment), or rash
• Not to increase or abruptly decrease dose; serious consequences may result
• That drug is not a cure, relieves symptoms

Treatment of overdose: Withdraw drug, administer tertiary anticholinergics, provide supportive care

---

dopamine (℞)

(doe′pa-meen)
dopamine HCl, Intropin, Revimine*

Func. class.: Adrenergic
Chem. class.: Catecholamine

Action: Causes increased cardiac output; acts on β_1- and α-receptors, causing vasoconstriction in blood vessels; low dose causes renal and mesenteric vasodilation; β_1 stimulation produces inotropic effects with increased cardiac output

Uses: Shock; increased perfusion; hypotension

Unlabeled uses: COPD, RDS in infants

Dosage and routes:
Shock
• *Adult:* **IV INF** 2-5 µg/kg/min, not to exceed 50 µg/kg/min, titrate to patient's response
• *Child:* **IV** 5-20 µg/kg/min adjust depending on response
COPD
• *Adult:* **IV** 4 µg/kg/min

CHF
• *Adult:* **IV** 2-5 µg/kg/min
RDS
• *Infant:* **IV** 5 µg/kg/min

Available forms: Inj 40 mg, 160 mg/ml conc for IV inf; 0.8, 1.6, 3.2 mg/ml in D_5W

Side effects/adverse reactions:
CNS: Headache
CV: Palpitations, tachycardia, hypertension, ectopic beats, angina, wide QRS complex, peripheral vasoconstriction
GI: Nausea, vomiting, diarrhea
INTEG: Necrosis, tissue sloughing with extravasation, ***gangrene***
RESP: Dyspnea

Contraindications: Hypersensitivity, ventricular fibrillation, tachydysrhythmias, pheochromocytoma

Precautions: Pregnancy (C), lactation, arterial embolism, peripheral vascular disease

Do not confuse:
dopamine/dobutamine

Pharmacokinetics:
IV: Onset 5 min, duration <10 min; metabolized in liver, kidney, plasma, excreted in urine (metabolites), half-life 2 min

Interactions:
• Do not use within 2 wk of MAOIs, phenytoin; hypertensive crisis may result
• Dysrhythmias: general anesthetics
• Severe hypertension: ergots
• Decreased action of dopamine: β-blockers, α-blockers
• Increased B/P: oxytocics
• Increased pressor effect: tricyclics, MAOIs

Lab test interferences:
Increased: Urinary catecholamine, serum glucose

NURSING CONSIDERATIONS
Assess:
• Hypovolemia; if present, correct first

Side effects: *italics* = common; ***bold italics*** = life-threatening

• Oxygenation/perfusion deficit (check B/P, chest pain, dizziness, loss of consciousness)
• Heart failure: S₃ gallop, dyspnea, neck vein distention, bibasilar crackles in patients with CHF, cardiomyopathy
• I&O ratio: if urine output decreases, without decrease in B/P, drug may need to be reduced
• ECG during administration continuously; if B/P increases, drug should be decreased
• B/P and pulse q5min after parenteral route
• CVP or PWP during infusion if possible
• Paresthesias and coldness of extremities; peripheral blood flow may decrease
• Injection site: tissue sloughing; if this occurs, administer phentolamine mixed with NS

Administer:
IV
• Plasma expanders or whole blood for hypovolemia
• IV after diluting 200-400 mg/250-500 ml of D_5W, D_5 0.45% NaCl, D_5 0.9% NaCl, D_5LR, LR
• Parenteral IV dose slowly; after reconstituting, use infusion pump; flush line before infusing; infuse as secondary IV line

Additive compatibilities: Aminophylline, atracurium, bretylium, calcium chloride, cephalothin, chloramphenicol, dobutamine, enalaprilat, flumazenil, heparin, hydrocortisone, kanamycin, lidocaine, meropenem, methylprednisolone, nitroglycerin, oxacillin, potassium chloride, ranitidine, verapamil

Syringe compatibilities: Doxapram, heparin, ranitidine

Y-site compatibilities: Aldesleukin, amifostine, amiodarone, amrinone, atracurium, aztreonam, cefmetazole, cefpirome, ciprofloxacin, cisatracurium, cladribine, diltiazem, dobutamine, doxorubicin liposome, enalaprilat, epinephrine, esmolol, famotidine, fentanyl, fluconazole, foscarnet, granisetron, haloperidol, heparin, hydrocortisone, hydromorphone, labetalol, lidocaine, lorazepam, meperidine, methylprednisolone, metronidazole, midazolam, milrinone, morphine, nicardipine, nitroglycerin, norepinephrine, ondansetron, pancuronium, piperacillin/tazobactam, potassium chloride, propofol, ranitidine, remifentanil, sargramostim, sodium nitroprusside, streptokinase, tacrolimus, theophylline, thiotepa, tolazoline, vecuronium, verapamil, vit B/C, warfarin, zidovudine

Perform/provide:
• Storage of reconstituted sol for up to 24 hr if refrigerated
• Do not use discolored sol; protect from light

Evaluate:
• Therapeutic response: increased B/P with stabilization; increased urine output

Teach patient/family:
• The reason for drug administration

Treatment of overdose: Discontinue IV, may give a short-acting α-adrenergic blocker

---

dornase alfa (℞)
Pulmozyme
Func. class.: Cystic fibrosis agent (orphan drug)

Action: May break down molecules in large amounts of infected sputum; improves airflow, lessens chance of bacterial infection
Uses: Management of cystic fibrosis

◆ = Nursing alert   ✔ = Herb-drug interaction   ⃠ = Do not crush

Dosage and routes:
• *Adult/child >5 yr:* **INH** 2.5 mg qd by nebulizer
Available forms: Neb 2.5 mg (1 mg/ml)
Side effects/adverse reactions:
RESP: Possibly laryngitis, hoarseness, hemoptysis, transient decrease in pulmonary function
INTEG: Urticaria, rash
MISC: Chest pain
Contraindications: Hypersensitivity to this drug or Chinese hamster ovary cell products
Precautions: Pregnancy (B)
NURSING CONSIDERATIONS
Assess:
• Resp function: B/P, pulse, lung sounds
Administer:
• By nebulization only
Perform/provide:
• Storage in refrigerator
Evaluate:
• Therapeutic response: decreased thick tenacious secretions, ease of respirations
Teach patient/family:
• To rinse mouth after use
• About all aspects of drug; avoid smoking, smoke-filled rooms, persons with respiratory infections

doxacurium (℞)

(dox-a-cure′ee-um)
Nuromax
Func. class.: Neuromuscular blocker (nondepolarizing)
Action: Inhibits transmission of nerve impulses by binding with cholinergic receptor sites, antagonizing action of acetylcholine
Uses: Facilitation of endotracheal intubation, skeletal muscle relaxation during mechanical ventilation, surgery, or general anesthesia

Dosage and routes:
• *Adult:* **IV** 0.05 mg/kg; 0.08 mg/kg is used for prolonged neuromuscular blockade; maintenance 0.025 mg/kg
• *Child 2-12 yr:* **IV** 0.03-0.05 mg/kg; may decrease for maintenance dose
Available forms: Inj 1 mg/ml
Side effects/adverse reactions:
*CV: **Decreased B/P, ventricular fibrillation, myocardial infarction, cardiovascular accident***
*RESP: **Prolonged apnea, bronchospasm, wheezing, respiratory depression***
EENT: Diplopia
MS: Weakness, prolonged skeletal muscle relaxation, ***paralysis***
INTEG: Rash, urticaria
Contraindications: Hypersensitivity, neonates
Precautions: Pregnancy (C), renal, hepatic disease, lactation, children <3 mo, fluid and electrolyte imbalances, neuromuscular disease, respiratory disease, obesity, elderly, severe burns
Pharmacokinetics: Not metabolized; excretion of unchanged drug in urine and bile
Interactions:
• Increased neuromuscular blockade: aminoglycosides, quinidine, local anesthetics, polymyxin antibiotics, enflurane, isoflurane, tetracyclines, inhalation anesthetics, magnesium, colistin, procainamide, bacitracin, lincomycin, clindamycin, lithium
• Longer onset and shorter duration of doxacurium: phenytoin, carbamazepine
NURSING CONSIDERATIONS
Assess:
• For electrolyte imblances (K, Mg); may lead to increased action of this drug

• Vital signs (B/P, pulse, respirations, airway) until fully recovered; rate, depth, pattern of respirations, strength of hand grip
• I&O ratio; check for urinary retention, frequency, hesitancy
• Recovery: decreased paralysis of face, diaphragm, leg, arm, rest of body
• Allergic reactions: rash, fever, respiratory distress, pruritus; drug should be discontinued

Administer:

IV

• Using nerve stimulator by anesthesiologist to determine neuromuscular blockade
• After succinylcholine effects subside
• Anticholinesterase to reverse neuromuscular blockade
• By slow IV over 1-2 min (only by qualified persons, usually an anesthesiologist); only fresh sol

Solution compatibilities: LR, D$_5$/LR, D$_5$/0.9% NaCl, 0.9% NaCl

Y-site compatibilities: Etomidate, thiopental

Perform/provide:

• Storage at room temperature; do not freeze; stable for 24 hr
• Reassurance if communication is difficult during recovery from neuromuscular blockade
• Frequent (q2h) instillation of artificial tears and covering eyes to prevent drying of cornea

Evaluate:

• Therapeutic response: paralysis of jaw, eyelid, head, neck, rest of body

Treatment of overdose: Neostigmine; monitor VS; may require mechanical ventilation

---

doxapram (℞)

(dox'a-pram)

Dopram

Func. class.: Analeptic

Action: Respiratory stimulation through activation of peripheral carotid chemoreceptor; with higher doses, medullary respiratory centers are stimulated; with progressive CNS stimulation

Uses: Chronic obstructive pulmonary disease (COPD), postanesthesia respiratory depression, prevention of acute hypercapnia, drug-induced CNS depression

Investigational uses:

• Treatment of apnea in premature infants when methylxanthines have failed

Dosage and routes:

Postanesthesia

• *Adult:* IV inj 0.5-1 mg/kg, not to exceed 1.5 mg/kg total as a single injection; IV INF 250 mg in 250 ml sol, not to exceed 4 mg/kg; run at 1-3 mg/min

Drug-induced CNS depression

• *Adult:* IV priming dose of 2 mg/kg, repeated in 5 min; repeat q1-2h till patient awakes; IV INF priming dose 2 mg/kg at 1-3 mg/min, not to exceed 3 g/day

COPD (Hypercapnia)

• *Adult:* IV INF 1-2 mg/min, not to exceed 3 mg/min for no longer than 2 hr

Apnea of premature infant

• *Infant:* 1-1.5 mg/kg/hr loading dose followed by infusion of 0.5-2.5 mg/kg/hr

Available forms: Inj 20 mg/ml

Side effects/adverse reactions:

*CNS: **Convulsions,** (clonus/generalized), headache,* restlessness, dizziness, confusion, paresthesias,

---

◆ = Nursing alert   ∥ = Herb-drug interaction   ⊘ = Do not crush

flushing, sweating, bilateral Babinski's sign, rigidity, depression

GI: Nausea, vomiting, diarrhea, desire to defecate

GU: Retention, incontinence, elevation of BUN, albuminuria

CV: Chest pain, hypertension, change in heart rate, lowered T waves, tachycardia, ***dysrhythmias***

INTEG: Pruritus, irritation at injection site

EENT: Pupil dilation, sneezing

*RESP: **Laryngospasm, bronchospasm,*** rebound hypoventilation, dyspnea, cough, tachypnea, hiccups

Contraindications: Hypersensitivity, seizure disorders, severe hypertension, severe bronchial asthma, severe dyspnea, severe cardiac disorders, pneumothorax, pulmonary embolism, severe respiratory disease

Precautions: Bronchial asthma, pheochromocytoma, severe tachycardia, dysrhythmias, pregnancy (B), hypertension, lactation, children

Pharmacokinetics:

IV: Onset 20-40 sec, peak 1-2 min, duration 5-10 min; metabolized by liver; excreted by kidneys (metabolites); half-life 2.5-4 hr

Interactions:

• Synergistic pressor effect: MAOIs, sympathomimetics

• Cardiac dysrhythmias: halothane, cyclopropane, enflurane; delay use of doxapram for at least 10 min after inhalation anesthetics

NURSING CONSIDERATIONS

Assess:

• BP, heart rate, deep tendon reflexes, ABGs, LOC before administration, q30min

• Po_2, Pco_2, O_2 saturation during treatment

• Hypertension, dysrhythmias, tachycardia, dyspnea, skeletal muscle hyperactivity; may indicate overdosage; discontinue drug

• Respiratory stimulation: increased rate, abnormal rhythm

• Extravasation; change IV site q48h

Administer:

IV

• Undiluted or diluted with equal parts of sterile H_2O for inj; may be diluted 250 mg/250 ml of D_5W, $D_{10}W$ and run as infusion

• IV undiluted over 5 min; IV inf at 1-3 mg/min; adjust for desired respiratory response, using infusion pump IV; if an inf is used after initial dose, start at 1-3 mg/min depending on patient response; D/C after 2 hr; wait 1-2 hr and repeat

• Only after adequate airway is established

• After O_2, IV barbiturates, resuscitative equipment available

Syringe compatibilities: Amikacin, bumetadine, chlorpromazine, cimetidine, cisplatin, cyclophosphamide, dopamine, doxycycline, epinephrine, hydroxyzine, imipramine, isoniazid, lincomycin, methotrexate, netilmicin, phytonadione, pyridoxine, terbutaline, thiamine, tobramycin, vincristine

Perform/provide:

• Placing patient in Sims' position to prevent aspiration of vomitus

• Discontinue infusion if side effects occur; narrow margin of safety

Evaluate:

• Therapeutic response: increased breathing capacity

Teach patient/family:

• Purpose of medication

doxazosin (℞)

(dox-ay'zoe-sin)
Cardura
Func. class.: Peripheral α₁-adrenergic blocker
Chem. class.: Quinazoline

Action: Peripheral blood vessels are dilated, peripheral resistance lowered; reduction in blood pressure results from α₁-adrenergic receptors being blocked

Uses: Hypertension, urinary outflow obstruction, symptoms of benign prostatic hyperplasia

Investigational uses: CHF with digoxin and diuretics

Dosage and routes:

BPH

• *Adult:* **PO** 1 mg qd, increase in stepwise manner to 2, 4, 8 mg qd as needed, max 8 mg
• *Adult:* **PO** 1 mg qd, increasing up to 16 mg qd if required; usual range 4-16 mg/day

HTN

• *Geriatric:* **PO** 0.5 mg qhs, gradually increase

Available forms: Tabs 1, 2, 4, 8 mg

Side effects/adverse reactions:

CV: Palpitations, *orthostatic hypotension*, tachycardia, edema, **dysrhythmias,** chest pain

CNS: Dizziness, headache, drowsiness, anxiety, depression, vertigo, weakness, fatigue, asthenia

GI: Nausea, vomiting, diarrhea, constipation, abdominal pain

GU: Incontinence, polyuria

EENT: Epistaxis, tinnitus, dry mouth, red sclera, pharyngitis, rhinitis

Contraindications: Hypersensitivity to quinazolines

Precautions: Pregnancy (C), children, lactation, hepatic disease

Do not confuse:
Cardura/Coumadin
Cardura/Ridaura

Pharmacokinetics:
PO: Onset 2 hr, peak 2-6 hr, duration 6-12 hr; half-life 22 hr; metabolized in liver; excreted via bile/feces (<63%) and in urine (9%); extensively protein bound (98%)

Interactions:
• Increased hypotensive effects: β-blockers, verapamil
• Decreased hypotensive effects: indomethacin, NSAIDs
• Decreased effects of clonidine
 Increased doxazosin effect: angelica

NURSING CONSIDERATIONS

Assess:
• B/P (lying, standing) and pulse 2-6 hr after each dose and with each increase; postural effects may occur, rales, dyspnea, orthopnea with B/P; pulse, jugular venous distention q4h
• BUN, uric acid if on long-term therapy
• I&O, weight daily
• Edema in feet, legs daily
• Skin turgor, dryness of mucous membranes for hydration status

Administer:
• Tablets broken, crushed or chewed; if chewed, will be bitter

Perform/provide:
• Storage in tight container in cool environment

Evaluate:
• Therapeutic response: decreased B/P; decreased symptoms of BPH

Teach patient/family:
• That fainting occasionally occurs after first dose; do not drive or operate machinery for 4 hr after first dose or after dosage increase or take first dose hs
• To take 1st dose at hs to decrease orthostatic B/P changes

Treatment of overdose: Administer volume expanders or vasopressors; discontinue drug; place in supine position

---

doxepin (℞)

(dox′e-pin)
Adepin, doxepin HCl, Novo-Doxepin*, Sinequan, Sinequan Concentrate, Triadapin*, Zonolon Topical Cream

Func. class.: Antidepressant, tricyclic
Chem. class.: Dibenzoxepin, tertiary amine

Action: Blocks reuptake of norepinephrine, serotonin into nerve endings, increasing action of norepinephrine, serotonin in nerve cells

Uses: Major depression, anxiety

Investigational uses: Chronic pain management, topical pruritus

Dosage and routes:

Depression/anxiety
• *Adult:* PO 25-75 mg/day, may increase to 300 mg/day for severely ill
• *Geriatric:* PO 10-25 mg hs, increase qwk by 10-25 mg to desired dose

Pruritus
• *Adult:* PO 10 mg hs, may increase to 25 mg hs; TOP apply thin film qid at least 3 hr apart

Available forms: Caps 10, 25, 50, 75, 100, 150 mg; oral conc 10 mg/ml; cream 5%

Side effects/adverse reactions:

HEMA: Agranulocytosis, thrombocytopenia, eosinophilia, leukopenia

CNS: Dizziness, drowsiness, confusion, headache, anxiety, tremors, stimulation, weakness, insomnia,

nightmares, EPS (elderly), increased psychiatric symptoms, paresthesia

GI: Diarrhea, dry mouth, nausea, vomiting, *paralytic ileus,* increased appetite, cramps, epigastric distress, jaundice, *hepatitis,* stomatitis, constipation

GU: Urinary retention, acute renal failure

INTEG: Rash, urticaria, sweating, pruritus, photosensitivity

CV: Orthostatic hypotension, ECG changes, tachycardia, hypertension, palpitations, *dysrhythmias*

EENT: Blurred vision, tinnitus, mydriasis, ophthalmoplegia, glossitis

Contraindications: Hypersensitivity to tricyclics, urinary retention, narrow-angle glaucoma, prostatic hypertrophy

Precautions: Suicidal patients, elderly, pregnancy (C), UK-PO lactation, seizures

Do not confuse:
Sinequan/Serentil

Pharmacokinetics:

PO: Steady state 2-8 days; metabolized by liver; excreted by kidneys; crosses placenta; excreted in breast milk; half-life 8-24 hr

Interactions:
• Increased hypertensive action: clonidine, epinephrine, norepinephrine
• Increased doxepin effect: cimetidine, fluoxetine, sertraline
• Increased CNS depression: other CNS depressants
• Hyperpyretic crisis, convulsions, hypertensive episode: MAOI
⚕ Increased anticholinergic effect: belladonna leaf/root, henbane leaf
⚕ Increased action of doxepin: scopolia root, kava

Lab test interferences:

Increase: Serum bilirubin, blood glucose, alk phosphatase

NURSING CONSIDERATIONS
Assess:

• B/P (lying, standing), pulse q4h; if systolic B/P drops 20 mm Hg, hold drug, notify prescriber; take vital signs q4h in patients with cardiovascular disease

• Blood studies: CBC, leukocytes, differential, cardiac enzymes if patient is receiving long-term therapy

• Hepatic studies: AST, ALT, bilirubin

• Weight qwk; appetite may increase with drug

• ECG for flattening of T wave, bundle branch block, AV block, dysrhythmias in cardiac patients; drug should be discontinued gradually several days before surgery

• EPS primarily in elderly: rigidity, dystonia, akathisia

• Mental status: mood, sensorium, affect, suicidal tendencies, increase in psychiatric symptoms: depression, panic

• Urinary retention, constipation; constipation most likely in children, elderly

• Withdrawal symptoms: headache, nausea, vomiting, muscle pain, weakness; not usual unless drug is discontinued abruptly

• Alcohol consumption; if alcohol is consumed, hold dose until morning

Administer:

• Oral conc should be diluted with 120 ml of water, milk, orange, grapefruit juice, tomato, prune, pineapple juice; do not mix with grape juice

• Increased fluids, bulk in diet for constipation

• With food, milk for GI symptoms, do not give with carbonated beverages

• Dosage hs for oversedation during day; may take entire dose hs; elderly may not tolerate qd dosing

• Gum, hard candy, or frequent sips of water for dry mouth

• Topically by applying to affected area, rub slightly

Perform/provide:

• Storage in tight container protected from direct sunlight

• Assistance with ambulation during beginning therapy, since drowsiness/dizziness occurs

• Safety measures primarily for elderly

• Checking to see PO medication swallowed

Evaluate:

• Therapeutic response: decreased anxiety, depression

Teach patient/family:

• That therapeutic effect (depressions) may take 2-3 wk, antianxiety effects sooner

• To use caution in driving, other activities requiring alertness, because of drowsiness, dizziness, blurred vision

• To avoid alcohol ingestion, other CNS depressants

• Not to discontinue medication quickly after long-term use; may cause nausea, headache, malaise

• To wear sunscreen or large hat, since photosensitivity occurs

Treatment of overdose: ECG monitoring; lavage, activated charcoal; administer anticonvulsant, sodium bicarbonate

---

doxercalciferol (℞)
Hectorol

Func. class.: Parathyroid agent (calcium regulator)
Chem. class.: Vit D hormone

Action: Synthetic vit D analog, reduces parathyroid hormone
Uses: To lower high parathyroid hormone levels in patients undergoing chronic kidney dialysis

---

◆ = Nursing alert   ⫽ = Herb-drug interaction   ⊘ = Do not crush

Research note: One study has shown the advantage of parenteral use of doxercalciferol in dialysis patients with hyperparathyroidism[9]

Dosage and routes:

• *Adult:* **PO** 10 µg 3×/wk at dialysis

Available forms: Caps 2.5 µg

Side effects/adverse reactions:

CNS: Drowsiness, headache, lethargy

GI: Nausea, diarrhea, vomiting, anorexia, dry mouth, constipation, cramps, metallic taste

MS: Myalgia, arthralgia, decreased bone development

GU: Polyuria, hypercalciuria, hyperphosphatemia, hematuria

RESP: SOB

Contraindications: Hypersensitivity, hyperphosphatemia, hypercalcemia, vit D toxicity

Precautions: Pregnancy (C), renal calculi, lactation, CV disease

Pharmacokinetics: Unknown

Interactions:

• Decreased absorption of doxercalciferol: cholestyramine, magnesium antacids, mineral oil, do not use together

NURSING CONSIDERATIONS

Assess:

• BUN, urinary calcium, AST, ALT, cholesterol, creatinine, albumin, uric acid, chloride, magnesium, electrolytes, urine pH, phosphate; may increase calcium, should be kept at 9-10 mg/dl, vit D 50-135 IU/dl, phosphate 70 mg/dl

• Alk phosphatase; may be decreased

• For increased drug level, since toxic reactions may occur rapidly

• For dry mouth, metallic taste, polyuria, bone pain, muscle weakness, headache, fatigue, change in LOC, dysrhythmias, increased respirations, anorexia, nausea, vomiting, cramps, diarrhea, constipation; may indicate hypercalcemia

• Renal status: decreased urinary output (oliguria, anuria), edema in extremities, weight gain 5-7 lb, periorbital edema

• Nutritional status, diet for sources of vit D (milk, some seafood); calcium (dairy products, dark green vegetables), phosphates (dairy products) must be avoided

Perform/provide:

• Storage protected from light, heat, moisture

• Restriction of sodium, potassium if required

• Restriction of fluids if required for chronic renal failure

Evaluate:

• Therapeutic response: calcium 9-10 mg/dl, decreasing symptoms of hypocalcemia, hypoparathyroidism

Teach patient/family:

• The symptoms of hypercalcemia

• About foods rich in calcium

• To avoid products with sodium: cured meats, dairy products, cold cuts, olives, beets, pickles, soups, meat tenderizers in chronic renal failure

• To avoid products with potassium: oranges, bananas, dried fruit, peas, dark green leafy vegetables, milk, melons, beans in chronic renal failure

• To avoid OTC products containing calcium, potassium, or sodium in chronic renal failure

• To avoid all preparations containing vit D

• To monitor weight weekly

○ Not to break, crush, or chew caps

---

doxorubicin (℞)
(dox-oh-roo'bi-sin)
Adriamycin PFS, Adriamycin
RDF, Rubex
doxorubicin liposome (℞)
Doxil
Func. class.: Antineoplastic,
antibiotic
Chem. class.: Anthracycline
glycoside

Action: Inhibits DNA synthesis
primarily; derived from *Streptomy-ces peucetius;* replication is de-creased by binding to DNA, which causes strand splitting; active throughout entire cell cycle; a ves-icant

Uses: Wilms' tumor; bladder, breast, cervical, head, neck, liver, lung, ovarian, prostatic, stomach, tes-ticular, thyroid cancer; Hodgkin's disease; acute lymphoblastic leu-kemia; myeloblastic leukemia; neuroblastomas; lymphomas; sar-comas

Dosage and routes:
Doxorubicin
• *Adult:* IV 60-75 mg/m² q3wk, or 30 mg/m² on days 1-3 of 4-wk cy-cle, not to exceed 550 mg/m² cu-mulative dose; Doxil: Adult **IV** 20 mg/m² q3wk
• *Child:* IV 30 mg/m²/day × 3 days, may repeat q4wk
Doxorubicin liposome
• *Adult:* IV 20 mg/m² q3wk
Available forms: Inj 10, 20, 50, 100, 150 mg; Doxil: liposomal disper-sion for inj: 20 mg/ml
Side effects/adverse reactions:
HEMA: ***Thrombocytopenia, leuko-penia, anemia***
GI: Nausea, vomiting, anorexia, mu-cositis, ***hepatotoxicity***

GU: Impotence, sterility, amenor-rhea, gynecomastia, hyperuricemia
INTEG: Rash, necrosis at injection site, dermatitis, reversible alopecia, cellulitis, thrombophlebitis at injec-tion site
CV: Increased B/P, *sinus tachycar-dia, PVCs,* chest pain, ***bradycardia, extrasystoles***
Contraindications: Hypersensitiv-ity, pregnancy (1st trimester) (D), lactation, systemic infections
Precautions: Renal, hepatic, car-diac disease; gout, bone marrow de-pression (severe)
Do not confuse:
Adriamycin/Aredia
Adriamycin/Indamycin
doxorubicin/idarubicin
doxorubicin/daunorubicin
Pharmacokinetics: Triphasic pat-tern of elimination; half-life 12 min, 3⅓ hr, 29⅔ hr; metabolized by liver; crosses placenta; excreted in urine, bile, breast milk
Interactions:
• Increased toxicity: other antineo-plastics or radiation, mercaptopu-rine
• Increased risk of hemorrhagic cys-titis
• Cardiac toxicity: cyclophospha-mide
• Decreased antibody response: live virus vaccine
Lab test interferences:
Increase: Uric acid
NURSING CONSIDERATIONS
Assess:
• CBC, differential, platelet count weekly; withhold drug if WBC is <4000/mm³ or platelet count is <75,000/mm³; notify prescriber of these results
• Blood, urine uric acid levels
• Renal function studies: BUN, serum uric acid, urine CrCl, electrolytes before, during ther-apy

⬥ = Nursing alert   🗲 = Herb-drug interaction   ⊘ = Do not crush

• I&O ratio; report fall in urine output to <30 ml/hr
• Monitor temp q4h; fever may indicate beginning infection
• Liver function tests before, during therapy: bilirubin, AST, ALT, alk phosphatase as needed or monthly; check for jaundice of skin and sclera, dark urine, clay-colored stools, itchy skin, abdominal pain, fever, diarrhea
• ECG; watch for ST-T wave changes, low QRS and T, possible dysrhythmias (sinus tachycardia, heart block, PVCs)
• Bleeding: hematuria, guaiac, bruising, or petechiae, mucosa or orifices q8h
• Effects of alopecia on body image; discuss feelings about body changes
• Inflammation of mucosa, breaks in skin
• Buccal cavity q8h for dryness, sores, ulceration, white patches, oral pain, bleeding, dysphagia
• Alkalosis if severe vomiting is present
• Local irritation, pain, burning at injection site
• GI symptoms: frequency of stools, cramping
• Acidosis, signs of dehydration: rapid respirations, poor skin turgor, decreased urine output, dry skin, restlessness, weakness
• Cardiac status: B/P, pulse, character, rhythm, rate, ABGs, ECG

Administer:
• Antiemetic 30-60 min before giving drug to prevent vomiting
• Allopurinol or sodium bicarbonate to maintain uric acid levels, alkalinization of urine
• Topical or systemic analgesics for pain
• Transfusion for anemia
• Antispasmodic for GI symptoms

IV
◆ Do not interchange doxorubicin with doxorubicin liposome
• Hydrocortisone, dexamethasone, or sodium bicarbonate (1 mEq/1 ml) for extravasation; apply ice compresses
• IV after diluting 10 mg/5 ml of NaCl for inj; another 5 ml of diluent/10 mg is recommended; shake; give over 3-5 min; give through Y-tube of free-flowing 5% dextrose INF or NS

Additive compatibilities: Ondansetron

Syringe compatibilities: Bleomycin, cisplatin, cyclophosphamide, droperidol, leucovorin, methotrexate, metoclopramide, mitomycin, vincristine

Y-site compatibilities: Amifostine, aztreonam, bleomycin, chlorpromazine, cimetidine, cisplatin, cladribine, cyclophosphamide, dexamethasone, diphenhydramine, droperidol, famotidine, filgrastim, fludarabine, fluorouracil, granisetron, hydromorphone, leucovorin, lorazepam, melphalan, methotrexate, methylprednisolone, metoclopramide, mitomycin, morphine, ondansetron, paclitaxel, prochlorperazine, promethazine, propofol, ranitidine, sargramostim, sodium bicarbonate, teniposide, thiotepa, vinblastine, vincristine, vinorelbine
• IV liposome inj (Doxil): dilute dose up to 90 mg/250 ml D_5W, give over ½ hr; do not admix with other sol or meds

Perform/provide:
• Liquid diet: carbonated beverages, geletin may be added if patient is not nauseated or vomiting
• Increased fluid intake to 2-3 L/day to prevent urate, calculi formation
• Rinsing of mouth tid-qid with water, club soda; brushing of teeth bid-

tid with soft brush or cotton-tipped applicators for stomatitis; use unwaxed dental floss

• Storage at room temperature for 24 hr after reconstituting or 48 hr refrigerated

Evaluate:

• Therapeutic response: decreased tumor size, spread of malignancy

Teach patient/family:

• To report any complaints, side effects to nurse or prescriber

• That hair may be lost during treatment and wig or hairpiece may make patient feel better; tell patient that new hair may be different in color, texture

• To avoid foods with citric acid, hot or rough texture

• To report any bleeding, white spots, ulcerations in mouth to prescriber; tell patient to examine mouth qd

• That urine and other body fluids may be red-orange for 48 hr

• To avoid crowds and persons with infections when granulocyte count is low

• That contraceptive measures are recommended during therapy and 4 mo after

• To avoid vaccinations; reactions may occur

---

doxycycline (R)

(dox-i-sye'kleen)

Apo-Doxy*, Doryx, Doxy, Doxy-Caps, Doxycin*, doxycycline, Monodox, Novodoxyclin*, Periostat, Vibramycin, Vibramycin IV, Vibra-Tabs

Func. class.: Antiinfective

Chem. class.: Tetracycline

Action: Inhibits protein synthesis, prosphorylation in microorganisms by binding to 30S ribosomal subunits, reversibly binding to 50S ribosomal subunits; bacteriostatic

Uses: Syphilis, *Chlamydia trachomatis,* gonorrhea, *Rickettsia,* lymphogranuloma venereum, uncommon gram-negative/positive organisms, malaria prophylaxis, chronic periodontitis, acne

Investigational uses: Traveler's diarrhea, Lyme disease, prevention of chronic bronchitis

Dosage and routes:

• *Adult:* **PO/IV** 100 mg q12h on day 1, then 100 mg/day; **IV** 200 mg in 1-2 inf on day 1, then 100-200 mg/day; delivery syst: 10% for cont rel

• *Child >8 yr:* **PO/IV** 2.2-4.4 mg/kg/day in divided doses q12h

Gonorrhea (uncomplicated) in patients allergic to penicillin

• *Adult:* **PO** 200 mg, then 100 mg hs and 100 mg bid × 3 days or 300 mg, then 300 mg in 1 hr; disseminated; 100 mg **PO** bid × at least 7 days

Malaria prophylaxis

• *Adult:* 100 mg qd 1-2 days prior to travel and daily during travel

C. trachomatis

• *Adult:* **PO** 100 mg bid × 7 days

Syphilis

• *Adult:* **PO** 300 mg/day in divided doses × 10 days

Periodontitis

• *Adult:* 20 mg bid after scaling and root planing for ≤9 mo; give ≥1 hr prior to meal AM or PM

Available forms: Tabs 100 mg; caps 50, 100 mg; syr 25 mg/5 ml, 50 mg/5 ml; pwd for inj 100, 200 mg; pwd for oral susp 25, 50 mg/5 ml

Side effects/adverse reactions:

CNS: Fever

HEMA: Eosinophilia, neutropenia, thrombocytopenia, hemolytic anemia

EENT: Dysphagia, glossitis, de-

---

creased calcification of deciduous teeth, oral candidiasis

GI: Nausea, abdominal pain, vomiting, diarrhea, anorexia, enterocolitis, ***hepatotoxicity,*** flatulence, abdominal cramps, gastric burning, stomatitis

CV: Pericarditis

GU: Increased BUN

*INTEG: Rash, urticaria, photosensitivity, increased pigmentation, **exfoliative dermatitis,** pruritus, **angioedema***

Contraindications: Hypersensitivity to tetracyclines, children <8 yr, pregnancy (D)

Precautions: Hepatic disease, lactation

Pharmacokinetics:

PO: Well absorbed, widely distributed peak 1½-4 hr, half-life 14-17 hr; excreted in urine, feces, bile, 90% protein bound, crosses placenta, enters breast milk

Interactions:

• Decreased effects of doxycycline: antacids, NaHCO₃, dairy products, alkali products, iron, kaolin/pectin, barbiturates, carbamazepine, phenytoin, cimetidine sucralfate, cholestyramine, colestipol

• Increased effect: warfarin

• Decreased effects: penicillins, oral contraceptives

⬛ Increased action: bromelain

Lab test interferences:

False increase: Urinary catecholamines; ALT, AST

NURSING CONSIDERATIONS

Assess:

• I&O ratio

• Blood studies: PT, CBC, AST, ALT, BUN, creatinine

• Signs of infection

• Allergic reactions: rash, itching, pruritus, angioedema

• Nausea, vomiting, diarrhea; administer antiemetic, antacids as ordered

• Overgrowth of infection: fever, malaise, redness, pain, swelling, drainage, perineal itching, diarrhea, changes in cough or sputum

• IV site for phlebitis/thrombosis; drug is highly irritating

Administer:

• After C&S

• 2 hr before or after laxative or iron products; 3 hr after antacid or kaolin-pectin products

IV

• After diluting 100 mg or less/10 ml of sterile H₂O or NS for inj; further dilute with 100-1000 ml of NaCl, D₅, Ringer's LR D₅LR, Normosol-M, Normosol-R in D₅W; run 100 mg or less over 1-4 hr; do not give IM/SC; inf must be completed in 6 hr, when diluted in LR sol, or 12 hr in other sol

Additive compatibilities: Ranitidine

Syringe compatibilities: Doxapram

Y-site compatibilities: Acyclovir, amifostine, amiodarone, aztreonam, cisatracurium, cyclophosphamide, diltiazem, filgrastim, fludarabine, granisetron, hydromorphone, magnesium sulfate, melphalan, meperidine, morphine, ondansetron, perphenazine, propofol, remifentanil, sargramostim, tacrolimus, teniposide, theophylline, thiotepa, vinorelbine

Perform/provide:

• Storage in tight, light-resistant container at room temperature; IV stable for 12 hr at room temperature, 72 hr refrigerated; discard if precipitate forms

Evaluate:

• Therapeutic response: decreased temp, absence of lesions, negative C&S

Teach patient/family:

• To avoid sun, since burns may occur; sunscreen does not seem to decrease photosensitivity

• That all prescribed medication must be taken to prevent superinfection

🚫 Not to break, crush, or chew caps

• To take with a full glass of water; may take with food

RARELY USED

D-penicillamine (℞)
(pen-i-sill'a-meen)
Cuprimine, Depen
Func. class.: Heavy metal antagonist
Chem. class.: Chelating agent

Uses: Wilson's disease, rheumatoid arthritis, cystinuria, heavy metal poisoning (lead, mercury, gold)
Dosage and routes:
Cystinuria
• *Adult:* **PO** 250 mg qid ac, not to exceed 5 g/day
• *Child:* **PO** 30 mg/kg/day in divided doses qid ac
Wilson's disease
• *Adult:* **PO** 250 mg qid ac
• *Child:* **PO** 20 mg/kg/day in divided doses ac
Rheumatoid arthritis
• *Adult:* **PO** 125-250 mg/day, then increase 250 mg q2-3mo if needed, not to exceed 1 g/day
• *Child:* **PO** 3 mg/kg/day × 3 mo, then 6 mg/kg/day in divided doses for 3 mo, then increase to max 10 mg/kg/day
Contraindications: Hypersensitivity to penicillins, anuria, agranulocytosis, severe renal disease, pregnancy (D), lactation

droperidol (℞)
(droe-per'i-dole)
droperidol, Inapsine
Func. class.: Neuroleptic
Chem. class.: Butyrophenone
Action: Acts on CNS at subcortical levels, produces tranquilization, sleep; antiemetic
Uses: Premedication for surgery; induction, maintenance in general anesthesia; postoperatively for nausea, vomiting
Dosage and routes:
Induction
• *Adult:* **IV/IM** 0.22-0.275 mg/kg given with analgesic or general anesthetic; may give 1.25-2.5 mg additionally
• *Child 2-12 yr:* **IV** 88-165 µg/kg, titrated to response needed
Premedication
• *Adult:* **IM** 2.5-10 mg ½-1 hr before surgery, may give 1.25-2.5 mg additionally
• *Child 2-12 yr:* **IM** 1-1.5 mg/20-25 lb
Maintaining general anesthesia
• *Adult:* **IV** 1.25-2.5 mg
Regional anesthesia adjunct
• *Adult:* **IV/IM** 2.5-5 mg
Diagnostic procedures without general anesthesia
• *Adult:* **IM** 2.5-10 mg ½-1 hr prior to procedure; 1.25-2.5 mg may be needed
Antiemetic
• *Adult:* **IV** 0.5-1.25 mg q4h prn (unlabeled)
Available forms: Inj 2.5 mg/ml
Side effects/adverse reactions:
*RESP: **Laryngospasm, bronchospasm***
CNS: Dystonia, akathisia, flexion of arms, fine tremors, dizziness, anxiety, drowsiness, restlessness, hallucination, depression, *seizures*

◆ = Nursing alert 🌿 = Herb-drug interaction 🚫 = Do not crush

CV: Tachycardia, hypotension
EENT: Upward rotation of eyes, oculogyric crisis
INTEG: Chills, facial sweating, shivering

Contraindications: Hypersensitivity, child <2 yr, pregnancy (C), lactation

Precautions: Elderly, cardiovascular disease (hypotension, bradydysrhythmias), renal disease, liver disease, Parkinson's disease

Pharmacokinetics:

IM/IV: Onset 3-10 min, peak ½ hr, duration 3-6 hr; metabolized in liver; excreted in urine as metabolites; crosses placenta, half-life 2-3 hr

Interactions:
• Increased CNS depression: alcohol, opiates, barbiturates, antihistamines, antipsychotics, or other CNS depressants
• Increased hypotension: nitrates, antihypertensives
• Increased side effects of lithium
⚕ Increased action: kava

NURSING CONSIDERATIONS
Assess:
• VS q10min during IV administration, q30min after IM dose
• EPS: dystonia, akathisia
◆ For increasing heart rate or decreasing B/P, notify prescriber at once; do not place patient in Trendelenburg position, or sympathetic blockade may occur, causing respiratory arrest
Administer:
• Anticholinergics (benztropine, diphenhydramine) for EPS
• Only with crash cart, resuscitative equipment nearby
• IM deep in large muscle mass
IV, direct
• Undiluted; give through Y-tube at 10 mg or less/min; titrate to patient response

INT INF
• May be given as an infusion by adding dose to 250 ml LR, D_5W, 0.9% NaCl, give slowly, titrate to patient response

Syringe compatibilities: Atropine, bleomycin, butorphanol, chlorpromazine, cimetidine, cisplatin, cyclophosphamide, dimenhydrinate, diphenhydramine, doxorubicin, fentanyl, glycopyrrolate, hydroxyzine, meperidine, metoclopramide, midazolam, mitomycin, morphine, nalbuphine, pentazocine, perphenazine, prochlorperazine, promazine, promethazine, scopolamine, vinblastine, vincristine

Y-site compatibilities: Amifostine, aztreonam, bleomycin, cisatracurium, cisplatin, cladribine, cyclophosphamide, cytarabine, doxorubicin, doxorubicin liposome, famotidine, filgrastim, fluconazole, fludarabine, granisetron, hydrocortisone, idarubicin, melphalan, meperidine, metoclopramide, mitomycin, ondansetron, paclitaxel, potassium chloride, propofol, remifentanil, sargramostim, teniposide, thiotepa, vinblastine, vincristine, vinorelbine, vit B/C

Evaluate:
• Therapeutic response: decreased anxiety, absence of vomiting during and after surgery

Teach patient/family:
• To rise slowly from sitting or standing to minimize orthostatic hypotension
• To avoid ambulation without assistance

---

drotrecogin alfa
See appendix a—selected new drugs

---

dutasteride
See appendix a—selected new drugs

dyphylline (R)
(dye'fi-lin)
Dilor, Dyflex-200, Dylline, dyphylline, Lufyllin, Neothylline

Func. class.: Bronchodilator
Chem. class.: Xanthine, theophylline derivative

Action: Relaxes smooth muscle of respiratory system by blocking phosphodiesterase, which increases cyclic AMP; cyclic AMP results in positive inotropic, chronotropic effects, bronchodilation, stimulation of CNS

Uses: Bronchial asthma, bronchospasm in chronic bronchitis and emphysema, COPD

Dosage and routes:
• *Adult:* **PO** 200-800 mg q6h; **IM** 250-500 mg q6h injected slowly, max 15 mg/kg/dose
• *Child >6 yr:* **PO** 4-7 mg/kg/day in 4 divided doses

Available forms: Tabs 200, 400 mg; elix 33.3, 53.3 mg/5 ml; inj 250 mg/ml

Side effects/adverse reactions:
CNS: Anxiety, restlessness, insomnia, dizziness, **convulsions,** headache, light-headedness, muscle twitching
CV: Palpitations, **circulatory failure,** sinus tachycardia, hypotension, flushing, **dysrhythmias**
GI: Nausea, vomiting, anorexia, dyspepsia, epigastric pain, rectal irritation, bleeding
INTEG: Flushing, urticaria
RESP: Tachypnea, **respiratory arrest**

OTHER: Fever, dehydration, **albuminuria,** hyperglycemia, increased diuresis

Contraindications: Hypersensitivity to xanthines, tachydysrhythmias, hyperthyroidism, peptic ulcer

Precautions: Elderly, CHF, cor pulmonale, hepatic disease, diabetes mellitus, hypertension, children, renal disease, pregnancy (B), lactation, glaucoma

Pharmacokinetics: Well absorbed, peak 1 hr, duration 6 hr, half-life 2 hr, excreted in urine (85%) unchanged, and in breast milk

Interactions:
• Increased action of dyphylline: cimetidine, propranolol, erythromycin, troleandomycin
• Cardiotoxicity: β-blockers
• Increased metabolism of dyphylline: barbiturates, phenytoin
• Decreased elimination of dyphylline: uricosurics
• Decreased levels of phenytoin

NURSING CONSIDERATIONS
Assess:
• Dyphylline blood levels; toxicity may occur with small increase above 20 μg/ml; assess for drug toxicity: nausea, vomiting, anorexia, cramping, diarrhea, confusion, dysrhythmias, seizures, diuresis, flushing, headache
• Monitor I&O; diuresis occurs; dehydration may be the result in elderly or children
• Whether theophylline was given recently
• Auscultate lung fields bilaterally; notify prescriber of abnormalities, monitor pulmonary function studies baseline and periodically
• Allergic reactions: rash, urticaria; drug should be discontinued

Administer:
• Give around the clock to maintain blood levels, give qd dose each AM

 = Nursing alert   = Herb-drug interaction   ⊘ = Do not crush

• PO after meals to decrease GI symptoms; absorption may be affected
• Avoid IM injection; pain occurs, do not use if precipitate occurs
Perform/provide:
• Storage protected from light, at room temperature
Evaluate:
• Therapeutic response: decreased dyspnea, respiratory rate, rhythm
Teach patient/family:
• To check OTC medications, current prescription medications for ephedrine; will increase stimulation; not to drink alcohol, caffeine, or other xanthine products; not to change brands
• To avoid hazardous activities; dizziness, drowsiness, blurred vision may occur
• For GI upset, to take drug with 8 oz water and food
• To avoid smoking, condition may worsen
• To obtain blood levels 6-12 mo

RARELY USED

edetate calcium disodium (Ŗ)
(ee'de-tate)
calcium disodium versenate, calcium EDTA, edathamil calcium disodium, sodium calcium edetate
Func. class.: Heavy metal antagonist (antidote)
Chem. class.: Chelating agent

Uses: Lead poisoning, acute lead encephalopathy
Dosage and routes:
Acute lead encephalopathy
• *Adult and child:* 1.5 g/m^2/day × 3-5 days in 2-3 divided doses **IM** or

slow **IV** with dimercaprol; may be given again after 4 days off drug
Lead poisoning
• *Adult:* **IV** 1 g/250-500 ml D$_5$W or 0.9% NaCl over 1-2 hr or q12h × 3-5 days; may repeat after 2 days; not to exceed 50 mg/kg/day; may be given as **CONT INF** over 8-24 hr
• *Adult:* **IM** 35 mg/kg bid
• *Child:* **IM** 35 mg/kg/day in divided doses q8-12h, not to exceed 50 mg/kg/day; may give for 3-5 days, off 4 days before next course
Contraindications: Hypersensitivity, anuria, poisoning of other metals, severe renal disease, child <3 yr

---

RARELY USED

edetate disodium (Ŗ)
(ee'de-tate)
Chealamide, Disodium EDTA, Disotate, Endrate
Func. class.: Metal antagonist

Uses: Hypercalcemic crisis, control of ventricular dysrhythmias associated with digitalis toxicity
Dosage and routes: *Adult and child:* **IV INF** 15-50 mg/kg/day in 2 divided doses, diluted in 500 ml D$_5$W or 0.9% NaCl, given over 3-4 hr, not to exceed 3 g/day (adult) or 70 mg/kg/day (child); allow 5 days between courses (child), 2 days (adult)
Contraindications: Hypersensitivity, anuria, hepatic insufficiency, poisoning of other metals, severe renal disease, child <3 yr, seizure disorders, active/inactive TB

---

edrophonium (℞)

(ed-roh-fone'ee-um)

Enlon, Reversol, Tensilon

Func. class.: Cholinergics, anticholinesterase

Chem. class.: Quaternary ammonium compound

Action: Inhibits destruction of acetylcholine, which increases concentration at sites where acetylcholine is released; this facilitates transmission of impulses across myoneural junction

Uses: To diagnose myasthenia gravis; curare antagonist; differentiation of myasthenic crisis from cholinergic crisis

Dosage and routes:

Tensilon test (myasthenia gravis diagnosis)

• *Adult:* IV 1-2 mg over 15-30 sec, then 8 mg if no response; IM 10 mg; if cholinergic reaction occurs, retest after ½ hr with 2 mg IM

• *Child >34 kg:* IV 2 mg; if no response in 45 sec, then 1 mg q45sec, not to exceed 10 mg; IM 5 mg

• *Child <34 kg:* IV 1 mg; if no response in 45 sec, then 1 mg q45sec, not to exceed 5 mg; IM 2 mg

• *Infant:* IV 0.5 mg

Reversal of nondepolarizing neuromuscular blockers

• *Adult:* IV 10 mg over 30-45 sec, may repeat, not to exceed 40 mg

Differentiation of myasthenic crisis from cholinergic crisis

• *Adult:* IV 1 mg, if no response in 1 min, may repeat

Available forms: Inj 10 mg/ml

Side effects/adverse reactions:

INTEG: Rash, urticaria

CNS: Dizziness, headache, sweating, weakness, ***convulsions,*** incoordination, ***paralysis,*** drowsiness, ***loss of consciousness***

GI: Nausea, diarrhea, vomiting, cramps, increased salivary and gastric secretions, dysphagia, increased peristalsis

CV: Dysrhythmias, bradycardia, hypotension, ***AV block***, ECG changes, ***cardiac arrest,*** syncope

GU: Urinary frequency, incontinence, urgency

*RESP: **Respiratory depression, bronchospasm, constriction, laryngospasm, respiratory arrest,** dyspnea,* increased bronchial secretions

EENT: Miosis, blurred vision, lacrimation, visual changes

Contraindications: Obstruction of intestine, renal system, hypersensitivity

Precautions: Seizure disorders, bronchial asthma, coronary occlusion, hyperthyroidism, dysrhythmias, peptic ulcer, megacolon, poor GI motility, pregnancy (C), bradycardia, hypotension

Pharmacokinetics:

IV: Onset 30-60 sec, duration 6-15 min

IM: Onset 2-10 min, duration 12-45 min

Interactions:

• Decreased action of edrophonium: procainamide, quinidine, atropine, anesthetics, phenothiazines, antihistamines, haloperidol, magnesium, corticosteroids, antidysrhythmics

• Bradycardia: digitalis

• Prolonged action of: depolarizing muscle relaxants

NURSING CONSIDERATIONS

Assess:

• VS, respiration during test; muscle strength

• Diabetic patient carefully, since this drug lowers blood glucose

Administer:

 Only with atropine sulfate available for cholinergic crisis

 = Nursing alert   🌿 = Herb-drug interaction   🚫 = Do not crush

• Only after all other cholinergics have been discontinued

IV, direct

• 2 mg or less over 15-30 sec; as a curare antagonist, over 30-45 sec; or given as continuous infusion in myasthenic crisis

Y-site compatibilities: Heparin, hydrocortisone, potassium chloride, vit B/C

Perform/provide:

• Storage at room temperature

Evaluate:

• Therapeutic response: increased muscle strength, hand grasp; improved gait; absence of labored breathing (if severe)

Teach patient/family:

• To wear Medic Alert ID specifying myasthenia gravis, drugs taken

Treatment of overdose: Respiratory support, atropine 1-4 mg (IV)

---

efavirenz (℞)

(ef-ah-veer′enz)

Sustiva

Func. class.: Antiretroviral

Chem. class.: Nonnucleoside reverse transcriptase inhibitor (NNRTI)

Action: Binds directly to reverse transcriptase and blocks RNA, DNA causing a disruption of the enzyme's site

Uses: HIV-1 in combination with other antivirals

Dosage and routes:

Given in combination with protease inhibitor or nucleoside analog reverse transcriptase inhibitors (NARTIs)

• *Adult and child >40 kg:* **PO** 600 mg qd hs

• *Child: 10-15 kg:* **PO** 200 mg qd hs

• *Child: 15-20 kg:* **PO** 250 mg qd hs

• *Child: 20-25 kg:* **PO** 300 mg qd hs

• *Child: 25-32.5 kg:* **PO** 350 mg qd hs

• *Child: 32.5-40 kg:* **PO** 400 mg qd hs

Available forms: Caps 50, 100, 200 mg

Side effects/adverse reactions:

GU: Hematuria, kidney stones

CNS: Fatigue, impaired concentration, insomnia, abnormal dreams, depression, headache

GI: Diarrhea, abdominal pain, *nausea,* hyperlipidemia

INTEG: Rash, dizziness, ***erythema multiforme, Stevens-Johnson syndrome, toxic epidermal necrolysis***

Contraindication: Hypersensitivity

Precautions: Liver disease, pregnancy (C), lactation, children <3 yr, renal disease, myelosuppression

Pharmacokinetics: Well absorbed, metabolized by liver, terminal half-life 52-76 hr, >99% protein binding, metabolized by liver

Interactions:

• Decreased efavirenz levels: rifamycins

• Do not give together with benzodiazepines, ergots, midazolam, triazolam, cisapride

• Decreased levels of: indinavir, saquinavir, clarithromycin

• Increased levels of both drugs: ritonavir, estrogens

• Increased levels of: warfarin

• Drug/food: increased absorption: high-fat foods

Lab interferences:

Increase: ALT

False-positive: cannibinoids

NURSING CONSIDERATIONS

Assess:

• Signs of infection, anemia

• Liver studies: ALT, AST: renal studies

• Bowel pattern before, during treatment; if severe abdominal pain with

---

bleeding occurs, drug should be discontinued; monitor hydration
• Skin eruptions; rash, urticaria, itching
• Allergies before treatment, reaction to each medication
• CBC, blood chemistry, plasma HIV RNA, absolute CD4+/CD8+ cell counts/%, serum β_2 microglobulin, serum ICD+24 antigen levels, cholesterol, hepatic enzymes
• Signs of toxicity: severe nausea/vomiting, maculopapular rash

Administer:
• May be given without regard to meals, avoid high-fat foods
• HS to decrease CNS side effects

Evaluate:
• Therapeutic response: increased CD4 cell counts; decreased viral load; slowing progression of HIV

Teach patient/family:
• To take as prescribed; if dose is missed, take as soon as remembered; do not double dose; take with water, juice; may be taken with or without food
• To make sure health-care provider knows all the medications, supplements, or OTC drugs taken
• That if severe rash occurs, to notify health-care provider; that adverse reactions (rash, dizziness, abnormal dreams, insomnia) lessen after a month
• Not to breastfeed or become pregnant if taking this drug, use nonhormonal contraception
• To avoid hazardous activities if dizziness/drowsiness occur
• That drug does not cure disease, but controls symptoms, HIV can be transmitted to others even while taking this drug, to continue with safe-sex practices

---

**enalapril/
enalaprilat (R)**
(e-nal'a-pril)/(e-nal'a-pril-at)
Vasotec, Vasotec IV
Func. class.: Antihypertensive
Chem. class.: Angiotensin-converting enzyme inhibitor

Action: Selectively suppresses renin-angiotensin-aldosterone system; inhibits ACE; prevents conversion of angiotensin I to angiotensin II, dilation of arterial, venous vessels

Uses: Hypertension, systolic CHF, diabetic neuropathy, post MI, left ventricular dysfunction

Dosage and routes:
Hypertension
• *Adult:* PO 5 mg/day, may increase or decrease to desired response range 10-40 mg/day; IV 1.25 mg q6h over 5 min
• *Child:* PO 0.1 mg/kg/day in 1-2 divided doses, max 0.5 mg/kg/day
• *Child:* IV 5-10 µg/kg/dose q8-24h

Patients on diuretics
• *Adult:* IV 0.625 mg over 5 min, may give additional doses of 1.25 mg q6h

Renal impairment
• *Adult:* PO 2.5 mg qd (CrCl <30 ml/min) increase gradually; IV CrCl >30 ml/min 1.25 mg q6h; CrCl <30 ml/min 0.625 mg as one-time dose, increase as per B/P

CHF
• *Adult:* PO 5-20 mg/day in 2 divided doses

Available forms: enalapril: tabs 2.5, 5, 10, 20 mg; enalaprilat: inj 1.25 mg/ml

Side effects/adverse reactions:
CV: Hypotension, chest pain, tachycardia, *dysrhythmias,* syncope
CNS: Insomnia, dizziness, paresthesias, headache, fatigue, anxiety

---

 = Nursing alert   = Herb-drug interaction $\bigcirc$ = Do not crush

GI: Nausea, vomiting, colitis, cramps, diarrhea, constipation, flatulence, dry mouth, loss of taste

INTEG: Rash, purpura, alopecia, hyperhidrosis

*HEMA: **Agranulocytosis, neutropenia***

EENT: Tinnitus, visual changes, sore throat, double vision, dry burning eyes

*GU: **Proteinuria, renal failure,*** increased frequency of polyuria or oliguria

RESP: Dyspnea, dry cough, rales, angioedema

META: Hyperkalemia

Contraindications: Hypersensitivity, history of angioedema, pregnancy (D) 2nd and 3rd trimester

Precautions: Renal disease, hyperkalemia, pregnancy (C) 1st trimester, lactation, hepatic failure, dehydration, bilateral renal artery stenosis

Do not confuse:

enalapril/ramipril

enalapril/Eldepryl

Pharmacokinetics:

PO: Peak 4-6 hr; half-life 1½ hr; metabolized by liver to active metabolite, excreted in urine

IV: Onset 5-15 min, peak up to 4 hr

Interactions:

• Hypersensitivity: allopurinol

• Increased hypotension: diuretics, other antihypertensives, phenothiazines, nitrates, acute alcohol ingestion

• Decreased effects of enalapril: aspirin, antacids

• Increased potassium levels: salt substitutes, potassium-sparing diuretics, potassium supplements

• Increased levels of lithium, digoxin

Lab test interferences:

False-positive: ANA titer

Increase: ALT, AST, bilirubin, alk phosphatase, glucose, uric acid

NURSING CONSIDERATIONS

Assess:

• Blood studies: neutrophils, decreased platelets; WBC with diff baseline and q3mo, if neutrophils <1000/mm^3, discontinue treatment

• B/P, peak/trough level, orthostatic hypotension, syncope when used with diuretic, pulse q4h; note rate, rhythm, quality

• Electrolytes: K, Na, Cl during 1st 2 wk of therapy

• Baselines in renal, liver function tests before therapy begins and 1 wk into therapy

• Edema in feet, legs daily

• Skin turgor, dryness of mucous membranes for hydration status

• Symptoms of CHF: edema, dyspnea, wet rales

Administer:

IV, direct/int inf

• Undiluted over 5 min, use diluent provided or 50 ml D$_5$W, 0.9% NaCl, 0.9% NaCl in D$_5$W or LR, Isolyte E, give through Y-tube of free-flowing inf of 0.9% NaCl, D$_5$W, LR, Isolyte E

Additive compatibilities: Dobutamine, dopamine, heparin, meropenem, nitroglycerin, nitroprusside, potassium chloride

Y-site compatibilities: Allopurinol, amifostine, amikacin, aminophylline, ampicillin, ampicillin/sulbactam, aztreonam, butorphanol, calcium gluconate, cefazolin, cefoperazone, ceftazidime, ceftizoxime, chloramphenicol, cimetidine, cisatracurium, cladribine, clindamycin, dextran 40, dobutamine, dopamine, doxorubicin liposome, erythromycin, esmolol, famotidine, fentanyl, filgrastim, ganciclovir, gentamicin, granisetron, heparin, hetastarch, hydrocortisone, labetalol, lidocaine, magnesium sulfate, melphalan, meropenem, methylprednisolone, metronidazole, morphine, nafcillin, nicardipine, nitroprusside, penicillin G potassium, phenobarbital, piperacillin, piperacillin/tazobactam, potassium chloride, potassium phosphate, propofol, ranitidine, remifentanil, teniposide, thiotepa, tobramycin, trimethoprim-sulfamethoxazole, vancomycin, vinorelbine

Evaluate:
• Therapeutic response: decreased B/P

Teach patient/family:
• Not to use OTC (cough, cold, or allergy) products unless directed by prescriber; to avoid salt substitutes
• To avoid sunlight or wear sunscreen for photosensitivity
• To comply with dosage schedule, even if feeling better
• To notify prescriber of mouth sores, sore throat, fever, swelling of hands or feet, irregular heartbeat, chest pain, signs of angioedema
• That excessive perspiration, dehydration, vomiting, diarrhea may lead to fall in blood pressure; consult prescriber if these occur
• That drug may cause dizziness, fainting; light-headedness may occur during 1st few days of therapy
• That drug may cause skin rash or impaired perspiration; angioedema may occur and to D/C if it occurs
• Not to discontinue drug abruptly
• That CV adverse reactions may reoccur
• To rise slowly to sitting or standing position to minimize orthostatic hypotension

Treatment of overdose: Lavage, IV atropine for bradycardia, IV theophylline for bronchospasm, digitalis, O_2, diuretic for cardiac failure

enoxacin (℞)
(e-nox′a-sin)
Penetrex
Func. class.: Antiinfective
Chem. class.: Fluoroquinolone

Action: Inhibits the enzyme that repairs bacterial DNA, thereby preventing bacterial replication; DNA-gyrase inhibitor

Uses: Uncomplicated urethral or cervical gonorrhea, uncomplicated and complicated UTI; effective against staphylococci, *Aeromonas* sp., *Citrobacter* sp., *Enterobacter* sp., *Escherichia coli*, *Haemophilus ducreyi*, *Klebsiella* sp., *Morganella morganii*, *Neisseria gonorrheae*, *Proteus vulgaris*, *Proteus mirabilis*, *Providencia* sp., *Pseudomonas aeruginosa*, *Serratia*

Dosage and routes:
Gonorrhea
• *Adult:* **PO** 400 mg as a single dose
Uncomplicated UTI
• *Adult:* **PO** 200 mg q12h × 7 days
Complicated UTI
• *Adult:* **PO** 400 mg q12h × 14 days
Renal disease
• CrCl <30 ml/min give initial dose, then give 50% of dose q12h
Available forms: Tabs 200, 400 mg

Side effects/adverse reactions:
*SYST: **Anaphylaxis, Stevens-Johnson syndrome***

CNS: Dizziness, headache, fatigue, somnolence, depression, insomnia, anxiety, **seizures**

GI: Diarrhea, nausea, vomiting, anorexia, flatulence, heartburn, abdominal pain, dry mouth, increased AST, ALT, **pseudomembranous colitis**

INTEG: Rash, pruritus, photosensitivity

EENT: Visual disturbances, dizziness

◆ = Nursing alert   🖉 = Herb-drug interaction   Ⓢ = Do not crush

Contraindications: Hypersensitivity to quinolones

Precautions: Pregnancy (C), lactation, children, elderly, renal disease, seizure disorders

Do not confuse:

enoxacin/enoxaparin

Pharmacokinetics:

PO: Peak 1 hr, half-life 3-6 hr, steady state 2 days; excreted in urine as unchanged drug, metabolites

Interactions:

• Increased levels of: aminophylline, cimetidine, cyclosporine, oral anticoagulants, theophylline, use cautiously

• Decreased absorption of enoxacin: antacids with magnesium, aluminum; iron salts, sucralfate, bismuth subsalicylate

• Increased digoxin levels: digoxin, monitor for toxicity

• Drug/food: decreased absorption with food, dairy products

NURSING CONSIDERATIONS

Assess:

• Kidney, liver function studies: BUN, creatinine, AST, ALT, alk phosphatase

• I&O ratio, urine pH; <5.5 is ideal

• CNS symptoms: insomnia, vertigo, headache, agitation, confusion

• Allergic reactions and anaphylaxis: rash, flushing, urticaria, pruritus; may occur a few days after therapy begins, emergency equipment should be available

Administer:

• After clean-catch urine for C&S

• 2 hr before or 2 hr after antacids, zinc, iron, calcium

Perform/provide:

• Limited intake of alkaline foods, drugs; milk, dairy products, peanuts, vegetables, alkaline actacids, sodium bicarbonate

Evaluate:

• Therapeutic response: negative C&S, absence of symptoms of infection

Teach patient/family:

• That fluids must be increased to 2 L/day to avoid crystallization in kidneys

• If dizziness occurs, to ambulate, perform activities with assistance, do not perform hazardous activities

• Not to take within 2 hr of antacids, calcium, iron, milk, sucralfate; not to double or miss doses

• To use sunscreen, protective clothing for photosensitivity

• To complete full course of drug therapy, take 1 hr ac or 2 hr pc

• To contact prescriber if adverse reactions occur or if inflammation or pain of tendon occurs

• To avoid use with OTC medications unless approved by prescriber

---

enoxaparin (℞)

(ee-nox′a-par-in)

Lovenox

Func. class.: Anticoagulant, antithrombotic

Chem. class.: Unfractionated porcine heparin

Action: Prevents conversion of fibrinogen to fibrin and prothrombin to thrombin by enhancing inhibitory effects of antithrombin III; produces higher ratio of anti–factor Xa to IIa

Uses: Prevention of deep-vein thrombosis, pulmonary emboli in hip and knee replacement

Dosage and routes:

Hip/knee replacement

• *Adult:* **SC** 30 mg bid given 12-24 hr postop for 7-10 days, provided that hemostasis has been established

Abdominal surgery

• *Adult:* **SC** 40 mg qd × 7-10 days to prevent thromboembolic complications, start 2 hr before surgery

Prevention of ischemic complications in unstable angina/non-Q-wave MI with aspirin
• *Adult:* SC 1 mg/kg q12h until stable with aspirin 100-325 mg qd
Available forms: Inj 30 mg/0.3 ml, 40 mg/0.4 ml, 60 mg/0.6 ml, 80 mg/0.8 ml, 100 mg/1 ml
Side effects/adverse reactions:
CNS: Fever, confusion
GI: Nausea
SYST: Edema, peripheral edema
HEMA: **Hypochromic anemia, thrombocytopenia,** bleeding
CV: **Cardiac toxicity**
INTEG: Ecchymosis
Contraindications: Hypersensitivity to this drug, heparin, or pork; hemophilia, leukemia with bleeding, peptic ulcer disease, thrombocytopenic purpura, heparin-induced thrombocytopenia
Precautions: Alcoholism, elderly, pregnancy (B), hepatic disease (severe), renal disease (severe), blood dyscrasias, severe hypertension, subacute bacterial endocarditis, acute nephritis, lactation, children
Do not confuse:
enoxaparin/enoxacin
Pharmacokinetics:
SC: 90% absorbed, maximum antithrombin activity (3-5 hr), elimination half-life 4½ hr, excreted in urine
Interactions:
• Increased action of enoxaparin: anticoagulants, salicylates, NSAIDs, antiplatelets
• Increased hypoprothrombinemia: plicamycin, valproic acid
• Do not mix with other drugs or infusion fluids
🌿 Increased risk of bleeding: bromelain, cinchona bark
Lab test interferences:
Decrease: Platelet count
Increase: AST, ALT

NURSING CONSIDERATIONS
Assess:
• Blood studies (Hct, CBC, coagulation studies, platelets, occult blood in stools), anti–factor Xa; thrombocytopenia may occur
• For bleeding: gums, petechiae, ecchymosis, black tarry stools, hematuria; notify prescriber
• For neurologic symptoms in patients who have received spinal anesthesia
Administer:
• Only after screening patient for bleeding disorders
• SC only; do not give IM, begin 2 hr prior to surgery, do not aspirate, rotate sites, do not expel bubble from syringe before administration
• To recumbent patient; give SC; rotate inj sites (left/right anterolateral, left/right posterolateral abdominal wall)
• Insert whole length of needle into skin fold held with thumb and forefinger
◆ Only this drug when ordered; not interchangeable with heparin
• At same time each day to maintain steady blood levels
• Leave vascular access sheath in place for 6 hr after dose, then give next dose 6 hr after sheath removal
• Avoiding all IM injections that may cause bleeding
Perform/provide:
• Storage at 77° F (25° C); do not freeze
Evaluate:
• Therapeutic response: prevention of deep vein thrombosis
Teach patient/family:
• To use soft-bristle toothbrush to avoid bleeding gums, to use electric razor
• To report any signs of bleeding: gums, under skin, urine, stools
• To avoid OTC drugs containing aspirin

◆ = Nursing alert   🌿 = Herb-drug interaction   🚫 = Do not crush

Treatment of overdose: Protamine SO$_4$ 1% sol; dose should equal dose of enoxaparin

---

entacapone (R)
(en'ta-kah-pone)
Comtan
Func. class.: Antiparkinson agent
Chem. class.: COMT inhibitor

Action: Inhibits COMT (catechol *O*-methyltransferase) and alters the plasma pharmacokinetics of levodopa. Given with levodopa/carbidopa

Uses: Parkinsonism in those experiencing end of dose, decreased effect as adjunct to levodopa/carbidopa

Research note: Motor impairment was improved in patients with severe Parkinson's disease when entacapone was given to patients taking levodopa[10]

Dosage and routes:
• *Adult:* **PO** 200 mg given with carbidopa/levodopa, max 1600 mg/ day

Available forms: Tabs 200 mg film coated

Side effects/adverse reactions:
CNS: Involuntary choreiform movements, hand tremors, fatigue, headache, anxiety, twitching, numbness, dyskinesia, hypokinesia, hyperkinesia, weakness, confusion, agitation, nightmares, psychosis, hallucination, hypomania, severe depression, dizziness, **neuroleptic malignant syndrome**

GI: Nausea, vomiting, anorexia, abdominal distress, dry mouth, flatulence, bitter taste, diarrhea, constipation, dyspepsia, gastritis, GI disorder

INTEG: Rash, sweating, alopecia
CV: Orthostatic hypotension

MISC: Dark urine, back pain, dyspnea, purpura, fatigue, asthenia, infection-bacterial, **rhabdomyolysis**

Contraindications: Hypersensitivity

Precautions: Renal disease, hepatic disease, pregnancy (C), affective disorders, psychosis, lactation, children

Pharmacokinetics: Duration up to 8 hr; excreted in urine, feces; well absorbed, protein binding 98%, metabolized liver extensively, enters breast milk; half-life of levodopa is extended, half-life 0.5 hr initial, 2.5 hr second

Interactions:
• Increased B/P, tachycardia, dysrhythmias, avoid use: bitolterol, apomorphine, dopamine, dobutamine, epinephrine, methyldopa, isoetharine, norepinephrine
• Decreased excretion of entacapone: ampicillin, chloramphenicol, probenecid, erythromycin, rifampin
• Prevents catecholamine metabolism, do not use together: MAOIs

NURSING CONSIDERATIONS
Assess:
◆Neuroleptic malignant syndrome: high temp, increased CPK, rigidity, change in consciousness
• Involuntary movements in parkinsonism: akinesia, tremors, staggering gait, muscle rigidity, drooling when given with levodopa/carbidopa
• B/P, respiration during initial treatment
• Mental status: affect, mood, behavioral changes, depression; complete suicide assessment

Administer:
• Only after MAOIs have been discontinued for 2 wk

Perform/provide:
• Assistance with ambulation during beginning therapy

Side effects: *italics* = common; ***bold italics*** = life-threatening

Evaluate:
• Therapeutic response: decrease in akathisia, increased mood when given with levodopa/carbidopa

Teach patient/family:
• That hallucinations, mental changes, nausea, dyskinesia can occur
• To change positions slowly to prevent orthostatic hypotension; not to drive or operate machinery until stabilized on medication and mental performance is not affected
• To use drug exactly as prescribed
• That urine, sweat may darken
• To notify prescriber if pregnancy is suspected; or if lactating, drug is excreted in breast milk

---

ephedrine (℞)

(e-fed'rin)
ephedrine sulfate

Func. class.: Bronchodilator, nonselective adrenergic, mixed direct and indirect effects

Chem. class.: Phenylisopropylamine

Action: Causes increased contractility and heart rate by acting on β-receptors in the heart; also acts on α-receptors, causing vasoconstriction in blood vessels

Uses: Shock; increased perfusion; hypotension, bronchodilation

Dosage and routes:

Vasopressor
• *Adult:* **IM/SC** 25-50 mg, not to exceed 150 mg/24 hr; **IV** 10-25 mg, not to exceed 150 mg/24 hr
• *Child:* **SC/IV** 3 mg/kg/day or 25-100 mg/m²/day in divided doses q4-6h or 16.7 mg/m² q4-6h

Bronchodilator
• *Adult and child ≥12 yr:* **PO** 25-50 mg bid-qid, not to exceed 400 mg/day; **IM/SC** 12.5-25 mg
• *Child 6-12yr:* 6.25-12.5 mg q4h, max 75 mg/24 hr
• *Child >2 yr:* **PO** 2-3 mg/kg/day or 100 mg/m²/day in 4-6 divided doses

Orthostatic hypotension
• *Adult:* **PO** 25 mg qd-qid
• *Child:* **PO** 3 mg/kg/day in 4-6 divided doses

Stimulation
• *Adult:* **PO** 25-50 mg q3-4h prn
• *Child:* **PO** 3 mg/kg/day or 100 mg/m²/day in divided doses

Labor
• *Adult:* Administer **IV** dose to maintain B/P at or <130/80 mm Hg

Available forms: Inj 25, 30, 50 mg/ml; caps 25, 50 mg

Side effects/adverse reactions:
CNS: Tremors, *anxiety,* insomnia, sweating, headache, dizziness, confusion, hallucinations, *convulsions, CNS depression, cerebral hemorrhage*
GU: Dysuria, urinary retention
CV: Palpitations, tachycardia, hypertension, chest pain, *dysrhythmias*
GI: Anorexia, nausea, vomiting
RESP: **Dyspnea**

Contraindications: Hypersensitivity to sympathomimetics, narrow-angle glaucoma, nonanaphylactic shock during general anesthesia

Precautions: Pregnancy (C), lactation, cardiac disorders, hyperthyroidism, diabetes mellitus, prostatic hypertrophy, hypertension

Pharmacokinetics:
PO: Onset 15-60 min, duration 2-4 hr
IM: Onset 10-20 min, duration 1 hr
IV: Onset 5 min, duration 2 hr
Metabolized in liver; excreted in urine (unchanged), breast milk; crosses blood-brain barrier, placenta

Interactions:
• Severe hypertension: oxytocics

⬥ = Nursing alert   🌿 = Herb-drug interaction   🚫 = Do not crush

• Do not use with MAOIs; hypertensive crisis may occur
• Decreased effect of ephedrine: methyldopa, urinary acidifiers, rauwolfia alkaloids, α-adrenergic blockers, diuretics, tricyclics
• Increased effect of ephedrine: urinary alkalizers
• Dysrhythmia: halothane anesthetics, cardiac glycosides, levodopa
• Decreased effect of guanethidine
🍂 Increased action of ephedrine: ephedra

NURSING CONSIDERATIONS
Assess:
• I&O ratio
• ECG continuously during administration; if B/P increases, drug is decreased; B/P and pulse q5min after parenteral route; CVP or PWP during infusion if possible
• For paresthesias and coldness of extremities; peripheral blood flow may decrease; long-term use may produce a pseudoanxiety state requiring sedative; increased lactic acid with severe metabolic acidosis can occur
• Injection site: tissue sloughing; if this occurs, administer phentolamine mixed with 0.9% NaCl
Administer:
IV, direct
• Through Y-tube or 3-way stopcock; give 10-25 mg slowly; may repeat in 5-10 min, protect from light
• Plasma expanders for hypovolemia
Additive compatibilities: Chloramphenicol, lidocaine, metaraminol, nafcillin, penicillin G potassium
Solution compatibilities: D$_5$W, D$_{10}$W, LR, 0.9% NaCl, 0.45% NaCl, Ringer's
Syringe compatibilities: Pentobarbital
Y-site compatibilities: Etomidate, propofol

Perform/provide:
• Storage of reconstituted sol refrigerated no longer than 24 hr
• Do not use discolored sol
Evaluate:
• Therapeutic response: increased B/P with stabilization
Teach patient/family:
• The reason for drug administration

E

epinephrine (℞)
(ep-i-nef'rin)
Adrenalin Ana-Guard, AsthmaHaler Mist, AsthmaNefrin (racepinephrine), Bronitin Mist, Bronkaid Mist, Epinal, epinephrine, Epinephrine Pediatric, EpiPen, EpiPen Jr., Epitrate, Eppy/N, Medihaler microNefrin, Nephron, Primatene Mist, S-2, Sus-Phrine, Vaponefrin (racepinephrine)

Func. class.: Bronchodilator nonselective adrenergic agonist, vasopressor

Chem. class.: Catecholamine

Action: β$_1$- and β$_2$-agonist causing increased levels of cAMP producing bronchodilation, cardiac, and CNS stimulation; large doses cause vasoconstriction via α-receptors; small doses can cause vasodilation via β$_2$-vascular receptors

Uses: Acute asthmatic attacks, hemostasis, bronchospasm, anaphylaxis, allergic reactions, cardiac arrest, adjunct in anesthesia, shock

Dosage and routes:
Asthma
• *Adult and child:* INH 1-2 puffs of 1:100 or 2.25% racemic q15min
Bronchodilator
• *Adult:* SC 0.2-0.5 mg q20min-4h, max 1 mg/dose

Anaphylactic shock/vasopressor
- *Adult:* SC/IM 0.1-0.5 mg, repeat q5min if needed, then IV; IV 0.1-0.25 mg, repeat q5-15min or inf 1 µg/min, increase to 4 µg/min if needed
- *Child <30 kg:* SC/IM/IV 10 µg/kg, repeat q5-15min up to 0.3 mg

Anaphylactic reaction/asthma
- *Adult:* SC/IM 0.1-0.5 mg, repeat q10-15min, do not exceed 1 mg/dose; epinephrine susp 0.5 mg SC, may repeat 0.5-1.5 mg q6h
- *Child:* SC 0.01 mg/kg, repeat q15min, × 2 doses, then q4h, max 0.5 mg/dose; epinephrine susp 0.025 mg/kg SC, may repeat q6h, max 0.75 mg in child ≤30 kg

Cardiac arrest
- *Adult:* IC, IV, endotracheal 0.1-1 mg, repeat q5min prn
- *Child:* IC, IV, endotracheal 5-10 µg q5min, may use 0.1 µg/kg/min IV INF after initial dose

Available forms: Aerosol 0.16 mg/spray, 0.2 mg/spray, 0.25 mg/spray; inj 1:1000 (1 mg/ml), 1:200 (5 mg/ml), 0.01 mg/ml (1:100,000), 0.1 mg/ml (1:10,000), 0.5 mg/ml (1:2000); sol for nebulization 1:100, 1.25%, 2.25% (base)

Side effects/adverse reactions:
CNS: Tremors, anxiety, insomnia, headache, *dizziness,* confusion, hallucinations, *cerebral hemorrhage,* weakness, drowsiness, headache
CV: Palpitations, tachycardia, hypertension, *dysrhythmias,* increased T wave
GI: Anorexia, nausea, vomiting
RESP: Dyspnea

Contraindications: Hypersensitivity to sympathomimetics, narrow-angle glaucoma, nonanaphylactic shock during general anesthesia, OBS, local anesthesia of certain areas, labor, cardiac dilation, coronary insufficiency, cerebral arteriosclerosis, organic heart disease

Precautions: Pregnancy (C), lactation, cardiac disorders, hyperthyroidism, diabetes mellitus, prostatic hypertrophy, hypertension

Pharmacokinetics:
SC: Onset 3-5 min, duration 20 min
PO, INH: Onset 1 min
Crosses placenta; metabolized in liver

Interactions:
- Do not use with MAOIs or tricyclics; hypertensive crisis may occur
- Toxicity: other sympathomimetics
- Decreased hypertensive effects: α-adrenergic blockers
- Dysrhythmias: bretylium, cardiac glycosides, halothane anesthetics
- Decreased vascular response: diuretics, ergot alkaloids, phenothiazines
- Increased pressor response: guanethidine, antihistamines, levothyroxine
- Severe hypertension: oxytocics

🌿 Increased action of epinephrine: ephedra

NURSING CONSIDERATIONS
Assess:
- ECG during administration continuously; if B/P increases, drug is decreased; B/P and pulse q5min after parenteral route; CVP, ISVR, PCWP during infusion if possible; inadvertent high arterial B/P can result in angina, aortic rupture, cerebral hemorrhage
- Injection site: tissue sloughing; administer phentolamine with NS
- Sulfite sensitivity, which may be life-threatening

Administer:
- Increased dose of insulin in diabetic patients
- Check for correct concentration, route, dosage before administering IM/SC
- Rotate injection sites, massage after inj, shake before using

---

◆ = Nursing alert   🌿 = Herb-drug interaction   🚫 = Do not crush

IV

• Parenteral dose slowly, after reconstituting 1 mg (1:1000 sol)/10 ml or more 0.9% NaCl; to prepare a 1:10,000 sol for maintenance, may be further diluted in 500 ml D$_5$W; give 1 mg or less over 1 min or more through Y-tube or 3-way stopcock; 1 mg = 1 ml of 1:1000 or 10 ml of 1:10,000; protect from light

Additive compatibilities: Amikacin, cimetidine, dobutamine, floxacillin, furosemide, metaraminol, ranitidine, verapamil

Syringe compatibilities: Doxapram, heparin, milrinone

Y-site compatibilities: Amrinone, atracurium, calcium chloride, calcium gluconate, cisatracurium, diltiazem, dobutamine, dopamine, famotidine, fentanyl, furosemide, heparin, hydrocortisone sodium succinate, hydromorphone, labetalol, lorazepam, midazolam, milrinone, morphine, nicardipine, nitroglycerin, norepinephrine, pancuronium, phytonadione, potassium chloride, propofol, ranitidine, remifentanil, vecuronium, vit B/C, warfarin

Endotracheal
• Give directly via endrotracheal tube

Inhalation
• Place in nebulizer (10 gtts of a 1% base sol)
• Dilute racepinephrine 2.25% sol

Perform/provide:
• Storage of reconstituted sol refrigerated no longer than 24 hr
• Do not use discolored sol

Evaluate:
• Therapeutic response: increased B/P with stabilization or ease of breathing

Teach patient/family:
• The reason for drug administration

• To rinse mouth after use to prevent dryness after inhalation
• Not to take OTC preparations

Treatment of overdose: Administer an α-blocker and a β-blocker

epirubicin (℞)
(ep-ih-roo'bi-sin)
Ellence

Func. class.: Antineoplastic, antibiotic

Chem. class.: Anthracycline

Action: Inhibits DNA synthesis primarily; replication is decreased by binding to DNA, which causes strand splitting; maximum cytotoxic effects at S and G$_2$ phases, a vesicant

Uses: Breast cancer as an adjuvant therapy, with axillary node involvement following resection

Research note: One study has concluded that epirubicin produces mild subclinical myocardial damage with a decline in LVEF[11]

Dosage and routes:
• *Adult:* **IV Inf** 100-120 mg/m^2 initially, given with other antineoplastics; given in repeated cycles; 3-4 wk cycles

Hepatic dose
• *Adult:* **IV** bilirubin 1.2-3 mg/dl or AST 2-4 × normal upper limit 50% of starting dose; bilirubin >3 mg/dl or AST >4 × normal upper limit 25% of starting dose

Available forms: Inj 2 mg/ml

Side effects/adverse reactions:
*HEMA: **Thrombocytopenia, leukopenia, anemia, neutropenia, secondary AML***
GI: Nausea, vomiting, anorexia, mucositis, diarrhea
GU: Amenorrhea, hot flashes, hyperuricemia
INTEG: Rash, necrosis at injection site, reversible alopecia

MISC: Infection, febrile neutropenia, lethargy, fever, conjunctivitis
CV: Increased B/P, *sinus tachycardia, PVCs,* chest pain, *bradycardia, extrasystoles,* CHF

Contraindications: Hypersensitivity to this drug, anthracyclines, anthracenediones, severe hepatic disease, baseline neutrophil count <1500 cell/mm^3, severe myocardial insufficiency, recent MI, pregnancy (D), lactation, systemic infections

Precautions: Renal, hepatic, cardiac disease; gout, bone marrow depression (severe), elderly, children

Pharmacokinetics: Triphasic pattern of elimination; half-life 3 min, 2.5 hr, 33 hr; metabolized by liver; crosses placenta; excreted in urine, bile, breast milk

Interactions:
• Increased toxicity: other antineoplastics or radiation, cimetidine
• Decreased antibody response: live virus vaccine

NURSING CONSIDERATIONS
Assess:
• Bone marrow depression, infection: increased temp
• CBC, differential, platelet count weekly; withhold drug if baseline neutrophil ≤1500/mm^3; leukocyte nadir occurs 10-14 days after administration, recovery by 21st day; notify prescriber of these results
• Blood, urine uric acid levels; swelling, joint pain primarily in extremities, patient should be well hydrated to prevent urate deposits
• Renal function studies: BUN, serum uric acid, urine CrCl, electrolytes before, during therapy; I&O ratio; report fall in urine output to <30 ml/hr; dosage adjustment is needed if serum creatinine >5 mg/dl
• Liver function tests before, during therapy: bilirubin, AST, ALT, alk phosphatase as needed or monthly

• Cardiac status: B/P, pulse, character, rhythm, rate, ABGs, ECG, LVEF, MUGA scan, or ECHO; watch for ST-T wave changes, low QRS and T, possible dysrhythmias (sinus tachycardia, heart block, PVCs)
• Bleeding: hematuria, guaiac, bruising, or petechiae, mucosa or orifices q8h
• Effects of alopecia on body image; discuss feelings about body changes
• Alkalosis if severe vomiting is present
• Local irritation, pain, burning at injection site
• GI symptoms: frequency of stools, cramping
• Acidosis, signs of dehydration: rapid respirations, poor skin turgor, decreased urine output, dry skin, restlessness, weakness

Administer:
• Antiemetic 30-60 min before giving drug to prevent vomiting
• Allopurinol or sodium bicarbonate to maintain uric acid levels, alkalinization of urine
IV
• Hydrocortisone, dexamethasone, or sodium bicarbonate (1 mEq/1 ml) for extravasation; apply ice compresses
• Given into tubing of free-flowing IV infusion (0.9% NaCl or D_5) give over 3-5 min; do not mix with other drugs in syringe

Perform/provide:
• Strict hand-washing technique, gloves, protective clothing
• Liquid diet: carbonated beverages, gelatin may be added if patient is not nauseated or vomiting
• Increased fluid intake to 2-3 L/day to prevent urate, calculi formation

Evaluate:
• Therapeutic response: decreased tumor size, spread of malignancy

◆ = Nursing alert   ⫸ = Herb-drug interaction   ⊘ = Do not crush

Teach patient/family:
• To report any complaints, side effects to nurse or prescriber
• That hair may be lost during treatment and wig or hairpiece may make patient feel better; tell patient that new hair may be different in color, texture
• To avoid crowds and persons with infections when granulocyte count is low
• That contraceptive measures are recommended during therapy and 4 mo thereafter
• To avoid vaccinations, reactions may occur; to avoid cimetidine during therapy
• That urine may appear red for 2 days
• To avoid crowds, persons with known infections
• To avoid OTC medications, supplements unless approved by prescriber

epoetin (℞)

(ee-poe′e-tin)
EPO, Epogen, Eprex*, erythropoietin, Procrit
Func. class.: Antianemic, biologic modifier, hormone
Chem. class.: Amino acid polypeptide

Action: Erythropoietin is one factor controlling rate of red cell production; drug is developed by recombinant DNA technology
Uses: Anemia caused by reduced endogenous erythropoietin production, primarily end-stage renal disease; to correct hemostatic defect in uremia; anemia due to AZT treatment in HIV patients; anemia due to chemotherapy; reduction of allogeneic blood transfusion in surgery patients

Dosage and routes:
Anemia secondary to chemotherapy
• *Adult:* SC 150 U/kg 3 ×/wk, may increase after 2 mo up to 300 U/kg 3 ×/wk
Anemia in chronic renal failure
• *Adult:* SC/IV 50-100 U/kg 3 ×/wk, then adjust dose by 25 U/kg/dose to maintain Hct; maintenance: 12.5-25 U/kg, titrate to target Hct
Anemia secondary to zidovudine treatment
• *Adult:* SC/IV 100 U/kg 3 ×/wk × 2 mo, may increase by 50-100 U/kg q1-2mo, up to 300 U/kg 3 ×/wk
Surgery
• *Adult:* SC 300 U/kg/day × 10 days prior to surgery, the day of surgery, and for 4 days postsurgery or 600 U/kg at 3 wk, 2 wk, 1 wk, prior to and on day of surgery
Available forms: Inj 2000, 3000, 4000, 10,000, 20,000 U/ml
Side effects/adverse reactions:
CV: Hypertension, **hypertensive encephalopathy,** headache
CNS: **Seizures,** coldness, sweating
MS: Bone pain
Contraindications: Hypersensitivity to mammalian cell–derived products, or human albumin, uncontrolled hypertension
Precautions: Seizure disorder, porphyria, pregnancy (C)
Pharmacokinetics:
IV: Metabolized in body; extent of metabolism unknown; onset of increased reticulocyte count 1-6 wk; peak, immediate
Interactions:
• Need for increased anticoagulant during hemodialysis
NURSING CONSIDERATIONS
Assess:
• Renal studies: urinalysis, protein, blood, BUN, creatinine
• Blood studies: ferritin, transferrin monthly; transferrin sat ≥20%, fer-

ritin ≥100 ng/ml; Hct 2×/wk until stabilized in target range (30%-33%) then at regular intervals; those with endogenous erythropoietin levels of <500 U/L respond to this agent

• B/P; check for rising B/P as Hct rises, antihypertensives may be needed

• CV status: hypertension may occur rapidly leading to hypertensive encephalopathy

• I&O; report drop in output to <50 ml/hr

• For seizures if Hct is increased within 2 wk by 4 pts

• CNS symptoms: coldness, sweating, pain in long bones

Administer:

• Do not shake vial

IV

• Additional heparin to lower chance of clots

• By direct inj or bolus into IV tubing or venous line at end of dialysis

• Dialysis patients: thrill, bruit of shunts, monitor for circulation impairment

• Decrease dose by 25 U/kg, if Hct increases by 4% in 2 wk

Solution compatibilities: NaCl 0.9%, $D_{10}W$, $D_{10}W$/albumin, sterile water for inj, TPN

SC

• Used for patients not on dialysis; admix before giving, using 0.9% NaCl with benzyl alcohol 0.9% 1:1

Evaluate:

• Therapeutic response: increase in reticulocyte count in 1-6 wk, Hgb/Hct; increased appetite, enhanced sense of well-being

Teach patient/family:

• To avoid driving or hazardous activity during beginning of treatment To monitor B/P

• To take iron supplements, vitamin B_{12}, folic acid as directed

eprosartan mesylate

See appendix a—selected new drugs

eptifibatide (Ŗ)

(ep-tih-fib′ah-tide)
Integrilin
Func. class.: Antiplatelet agent
Chem. class.: Glycoprotein IIb/ IIIa inhibitor

Action: Platelet glycoprotein antagonist. this agent reversibly prevents fibrinogen, von Willebrand's factor from binding to the glycoprotein IIb/IIIa receptor, inhibitin platelet aggregation

Uses: Acute coronary syndrome including those with PCI (percutaneous coronary intervention)

Dosage and routes:

Acute coronary syndrome

• *Adult:* **IV BOL** 180 μg/kg as soon as diagnosed, then **IV CONT** 2 μg/ kg/min until discharge or CABG up to 72 hr; may decrease inf rate to 0.5 μg/kg/min if undergoing PCI; continue inf for 20-24 hr postprocedure, allowing up to 96 hr of treatment

PCI in patients without acute coronary syndrome

• *Adult:* **IV BOL** 135 μg/kg given immediately before PCI; then 0.5 μg/kg/min × 20-24 hr

Available forms: Sol for inj 2 mg/ml (10 ml), 0.75 mg/ml (100 ml)

Side effects/adverse reactions:

CV: Stroke, hypotension
SYST: Bleeding, anaphylaxis
GU: Hematuria
HEMA: Thrombocytopenia

Contraindications: Hypersensitivity, active internal bleeding; history of bleeding, stroke within 1 mo; major surgery with severe trauma, severe hypotension, history of intra-

◆ = Nursing alert   🖉 = Herb-drug interaction   Ⓢ = Do not crush

cranial bleeding, intracranial neoplasm, arteriovenous malformation/aneurysm, aortic dissection, dependence on renal dialysis

Precautions: Bleeding, pregnancy (B), lactation, children, elderly, renal function impairment

Interactions:
• Increased bleeding: aspirin, heparin, NSAIDs, anticoagulants, ticlopidine, clopidogrel, dipyridamole, thrombolytics, plicamycin, valproate, abciximab
• Do not give with platelet receptor inhibitors IIb, IIIa

Pharmacokinetics: half-life 2.5 hr, steady state 4-6 hr, metabolism limited, excretion via kidneys

NURSING CONSIDERATIONS
Assess:
◆ Platelets, Hgb, Hct, creatinine, PT/APTT baseline INR within 6 hr of loading dose and qd thereafter, patients undergoing PCI should have ACT monitored; maintain APTT 50-70 sec unless PCI is to be performed; during PCI, ACT should be 300-350 sec; if platelets drop <100,000/mm³, obtain additional platelet counts; if thrombocytopenia is confirmed, discontinue drug; also, draw Hct, Hgb, serum creatinine
◆ For bleeding: gums, bruising, ecchymosis, petechiae; from GI, GU tract, cardiac cath sites, IM inj sites

Administer:
• Aspirin and heparin may be given with this drug
• D/C heparin before removing femoral artery sheath, after PCI
IV
• After withdrawing bolus dose from 10 ml vial, give IV push over 1-2 min; follow bolus dose with continuous inf using pump, give drug undiluted directly from 100 ml vial, spike 100 ml vial with vented infusion set, use caution when centering spike on circle of stopper top

Y-site compatabilities: alteplase, atropine, dobutamine, heparin, lidocaine, meperidine, metoprolol, midazolam, morphine, nitroglycerin, verapamil

Solution compatibilities: 0.9% NaCl, D₅/0.9% NaCl

Perform/provide:
• Do not give discolored solutions or those with particulates, discard unused amount
• Discontinuing drug prior to CABG
• All medications PO if possible, avoid IM inj and all catheters

Teach patient/family:
• Reason for medication and expected results
• To report bruising, bleeding, chest pain immediately

---

ergonovine (℞)
(er-goe-noe'veen)
ergonovine, Ergotrate
Func. class.: Oxytocic
Chem. class.: Ergot alkaloid

Action: Stimulates uterine contractions and vascular smooth muscle, decreases bleeding

Uses: Postpartum or postabortion hemorrhage

Investigational uses: To induce a coronary artery spasm for diagnostic purposes

Dosage and routes:
Oxytocic
• *Adult:* **PO/SL** 0.2-0.4 mg q6-12h; **IM** 0.2 mg q2-4h, not to exceed 5 doses; **IV** 0.2 mg given over 1 min
Induced coronary artery spasm
• *Adult:* **IV** 50 µg q5min up to 400 µg or when chest pain occurs
Available forms: Inj 0.2, 0.25 mg/ml; tab 0.2 mg

Side effects/adverse reactions:
CNS: Headache, dizziness, fainting
CV: Hypertension, chest pain
GI: Nausea, vomiting, diarrhea
INTEG: Sweating
RESP: Dyspnea
EENT: Tinnitus
GU: Cramping
Contraindications: Hypersensitivity to ergot medication, augmentation of labor, before delivery of placenta, spontaneous abortion (threatened), pelvic inflammatory disease
Precautions: Hepatic disease, renal disease, cardiac disease, asthma, anemia, convulsive disorders, hypertension, glaucoma, obliterative vascular disease
Pharmacokinetics:
IM: Onset 2-5 min, duration 3 hr
IV: Onset immediate, duration 45 min
Metabolized in liver, excreted in urine
Interactions:
• Hypertension: sympathomimetics, ergots
 Hypertension: ephedra
NURSING CONSIDERATIONS
Assess:
• Ergotism: nausea, vomiting, weakness, muscular pain, insensitivity to cold, paresthesias of extremities; drug should be discontinued
• B/P, pulse; watch for change that may indicate hemorrhage
• Respiratory rate, rhythm, depth; notify prescriber of abnormalities
• Fundal tone, nonphasic contractions; check for relaxation
Administer:
• IM inj deep in large muscle mass; rotate injection sites if additional doses are given
• With emergency equipment available
IV, direct
• Dilute with 5 ml 0.9% NaCl, give

through Y-tube or 3-way stopcock over 1 min
Additive compatibilities: Amikacin, cephapirin, sodium bicarbonate
Evaluate:
• Therapeutic response: decreased blood loss, severe cramping
Teach patient/family:
• To report increased blood loss, increased temp, or foul-smelling lochia; that cramping is normal
• The importance of pad count
• To avoid nicotine products
Treatment of overdose: Stop drug, give vasodilators, heparin, dextran

---

ergotamine (Ꝛ)
(er-got′a-meen)
Ergomar*, Ergostat,
Gynergen*
dihydroergotamine
(dye-hye-droe-er-got′a-meen)
DHE45, Dihydroergotamine-
Sandoz*, Migranal
Func. class.: α-Adrenergic
blocker, vascular headache
suppressant
Chem. class.: Ergot alkaloid—
amino acid

Action: Constricts smooth muscle in peripheral, cranial blood vessels, relaxes uterine muscle; blocks serotonin release
Uses: Vascular headache (migraine, cluster histamine)
Dosage and routes:
ergotamine
• *Adult:* **SL** 1 tab, may use q30min, max 3 tabs/24 hr
dihydroergotamine
• *Adults:* **SC/IM** 1 mg, may repeat in 1 hr to 3 mg, max 3 mg/day or 6 mg/wk; **IV** 0.5 mg, may repeat in 1 hr, max 2 mg/day or 6 mg/wk
• *Child ≥6 yr:* **SC/IM** 0.5 mg, may repeat in 1 hr; **IV:** 0.25 mg, may repeat in 1 hr

---

 = Nursing alert   = Herb-drug interaction $\bigcirc$ = Do not crush

Severe acute migraine
• *Child 12-16 yr:* **IV** 0.25-0.5 mg, may repeat q20min for 1-2 doses
Available forms: ergotamine: SL tabs 2 mg; dihydroergotamine: inj 1 mg/ml; nasal spray 4 mg/ml
Side effects/adverse reactions:
CNS: Numbness in fingers, toes, headache, weakness
CV: Transient tachycardia, chest pain, bradycardia, edema, claudication, increase or decrease in B/P, ***MI***
GI: Nausea, vomiting, diarrhea, abdominal cramps
MS: Muscle pain
Contraindications: Hypersensitivity to ergot preparations, occlusion (peripheral, vascular), CAD, hepatic disease, renal disease, peptic ulcer, hypertension, pregnancy (X), Raynaud's disease, peripheral vascular disease, intermittent claudication
Precautions: Lactation, children, anemia, elderly
Pharmacokinetics:
IM/SC: Duration 8 hr
IV: Peak ¼-2 hr, duration 8 hr
PO: Peak 30 min-3 hr; metabolized in liver; excreted as metabolites in feces; crosses blood-brain barrier; excreted in breast milk
Interactions:
• Increased risk of ergot toxicity: macrolides
• Increased vasoconstriction: β-blockers
NURSING CONSIDERATIONS
Assess:
• Ergotism: nausea, vomiting, weakness, muscular pain, insensitivity to cold, paresthesia of extremities; drug should be discontinued
• Weight daily, check for peripheral edema in feet, legs
• For stress level, activity, recreation, coping mechanisms

• Neurologic status: LOC, blurring vision, nausea, vomiting, tingling in extremities that occurs preceding the headache
• Ingestion of tyramine foods (pickled products, beer, wine, aged cheese), food additives, preservatives, colorings, artificial sweeteners, chocolate, caffeine; may precipitate headaches
• Toxicity: dyspnea, hypotension or hypertension, rapid, weak pulse, delirium, nausea, vomiting
Administer:
• At beginning of headache; dose must be titrated to patient response
• Not to pregnant women; harm to fetus may occur
IV
• Give dihydroergotamine undiluted over 1 min
Perform/provide:
• Quiet, calm environment with decreased stimulation for noise, bright light, or excessive talking
Evaluate:
• Therapeutic response: decrease in frequency, severity of headache
Teach patient/family:
• Not to use OTC medications; serious drug interactions may occur
• To maintain dose at approved level; not to increase even if drug does not relieve headache
• To report side effects including increased vasoconstriction starting with cold extremities, then paresthesia, weakness
• That an increase in headaches may occur when this drug is discontinued after long-term use
◆ To keep drug out of reach of children; death may occur
Treatment of overdose: Induce emesis or gastric lavage if orally ingested; administer saline cathartic; keep warm

ertapenem
See appendix a—selected new drugs

erythromycin base (℞)
(eh-rith-roh-my'sin)
Apo-Erythro*, E-Mycin, Eramycin, Erybid*, Eryc, Ery-Tab, E-Base, Erythromid*, Erythromycin Base Filmtab, Erythromycin Delayed-Release, Novo-Rythro Encap*, PCE
erythromycin estolate (℞)
Ilosone, Novo-Rythro*
erythromycin ethylsuccinate (℞)
Apo-Erythro-Es*, E.E.S., Ery Ped, Novo-Rythro*
erythromycin gluceptate
erythromycin lactobionate (℞)
Erythrocin
erythromycin stearate (℞)
Apo-Erythro-S*, Novo-Rythro*
Func. class.: Antiinfective
Chem. class.: Macrolide

Action: Binds to 50S ribosomal subunits of susceptible bacteria and suppresses protein synthesis

Uses: Infections caused by *Neisseria gonorrhoeae;* mild to moderate respiratory tract, skin, soft tissue infections caused by *Streptococcus pneumoniae, Mycoplasma pneumoniae, Corynebacterium diphtheriae, Bordetella pertussis, Treponema pallidum, Borrelia burgdorferi, Listeria monocytogenes;* syphilis; Legionnaire's disease, *Legionella pneumophila, Chlamydia trachomatis; Haemophilus influenzae* (when used with sulfonamides)

Research note: Grapefruit juice increased erythromycin concentrations in a study of 6 people[12]

Dosage and routes:

Soft tissue infections
• *Adult:* **PO** 250-500 mg q6h (base, estolate, stearate); **PO** 400-800 mg q6h (ethylsuccinate); **IV INF** 15-20 mg/kg/day (lactobionate) divided q6h
• *Child:* **PO** 30-50 mg/kg/day in divided doses q6h (salts); **IV** 20-40 mg/kg/day in divided doses q6h (lactobionate)

N. gonorrhoeae/PID
• *Adult:* **IV** 500 mg q6h × 3 days (gluceptate, lactobionate), then **PO** 250 mg (base, estolate, stearate) or 400 mg (ethylsuccinate) q6h × 1 wk

Syphilis
• *Adult:* **PO** 30 g in divided doses over 15 days (base, estolate, stearate)

Chlamydia
• *Adult:* **PO** 500 mg q6h × 1 wk or 250 mg qid × 2 wk
• *Infant:* **PO** 50 mg/kg/day in 4 divided doses × 3 wk or more
• *Newborn:* **PO** 50 mg/kg/day in 4 divided doses × 2 wk or more

Intestinal amebiasis
• *Adult:* **PO** 250 mg q6h × 10-14 days (base, estolate, stearate)
• *Child:* **PO** 30-50 mg/kg/day in divided doses q6h × 10-14 days (base, estolate, stearate)

Available forms: Base: tabs, enteric-coated 250, 333 mg; tabs, film-coated 250, 500 mg; caps, enteric-coated 125, 250 mg; estolate: tabs, chewable 125, 250 mg; tabs 500 mg; caps 125, 250 mg; drops 100 mg/ml; susp 125, 250 mg/5 ml; stearate: tabs, film-coated 250, 500 mg; ethylsuccinate: tabs, chewable 200, 400 mg; 100 mg/2.5

ml, 200, 400 mg/5 ml; susp 200, 400 mg; powder for suspension: 100 mg/2.5 ml, 200 and 400 mg/5 ml; powder for inj: 500 mg and 1 g (lactobionate), 250 mg, 500 mg, 1 g (as gluceptate)

Side effects/adverse reactions:

CV: ***Dysrhythmias***

INTEG: Rash, urticaria, pruritus, thrombophlebitis (IV site)

GI: Nausea, vomiting, diarrhea, **hepatotoxicity,** abdominal pain, stomatitis, heartburn, anorexia, pruritus ani

GU: Vaginitis, moniliasis

EENT: Hearing loss, tinnitus

SYST: **Anaphylaxis**

Contraindications: Hypersensitivity, preexisting liver disease (estolate), hepatic disease

Precautions: Pregnancy (B), hepatic disease, lactation

Pharmacokinetics: Peak 4 hr (base): ½–2½ hr (ethylsuccinate), duration 6 hr, half-life 1-2 hr; metabolized in liver; excreted in bile, feces, protein binding 75%-90%

Interactions:

• Increased action, toxicity of: oral anticoagulants, digoxin, theophylline, methylprednisolone, cyclosporine, bromocriptine, disopyramide, ergots, triazolam, dihydropyridine, calcium antagonists, lovastatin, simvastatin, midazolam, clindamycin

◆ Serious dysrhythmias: pimozide, sparfloxacin; do not use together

Lab test interferences:

False increase: 17-OHCS/17-KS

Increase: AST/ALT

Decrease: Folate assay

NURSING CONSIDERATIONS

Assess:

• For infection: temp, characteristics of wounds, urine, stools, sputum, WBCs, baseline and periodically

• I&O ratio; report hematuria, oliguria in renal disease

• Liver studies: AST, ALT, if patient is on long-term therapy

• Renal studies: urinalysis, protein, blood

• C&S before drug therapy; drug may be given as soon as culture is taken; C&S may be repeated after treatment

• Bowel pattern before, during treatment

• Skin eruptions, itching

• Respiratory status: rate, character, wheezing, tightness in chest; discontinue drug if these occur

• Allergies before treatment, reaction of each medication

Administer:

• Do not give by IM or IV push

• Enteric-coated tablets may be given with food

🚫 Do not break, crush, or chew

• Chewable tabs should be chewed only

IV

• After diluting 500 mg or less/10 ml sterile H_2O without preservatives; dilute further in 80-250 ml of 0.9% NaCl, LR, Normosol-R; may be further diluted to 1 mg/ml and given as continuous infusion; run 1 g or less/100 ml over ½-1 hr; continuous infusion over 6 hr, may require buffers to neutralize pH if dilution is <250 ml, use infusion pump

Additive compatibilities: *Gluceptate:* Calcium gluconate, hydrocortisone, methicillin, penicillin G potassium, potassium chloride, sodium bicarbonate

Lactobionate: Aminophylline, ampicillin, cimetidine, diphenhydramine, hydrocortisone, lidocaine, methicillin, penicillin G potassium or sodium, pentobarbital, polymyxin B, potassium chloride, prednisolone, prochlorperazine, promazine, ranitidine, sodium bicarbonate, verapamil

Syringe compatibilities: *Lactobionate:* Methicillin

Y-site compatibilities: Acyclovir, amiodarone, cyclophosphamide, diltiazem, enalaprilat, esmolol, famotidine, foscarnet, heparin, hydromorphone, idarubicin, labetalol, lorazepam, magnesium sulfate, meperidine, midazolam, morphine, multivitamins, perphenazine, tacrolimus, theophylline, vit B/C, zidovudine

Perform/provide:

• Storage at room temperature; store susp in refrigerator

• Adequate intake of fluids (2 L) during diarrhea episodes

Evaluate:

• Therapeutic response: decreased symptoms of infection

Teach patient/family:

• To take oral drug with full glass of water; with food for GI symptoms

• Not to take with fruit juice

• To report sore throat, fever, fatigue (could indicate superinfection)

• To notify nurse of diarrhea stools, dark urine, pale stools, jaundice of eyes or skin, and severe abdominal pain

• To take at evenly spaced intervals; complete dosage regimen

Treatment of hypersensitivity: Withdraw drug; maintain airway; administer epinephrine, aminophylline, O₂, IV corticosteroids

---

esmolol (℞)

(ez'moe-lole)
Brevibloc
Func. class.: β-Adrenergic blocker (antidysrhythmic II)

Action: Competitively blocks stimulation of β_1-adrenergic receptors in the myocardium; produces negative chronotropic, inotropic activity (decreases rate of SA node discharge, increases recovery time), slows conduction of AV node, decreases heart rate, decreases O₂ consumption in myocardium; also decreases renin-aldosterone-angiotensin system at high doses; inhibits β_2-receptors in bronchial system slightly

Uses: Supraventricular tachycardia, noncompensatory tachycardia, hypertensive crisis

Dosage and routes:

• *Adult:* **IV** loading dose 500 μg/kg/min over 1 min; maintenance 50 μg/kg/min for 4 min; if no response in 5 min, give 2nd loading dose; then increase inf to 100 μg/kg/min for 4 min; if no response, repeat loading dose, then increase maintenance inf by 50 μg/kg/min (max of 200 μg/kg/min), titrate to patient response

• *Child:* **IV** 50 μg/kg/min, may increase q10min (max 300 μg/kg/min)

Available forms: Inj 10 mg, 250 mg/ml

Side effects/adverse reactions:

INTEG: Induration, inflammation at site, discoloration, edema, erythema, burning pallor, flushing, rash, pruritus, dry skin, alopecia

CNS: Confusion, light-headedness, paresthesia, somnolence, fever, dizziness, fatigue, headache, depression, anxiety, *seizures*

GI: Nausea, vomiting, anorexia, gastric pain, flatulence, constipation, heartburn, bloating

CV: Hypotension, bradycardia, chest pain, peripheral ischemia, shortness of breath, *CHF,* conduction disturbances

GU: Urinary retention, impotence, dysuria

RESP: Bronchospasm, dyspnea, cough, wheeziness, nasal stuffiness

---

◆ = Nursing alert   ∥ = Herb-drug interaction   ⊘ = Do not crush

Contraindications: 2nd- or 3rd-degree heart block, cardiogenic shock, CHF, cardiac failure, hypersensitivity

Precautions: Hypotension, pregnancy (C), peripheral vascular disease, diabetes, hypoglycemia, thyrotoxicosis, renal disease, lactation

Do not confuse:

Brevibloc/Brevital

Pharmacokinetics:

Onset very rapid, duration short, half-life 9 min; metabolized by hydrolysis of the ester linkage; excreted via kidneys

Interactions:

• Increased digoxin levels: digoxin
• Increased α-adrenergic stimulation: ephedrine, epinephrine, amphetamine, norepinephrine, phenylephrine, pseudoephedrine
• Decreased action of: thyroid hormones, theophylline, dopamine, dobutamine
• Avoid use with MAOIs
🌿 Potassium deficiency: aloe, buckthorn bark/berry, cascara sagrada bark, senna pod/leaf

Lab test interferences:

Interference: Glucose/insulin tolerance test

NURSING CONSIDERATIONS

Assess:

• I&O ratio, weight daily, watch for signs of CHF (jugular vein distension, weight gain, rales or crackles, edema)
• B/P, pulse q4h; note rate, rhythm, quality; rapid changes can cause shock; if systolic <100 or diastolic <60, notify prescriber before giving drug
• ECG continuously during inf, hypotension is common
• Baselines in renal, LFTs before therapy begins
• Breath sounds and respiratory pattern: wheezing from bronchospasm

Administer:

• Reduced dosage in cool environment

IV

• IV diluted 5 g/20 ml of D_5W, D_5R, D_5 0.9% NaCl, 0.45% NaCl, LR, D_5 0.45% NaCl, 0.9% NaCl further dilute in the remaining 480 ml (10 mg/ml) and give as infusion; give loading dose over 1 min, then maintenance over 4 min; may repeat loading dose q5min with increased maintenance dose; maintenance dose should not be >200 µg/kg/min and be given up to 48 hr; dose should be tapered at 25 µg/kg/min; use infusion pump

Additive compatibilities: Aminophylline, atracurium, bretylium, heparin

Y-site compatibilities: Amikacin, aminophylline, amiodarone, ampicillin, atracurium, butorphanol, calcium chloride, cefazolin, cefmetazole, cefoperazone, ceftazidime, ceftizoxime, chloramphenicol, cimetidine, cisatracurium, clindamycin, diltiazem, dopamine, enalaprilat, erythromycin, famotidine, fentanyl, gentamicin, heparin, hydrocortisone, insulin (regular), labetalol, magnesium sulfate, methyldopate, metronidazole, midazolam, morphine, nafcillin, nitroglycerin, nitroprusside, norepinephrine, pancuronium, penicillin G potassium, phenytoin, piperacillin, polymyxin B, potassium chloride, potassium phosphate, propofol, ranitidine, remifentanil, streptomycin, tacrolimus, tobramycin, trimethoprim-sulfamethoxazole, vancomycin, vecuronium

Perform/provide:

• Storage protected from light, moisture; in cool environment

Evaluate:

• Therapeutic response: lower B/P immediately, lower heart rate

Teach patient/family:
• To notify prescriber if pain, swelling occurs at IV site
Treatment of overdose: Discontinue drug

---

esomeprazole
See appendix a—selected new drugs

---

estradiol
(es-tra-dye'ole)
Estrace
estradiol cypionate
depGynogen, Depo-Estradiol, Depogen, Dura-Estrin, E-Cypionate, Estragyn LA5, Estro-Cyp, Estrofem, Estroject-LA, Estrol-L.A.
estradiol valerate
Clinigen LA, Delestrogen, Dioval, Duragen, Estra-L, Estro-span, Femogex*, Gynogen LA, Menaval, Valergen
estradiol transdermal system
Alora, Climera, Esclim, Estraderm, FemPatch, Vivelle
estradiol vaginal tablet
Vagifem
estradiol vaginal ring
Estring
Func. class.: Estrogen, progestins

Action: Needed for adequate functioning of female reproductive system; affects release of pituitary gonadotropins, inhibits ovulation, adequate calcium use in bone
Uses: Menopause, inoperable breast cancer (selected cases), prostatic cancer, atrophic vaginitis, kraurosis vulvae, hypogonadism, primary ovarian failure, prevention of osteoporosis

Dosage and routes:
Hormone replacement
• *Adult:* **TD** 0.05-0.1 mg/24 hr, apply 2 ×/wk
Menopause/hypogonadism/castration/ovarian failure
• *Adult:* **PO** 1-2 mg qd 3 wk on, 1 wk off or 5 days on, 2 days off **IM** 1-5 mg q3-4wk (cypionate); 10-20 mg q4wk (valerate)
• *Adult:* **TOP** Estraderm 0.05 mg/24 hr applied 2 ×/wk Climera 0.05 mg/hr applied 1 ×/wk in a cyclic regimen; women with hysterectomy may use continuously
Prostatic cancer
• *Adult:* **IM** 30 mg q1-2wk (valerate); **PO** 1-2 mg tid (oral estradiol)
Breast cancer
• *Adult:* **PO** 10 mg tid × 3 mo or longer
Atropic vaginitis/kraurosis vulvae
• *Adult:* **VAG CREAM** 2-4 g qd × 1-2 wk, then 1 g 1-3 ×/wk cycled; vag tab 1 qd × 2 wk, maintenance 1 tab 2 ×/wk
Available forms: Estradiol tabs 0.5, 1, 2 mg; cypionate inj 5 mg/ml; valerate inj 10, 20, 40 mg/ml; transderm 0.025, 0.0375, 0.05, 0.075, 0.1 mg/24 hr release rate; vag cream 100 µg/g; vag tab 25 µg; vag ring 2 mg/90 days
Side effects/adverse reactions:
CNS: Dizziness, headache, migraines, depression, *seizures*
CV: Hypotension, thrombophlebitis, edema, *thromboembolism, stroke, pulmonary embolism, myocardial infarction*
GI: Nausea, vomiting, diarrhea, anorexia, pancreatitis, cramps, constipation, increased appetite, increased weight, *cholestatic jaundice, hepatic adenoma*
EENT: Contact lens intolerance, increased myopia, astigmatism

---

◆ = Nursing alert   ∥ = Herb-drug interaction   ⊘ = Do not crush

GU: Amenorrhea, cervical erosion, breakthrough bleeding, dysmenorrhea, vaginal candidiasis, breast changes, *gynecomastia, testicular atrophy, impotence,* **increased risk of breast cancer, endometrial cancer**

INTEG: Rash, urticaria, acne, hirsutism, alopecia, oily skin, seborrhea, purpura, melasma

META: Folic acid deficiency, hypercalcemia, hyperglycemia

Contraindications: Breast cancer, thromboembolic disorders, reproductive cancer, genital bleeding (abnormal, undiagnosed), pregnancy (X)

Precautions: Hypertension, asthma, blood dyscrasias, gallbladder disease, CHF, diabetes mellitus, bone disease, depression, migraine headache, convulsive disorders, hepatic disease, renal disease, family history of cancer of breast or reproductive tract

Pharmacokinetics:

PO/INJ/TD: Degraded in liver; excreted in urine; crosses placenta; excreted in breast milk

Interactions:

• Decreased action of anticoagulants, oral hypoglycemics, tamoxifen

• Decreased action of estradiol: anticonvulsants, barbiturates, phenylbutazone, rifampin, calcium

• Increased action of: corticosteroids

• Increased toxicity: cyclosporine, dantrolene

🍴 Increased estrogen level: grapefruit juice

Lab test interferences:

Increase: BSP retention test, PBI, T_4, serum sodium, platelet aggregation, thyroxine-binding globulin (TBG), prothrombin, factors VII, VIII, IX, X, triglycerides

Decrease: Serum folate, serum triglyceride, T_3 resin uptake test, glucose tolerance test, antithrombin III, pregnanediol, metyrapone test

False positive: LE prep, antinuclear antibodies

NURSING CONSIDERATIONS

Assess:

• Blood glucose of diabetic patient

• Weight daily, notify prescriber of weekly weight gain >5 lb; if increase, diuretic may be ordered

• B/P q4h, watch for increase caused by H_2O and Na retention

• I&O ratio; decreasing urinary output, increasing edema, report changes

• Liver function studies, including AST, ALT, bilirubin, alk phosphatase baseline, periodically

• Hypertension, cardiac symptoms, jaundice, hypercalcemia

• Mental status: affect, mood, behavioral changes, aggression

• Female patient for intact uterus, if so, progesterone should be added to estrogen therapy to decrease risk of endometrial cancer

Administer:

• Titrated dose; use lowest effective dose

• IM inj deeply in large muscle mass

PO

• With food or milk to decrease GI symptoms

Transdermal

• Apply to trunk of body 2 ×/wk

• On intermittent cycle schedule: 3 wk on, then 1 wk off; if patch falls off, reapply

Vaginal

• Use applicator provided

Evaluate:

• Therapeutic response: reversal of menopause symptoms or decrease in tumor size in prostatic cancer

Teach patient/family:

• To weigh weekly, report gain >5 lb

◆ To report breast lumps, vaginal bleeding, edema, jaundice, dark

---

urine, clay-colored stools, dyspnea, headache, blurred vision, abdominal pain, numbness or stiffness in legs, chest pain, tenderness, redness, and swelling in extremities; male to report impotence or gynecomastia

---

RARELY USED

estramustine
(ess-tra-muss'teen)
Emcyt
Func. class.: Antineoplastic

Uses: Metastatic prostate cancer
Dosage and routes:
• *Adult:* **PO** 10-16 mg/kg in 3-4 divided doses/day; treatment may continue for ≥3 mo or 600 mg/m²/day in 3 divided doses
Contraindications: Hypersensitivity to estradiol, thromboembolic disorders, pregnancy (D)

---

estrogens, conjugated
Cenestin, C.E.S.*, Congest, Premarin
estrogens, conjugated synthetic A
Cenestin
Func. class.: Estrogen, hormone

Action: Needed for adequate functioning of female reproductive system; it affects release of pituitary gonadotropins, inhibits ovulation, adequate calcium use in bone
Uses: Menopause, inoperable breast cancer, prostatic cancer, abnormal uterine bleeding, hypogonadism, primary ovarian failure, osteoporosis
Research notes: Women who take thyroxine and estrogen concurrently may need to have their thyroxine dose increased.[13]
When thyroid replacement is used with estrogens, a dosage adjustment increase may be required in the thyroid agent.[14]
Dosage and routes:
Menopause
• *Adult:* **PO** 0.3-1.25 mg qd 3 wk on, 1 wk off
Osteoporosis
• *Adult:* **PO** 0.625 mg qd or in cycle
Atrophic vaginitis
• *Adult:* **VAG CREAM** 2-4 g ml qd × 21 days, off 7 days, repeat
Prostatic cancer
• *Adult:* **PO** 1.25-2.5 mg tid
Breast cancer
• *Adult:* **PO** 10 mg tid × 3 mo or longer
Abnormal uterine bleeding
• *Adult:* **IV/IM** 25 mg, repeat in 6-12 hr
Castration/primary ovarian failure
• *Adult:* **PO** 1.25 mg qd 3 wk on, 1 wk off
Hypogonadism
• *Adult:* **PO** 2.5 mg bid-tid × 20 days/mo
Available forms: Tabs 0.3, 0.625, 0.9, 1.25, 2.5 mg; inj 25 mg/vial; vag cream 0.625 mg/g; synthetic A tabs 0.625, 0.9 mg
Side effects/adverse reactions:
CNS: Dizziness, headache, migraine, depression, *seizures*
CV: Hypotension, thrombophlebitis, edema, *thromboembolism, stroke, pulmonary embolism, myocardial infarction*
GI: Nausea, vomiting, diarrhea, anorexia, pancreatitis, cramps, constipation, increased appetite, increased weight, *cholestatic jaundice, hepatic adenoma*
EENT: Contact lens intolerance, increased myopia, astigmatism
GU: Amenorrhea, cervical erosion, breakthrough bleeding, dysmenorrhea, vaginal candidiasis, breast changes, *gynecomastia, testicular*

---

*atrophy, impotence, **increased risk of breast cancer, endometrial cancer***

INTEG: Rash, urticaria, acne, hirsutism, alopecia, oily skin, seborrhea, purpura, melasma

META: Folic acid deficiency, hypercalcemia, hyperglycemia

Contraindications: Breast cancer, thromboembolic disorders, reproductive cancer, genital bleeding (abnormal, undiagnosed), pregnancy (X), lactation

Precautions: Hypertension, asthma, blood dyscrasias, gallbladder disease, CHF, diabetes mellitus, bone disease, depression, migraine headache, convulsive disorders, hepatic disease, renal disease, family history of cancer of breast or reproductive tract

Do not confuse:
Premarin/Provera

Pharmacokinetics:

PO/IV/IM: Degraded in liver, excreted in urine, crosses placenta, excreted in breast milk

Interactions:

• Increased toxicity: cyclosporine, dantrolene

• Decreased action of anticoagulants, oral hypoglycemics, tamoxifen

• Decreased action of estrogens: anticonvulsants, barbiturates, phenylbutazone, rifampin

• Increased action of corticosteroids

🥄 Increased estrogen level: grapefruit juice

NURSING CONSIDERATIONS
Assess:

• Blood glucose if diabetic patient

• Weight daily; notify prescriber of weekly weight gain >5 lb; if increase, diuretic may be ordered

• B/P q4h; watch for increase caused by H_2O and Na retention

• I&O ratio; be alert for decreasing urinary output, increasing edema

• Liver function studies: AST, ALT, bilirubin, alk phosphatase

• Hypertension, cardiac symptoms, jaundice, hypercalcemia

• Mental status: affect, mood, behavioral changes, aggression

• Female patient for intact uterus, if so, progesterone should be added to estrogen therapy to decrease risk of endometrial cancer

Administer:

• Titrated dose, use lowest effective dose

IM

• IM reconstitute after withdrawing >5 ml of air from container and inject sterile diluent on vial side, rotate to dissolve; give injection deep in large muscle mass

• With food or milk to decrease GI symptoms (PO)

IV, direct

• IV, after reconstituting as for IM, inject into distal port of running IV line of D_5W, 0.9% NaCl, LR at 5 mg/min or less

Y-site compatibilities: Heparin/hydrocortisone, potassium chloride, vit B/C

Vaginal

• Use applicator provided

Evaluate:

• Therapeutic response: absence of breast engorgement, reversal of menopause symptoms, or decrease in tumor size in prostatic cancer

Teach patient/family:

• To avoid breastfeeding, since drug is excreted in breast milk

• To weigh weekly, report gain >5 lb

◆ To report breast lumps, vaginal bleeding, edema, jaundice, dark urine, clay-colored stools, dyspnea, headache, blurred vision, abdominal pain, leg pain and redness, numbness or stiffness in legs, chest pain; male to report impotence or gynecomastia

• To avoid sunlight or wear sunscreen; burns may occur

• To notify prescriber if pregnancy is suspected

---

etanercept (℞)
(eh-tan'er-sept)
Enbrel
Func. class.: Antirheumatic agent (disease modifying)

Action: Binds tumor necrosis factor (TNF), which is involved in immune and inflammatory reactions

Uses: Acute, chronic rheumatoid arthritis that has not responded to other disease-modifying agents, polyarticular course juvenile rheumatoid arthritis (JRA)

Investigational uses: CHF, psoriasis/psoriatic arthritis

Dosage and routes:

• *Adult:* SC 25 mg 2×/wk, may be given with other drugs for rheumatoid arthritis

• *Child 4-17 yr:* SC 0.4 mg/kg 2×/wk, max 25 mg 1 dose

CHF

• *Adult:* SC 5-12 mg/m² 2×/wk × 3 mo

Psoriasis/psoriatic arthritis

• *Adult:* SC 25 mg 2×/wk × 12 wk

Available forms: Powder for inj: 25 mg

Side effects/adverse reactions:
GI: Abdominal pain, dyspepsia
CNS: Headache, asthenia, dizziness
INTEG: Rash, *inj site reaction*
RESP: Pharyngitis, cough, URI, non-URI, sinusitis, *rhinitis*

Contraindications: Hypersensitivity, sepsis

Precautions: Pregnancy (B), lactation, children <4 yr, elderly

Pharmacokinetics: Elimination half-life 115 hr, 60% absorbed SC

Interactions:

• Do not give concurrently with vaccines, immunizations should be brought up to date before treatment

NURSING CONSIDERATIONS
Assess:

• Pain, stiffness, ROM, swelling of joints during treatment

• For injection site pain, swelling, usually occur after 2 inj (4-5 days)

Administer:

• After reconstituting 1 ml of supplied diluent, slowly inject diluent into vial, swirl contents, do not shake, sol should be clear/colorless, do not use if cloudy or discolored

• Do not admix with other sol or medications, do not use filter

• May be injected SC into upper arm, abdomen, or thigh, rotate injection sites

Evaluate:

• Therapeutic response: decreased inflammation, pain in joints

Teach patient/family:

• That drug must be continued for prescribed time to be effective

• To use caution when driving; dizziness may occur

• About self-administration if appropriate: inj should be made in thigh, abdomen, upper arm; rotate sites at least 1 in from old site

---

ethambutol (℞)
(e-tham'byoo-tole)
Etibi*, Myambutol
Func. class.: Antitubercular
Chem. class.: Diisopropylethylene diamide derivative

Action: Inhibits RNA synthesis, decreases tubercle bacilli replication

---

◆ = Nursing alert   ∥ = Herb-drug interaction   ⊘ = Do not crush

Uses: Pulmonary tuberculosis, as an adjunct, other mycobacterial infections

Dosage and routes:
• *Adult and child >13 yr:* **PO** 15-25 mg/kg/day as a single dose or 50 mg/kg 2×/wk or 25-30 mg/kg 3 ×/wk
Renal disease
• CrCl 10-50 ml/min dose q24-36h; CrCl <10 ml/min dose q48h
Retreatment
• *Adult:* **PO** 25 mg/kg/day as single dose × 2 mo with at least 1 other drug, then decrease to 15 mg/kg/day as single dose, max 2.5 g/day
• *Child:* 15 mg/kg/day
Available forms: Tabs 100, 400 mg
Side effects/adverse reactions:
GI: Abdominal distress, anorexia, nausea, vomiting
INTEG: Dermatitis, pruritus, *toxic epidermal necrolysis*
CNS: Headache, confusion, fever, malaise, dizziness, disorientation, hallucinations
EENT: Blurred vision, optic neuritis, photophobia, decreased visual acuity
META: Elevated uric acid, acute gout, liver function impairment
MISC: **Thrombocytopenia,** joint pain, bloody sputum, **anaphylaxis**
Contraindications: Hypersensitivity, optic neuritis, child <13 yr
Precautions: Pregnancy (B), lactation, renal disease, diabetic retinopathy, cataracts, ocular defects, hepatic and hematopoietic disorders

Pharmacokinetics:
PO: Peak 2-4 hr, half-life 3 hr; metabolized in liver; excreted in urine (unchanged drug/inactive metabolites, unchanged drug in feces)

Interactions:
• Delayed absorption of ethambutol: aluminum salts
• Neurotoxicity: other neurotoxics
NURSING CONSIDERATIONS
Assess:
• Liver studies qwk × 2 wk, then q2mo: ALT, AST, bilirubin
• Signs of anemia: Hct, Hgb, fatigue
• Mental status often: affect, mood, behavioral changes; psychosis may occur
• Hepatic status: decreased appetite, jaundice, dark urine, fatigue
• C&S, including sputum, before treatment
• Visual status: decreased activity, altered color perception
Administer:
PO
• With meals to decrease GI symptoms
• Antiemetic if vomiting occurs
• After C&S is completed; qmo to detect resistance
• 2 hr before antacids
Evaluate:
• Therapeutic response: decreased symptoms of TB, decrease in acid-fast bacteria
Teach patient/family:
• To avoid alcohol products
• That compliance with dosage schedule, duration is necessary
• That scheduled appointments must be kept or relapse may occur
• To report any visual changes, rash, hot, swollen, painful joints, numbness or tingling of extremities to prescriber

---

RARELY USED

ethosuximide (Ɍ)
(eth-oh-sux′i-mide)
Zarontin
Func. class.: Anticonvulsant

Uses: Absence seizures, partial seizures, tonic-clonic seizures
Dosage and routes:
• *Adult and child >6 yr:* **PO** 250 mg bid initially; may increase by 250 mg q4-7d, not to exceed 1.5 g/day
• *Child 3-6 yr:* **PO** 250 mg/day or 125 mg bid; may increase by 250 mg q4-7d, not to exceed 1.5 g/day
Contraindications: Hypersensitivity to succinimide derivatives

---

etidronate (Ɍ)
(eh-tih-droe′nate)
Didronel, Didronel IV
Func. class.: Parathyroid agent (calcium regulator)
Chem. class.: Diphosphate

Action: Decreases bone resorption and new bone development (accretion)
Uses: Paget's disease, heterotopic ossification, hypercalcemia of malignancy
Dosage and routes:
Paget's disease
• *Adult:* **PO** 5-10 mg/kg/day, 2 hr ac with H₂O, not to exceed 20 mg/kg/day, max 6 mo or 11-20 mg/kg/day for max of 3 mo
Heterotopic ossification
• *Adult:* **PO** 20 mg/kg qd × 2 wk, then 10 mg/kg/day for 10 wk, total 12 wk

Hypercalcemia
• *Adult:* **IV** 7.5 mg/kg/day × 3 days, then **PO** 20 mg/kg/day
Heterotopic ossification/hip replacement
• *Adult:* **PO** 20 mg/kg/day × 4 wk before and 3 mo after surgery
Available forms: Tabs 200, 400 mg; inj 50 mg/ml
Side effects/adverse reactions:
GI: Nausea, diarrhea; metallic taste (IV)
MS: Bone pain, hypocalcemia, decreased mineralization of nonaffected bones
GU: **Nephrotoxicity**
CNS: **Seizures**
Contraindications: Pathologic fractures, children, colitis, severe renal disease with creatinine >5 mg/dl
Precautions: Pregnancy (C), renal disease, lactation, restricted vit D/calcium
Do not confuse:
etidronate/etretinate
etidronate/etomidate
Pharmacokinetics: Absorbed poorly (PO), not metabolized; excreted in urine/feces; therapeutic response: 1-3 mo
Interactions:
• Decreased absorption: calcium, aluminum, magnesium antacids/supplements, iron products
• Drug/food: dairy products: decreased absorption
NURSING CONSIDERATIONS
Assess:
• I&O ratio; check for decreased output in renal patients
• BUN, creatinine, uric acid, phosphate chloride, albumin, pH, urine Ca, Mg, alk phosphatase, urinalysis; Ca should be kept at 9-10 mg/dl; vit D 50-135 IU/dl
• Muscle spasm, laryngospasm, paresthesias, facial twitching, colic; may indicate hypocalcemia

---

◆ = Nursing alert   = Herb-drug interaction   ⊘ = Do not crush

- Nutritional status, diet for sources of vit D (milk, some seafood), Ca (dairy products, dark green vegetables), phosphates—adequate intake is necessary
- Persistent nausea or diarrhea

Administer:

PO

- Drug therapy should not last longer than 6 mo
- On empty stomach with H_2O 2 hr ac

IV

- IV after diluting in 250 ml or more 0.9% NaCl; give over 2 hr or longer
- Food, especially high in Ca; vitamins with mineral supplements or antacids high in metals should not be given within 2 hr of dose

Evaluate:

- Therapeutic response: management of bone deficiencies, Paget's disease

Teach patient/family:

- To avoid OTC products
- That therapeutic response may take 1-3 mo; effects persist for months after drug is discontinued
- That adequate intake of Ca^+, vit D is necessary
- To report sudden onset of unexplained pain, restricted mobility, heat over bone; hypercalcemic relapse

---

etodolac (℞)

(ee-toe'doe-lak)
Lodine, Lodine XL
Func. class.: Nonsteroidal antiinflammatory/nonopioid analgesic

Action: Inhibits prostaglandin synthesis by decreasing an enzyme needed for biosynthesis; analgesic, antiinflammatory, antipyretic

Uses: Mild to moderate pain, osteoarthritis

Dosage and routes:

Osteoarthritis

- *Adult:* **PO** 800-1200 mg/day in divided doses q6-8h initially, then adjust dose to 600-1200 mg/day in divided doses; do not exceed 1200 mg/day; patients <60 kg not to exceed 20 mg/kg

Analgesia

- *Adult:* **PO** 200-400 mg q6-8h prn for acute pain; do not exceed 1200 mg/day; patients <60 kg, not to exceed 20 mg/kg

Available forms: Caps 200, 300 mg; tabs 400, 500 mg; ext rel 400, 600 mg

Side effects/adverse reactions:

CV: Tachycardia, peripheral edema, fluid retention, palpitations, dysrhythmias, CHF

GU: **Nephrotoxicity:** *dysuria,* **hematuria,** *oliguria, azotemia,* cystitis, urinary tract infection

HEMA: **Blood dyscrasias**

INTEG: Erythema, urticaria, purpura, rash, pruritus, sweating, **Stevens-Johnson syndrome**

GI: Nausea, anorexia, vomiting, diarrhea, jaundice, **cholestatic hepatitis,** constipation, flatulence, cramps, dry mouth, peptic ulcer, dyspepsia, **GI bleeding**

CNS: Dizziness, headache, drowsiness, fatigue, tremors, confusion, insomnia, anxiety, depression, lightheadedness, vertigo

EENT: Tinnitus, hearing loss, blurred vision, photophobia

SYST: **Angioedema, anaphylaxis**

Contraindications: Hypersensitivity; patients in whom aspirin, iodides, or other nonsteroidal antiinflammatories have produced asthma; rhinitis, urticaria, nasal polyps, angioedema, bronchospasm

Precautions: Pregnancy (C); lacta-

Side effects: *italics* = common; **bold italics** = life-threatening

tion; children; bleeding; GI, cardiac disorders; elderly; renal, hepatic disorders

Do not confuse:

Lodine/codeine

Pharmacokinetics:

PO: Peak 1-2 hr, serum protein binding >90%, half-life 7 hr; metabolized by liver (metabolites excreted in urine)

Interactions:

• Increased toxicity: cyclosporine, digoxin, lithium, methotrexate, phenytoin

• May increase GI toxicity: aspirin

• Decreased effect of etodolac: antacids

• Decreased effect of: β-blockers, diuretics

NURSING CONSIDERATIONS

Assess:

• Pain: location, frequency, characteristics; relief after med

• Blood, renal, liver studies: BUN, creatinine, AST, ALT, Hgb, before treatment, periodically thereafter

• For GI bleeding: black stools, hematemesis

• Audiometric, ophthalmic examination before, during, after treatment

• For eye, ear problems: blurred vision, tinnitus; may indicate toxicity

• For asthma, aspirin hypersensitivity, nasal polyps that may be hypersensitive to etodolac

Administer:

PO

• With food to decrease GI symptoms, since extent of absorption is not affected by food

Perform/provide:

• Storage at room temperature

Evaluate:

• Therapeutic response: decreased pain, stiffness, swelling in joints, ability to move more easily

Teach patient/family:

• To report blurred vision or ringing, roaring in ears; may indicate toxicity

🚫 Not to break, crush, or chew ext rel tabs

• To avoid driving, other hazardous activities if dizziness or drowsiness occurs

◆ To report change in urine pattern, weight increase, edema, pain increase in joints, fever, blood in urine; indicates nephrotoxicity

• That therapeutic effects may take up to 1 mo

• To avoid aspirin, NSAIDs, acetaminophen, alcoholic beverages while taking this medication

---

RARELY USED

etomidate (℞)

(e-tom′i-date)

Amidate

Func. class.: General anesthetic

Uses: Induction of general anesthesia

Dosage and routes:

• *Adult and child >10 yr:* **IV** 0.2-0.6 mg/kg over ½-1 min

Contraindications: Hypersensitivity, labor/delivery

---

etoposide (℞)

(e-toe-poe′side)

Etopophos, VePesid, VP-16

Func. class.: Antineoplastic-misc.

Chem. class.: Semisynthetic podophyllotoxin

Action: Inhibits mitotic activity through metaphase to mitosis; also inhibits cells from en-

---

◆ = Nursing alert   🌿 = Herb-drug interaction   🚫 = Do not crush

tering mitosis, depresses DNA, RNA synthesis, cell cycle specific S and G_2

Uses: Leukemias, lung, testicular cancer, lymphomas, neuroblastoma, melanoma, ovarian cancer

Research note: A study showed an increase in etoposide when combined with atovaquone[15]

Dosage and routes:
Testicular cancer
• *Adult:* **IV** 50-100 mg/m^2/day × 3-5 days given q3-5wk or 200-250 mg/m^2/wk, or 125-140 mg/m^2/day 3 × wk, q5wk

Lung cancer
• *Adult:* **PO** 35 mg/m^2/day × 4 days, given q3-4wk, **IV** 35 mg/m^2/day × 4 days

Available forms: Inj 20 mg/ml; caps 50, 100 mg; 113.6 etoposide phosphate = 100 etoposide

Side effects/adverse reactions:
*HEMA: **Thrombocytopenia, leukopenia, myelosuppression, anemia***
*GI: Nausea, vomiting, anorexia, **hepatotoxicity,** dyspepsia, diarrhea, constipation*
INTEG: Rash, alopecia, phlebitis at IV site, radiation recall
*RESP: **Bronchospasm,** pleural effusion*
*CV: Hypotension, **MI, dysrhythmias***
CNS: Headache, *fever,* peripheral neuropathy, paresthesias, confusion
*GU: **Nephrotoxicity***
*SYST: **Anaphylaxis***

Contraindications: Hypersensitivity, bone marrow depression, severe hepatic disease, severe renal disease, bacterial infection, pregnancy (D), viral infection

Precautions: Renal disease, hepatic disease, lactation, children, gout

Pharmacokinetics: Half-life 3 hr, terminal 15 hr; metabolized in liver; excreted in urine; crosses placental barrier

Do not confuse:
VePesid/Versed
Interactions:
• Increased PT: warfarin

NURSING CONSIDERATIONS
Assess:
• CBC, differential, platelet count weekly; withhold drug if WBC is <1000 or platelet count is <50,000; notify prescriber
• Renal function studies: BUN, serum uric acid, urine CrCl, electrolytes before, during therapy
• I&O ratio; report fall in urine output to <30 ml/hr; check blood pressure bid and report any significant decrease
• Monitor temp q4h; may indicate beginning infection
• Liver function tests before, during therapy (bilirubin, AST, ALT, LDH) as needed or monthly
• RBC, Hct, Hgb; may be decreased
• Bleeding: hematuria, guaiac stools, bruising or petechiae, mucosa or orifices q8h
• Effects of alopecia on body image; discuss feelings about body changes
• Jaundice of skin and sclera, dark urine, clay-colored stools, itchy skin, abdominal pain, fever, diarrhea
• B/P q15 min during inf, if systolic reading <90 mm Hg, discontinue inf and notify prescriber
• Buccal cavity q8h for dryness, sores or ulceration, white patches, oral pain, bleeding, dysphagia
• Local irritation, pain, burning, discoloration at injection site
◆ Symptoms indicating severe allergic reaction: rash, pruritus, urticaria, purpuric skin lesions, itching, flushing
◆ Symptoms of anaphylaxis: flushing, restlessness, coughing, difficulty breathing
• Frequency of stools, charac-

E

teristics: cramping, acidosis; signs of dehydration: rapid respirations, poor skin turgor, decreased urine output, dry skin, restlessness, weakness

Administer:
• Antiemetic 30-60 min before giving drug and prn to prevent vomiting
• Allopurinol or sodium bicarbonate to maintain uric acid levels, alkalinization of urine
• Hyaluronidase 150 U/ml to 1 ml NaCl to infiltration area, ice compress for vesicant activity
• Antispasmodic, epinephrine, corticosteroids, antihistamines for reactions

IV (VePesid)
• After diluting 100 mg/250 ml or more D_5W or NaCl to 0.2-0.4 mg/ml, infuse over 30-60 min; phosphate may be given over 5 min-3½ hr; may dilute further to 0.1 mg/ml in 0.9% NaCl, D_5W

Additive compatibilities: Carboplatin, cisplatin, cytarabine, floxuridine, fluorouracil, hydroxyzine, ifosfamide, ondansetron

Y-site compatibilities: Allopurinol, amifostine, aztreonam, cladribine, doxorubicin liposome, fludarabine, granisetron, melphalan, ondansetron, paclitaxel, piperacillin/tazobactam, sargramostim, sodium bicarbonate, teniposide, thiotepa, vinorelbine

Perform/provide:
• Liquid diet: carbonated beverages, Jell-O; dry toast or crackers may be added if patient is not nauseated or vomiting
• Increase fluid intake to 2-3 L/day to prevent urate deposits, calculi formation
• Diet low in purines: organ meats (kidney, liver), dried beans, peas to maintain alkaline urine
• Nutritious diet with iron, vitamin supplements

Evaluate:
• Therapeutic response: decreased tumor size, spread of malignancy

Teach patient/family:
• To report any complaints or side effects to nurse or prescriber
• To report any changes in breathing or coughing
• That hair may be lost during treatment; a wig or hairpiece may make patient feel better; tell patient that new hair may be different in color, texture

---

exemestane (Rx)

(ex-em'eh-stane)
Aromasin
Func. class.: Antineoplastic
Chem. class.: Aromatase inhibitor

Action: Lowers serum estradiol concentrations; many breast cancers have strong estrogen receptors

Uses: Advanced breast carcinoma not responsive to other therapy in estrogen-receptor-positive patients (postmenopausal)

Research note: One study showed that this drug produced no change in parturition and was not teratogenic in rats and rabbits[16]

Dosage and routes:
• *Adult:* **PO** 25 mg qd pc
Available forms: Tabs 25 mg

Side effects/adverse reactions:
GI: Nausea, vomiting, fatigue, diarrhea, constipation, abdominal pain, increased appetite
CV: Hypertension
CNS: Hot flashes, headache, depression, insomnia, anxiety
RESP: Cough, dyspnea

Contraindications: Hypersensitiv-

 = Nursing alert   = Herb-drug interaction   ⃠ = Do not crush

ity, pregnancy (D), premenopausal women

Precautions: Lactation, children, elderly, liver disease, renal disease

Pharmacokinetics: Half-life 24 hr, excreted in feces, urine

NURSING CONSIDERATIONS
Assess:
• B/P, hypertension may occur
Perform/provide:
• Liquid diet, if needed including cola, gelatin; dry toast or crackers may be added if patient is not nauseated or vomiting
• Increase fluid intake to 2-3 L/day to prevent dehydration
• Nutritious diet with iron, vitamin supplements as ordered
• Storage in light-resistant container at room temperature
Evaluate:
• Therapeutic response: decreased tumor size, spread of malignancy
Teach patient/family:
• To report any complaints, side effects to prescriber
• That hot flashes are reversible after discontinuing treatment

---

factor IX complex (human)/factor IV
(℞)

Alpha-Nine SD, Benefix, Konyne 80, Mononine, Profilnine/Alpha Nine, Proplex SX-T, Proplex T

Func. class.: Hemostatic
Chem. class.: Factors II, VII, IX, X

Action: Causes an increase in blood levels of clotting factors II, VII, IX, X; factor IX (human) has IX activity

Uses: Hemophilia B (Christmas disease), factor IX deficiency, anticoagulant reversal, control of bleeding in patients with factor VIII inhibitors, reversal of overdose of anticoagulants in emergencies

Dosage and routes:
Factor IX complex (human) bleeding in hemophilia B
• *Adult and child:* **IV** establish 25% of normal factor IX or 60-75 U/kg, then 10-20 U/kg/day 1-2 ×/wk
Prophylaxis for bleeding in hemophilia B
• *Adult and child:* **IV** 10-20 U/kg 1-2 ×/wk
Bleeding in hemophilia A/inhibitors of factor VIII (Proplex T, Konyne 80)
• *Adult and child:* **IV** 75 U/kg, repeat in 12 hr
Oral anticoagulant reversal
• *Adult and child:* **IV** 15 U/kg
Factor VII deficiency (use Proplex T only)
• *Adult and child:* **IV** 0.5 U/kg × weight (kg) × desired factor IX increase (% of normal); repeat q4-6h if needed
Factor IX (human) minor-moderate hemorrhage
Use only Alpha Nine, Alpha-Nine SD
• *Adult and child:* **IV** dose to increase factor IX level to 20%-30% in one dose
Serious hemorrhage
• *Adult and child:* **IV** dose to increase factor IX to 30%-50% as daily inf
Minor hemorrhage (mononine only)
• *Adult and child:* **IV** dose to increase factor IX to 15%-25% (20-30 U/kg), repeat in 24 hr if needed
Major hemorrhage
• *Adult and child:* **IV** dose to increase factor IX to 25%-50% (75 U/kg) q18-30h × 10 days or less
Available forms: Inj (number of units noted on label)

Side effects/adverse reactions:
GI: Nausea, vomiting, abdominal cramps, jaundice, ***viral hepatitis***
INTEG: Rash, flushing, *urticaria*
CNS: Headache, dizziness, malaise, paresthesia, *lethargy, chills, fever, flushing*
HEMA: ***Thrombosis, hemolysis, AIDS, DIC***
CV: Hypotension, tachycardia, *MI,* ***venous thrombosis, pulmonary embolism***
RESP: ***Bronchospasm***

Contraindications: Hypersensitivity to mouse protein, hepatic disease, DIC, elective surgery, mild factor IX deficiency

Precautions: Neonates/infants, pregnancy (C)

Pharmacokinetics:
IV: Half-life factor VII–3-6 hr, factor IX–24-36 hr; rapidly cleared from plasma

Interactions:
• Incompatible with protein products
⬥ Increased risk of thrombosis: aminocaproic acid; do not administer

NURSING CONSIDERATIONS
Assess:
• Blood studies (coagulation factors assays by % normal: 5% prevents spontaneous hemorrhage, 30%-50% for surgery, 80%-100% for severe hemorrhage)
• Increased B/P, pulse
• For bleeding q15-30min, immobilize and apply ice to affected joints
• I&O; if urine becomes orange or red, notify prescriber
• Allergic or pyrogenic reaction: fever, chills, rash, itching, slow infusion rate if not severe
⬥ DIC: bleeding, ecchymosis, hypersensitivity, changes in coagulation tests

Administer:
• Hepatitis B vaccine before administration
• IV after warming to room temperature 3 ml/min or less, with plastic syringe only; do not admix
• After dilution with provided diluent, 50 U/ml or 25 U/ml; do not exceed 10 ml/min; decrease rate if fever, headache, flushing, tingling occur
• After crossmatch if patient has blood type A, B, AB, to determine incompatibility with factor

Perform/provide:
• Storage of reconstituted sol for 3 hr at room temperature or up to 2 yr refrigeration (powder); check expiration date

Evaluate:
• Therapeutic response: prevention of hemorrhage

Teach patient/family:
• To report any signs of bleeding: gums, under skin, urine, stools, emesis
• The risk of viral hepatitis, AIDS; to be tested q2-3mo for HIV, even though risk is low
• That immunization for hepatitis B may be given first
• To carry ID identifying disease; avoid salicylates, NSAIDs; inform other health professionals of condition

---

famciclovir (℞)

(fam-cy'clo-veer)
Famvir
Func. class.: Antiviral
Chem. class.: Guanosine nucleoside

Action: Inhibits DNA polymerase and viral DNA synthesis by conversion of this guanosine nucleoside to penciclovir
Uses: Treatment of acute herpes zoster (shingles), genital herpes; re-

---

⬥ = Nursing alert   ▮ = Herb-drug interaction   🚫 = Do not crush current mucocutaneous herpes simplex virus (HSV) in HIV patients

Dosage and routes:

Herpes zoster

• *Adult:* PO 500 mg q8h

Renal dose: CrCl ≥60 ml/min, 500 mg q8h; 40-59 ml/min, 500 mg q12h; 20-39 ml/min, 500 mg q24h

Recurrent mucocutaneous herpes simplex

• *Adult:* PO 500 mg q12h × 1 wk

Recurrent herpes simplex virus

• *Adult:* PO 125 mg q12h × 5 days

Suppression of recurrent herpes simplex virus

• *Adult:* PO 250 mg q12h up to 1 yr

Available forms: Tabs 125, 250, 500 mg

Side effects/adverse reactions:

MS: Back pain, arthralgia

GU: Decreased sperm count

CNS: Headache, fatigue, dizziness, paresthesia, somnolence, fever

RESP: Pharyngitis, sinusitis

GI: Nausea, vomiting, diarrhea, constipation, abdominal pain, anorexia

INTEG: Pruritus

Contraindications: Hypersensitivity to this drug, penciclovir

Precautions: Renal disease, pregnancy (B), hypersensitivity to acyclovir, ganciclovir, lactation

Pharmacokinetics: Unknown

Interactions:

• Decreased renal excretion: theophylline, probenecid, digoxin

• Decreased metabolism: cimetidine

NURSING CONSIDERATIONS

Assess:

• For number, distribution of lesions; burning, itching, pain, which are early symptoms of herpes infection

• Renal function studies: urine CrCl, BUN before and during treatment if decreased renal function; dose may have to be lowered

• Bowel pattern before, during treatment; diarrhea may occur

• Posttherapeutic neuralgia during and after treatment

Administer:

• With or without meals; absorption does not appear to be lowered when taken with food

• Within 72 hr of the appearance of rash in herpes zoster

Evaluate:

• Therapeutic response: decreased size, spread of lesions

Teach patient/family:

• How to recognize beginning infection

• How to prevent spread of infection; that this medication does not prevent the spread to others, that condoms should be used

• The reason for medication, expected results

• That women with genital herpes should have yearly Pap smears, cervical cancer is more likely

---

famotidine (OTC, ℞)

(fa-moe′ti-deen)

Mylanta AR, Pepcid, Pepcid AC, Pepcid IV, Pepcid RPD*

Func. class.: H$_2$-histamine receptor antagonist

Action: Competitively inhibits histamine at histamine H$_2$-receptor site, decreasing gastric secretion while pepsin remains at a stable level

Uses: Short-term treatment of active duodenal ulcer, maintenance therapy for duodenal ulcer, Zollinger-Ellison syndrome, multiple endocrine adenomas, gastric ulcers; gastroesophageal reflux disease, heartburn

Investigational uses: GI disorders in those taking NSAIDs; urticaria; prevention of stress ulcers, aspiration pneumonitis, inactivation of oral pancreatic enzymes in pancreatic disorders, prevention of paclitaxel hypersensitivity reactions

Dosage and routes:

Active ulcer

• *Adult:* **PO** 40 mg qd hs × 4-8 wk, then 20 mg qd hs if needed (maintenance); **IV** 20 mg q12h if unable to take **PO**

• *Child 1-16 yr:* 0.5 mg/kg/day hs or divided bid, max 40 mg qd

Hypersecretory conditions

• *Adult:* **PO** 20 mg q6h; may give 160 mg q6h if needed; **IV** 20 mg q12h if unable to take **PO**

• *Child* 1-16 yr: 1 mg/kg/day divide bid, max 40 mg bid

Heartburn relief/prevention

• *Adult:* **PO** 10 mg with water or 1 hr before eating

Paclitaxel hypersensitivity reactions

• *Adult:* **IV** 20 mg ½ hr prior to infusion

Renal disease

• CrCl <10 ml/min 20 mg hs or dose q36-48h

Available forms: Tabs 10, 20, 40 mg; powder for oral susp 40 mg/5 ml; inj 10 mg/ml, 20 mg/50 ml 0.9% NaCl; orally disintegrating tabs (RPD) 20, 40 mg; chew tabs 10 mg

Side effects/adverse reactions:

*HEMA: **Thrombocytopenia, aplastic anemia***

CNS: Headache, dizziness, paresthesia, depression, anxiety, somnolence, insomnia, fever

EENT: Taste change, tinnitus, orbital edema

GI: Constipation, nausea, vomiting, anorexia, cramps, abnormal liver enzymes, diarrhea

INTEG: Rash

MS: Myalgia, arthralgia

*CV: **Dysrhythmias***

Contraindications: Hypersensitivity

Precautions: Pregnancy (B), lactation, children <12 yr, severe renal disease, severe hepatic function, elderly

Pharmacokinetics: Absorption 50% (PO)

PO: Onset 30-60 min, duration 6-12 hr, peak 1-3 hr

IV: Onset immediate, peak 30-60 min, duration 8-15 hr, plasma protein-binding 15%-20%; metabolized in liver 30% (active metabolites), 70% excreted by kidneys, half-life 2½-3½ hr

Interactions:

• Decreased absorption: ketoconazole

• Decreased absorption of famotidine: antacids

NURSING CONSIDERATIONS

Assess:

• For epigastric pain, adominal pain, frank or occult blood in emesis, stools

• Blood counts during therapy; watch for decreasing platelets; if low, therapy may have to be discontinued and restarted after hematologic recovery

• For bleeding, hematuria, hematuresis, occult blood in stools; abdominal pain

• Blood dyscrasias (thrombocytopenia): bruising, fatigue, bleeding, poor healing

Administer:

• Antacids 1 hr before or 2 hr after famotidine; may be given with foods or liquids

• After shaking oral suspension

IV, direct

• After diluting 2 ml of drug (10 mg/ml) in 0.9% NaCl to total volume of 5-10 ml; inject over 2 min to prevent hypotension

IV, int inf

• After diluting 20 mg (2 ml) of drug in 100 ml of LR, 0.9% NaCl, D_5W, $D_{10}W$; run over 15-30 min

---

Additive compatibilities: Cefazolin, cefmetazole, flumazenil, vancomycin

Y-site compatibilities: Acyclovir, allopurinol, amifostine, aminophylline, amphotericin, ampicillin, ampicillin/sulbactam, amrinone, amsacrine, atropine, aztreonam, bretylium, calcium gluconate, cefazolin, cefoperazone, cefotaxime, cefotetan, cefoxitin, ceftazidime, ceftizoxime, ceftriaxone, cefuroxime, cephalothin, cephapirin, chlorpromazine, cisatracurium, cisplatin, cladribine, cyclophosphamide, cytarabine, dexamethasone, dextran 40, digoxin, diphenhydramine, dobutamine, dopamine, doxorubicin, doxorubicin liposome, droperidol, enalaprilat, epinephrine, erythromycin, esmolol, filgrastim, fluconazole, fludarabine, folic acid, gentamicin, granisetron, haloperidol, heparin, hydrocortisone, hydromorphone, hydroxyzine, imipenem/cilastatin, insulin (regular), isoproterenol, labetalol, lidocaine, lorazepam, magnesium sulfate, melphalan, meperidine, methotrexate, methylprednisolone, metoclopramide, mezlocillin, midazolam, morphine, nafcillin, nitroglycerin, nitroprusside, norepinephrine, ondansetron, oxacillin, paclitaxel, perphenazine, phenylephrine, phenytoin, phytonadione, piperacillin, potassium chloride/phosphate, procainamide, propofol, remifentanil, sargramostim, sodium bicarbonate, teniposide, theophylline, thiamine, thiotepa, ticarcillin, ticarcillin/clavulanate, verapamil, vinorelbine

Perform/provide:
• Storage in cool environment (oral); IV sol is stable for 48 hr at room temperature; do not use discolored sol; discard unused oral sol after 1 mo

Evaluate:
• Therapeutic response: decreased abdominal pain

Teach patient/family:
• That drug must be continued for prescribed time in prescribed method to be effective; do not double dose
• To report bleeding, bruising, fatigue, malaise, since blood dyscrasias occur
• About possibility of decreased libido, reversible after discontinuing therapy
• To avoid irritating foods, alcohol, aspirin, and extreme temperature of foods that may irritate GI system
• That smoking should be avoided; diminishes effectiveness of drug
• To avoid tasks requiring alertness; dizziness, drowsiness may occur
• To increase bulk and fluids in the diet to prevent constipation

---

fat emulsions (℞)

Intralipid 10%, Intralipid 20%, Liposyn II 10%, Liposyn II 20%, Liposyn III 10%, Liposyn III 20%, Soyacal 20%

Func. class.: Caloric

Chem. class.: Fatty acid, long chain

Action: Needed for energy, heat production; consist of neutral triglycerides, primarily unsaturated fatty acids

Uses: Increase calorie intake, fatty acid deficiency, prevention

Dosage and routes:

Deficiency
• *Adult and child:* IV 8%-10% of required calorie intake (intralipid)

Adjunct to TPN
• *Adult:* IV 1 ml/min over 15-30 min (10%) or 0.5 ml/min over 15-30 min (20%); may increase to 500 ml over 4-8 hr if no adverse reactions occur; not to exceed 2.5 g/kg

---

• *Child:* IV 0.1 ml/min over 10-15 min (10%) or 0.05 ml/min over 10-15 min (20%); may increase to 1 g/kg over 4 hr if no adverse reactions occur; not to exceed 4 g/kg

Prevention of deficiency

• *Adult:* IV 500 ml 2 ×/wk (10%), given 1 ml/min for 30 min, not to exceed 500 ml over 6 hr

• *Child:* IV 5-10 ml/kg/day (10%), given 0.1 ml/min for 30 min, not to exceed 100 ml/hr

Available forms: Inj 10% (50, 100, 200, 250, 500 ml), 20% (50, 100, 200, 250, 500 ml)

Side effects/adverse reactions:

CNS: Dizziness, headache, drowsiness, *focal seizures*

CV: Shock

GI: Nausea, vomiting, *hepatomegaly*

RESP: Dyspnea, *fat in lung tissue*

HEMA: Hyperlipemia, hypercoagulation, thrombocytopenia, leukopenia, leukocytosis

Contraindications: Hypersensitivity, hyperlipemia, lipid necrosis, acute pancreatitis accompanied by hyperlipemia, hyperbilirubinemia of the newborn

Precautions: Severe liver disease, diabetes mellitus, thrombocytopenia, gastric ulcers, premature and term newborns, pregnancy (C), sepsis

NURSING CONSIDERATIONS
Assess:

• Triglycerides, free fatty acid levels, platelet counts daily to prevent fat overload, thrombocytopenia

• Liver function studies: AST, ALT Hct, Hgb; notify prescriber if abnormal

• Nutritional status: calorie count by dietitian; monitor weight daily

Administer:

IV, int inf

• At 10% (1 ml/min); 20% (0.5 ml/min) initially × 15-30 min, may increase 10% (120 ml/hr); 20% (62.5 ml/hr) if no adverse reaction; do not give more than 500 ml on first day

• After changing IV tubing at each infusion: infection may occur with old tubing

• With infusion pump at prescribed rate; do not use in-line filter sized for lipid emulsion; clogging will occur

Additive compatibilities: Cefamandole, chloramphenicol, cimetidine, cyclosporine, diphenhydramine, famotidine, heparin, hydrocortisone, multivitamins, nizatidine, penicillin G potassium

Y-site compatibilities: Ampicillin, cefamandole, cefazolin, cefoxitin, cephapirin, clindamycin, digoxin, dopamine, erythromycin, furosemide, gentamicin, IL-2, isoproterenol, kanamycin, lidocaine, norepinephrine, oxacillin, penicillin G potassium, ticarcillin, tobramycin

Perform/provide:

• Do not use mixed sol if separated or oily looking

Evaluate:

• Therapeutic response: increased weight

Teach patient/family:

• The reason for use of lipids

RARELY USED

felbamate (℞)

(fell′ba-mate)

Felbatol

Func. class.: Anticonvulsant

Uses: Partial seizures, with or without generalization in adults; partial and generalized seizures in children with Lennox-Gastaut syndrome

Dosage and routes:

Adjunctive therapy

• *Adult:* **PO** add 1.2 g/day in 3-4

divided doses; reduce other anticonvulsants (valproic acid, phenytoin, carbamazepine and derivatives) by 20% to control plasma concentrations; may increase felbamate 1.2 g/day increments qwk, up to 3.6 g/day

Monotherapy
• *Adult:* **PO** 1.2 g/day in 3-4 divided doses; titrate with close supervision; increase dose by 600-mg increments q2wk to 3.6 g/day if needed

Lennox-Gastaut syndrome adjunctive therapy
• *Child 2-14 yr:* **PO** add 15 mg/kg/day in 3-4 divided doses; reduce other anticonvulsants (valproic acid, phenytoin, carbamazepine and derivatives) by 20% to control plasma concentrations; may increase felbamate 15 mg/kg/day qwk up to 45 mg/day

Contraindications: Hypersensitivity to this drug, other carbamates, blood dyscrasia, hepatic disease

---

felodipine (℞)
(fe-loe′-di-peen)
Plendil, Renedil*
Func. class.: Antihypertensive, calcium channel blocker, antianginal
Chem. class.: Dihydropyridine

Action: Inhibits calcium ion influx across cell membrane, resulting in inhibition of excitation/contraction
Uses: Essential hypertension, alone or with other antihypertensives, angina pectoris, Prinzmetal's angina (vasospastic)
Dosage and routes:
• *Adult:* **PO** 5 mg qd initially, usual range 5-10 mg qd; max 20 mg qd; do not adjust dosage at intervals of <2 wk
• *Geriatric:* **PO** 2.5 mg qd

Hepatic disease
• **PO** 2.5-5 mg, max 10 mg/day
Available forms: Ext rel tabs 2.5, 5, 10 mg
Side effects/adverse reactions:
*CV: **Dysrhythmia,** edema, **CHF,** hypotension, palpitations, **MI, pulmonary edema,** tachycardia, syncope, AV block, angina*
GI: Nausea, vomiting, diarrhea, gastric upset, constipation, increased liver function studies, dry mouth
GU: Nocturia, polyuria
INTEG: Rash, pruritus
MISC: Flushing, sexual difficulties, cough, nasal congestion, shortness of breath, wheezing, epistaxis, respiratory infection, chest pain, ***Stevens-Johnson syndrome,*** gingival hyperplasia
CNS: Headache, fatigue, drowsiness, dizziness, anxiety, depression, nervousness, insomnia, lightheadedness, paresthesia, tinnitus, psychosis, somnolence
HEMA: Anemia
Contraindications: Hypersensitivity, sick sinus syndrome, 2nd- or 3rd-degree heart block
Precautions: CHF, hypotension <90 mm Hg systolic, hepatic injury, pregnancy (C), lactation, children, renal disease, elderly
Do not confuse:
Plendil/pindolol
Plendil/Prinivil
Pharmacokinetics: Peak plasma levels 2.5-5 hr; highly protein bound, >99% metabolized in liver, 0.5% excreted unchanged in urine; elimination half-life 11-16 hr
Interactions:
• Decreased felodipine levels: anticonvulsants
• Decreased theophylline level: theophylline
• Increased felodipine level: cimetidine, ranitidine

🌿 Increased felodipine level: grapefruit juice

NURSING CONSIDERATIONS
Assess:
• I&O, weight daily; for CHF: weight gain, rales, crackles, dyspnea, edema, jugular venous distension
• Renal, hepatic studies; potassium
• Cardiac status: B/P, pulse, respiration; ECG periodically
• For angina pain: location, duration, intensity; ameliorating, aggravating factors

Administer:
• Once daily as whole tab without regard to meals

Evaluate:
• Therapeutic response: decreased B/P

Teach patient/family:
🚫 To swallow whole; do not break, crush, or chew sus rel products
• To avoid hazardous activities until stabilized on drug, dizziness is no longer a problem
• To avoid OTC drugs unless directed by a prescriber, to limit caffeine consumption
• The importance of complying with all areas of medical regimen: diet, exercise, stress reduction, drug therapy
• That capsules may appear in stools, but are insignificant

Treatment of overdose: Atropine for AV block, vasopressor for hypotension

---

fenofibrate (℞)
(fen-oh-fee′brate)
Tricor
Func. class.: Antilipemic
Chem. class.: Fibric acid derivative

Action: Inhibits biosynthesis of low-density and very low-density lipoproteins, which are responsible for triglyceride development; mobilizes triglycerides from tissue; increases excretion of neutral sterols

Uses: Hypercholesterolemia, types IV, V hyperlipidemia that do not respond to other treatment and are at risk for pancreatitis

Investigational uses: Polymetabolic syndrome X

Dosage and routes:
Hypertriglyceridemia
• *Adult:* PO 54-160 mg/day, may increase q4-8wk, max 160 mg/day
Primary hypercholesterolemia/ mixed hyperlipidemia
• *Adult:* PO 160 mg/day
Renal and geriatric dose
• PO 54 mg/day (CrCl <50 ml/min)
Available forms: Tabs 54, 160 mg

Side effects/adverse reactions:
CNS: Fatigue, weakness, drowsiness, dizziness
CV: Angina, *dysrhythmias*
GI: Nausea, vomiting, dyspepsia, increased liver enzymes, flatulence, hepatomegaly, gastritis
GU: Dysuria, proteinuria, oliguria
INTEG: Rash, urticaria, pruritus
MISC: Polyphagia, weight gain
MS: Myalgias, arthralgias

Contraindications: Severe hepatic disease, severe renal disease, primary biliary cirrhosis

Precautions: Peptic ulcer, pregnancy (C), lactation, pancreatitis

Pharmacokinetics: Peak 6-8h; protein binding 99%, converted to fenofibric acid, metabolized in liver, excreted in urine (60%), half-life 20 hr

Interactions:
• Increased fenofibrate effect: cyclosporine
• Decreased absorption of fenofibrate: bile acid sequestrants

---

◆ = Nursing alert   🌿 = Herb-drug interaction   🚫 = Do not crush

• Do not use with HMG-CoA reductase inhibitors, rhabdomyolysis may occur
• Increased anticoagulant effects: oral anticoagulants
• Drug/food: increased absorption

NURSING CONSIDERATIONS

Assess:
• Lipid levels, LFTs baseline and periodically during treatment, CPK if muscle pain occurs, CBC, Hct, Hgb; PT with anticoagulant therapy
• Pancreatitis, cholelithiasis renal failure, rhabdomyolyis, myositis, drug should be discontinued

Administer:
• Drug with meals; may increase q4-8wk
• Bowel pattern daily; increase bulk, water in diet if constipation develops

Evaluate:
• Therapeutic response: decreased triglycerides, diarrhea, pruritus (excess bile acids)

Teach patient/family:
• That compliance is needed
• That risk factors should be decreased: high-fat diet, smoking, alcohol consumption, absence of exercise
• To notify prescriber if pregnancy is suspected or planned
• To report GU symptoms: decreased libido, impotence, dysuria, proteinuria, oliguria, hematuria
• To notify prescriber of muscle pain, weakness, fever, fatigue; epigastric pain

fenoldopam (Rx)
(feh-nahl'doh-pam)
Corlopam
Func. class.: Antihypertensive, vasodilator

Action: Antagonizes D_1-like dopamine receptors; binds to α_2-adrenoceptors; increases renal blood flow

Uses: Hypertensive crisis, malignant hypertension

Dosage and routes:
• *Adult:* IV 0.01-1.6 µg/kg/min

Available forms: Inj conc 10 mg/ml

Side effects/adverse reactions:
CNS: Headache, anxiety, dizziness
CV: **Hypotension,** ST-T-wave changes, angina pectoris, palpitations, *MI, ischemic heart disease*
GI: Nausea, vomiting, constipation, diarrhea
HEMA: **Leukocytosis,** bleeding
META: Increased BUN, glucose, LDH, creatinine, hypokalemia

Contraindications: Hypersensitivity, sulfite sensitivity

Precautions: Tachycardia, pregnancy (B), lactation, children, intraocular pressure, hypokalemia

Pharmacokinetics: Elimination half-life 5 min, steady state 20 min

Interactions:
• Increased hypotension: avoid use with β-blockers

NURSING CONSIDERATIONS

Assess:
• B/P q5min until stabilized, then q1h × 2 hr, then q4h; pulse, jugular venous distension q4h
• Electrolytes, blood studies: K, Na, Cl, CO_2, CBC, serum glucose
• Skin turgor, dryness of mucous membranes for hydration status
• IV site for extravasation, rate

Administer:
IV
• After diluting contents of ampules in 0.9% NaCl, or 5% dextrose inj

---

(40 µg/ml); then add 4 ml of conc (40 mg of drug/1000 ml); 2 ml of conc (20 mg of drug/500 ml); 1 ml of conc (10 mg of drug/250 ml); do not admix
• To patient in recumbent position; keep in that position for 1 hr after administration

Perform/provide:
• Diluted sol is stable in normal light/ temperature for 24 hr

Evaluate:
• Therapeutic response: decreased B/P

Teach patient/family:
• To report dyspnea, chest pain, bleeding
• Reason for medication and expected results

RARELY USED

fenoprofen (℞)
(fen-oh-proe'fen)
Fenoprofen, Nalfon
Func. class.: Nonsteroidal antiinflammatory/nonopioid analgesic

Uses: Mild to moderate pain, osteoarthritis, rheumatoid arthritis, acute gout, arthritis, ankylosing spondylitis, inflammation, dysmenorrhea

Dosage and routes:
Pain
• *Adult:* **PO** 200 mg q4-6h prn
Arthritis
• *Adult:* **PO** 300-600 mg qid, not to exceed 3.2 g/day

Contraindications: Hypersensitivity, asthma, severe renal disease, severe hepatic disease

fentanyl (℞)
(fen'ta-nill)
Actiq, Fentanyl, Fentanyl Oralet, Sublimaze
Func. class.: Opioid analgesic
Chem. class.: Synthetic phenylpiperidine
Controlled Substance Schedule II

Action: Inhibits ascending pain pathways in CNS, increases pain threshold, alters pain perception by binding to opiate receptors

Uses: Preoperatively, postoperatively; adjunct to general anesthetic, when combined with droperidol; Fentanyl Oralet—anesthesia as premedication, conscious sedation; Actiq—breakthrough cancer pain

Dosage and routes:
Anesthetic
• *Adult:* **IV** 0.05-0.1 mg q2-3 min prn
Preoperatively
• *Adult:* **IM** 0.05-0.1 mg q30-60 min before surgery
Postoperatively
• *Adult:* **IM** 0.05-0.1 mg q1-2h prn
Fentanyl Oralet
• *Adult:* Transmucosal 5 µg/kg = fentanyl IM 0.75-1.25 µg/kg, do not exceed 5 µg/kg
• *Child:* Transmucosal may need doses of 5-15 µg/kg; must be watched continuously for hypoventilation
Actiq
• *Adult:* Transmucosal 200 µg, redose if needed 15 min after completion of 1st dose, do not give more than 2 doses during titration period
Available forms: Inj 0.05 mg/ml; lozenges 100, 200, 300, 400 µg; lozenges on a stick 200, 400, 600, 800, 1200, 1600 µg
Side effects/adverse reactions:
CNS: Dizziness, delirium, euphoria

◆ = Nursing alert   ∥ = Herb-drug interaction   ⊘ = Do not crush

GI: Nausea, vomiting
MS: Muscle rigidity
EENT: Blurred vision, miosis
CV: ***Bradycardia, arrest,*** hypotension or hypertension
RESP: ***Respiratory depression, arrest, laryngospasm***
GU: Urinary retention
INTEG: Rash, diaphoresis
Contraindications: Hypersensitivity to opiates, myasthenia gravis
Precautions: Elderly, respiratory depression, increased intracranial pressure, seizure disorders, severe respiratory disorders, cardiac dysrhythmias, pregnancy (C), lactation
Pharmacokinetics:
IM: Onset 7-8 min, peak 30 min, duration 1-2 hr
IV: Onset immediate, peak 3-5 min, duration ½-1 hr; metabolized by liver; excreted by kidneys; crosses placenta; excreted in breast milk; half-life 1½-6 hr; 80% bound to plasma proteins
Interactions:
• Effects may be increased with other CNS depressants: alcohol, opioids, sedative/hypnotics, antipsychotics, skeletal muscle relaxants
🌿 Increased action: kava
NURSING CONSIDERATIONS
Assess:
• VS after parenteral route; note muscle rigidity, drug history, liver, kidney function test
• CNS changes: dizziness, drowsiness, hallucinations, euphoria, LOC, pupil reaction
• Allergic reactions: rash, urticaria
• Respiratory dysfunction: respiratory depression, character, rate, rhythm; notify prescriber if respirations are <10/min
Administer:
• By injection (IM, IV); give slowly to prevent rigidity

• Only with resuscitative equipment available
IV
• IV undiluted by anesthesiologist or diluted with 5 ml or more sterile H_2O or 0.9% NaCl given through Y-tube or 3-way stopcock at 0.1 mg or less/1-2 min
Additive compatibilities: Bupivacaine
Solution compatibilities: D_5W, 0.9% NaCl
Syringe compatibilities: Atracurium, atropine, bupivacaine/ketamine, butorphanol, chlorpromazine, cimetidine, clonidine/lidocaine, dimenhydrinate, diphenhydramine, droperidol, heparin, hydromorphone, hydroxyzine, meperidine, metoclopramide, midazolam, morphine, pentazocine, perphenazine, prochlorperazine, promazine, promethazine, ranitidine, scopolamine
Y-site compatibilities: Amphotericin B cholesteryl, atracurium, cisatracurium, diltiazem, dobutamine, dopamine, enalaprilat, epinephrine, esmolol, etomidate, furosemide, heparin, hydrocortisone, hydromorphone, labetalol, lorazepam, midazolam, milrinone, morphine, nafcillin, nicardipine, nitroglycerin, norepinephrine, pancuronium, potassium chloride, propofol, ranitidine, remifentanil, sargramostim, thiopental, vecuronium, vit B/C
Transmucosal
• Remove foil just before administration, instruct patient to place under tongue and suck, not chew (Oralet); place between cheek and lower gum, moving it back and forth and suck, not chew (Actiq); all products not used or partially used should be flushed down the toilet
Perform/provide:
• Storage in light-resistant area at room temperature

Teach patient/family:
• Coughing, turning, deep breathing for postoperative patients
• Safety measures: side rails, nightlight, call bell within reach
Evaluate:
• Therapeutic response: induction of anesthesia, breakthrough cancer pain

---

fentanyl/droperidol combination (℞)

(fen'ta-nil)/(droe-per'i-dole)
Innovar

Func. class.: General anesthetic, opioid analgesic
Chem. class.: Phenylpiperone derivative

Controlled Substance Schedule II

Action: Action at subcortical levels to reduce motor activity, produces analgesia

Uses: Premedication, adjunct to general anesthesia, maintenance of anesthesia

Dosage and routes:
Induction
• *Adult:* IV 1 ml/20-25 lb
• *Child:* IV 0.5 ml/20 lb
Premedication
• *Adult:* IM 0.5-2 ml 45-60 min before surgery or procedure
• *Child:* IM 0.25 ml/20 lb 45-60 min before surgery or procedure
Available forms: Inj 0.05 mg fentanyl, 2.5 mg droperidol/ml

Side effects/adverse reactions:
RESP: **Laryngospasm, bronchospasm, respiratory arrest**
CNS: Dystonia, akathisia, flexion of arms, fine tremors, dizziness, anxiety, drowsiness, restlessness, hallucination, depression, muscular rigidity, EPS
CV: Tachycardia, hypotension, circulatory depression

EENT: Upward rotation of eyes, oculogyric crisis, blurred vision
INTEG: Chills, facial sweating, shivering, diaphoresis
GI: Nausea, vomiting

Contraindications: Hypersensitivity, child <2 yr, myasthenia gravis
Precautions: Elderly, increased intracranial pressure, cardiovascular disease (bradydysrhythmias), renal disease, liver disease, Parkinson's disease, COPD, pregnancy (C)

Pharmacokinetics:
IV: Onset 20 sec, peak 2-10 min, duration ½-2 hr; tranquilizing effect may last up to 12 hr
IM: Onset 7 min, duration 1-2 hr; metabolized in liver; excreted in urine metabolites (90%)

Interactions:
• Increased CNS depression: alcohol, opioids, barbiturates, antipsychotics, other CNS depressants
• Decreased effects of amphetamines, anticonvulsants, anticoagulants
• Increased intraocular pressure: anticholinergics, antiparkinson drugs
• Increased side effects of lithium
⫟ Increased action: kava

NURSING CONSIDERATIONS
Assess:
• VS q10min during IV administration, q30min after IM dose
• LFTs and BUN, creatinine, Paco$_2$
• Rigidity of skeletal muscles
• EPS: dystonia, akathisia
• Increasing heart rate or decreasing B/P by >10% from baseline; notify prescriber at once; do not place patient in Trendelenburg position or sympathetic blockade may occur, causing respiratory arrest

Administer:
• Anticholinergics (benztropine, diphenhydramine) for EPS

◆ = Nursing alert   ⫟ = Herb-drug interaction   ⊘ = Do not crush

• Only with crash cart, resuscitative equipment nearby; narcotic antagonist for severe respiratory depression, cardiac monitor

IV

• IV direct undiluted through Y-tube or 3-way stopcock; give each 1 ml undiluted drug/1min or more; 0.1 ml/kg may be diluted in 250 ml D$_5$W and given as IV INF over 5-10 min; titrate to response

Additive compatibilities: Sodium bicarbonate

Syringe compatibilities: Benzquinamide, glycopyrrolate

Y-site compatibilities: Hydrocortisone, potassium chloride, vit B/C

Perform/provide:

• Slow movement of patient to avoid orthostatic hypotension

Evaluate:

• Therapeutic response: decreased anxiety, absence of vomiting, maintenance of anesthesia

Teach patient/family:

• To use deep breathing, turning, coughing after surgery to prevent increased secretions in lungs

---

fentanyl
transdermal (℞)
Duragesic

Func. class.: Opioid analgesic
Chem. class.: Synthetic phenylpiperidine

Controlled Substance Schedule II

Action: Inhibits ascending pain pathways in CNS, increases pain threshold, alters pain perception by binding to opiate receptors

Uses: Management of chronic pain for those requiring opioid analgesia

Dosage and routes:

• *Adult:* 25 µg/hr; may increase until pain relief occurs; apply patch to flat surface on upper torso and wear for 72 hr; apply new patch on different site for continued relief

Available forms: Patch 25, 50, 75, 100 µg/hr

Side effects/adverse reactions:

MS: Asthenia

GU: Urinary retention, urgency, dysuria, frequency, oliguria

INTEG: Sweating, pruritus, rash, erythema, papules

CNS: Dizziness, delirium, euphoria, light-headedness, sedation, dysphoria, agitation, anxiety, confusion, headache, depression

GI: Nausea, vomiting, diarrhea, cramps, anorexia, constipation, dyspepsia

EENT: Blurred vision, miosis

CV: Bradycardia, **cardiac arrest,** hypotension or hypertension, facial flushing, chills, chest pain, dysrhythmias

RESP: **Respiratory depression, laryngospasm, bronchospasm,** depresses cough, hypoventilation, dyspnea, hiccups, apnea

Contraindications: Hypersensitivity to opiates, myasthenia gravis, children <12 yr, patient <18 yr with weight <110 lb

Precautions: Elderly, respiratory depression, increased intracranial pressure, seizure disorders, severe respiratory disorders, cardiac dysrhythmias, pregnancy (C), fever

Interactions:

• Effects may be increased with other CNS depressants: alcohol, opioids, sedative/hypnotics, antipsychotics, skeletal muscle relaxants

🍃 Increased action: kava

NURSING CONSIDERATIONS

Assess:

• Pain control; check for duration, site, character of pain, fever; use pain and sedation scoring

• CNS changes: dizziness, drowsiness, hallucinations, euphoria, LOC, pupil reaction
• Allergic reactions: rash, urticaria
• Respiratory dysfunction: respiratory depression, character, rate, rhythm; notify prescriber if respirations are <10/min
Administer:
• q72h for continuous pain relief; dosage is adjusted after at least two applications, apply to clean, dry skin, press firmly
• Give short-acting analgesics until patch takes effect (24 hr)
Perform/provide:
• Safety measures: side rails, nightlight, call bell within reach
Evaluate:
• Therapeutic response: decreased pain
Teach patient/family:
• To avoid activities that require alertness
• That excessive heat may increase absorption
• That excessive perspiration may alter adhesiveness
• To dispose of patch by placing sticky sides together and flushing in toilet
• That patient may need to clip hair before applying to ensure adhesion

ferrous fumarate (℞)
Femiron, Feostat, Feostat Drops, Hemocyte, Ircon, Nephro-Fer, Novofumar*, Palafer*, Span-FF
ferrous gluconate (℞)
Fergon, Fertinic*, Novoferrogluc*
ferrous sulfate (℞)
Apo-Ferrous Sulfate*, ED-IN-SOL, Feosol, Fer-gen-sol, Fer-Iron Drops, Fero-Grad, Mol-Iron
ferrous sulfate, dried (℞)
Fe⁵⁰, Feosol, Feratab, Novoferrosulfa*, PMS-Ferrous Sulfate, Slow Fe
ferric gluconate complex (℞)
Ferrlecit
carbonyl iron
(kar'bo-nil)
Feosol
iron polysaccharide
Hytinic, Niferex, Nu-Iron, Nu-Iron 150
Func. class.: Hematinic
Chem. class.: Iron preparation

Action: Replaces iron stores needed for red blood cell development, energy and O_2 transport, utilization; fumarate contains 33% elemental iron; gluconate, 12%; sulfate, 20%; iron, 30%; ferrous sulfate exsiccated
Uses: Iron deficiency anemia, prophylaxis for iron deficiency in pregnancy
Dosage and routes:
Fumarate
• *Adult:* **PO** 200 mg tid-qid
• *Child 2-12 yr:* **PO** 3 mg/kg/day (elemental iron) tid-qid
• *Child 6 mo-2 yr:* **PO** up to 6 mg/kg/day (elemental iron) tid-qid;

◆ = Nursing alert   〽 = Herb-drug interaction   ⊘ = Do not crush

PO 6 mg/kg/day in 3-4 divided doses
• *Infant:* **PO** 10-25 mg/day (elemental iron) in 3-4 divided doses
Gluconate
• *Adult:* **PO** 200-600 mg tid
• *Child 6-12 yr:* **PO** 300-900 mg qd
• *Child <6 yr:* **PO** 100-300 mg qd
Sulfate
• *Adult:* **PO** 0.75-1.5 g/day in divided doses tid
• *Child 6-12 yr:* **PO** 600 mg/day in divided doses
Pregnancy
• *Adult:* **PO** 300-600 mg/day in divided doses
Complex
Adult IV Inf (125 mg) 10 ml/100 ml of NaCl for Inj given over 1 hr
Iron polysaccharide
• *Adult:* **PO** 100-200 mg tid
• *Child:* **PO** 4-6 mg/kg/day in 3 divided doses
Available forms:
Fumarate
Tabs 63, 195, 200, 324, 325 mg; tabs chewable 100 mg; tabs cont rel 300 mg; oral susp 100 mg/5 ml, 45 mg/0.6 ml
Gluconate
Tabs 300, 320, 325 mg; caps 86, 325, 435 mg; tabs film-coated 300 mg; elix 300 mg/5 ml
Sulfate
Tabs, 195, 300, 325 mg; tabs enteric-coated 325 mg; tabs ext rel, time-rel caps, 525 mg
Dried
Tabs, 200 mg; tabs ext rel 160 mg; caplets ext rel 160 mg
Complex
Inj. 62.5 mg/5 ml (12.5 mg/ml)
Iron polysaccharide
Tabs 50 mg, caps 150 mg, sol 100 mg/5 ml
Side effects/adverse reactions:
GI: Nausea, constipation, epigas-

tric pain, black and red tarry stools, vomiting, diarrhea
INTEG: Temporarily discolored tooth enamel and eyes
Contraindications: Hypersensitivity, ulcerative colitis/regional enteritis, hemosiderosis/hemochromatosis, peptic ulcer disease, hemolytic anemia, cirrhosis
Precautions: Anemia (long-term), pregnancy (B) (ferric gluconate complex), (C) (iron dextran, oral products)
Pharmacokinetics:
PO: Excreted in feces, urine, skin, breast milk; enters bloodstream; bound to transferrin; crosses placenta
Interactions:
• Decreased absorption of: penicillamine, levodopa, methyldopa, fluoroquinolones, L-thyroxine, tetracycline
• Decreased absorption of iron preparations: antacids, cimetidine, cholestyramine, vit E
• Increased action of iron preparation: ascorbic acid, chloramphenicol
• Drug/food: decreased absorption: dairy products, caffeine, eggs
Lab test interferences:
False positive: Occult blood
NURSING CONSIDERATIONS
Assess:
• Blood studies: Hct, Hgb, reticulocytes, bilirubin before treatment, at least monthly
◆ Toxicity: nausea, vomiting, diarrhea (green, then tarry stools), hematemesis, pallor, cyanosis, shock, coma
• Elimination; if constipation occurs, increase water, bulk, activity
• Nutrition: amount of iron in diet (meat, dark green leafy vegetables, dried beans, dried fruits, eggs)
• Cause of iron loss or anemia, in-

cluding salicylates, sulfonamides, antimalarials, quinidine

Administer:
• Between meals for best absorption; may give with juice; do not give with antacids or milk, delay at least 1 hr; if GI symptoms occur, give pc even if absorption is decreased; eggs, milk products, chocolate, caffeine interfere with absorption
• Liquid through plastic straw to avoid discoloration of tooth enamel; dilute thoroughly
• At least 1 hr before hs, since corrosion may occur in stomach
• For <6 mo for anemia

Perform/provide:
• Storage in tight, light-resistant container

Evaluate:
• Therapeutic response: improvement in Hct, Hgb, reticulocytes; decreased fatigue, weakness

Teach patient/family:
• That iron will change stools black or dark green
• That iron poisoning may occur if increased beyond recommended level
🚫 To swallow tab whole; not to break, crush, or chew unless labeled as chewable
• To keep out of reach of children
• Not to substitute one iron salt for another; elemental iron content differs (e.g., 300 mg ferrous fumarate contains about 100 mg elemental iron; 300 mg ferrous gluconate contains only about 30 mg elemental iron)
• To avoid reclining position for 15-30 min after taking drug to avoid esophageal corrosion
• To follow diet high in iron

Treatment of overdose: Induce vomiting; give eggs, milk until lavage can be done

---

fexofenadine (℞)
(fex-oh-fi′na-deen)
Allegra
Func. class.: Antihistamine
Chem. class.: Piperidine, peripherally selective

Action: Acts on blood vessels, GI, respiratory system by competing with histamine for H_1-receptor site; decreases allergic response by blocking pharmacologic effects of histamine

Uses: Rhinitis, allergy symptoms, chronic idiopathic urticaria

Dosage and routes:
• *Adult and child >12 yr:* 60 mg bid
• *Child 6-11 yr:* **PO** 30 mg bid
Renal dose:
• CrCl <80 ml/min 60 mg qd

Available forms: Caps 60 mg; ext rel tab 180 mg; tab 30 mg

Side effects/adverse reactions:
GU: Frequency, dysuria, urinary retention, impotence
HEMA: **Hemolytic anemia, thrombocytopenia, leukopenia, agranulocytosis, pancytopenia**
RESP: Thickening of bronchial secretions, dry nose, throat
GI: Nausea, diarrhea, abdominal pain, vomiting, constipation
CNS: Headache, stimulation, drowsiness, sedation, fatigue, confusion, blurred vision, tinnitus, restlessness, tremors, paradoxical excitation in children or elderly
INTEG: Rash, eczema, photosensitivity, urticaria
CV: Hypotension, palpitations, bradycardia, tachycardia, *dysrhythmias* (rare)

Contraindications: Hypersensitivity, newborn or premature infants, lactation, severe hepatic disease

Precautions: Pregnancy (C), elderly, children, respiratory disease,

---

◆ = Nursing alert   🌿 = Herb-drug interaction   🚫 = Do not crush

narrow-angle glaucoma, prostatic hypertrophy, bladder neck obstruction, asthma

Pharmacokinetics: Well absorbed; onset 3-5 min, peak 1-2 hr, duration 8-12 hr

Interactions:

• Increased CNS depression: alcohol, other CNS depressants

🌿 Increased anticholinergic effect: henbane leaf

Lab test interferences:

False negative: Skin allergy tests

NURSING CONSIDERATIONS

Assess:

• I&O ratio: be alert for urinary retention, frequency, dysuria, especially elderly; drug should be discontinued if these occur

• Respiratory status: rate, rhythm, increase in bronchial secretions, wheezing, chest tightness

Administer:

• On empty stomach 1 hr before or 2 hr after meals

Perform/provide:

• Hard candy, gum, frequent rinsing of mouth for dryness

• Storage in tight, light-resistant container

Evaluate:

• Therapeutic response: absence of running or congested nose or rashes

Teach patient/family:

• All aspects of drug use; to notify prescriber if confusion, sedation, hypotension occur

• To avoid driving, other hazardous activity if drowsiness occurs

• To avoid alcohol, other CNS depressants

• Not to exceed recommended dose; dysrhythmias may occur

🚫 Not to break, crush, or chew caps, ext rel tabs

Treatment of overdose: Administer ipecac syrup or lavage, diazepam, vasopressors, barbiturates (short-acting)

---

fibrinolysin/ desoxy- ribonuclease (℞)

(fye-brin-oh-lye′sin)/(dez-ox-ee- rye-boo-nuke′lee-ase)

Elase

Func. class.: Enzyme

Chem. class.: Proteolytic, bovine

Action: Dissolves fibrin in clots and fibrinous exudates; attacks DNA in areas of disintegrating cells

Uses: Debridement of wounds, vaginitis, cervicitis, ulcerative colitis; 2nd-, 3rd-degree burns; irrigating wounds, topically

Dosage and routes:

Debridement/intravaginally

• *Adult:* **OINT** 5 g × 5 applications

Irrigating

• *Adult:* **IRIG** dilution depends on type of wound

Available forms: Fibrinolysin with desoxyribonuclease 666.6 U/g; powder for reconstitution fibrinolysin 25 U/desoxyribonuclease 15,000 U

Side effects/adverse reactions:

INTEG: Hyperemia

Contraindications: Hypersensitivity to bovine or mercury products, hematoma

Precautions: Pregnancy (C)

NURSING CONSIDERATIONS

Assess:

• For signs of irritation and inflammation; drug should be discontinued

• Wound: drainage, color, odor, size, depth

Administer:

• After reconstituting with 10 ml sterile NaCl sol; use only fresh sol

• After removing necrotic debris, dry eschar

• Wet dressing by mixing 1 vial

Elase/10-50 ml NS; saturate gauze with sol; pack area; remove in 6-8 hr; repeat tid-qid

Perform/provide:

• Cleansing of wound using aseptic technique; cover with drug, then dressing; change at least qid

Evaluate:

• Therapeutic response: decrease in wound scarring, tissue necrosis

---

filgrastim (℞)

(fill-grass'stim)

G-CSF, granulocyte colony stimulator, Neupogen

Func. class.: Biologic modifier

Chem. class.: Granulocyte colony-stimulating factor

Action: Stimulates proliferation and differentiation of neutrophils

Uses: To decrease infection in patients receiving antineoplastics that are myelosuppressive; to increase WBC in patients with drug-induced neutropenia; bone marrow transplantation

Investigational uses: Neutropenia in HIV infection

Dosage and routes:

After myelosuppressive chemotherapy

• *Adult and child:* **IV/SC** 5 µg/kg/day in a single dose × 14 days; may increase by 5 µg/kg in each cycle; give qd for up to 2 wk until the absolute neutrophil count (ANC) is 10,000/mm^3; response to G-CSF is much greater with **SC** than **IV** therapy

After bone marrow transplantation

• **IV/SC** 10 µg/kg/day as an **INF (IV)** over 4 hr or 24 hr, begin 24 hr after chemotherapy and 24 hr after bone marrow transplantation

Peripheral blood progenitor cell collection/therapy

• 10 µg/kg/day as a bolus or **CONT INF** × 4 days or more before leukapheresis, continue to last leukapheresis; may alter dose if WBC >100,000 cells/mm^3

Severe neutropenia (chronic)

• *Adult:* **SC** 5 µg qd-bid

Available forms: Inj 300 µg/ml

Side effects/adverse reactions:

RESP: Respiratory distress syndrome

CNS: Fever

HEMA: **Thrombocytopenia**

INTEG: Alopecia, exacerbation of skin conditions

MS: Osteoporosis, skeletal pain

GI: Nausea, vomiting, diarrhea, mucositis, anorexia

Contraindications: Hypersensitivity to proteins of *E. coli*

Precautions: Pregnancy (C), lactation, cardiac conditions, children, myeloid malignancies

Pharmacokinetics:

IV: Onset 5-60 min, peak 24 hr, duration up to a week

SC: Onset 5-60 min, peak 2-8 hr, duration up to a week

Interactions:

• Do not use this drug concomitantly with antineoplastics

Lab test interferences:

Increase: Uric acid, lactate dehydrogenase, alk phosphatase

NURSING CONSIDERATIONS

Assess:

• Blood studies: CBC, platelet count before treatment and twice weekly; neutrophil counts may be increased for 2 days after therapy

• B/P, respirations, pulse before and during therapy

• Bone pain, give mild analgesics

Administer:

• Using single-use vials; after dose is withdrawn, do not reenter vial

• For 2 wk or until ANC is 10,000/

◆ = Nursing alert   ⧸ = Herb-drug interaction   ⊘ = Do not crush mm^3 after the expected chemotherapy neutrophil nadir

Cont IV inf

• Dilute in D$_5$W to a conc of >15 µg/ml, vial is for one-time use; give over 15-30 min (chemotherapy); over 4-24 hr (bone marrow transplantation); do not use 0.9% NaCl to dilute drug

Y-site compatibilities: Acyclovir, allopurinol, amikacin, aminophylline, ampicillin, ampicillin/sulbactam, aztreonam, bleomycin, bumetanide, buprenorphine, butorphanol, calcium gluconate, carboplatin, carmustine, cefazolin, cefotetan, ceftazidime, chlorpromazine, cimetidine, cisplatin, cyclophosphamide, cytarabine, dacarbazine, daunorubicin, dexamethasone, diphenhydramine, doxorubicin, doxycycline, droperidol, enalaprilat, famotidine, floxuridine, fluconazole, fludarabine, gallium, ganciclovir, granisetron, haloperidol, hydrocortisone, hydromorphone, hydroxyzine, idarubicin, ifosfamide, leucovorin, lorazepam, mechlorethamine, melphalan, meperidine, mesna, methotrexate, metoclopramide, miconazole, minocycline, mitoxantrone, morphine, nalbuphine, netilmicin, ondansetron, plicamycin, potassium chloride, promethazine, ranitidine, sodium bicarbonate, streptozocin, ticarcillin, ticarcillin/clavulanate, tobramycin, trimethoprim-sulfamethoxazole, vancomycin, vinblastine, vincristine, vinorelbine, zidovudine

Perform/provide:

• Storage in refrigerator; do not freeze; may store at room temperature up to 6 hr

• Avoid shaking

Evaluate:

• Therapeutic response: absence of infection

Teach patient/family:

• The technique for self-administration: dose, side effects, disposal of containers and needles; provide instruction sheet

---

finasteride (R)

(fin-ass′te-ride)

Propecia, Proscar

Func. class.: Hormone, androgen inhibitor, hair stimulant

Chem. class.: 5-α-Reductase inhibitor

Action: Inhibits 5-α-reductase and reduction in DHT; DHT induces androgenic effects by binding to androgen receptors in the cell nuclei of the prostate gland, liver, skin; prevents development of BHP

Uses: Symptomatic benign prostatic hyperplasia (Proscar); male-pattern baldness (Propecia)

Dosage and routes:

BPH

• *Adult:* **PO** 5 mg qd × 6-12 mo

Male pattern baldness

• *Adult:* **PO** 1 mg qd

Available forms: Tabs 1, 5 mg

Side effects/adverse reactions:

GU: Impotence, decreased libido, decreased volume of ejaculate

Contraindications: Hypersensitivity, children, women who are pregnant or may become pregnant should not handle tabs, pregnancy (X)

Precautions: Large residual urinary volume, severely diminished urinary flow, liver function abnormalities

Do not confuse:

Proscar/Prosom

Proscar/Prozac

Pharmacokinetics: Bioavailability 63%, readily absorbed from GI tract, plasma protein binding 90%; metabolized in the liver; excreted in urine (metabolites) 39%, feces

---

(57%); crosses blood-brain barrier; peak 1-2 hr, duration 24 hr
Interactions:
• Decreased effect of finasteride: theophylline, adrenergic broncholdilators, anticholinergics
NURSING CONSIDERATIONS
Assess:
• Urinary patterns, residual urinary volume, severely diminished urinary flow
• PSA levels and digital rectal exam prior to initiating therapy and periodically thereafter
• Liver function studies prior to treatment; extensively metabolized in liver
Administer:
• Without regard to meals
• For a minimum of 6 mo; not all patients will respond
Perform/provide:
• Storage <86° F (30° C); protect from light; keep container tightly closed
Evaluate:
• Therapeutic response: increased urinary flow, decreased postvoiding dribbling, frequency, nocturia or hair growth within 3-6 mo
Teach patient/family:
◆ Pregnant women or women who may become pregnant should not touch crushed tabs or come into contact with semen of a patient taking this drug; may adversely affect developing male fetus
• That volume of ejaculate may be decreased during treatment; impotence and decreased libido may also occur
• Propecia results may not occur for 3 mo
• Proscar results may not occur for 6-12 mo

RARELY USED

flavoxate (Ŗ)
(fla-vox′ate)
Func. class.: Spasmolytic

Uses: Relief of nocturia, incontinence, suprapubic pain, dysuria, frequency associated with urologic conditions (symptomatic only)
Dosage and routes:
• *Adult and child >12 yr:* **PO** 100-200 mg tid-qid
Contraindications: Hypersensitivity, GI obstruction, GI hemorrhage, GU obstruction

flecainide (Ŗ)
(flek-ay′nide)
Tambocor
Func. class.: Antidysrhythmic (Class IC)

Action: Decreases conduction in all parts of the heart, with greatest effect on His-Purkinje system, which stabilizes cardiac membrane
Uses: Life-threatening ventricular dysrhythmias, sustained ventricular tachycardia, supraventricular tachydysrhythmias
Dosage and routes:
• *Adult:* **PO** 50-100 mg q12h; may increase q4d by 50 mg q12h to desired response, not to exceed 400 mg/day
Renal disease
• CrCl <35 ml/min dose 50%-75%
Available forms: Tabs 50, 100, 150 mg
Side effects/adverse reactions:
CNS: Headache, dizziness, involuntary movement, confusion, psychosis, restlessness, irritability, paresthesias, ataxia, flushing, somnolence, depression, anxiety, malaise

---

◆ = Nursing alert   🍃 = Herb-drug interaction   🚫 = Do not crush

EENT: Tinnitus, *blurred vision,* hearing loss

GI: Nausea, vomiting, anorexia, constipation, abdominal pain, flatulence, change in taste

CV: Hypotension, bradycardia, angina, PVCs, ***heart block, cardiovascular collapse, arrest,*** dysrhythmias, ***CHF, fatal ventricular tachycardia***

RESP: Dyspnea, ***respiratory depression***

INTEG: Rash, urticaria, edema, swelling

HEMA: Leukopenia, thrombocytopenia

GU: Impotence, decreased libido, polyuria, urinary retention

Contraindications: Hypersensitivity, severe heart block, cardiogenic shock, nonsustained ventricular dysrhythmias, frequent PVCs, non–life-threatening dysrhythmias

Precautions: Pregnancy (C), lactation, children, renal disease, liver disease, CHF, respiratory depression, myasthenia gravis

Pharmacokinetics:

PO: Peak 3 hr; half-life 12-27 hr; metabolized by liver; excreted unchanged by kidneys (10%); excreted in breast milk

Interactions:

• Increased CV depressant action: β-blockers, disopyramide, verapamil

• Increased level of flecainide: amiodarone, cimetidine

• Increased digoxin level: digoxin

• Increased or decreased effect: alkalinizing agents, acidifying agents

🍃 Potassium deficiency: aloe, buckthorn bark/berry, cascara sagrada bark, senna pod/leaf

Lab test interferences:

Increase: CPK

NURSING CONSIDERATIONS
Assess:

• I&O, daily weight; CHF: edema, weight gain, dyspnea, jugular vein distention, rales, crackles

• For hypokalemia, hyperkalemia before administration; correct electrolytes

• Blood levels: trough (0.2-1 μg/ml)

• B/P, ECG continuously for fluctuations, watch for QRS widening, prolongation of QT and PR

• CNS effects: dizziness, confusion, psychosis, paresthesias, convulsions; drug should be discontinued

• Increased respiration, increased pulse; drug should be discontinued

Administer:

• Reduced dosage as soon as dysrhythmia is controlled

• May give with meals for GI upset

Evaluate:

• Therapeutic response: decreased dysrhythmias

Teach patient/family:

• To change position slowly from lying or sitting to standing to minimize orthostatic hypotension

• To take as prescribed, not to skip or double dose

• To avoid hazardous activities that require alertness until response is known

• To carry ID with disorder, medications taken

• To notify all health care providers of treatment

Treatment of overdose: O_2, artificial ventilation, ECG, dopamine for circulatory depression, diazepam or thiopental for convulsions, treat ventricular dysrhythmias

---

RARELY USED

floxuridine (Ŗ)

(flox-yoor'i-deen)
Floxuridine, FUDR
Func. class.: Antineoplastic,
antimetabolite

Uses: GI adenocarcinoma metastatic
to liver; cancer of breast, head, neck,
liver, brain, gallbladder, bile duct
Dosage and routes:
• *Adult:* **INTRAARTERIAL** by
cont inf 0.1-0.6 mg/kg/day × 1-6
wk; **HEPATIC ARTERY INJ**
0.4-0.6 mg/kg/day × 1-6 wk
Contraindications: Hypersensitivity, myelosuppression, pregnancy
(D), poor nutritional status, serious
infections

---

fluconazole (Ŗ)

(floo-kon'a-zole)
Diflucan
Func. class.: Antifungal

Action: Inhibits ergosterol biosyn-
thesis, causes direct damage to mem-
brane phospholipids
Uses: Oropharyngeal candidiasis in
AIDS patients, chronic mucocuta-
neous candidiasis, urinary candidi-
asis, cryptococcal meningitis
Dosage and routes:
Renal disease
• CrCl 11-50 ml/min dose 50%
Vaginal candidiasis
• *Adult:* PO 150 mg as a single dose
Serious fungal infections
• *Adult:* PO/IV 50-400 mg initially,
then 200 mg qd for 4 wk
• *Child:* 6-12 mg/kg/day
Oropharyngeal candidiasis
• *Adult:* PO/IV 200 mg initially, then
100 mg qd for at least 2 wk
• *Child:* 3 mg/kg/day
Available forms: Tabs 50, 100, 150,

200 mg; inj 2 mg/ml; powder for
oral susp 50, 200 mg/ml
Side effects/adverse reactions:
GI: Nausea, vomiting, diarrhea,
cramping, flatus, increased AST,
ALT, ***hepatotoxicity***
CNS: Headache
INTEG: ***Stevens-Johnson syndrome***
Contraindications: Hypersensitiv-
ity
Precautions: Renal disease, preg-
nancy (C), lactation
Do not confuse:
Diflucan/Diprivan
Pharmacokinetics: Peak 2-4 hr, bio-
availability (PO) 90%, excreted un-
changed in urine 80%
Interactions:
• Potentiation of anticoagulation:
warfarin
• Increased plasma concentrations:
cyclosporine, phenytoin, theophyl-
line, rifabutin, tacrolimus
• Hypoglycemia: oral antidiabetics
• Increased effect of zidovudine
NURSING CONSIDERATIONS
Assess:
• For infection: clearing of CSF cul-
ture during treatment, obtain C&S
baseline and throughout, drug may
be started as soon as culture is taken
◆ For hepatotoxicity: increasing
AST, ALT, periodically alk phos-
phatase, bilirubin
Administer:
PO
• Shake oral susp before each use
IV
• After diluting according to package directions; run at 200 mg/hr or
less; do not use plastic containers in
connections; check for bag leaks
• Using an infusion pump check for
extravasation and necrosis q2h
Additive compatibilities: Acyclovir, amikacin, amphotericin B, cefazolin, ceftazidime, clindamycin,
gentamicin, heparin, meropenem,
metronidazole, morphine, piperacil-

◆ = Nursing alert   ∦ = Herb-drug interaction   ⊘ = Do not crush lin, potassium chloride, theophylline

Y-site compatibilities: Acyclovir, aldesleukin, allopurinol, amifostine, amikacin, aminophylline, ampicillin/sulbactam, aztreonam, benztropine, cefazolin, cefepime, cefotetan, cefoxitin, chlorpromazine, cimetidine, cisatracurium, dexamethasone, diphenhydramine, dobutamine, dopamine, doxorubicin liposome, droperidol, famotidine, filgrastim, fludarabine, foscarnet, gallium, ganciclovir, gentamicin, granisetron, heparin, hydrocortisone, immune globulin, leucovorin, lorazepam, melphalan, meperidine, meropenem, metoclopramide, metronidazole, midazolam, morphine, nafcillin, nitroglycerin, ondansetron, oxacillin, paclitaxel, pancuronium, penicillin G potassium, phenytoin, piperacillin/tazobactam, prochlorperazine, promethazine, propofol, ranitidine, remifentanil, sargramostim, tacrolimus, teniposide, theophylline, thiotepa, ticarcillin/clavulanate, tobramycin, vancomycin, vecuronium, vinorelbine, zidovudine

Perform/provide:
• Storage protected from moisture and light, diluted sol is stable 24 hr

Evaluate:
• Therapeutic response: decreasing oral candidiasis, fever, malaise, rash; negative C&S for infection organism

Teach patient/family:
• That long-term therapy may be needed to clear infection
• That medication may be taken with food to reduce GI effects
• To notify prescriber of nausea, vomiting, diarrhea, jaundice, anorexia, clay-colored stools, dark urine

RAREY USED

fludarabine (℞)

(floo-dar′a-been)
Fludara
Func. class.: Antineoplastic, antimetabolite

Uses: Chronic lymphocytic leukemia, non-Hodgkin's lymphoma
Dosage and routes:
• *Adult:* IV 25 mg/m^2 over 30 min qd × 5 days, may repeat q28d; reconstitute with 2 ml of sterile water for inj; dissolution should occur in <15 sec
Contraindications: Hypersensitivity, pregnancy (D), lactation

fludrocortisone (℞)

(floo-droe-kor′ti-sone)
Florinef
Func. class.: Corticosteroid
Chem. class.: Mineralocorticoid

Action: Promotes increased reabsorption of sodium and loss of potassium, water, hydrogen from distal renal tubules
Uses: Adrenal insufficiency, salt-losing adrenogenital syndrome
Investigational uses: Renal tubular acidosis (type IV) idiopathic orthostatic hypotension
Dosage and routes:
• *Adult:* PO 0.1-0.2 mg qd
• *Child:* PO 0.05-0.1 mg/day
Available forms: Tabs 0.1 mg
Side effects/adverse reactions:
CNS: Flushing, sweating, headache, paralysis
CV: Hypertension, ***circulatory collapse, thrombophlebitis, embolism,*** tachycardia, ***CHF***
MS: Fractures, osteoporosis, weakness

ENDO: Weight gain, adrenal suppression
MISC: Hypersensitivity
META: Hypokalemia
Contraindications: Hypersensitivity, acute glomerulonephritis, amebiasis, psychoses, Cushing's syndrome
Precautions: Pregnancy (C), osteoporosis, CHF, lactation
Pharmacokinetics:
PO: Half-life 3.5 hr, metabolized by liver, excreted in urine
Interactions:
• Decreased action of fludrocortisone: barbiturates, rifampin
• Decreased potassium levels: thiazides, potassium-wasting drugs, loop diuretics, amphotericin B, piperacillin, mezlocillin
• Increased B/P: sodium-containing food or medication
🔏 Potassium deficiency: aloe, buckthorn, cascara sagrada, senna
Lab test interferences:
Increase: Potassium, sodium
Decrease: Hct
NURSING CONSIDERATIONS
Assess:
• Weight daily; notify prescriber of weekly gain >5 lb; I&O ratio; be alert for decreasing urinary output, increasing edema
• B/P q4h, pulse; notify prescriber if chest pain occurs
• K depletion: paresthesias, fatigue, nausea, vomiting, depression, polyuria, dysrhythmias, weakness
• Electrolytes: sodium, potassium, chloride, hypokalemia is common
Administer:
• Titrated dose; use lowest effective dose
• With food or milk to decrease GI symptoms
Perform/provide:
• Assistance with ambulation in patient with bone tissue disease to prevent fractures

Evaluate:
• Therapeutic response: correction of adrenal insufficiency
Teach patient/family:
• That ID as steroid user should be carried
• Not to discontinue this medication abruptly
• To notify health-care provider of muscle cramps, weight gain, edema, nausea

---

flumazenil (℞)
(flu-maz'e-nill)
Anexate*, Romazicon
Func. class.: Antidote: Benzodiazepine receptor antagonist
Chem. class.: Imidazobenzodiazepine derivative

Action: Antagonizes actions of benzodiazepines on CNS, competitively inhibits activity at benzodiazepine recognition site on GABA/benzodiazepine receptor complex
Uses: Reversal of sedative effects of benzodiazepines
Dosage and routes:
Reversal of conscious sedation or in general anesthesia
• *Adult:* **IV** 0.2 mg given over 15 sec; wait 45 sec, then give 0.2 mg if consciousness does not occur; may be repeated at 60-sec intervals prn (max 3 mg/hr)
• *Child:* **IV** 10 μg (0.01 mg)/kg; cumulative dose of 1 mg or less
Management of suspected benzodiazepine overdose
• *Adult:* **IV** 0.2 mg given over 30 sec; wait 30 sec, then give 0.3 mg over 30 sec if consciousness does not occur; further doses of 0.5 mg can be given over 30 sec at intervals of 1 min up to cumulative dose of 3 mg

---

◆ = Nursing alert 🔏 = Herb-drug interaction 🚫 = Do not crush

• *Child:* **IV** 100 μg (0.1 mg)/kg; cumulative dose of 1 mg or less
Available forms: Inj 0.1 mg/ml
Side effects/adverse reactions:
EENT: Abnormal vision, blurred vision, tinnitus
CV: Hypertension, palpitations, cutaneous vasodilation, ***dysrhythmias,*** bradycardia, tachycardia, chest pain
GI: Nausea, vomiting, hiccups
CNS: Dizziness, agitation, emotional lability, confusion, ***seizures,*** somnolence
SYST: Headache, injection site pain, increased sweating, fatigue, rigors
Contraindications: Hypersensitivity to this drug or benzodiazepines, serious cyclic antidepressant overdose, patients given benzodiazepine for control of life-threatening condition
Precautions: Pregnancy (C), lactation, children, elderly, renal disease, seizure disorders, head injury, labor/delivery, hepatic disease, hypoventilation, panic disorder, drug and alcohol dependency, ambulatory patients
Do not confuse:
Mazicon/Mivacron
Pharmacokinetics: Terminal half-life 41-79 min; metabolized in liver
Interactions:
• Toxicity: mixed drug overdosage
NURSING CONSIDERATIONS
Assess:
• Cardiac status using continuous monitoring
• For seizures; protect patient from injury; most likely those that have withdrawals from sedatives
• GI symptoms: nausea, vomiting; place in side-lying position to prevent aspiration
• Allergic reactions: flushing, rash, urticaria, pruritus
Administer:
• Check airway and IV access before administration

IV, direct
• Give undiluted or diluted with 0.9% NaCl, D_5W, LR, give over 15 sec into running IV
Additive compatibilities: Aminophylline, cimetidine, dobutamine, dopamine, famotidine, heparin, lidocaine, procainamide, ranitidine
Solution compatibilities: D_5W
Evaluate:
• Therapeutic response: decreased sedation, respiratory depression, toxicity
Teach patient/family:
• That amnesia may continue
• Not to engage in hazardous activities for 18-24 hr after discharge
• Not to take any alcohol or nonprescription drugs for 18-24 hr

---

fluoride (PO) (℞)
(floor'ide)
Fluor-A-Day*, Fluoride Loz, Fluoritab, Flura-Loz, Karidium, Luride, Pediaflor, Pharmaflur, Phos-Flur, Solu-Flur*
fluoride (top) (℞)
ACT, Fluorigard, Fluorinse, Gel Kam, Gel-Tin, Karigel, MouthKote, Stop, Thera-Flur
Func. class.: Trace elements
Chem. class.: Fluoride ion

Action: Needed for hard tooth enamel and for resistance to periodontal disease; reduces acid production by dental bacteria
Uses: Prevention of dental caries, osteoporosis
Dosage and routes:
• *Adult and child >12 yr:* **Top** 10 ml 0.2% sol qd after brushing teeth, rinse mouth for >1 min with sol
• *Child 6-12 yr:* **Top** 5 ml 0.2% sol
• *Child >3 yr:* **PO** 1 mg qd
• *Child <3 yr:* **PO** 0.5 mg qd

Available forms: Tabs chewable 0.5, 1 mg; tabs 1 mg, tabs effervescent 10 mg; drops 0.125, 0.25, 0.5 mg/drop; rinse supplements 0.2 mg/ml, rinse 0.01%, 0.02%, 0.04%, 0.09%; gel 0.1%, 0.5%; lozenges 1 mg; sol 0.2 mg/ml

Side effects/adverse reactions:

ACUTE OVERDOSE: **Black tarry stools, bloody vomit, diarrhea, decreased respiration, increased salivation, watery eyes**

CHRONIC OVERDOSE: **Hypocalcemia and tetany, respiratory arrest, sores in mouth, constipation, loss of appetite, nausea, vomiting, weight loss, discoloration of teeth** (white, black, brown)

Contraindications: Hypersensitivity, pregnancy (NR)

Precautions: Child <6 yr

Pharmacokinetics:

PO: Excreted in urine and feces; crosses placenta, breast milk

Interactions:

• Drug/food: avoid use with dairy products

NURSING CONSIDERATIONS

Assess:

• For mottling of teeth, during treatment

Administer:

• Drops after meals with fluids or undiluted tabs; may be chewed; do not swallow whole; may be given with water or juice; avoid milk

Evaluate:

• Therapeutic response: absence of dental caries

Teach patient/family:

• To monitor children using gel or rinse; not to be swallowed

• Not to drink, eat, or rinse mouth for at least ½ hr

• Not to use during pregnancy

• To apply after brushing and flossing hs

• To store out of children's reach

---

fluorouracil (R)

(flure-oh-yoor′a-sil)

Adrucil, Efudex, 5-FU

Func. class.: Antineoplastic, antimetabolite

Chem. class.: Pyrimidine antagonist

Action: Inhibits DNA, RNA synthesis; interferes with cell replication by competitively inhibiting thymidylate synthesis, S phase of cell cycle–specific, a vesicant

Uses:

Systemic: Cancer of breast, colon, rectum, stomach, pancreas; Topical: Multiple actinic keratoses, superficial basal cell carcinomas

Dosage and routes:

• *Adult:* **IV** 12 mg/kg/day × 4 days, not to exceed 800 mg/day; may repeat with 6 mg/kg on day 6, 8, 10, 12; maintenance is 10-15 mg/kg/wk as a single dose, not to exceed 1 g/wk

Actinic/solar keratoses

• *Adult:* **Top** 1% cream/sol 1-2 ×/day

Superficial basal cell carcinoma

• *Adult:* **Top** 5% sol 2 ×/day × 3-12 wk

Available forms: Inj 50 mg/ml; cream 1%, 5%; sol 1%, 2%, 5%

Side effects/adverse reactions:

Systemic use

CV: Myocardial ischemia, angina

HEMA: **Thrombocytopenia, leukopenia, myelosuppression, anemia, agranulocytosis**

GI: Anorexia, stomatitis, diarrhea, nausea, vomiting, **hemorrhage,** enteritis glossitis

EENT: Epistaxis

INTEG: Rash, fever, photosensitivity

CNS: Lethargy, malaise, weakness, acute cerebellar dysfunction

---

Contraindications: Hypersensitivity, myelosuppression, pregnancy (D), poor nutritional status, serious infections

Precautions: Renal disease, hepatic disease, bone marrow depression, angina, lactation, children

Do not confuse:

fluorouracil/flucytosine

Pharmacokinetics: Half-life 20 hr terminal; metabolized in the liver; excreted in the urine; crosses blood-brain barrier

Interactions:

• Increased toxicity, bone marrow depression: radiation or other antineoplastics

• Decreased antibody response: live virus vaccines

Lab test interferences:

Increase: Liver function studies, 6-HIAA

Decrease: Albumin

NURSING CONSIDERATIONS

Assess:

• CBC, differential, platelet count qd (IV); withhold drug if WBC is <3500/mm^3 or platelet count is <100,000/mm^3; notify prescriber of these results; drug should be discontinued; nadir of leukopenia within 2 wk, recovery 1 mo

• Renal function studies: BUN, serum uric acid, urine CrCl, electrolytes before, during therapy

• Temp q4h; fever may indicate beginning infection

• Liver function tests before, during therapy: bilirubin, alk phosphatase, AST, ALT, LDH; before and during therapy

• Bleeding: hematuria, guaiac, bruising or petechiae, mucosa or orifices q8h

• Inflammation of mucosa, breaks in skin; buccal cavity q8h for dryness, sores or ulceration, white patches, oral pain, bleeding, dysphagia

• GI symptoms: frequency of stools, cramping

Administer:

• Antiemetic 30-60 min before giving drug to prevent vomiting and for several days thereafter

IV

• Prepared in biologic cabinet using gloves, gown, mask

• Undiluted; may inject through Y-tube or 3-way stopcock; give over 1-3 min; may be diluted in NS, D$_5$W, given over 2-8 hr as IV INF

Additive compatibilities: Bleomycin, cephalothin, cyclophosphamide, etoposide, floxuridine, hydromorphone, ifosfamide, methotrexate, mitoxantrone, prednisolone, vincristine

Solution compatibilities: Amino acids 4.25%/D$_{25}$, D$_5$/LR, D$_{3.3}$/0.3 NaCl, D$_5$W, 0.9% NaCl, TPN #23

Syringe compatibilities: Bleomycin, cisplatin, cyclophosphamide, furosemide, heparin, leucovorin, methotrexate, metoclopramide, mitomycin, vinblastine, vincristine

Y-site compatibilities: Allopurinol, amifostine, aztreonam, bleomycin, cefepime, cisplatin, cyclophosphamide, doxorubicin, doxorubicin liposome, fludarabine, furosemide, granisetron, heparin, hydrocortisone, leucovorin, mannitol, melphalan, methotrexate, metoclopramide, mitomycin, paclitaxel, piperacillin/tazobactam, potassium chloride, propofol, sargramostim, teniposide, thiotepa, vinblastine, vincristine, vit B/C

Topical

• Wear gloves when applying; may use with a loose dressing; use a plastic or wooden applicator

Perform/provide:

• Strict asepsis, protective isolation if WBC levels are low

• Changing of IV site q48h

• Rinsing of mouth tid-qid with water, club soda; brushing of teeth bid-

tid with soft brush or cotton-tipped applicator for stomatitis; use unwaxed dental floss
• Nutritious diet with iron, vitamin supplements, low fiber, few dairy products, especially when combined with radiotherapy as ordered

Evaluate:
• Therapeutic response: decreased tumor size, spread of malignancy

Teach patient/family:
• To avoid crowds, persons with known infections
• To avoid foods with citric acid, hot or rough texture if stomatitis is present; to drink adequate fluids
• To report stomatitis: any bleeding, white spots, ulcerations in mouth; tell patient to examine mouth qd, report symptoms; viscous lidocaine may be used
• To report signs of infection: fever, sore throat, flulike symptoms
• To report signs of anemia: fatigue, headache, faintness, shortness of breath, irritability
• To report bleeding: avoid use of razors, commercial mouthwash
• To avoid use of aspirin products, or NSAIDs
• To use contraception during therapy (men and women)
• Not to receive vaccinations during therapy
• To use sunscreen or stay out of the sun to prevent photosensitivity
• About hair loss, explore use of wigs or other products

fluoxetine (R)

(floo-ox'eh-teen)
Prozac, Prozac Weekly
Func. class.: Antidepressant, SSRI (selective serotonin reuptake inhibitor)

Action: Inhibits CNS neuron uptake of serotonin but not of norepinephrine

Uses: Major depressive disorder, obsessive-compulsive disorder (OCD), bulimia nervosa

Investigational uses: Alcoholism, anorexia nervosa, ADHD, bipolar II affective disorder, borderline personality disorder, cataplexy, narcolepsy, kleptomania, migraine, obesity, posttraumatic stress disorder, schizophrenia, Tourette's syndrome, trichotillomania, levodopa-induced dyskinesia, social phobia

Dosage and routes:

Depression/obsessive-compulsive disorder
• *Adult:* **PO** 20 mg qd in AM; after 4 wk if no clinical improvement is noted, dose may be increased to 20 mg bid in AM, PM, not to exceed 80 mg/day; **PO** weekly
• *Geriatric:* **PO** 10 mg/day, increase as needed
• *Child 5-18 yr:* **PO** 5-10 mg/kg/day, max 20 mg/day

Bulimia nervosa
• *Adult:* **PO** 60 mg/day in AM
Available forms: Pulvules 10, 20, 40 mg; tabs 10, liq 20 mg/5 ml; Prozac Weekly

Side effects/adverse reactions:
*CNS: Headache, nervousness, insomnia, drowsiness, anxiety, tremor, dizziness, fatigue, sedation, poor concentration, abnormal dreams, agitation, **seizures,** apathy, euphoria, hallucinations, delusions, psychosis*

 = Nursing alert   🖋 = Herb-drug interaction   🚫 = Do not crush

GI: Nausea, diarrhea, dry mouth, anorexia, dyspepsia, constipation, cramps, vomiting, taste changes, flatulence, decreased appetite
INTEG: Sweating, rash, pruritus, acne, alopecia, urticaria
RESP: Infection, pharyngitis, nasal congestion, sinus headache, sinusitis, cough, dyspnea, bronchitis, asthma, hyperventilation, pneumonia
CV: Hot flashes, palpitations, angina pectoris, ***hemorrhage,*** hypertension, ***tachycardia,*** first-degree AV block, ***bradycardia, MI, thrombophlebitis***
MS: Pain, arthritis, twitching
GU: Dysmenorrhea, decreased libido, urinary frequency, UTI, amenorrhea, cystitis, impotence, urine retention
EENT: Visual changes, ear/eye pain, photophobia, tinnitus
SYST: Asthenia, viral infection, fever, allergy, chills
Contraindications: Hypersensitivity
Precautions: Pregnancy (B), lactation, children, elderly, diabetes mellitus
Do not confuse:
Prozac/Proscar
Prozac/Prosom
Prozac/Prilosec
Pharmacokinetics:
PO: Peak 6-8 hr; metabolized in liver; excreted in urine; half-life 1-384 hr; steady state 28-35 days, protein binding 94%
Interactions:
◆ Do not use MAOIs with or 14 days prior to fluoxetine
• Increased side effects: highly protein-bound drugs
• Increased effect: haloperidol
• Decreased fluoxetine effect: cyproheptadine
• Increased half-life of: diazepam
• Increased levels or toxicity of: car-

bamazepine, lithium, digoxin, warfarin, phenytoin
• Increased levels of: tricyclics, phenothiazines
• Paradoxical worsening of OCD: buspirone
• Increased CNS depression: alcohol, antidepressants, opioids, sedatives
🌿 Increased action: kava
🌿 St. John's wort: Do not use together
Lab test interferences:
Increase: Serum bilirubin, blood glucose, alk phosphatase
Decrease: VMA, 5-HIAA
False increase: Urinary catecholamines

NURSING CONSIDERATIONS
Assess:
• Mental status: mood, sensorium, affect, suicidal tendencies, increase in psychiatric symptoms, depression, panic
• Appetite in bulimia nervosa, weight qd, increase nutritious foods in diet, watch for binging and vomiting
• Allergic reactions: itching, rash urticaria, drug should be discontinued, may need to give antihistamine
• B/P (lying/standing), pulse q4h; if systolic B/P drops 20 mm Hg, hold drug, notify prescriber; take vital signs q4h in patients with cardiovascular disease
• Blood studies: CBC, leukocytes, differential, cardiac enzymes if patient is receiving long-term therapy; check platelets; bleeding can occur
• Hepatic studies: AST, ALT, bilirubin, creatinine
• Weight qwk; appetite may decrease with drug
• ECG for flattening of T wave, bundle branch, AV block, dysrhythmias in cardiac patients
• Alcohol consumption; if alcohol is consumed, hold dose until AM

Administer:

• With food or milk for GI symptoms

• Crushed if patient is unable to swallow medication whole (tab only)

• Dosage hs if oversedation occurs during the day; may take entire dose hs; elderly may not tolerate once/day dosing

• Gum, hard candy, frequent sips of water for dry mouth

Perform/provide:

• Storage at room temperature; do not freeze

• Assistance with ambulation during therapy, since drowsiness, dizziness occur

• Safety measures primarily in elderly

• Checking to see if PO medication swallowed

Evaluate:

• Therapeutic response: decreased depression, symptoms of OCD

Teach patient/family:

• That therapeutic effect may take 1-4 wk

• To use caution in driving, other activities requiring alertness because of drowsiness, dizziness, blurred vision

• To use sunscreen to prevent photosensitivity

• To avoid alcohol ingestion, other CNS depressants

• To notify prescriber if pregnant or plan to become pregnant or breastfeed

• To change positions slowly, orthostatic hypotension may occur

• To avoid all OTC drugs unless approved by prescriber

---

fluphenazine decanoate (R)
(floo-fen′a-zeen)
Modecate*, Modecate Concentrate*, Prolixin Decanoate
fluphenazine enanthate (R)
Moditen Enanthate*, Prolixin Enanthate
fluphenazine hydrochloride (R)
Apo-Fluphenazine*, Moditen HCL*, Moditen HCl-H.P.*, Permitil*, Prolixin
Func. class.: Antipsychotic
Chem. class.: Phenothiazine, piperazine

Action: Depresses cerebral cortex, hypothalamus, limbic system, which control activity and aggression; blocks neurotransmission produced by dopamine at synapse; exhibits strong α-adrenergic and anticholinergic blocking action; mechanism for antipsychotic effects is unclear

Uses: Psychotic disorders, schizophrenia

Dosage and routes:

decanoate

• *Adult and child >16 yr:* **SC/IM** 12.5-25 mg q1-3wk, may increase slowly

• *Child 12-16 yr:* **IM/SC** 6.25-18.75 mg, then repeat q1-3wk, then increase slowly, max 25 mg

• *Child 5-12 yr:* **IM/SC** 3.125-12.5 mg, then repeat q1-3wk, increase slowly

HCl

• *Adult:* **PO** 2.5-10 mg, in divided doses q6-8h, not to exceed 20 mg qd; **IM** initially 1.25 mg then 2.5-10 mg in divided doses q6-8h

---

◆ = Nursing alert   ∥ = Herb-drug interaction   ⊘ = Do not crush

• *Child:* **PO** 0.25-3.5 mg qd in divided doses q4-6h, max 10 mg/qd
enanthate
• *Adult:* **IM/SC** 25 mg q1-3wk, may increase slowly, max 100 mg/dose
Available forms: HCl tabs 1, 2.5, 5, 10 mg; elix 2.5 mg/5 ml; conc 5 mg/ml; inj 2.5, 10 mg/ml; enanthate, decanoate inj 25 mg/ml

Side effects/adverse reactions:

*RESP: **Laryngospasm,** dyspnea, **respiratory depression***

*CNS: EPS: pseudoparkinsonism, akathisia, dystonia, tardive dyskinesia, drowsiness, headache, **seizures, neuroleptic malignant syndrome***

HEMA: Anemia, ***leukopenia, leukocytosis, agranulocytosis, aplastic anemia, thrombocytopenia***

INTEG: Rash, photosensitivity, dermatitis

EENT: Blurred vision, glaucoma, dry eyes

GI: Dry mouth, nausea, vomiting, anorexia, constipation, diarrhea, jaundice, weight gain, ***paralytic ileus, hepatitis***

GU: Urinary retention, urinary frequency, enuresis, impotence, amenorrhea, gynecomastia

CV: Orthostatic hypotension, hypertension, ***cardiac arrest,*** ECG changes, ***tachycardia***

Contraindications: Hypersensitivity, circulatory collapse, liver damage, cerebral arteriosclerosis, coronary disease, severe hypertension/hypotension, blood dyscrasias, coma, child <12 yr, brain damage, narrow-angle glaucoma, bone marrow depression, alcohol and barbiturate withdrawal

Precautions: Pregnancy (C), lactation, seizure disorders, hypertension, hepatic disease, cardiac disease, elderly

Do not confuse:
Prolixin/Proloid

Pharmacokinetics:

PO/IM (HCl): Onset 1 hr, peak 2-4 hr, duration 6-8 hr

SC (enanthate): Onset 1-2 days, peak 2-3 days, duration 1-3 wk, half-life 3.5-4 days; decanoate: onset 1-3 days, peak 1-2 days, duration over 4 wk, single-dose half-life 6.8-9.6 days; multiple dose, 14.3 days; metabolized by liver; excreted in urine (metabolites); crosses placenta; enters breast milk

Interactions:

• Oversedation: other CNS depressants, alcohol, barbiturate anesthetics

• Toxicity: epinephrine

• Decreased effects of levodopa, lithium

• Decreased effects of fluphenazine: smoking, barbiturates

• Increased anticholinergic effects: anticholinergics

� Increased anticholinergic effect: henbane leaf

🌿 Possible increased action: kava

Lab test interferences:

Increase: Liver function tests, cardiac enzymes, cholesterol, blood glucose, prolactin, bilirubin, PBI, cholinesterase

Decrease: Hormones (blood and urine)

False positive: Pregnancy tests, PKU urinary steroids, 17-OHCS, pregnancy tests

NURSING CONSIDERATIONS
Assess:

• Swallowing of PO medication; check for hoarding, giving of medication to other patients

• I&O ratio; palpate bladder if low urinary output occurs

• Bilirubin, CBC, liver function studies monthly

• Urinalysis is recommended before and during prolonged therapy

• Affect, orientation, LOC, reflexes,

gait, coordination, sleep pattern disturbances

• B/P standing and lying; take pulse and respirations q4h during initial treatment; establish baseline before starting treatment; report drops of 30 mm Hg

• Dizziness, faintness, palpitations, tachycardia on rising

• EPS including akathisia (inability to sit still, no pattern to movements), tardive dyskinesia (bizarre movements of jaw, mouth, tongue, extremities), pseudoparkinsonism (rigidity, tremors, pill rolling, shuffling gait)

• Skin turgor qd

• Constipation, urinary retention qd; if these occur, increase bulk, H_2O in diet

Administer:

• Concentrate with juice, milk, or uncaffeinated drinks

• Antiparkinsonian agent if EPS occur

• IM inj into large muscle mass; to minimize postural hypotension, give injection and have patient remain seated or recumbent for ½ hr

• Use dry needle, or solution will become cloudy; use 21G or larger due to viscosity

Syringe compatibilities: Benztropine, diphenhydramine, hydroxyzine

Perform/provide:

• Decreased sensory input by dimming lights, avoiding loud noises

• Supervised ambulation until stabilized on medication; do not involve in strenuous exercise; fainting is possible; patient should not stand still for long periods

• Increased fluids to prevent constipation

• Sips of water, candy, gum for dry mouth

• Storage in tight, light-resistant container in cool environment

Evaluate:

• Therapeutic response: decrease in emotional excitement, hallucinations, delusions, paranoia, reorganization of patterns of thought, speech

Teach patient/family:

• That orthostatic hypotension occurs often; to rise from sitting or lying position gradually; avoid hazardous activities until stabilized on medication

• To avoid hot tubs, hot showers, tub baths, since hypotension may occur; that in hot weather, heat stroke may occur; take extra precautions to stay cool

◆ To avoid abrupt withdrawal of this drug, or EPS may result; drug should be withdrawn slowly

• To avoid OTC preparations (cough, hay fever, cold) unless approved by prescriber; serious drug interactions may occur; avoid use with alcohol, CNS depressants; increased drowsiness may occur

• To use a sunscreen to prevent burns

• About importance of compliance with drug regimen

• About EPS and necessity for meticulous oral hygiene, since oral candidiasis may occur

• To report sore throat, malaise, fever, bleeding, mouth sores; if these occur, CBC should be drawn and drug discontinued

• That urine may turn pink to reddish-brown

Treatment of overdose: Lavage; if orally ingested, provide an airway; *do not induce vomiting*

---

flurazepam (℞)

(flure-az'e-pam)
Apo-Flurazepam*, Dalmane, flurazepam, Novoflupam*, Somnol*

Func. class.: Sedative/hypnotic
Chem. class.: Benzodiazepine derivative

Controlled Substance Schedule IV (USA), Schedule F (Canada)

Action: Produces CNS depression at the limbic, thalamic, hypothalamic levels of CNS; may be mediated by neurotransmitter γ-aminobutyric acid (GABA); results are sedation, hypnosis, skeletal muscle relaxation, anticonvulsant activity, anxiolytic action

Uses: Insomnia

Dosage and routes:
• *Adult:* PO 15-30 mg hs; may repeat dose once if needed
• *Elderly:* PO 15 mg hs; may increase if needed

Available forms: Caps 15, 30 mg

Side effects/adverse reactions:
*HEMA: **Leukopenia, granulocytopenia** (rare)*
CNS: Lethargy, drowsiness, daytime sedation, dizziness, confusion, lightheadedness, headache, anxiety, irritability
GI: Nausea, vomiting, diarrhea, heartburn, abdominal pain, constipation
CV: Chest pain, pulse changes, palpitations
MISC: Physical, psychological dependence

Contraindications: Hypersensitivity to benzodiazepines, pregnancy, lactation, intermittent porphyria, uncontrolled pain, pregnancy (UK)

Precautions: Anemia, hepatic disease, renal disease, suicidal individuals, drug abuse, elderly, psychosis, child <15 yr

Pharmacokinetics:
PO: Onset 15-45 min, duration 7-8 hr; metabolized by liver; excreted by kidneys (inactive/active metabolites); crosses placenta; excreted in breast milk; half-life 47-100 hr

Interactions:
• Increased effects of flurazepam: cimetidine, disulfiram, probenicid, isoniazid, oral contraceptives, fluoxetine, ketoconazole, propranolol, valproic acid
• Increased CNS depression: alcohol, CNS depressants
• Decreased effect of flurazepam: rifampin, barbiturates, theophylline
🌿 Increased action: kava

Lab test interferences:
Increase: AST, ALT, serum bilirubin
False increase: Urinary 17-OHCS
Decrease: RAI uptake

NURSING CONSIDERATIONS
Assess:
• Blood studies: Hct, Hgb, RBC (if on long-term therapy)
• Hepatic studies: AST, ALT, bilirubin
• Mental status: mood, sensorium, affect, memory (long, short), physical, psychological dependence or tolerance
• Type of sleep problem: falling asleep, staying asleep

Administer:
• After removal of cigarettes to prevent fires
• After trying conservative measures for insomnia
• ½-1 hr before hs for sleeplessness
• Caps may be opened and mixed with food

Perform/provide:
• Assistance with ambulation after receiving dose
• Safety measures: night-light, call bell within easy reach

• Checking to see if PO medication has been swallowed
• Storage in tight container in cool environment

Evaluate:
• Therapeutic response: ability to sleep at night, decreased amount of early morning awakening if taking drug for insomnia

Teach patient/family:
• To avoid driving or other activities requiring alertness until drug is stabilized
• To avoid alcohol ingestion or CNS depressants; serious CNS depression may result
• That effects may take 2 nights for benefits to be noticed
• Alternative measures to improve sleep: reading, exercise several hr before hs, warm bath, warm milk, TV, self-hypnosis, deep breathing
• That hangover is common in elderly

Treatment of overdose: Lavage, activated charcoal; monitor electrolytes, vital signs

---

flutamide (R)

(floo'-ta-mide)
Eulexin
Func. class.: Antineoplastic, hormone
Chem. class.: Antiandrogen

Action: Interferes with testosterone uptake in the nucleus or testosterone activity in target tissues; arrests tumor growth in androgen-sensitive tissue, i.e., prostate gland

Uses: Metastatic prostatic carcinoma, stage D_2 in combination with LHRH agonistic analogs (leuprolide)

Dosage and routes:
• *Adult:* PO 250 mg q8h tid, for a daily dosage of 750 mg

Stage B_2-C prostatic carcinoma
• *Adult:* Start 8 wk prior to radiation therapy and continue during radiation therapy; give with goserelin

Stage D_2 metastatic carcinoma
• *Adult:* Give with LHRH agonist and continue until progression

Available forms: Caps 125 mg

Side effects/adverse reactions:
CNS: Hot flashes, drowsiness, confusion, depression, anxiety, paresthesia
GU: Decreased libido, impotence, gynecomastia
GI: Diarrhea, nausea, vomiting, increased liver function studies, ***hepatitis,*** anorexia
*HEMA: **Leukopenia, thrombocytopenia, hemolytic anemia***
INTEG: Irritation at site, rash, photosensitivity
MISC: Edema, neuromuscular and pulmonary symptoms, hypertension

Contraindications: Hypersensitivity, pregnancy (D)

Pharmacokinetics: Rapidly and completely absorbed; excreted in urine and feces as metabolites; half-life 6 hr, geriatric half-life 8 hr; 94% bound to plasma proteins

NURSING CONSIDERATIONS

Assess:
◆ Liver function studies: AST, ALT, alk phosphatase, which may be elevated; if LFTs are elevated, drug may need to be discontinued; monitor CBC, bilirubin, creatinine
• For CNS symptoms including: drowsiness, confusion, depression, anxiety

Evaluate:
• Therapeutic response: decrease in prostatic tumor size, decrease in spread of cancer

Teach patient/family:
🚫 Not to break, crush, or chew caps
• That flutamide must be taken with leuprolide, do not change dosing

---

◆ = Nursing alert   🌿 = Herb-drug interaction   🚫 = Do not crush

• To report side effects: decreased libido, impotence, breast enlargement, hot flashes, diarrhea
• To report nausea, vomiting, yellow eyes or skin, dark urine, clay-colored stools, hepatotoxicity may be the cause

---

fluvastatin (℞)

(flu′vah-stay-tin)
Lescol
Func. class.: Antilipidemic
Chem. class.: HMG-CoA reductase inhibitor

Action: Inhibits HMG-CoA reductase enzyme, which reduces cholesterol synthesis

Uses: As an adjunct in primary hypercholesterolemia (types Ia, Ib), coronary atherosclerosis in CAD

Dosage and routes:
• *Adult:* **PO** 20-40 mg qd in PM initially, usual range 20-80 mg, not to exceed 80 mg; should be given in 2 doses (40 mg AM, 40 mg PM); dosage adjustments may be made in 4 wk intervals or more

Available forms: Caps 20, 40 mg

Side effects/adverse reactions:
INTEG: Rash, pruritus
GI: Nausea, constipation, diarrhea, dyspepsia, flatus, *liver dysfunction,* pancreatitis
EENT: Lens opacities
MS: Myalgia, *myositis, rhabdomyolysis*
CNS: Headache, dizziness, insomnia
MISC: Fatigue, influenza
HEMA: ***Thrombocytopenia, hemolytic anemia, leukopenia***
RESP: Upper respiratory infection, rhinitis, cough, pharyngitis, sinusitis

Contraindications: Hypersensitivity, pregnancy (X), lactation, active liver disease

Precautions: Past liver disease, alcoholism, severe acute infections, trauma, hypotension, uncontrolled seizure disorders, severe metabolic disorders, electrolyte imbalance

Pharmacokinetics: Metabolized in liver, highly protein bound, excreted primarily in feces, half-life <1 hr

Interactions:
• Increased effects of warfarin
• Increased myalgia, myositis: cyclosporine, gemfibrozil, niacin, erythromycin, clofibrate; azole antiinfectives given with clofibrate
• Decreased effects of fluvastatin: propranolol, nicotinic acid, digoxin, rifampin, alcohol

NURSING CONSIDERATIONS
Assess:
• Fasting lipid profile (cholesterol, LDL, HDL, TG) q8wk, then q3-6 mo when stable
• Liver function studies q1-2mo during the first 1½ yr of treatment; AST, ALT, LFTs may be increased
• Renal studies in patients with compromised renal system: BUN, I&O ratio, creatinine
• Ophthalmic examination before, 1 mo after treatment begins, annually; lens opacities may occur

Perform/provide:
• Storage in cool environment in tight container protected from light

Evaluate:
• Therapeutic response: decrease in LDL, VLDL, total cholesterol; increased HDL, decreased triglycerides

Teach patient/family:
• That blood work will be necessary during treatment, to take as prescribed
• To report severe GI symptoms, headache, muscle pain, weakness, tenderness
• That previously prescribed regimen will continue: low-cholesterol

F

Side effects: *italics* = common; ***bold italics*** = life-threatening

diet, exercise program, smoking cessation

🚫 Not to break, crush, or chew caps

• To report suspected pregnancy, not to use during pregnancy

• To use sunscreen or stay out of sun to prevent photosensitivity

• To notify all health care providers of drugs taken

---

fluvoxamine (℞)

(flu-vox′a-meen)
Luvox
Func. class.: Antidepressant SSRI (selective serotonin reuptake inhibitor)

Action: Inhibits CNS neuron uptake of serotonin but not of norepinephrine

Uses: Obsessive-compulsive disorder

Research note: A study showed that increased plasma concentrations of olanzapine occurred when the drug was given with fluvoxamine[17]

Investigational uses: Depression

Dosage and routes:

• *Adult:* **PO** 50 mg hs, increase by 50 mg at 4-7 day intervals, max 300 mg, doses over 100 mg should be divided

• *Child 8-17 yr:* **PO** 25 mg hs, increase by 25 mg/day q4-7 days, max 200 mg/day, doses over 50 mg should be divided

Available forms: Tabs 25, 50, 100 mg

Side effects/adverse reactions:

CNS: Headache, drowsiness, dizziness, convulsions, sleep disorders

GI: Nausea, anorexia, constipation, **hepatotoxicity,** *vomiting, diarrhea*

INTEG: Rash, sweating

GU: Decreased libido

Contraindications: Hypersensitivity

Precautions: Pregnancy (C), lactation, children, elderly

Pharmacokinetics: Crosses blood-brain barrier, 77% protein binding, metabolism by the liver, terminal half-life 16.9 hr, peak 2-8 hr

Interactions:

• Decreased metabolism, increased action of: propranolol, diazepam, lithium, theophylline, carbamazepine, warfarin

• Increased CNS depression: alcohol, barbiturates, benzodiazepines

• Increased levels of fluvoxamine, toxicity: tricyclics, clozapine

◆ Fatal reaction: MAO inhibitors

• Drug/smoking: Increased metabolism, decreased effects

◆🌿 Increased effect, possible fatal reaction: St. John's wort

🌿 Increased effect: kava

NURSING CONSIDERATIONS

Assess:

• Hepatic studies: AST, ALT, bilirubin

• Mental status: mood, sensorium, affect, suicidal tendencies; increase in psychiatric symptoms: depression, panic, obsessive-compulsive symptoms

• Constipation; most likely in elderly

◆ For toxicity: nausea, vomiting, diarrhea, syncope, increased pulse, seizures

Administer:

• With food, milk for GI symptoms

Perform/provide:

• Storage at room temperature; do not freeze

Evaluate:

• Therapeutic response: decrease in depression

Teach patient/family:

• That therapeutic effects may take 2-3 wk

◆ = Nursing alert   🌿 = Herb-drug interaction   🚫 = Do not crush

- To use caution in driving, other activities requiring alertness because of drowsiness, dizziness that may occur
- Not to use other CNS depressants, alcohol, barbiturates, benzodiazepines, St. John's wort, kava
- To notify prescriber if pregnancy is suspected or planned
- To notify prescriber of allergic reaction
- To increase bulk in diet if constipation occurs, especially elderly

---

folic acid (vit B₉) (OTC)
(foe'lik a'sid)
Apo-Folic*, Folate, Folvite, Novofolacid*, Vitamin B₉
Func. class.: Vit B complex group

Action: Needed for erythropoiesis; increases RBC, WBC, platelet formation in megaloblastic anemias
Uses: Megaloblastic or macrocytic anemia caused by folic acid deficiency; liver disease, alcoholism, hemolysis, intestinal obstruction, pregnancy
Dosage and routes:
Therapeutic dose
- *Adult and child:* **PO/IM/SC/IV** up to 1 mg qd
Maintenance dose
- *Adult and child >4 yr:* **PO/IM/IV/SC** 0.4 mg/day
- *Pregnant and lactating:* **PO/IM/IV/SC** 0.8 mg/day
- *Child <4 yr:* **PO/IM/IV/SC** up to 0.3 mg/day
- *Infants:* **PO/IM/IV/SC** up to 0.1 mg/day
Available forms: Tabs 0.1, 0.4, 0.8, 1, 5 mg; inj 5, 10 mg/ml
Side effects/adverse reactions:
RESP: **Bronchospasm**
INTEG: Flushing

Contraindications: Hypersensitivity, anemias other than megaloblastic/macrocytic anemia, vit B₁₂ deficiency anemia, uncorrected pernicious anemia
Precautions: Pregnancy (A)
Pharmacokinetics:
PO: Peak ½-1 hr; bound to plasma proteins; excreted in breast milk; metabolized by liver; excreted in urine (small amounts)
Interactions:
- Decreased folate levels: methotrexate, sulfonamides, sulfasalazine
- Increased need for folic acid: estrogen, hydantoins, carbamazepine, glucocorticoids

NURSING CONSIDERATIONS
Assess:
- For fatigue, dyspnea, weakness, dyspnea that are signs of megaloblastic anemia
- Folate levels: 6-15 µg/ml, Hgb, Hct, and reticulocyte count
- Nutritional status: bran, yeast, dried beans, nuts, fruits, fresh vegetables, asparagus
- Drugs currently taken: estrogen, carbamazepine, glucocorticoids, hydantoins; these drugs may cause increased folic acid use by body and contribute to a deficiency
Administer:
IV
- Direct undiluted 5 mg or less/1 min or more; or may be added to most IV sol or TPN
Solution compatibilities: D₂₀W
Y-site compatibilities: Famotidine
Perform/provide:
- Storage in light-resistant container
Evaluate:
- Therapeutic response: increased weight, oriented, well-being; absence of fatigue; increase in reticulocyte count within 5 days of beginning treatment

Teach patient/family:
• To take drug exactly as prescribed; periodic lab work is required
• To alter nutrition to include high-folic-acid foods: organ meats, vegetables, fruit
• That urine will turn bright yellow
• To notify prescriber of allergic reaction

---

fondaparinux sodium
See appendix a—selected new drugs

---

formoterol
See appendix a—selected new drugs

---

foscarnet (℞)
(foss-kar'net)
Foscavir
Func. class.: Antiviral
Chem. class.: Inorganic pyrophosphate organic analog

Action: Antiviral activity is produced by selective inhibition at the pyrophosphate binding site on virus-specific DNA polymerases and reverse transcriptases at concentrations that do not affect cellular DNA polymerases

Uses: Treatment of CMV retinitis, HSV infections, used with ganciclovir for relapsing patients

Dosage and routes:
CMV retinitis
• *Adult:* IV INF 60 mg/kg given over at least 1 hr, q8h × 2-3 wk initially, then 90-120 mg/kg/day over 2 hr, usually give with at least 750-1000 ml NS qd

HSV
• *Adult:* IV 40 mg/kg q8-12h × 2-3 wk

In renal abnormalities:
• *Adult:* IV
Male:

$$\frac{140 - age}{serum\ creatinine \times 72} = CrCl$$

Female: $0.85 \times$ above value
Dose based on table provided in package insert
Available forms: Inj 24 mg/ml
Side effects/adverse reactions:
CNS: Fever, dizziness, *headache*, **seizures,** *fatigue*, neuropathy, tremor, ataxia, dementia, stupor, EEG abnormalities, vertigo, **coma,** abnormal gait, hypertonia, EPS, hemiparesis, **paralysis,** hyperreflexia, paraplegia, **tetany,** hyporeflexia, neuralgia, neuritis, **cerebral edema,** *paresthesia*, depression, *confusion, anxiety*, insomnia, somnolence, amnesia, hallucinations, agitation
GI: Nausea, vomiting, diarrhea, anorexia, abdominal pain, constipation, dysphagia, rectal hemorrhage, dry mouth, melena, flatulence, ulcerative stomatitis, pancreatitis, enteritis, enterocolitis, glossitis, proctitis, stomatitis, increased amylases, gastroenteritis, ***pseudomembranous colitis,*** duodenal ulcer, **paralytic ileus, esophageal ulceration,** abnormal A-G ratio, increased AST, ALT, cholecystitis, **hepatitis,** dyspepsia, tenesmus, hepatosplenomegaly, jaundice
INTEG: Rash, sweating, pruritus, skin ulceration, seborrhea, skin discoloration, alopecia, acne, dermatitis, pain/inflammation at injection site, facial edema, dry skin, urticaria
*HEMA: Anemia, **granulocytopenia, leukopenia, thrombocytopenia,** platelet abnormalities, **thrombosis, pulmonary embolism, coagulation disorders, decreased prothrombin, hypochromic anemia, pancytopenia, hemolysis, leukocytosis,** lymphadenopathy, epistaxis, lymphopenia*

◆ = Nursing alert   𝟙 = Herb-drug interaction   ⊘ = Do not crush

SYST: *Hypokalemia, hypocalcemia, hypomagnesemia*; increased alk phosphatase, LDH, BUN; acidosis, hypophosphatemia, hyperphosphatemia, dehydration, glycosuria, increased CPK, hypervolemia, infection, *sepsis, death, ascites,* hyponatremia, hypochloremia, hypercalcemia

GU: *Acute renal failure,* decreased CrCl and increased serum creatinine, *glomerulonephritis, toxic nephropathy, nephrosis, renal tubular disorders, pyelonephritis, uremia, hematuria, albuminuria,* dysuria, polyuria

RESP: *Coughing*, *dyspnea*, pneumonia, sinusitis, pharyngitis, *pulmonary infiltration,* stridor, *pneumothorax, hemoptysis, bronchospasm,* bronchitis, *respiratory depression, pleural effusion, pulmonary hemorrhage,* rhinitis

EENT: Visual field defects, vocal cord paralysis, speech disorders, taste perversion, eye pain, conjunctivitis, tinnitus, otitis

CV: Hypertension, palpitations, ECG abnormalities, 1st degree AV block, nonspecific ST-T segment changes, hypotension, cerebrovascular disorder, cardiomyopathy, *cardiac arrest,* bradycardia, dysrhythmias

MS: Arthralgia, myalgia

Contraindications: Hypersensitivity, CrCl <0.4 ml/min/kg

Precautions: Pregnancy (C), lactation, children, elderly, renal disease, seizure disorders, electrolyte/mineral imbalances, severe anemia

Pharmacokinetics: 14%-17% plasma protein bound, half-life 2-8 hr in normal renal function

Interactions:
• Nephrotoxicity: aminoglycosides, amphotericin B
• Hypocalcemia: pentamidine

NURSING CONSIDERATIONS
Assess:
General
• Kidney, liver function studies: BUN, creatinine, AST, ALT
• I&O ratio, urine pH, serum creatinine baseline, 3×/wk during initial therapy, then 2×/wk thereafter; CrCl baseline, throughout treatment; if CrCl <0.4 ml/min/kg, discontinue
• Blood counts q2wk; watch for decreasing granulocytes, Hgb; if low, therapy may have to be discontinued and restarted after hematologic recovery; blood transfusions may be required
• Electrolytes and minerals: Ca, P, Mg, Na, K; watch closely for tetany during first administration
• GI symptoms: nausea, vomiting, diarrhea; severe symptoms may necessitate discontinuing drug
◆ Blood dyscrasias (anemia, granulocytopenia); bruising, fatigue, bleeding, poor healing
• Allergic reactions: flushing, rash, urticaria, pruritus
CMV retinitis
• Culture should be done prior to treatment (blood, urine, throat)
• Ophthalmic exam should confirm diagnosis
Administer:
• Increased fluids before and during drug administration to induce diuresis and minimize renal toxicity
IV, int inf
• Using infusion device, at no more than 1 mg/kg/min; do not give by rapid or bolus IV; give by CVP or peripheral vein; standard 24 mg/ml sol may be used without dilution if using by CVP; dilute the 24 mg/ml sol to 12 mg/ml with D_5W or NS if using peripheral vein
Y-site compatibilities: Aldesleukin, amikacin, aminophylline, ampicillin, aztreonam, benzquinamide, cefazolin, cefoperazone, cefoxitin,

ceftazidime, ceftizoxime, ceftriaxone, cefuroxime, chloramphenicol, cimetidine, clindamycin, dexamethasone, dopamine, erythromycin, fluconazole, flucytosine, furosemide, gentamicin, heparin, hydrocortisone, hydromorphone, hydroxyzine, imipenem-cilastatin, metoclopramide, metronidazole, miconazole, morphine, nafcillin, oxacillin, penicillin G potassium, phenytoin, piperacillin, ranitidine, ticarcillin/clavulanate, tobramycin

Perform/provide:
• Regular ophthalmologic exams
• Close monitoring during therapy for tingling, numbness, paresthesias; if these occur, stop infusion, obtain lab sample for electrolytes

Evaluate:
• Therapeutic response: improvement in CMV retinitis

Teach patient/family:
• To call prescriber if sore throat, swollen lymph nodes, malaise, fever occur, since other infections may occur
• To report perioral tingling, numbness in extremities, and paresthesias
• That serious drug interactions may occur if OTC products are ingested; check first with prescriber
• That drug is not a cure but will control symptoms

---

fosinopril (℞)
(foss'in-oh-pril)
Monopril
Func. class.: Antihypertensive
Chem. class.: Angiotensin-converting enzyme (ACE) inhibitor

Action: Selectively suppresses renin-angiotensin-aldosterone system; inhibits ACE; prevents conversion of angiotensin I to angiotensin II; results in dilation of arterial, venous vessels

Uses: Hypertension, alone or in combination with thiazide diuretics, systolic CHF

Dosage and routes:
CHF
• *Adult:* **PO** 10 mg qd, then up to 40 mg/day increased over several wk; use lower dose in those diuresed before fosinopril
Hypertension
• *Adult:* **PO** 10 mg qd initially, then 20-40 mg/day divided bid or qd
Renal dose
5 mg qd

Available forms: Tabs 10, 20 mg
Side effects/adverse reactions:
CV: Hypotension, chest pain, palpitations, angina, orthostatic hypotension
GU: **Proteinuria,** increased BUN, creatinine, decreased libido
HEMA: Decreased Hct, Hgb; *eosinophilia, leukopenia, neutropenia*
INTEG: **Angioedema,** rash, flushing, sweating, photosensitivity, pruritus
RESP: Cough, sinusitis, dyspnea, **bronchospasm**
META: Hyperkalemia
GI: Nausea, constipation, vomiting, diarrhea
CNS: Insomnia, paresthesia, headache, dizziness, fatigue, memory disturbance, tremor, mood change
MS: Arthralgia, myalgia

Contraindications: Hypersensitivity to ACE inhibitors, pregnancy (D) 2nd/3rd trimester, lactation, children
Precautions: Impaired liver function, hypovolemia, blood dyscrasias, CHF, COPD, asthma, elderly
Do not confuse:
Monopril/minoxidil

◆ = Nursing alert　　🌿 = Herb-drug interaction　　🚫 = Do not crush

Pharmacokinetics:
PO: Peak 3 hr; serum protein binding 97%; half-life 12 hr; metabolized by liver (metabolites excreted in urine, feces)

Interactions:
• Increased hypotension: diuretics, other antihypertensives, ganglionic blockers, adrenergic blockers, phenothiazines, nitrates, acute alcohol ingestion
• Increased toxicity: vasodilators, hydralazine, prazosin, K-sparing diuretics, sympathomimetics, digoxin, lithium
• Decreased absorption: antacids
• Decreased antihypertensive effect: indomethacin

Lab test interferences:
False-positive: Urine acetone
Positive: ANA titer
Increase: AST, ALT, alk phosphatase, glucose, bilirubin, uric acid

NURSING CONSIDERATIONS
Assess:
• Blood studies: neutrophils, decreased platelets; obtain WBC with diff baseline and qmo × 6 mo, then q2-3 mo × 1 yr; if neutrophils <1000/mm^3, discontinue
• B/P, orthostatic hypotension, syncope
• Renal studies: protein, BUN, creatinine; increased levels may indicate nephrotic syndrome
• Baselines in renal, liver function tests before therapy begins
• K levels, although hyperkalemia rarely occurs
• Edema in feet, legs daily, weigh daily in CHF
• Allergic reactions: rash, fever, pruritus, urticaria; drug should be discontinued if antihistamines fail to help

Administer:
• IV infusion of 0.9% NaCl (as ordered) to expand fluid volume if severe hypotension occurs

Perform/provide:
• Storage in tight container at 86° F (30° C) or less
• Supine position for severe hypotension

Evaluate:
• Therapeutic response: decrease in B/P

Teach patient/family:
• Not to discontinue drug abruptly
• Not to use OTC products (cough, cold, allergy) unless directed by prescriber; not to use salt substitutes containing potassium without consulting prescriber
• The importance of complying with dosage schedule, even if feeling better
• To rise slowly to sitting or standing position to minimize orthostatic hypotension
• To notify prescriber of mouth sores, sore throat, fever, swelling of hands or feet, irregular heartbeat, chest pain
• To report excessive perspiration, dehydration, vomiting, diarrhea; may lead to fall in B/P
• That drug may cause dizziness, fainting, light-headedness during first few days of therapy
• That drug may cause skin rash or impaired perspiration
• How to take B/P; normal readings for age group
• To notify prescriber if pregnancy is planned or suspected

Treatment of overdose: 0.9% NaCl IV INF, hemodialysis

fosphenytoin (℞)

(foss-fen'i-toy-in)
Cerebyx
Func. class.: Anticonvulsant
Chem. class.: Hydantoin

Action: Inhibits spread of seizure activity in motor cortex by altering ion transport; increases AV conduction

Uses: Generalized tonic-clonic seizures; status epilepticus

Dosage and routes:

Status epilepticus

• *Adult and child:* **IV** loading dose 15-20 mg PE/kg given at 100-150 mg PE/min

Nonemergent/maintenance dosing

• *Adult and child:* **IV** loading dose 10-20 mg PE/kg; maintenance dosing 4-6 mg PE/kg/day given at a rate of <150 mg PE/min

Available forms: Inj 150 mg (100 mg phenytoin equiv), 750 mg (500 mg phenytoin equiv)

Side effects/adverse reactions:

CNS: Drowsiness, dizziness, insomnia, paresthesias, depression, suicidal tendencies, aggression, headache, confusion

CV: Hypotension, *ventricular fibrillation*

EENT: Nystagmus, diplopia, blurred vision

GI: Nausea, vomiting, constipation, anorexia, weight loss, hepatitis, jaundice, gingival hyperplasia

GU: Nephritis, urine discoloration

HEMA: Agranulocytosis, leukopenia, aplastic anemia, thrombocytopenia, megaloblastic anemia

INTEG: Rash, lupus erythematosus, *Stevens-Johnson syndrome,* hirsutism

SYST: Hypocalcemia, hypokalemia, hyperglycemia

Contraindications: Hypersensitivity, psychiatric conditions, pregnancy (D), bradycardia, SA and AV block, Stokes-Adams syndrome

Precautions: Allergies, hepatic disease, renal disease

Pharmacokinetics: Metabolized by liver, excreted by kidneys

Interactions:

• Decreased effects of fosphenytoin: alcohol (chronic use), antihistamines, antacids, antineoplastics, CNS depressants, rifampin, folic acid, carbamazepine, reserpine, tricyclics

• Increased fosphenytoin level: cimetidine, amiodarone, chloramphenicol, estrogens, H_2 antagonists, phenothiazines, salicylates, sulfonamides

• Drug/food: decreased folic acid absorption: methylphenidate, trazodone, benzodiazepines, isoniazid, azole antiinfectives

Lab test interferences:

Decrease: Dexamethasone, metyrapone test serum, PBI, urinary steroids

Increase: Glucose, alk phosphatase

NURSING CONSIDERATIONS

Assess:

• Drug level: toxic level 30-50 μg/ml

• Blood studies: CBC, platelets q2 wk until stabilized, then qmo × 12 mo, then q3mo; discontinue drug if neutrophils <1600/mm³

• Mental status: mood, sensorium, affect, memory (long, short)

• Seizure activity including type, location, duration, and character; provide seizure precaution

• Renal studies; urinalysis, BUN, urine creatine

• Hepatic studies: ALT, AST, bilirubin, creatinine

• Allergic reaction: red raised rash; if this occurs, drug should be discontinued

 = Nursing alert   = Herb-drug interaction   🚫 = Do not crush

• For toxicity: bone marrow depression, nausea, vomiting, ataxia, diplopia, cardiovascular collapse, slurred speech, confusion

• Respiratory depression; rate, depth, character of respirations

◆ Blood dyscrasias: fever, sore throat, bruising, rash, jaundice

• Continuous monitoring of ECG, B/P, respiratory function

• Rash, discontinue as soon as rash develops, serious adverse reactions such as Stevens-Johnson syndrome can occur

Administer:

IV

• Dilute in D$_5$ or 0.9% NaCl 1.5-25 mg PE/ml, give <150 mg PE/min

Y-site compatibilities: Esmolol, famotidine, foscarnet

Additive compatibilities: Potassium chloride

Solution compatibilities: D$_5$W, D$_{10}$W, amino acid inj 10%, D$_5$LR, D$_5$/0.9% NaCl, Plasmalyte A, LR, sterile water for inj

Evaluate:

• Therapeutic response: decrease in severity of seizures

Teach patient/family:

• The reason for and expected outcome of treatment

• Not to use machinery or engage in hazardous activity, as drowsiness, dizziness may occur

• To carry medical ID denoting drug use, name of prescriber

• To notify prescriber of rash, bleeding, bruising, slurred speech, jaundice of skin or eyes, joint pain, nausea, vomiting, severe headaches

• To keep all medical appointments, including lab work, physical assessment

• To notify prescriber if pregnancy is planned, suspected

• To use contraception while using this product

---

frovatriptan
See appendix a—selected new drugs

---

furosemide (R)
(fur-oh'se-mide)
Apo-Furosemide*, Furoside*, Lasix, Lasix Special*, Myrosemide*, Novosemide*, Uritol*
Func. class.: Loop diuretic
Chem. class.: Sulfonamide derivative

Action: Inhibits reabsorption of sodium and chloride at proximal and distal tubule and in the loop of Henle

Uses: Pulmonary edema; edema in CHF, liver disease, nephrotic syndrome, ascites, hypertension

Investigational uses: Hypercalcemia in malignancy

Dosage and routes:

• *Adult:* **PO** 20-80 mg/day in AM; may give another dose in 6 hr up to 600 mg/day; **IM/IV** 20-40 mg, increased by 20 mg q2h until desired response

• *Child:* **PO/IM/IV** 2 mg/kg; may increase by 1-2 mg/kg/q6-8h up to 6 mg/kg

Pulmonary edema

• *Adult:* **IV** 40 mg given over several min, repeated in 1 hr; increase to 80 mg if needed

Hypertensive crisis/acute renal failure

• *Adult:* **IV** 100-200 mg over 1-2 min

Antihypercalcemia

• *Adult:* **IM/IV** 80-100 mg q1-4h or **PO** 120 mg qd or divided bid

• *Child:* **IM/IV** 25-50 mg, repeat q4h if needed

Available forms: Tabs 20, 40, 80

---

mg; oral sol 10 mg/ml, 40 mg/5 ml; inj 10 mg/ml

Side effects/adverse reactions:

CNS: Headache, fatigue, weakness, vertigo, paresthesias

CV: Orthostatic hypotension, chest pain, ECG changes, ***circulatory collapse***

EENT: **Loss of hearing,** ear pain, tinnitus, blurred vision

ELECT: Hypokalemia, hypochloremic alkalosis, hypomagnesemia, hyperuricemia, hypocalcemia, hyponatremia, metabolic alkalosis

ENDO: Hyperglycemia

GI: Nausea, diarrhea, dry mouth, vomiting, anorexia, cramps, oral, gastric irritations, pancreatitis

GU: Polyuria, **renal failure,** glycosuria

*HEMA: **Thrombocytopenia, agranulocytosis, leukopenia, neutropenia, anemia***

INTEG: Rash, pruritus, purpura, ***Stevens-Johnson syndrome,*** sweating, photosensitivity, urticaria

MS: Cramps, stiffness

Contraindications: Hypersensitivity to sulfonamides, anuria, hypovolemia, infants, lactation, electrolyte depletion

Precautions: Diabetes mellitus, dehydration, severe renal disease, pregnancy (C), cirrhosis, ascites

Do not confuse:

Lasix/Lomotil

Lasix/Luvox

Lasix/Lanoxin

Pharmacokinetics:

PO: Onset 1 hr, peak 1-2 hr, duration 6-8 hr; absorbed 70%

IV: Onset 5 min, peak ½ hr, duration 2 hr (metabolized by the liver 30%) Excreted in urine, some as unchanged drug, feces; crosses placenta; excreted in breast milk; half-life ½-1 hr

Interactions:

• Increased toxicity: lithium, nondepolarizing skeletal muscle relaxants, digitalis

• Increased hypotensive action of antihypertensives, nitrates

• Increased ototoxicity: aminoglycosides, cisplatin, vancomycin

Lab test interferences:

Interference: GTT

NURSING CONSIDERATIONS

Assess:

• Signs of metabolic alkalosis: drowsiness, restlessness

• Signs of hypokalemia: postural hypotension, malaise, fatigue, tachycardia, leg cramps, weakness

• Rashes, temp elevation qd

• Confusion, especially in elderly; take safety precautions if needed

• Hearing, including tinnitus and hearing loss, when giving high doses for extended periods

• Weight, I&O qd to determine fluid loss; effect of drug may be decreased if used qd

• Rate, depth, rhythm of respiration, effect of exertion, lung sounds

• B/P lying, standing; postural hypotension may occur

• Electrolytes: K, Na, Cl; include BUN, blood sugar, CBC, serum creatinine, blood pH, ABGs, uric acid, Ca, Mg

• Skin turgor, edema, condition of mucous membranes in mouth and nose

• Glucose in urine if patient is diabetic

• Allergies to sulfonamides, thiazides

Administer:

• In AM to avoid interference with sleep if using drug as a diuretic

• K replacement if K <3 mg/dL

• PO with food if nausea occurs; absorption may be decreased slightly; tabs may be crushed

◆ = Nursing alert   ⫘ = Herb-drug interaction   ⊘ = Do not crush

IV

• Undiluted; may be given through Y-tube or 3-way stopcock; give 20 mg or less/min; may be added to NS or D_5W if large doses are required and given as IV INF, not to exceed 4 mg/min; use infusion pump

Additive compatibilities: Amikacin, aminophylline, ampicillin, atropine, bumetanide, calcium gluconate, cefamandole, cefoperazone, cefuroxime, cimetidine, cloxacillin, dexamethasone, diamorphine, digoxin, epinephrine, heparin, isosorbide, kanamycin, lidocaine, meropenem, morphine, nitroglycerin, penicillin G, potassium chloride, ranitidine, scopolamine, sodium bicarbonate, theophylline, tobramycin, verapamil

Syringe compatibilities: Bleomycin, cisplatin, cyclophosphamide, fluorouracil, heparin, leucovorin, methotrexate, mitomycin

Y-site compatibilities: Allopurinol, amifostine, amikacin, amphotericin B cholesteryl, aztreonam, bleomycin, cefepime, cefmetazole, cisplatin, cladribine, cyclophosphamide, cytarabine, doxorubicin liposome, epinephrine, fentanyl, fludarabine, fluorouracil, foscarnet, gallium, granisetron, heparin, hydrocortisone, hydromorphone, indomethacin, kanamycin, leucovorin, lorazepam, melphalan, meropenem, methotrexate, mitomycin, nitroglycerin, norepinephrine, paclitaxel, piperacillin/tazobactam, potassium chloride, propofol, ranitidine, remifentanil, sargramostim, tacrolimus, teniposide, thiotepa, tobramycin, tolazoline, vit B/C

Evaluate:

• Therapeutic response: improvement in edema of feet, legs, sacral area daily if medication is being used for CHF

Teach patient/family:

• To discuss the need for a high-K diet or K replacement with prescriber

• To increase fluid intake 2-3 L/day unless contraindicated

• To rise slowly from lying or sitting position; orthostatic hypotension may occur

• To recognize adverse reactions that may occur: muscle cramps, weakness, nausea, dizziness

• Regarding entire regimen, including exercise, diet, stress relief for hypertension

• To take with food or milk for GI symptoms

• To use sunscreen or protective clothing to prevent photosensitivity

• To take early in day to prevent sleeplessness

• To avoid OTC medication unless directed by prescriber

Treatment of overdose: Lavage if taken orally; monitor electrolytes; administer dextrose in saline; monitor hydration, CV, renal status

---

gabapentin (℞)

(gab'a-pen-tin)

Neurontin

Func. class.: Anticonvulsant

Action: Mechanism unknown; may increase seizure threshold; structurally similar to GABA; gabapentin binding sites in neocortex, hippocampus

Uses: Adjunct treatment of partial seizures, with or without generalization in patients >12 yr; adjunct in partial seizures in children 3-12 yr

Investigational uses: Tremors in ms, neuropathic pain, bipolar disorder, migraine prophylaxis, alcohol/cocaine withdrawal, diabetic neuropathy

G

Dosage and routes:
• *Adult and child >12 yr:* **PO** 900-1800 mg/day in 3 divided doses; may titrate by giving 300 mg on the first day, 300 mg bid on second day, 300 mg tid on third day; may increase to 1800 mg/day by adding 300 mg on subsequent days
• *Child 5-12 yr:* **PO** 10-15 mg/kg/day in 3 divided doses, initially titrate dose upward over approximately 3 days; 40 mg/kg/day; all given in 3 divided doses; rect 200 mg as single dose
• *Child 3-4 yr:* **PO** 10-15 mg/kg/day in 3 divided doses, initially titrate dose upward over approximately 3 days; 25-35 mg/kg/day; all given in 3 divided doses; rect 200 mg as single dose
Renal dose
• *Adult and child >12 yr:* CrCl 30-60 ml/min 300 mg bid, CrCl 15-30 ml/min 300 mg qd, CrCl <15 ml/min 300 mg qod
Available forms: Caps 100, 300, 400 mg; tabs 600, 800 mg; oral sol 250 mg/5 ml
Side effects/adverse reactions:
CNS: Dizziness, fatigue, anxiety, somnolence, ataxia, amnesia, abnormal thinking, unsteady gait, depression
CV: Vasodilation, peripheral edema
EENT: Dry mouth, blurred vision, diplopia
GI: Constipation, increased appetite, dental abnormalities
GU: Impotence, bleeding, *UTI*
HEMA: **Leukopenia,** decreased WBC
INTEG: Pruritus, abrasion
MS: Myalgia
RESP: Rhinitis, pharyngitis, coughing
Contraindications: Hypersensitivity to this drug
Precautions: Hepatic disease, renal disease, pregnancy (C), lactation, children <12 yr, elderly

Pharmacokinetics: Largely unbound to plasma proteins; not metabolized; excreted in urine (unchanged); elimination half-life 5-7 hr
Interactions:
• Decreased levels of gabapentin: antacids
Lab test interferences:
False-positive: Urinary protein using Ames N-multistix SG
NURSING CONSIDERATIONS
Assess:
• Renal studies: urinalysis, BUN, urine creatinine q3mo
• Hepatic studies: ALT, AST, bilirubin
• Description of seizures; location, duration, characteristics
• Mental status: mood, sensorium, affect, behavioral changes; if mental status changes, notify prescriber
• Eye problems, need for ophthalmic examinations before, during, after treatment (slit lamp, fundoscopy, tonometry)
• Allergic reaction: purpura, red raised rash; if these occur, drug should be discontinued
• Pain: location, duration, characteristics if using for chronic pain
Administer:
• 2 hr apart when giving antacids
• Caps may be opened and contents put in applesauce or dissolved in juice
Perform/provide:
• Storage at room temperature away from heat and light
• Hard candy, frequent rinsing of mouth, gum for dry mouth
• Assistance with ambulation during early part of treatment; dizziness occurs
• Seizure precautions: padded side rails; move objects that may harm patient
• Increased fluids, bulk in diet for constipation

◆ = Nursing alert   ∥ = Herb-drug interaction   ⊘ = Do not crush

Evaluate:
• Therapeutic response: decreased seizure activity; decrease in chronic pain

Teach patient/family:
• To carry ID stating patient's name, drugs taken, condition, prescriber's name and phone number
• To avoid driving, other activities that require alertness: dizziness, drowsiness may occur
• Not to discontinue medication quickly after long-term use, taper over ≥1 wk; withdrawal-precipitated seizures may occur
🚫 Not to crush or chew caps
• To notify prescriber if pregnancy planned or suspected, avoid breast-feeding

Treatment of overdose: Lavage, VS

galantamine
See appendix a—selected new drugs

gallamine (R)
(gal'a-meen)
Flaxedil

Func. class.: Neuromuscular blocker (nondepolarizing)

Action: Inhibits transmission of nerve impulses by binding with cholinergic receptor sites, antagonizing action of acetylcholine

Uses: Facilitation of endotracheal intubation, skeletal muscle relaxation during mechanical ventilation, surgery, general anesthesia

Dosage and routes:
• *Adult and child >1 mo:* **IV** 1 mg/kg, not to exceed 100 mg, then 0.5-1 mg/kg q30-40min
• *Child <1 mo, >5 kg:* **IV** 0.25-0.75 mg/kg, then 0.01-0.05 mg/kg q30-40min

Available forms: Inj 20 mg/ml

Side effects/adverse reactions:
CV: Bradycardia, tachycardia, increased, decreased B/P
*RESP: **Prolonged apnea, bronchospasm, cyanosis, respiratory depression***
EENT: Increased secretions
INTEG: Rash, flushing, pruritus, urticaria
*CNS: **Malignant hyperthermia***
GI: Decreased motility

Contraindications: Hypersensitivity to iodides
Precautions: Pregnancy (C), thyroid disease, collagen disease, cardiac disease, lactation, children <2 yr, electrolyte imbalances, dehydration, neuromuscular disease (myasthenia gravis), respiratory disease, renal disease

Pharmacokinetics:
IV: Onset 2 min, duration 20-30 min; half-life 2 min, 29 min (terminal); excreted in urine, feces (metabolites); crosses placenta

Interactions:
• Increased neuromuscular blockade: aminoglycosides, clindamycin, lincomycin, quinidine, local anesthetics, polymyxin antibiotics, lithium, narcotic analgesics, thiazides, enflurane, isoflurane; used with cyclopropane, may provoke ventricular dysrhythmias
• Dysrhythmias: theophylline
• Incompatible with anesthetics, barbiturates in sol; incompatible with any other drug in syringe

NURSING CONSIDERATIONS
Assess:
• For electrolyte imbalances (K, Mg); may lead to increased action of this drug
• Vital signs (B/P, pulse, respirations, airway) q15min until fully recovered; rate, depth, pattern of respirations, strength of hand grip
• I&O ratio; check for urinary retention, frequency, hesitancy

• Recovery: decreased paralysis of face, diaphragm, leg, arm, rest of body

• Allergic reactions: rash, fever, respiratory distress, pruritus; drug should be discontinued

Administer:

• Using nerve stimulator by anesthesiologist to determine neuromuscular blockade

• Anticholinesterase to reverse neuromuscular blockade

• IV undiluted over 1-2 min (only by qualified person, usually an anesthesiologist)

• Only slightly discolored sol

Perform/provide:

• Storage in light-resistant, cool area

• Reassurance if communication is difficult during recovery from neuromuscular blockade

Evaluate:

• Therapeutic response: paralysis of jaw, eyelid, head, neck, rest of body

Treatment of overdose: Edrophonium or neostigmine, atropine; monitor VS; may require mechanical ventilation

---

gallium (℞)

(gal′ee-um)

Ganite

Func. class.: Electrolyte modifier

Chem. class.: Hypocalcemic drug

Action: Lowers serum calcium levels by inhibiting calcium resorption from bone

Uses: Cancer-related hypercalcemia

Dosage and routes:

• *Adult:* **IV** 100-200 mg/m^2 qd × 5 days; infuse over 24 hr, rest period of 2-4 wk between courses

Available forms: 25 mg/ml inj

Side effects/adverse reactions:

*HEMA: **Anemia, leukopenia, thrombocytopenia***

CV: Tachycardia, hypotension

EENT: Blurred vision, optic neuritis, hearing loss

*GU: **Nephrotoxicity,** increased BUN, creatinine*

GI: Nausea, vomiting, diarrhea, constipation, mucositis, metallic taste

META: Hypophosphatemia, hypocalcemia, decreased serum bicarbonate

Contraindications: Hypersensitivity, severe renal disease

Precautions: Pregnancy (C), lactation, children, mild renal disease

Pharmacokinetics:

IV: Onset 12-48 hr, peak 5 days, duration 4-14 days, excreted by kidneys

Interactions:

• Increased nephrotoxicity: aminoglycosides, amphotericin B

NURSING CONSIDERATIONS

Assess:

• Renal status: BUN, creatinine, urine output; if creatinine level is 2.5 mg/dl or more, drug should be discontinued

• Monitor Ca, phosphate, bicarbonate, since all levels may be decreased and supplements of phosphate may be needed

• For hypercalcemia: nausea, vomiting, fatigue, weakness, thirst, dehydration, dysrhythmias, change in mental status

• For hypocalcemia: dysrhythmias; paresthesia; twitching; colic; laryngospasm; Trousseau's, Chvostek's sign; tremors

• For hypophosphatemia: confusion, decreased reflexes, joint stiffness and pain, portal hypotension

Administer:

IV

• Adequate hydration with IV saline, 2 L/day during treatment

---

◆ = Nursing alert   ⫽ = Herb-drug interaction   ⊘ = Do not crush

• After dilution of dose/1 L 0.9% NaCl or D_5W, run over 24 hr, use infusion pump

Y-site compatibilities: Acyclovir, allopurinol, amifostine, aminophylline, ampicillin/sulbactam, aztreonam, cefazolin, ceftazidime, ceftriaxone, cimetidine, ciprofloxacin, cladribine, cyclophosphamide, dexamethasone, diphenhydramine, filgrastim, fluconazole, furosemide, granisetron, heparin, hydrocortisone, ifosfamide, magnesium sulfate, mannitol, melphalan, meperidine, mesna, methotrexate, metoclopramide, ondansetron, piperacillin, piperacillin/tazobactam, potassium chloride, ranitidine, sodium bicarbonate, teniposide, thiotepa, ticarcillin/clavulanate, trimethoprim-sulfamethoxazole, vancomycin, vinorelbine

Perform/provide:

• Storage of solution 48 hr at room temperature, 1 wk in refrigerator

Evaluate:

• Therapeutic response: decreased serum Ca levels

Teach patient/family:

• To follow dietary guidelines given by prescriber, including avoiding Ca (dairy products, broccoli) and vit D (fortified milk, grain products, fish oil)

---

ganciclovir (R)

(gan-sye'kloe-vir)
Cytovene, Vitrasert
Func. class.: Antiviral
Chem. class.: Synthetic nucleoside analog

Action: Inhibits replication of herpesviruses in vitro, in vivo by selective inhibition of the human CMV DNA polymerase and by direct incorporation into viral DNA

Uses: Cytomegalovirus (CMV) retinitis in immunocompromised persons, including those with AIDS, after indirect ophthalmoscopy confirms diagnosis

Investigational uses: CMV pneumonia in organ transplant patients, CMV gastroenteritis in patients with IBS, CMV pneumonitis

Dosage and routes:

• Reduce dose in renal disease CrCl <70 ml/min

Prevention of CMV

• *Adult:* IV 5 mg/kg q12h × 1-2 wk, then 5 mg/kg/day, then 5 mg/kg/day or 6 mg/kg × 5 days/wk; **PO** 1000 mg tid

Induction treatment

• *Adult:* IV 5 mg/kg given over 1 hr, q12h × 2-3 wk

Maintenance treatment

• *Adult:* IV INF 5 mg/kg given over 1 hr, qd × 7 days/wk; or 6 mg/kg qd × 5 days/wk; **PO** 1000 mg tid with food or 500 mg q3h while awake; **INTRAVITREAL:** 4.5 mg implant

Available forms: Powder for inj 500 mg/vial; caps 250, 500 mg; implant, intravitreal 4.5 mg

Side effects/adverse reactions:

*HEMA: **Granulocytopenia, thrombocytopenia, irreversible neutropenia, anemia,** eosinophilia*

*GI: Abnormal LFTs, nausea, vomiting, anorexia, diarrhea, abdominal pain, **hemorrhage***

INTEG: Rash, alopecia, pruritus, urticaria, pain at site, phlebitis

*CNS: Fever, chills, **coma, confusion,** abnormal thoughts, dizziness, bizarre dreams, headache, psychosis, tremors, somnolence, paresthesia, weakness, **seizures***

CV: Dysrhythmia, hypertension/hypotension

RESP: Dyspnea

EENT: Retinal detachment in CMV retinitis

GU: ***Hematuria,*** increased creatinine, BUN

Contraindications: Hypersensitivity to acyclovir or ganciclovir, absolute neutrophil count <500, platelet count <25,000

Precautions: Preexisting cytopenias, renal function impairment, pregnancy (C), lactation, children <6 mo, elderly

Do not confuse:

Cytovene/Cytosar

Pharmacokinetics: Half-life 3-4½ hr; excreted by kidneys (unchanged); crosses blood-brain barrier, CSF

Interactions:

• Decreased renal clearance of ganciclovir: probenecid

• Increased toxicity: dapsone, pentamidine, flucytosine, vincristine, vinblastine, adriamycin, doxorubicin, amphotericin B, trimethoprim-sulfa combinations, or other nucleoside analogs, cyclosporine

• Severe granulocytopenia: zidovudine, antineoplastics, radiation; do not give together

• Increased seizures: imipenem/cilastatin

NURSING CONSIDERATIONS

Assess:

• For leukopenia/neutropenia/thrombocytopenia: WBCs, platelets q2d during 2 ×/d dosing and then q1wk

• For leukopenia with qd WBC count in patients with prior leukopenia with other nucleoside analogs or for whom leukopenia counts are <1000 cells/mm^3 at start of treatment

• Serum creatinine or CrCl ≥q2wk

Administer:

PO

• With food

IV

• Mixed in biologic cabinet, using gown, gloves, mask

• IV after diluting 500 mg/10 ml sterile H_2O for inj (50 mg/ml); shake; further dilute in 100 ml D_5W, 0.9% NaCl, LR and run over 1 hr; use infusion pump, in-line filter

• Slowly; do not give by bolus IV, IM, SC inj

• Using diluted sol within 12 hr; do not refrigerate or freeze

Y-site compatibilities: Allopurinol, amphotericin B cholesteryl, cisplatin, cyclophosphamide, doxorubicin liposome, enalaprilat, filgrastim, fluconazole, granisetron, melphalan, methotrexate, paclitaxel, propofol, remifentanil, tacrolimus, teniposide, thiotepa

Evaluate:

• Therapeutic response: decreased symptoms of CMV

Teach patient/family:

• That drug does not cure condition, that regular ophthalmologic examinations are necessary

• That major toxicities may necessitate discontinuing drug

• To use contraception during treatment and that infertility may occur; men should use barrier contraception for 90 days after treatment

• To take PO with food

◆ To report infection: fever, chills, sore throat; blood dyscrasias: bruising, bleeding, petechiae

• To avoid crowds, persons with respiratory infections

• To use sunscreen to prevent burns

---

ganirelix (℞)

Antagon

Func. class.: Gonadotropin-releasing hormone antagonist

Chem. class.: Synthetic decapeptide

Action: Inhibitor of pituitary gonadotropin secretion; initially increases LH and FSH, induces a rapid

◆ = Nursing alert   ∅ = Herb-drug interaction   ⊘ = Do not crush

suppression of gonadotropin secretion

Uses: For inhibition of premature LH surges in women undergoing controlled ovarian hyperstimulation

Dosage and routes:

• *Adult:* **SC** 250 μg qd during early to mid follicular phase, continue until the day of hCG administration

Available forms: Inj 250 μg/0.5 ml

Side effects/adverse reactions:

CNS: Headache

ENDO: Ovarian hyperstimulation syndrome, abdominal pain (gyn)

GI: Nausea

GU: Spotting, breakthrough bleeding

INTEG: Pain on injection

SYST: ***Fetal death***

Contraindications: Hypersensitivity, pregnancy (X), latex allergy, lactation

Pharmacokinetics: Excreted in feces/urine, half-life 13-16 hr, metabolized to metabolites, protein binding 82%

NURSING CONSIDERATIONS

Assess:

• For suspected pregnancy, drug should not be used

• For latex allergy, drug should not be used

Administer:

• SC using abdomen, around navel or upper thigh, swab inj area with disinfectant, clean a 2 in circle and allow to dry, pinch up area between thumb and finger, insert needle at 45°-90° to surface, if positioned correctly, no blood will be drawn back into syringe, if blood is drawn into syringe, reposition needle without removing it

Perform/provide:

• Protection from light

Evaluate:

• Therapeutic response: pregnancy

Teach patient/family:

• To report abdominal pain, vaginal bleeding

---

gatifloxacin (℞)

(gat-ih-floks'ah-sin)

Tequin

Func. class.: Broad-spectrum antiinfective

Chem. class.: Fluoroquinolone antibacterial

G

Action: Interferes with conversion of intermediate DNA fragments into high–molecular weight DNA in bacteria; DNA gyrase inhibitor

Uses: Infection caused by susceptible *Escherichia coli, Staphylococcus aureus, Haemophilus influenzae, Haemophilus parainfluenzae, Klebsiella pneumoniae, Moraxella catarrhalis, Neisseria gonorrhoeae, Proteus mirabilis,* and other microorganisms: *Chlamydia pneumoniae, Legionella pneumophila, Mycoplasma pneumoniae,* acute bacterial exacerbation of chronic bronchitis, acute sinusitis, community-acquired respiratory tract infections, gonorrhea

Investigational uses: Multidrug-resistant *Staphylococcus pneumoniae* in children with acute otitis media, sinusitis; *Mycobacterium leprae*

Dosage and routes:

Renal dose

• CrCl ≥40 ml/min 400 mg qd; <40 ml/min 200 mg qd after 400 mg initially; hemodialysis 200 mg qd after 400 mg initially

Uncomplicated urinary tract infections

• *Adult:* **PO/IV** 400 mg single dose

Complicated/severe urinary tract infections
• *Adult:* **PO/IV** 400 mg × 7-10 days
Chronic bronchitis
• *Adult:* **PO/IV** 400 mg × 7-10 days
Acute sinusitis
• *Adult:* **PO/IV** 400 mg × 10 days
Community-acquired pneumonia
• *Adult:* **PO/IV** 400 mg × 7-14 days
Gonorrhea
• *Adult:* **PO/IV** 400 mg single dose
Available forms: Tabs 200, 400 mg; inj 20 ml (200 mg), 40 ml (400 mg)
Side effects/adverse reactions:
CNS: Headache, dizziness, insomnia, paresthesia, tremor, vasodilation
GI: Nausea, diarrhea, increased ALT, AST, *pseudomembranous colitis*
INTEG: Rash, pruritus, urticaria, photosensitivity, flushing, fever, chills
RESP: Dyspnea, pharyngitis
SYST: Anaphylaxis, Stevens-Johnson syndrome
ENDO: Increased blood glucose
Contraindications: Hypersensitivity to quinolones
Precautions: Pregnancy (C), lactation, children, renal disease
Pharmacokinetics: Half-life 6½-14 hr; excreted in urine unchanged, protein binding 20%, peak 2-5 hr depending on dose
Interactions:
• Decreased absorption of gatifloxacin: magnesium antacids, aluminum hydroxide, sucralfate, calcium
• Increased serum levels of gatifloxacin: probenecid, cimetidine
• May increase warfarin level
NURSING CONSIDERATIONS
Assess:
• CNS symptoms: headache, dizziness, insomnia
• Kidney, liver function studies, blood glucose: BUN, creatinine, AST, ALT
• I&O ratio, urine pH <5.5 is ideal

• Allergic reactions and anaphylaxis: fever, flushing, rash, urticaria, pruritus, emergency equipment should be nearby
Administer:
PO
• 2 hr before or 2 hr after antacids, zinc, iron, calcium
IV
• Do not use flexible containers in series connections, air embolism may occur
• Do not use if particulate matter is present
• Do not admix with other drugs
• Dilute with compatible sol to 2 mg/ml before administration
Solution compatibilities: D_5, 0.9% NaCl, D_5/0.9% NaCl, LR/D_5, water for inj
Perform/provide:
• Limited intake of alkaline foods, drugs: milk, dairy products, alkaline antacids, sodium bicarbonate
Evaluate:
• Therapeutic response: decreased pain, frequency, urgency, C&S; absence of infection
Teach patient/family:
• Not to take any products containing magnesium or calcium (such as antacids), iron, or aluminum with this drug or within 4 hr of drug; to increase fluid intake to 2 L/day to prevent crystalluria
• That photosensitivity may occur; patient should avoid sunlight or use sunscreen to prevent burns
• If dizziness occurs, to ambulate, perform activities with assistance
• To contact prescriber if adverse reaction occurs or if inflammation or pain in tendon occurs
• To use frequent rinsing of mouth, sugarless candy, or gum for dry mouth
• To avoid other medications unless approved by prescriber

◆ = Nursing alert   ∥ = Herb-drug interaction   ⊘ = Do not crush

• Not to use theophylline with this product, will cause toxicity; contact prescriber if taking theophylline

• To take as prescribed, not to double or miss doses, to take all medications

---

gemcitabine (R)

(jem-sit'a-been)

Gemzar

Func. class.: Misc. antineoplastic

Chem. class.: Nucleoside analog

Action: Exhibits antitumor activity by killing cells undergoing DNA synthesis (S-phase) and blocking G1/S-phase boundary

Uses: Adenocarcinoma of the pancreas (nonresectable stage II, III, or metastatic stage IV); non–small cell lung cancer (stage IIIA or B, IV); in combination with cisplatin for inoperable, advanced, or metastatic non–small cell lung cancer

Dosage and routes:

Pancreatic carcinoma

• *Adult:* IV 1000 mg/m² given over ½ hr qwk × 7 wk, then 1 wk rest period; subsequent cycles should be infused once qwk × 3 wk out of every 4 wk

Non–small cell lung cancer

4-wk schedule:

• *Adult:* IV 1000 mg/m² given over ½ hr on days 1, 8, 15, of each 28-day cycle. Give cisplatin IV 100 mg/m² on day 1 after gemcitabine

3-wk schedule:

• *Adult:* IV 1250 mg/m² given over ½ hr on days 1, 8 of each 21-day cycle. Give cisplatin 100 mg/m² after the inf of gemcitabine on day 1

Available forms: Lyophilized pwd for inj 20 mg/ml

Side effects/adverse reactions:

GI: Diarrhea, nausea, vomiting, anorexia, constipation, stomatitis

INTEG: Irritation at site, rash, alopecia

HEMA: **Leukopenia, anemia, neutropenia, thrombocytopenia**

GU: Proteinuria, hematuria

OTHER: Dyspnea, fever, **hemorrhage,** infection, flulike symptoms, paresthesia

Contraindications: Hypersensitivity, pregnancy (D)

Precautions: Lactation, children, elderly, myelosuppression, irradiation

Pharmacokinetics: Half-life 42-79 min, crosses placenta

Interactions:

• Increased bleeding: NSAIDs, alcohol, salicylates

• Increased myelosuppression, diarrhea: other antineoplastics, radiation

• Decreased antibody response: live virus vaccines

NURSING CONSIDERATIONS

Assess:

• CBC, differential, platelet count before each dose; absolute granulocyte count >1000, platelets >100,000, give complete dose; absolute granulocyte count 500-1000, platelets 50,000-100,000, give 75%; absolute granulocyte count <500, platelets <50,000, do not give

• Blood dyscrasias: bruising, bleeding, petechiae

• I&O, nutritional intake; food preferences: list likes, dislikes

• Hepatic/renal studies

• Buccal cavity q8h for dryness, sores, or ulceration, white patches, oral pain, bleeding, dysphagia

• GI symptoms: frequency of stools; cramping

• Signs of dehydration: rapid respirations, poor skin turgor, decreased urine output, dry skin, restlessness, weakness

Administer:

IV

• Prepare in biologic cabinet using gown, mask, gloves

• After reconstituting with 0.9% NaCl 5 ml/200 mg vial of drug or 25 ml/1 g of drug, shake = 40 mg/ml may be further diluted with 0.9% NaCl to conc as low as 0.1 mg/ml; discard unused portions, give over ½ hr, do not admix

Perform/provide:

• Increased fluid intake to 2-3 L/day to prevent dehydration, unless contraindicated

• Changing of IV site q48h

• Rinsing of mouth tid-qid with water, club soda; brushing of teeth bid-tid with soft brush or cotton-tipped applicator for stomatitis; use unwaxed dental floss

• Nutritious diet with iron, vitamin supplement, low fiber, few dairy products

Evaluate:

• Therapeutic response: decrease in tumor size, decrease in spread of cancer

Teach patient/family:

• To avoid foods with citric acid or hot or rough texture if stomatitis is present; to drink adequate fluids

• To avoid use with NSAIDs, alcohol, salicylates

• To report stomatitis; any bleeding, white spots, ulcerations in mouth; tell patient to examine mouth qd, report symptoms

• To report signs of anemia: fatigue, headache, faintness, shortness of breath, irritability; hematuria, dysuria

• To use contraception during therapy

• Not to receive vaccinations during treatment

gemfibrozil (℞)
(jem-fi'broe-zil)
gemfibrozil, Lopid
Func. class.: Antilipemic
Chem. class.: Fibric acid derivative

Action: Inhibits biosynthesis of VLDL, decreases triglycerides, increases HDL

Uses: Type IIb, III/IV, V hyperlipidemia as adjunct with diet therapy

Dosage and routes:
• *Adult:* **PO** 1200 mg in divided doses bid 30 min before meals

Available forms: Tabs 600 mg; caps 300 mg

Side effects/adverse reactions:

GI: Nausea, vomiting, *dyspepsia, diarrhea, abdominal pain, flatulence*

INTEG: Rash, urticaria, pruritus

HEMA: **Leukopenia, anemia, eosinophilia, thrombocytopenia**

CNS: Dizziness, blurred vision

MISC: Taste perversion

Contraindications: Severe hepatic disease, preexisting gallbladder disease, severe renal disease, primary biliary cirrhosis, hypersensitivity

Precautions: Monitor hematologic and hepatic function, pregnancy (C), lactation

Pharmacokinetics:

PO: Peak 1-2 hr; plasma protein binding >90%; half-life 1½ hr; 70% unchanged, excreted in urine; metabolized in liver (minimal)

Interactions:
• Increased hypoglycemic effect: sulfonylureas

• May increase anticoagulant properties: oral anticoagulants
• Increased risk of myositis, myalgia: HMG-CoA reductase inhibitors
• Decreased gemfibrozil effect: cyclosporine

Lab test interferences:
Increase: Liver function studies, CPK, BSP, thymol turbidity, glucose
Decrease: Hgb, Hct, WBC

NURSING CONSIDERATIONS
Assess:
• Triglycerides, cholesterol; if lipids increase, drug should be discontinued; LDL, VLDL baseline and periodically
• Renal studies, LFTs, CBC, blood glucose if patient is on long-term therapy; if LFTs increase, therapy should be discontinued
• Bowel pattern daily; watch for increasing diarrhea, which is common

Administer:
PO
• 30 min before morning and evening meals

Evaluate:
• Therapeutic response: decreased cholesterol, triglyceride levels, HDL, cholesterol ratios improved

Teach patient/family:
• That compliance is needed for positive results; do not double or skip dose
• That risk factors should be decreased: high-fat diet, smoking, alcohol consumption, absence of exercise
• To notify prescriber of diarrhea, nausea, vomiting, chills, fever, sore throat, muscle cramps, abdominal cramps, severe flatulence
🚫 Not to break, crush, or chew caps
• That drug may be discontinued, if no improvement in 3 mo

gemtuzumab (℞)
(gem-tue-zue'mab)
Mylotarg
Func. class.: Misc. antineoplastic
Chem. class.: Monoclonal antibody

Action: Composed of recombinant humanized IgG$_4$ kappa antibody, binds to CD33 antigen that is released in myeloid cells

Uses: Acute myeloid leukemia (AML)

Dosage and routes:
• *Adult:* **IV** 9 mg/m^2 as a 2 hr inf; before giving inf, give diphenhydramine 50 mg **PO,** acetaminophen 650-1000 mg **PO** 1 hr prior to inf; then use acetaminophen 650-1000 mg q1-4h prn

Available forms: Pwd for inj, lyophilized 5 mg

Side effects/adverse reactions:
CNS: Dizziness, insomnia, depression
CV: Hypertension, hemorrhage, tachycardia, hypotension
INTEG: Rash, herpes simplex, local reaction, petechiae
GI: Anorexia, diarrhea, constipation, nausea, stomatitis, vomiting
GU: Hematuria, vaginal hemorrhage
MISC: Fever, myalgias, headache, chills
RESP: Cough, pneumonia, epistaxis, rhinitis
META: Hypokalemia, hypomagnesemia

Contraindications: Hypersensitivity, pregnancy (D), severe myelosuppression

Precautions: Lactation, children, severe renal or hepatic disease

Pharmacokinetics: Half-life 45 and 100 hr, respectively

NURSING CONSIDERATIONS
Assess:
• For symptoms of infection; chills, fever, headache, may be masked by drug fever
• CNS reaction: LOC, mental status, dizziness, confusion
• Cardiac status: Lung sounds; ECG before and during treatment, especially in those with cardiac disease
• Bone marrow depression: bruising, bleeding, blood in stools, urine, sputum, emesis
Administer:
• Do not give IV push or bolus
• Protect from light, use biologic safety hood, allow to come to room temp
• Reconstitute each vial with 5 ml sterile water for inj using sterile syringes, swirl each vial, check for discoloration or particulate matter, give over 2 hr, use a separate line with 1.2 micron terminal filter
Perform/provide:
• Storage of reconstituted sol for ≤8 hr in refrigerator
Evaluate:
• Therapeutic response: decrease in size, number of lesions
Teach patient/family:
• To take acetaminophen for fever
• To avoid hazardous tasks, since confusion, dizziness may occur; avoid prolonged sunlight, use sunscreen
• To report signs of infection: sore throat, fever, diarrhea, vomiting

gentamicin (℞)
(jen-ta-mye′sin)
Cidomycin*, Garamycin, gentamicin sulfate, G-Mycin, Jenamicin
Func. class.: Antiinfective
Chem. class.: Aminoglycoside

Action: Interferes with protein synthesis in bacterial cell by binding to ribosomal subunit, causing misreading of genetic code; inaccurate peptide sequence forms in protein chain, causing bacterial death
Uses: Severe systemic infections of CNS, respiratory, GI, urinary tract, bone, skin, soft tissues caused by susceptible strains of *Proteus aeruginosa, Proteus, Klebsiella, Serratia, Escherichia coli, Enterobacter, Citrobacter, Staphylococcus, Shigella, Salmonella, Acinetobacter*, acute PID
Dosage and routes:
Severe systemic infections
• *Adult:* **IV INF** 3-5 mg/kg/day in 3 divided doses q8h; dilute in 50-200 ml 0.9% NaCl or D₅W given over 30 min-1 hr; **IM** 3 mg/kg/day in divided doses q8h
• *Child:* **IV/IM** 2-2.5 mg/kg q8h
• *Neonate and infant:* **IV/IM** 2.5 mg/kg q8-12h
• *Neonate <1 wk:* 2.5 mg/kg q12-24h
Once daily dosing/extended interval dosing (unlabeled)
• *Adult:* **IV** 4-7 mg/kg/q24h, adjust according to levels
Renal dose
• *Adult:* **IV/IM** 1-1.7 mg/kg initially, then adjust according to levels
Available forms: Inj 10, 40 mg/ml; premixed inj 40, 60, 70, 80, 100 mg/50 ml; 40, 60, 80, 90, 100, 120, 160, 180 mg/ml

⬦ = Nursing alert   🖊 = Herb-drug interaction   🚫 = Do not crush

Side effects/adverse reactions:
*GU: **Oliguria, hematuria, renal damage, azotemia, renal failure, nephrotoxicity***

CNS: Confusion, depression, numbness, tremors, ***convulsions,*** muscle twitching, ***neurotoxicity,*** dizziness, vertigo

*EENT: **Ototoxicity,** deafness,* visual disturbances, tinnitus

*HEMA: **Agranulocytosis, thrombocytopenia, leukopenia, eosinophilia,*** anemia

GI: Nausea, vomiting, anorexia; increased ALT, AST, bilirubin; hepatomegaly, ***hepatic necrosis,*** splenomegaly

CV: Hypotension, hypertension, palpitations

INTEG: Rash, burning, urticaria, dermatitis, alopecia

Contraindications: Severe renal disease, hypersensitivity

Precautions: Neonates, mild renal disease, pregnancy (C), hearing deficits, myasthenia gravis, lactation, elderly, Parkinson's disease

Do not confuse:
Geramycin/kanamycin

Pharmacokinetics:
IM: Onset rapid, peak 1-2 hr
IV: Onset immediate, peak 1-2 hr; plasma half-life 1-2 hr, infants 6-7 hr; duration 6-8 hr; not metabolized; excreted unchanged in urine; crosses placental barrier; poor penetration into CSF

Interactions:
• Increased ototoxicity, neurotoxicity, nephrotoxicity: other aminoglycosides, amphotericin B, polymyxin, vancomycin, ethacrynic acid, furosemide, mannitol, methoxyflurane, cisplatin, cephalosporins, penicillins
• Increased effects: nondepolarizing neuromuscular blockers

NURSING CONSIDERATIONS
Assess:
• Weight before treatment; calculation of dosage is usually based on ideal body weight, but may be calculated on actual body weight
• I&O ratio, urinalysis daily for proteinuria, cells, casts; report sudden change in urine output; toxicity is increased in patients with decreased renal function if high doses are given
• VS during infusion; watch for hypotension, change in pulse
• IV site for thrombophlebitis, including pain, redness, swelling, q30min, change site if needed; discontinue, apply warm compresses to site
• Serum peak, drawn at 30-60 min after IV inf or 60 min after IM inj, and trough level drawn just before next dose; blood level should be 2-4 times bacteriostatic level; peak = 4-12 µg/ml, trough = 1-2 µg/ml
• Urine pH if drug is used for UTI; urine should be kept alkaline
• Renal impairment by securing urine for CrCl testing, BUN, serum creatinine; lower dosage should be given in renal impairment (CrCl <80 ml/min)
• Deafness by audiometric testing, ringing, roaring in ears, vertigo; assess hearing before, during, after treatment
• Dehydration: high specific gravity, decrease in skin turgor, dry mucous membranes, dark urine
• Overgrowth of infection including fever, malaise, redness, pain, swelling, perineal itching, diarrhea, stomatitis, change in cough or sputum
• C&S before starting treatment to identify infecting organism
• Vestibular dysfunction: nausea, vomiting, dizziness, headache; drug should be discontinued if severe

• Injection sites for redness, swelling, abscesses; use warm compresses at site

Administer:

• IM inj in large muscle mass; rotate injection sites

• Drug in evenly spaced doses to maintain blood level

• Bicarbonate to alkalinize urine if ordered for UTI, as drug is most active in alkaline environment

IV

• After diluting in 50-200 ml NS or D_5W; sol concentration should be 1 mg/ml or less; decrease vol of diluent in child; maintain 0.1% sol run over ½-1 hr (adults) or up to 2 hr (children); flush IV line with NS or D_5W after administration

Additive compatibilities: Atracurium, aztreonam, bleomycin, cefoxitin, cimetidine, ciprofloxacin, fluconazole, meropenem, methicillin, metronidazole, ofloxacin, penicillin G sodium, ranitidine, verapamil

Syringe compatibilities: Clindamycin, methicillin, penicillin G sodium

Y-site compatibilities: Acyclovir, amifostine, amiodarone, amsacrine, atracurium, aztreonam, cefpirome, ciprofloxacin, cyclophosphamide, cytarabine, diltiazem, enalaprilat, esmolol, famotidine, filgrastim, fluconazole, fludarabine, foscarnet, granisetron, hydromorphone, IL-2, insulin, labetalol, lorazepam, magnesium sulfate, melphalan, meperidine, meropenem, midazolam, morphine, multivitamins, ondansetron, paclitaxel, pancuronium, perphenazine, sargramostim, tacrolimus, teniposide, theophylline, thiotepa, tolazine, vecuronium, vinorelbine, vit B/C, zidovudine

Perform/provide:

• Adequate fluids of 2-3 L/day, unless contraindicated, to prevent irritation of tubules

• Supervised ambulation, other safety measures with vestibular dysfunction

Evaluate:

• Therapeutic response: absence of fever, draining wounds, negative C&S after treatment

Teach patient/family:

• To report headache, dizziness, symptoms of overgrowth of infection, renal impairment

• To report loss of hearing, ringing, roaring in ears, or feeling of fullness in head

---

glatiramer (℞)
(glah-tear′a-meer)
Copaxone
Func. class.: Multiple sclerosis agent

Action: Unknown, may modify the immune responses responsible for multiple sclerosis (MS)

Uses: Reduction of the frequency of relapses in patients with relapsing-remitting MS

Dosage and routes:

• *Adult:* **SC** 20 mg/day

Available forms: Inj 20 mg/ml

Side effects/adverse reactions:

CV: Migraine, palpitations, syncope, tachycardia, vasodilation

GI: Nausea, vomiting, diarrhea, anorexia, gastroenteritis

HEMA: Ecchymosis, lymphadenopathy

META: Edema, weight gain

MS: Arthralgia

CNS: Anxiety, hypertonia, tremor, vertigo, speech disorder, agitation, confusion

RESP: Bronchitis, dyspnea

INTEG: Pruritus, rash, sweating, urticaria, erythema

EENT: Ear pain

GU: Urinary urgency, dysmenorrhea, vaginal moniliasis

 = Nursing alert   = Herb-drug interaction   = Do not crush

Contraindications: Hypersensitivity to this drug or mannitol

Precautions: Immune disorders, renal disease, pregnancy (B), lactation

Pharmacokinetics: Unknown

NURSING CONSIDERATIONS
Assess:
• Blood, renal, hepatic studies: prior to treatment
• For CNS symptoms: anxiety, confusion, vertigo
• GI status: diarrhea, vomiting, abdominal pain, gastroenteritis
• Cardiac status: tachycardia, palpitations, vasodilation, chest pain

Administer:
• SC route
• Using a sterile syringe/needle to transfer the supplied diluent into the vial, rotate vial gently, do not shake; withdraw medication using a syringe with 27G needle; administer SC into hip, thigh, arm; discard unused portion
• Use SC route only; do not give IM or IV
• Do not use sol that contains precipitate or is discolored
• Use immediately

Evaluate:
• Therapeutic response: decreased symptoms of MS

Teach patient/family:
• Give written, detailed instructions about the drug; provide initial and return demonstrations on inj procedure; give information on use and disposal of drug
• That blurred vision, sweating may occur
• That irregular menses, dysmenorrhea, or metrorrhagia as well as breast pain may occur; use contraception during treatment
• That if pregnancy is suspected, or if nursing, notify prescriber

• Not to change dosing or to stop taking drug without advice of prescriber

glipizide (℞)
(glip-i′zide)
Glucotrol, Glucotrol XL
glimepiride
(glye-me′pi-ride)
Amaryl
Func. class.: Antidiabetic
Chem. class.: Sulfonylurea (2nd generation)

Action: Causes functioning β-cells in pancreas to release insulin, leading to drop in blood glucose levels; may improve insulin binding to insulin receptors or increase the number of insulin receptors with prolonged administration; may also reduce basal hepatic glucose secretion; not effective if patient lacks functioning β-cells

Uses: Stable adult-onset diabetes mellitus (type II) NIDDM

Dosage and routes:
Glipizide
• *Adult:* PO 5 mg initially, then increase to desired response; max 40 mg/day in divided doses or 15 mg/dose
• *Elderly/hepatic disease:* PO 2.5 mg initially, then increase to desired response; max 40 mg/day in divided doses or 15 mg/dose
Glimepiride
• *Adult:* PO 1-2 mg qd, then increase q1-2wk up to 8 mg/day
Renal dose
Adult: PO CrCl <20 ml/min, 1 mg qd with breakfast, may titrate upward as needed
Available forms: glipizide: tabs 5, 10 mg scored; ext rel tab 5, 10 mg; glimepiride: tabs 1, 2, 4 mg

Side effects/adverse reactions:

CNS: Headache, weakness, dizziness, drowsiness, tinnitus, fatigue, vertigo

*GI: **Hepatotoxicity, cholestatic jaundice,*** nausea, vomiting, diarrhea, heartburn

*HEMA: **Leukopenia, thrombocytopenia, agranulocytosis, aplastic anemia;*** increased AST, ALT, alk phosphatase; ***pancytopenia, hemolytic anemia***

INTEG: Rash, allergic reactions, pruritus, urticaria, eczema, photosensitivity, erythema

*ENDO: **Hypoglycemia***

Contraindications: Hypersensitivity to sulfonylureas, juvenile or type 1 diabetes

Precautions: Pregnancy (C), elderly, cardiac disease, severe renal disease, severe hepatic disease, thyroid disease

Do not confuse:

Glucotrol/glyburide

Pharmacokinetics:

PO: Completely absorbed by GI route, onset 1-1½ hr, peak 1-3 hr, duration 10-24 hr, half-life 2-4 hr; metabolized in liver; excreted in urine; 90%-95% is plasma protein bound

Interactions:

• Increased action of: digitalis, glycosides

• Increased hypoglycemic effects: insulin, MAOIs, cimetidine, chloramphenicol, guanethidine, methyldopa, nonsteroidal antiinflammatories, salicylates, probenecid, androgens, anticoagulants, clofibrate, fenfluramine, fluconazole, gemfibrozil, histamine H_2 antagonists, magnesium salts, phenylbutazone, sulfinpyrazone, sulfonamides, tricyclics, urinary acidifiers

• Effectiveness may be decreased: thiazide diuretics, rifampin, isoniazid, β-blockers, cholestyramine, diazoxide, hydantoins, urinary alkalinizers, charcoal

🌿 Decreased hypoglycemic effect: broom, buchu, dandelion, juniper

🌿 Increased or decreased hypoglycemic effect: chromium, fenugreek, ginseng

🌿 Increased glucose tolerance: karela

NURSING CONSIDERATIONS

Assess:

• Blood, urine glucose, glycosylated Hgb levels during treatment to determine diabetes control

• CBC baseline and throughout treatment

• Hypo/hyperglycemic reaction that can occur soon after meals; for severe hypoglycemia give IV $D_{50}W$, then IV dextrose solution

Administer:

• Drug 30 min before meals; if patient is NPO, may need to hold dose to prevent hypoglycemia

• May crush tabs and mix with fluids, if unable to swallow whole

Perform/provide:

• Storage in tight, light-resistant container at room temperature

Evaluate:

• Therapeutic response: decrease in polyuria, polydipsia, polyphagia, clear sensorium, absence of dizziness, stable gait

Teach patient/family:

• Not to drink alcohol; explain disulfiram reaction (nausea, headache, cramps, flushing, hypoglycemia)

• To check for symptoms of cholestatic jaundice: dark urine, pruritus, yellow sclera; prescriber should be notified

• The symptoms of hypo/hyperglycemia, what to do about each; to have glucagon emergency kit available

---

◆ = Nursing alert   🌿 = Herb-drug interaction   🚫 = Do not crush

• That drug must be continued on daily basis; explain consequence of discontinuing drug abruptly
• To take drug in morning to prevent hypoglycemic reactions at night
• To use sunscreen or stay out of the sun to prevent photosensitivity
• To avoid OTC medications unless ordered by prescriber
• That diabetes is a lifelong illness; drug will not cure disease
• That all food in diet plan must be eaten to prevent hypoglycemia
• To carry ID for emergency purposes with prescriber and medications
• To test urine for glucose/ketones tid if this drug is replacing insulin; to use a capillary blood glucose test while on this drug
• To continue weight control, dietary restrictions, exercise, hygiene

Treatment of overdose: Glucose 25 g IV via dextrose 50% solution 50 ml or 1 mg glucagon

glyburide (℞)

(glye′byoor-ide)
DiaBeta*, Euglucon*, Glynase PresTab, Micronase
Func. class.: Antidiabetic
Chem. class.: Sulfonylurea (2nd generation)

Action: Causes functioning β-cells in pancreas to release insulin, leading to drop in blood glucose levels; may improve insulin binding to insulin receptors and increase number of insulin receptors with prolonged administration; may also reduce basal hepatic glucose secretion; not effective if patient lacks functioning β-cells

Uses: Stable adult-onset diabetes mellitus (type II) NIDDM

Dosage and routes:
DiaBeta/Micronase
• *Adult:* **PO** 1.25-5 mg initially, then increased to desired response at weekly intervals up to 20 mg/day
• *Elderly:* **PO** 1.25 mg initially, then increased to desired response; max 20 mg/day, maintenance 1.25-20 mg/qd

Glynase PresTab (micronized)
• *Adult:* **PO** 1.5-3 mg/day initially, may increase by 1.5 mg/wk, max 12 mg/day
• *Elderly:* **PO** 0.75-3 mg/day, may increase by 1.5 mg/wk

Available forms: Tabs 1.25, 2.5, 5 mg; (Glynase PresTab) 1.5, 3, 6 mg

Side effects/adverse reactions:
CNS: Headache, weakness, paresthesia, tinnitus, fatigue, vertigo
GI: Nausea, fullness, heartburn, **hepatotoxicity, cholestatic jaundice,** vomiting, diarrhea
HEMA: Leukopenia, thrombocytopenia, agranulocytosis, aplastic anemia, increased AST, ALT, alk phosphatase
INTEG: Rash, allergic reactions, pruritus, urticaria, eczema, photosensitivity, erythema
ENDO: Hypoglycemia
MS: Joint pain

Contraindications: Hypersensitivity to sulfonylureas, juvenile or type I diabetes

Precautions: Pregnancy (C), elderly, cardiac disease, severe renal disease, severe hepatic disease, thyroid disease, severe hypoglycemic reactions

Do not confuse:
glyburide/Glucotrol
DiaBeta/Zebeta

Pharmacokinetics:
PO: Completely absorbed by GI route; onset 2-4 hr, peak 4 hr, duration 24 hr; half-life 10 hr; metabolized in liver; excreted in urine,

feces (metabolites); crosses placenta; 99% is plasma protein bound

Interactions:

• Both drugs' effects may be decreased: diazoxide

• Increased level: digoxin

• Increased hypoglycemic effects: insulin, MAOIs, oral anticoagulants, chloramphenicol, guanethidine, methyldopa, NSAIDs, salicylates, probenecid, androgens, fenfluramine, fluconazole, gemfibrozil, histamine H_2 antagonists, magnesium salts, phenylbutazone, sulfinpyrazone, sulfonamides, tricyclics, urinary acidifiers

• Decreased action of glyburide: thiazide diuretics, rifampin, isoniazid, cholestyramine, diazoxide, hydantoins, urinary alkalinizers, charcoal

• Mask symptoms of hypoglycemia: β-blockers

🍃 Decreased hypoglycemic effect: broom, buchu, dandelion, juniper

🍃 Increased or decreased hypoglycemic effect: chromium, fenugreek, ginseng

🍃 Increased glucose tolerance: karela

NURSING CONSIDERATIONS

Assess:

• Hypo/hyperglycemic reaction that can occur soon after meals; for severe hypoglycemia, give IV $D_{50}W$, then IV dextrose sol

• Blood, urine glucose; glycosylated Hgb levels during treatment

• CBC baseline and throughout treatment

Administer:

• With breakfast, hold dose if NPO to avoid hypoglycemia

Perform/provide:

• Storage in tight container in cool environment

Evaluate:

• Therapeutic response: decrease in polyuria, polydipsia, polyphagia, clear sensorium, absence of dizziness, stable gait

Teach patient/family:

• To check for symptoms of cholestatic jaundice: dark urine, pruritus, jaundiced sclera; if these occur, notify prescriber

• To use a capillary blood glucose test while on this drug

• The symptoms of hypo/hyperglycemia, what to do about each

• That drug must be continued on daily basis; explain consequence of discontinuing drug abruptly

• To take drug in morning to prevent hypoglycemic reactions at night

• To avoid OTC medications unless ordered by prescriber

• That diabetes is a lifelong illness; drug will not cure disease

• That all food included in diet plan must be eaten to prevent hypoglycemia; to have glucagon emergency kit available

• To use sunscreen or stay out of the sun to prevent photosensitivity

• To carry an ID for emergency purposes with prescriber and medications

Treatment of overdose: Glucose 25 g IV via dextrose 50% sol, 50 ml or 1 mg glucagon

---

glycerin (OTC)

(gli′ser-in)

Fleet Babylax, Glycerin USP, Glycerol, Osmoglyn, Sani-Supp

Func. class.: Laxative, hyperosmotic

Chem. class.: Trihydric alcohol

Action: Increases osmotic pressure, draws fluid into colon, lumen from extravascular spaces to intravascular

---

◆ = Nursing alert   🍃 = Herb-drug interaction   🚫 = Do not crush

Uses: Constipation, intraocular pressure reduction

Dosage and routes:

Laxative

• *Adult and child >6 yr:* **RECT SUPP** 3 g; **ENEMA** 5-15 ml

• *Child <6 yr:* **RECT SUPP** 1-1.5 g; **ENEMA** 2-5 ml

Intraocular pressure reduction

• *Adult:* **PO** 1-1.5 g/kg once, then may be given 500 mg/kg q6h

• *Child:* **PO** 1-1.5 g/kg once, then 500 mg/kg 4-8 hr after first dose

Available forms: Rect sol 4 ml/ applicator; supp; oral sol 0.6 g/ml

Side effects/adverse reactions:

CNS: Headache, confusion, ***convulsions***

GI: Nausea, vomiting, diarrhea

META: Dehydration

Contraindications: Hypersensitivity

Precautions: Pregnancy (C)

NURSING CONSIDERATIONS

Assess:

• Cause of constipation; identify whether fluids, bulk, or exercise is missing from lifestyle

• Cramping, rectal bleeding, nausea, vomiting; if these symptoms occur, drug should be discontinued

Administer:

• Insert supp; may cause evacuation in ½ hr

• Enema: use 4 ml applicator; patient should be in side-lying position

• Pour oral sol over cracked ice and sip through a straw

• To prevent cerebral dehydration, headache, patient should be recumbent during and after administration

Perform/provide:

• Storage in cool environment; do not freeze

Evaluate:

• Therapeutic response: decrease in constipation

Teach patient/family:

• Not to use laxatives for long-term therapy; bowel tone will be lost

• That normal bowel movements do not always occur daily

• Not to use in presence of abdominal pain, nausea, vomiting

• To notify prescriber if constipation unrelieved or if symptoms of electrolyte imbalance occur: muscle cramps, pain, weakness, dizziness, excessive thirst

G

RARELY USED

glycerin, anhydrous (℞)

(gli′ser-in, an-hye′drus)

Func. class.: Ophthalmic

Uses: Reduce corneal edema

Dosage and routes:

• *Adult:* **INSTILL** 1-2 gtt after local anesthetic

Contraindications: Hypersensitivity

---

glycopyrrolate (℞)

(glye-koe-pye′roe-late)

glycopyrrolate, Robinul, Robinul-Forte

Func. class.: Cholinergic blocker

Chem. class.: Quaternary ammonium compound

Action: Inhibits the action of acetylcholine at receptor sites in autonomic nervous system, which controls secretions, free acids in stomach

Uses: Decreased secretions before surgery, reversal of neuromuscular blockade, peptic ulcer disease, irritable bowel syndrome

Investigational uses: Drooling

Dosage and routes:
Preoperatively
• *Adult:* IM 4.4 µg/kg ½-1 hr before surgery, max 0.1 mg
• *Child:* IM 4.4-8.8 µg/kg
Reversal of neuromuscular blockade
• *Adult and child:* IV 200 µg for each 1 mg of neostigmine or 5 mg IV of pyridostigmine simultaneously
GI disorders
• *Adult:* PO 1-2 mg bid-tid; IM/IV 100-200 µg tid-qid, titrated to patient response
Antidysrhythmic
• *Adult:* IV 100 µg, may repeat q2min
• *Child:* IV 4.4 µ/kg, may repeat q2min, max 100 µg
Drooling
• *Adult:* PO doses vary widely
Available forms: Tabs 1, 2 mg; inj 200 µg (0.2 mg)/ml
Side effects/adverse reactions:
INTEG: Urticaria, allergic reactions
MISC: Suppression of lactation, nasal congestion, decreased sweating
CNS: Confusion, anxiety, restlessness, irritability, delusions, hallucinations, headache, sedation, depression, incoherence, dizziness, lethargy, flushing, weakness
EENT: Blurred vision, photophobia, dilated pupils, difficulty swallowing, increased intraocular pressure, mydriasis, cycloplegia
CV: Palpitations, tachycardia, postural hypotension, paradoxical bradycardia
GI: Dryness of mouth, constipation, nausea, vomiting, abdominal distress, paralytic ileus, altered taste perception
SYST: Anaphylaxis
GU: Urinary hesitancy, retention, impotence
Contraindications: Hypersensitivity, narrow-angle glaucoma, myasthenia gravis, GI/GU obstruction, child <3 yr, tachycardia, myocardial ischemia, hepatic disease, ulcerative colitis, toxic megacolon
Precautions: Pregnancy (B), elderly, lactation, prostatic hypertrophy, renal disease, CHF, pulmonary disease, hyperthyroidism
Pharmacokinetics:
PO: Peak 1 hr, duration 8-12 hr
IM: Peak 30-45 min, duration 2-7 hr
IV: Peak 10-15 min, duration 2-7 hr; excreted in urine (50%) (unchanged); half-life 1-2 hr
Interactions:
• Increased anticholinergic effect: alcohol, antihistamines, phenothiazines, amantadine, tricyclics
• Decreased absorption of glycopyrrolate: antacids, antidiarrheals
NURSING CONSIDERATIONS
Assess:
• I&O ratio; retention commonly causes decreased urinary output
• Urinary hesitancy, retention: palpate bladder if retention occurs
• Constipation; increase fluids, bulk, exercise if this occurs
• Mental status: affect, mood, CNS depression, worsening of mental symptoms during early therapy
Administer:
• Parenteral dose with patient recumbent to prevent postural hypotension
• Parenteral dose slowly; keep in bed for at least 1 hr after dose; monitor vital signs
• After checking dose carefully; even slight overdose may lead to toxicity
• With or after meals to prevent GI upset; may give with fluids other than water
IV
• Undiluted, give through a Y-tube or 3-way stopcock; give 0.2 mg or less over 1-2 min
Syringe compatibilities: Atropine, benzquinamide, chlorpromazine,

cimetidine, codeine, diphenhydramine, droperidol, droperidol/fentanyl, hydromorphone, hydroxyzine, levorphanol, lidocaine, meperidine, meperidine/promethazine, midazolam, morphine, nalbuphine, neostigmine, oxymorphone, procaine, prochlorperazine, promazine, promethazine, pyridostigmine, ranitidine, scopolamine, triflupromazine, trimethobenzamide

Solution compatibilities: D$_5$W, 0.9% NaCl, Ringer's, D$_5$/0.45% NaCl

Perform/provide:
• Storage at room temperature

Evaluate:
• Therapeutic response: decreased secretions; decreased pain in GI disorders; reversal of neuromuscular blockers

Teach patient/family:
• Hard candy, frequent drinks, sugarless gum to relieve dry mouth
• Not to discontinue this drug abruptly; to taper off over 1 wk; to take PO ½-1 hr ac
• To avoid driving, other hazardous activities; drowsiness, blurred vision may occur
• To avoid OTC medication: cough, cold preparations with alcohol, antihistamines unless directed by prescriber
• To avoid hot temperatures, since sweating is decreased, heat stroke is possible
• To change positions slowly to prevent orthostatic hypotension
• To notify prescriber of eye pain, blurred vision, light sensitivity

---

goserelin (℞)

(goe′se-rel-lin)

Zoladex

Func. class.: Gonadotropin-releasing hormone, antineoplastic (hormone)

Chem. class.: Synthetic decapeptide analog of LHRH

Action: Inhibitor of pituitary gonadotropin secretion; initially increases LH and FSH, with increases in testosterone, reduction in sex steroid levels

Uses: Advanced prostate cancer (10.8 mg), endometriosis, advanced breast cancer, endometrial thinning (3.6 mg)

Dosage and routes:
• *Adult:* SC 3.6 mg q4wk or 10.8 mg q12wk

Endometrial thinning
• *Adult:* SC 1-2 depot inj, usually 1 depot, surgery performed at 4 wk, if 2 depots, surgery performed 2-4 wk after 2nd depot

Available forms: Depot inj 3.6, 10.8 mg

Side effects/adverse reactions:
CNS: Headaches, **spinal cord compression,** anxiety, depression
CV: **Dysrhythmia, cerebrovascular accident,** hypertension, **MI,** chest pain
ENDO: Gynecomastia, breast tenderness, hot flashes
GI: Nausea, vomiting, constipation, diarrhea, ulcer
GU: Spotting, breakthrough bleeding, decreased libido, renal insufficiency, urinary obstruction, urinary tract infection
INTEG: Rash, pain on injection
MS: Osteoneuralgia

Contraindications: Hypersensitivity to LHRH, LHRH-agonist analogs, pregnancy (D)—breast can-

---

cer, (X)—endometriosis, lactation, nondiagnosed vaginal bleeding

Pharmacokinetics: Peak serum concentrations in 14-28 days; half-life 4½ hr

Lab test interferences:

Increase: Alk phosphatase, estradiol, FSH, LH, testosterone levels

Decrease: Testosterone levels, progesterone

NURSING CONSIDERATIONS
Assess:

• I&O ratios; palpate bladder for distention in urinary obstruction

• For relief of bone pain (back pain), change in motor function

• Acid phosphatase PSA baseline and periodically

Administer:

• SC using implant, inserted by qualified person into upper subcutaneous tissue in abdominal wall q28d or q12wk (10.8 mg)

Evaluate:

• Therapeutic response: more normal levels of prostate-specific antigen, acid phosphatase, alk phosphatase; testosterone level of <25 ng/dl

Teach patient/family:

• That gynecomastia and postmenopausal symptoms may occur but will decrease after treatment is discontinued

• That bone pain may increase, then decrease

• To notify prescriber of difficulty urinating, hot flashes

• To keep appointments

---

granisetron (℞)
(grane-iss'e-tron)
Kytril
Func. class.: Antiemetic
Chem. class.: 5-HT$_3$ receptor antagonist

Action: Prevents nausea, vomiting by blocking serotonin peripherally, centrally, and in the small intestine

Uses: Prevention of nausea, vomiting associated with cancer chemotherapy including high-dose cisplatin

Investigational uses: Acute nausea, vomiting following surgery

Dosage and routes:

Nausea, vomiting in chemotherapy

• *Adult and child:* **IV** 10 µg/kg over 5 min, 30 min before the start of cancer chemotherapy

• *Adult:* **PO** 1 mg bid, give first dose 1 hr before chemotherapy and next dose 12 hr after first

Nausea, vomiting in radiation therapy

• *Adult:* **PO** 2 mg qd 1 hr prior to radiation

Available forms: Inj 1 mg/ml; tab 1 mg

Side effects/adverse reactions:

CNS: Headache, asthenia, anxiety, dizziness

CV: Hypertension

GI: Diarrhea, *constipation,* increased AST, ALT, *nausea*

HEMA: Leukopenia, anemia, *thrombocytopenia*

MISC: Rash, *bronchospasm*

Contraindications: Hypersensitivity

Precautions: Pregnancy (B), lactation, children, elderly

Pharmacokinetics: Metabolized in

---

liver to an active metabolite, half-life 10-12 hr

NURSING CONSIDERATIONS

Assess:

• For absence of nausea, vomiting during chemotherapy

• Hypersensitive reaction: rash, bronchospasm

Administer:

IV, direct

• Dilute in 0.9% NaCl for inj or D_5W (20-50 ml); give over 5-15 min; ½ hr before chemotherapy

Additive compatibilities: Dexamethasone, methylprednisolone

Solution compatibilities: D_5W, 0.9% NaCl

Y-site compatibilities: Acyclovir, allopurinol, amifostine, amikacin, aminophylline, amphotericin B cholesteryl, ampicillin, ampicillin/sulbactam, amsacrine, aztreonam, bleomycin, bumetanide, buprenorphine, butorphanol, calcium gluconate, carboplatin, carmustine, cefazolin, cefepime, cefonicid, cefoperazone, cefotaxime, cefotetan, cefoxitin, ceftazidime, ceftizoxime, ceftriaxone, cefuroxime, chlorpromazine, cimetidine, ciprofloxacin, cisplatin, cladribine, clindamycin, cyclophosphamide, cytarabine, dacarbazine, dactinomycin, daunorubicin, dexamethasone, diphenhydramine, dobutamine, dopamine, doxorubicin, doxorubicin liposome, doxycycline, droperidol, enalaprilat, etoposide, famotidine, filgrastim, fluconazole, fluorouracil, floxuridine, fludarabine, furosemide, gallium, ganciclovir, gentamicin, haloperidol, heparin hydrocortisone, hydromorphone, hydroxyzine, idarubicin, ifosfamide, imipenem-cilastatin, leucovorin, lorazepam, magnesium sulfate, melphalan, meperidine, mesna, methotrexate, methylprednisolone, metoclopramide, metronidazole, mezlocillin, miconazole, minocycline, mitomycin, mitoxantrone, morphine, nalbuphine, netilmicin, ofloxacin, paclitaxel, piperacillin, piperacillin/tazobactam, plicamycin, potassium chloride, prochlorperazine, promethazine, propofol, ranitidine, sargramostim, sodium bicarbonate, streptozocin, teniposide, thiotepa, ticarcillin, ticarcillin/clavulanate, tobramycin, trimethoprim - sulfamethoxazole, vancomycin, vinblastine, vincristine, vinorelbine, zidovudine

Perform/provide:

• Storage at room temperature for 24 hr after dilution

Evaluate:

• Therapeutic response: absence of nausea, vomiting during cancer chemotherapy

Teach patient/family:

• To report diarrhea, constipation, rash, changes in respirations

---

griseofulvin microsize (℞)
(gris-ee-oh-ful'vin)
Fulvicin-U/F, Grifulvin V,
Grisactin, Grisovin-FP*

griseofulvin ultramicrosize (℞)
Fulvicin P/G, Grisactin Ultra,
Gris-PEG
Func. class.: Antifungal
Chem. class.: Penicillium
griseofulvum derivative

Action: Arrests fungal cell division at metaphase; binds to human keratin, making it resistant to disease

Uses: Mycotic infections: tinea corporis, tinea pedis, tinea cruris, tinea barbae, tinea capitis, tinea unguium if caused by *Epidermophyton, Microsporum, Trichophyton*

Dosage and routes:
• *Adult:* **PO** 500-1000 mg qd in single or divided doses (microsize), 125-165 mg bid (ultramicrosize) or 250-330 mg qd; may need 500-660 mg in divided doses for severe infections
• *Child:* **PO** 10 mg/kg/day or 30 mg/m^2/day (microsize) or 5 mg/kg/day (ultramicrosize)
Available forms: Microcaps 125, 250 mg; tabs 250, 500 mg; oral susp 125 mg/ml; ultratabs 125, 165, 250, 330 mg

Side effects/adverse reactions:
INTEG: Rash, urticaria, photosensitivity, lichen planus
CNS: Headache, peripheral neuritis, paresthesias, confusion, dizziness, fatigue
EENT: Transient hearing loss
GU: Proteinuria, cylinduria, precipitate porphyria, increased thirst
GI: Nausea, vomiting, anorexia, diarrhea, cramps, dry mouth, flatulence, ***bleeding***
*HEMA: **Leukopenia, granulocytopenia, neutropenia, monocytosis***
*SYST: **Serum sickness***
Contraindications: Hypersensitivity, porphyria, hepatic disease, lupus erythematosus
Precautions: Penicillin sensitivity, pregnancy (C)
Pharmacokinetics:
PO: Peak 4 hr, half-life 9-24 hr, metabolized in liver; excreted in urine (inactive metabolites), feces, perspiration
Interactions:
• Tachycardia: alcohol
• Decreased action of griseofulvin: barbiturates
• Decreased action of warfarin, cyclosporine, salicylates, oral contraceptives
• Drug/food: increased absorption: High-fat foods

NURSING CONSIDERATIONS
Assess:
• I&O ratio, urinalysis
• Liver studies qwk (ALT, AST, bilirubin, alk phosphatase)
• Renal studies: BUN, serum creatinine
• Blood studies: CBC, platelets, q2wk
• For history of penicillin allergy; may be cross-sensitive to this drug
◆ For renal toxicity: increasing BUN, serum creatinine, proteinuria, cylindruria
• For blood dyscrasias: fatigue, malaise, dark urine, bruising
• Use only when topical treatment is ineffective
Administer:
• Drug carefully, making sure there is no confusion with dosage form (microsize vs ultramicrosize)
• With meals to decrease GI symptoms; fatty meals for better absorption
• Until three separate cultures are negative for infective organism
Perform/provide:
• Storage in tight, light-resistant container at room temperature
Evaluate:
• Therapeutic response: decreased rash, negative C&S for infecting organism
Teach patient/family:
• That long-term therapy may be needed to clear infection (2 wk-6 mo depending on organism)
• Proper hygiene: hand-washing technique, nail care, use of concomitant topical agents if prescribed
• The importance of compliance even after feeling better
• To avoid alcohol, since nausea, vomiting, hypertension may occur
• To use sunscreen or avoid direct sunlight to prevent photosensitivity
• To notify prescriber of sore throat,

◆ = Nursing alert   🌿 = Herb-drug interaction   🚫 = Do not crush

fever, skin rash, which may indicate overgrowth of organisms
• To use nonhormonal contraception

guaifenesin (OTC, R)
(gwye-fen'e-sin)
Anti-Tuss, Benylin-E*, Breonesin, Calmylin Expectorant*, Diabetic Tussin Ex, Duratuss-G, Fenesin, Gee-Gee, Genatuss, GG-Cen, Glyate, Glycotuss, Glytuss, guaifenesin, Guaifenex LA, Guiatuss, Halotussin, Humibid, Humibid L.A., Hytuss, Hytuss 2X, Liquibid, Monafed, Muco-Fen-LA, Mytussin, Naldecon Senior EX, Organidin NR, Pneumomist, Respa-GF, Resyl*, Robitussin, Scot-Tussin Expectorant, Sinumist-SR, Unitussin
Func. class.: Expectorant

Action: Acts as an expectorant by stimulating a gastric mucosal reflex to increase the production of lung mucus

Uses: Dry, nonproductive cough

Dosage and routes:
• *Adult:* **PO** 200-400 mg q4-6h, not to exceed 1.2 g/day; **EXT REL** 600-1200 mg q12h, not to exceed 2.4 g/day
• *Child 6-12 yr:* **PO** 100-200 mg q4h; 600 mg q12h (**EXT REL**) not to exceed 1.2 g/day
• *Child 2-6 yr:* **PO** 50-100 mg q4h; not to exceed 600 mg/day

Available forms: Tabs 100, 200 mg; tabs, ext rel 600, 1200 mg; caps 200 mg; caps, ext rel 300 mg; syr 100, 200 mg/5 ml

Side effects/adverse reactions:
CNS: Drowsiness
GI: Nausea, anorexia, vomiting

Contraindications: Hypersensitivity, persistent cough

Precautions: Pregnancy (C)

NURSING CONSIDERATIONS
Assess:
• Cough: type, frequency, character, including sputum; fluids should be increased to 2 L/day

Perform/provide:
• Storage at room temperature
• Increased fluids, room humidification to liquefy secretions

Evaluate:
• Therapeutic response: absence of cough

Teach patient/family:
• To avoid driving, other hazardous activities if drowsiness occurs (rare)
• To avoid smoking, smoke-filled room, perfumes, dust, environmental pollutants, cleansers

RARELY USED

guanabenz (R)
(gwan'a-benz)
Func. class.: Antihypertensive

Uses: Hypertension

Dosage and routes:
• *Adult:* **PO** 4 mg bid, increasing in increments of 4-8 mg/day q1-2wk, not to exceed 32 mg bid

Contraindications: Hypersensitivity to guanabenz

RARELY USED

guanadrel (R)
(gwahn'a-drel)
Func. class.: Antihypertensive

Uses: Hypertension (moderate to severe as an adjunct)

Dosage and routes:
• *Adult:* **PO** 5 mg bid, adjusted to

desired response weekly or monthly; may need 20-75 mg/day in divided doses; higher doses are given tid or qid

• *Geriatric:* **PO** 5 mg/day, titrate as needed

Renal dose

• CrCl 10-50 ml/min dose q12-24h; CrCl <10 ml/min dose q24-48h

Contraindications: Hypersensitivity, pheochromocytoma, lactation, CHF, child <18 yr

---

RARELY USED

guanethidine (℞)
(gwahn-eth'i-deen)
Func. class.: Antihypertensive

Uses: Moderate to severe hypertension

Dosage and routes:
• *Adult:* **PO** 10-12.5 mg qd, increase by 10 mg qwk; may require 25-50 mg qd
• *Adult:* (hospitalized) 25-50 mg; may increase by 25-50 mg/day or every other day
• *Child:* **PO** 0.2 mg/kg/day; (6 mg/m^2/day) increase q7-10d, 0.2 mg/kg or 6 mg/m^2/day not to exceed 3000 µg/kg/24 hr

Contraindications: Hypersensitivity, pheochromocytoma, recent MI, CHF, cardiac failure, sinus bradycardia

---

RARELY USED

guanfacine (℞)
(gwahn'fa-seen)
Func. class.: Antihypertensive

Uses: Hypertension in individual using a thiazide diuretic
Investigational uses: ADHD

Dosage and routes:
• *Adult:* **PO** 1 mg/day hs; may increase dose in 2-3 wk to 2-3 mg/day

Contraindications: Hypersensitivity

RARELY USED

halcinonide (℞)
(hal-sin'oh-nide)
Func. class.: Corticosteroid, synthetic

Uses: Inflammation of corticosteroid-responsive dermatoses
Dosage and routes:
• *Adult:* **TOP** apply to affected area bid-tid (not around eyes)
Contraindications: Hypersensitivity, viral infections, fungal infections

---

RARELY USED

halofantrine (℞)
(hay-loh-fan'trin)
Func. class.: Antimalarial

Uses: Mild to moderate malaria
Dosage and routes:
• *Adult:* **PO** 500 mg q6h × 3 doses; may need to repeat after 1 wk
Contraindications: Hypersensitivity, pregnancy, lactation, QT prolongation, AV conduction disorders, thiamine deficiency, ventricular dysrhythmias

---

◆ = Nursing alert   / = Herb-drug interaction   ⊘ = Do not crush

haloperidol (R)
(hal-oh-pehr'ih-dol)
Apo-Haloperidol*, Haldol,
Novo-Peridol*, Peridol*
haloperidol decanoate (R)
Haldol Decanoate, Haldol
LA*
haloperidol lactate (R)
Haldol, Haloperidol Injection,
Haloperidol Intensol
Func. class.: Antipsychotic,
neuroleptic
Chem. class.: Butyrophenone

Action: Depresses cerebral cortex, hypothalamus, limbic system, which control activity and aggression; blocks neurotransmission produced by dopamine at synapse; exhibits strong α-adrenergic, anticholinergic blocking action; mechanism for antipsychotic effects unclear

Uses: Psychotic disorders, control of tics, vocal utterances in Gilles de la Tourette's syndrome, short-term treatment of hyperactive children showing excessive motor activity, prolonged parenteral therapy in chronic schizophrenia, control of severe nausea and vomiting in chemotherapy, organic mental syndrome with psychotic features, hiccups (short-term)

Investigational uses: Nausea, vomiting in chemotherapy, surgery

Dosage and routes:
Psychosis
• *Adult:* **PO** 0.5-5 mg bid or tid initially depending on severity of condition; dose is increased to desired dose, max 100 mg/day; **IM** 2-5 mg q4-8h or bid-tid
• *Geriatric:* 0.25-0.5 mg qd-bid, titrate q3-4 days by 0.25-0.5 mg/dose

• *Child 3-12 yr:* **PO/IM** 0.05-0.15 mg/kg/day
• *Decanoate:* Initial dose **IM** is 10-15 mg × daily oral dose at 4 wk interval; do not administer **IV**; not to exceed 100 mg
Chronic schizophrenia
• *Adult:* **IM** 50-100 mg q4wk (decanoate)
• *Child 3-12 yr:* **PO/IM** 0.05-0.15 mg/kg/day
Tics/vocal utterances
• *Adult:* **PO** 0.5-5 mg bid or tid, increased until desired response occurs
• *Child 3-12 yr:* **PO** 0.05-0.075 mg/kg/day
Hyperactive children
• *Child 3-12 yr:* **PO** 0.05-0.075 mg/kg/day
Available forms: Tabs 0.5, 1, 2, 5, 10, 20 mg; lactate conc 2 mg/ml; inj 5 mg/ml, decanoate 50 mg base/ml, 100 mg base/ml
Side effects/adverse reactions:
*RESP: **Laryngospasm,** dyspnea, **respiratory depression***
*CNS: EPS: pseudoparkinsonism, akathisia, dystonia, tardive dyskinesia, drowsiness, headache, **seizures, neuroleptic malignant syndrome,** confusion*
INTEG: Rash, photosensitivity, dermatitis
EENT: Blurred vision, glaucoma, dry eyes
*GI: Dry mouth, nausea, vomiting, anorexia, constipation, diarrhea, jaundice, weight gain, **ileus, hepatitis***
GU: Urinary retention, urinary frequency, enuresis, impotence, amenorrhea, gynecomastia
*CV: Orthostatic hypotension, hypertension, **cardiac arrest,** ECG changes, **tachycardia***
Contraindications: Hypersensitivity, blood dyscrasias, coma,

child <3 yr, brain damage, bone marrow depression, alcohol and barbiturate withdrawal states, Parkinson's disease, angina, epilepsy, urinary retention, narrow-angle glaucoma

Precautions: Pregnancy (C), lactation, seizure disorders, hypertension, hepatic disease, cardiac disease, elderly

Do not confuse:

haloperidol/Halotestin
Haldol/Stadol

Pharmacokinetics:

PO: Onset erratic, peak 2-6 hr, half-life 24 hr

IM: Onset 15-30 min, peak 15-20 min, half-life 21 hr

IM (Decanoate): Peak 4-11 days, half-life 3 wk

Metabolized by liver; excreted in urine, bile; crosses placenta; enters breast milk

Interactions:

• Oversedation: other CNS depressants, alcohol, barbiturate anesthetics

• Toxicity: epinephrine

• Toxicity: lithium

• Decreased effects of lithium, levodopa

• Increased effects of both drugs: β-adrenergic blockers, alcohol

• Increased anticholinergic effects: anticholinergics

• Decreased effects of haloperidol: phenobarbital

🍃 Increased action: kava

Lab test interferences:

Increase: LFTs, cardiac enzymes, cholesterol, blood glucose, prolactin, bilirubin, PBI, cholinesterase, alk phosphatase

Decrease: Hormones (blood, urine), PT

False positive: Pregnancy tests, PKU

False negative: Urinary steroids

NURSING CONSIDERATIONS
Assess:

• Swallowing of PO medication; check for hoarding or giving of medication to other patients

• I&O ratio; palpate bladder if low urinary output occurs

• Bilirubin, CBC, liver function studies monthly

• Urinalysis is recommended before and during prolonged therapy

• For depression in bipolar patients; rapid mood swings may occur with this drug

• Affect, orientation, LOC, reflexes, gait, coordination, sleep pattern disturbances

• B/P standing and lying; take pulse and respirations q4h during initial treatment; establish baseline before starting treatment; report drops of 30 mm Hg

• Dizziness, faintness, palpitations, tachycardia on rising

• EPS including akathisia (inability to sit still, no pattern to movements), tardive dyskinesia (bizarre movements of jaw, mouth, tongue, extremities), pseudoparkinsonism (rigidity, tremors, pill rolling, shuffling gait)

• Skin turgor daily

◆ For neuroleptic malignant syndrome: hyperthermia, muscle rigidity, altered mental status, increased CPK, seizures, hyper/hypotension, tachycardia, notify prescriber immediately

• Constipation, urinary retention daily; if these occur, increase bulk, water in diet

Administer:

• Reduced dose to elderly

• Antiparkinsonian agent, to be used if EPS occur

• IM inj into large muscle mass, use 21G, 2-in needle; give no more than 3 ml/inj site; patient should remain recumbent for ½ hr

◆ = Nursing alert   🍃 = Herb-drug interaction   🚫 = Do not crush

• Oral liquid: use calibrated dropper; do not mix in coffee or tea
• PO with food or milk

Solution compatibilities: D_5W

Syringe compatibilities: Hydromorphone, sufentanil

Y-site compatibilities: Amifostine, amsacrine, aztreonam, cimetidine, cisatracurium, cladribine, dobutamine, dopamine, doxorubicin liposome, famotidine, filgrastim, fludarabine, granisetron, lidocaine, lorazepam, melphalan, midazolam, nitroglycerin, norepinephrine, ondansetron, paclitaxel, phenylephrine, propofol, remifentanil, sufentanil, tacrolimus, teniposide, theophylline, thiotepa, vinorelbine

Perform/provide:

• Decreased sensory input by dimming lights, avoiding loud noises
• Supervised ambulation until stabilized on medication; do not involve in strenuous exercise program because fainting is possible; patient should not stand still for long periods
• Increased fluids to prevent constipation
• Sips of water, candy, gum for dry mouth
• Storage in tight, light-resistant container

Evaluate:

• Therapeutic response: decrease in emotional excitement, hallucinations, delusions, paranoia, reorganization of patterns of thought, speech, improvement in specific behaviors

Teach patient/family:

• That orthostatic hypotension occurs often and to rise from sitting or lying position gradually
• To avoid hazardous activities until stabilized on medication
• To remain lying down after IM inj for at least 30 min
• To avoid hot tubs, hot showers, tub baths, since hypotension may occur
• To avoid abrupt withdrawal of this drug, or EPS may result; drug should be withdrawn slowly
• To avoid OTC preparations (cough, hay fever, cold) unless approved by prescriber, since serious drug interactions may occur; avoid use with alcohol, CNS depressants; increased drowsiness may occur
• To use a sunscreen to prevent burns
• Regarding compliance with drug regimen
• About EPS and necessity for meticulous oral hygiene, since oral candidiasis may occur
• To report impaired vision, jaundice, tremors, muscle twitching
• That in hot weather, heat stroke may occur; take extra precautions to stay cool

Treatment of overdose: Activated charcoal, lavage if orally ingested; provide an airway; do not induce vomiting

H

---

heparin (℞)

(hep′a-rin)
Calcilean*, Calciparine*, Hepalean*, Heparin Leo*, Heparin Lock Flush, heparin sodium, Heparin Sodium and 0.45% Sodium Chloride, Heparin Sodium and 0.9% Sodium Chloride , Hep-Lock, Hep-Lock U/P, Liquaemin Sodium

Func. class.: Anticoagulant, antithrombotic

Action: Prevents conversion of fibrinogen to fibrin and prothrombin to thrombin by enhancing inhibitory effects of antithrombin III

Uses: Deep-vein thrombosis, pulmonary emboli, myocardial infarction, open heart surgery, dissemi-

---

nated intravascular clotting syndrome, atrial fibrillation with embolization, as an anticoagulant in transfusion and dialysis procedures, prevention of DVT/PE

Dosage and routes:

Deep-vein thrombosis/MI

• *Adult:* **IV PUSH** 5000-7000 U q4h then titrated to PTT or ACT level; **IV BOL** 5000-7500 U, then **IV INF**; **IV INF** after bolus dose, then 1000 U/hr titrated to PTT or ACT level

• *Child:* **IV INF** 50 U/kg, maintenance 100 U/kg q4h or 20,000 U/m² qd

Pulmonary embolism

• *Adult:* **IV PUSH** 7500-10,000 U q4h then titrated to PTT or ACT level; **IV BOL** 7500-10,000, then **IV INF**; **IV INF** after bolus dose, then 1000 U/hr titrated to PTT or ACT level

• *Child:* **IV INF** 50 U/kg, maintenance 100 U/kg q4h or 20,000 U/m² qd

Cardiovascular surgery

• *Adult:* **IV INF** 150-300 U/kg

Prophylaxis for DVT/PE

• *Adult:* **SC** 5,000 U q8-12h

Heparin flush

• *Adult and child:* **IV** 10-100 U

Available forms:

Sodium carpaject: 5000 U/ml; disposable inj: 1000, 2500, 5000, 7500, 10,000, 15,000, 20,000, 40,000 U/ml; unit dose: 1000, 5000, 10,000, 20,000, 40,000 U/ml; vials: 1000, 2000, 2500, 5000, 7500, 10,000, 20,000, 40,000 U/ml; disposable syringes flush: 10 U/ml; vials: 100 U/ml; Ca inj: 5000 U/0.2 ml; ampules: 12,500 U/0.5 ml; 20,000 U/0.8 ml

Side effects/adverse reactions:

CNS: Fever, chills

GI: Diarrhea, nausea, vomiting, anorexia, stomatitis, abdominal cramps, *hepatitis*

GU: Hematuria

HEMA: Hemorrhage, thrombocytopenia

SYST: Anaphylaxis

INTEG: Rash, dermatitis, urticaria, alopecia, pruritus

Contraindications: Hypersensitivity, hemophilia, leukemia with bleeding, peptic ulcer disease, thrombocytopenic purpura, hepatic disease (severe), renal disease (severe), blood dyscrasias, severe hypertension, subacute bacterial endocarditis, acute nephritis

Precautions: Alcoholism, elderly, pregnancy (C)

Pharmacokinetics: Well absorbed (SC)

IV: Peak 5 min, duration 2-6 hr

SC: Onset 20-60 min, duration 8-12 hr

Half-life 1½ hr, excreted in urine, 95% bound to plasma proteins, does not cross placenta or alter breast milk; removed from the system via the lymph and spleen

Interactions:

• Decreased action of corticosteroids

• Increased action of diazepam

• Decreased action of heparin: digitalis, tetracyclines, antihistamines

• Increased action of heparin: oral anticoagulants, salicylates, dextran, steroids, nonsteroidal antiinflammatories

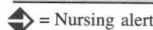 Increased risk of bleeding: bromelain, cinchona bark

Lab test interferences:

False increase: T_3 uptake, serum thyroxine, BSP

Decrease: Uric acid

False negative: ^{125}I fibrinogen uptake

NURSING CONSIDERATIONS

Assess:

• Blood studies (Hct, occult blood in stools) q3mo

 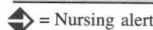

• Partial prothrombin time, which should be 1.5-2 × control, PTT often done qd, also APTT, ACT
• Platelet count q2-3d; thrombocytopenia may occur on 4th day of treatment
◆ Bleeding gums, petechiae, ecchymosis, black tarry stools, hematuria, epistaxis, decrease in Hct, B/P; indicate bleeding and possible hemorrhage
• Fever, skin rash, urticaria
• Needed dosage change q1-2wk

Administer:
• At same time each day to maintain steady blood levels
• SC deep with 25G ⅜-in needle; do not massage area or aspirate when giving SC inj; give in abdomen between pelvic bones, rotate sites; do not pull back on plunger, leave in for 10 sec; apply gentle pressure for 1 min
• Changing needles is not recommended
• Avoiding all IM injections that may cause bleeding

IV
• Diluted in 0.9% NaCl, dextrose, Ringer's sol and given by direct, intermittent, or continuous infusion; give 1000 U or less over 1 min; then 5000 U or less over 1 min; infusion may run from 4-24 hr; use infusion pump
• Blood after adding 7500 U/100 ml NaCl inj, add 6-8 ml of this sol/100 ml of whole blood

Additive compatibilities: Aminophylline, amphotericin, ascorbic acid, bleomycin, calcium gluconate, cefepime, cephapirin, chloramphenicol, clindamycin, cloxacillin, colistimethate, dimenhydrinate, dopamine, enalaprilat, erythromycin gluceptate, esmolol, floxacillin, fluconazole, flumazenil, furosemide, hydrocortisone, isoproterenol, lidocaine, lincomycin, magnesium sulfate, meropenem, methyldopate, methylprednisolone, metronidazole/sodium bicarbonate, nafcillin, norepinephrine, octreotide, penicillin G, potassium chloride, prednisolone, promazine, ranitidine, sodium bicarbonate, verapamil, vit B, vit B/C

Syringe compatibilities: Aminophylline, amphotericin B, ampicillin, atropine, azlocillin, bleomycin, cefamandole, cefazolin, cefoperazone, cefotaxime, cefoxitin, chloramphenicol, cimetidine, cisplatin, clindamycin, cyclophosphamide, diazoxide, digoxin, dimenhydrinate, dobutamine, dopamine, epinephrine, fentanyl, fluorouracil, furosemide, leucovorin, lidocaine, lincomycin, methotrexate, metoclopramide, mezlocillin, mitomycin, moxalactam, nafcillin, naloxone, neostigmine, nitroglycerin, norepinephrine, pancuronium, penicillin G, phenobarbital, piperacillin, sodium nitroprusside, succinylcholine, trimethoprim-sulfamethoxazole, verapamil, vincristine

Y-site compatibilities: Acyclovir, aldesleukin, allopurinol, amifostine, aminophylline, ampicillin, ampicillin/sulbactam, atracurium, atropine, aztreonam, betamethasone, bleomycin, calcium gluconate, cefazolin, cefotetan, cefotiam, ceftazidime, ceftriaxone, cephalothin, cephapirin, chlordiazepoxide, chlorpromazine, cimetidine, cisplatin, cladribine, clindamycin, conjugated estrogens, cyanocobalamin, cyclophosphamide, cytarabine, dexamethasone, digoxin, diphenhydramine, dopamine, doxorubicin liposome, edrophonium, enalaprilat, epinephrine, erythromycin, esmolol, ethacrynate, famotidine, fentanyl, fluconazole, fludarabine, fluorouracil, foscarnet, furosemide, gallium, gra-

H

Side effects: *italics* = common; ***bold italics*** = life-threatening

nisetron, hydralazine, hydrocortisone, hydromorphone, insulin (regular), isoproterenol, kanamycin, leucovorin, lidocaine, lorazepam, magnesium sulfate, melphalan, menadiol, meperidine, meropenem, methicillin, methotrexate, methoxamine, methyldopa, methylergonovine, metoclopramide, metronidazole, midazolam, milrinone, minocycline, mitomycin, morphine, nafcillin, neostigmine, nitroglycerin, nitroprusside, norepinephrine, ondansetron, oxacillin, oxytocin, paclitaxel, pancuronium, penicillin G potassium, pentazocine, phytonadione, piperacillin, piperacillin/tazobactam, potassium chloride, prednisolone, procainamide, prochlorperazine, propofol, propranolol, pyridostigmine, ranitidine, remifentanil, sargramostim, scopolamine, sodium bicarbonate, streptokinase, succinylcholine, tacrolimus, teniposide, theophylline, thiopental, thiotepa, ticarcillin, ticarcillin/clavulanate, trimethobenzamide, vecuronium, vinblastine, vincristine, vinorelbine, warfarin, zidovudine

Perform/provide:
• Storage in tight container

Evaluate:
• Therapeutic response: decrease of deep-vein thrombosis, PTT 1.5-2.5 × control, free flowing IV

Teach patient/family:
• To avoid OTC preparations that may cause serious drug interactions unless directed by prescriber
• That drug may be held during active bleeding (menstruation), depending on condition
• To use soft-bristle toothbrush to avoid bleeding gums, avoid contact sports, use electric razor, avoid IM injection
• To carry a Medic Alert ID identifying drug taken

• To report any signs of bleeding: gums, under skin, urine, stools
Treatment of overdose: Withdraw drug, protamine SO_4 1:1 solution

---

hepatitis B immune globulin (R)
Bay Hep B, Nabi-HB
Func. class.: Immune globulin

Action: Provides passive immunity to hepatitis B

Uses: Prevention of hepatitis B virus in exposed patients, including passive immunity in neonates born to HBsAg-positive mother

Dosage and routes:
Acute exposure to blood with HBsAg
• *Adult:* 2 doses, given after exposure and 1 mo later

Perinatal exposure of infants born to HBsAg-positive mothers
• *Infant:* 1 dose at birth, then start hepatitis B vaccine series soon after birth

Sexual exposure to HBsAg
• *Adult:* Administer 1 dose within 2 wk of exposure

Available forms:
Bay Hep B: Sol for inj 15%-18% protein
Nabi-HB: Sol for inj 5% ± 1% protein

Side effects/adverse reactions:
INTEG: Soreness at injection site, urticaria, erythema, swelling
SYST: Induration
CNS: Headache, dizziness, fever
GI: Nausea, vomiting
SYST: **Anaphylaxis, angioedema**

Contraindications: Hypersensitivity to immune globulins, coagulation disorders

Precautions: Pregnancy (C), elderly, lactation, children; active infection, IgA deficiency

---

NURSING CONSIDERATIONS
Assess:
• For history of allergies, skin conditions (eczema, psoriasis, dermatitis), reactions to vaccinations
• For skin reactions: rash, induration, urticaria
◆ For anaphylaxis: inability to breathe, bronchospasm, hypotension, wheezing, diaphoresis, fever, flushing

Administer:
• After rotating vial; do not shake
• Only with epinephrine 1:1000 on unit to treat laryngospasm
• In deltoid for better absorption (adult)

Perform/provide:
• Written record of immunization
• Comfort measures

Evaluate:
• Prevention of hepatitis B

Teach patient/family:
• That discomfort may occur at site
• To report any rash, wheezing, inability to breathe immediately

---

hetastarch (℞)
(het'a-starch)
Hespan
Func. class.: Plasma expander
Chem. class.: Synthetic polymer

Action: Similar to human albumin, which expands plasma volume by colloidal osmotic pressure

Uses: Plasma volume expander, leukapheresis

Dosage and routes:
• *Adult:* **IV INF** 500-1000 ml (30-60 g), total dose not to exceed 1500 ml/day, not to exceed 20 ml/kg/hr (hemorrhagic shock)

Leukapheresis
• *Adult:* **IV INF** 250-700 ml infused at 1:8 ratio with whole blood, may be repeated 2/wk up to 10 treatments

Available forms: 6% hetastarch/ 0.9% NaCl inj

Side effects/adverse reactions:
HEMA: Decreased hematocrit, platelet function, increased bleeding/ coagulation times, increased sed rate
INTEG: Rash, urticaria, pruritus, angioedema, chills, fever, flushing, peripheral edema
RESP: Wheezing, dyspnea, ***bronchospasm, pulmonary edema***
GI: Nausea, vomiting
EENT: Periorbital edema
SYST: ***Anaphylaxis***
CNS: Headache

Contraindications: Hypersensitivity, severe bleeding disorders, renal failure, CHF (severe)

Precautions: Pregnancy (C), liver disease, pulmonary edema

Pharmacokinetics:
IV: Expands blood volume 1-2 × amount infused, excreted in urine

Lab test interferences:
False increase: Bilirubin

NURSING CONSIDERATIONS
Assess:
• VS q5min × 30 min; CVP during infusion (5-10 cm H$_2$O normal range), PCWP
• Monitor CBC with differential, Hgb, Hct, PT, PTT, platelet count, clotting time during treatment; Hct may drop; do not allow to drop >30% by vol
• Urine output q1h, watch for increase in urinary output, which is common; if output does not increase, infusion should be decreased or discontinued
• I&O ratio and specific gravity, urine osmolarity; if specific gravity is very low, renal clearance is low; drug should be discontinued

---

Side effects: *italics* = common; ***bold italics*** = life-threatening

• Allergy: rash, urticaria, pruritus, wheezing, dyspnea, bronchospasm; drug should be discontinued immediately

◆ For circulatory overload: increased pulse, respirations, dyspnea, wheezing, chest tightness, chest pain
• For dehydration after infusion: decreased output, fever, poor skin turgor, increased specific gravity, dry skin

Administer:
IV
• INF undiluted, run at 20 ml/kg/hr (1.2 g/kg); reduced rate in septic shock, burns

Additive compatibilities: Cloxacillin, fosphenytoin

Y-site compatibilities: Cimetidine, diltiazem, enalaprilat
• Storage at room temperature; discard unused portion, do not freeze, do not use if turbid or deep brown or if precipitate forms

Evaluate:
• Therapeutic response: increased plasma volume

Teach patient/family:
• When to notify prescriber

RARELY USED

hyaluronidase (℞)
(hye-al-yoor-on'i-dase)
Wydase
Func. class.: Enzyme

Uses: Hypodermoclysis, subcutaneous urography; adjunct to dispersion of other drugs
Dosage and routes:
Adjunct
• *Adult and child:* **INJ** 150 U with other drug
Urography
• *Adult and child:* **SC** 75 U over

scapula, then contrast medium injected at same site
Hypodermoclysis
• *Adult and child >3 yr:* **SC** 150 U/L of lysis sol

Contraindications: Hypersensitivity to bovine products, CHF, hypoproteinemia, around infected/inflamed or cancerous area

---

hydralazine (℞)
(hye-dral'a-zeen)
Alazine, Apresoline,
hydralazine HCl, Novo-
Hylazin*, Pralzine, Rolzine,
Supres*
Func. class.: Antihypertensive, direct-acting peripheral vasodilator
Chem. class.: Phthalazine

Action: Vasodilates arteriolar smooth muscle by direct relaxation; reduction in blood pressure with reflex increases in cardiac function

Uses: Essential hypertension; severe essential hypertension, CHF
Dosage and routes:
• *Adult:* **PO** 10 mg qid 2-4 days, then 25 mg for rest of first wk, then 50 mg qid individualized to desired response, not to exceed 300 mg qd; **IV/IM BOL** 20-40 mg q4-6h, administer **PO** as soon as possible; **IM** 20-40 mg q4-6h
• *Child:* **PO** 0.75-3 mg/kg/day in 4 divided doses, max 7.5 mg/kg/24 hr; **IV BOL** 0.1-0.2 mg/kg q4-6h; **IM** 0.1-0.2 mg/kg q4-6h
Available forms: Inj 20 mg/ml; tabs 10, 25, 50, 100 mg
Side effects/adverse reactions:
MISC: Nasal congestion, muscle cramps, *lupuslike symptoms*
CV: Palpitations, reflex tachycar-

*dia, angina, **shock,*** edema, rebound hypertension

CNS: Headache, tremors, dizziness, anxiety, peripheral neuritis, depression

GI: Nausea, vomiting, anorexia, diarrhea, constipation

INTEG: Rash, pruritus

*HEMA: **Leukopenia, agranulocytosis,*** anemia, ***thrombocytopenia***

GU: Impotence, urinary retention, Na, H_2O retention

Contraindications: Hypersensitivity to hydralazines, coronary artery disease, mitral valvular rheumatic heart disease, rheumatic heart disease

Precautions: Pregnancy (C), CVA, advanced renal disease, elderly

Do not confuse:
Apresoline/allopurinol

Pharmacokinetics:
PO: Onset 20-30 min, peak 1 hr, duration 2-4 hr
IM: Onset 5-10 min, peak 1 hr, duration 2-4 hr
IV: Onset 5-20 min, peak 10-80 min, duration 2-6 hr; half-life 2-8 hr; metabolized by liver; less than 10% present in urine

Interactions:
• Increased tachycardia, angina: sympathomimetics (epinephrine, norepinephrine)
• Increased effects of β-blockers
• Severe hypotension: MAOIs

NURSING CONSIDERATIONS
Assess:
• B/P q5min × 2 hr, then q1h × 2 hr, then q4h
• Pulse, jugular venous distention q4h
• Electrolytes, blood studies: K, Na, Cl, CO_2, CBC, serum glucose
• Weight daily, I&O
• LE prep, ANA titer before starting therapy and during treatment; assess for fever, joint pain, rash, sore throat (lupuslike symptoms); notify prescriber
• Edema in feet, legs daily
• Skin turgor, dryness of mucous membranes for hydration status
• Rales, dyspnea, orthopnea
• IV site for extravasation, rate
• Fever, joint pain, tachycardia, palpitations, headache, nausea
• Mental status: affect, mood, behavior, anxiety; check for personality changes

Administer:
• Give with meals (PO) to enhance absorption
• To recumbent patient, keep for 1 hr after administration

IV
• IV undiluted; give through Y-tube or 3-way stopcock each 10 mg ≤min

Additive compatibilities: Dobutamine

Y-site compatibilities: Heparin, hydrocortisone, potassium chloride, verapamil, vit B/C

Evaluate:
• Therapeutic response: decreased B/P

Teach patient/family:
• To take with food to increase bioavailability (PO)
• To avoid OTC preparations unless directed by prescriber
• To notify prescriber if chest pain, severe fatigue, fever, muscle or joint pain occurs
• To rise slowly to prevent orthostatic hypotension
• To notify prescriber if pregnancy is suspected

Treatment of overdose: Administer vasopressors, volume expanders for shock; if PO, lavage or give activated charcoal, digitalization

hydrochlorothiazide (℞)

(hye-droe-klor-oh-thye'a-zide)
Diaqua, Diuchlor H*, Esidrix, Ezide, Hydro-Chlor, hydrochlorothiazide, HydroDiuril, Hydromal, Hydro-Par, Hydro-T, Hydrozide*, Microzide, Neo-Codema*, Novohydrazide*, Oretic, Thiuretic, Urozide*

Func. class.: Thiazide diuretic, antihypertensive

Chem. class.: Sulfonamide derivative

Action: Acts on distal tubule and ascending limb of loop of Henle by increasing excretion of water, sodium, chloride, potassium

Uses: Edema, hypertension, diuresis, CHF; edema in corticosteroid, estrogen, NSAIDs, idiopathic lower extremity edema therapy

Dosage and routes:

• *Adult:* **PO** 25-100 mg/day
• *Geriatric:* **PO** 12.5 mg/day, initially
• *Child >6 mo:* **PO** 2 mg/kg/day in divided doses
• *Child <6 mo:* **PO** up to 4 mg/kg/day in divided doses

Available forms: Tabs 25, 50, 100 mg; sol 50 mg/5 ml, 100 mg/ml

Side effects/adverse reactions:

GU: Urinary frequency, polyuria, **uremia, glucosuria,** hyperurecemia
CNS: Drowsiness, paresthesia, depression, headache, *dizziness, fatigue, weakness,* fever
GI: Nausea, vomiting, anorexia, constipation, diarrhea, cramps, pancreatitis, GI irritation, **hepatitis**
EENT: Blurred vision
INTEG: Rash, urticaria, purpura, photosensitivity, alopecia, erythema multiforme
META: Hyperglycemia, hyperuricemia, increased creatinine, BUN
HEMA: **Aplastic anemia, hemolytic anemia, leukopenia, agranulocytosis, thrombocytopenia, neutropenia**
CV: Irregular pulse, orthostatic hypotension, palpitations, volume depletion, allergic myocarditis
ELECT: **Hypokalemia,** hypercalcemia, hyponatremia, hypochloremia, hypomagnesemia

Contraindications: Hypersensitivity to thiazides or sulfonamides, anuria, renal decompensation, hypomagnesemia

Precautions: Hypokalemia, renal disease, pregnancy (B), lactation, hepatic disease, gout, COPD, LE, diabetes mellitus, hyperlipidemia, CrCl <25 ml/min

Pharmacokinetics:

PO: Onset 2 hr, peak 4 hr, duration 6-12 hr, half-life 6-15 hr; excreted unchanged by kidneys; crosses placenta; enters breast milk

Interactions:

• Increased toxicity of lithium, nondepolarizing skeletal muscle relaxants, cardiac glycosides
• Decreased effects of antidiabetics
• Decreased absorption of thiazides: cholestyramine, colestipol
• Increased risk of renal failure: NSAIDs
• Hyperglycemia, hyperuricemia, increased antihypertensives: diazoxide
• Hypokalemia: glucocorticoids, amphotericin B
• Increased effects: loop diuretics
🍃 Potassium deficiency: aloe, buckthorn bark/berry, cascara sagrada bark, licorice root, senna pod/leaf

Lab test interferences:

Increase: BSP retention, amylase, parathyroid test
Decrease: PBI, PSP

◆ = Nursing alert   🍃 = Herb-drug interaction   🚫 = Do not crush

hydrocodone 493

NURSING CONSIDERATIONS
Assess:
• Weight, I&O daily to determine fluid loss; effect of drug may be decreased if used qd
• Rate, depth, rhythm of respiration, effect of exertion
• B/P lying, standing; postural hypotension may occur
• Electrolytes: K, Mg, Na, Cl; include BUN, blood sugar, CBC, serum creatinine, blood pH, ABGs, uric acid, Ca; renal function
• Glucose in urine if patient is diabetic
• Signs of metabolic alkalosis: drowsiness, restlessness
• Signs of hypokalemia: postural hypotension, malaise, fatigue, tachycardia, leg cramps, weakness, dehydration
• Rashes, temp qd
• Confusion, especially in elderly; take safety precautions if needed
Administer:
• In AM to avoid interference with sleep if using drug as a diuretic
• K replacement if K <3 mg/dl
• With food; if nausea occurs, absorption may be decreased slightly
Evaluate:
• Therapeutic response: improvement in edema of feet, legs, sacral area qd, decreased B/P
Teach patient/family:
• To increase fluid intake to 2-3 L/day unless contraindicated; to rise slowly from lying or sitting position
• To notify prescriber of muscle weakness, cramps, nausea, dizziness
• That drug may be taken with food or milk
• To use sunscreen for photosensitivity
• That blood sugar may be increased in diabetics
• To take early in day to avoid nocturia

Treatment of overdose: Lavage if taken orally; monitor electrolytes; administer dextrose in saline; monitor hydration, CV, renal status

---

hydrocodone (℞)
(hye-droe-koe'done)
Hycodan, Robidone*, Tussigon
hydrocodone/acetaminophen
Allay, Anexsia, Anolor DH, Bancap HC, Co-Gesic, Dolacet, Dolagesic, Duocet, Hycomed, Hyco-Pap, Hydrocet, Hydrogesic, Lorcet, Lortab, Onset, Pancet, Panlor, Polygesic, Stagesic, T-Gesic, Ugesic, Vanacet, Vandone, Vicodin, Zydone
hydrocodone/aspirin
Azdone, Damason-P, Lortab ASA, Panasal
hydrocodone/ibuprofen
Vicoprofen
Func. class.: Antitussive opioid analgesic

Controlled Substance Schedule III
Action: Acts directly on cough center in medulla to suppress cough; binds to opiate receptors in CNS to reduce pain
Uses: Hyperactive and nonproductive cough, mild pain
Dosage and routes:
• *Adult:* **PO** 5-10 mg q4h prn
• *Child:* **PO** 1.25-5 mg q4h prn or 0.2 mg/kg q3-4h
Available forms: Syr 5 mg/5 ml; tabs 5 mg (long-acting)
Side effects/adverse reactions:
CNS: Drowsiness, dizziness, lightheadedness, confusion, headache, se-

* = Canada only   Side effects: *italics* = common; ***bold italics*** = life-threatening

dation, euphoria, dysphoria, weakness, hallucinations, disorientation, mood changes, dependence, ***convulsions***

GI: Nausea, vomiting, anorexia, constipation, cramps, dry mouth

GU: Increased urinary output, dysuria, urinary retention

INTEG: Rash, urticaria, flushing, pruritus

EENT: Tinnitus, blurred vision, miosis, diplopia

CV: Palpitations, tachycardia, bradycardia, change in B/P, ***circulatory depression,*** syncope

*RESP: **Respiratory depression***

Contraindications: Hypersensitivity, addiction (narcotic)

Precautions: Addictive personality, pregnancy (C), lactation, increased intracranial pressure, MI (acute), severe heart disease, respiratory depression, hepatic disease, renal disease

Do not confuse:

hydrocodone/hydrocortisone
Hycodan/Vicodin

Pharmacokinetics: Onset 10-20 min, duration 4-6 hr, half-life 3½-4½ hr; metabolized in liver; excreted in urine; crosses placenta

Interactions:

• Increased CNS depression: alcohol, opioids, sedative/hypnotics, phenothiazines, skeletal muscle relaxants, general anesthetics, tricyclics

Lab test interferences:

Increase: Amylase, lipase

NURSING CONSIDERATIONS

Assess:

• Pain: intensity, type, location, and other characteristics

• CNS changes: dizziness, drowsiness, hallucinations, euphoria, LOC, pupil reaction

• Allergic reactions: rash, urticaria

• Cough and respiratory dysfunction: respiratory depression, character, rate, rhythm; notify prescriber if respirations are <10/min

• Need for pain medication, physical dependence

Administer:

• With antiemetic after meals if nausea or vomiting occurs

Perform/provide:

• Storage in light-resistant area at room temperature

• Assistance with ambulation

• Safety measures: night-light, call bell within easy reach

Evaluate:

• Therapeutic response: decrease in pain or cough

Teach patient/family:

• To report any symptoms of CNS changes, allergic reactions

• That physical dependency may result when used for extended periods

• That withdrawal symptoms may occur: nausea, vomiting, cramps, fever, faintness, anorexia

🚫 Not to break, crush, or chew tabs

• To avoid driving, other hazardous activities, drowsiness occurs

• To avoid other CNS depressants, will enhance sedating properties of this drug

Treatment of overdose: Naloxone HCl (Narcan) 0.2-0.8 mg IV, O_2, IV fluids, vasopressors

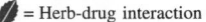

hydrocortisone (R)
(hy-dro-kor'tih-sone)
Cortef, Cortenema, Hydrocortone
hydrocortisone acetate (R)
Cortifoam, Hydrocortone Acetate
hydrocortisone cypionate (R)
Cortef
hydrocortisone sodium phosphate (R)
Hydrocortone Phosphate
hydrocortisone sodium succinate (R)
A-hydroCort, Solu-Cortef
Func. class.: Corticosteroid
Chem. class.: Short-acting glucocorticoid

Action: Decreases inflammation by suppression of migration of polymorphonuclear leukocytes, fibroblasts, reversal of increased capillary permeability and lysosomal stabilization

Uses: Severe inflammation, septic shock, adrenal insufficiency, ulcerative colitis, collagen disorders

Dosage and routes:
Adrenal insufficiency/inflammation
• *Adult:* **PO** 5-30 mg bid-qid; **IM/IV** 100-250 mg (succinate), then 50-100 mg **IM** as needed; **IM/IV** 15-240 mg q12h (phosphate)

Shock
• *Adult:* 500 mg-2 g q2-6h (succinate)
• *Child:* **IM/IV** 0.186-1 mg/kg bid-tid (succinate)

Colitis
• *Adult:* **ENEMA** 100 mg nightly for 21 days

Available forms: Tabs 5, 10, 20 mg; inj 25, 50 mg/ml; enema 100 mg/60 ml; acetate—inj 25*, 50 mg/ml*,

enema 10% aerosol foam; supp 25 mg; cypionate—oral susp 10 mg/5 ml; phosphate—inj 50 mg/ml; succinate inj 100 mg*, 250 mg*, 500 mg*, 1000 mg/vial*

Side effects/adverse reactions:
CNS: Depression, flushing, sweating, headache, mood changes
CV: Hypertension, **circulatory collapse, thrombophlebitis, embolism,** tachycardia, edema
EENT: Fungal infections, increased intraocular pressure, blurred vision
GI: Diarrhea, nausea, abdominal distention, **GI hemorrhage,** increased appetite, *pancreatitis*
HEMA: **Thrombocytopenia**
INTEG: Acne, poor wound healing, ecchymosis, petechiae
MS: Fractures, osteoporosis, weakness

Contraindications: Psychosis, hypersensitivity, idiopathic thrombocytopenia, acute glomerulonephritis, amebiasis, fungal infections, nonasthmatic bronchial disease, child <2 yr, AIDS, TB

Precautions: Pregnancy (C), lactation, diabetes mellitus, glaucoma, osteoporosis, seizure disorders, ulcerative colitis, CHF, myasthenia gravis, renal disease, esophagitis, peptic ulcer

Do not confuse:
hydrocortisone/hydrocodone

Pharmacokinetics:
PO: Onset 1-2 hr, peak 1 hr, duration 1-1½ days
IM/IV: Onset 20 min, peak 4-8 hr, duration 1-1½ days
RECT: Onset 3-5 days
Metabolized by liver, excreted in urine (17-OHCS, 17-KS), crosses placenta

Interactions:
• Decreased action of hydrocortisone: cholestyramine, colestipol, barbiturates, rifampin, ephedrine, phenytoin, theophylline

• Decreased effects of anticoagulants, anticonvulsants, antidiabetics, toxoids, vaccines

• Increased side effects: alcohol, amphotericin B, digitalis, cyclosporine, diuretics

• Risk of GI bleeding: salicylates, NSAIDs

 Potassium deficiency: aloe, buckthorn, cascara sagrada, senna

Lab test interferences:

Increase: Cholesterol, Na, blood glucose, uric acid, Ca, urine glucose

Decrease: Ca, K, T_4, T_3, thyroid ^{131}I uptake test, urine 17-OHCS, 17-KS

False negative: Skin allergy tests

NURSING CONSIDERATIONS

Assess:

• K, blood sugar, urine glucose while on long-term therapy; hypokalemia and hyperglycemia

• Weight daily, notify prescriber of weekly gain >5 lb

• B/P q4h, pulse; notify prescriber of chest pain

• I&O ratio; be alert for decreasing urinary output, increasing edema

• Plasma cortisol levels during long-term therapy (normal level: 138-635 nmol/L SI units when drawn at 8 AM)

• Infection: increased temp, WBC, even after withdrawal of medication; drug masks infection

• K depletion: paresthesias, fatigue, nausea, vomiting, depression, polyuria, dysrhythmias, weakness

• Edema, hypertension, cardiac symptoms

• Mental status: affect, mood, behavioral changes, aggression

Administer:

• Daily dose in AM for better results

• IM inj deep in large muscle mass; rotate sites; avoid deltoid; use 21G needle

• In one dose in AM to prevent adrenal suppression; avoid SC administration; may damage tissue

• With food or milk for GI symptoms (PO)

• Rectal: telling patient to retain for 20 min if possible

IV

• Phosphate: IV undiluted or added to dextrose or saline inj and given by infusion; give 25 mg or less/min

• Succinate: IV in mix-o-vial, or reconstitute 250 mg or less/2 ml bacteriostatic H_2O for inj; mix gently; give direct IV over 1 min or more; may be further diluted in 100, 250, 500, or 1000 ml of D_5W, D_5 0.9%, NaCl 0.9% given over ordered rate

Sodium phosphate preparations

Additive compatibilities: Amikacin, amphotericin B, bleomycin, cephapirin, metaraminol, sodium bicarbonate, verapamil

Syringe compatibilities: Metoclopramide

Y-site compatibilities: Allopurinol, amifostine, aztreonam, cefepime, cladribine, famotidine, filgrastim, fluconazole, fludarabine, granisetron, melphalan, ondansetron, paclitaxel, piperacillin/tazobactam, teniposide, thiotepa, vinorelbine

Sodium succinate preparations

Additive compatibilities: Amikacin, aminophylline, amphotericin B, calcium chloride, calcium gluconate, cephalothin, cephapirin, chloramphenicol, clindamycin, cloxacillin, corticotropin, daunorubicin, diphenhydramine, dopamine, erythromycin, floxacillin, lidocaine, magnesium sulfate, mephentermine, metronidazole/sodium bicarbonate, mitomycin, mitoxantrone, netilmicin, netilmicin/potassium chloride, norepinephrine, penicillin G potassium/sodium, piperacillin, polymyxin B, potassium chloride, sodium bicarbonate, theophylline, thiopental, vancomycin, verapamil, vit B/C

Syringe compatibilities: Metoclopramide, thiopental

Y-site compatibilities: Acyclovir, allopurinol, amifostine, aminophylline, amphotericin B cholesteryl, ampicillin, amrinone, amsacrine, atracurium, atropine, aztreonam, betamethasone, calcium gluconate, cefepime, cefmetazole, cephalothin, cephapirin, chlordiazepoxide, chlorpromazine, cisatracurium, cladribine, cyanocobalamin, cytarabine, dexamethasone, digoxin, diphenhydramine, dopamine, doxorubicin liposome, droperidol, edrophonium, enalaprilat, epinephrine, esmolol, estrogens conjugated, ethacrynate, famotidine, fentanyl, fentanyl/droperidol, filgrastim, fludarabine, fluorouracil, foscarnet, furosemide, gallium, granisetron, heparin, hydralazine, insulin (regular), isoproterenol, kanamycin, lidocaine, lorazepam, magnesium sulfate, melphalan, menadiol, meperidine, methicillin, methoxamine, methylergonovine, minocycline, morphine, neostigmine, norepinephrine, ondansetron, oxacillin, oxytocin, paclitaxel, pancuronium, penicillin G potassium, pentazocine, phytonadione, piperacillin/tazobactam, prednisolone, procainamide, prochlorperazine, propofol, propranolol, pyridostigmine, remifentanil, scopolamine, sodium bicarbonate, succinylcholine, tacrolimus, teniposide, theophylline, thiotepa, trimethaphan, trimethobenzamide, vecuronium, vinorelbine

Perform/provide:

• Assistance with ambulation in patient with bone tissue disease to prevent fractures

Evaluate:

• Therapeutic response: ease of respirations, decreased inflammation

Teach patient/family:

• That ID as steroid user should be carried

• To notify prescriber if therapeutic response decreases; dosage adjustment may be needed; of signs of infection

• Not to discontinue abruptly, or adrenal crisis can result; drug should be tapered off

• To avoid OTC products: salicylates, alcohol in cough products, cold preparations unless directed by prescriber

• About cushingoid symptoms of adrenal insufficiency: nausea, anorexia, fatigue, dizziness, dyspnea, weakness, joint pain

H

---

hydromorphone (℞)

(hye-droe-mor'fone)
Dilaudid, Dilaudid HP, hydromorphone HCl, PMS-Hydromorphone
Func. class.: Opiate analgesic
Chem. class.: Semisynthetic phenanthrene

Controlled Substance Schedule II

Action: Inhibits ascending pain pathways in CNS, increases pain threshold, alters pain perception

Uses: Moderate to severe pain, nonproductive cough

Dosage and routes:

• *Adult:* **PO** 1-6 mg q4-6h prn; **IM/SC/IV** 2-4 mg q4-6h; **RECT** 3 mg q4-6h prn

• *Geriatric:* **PO** 1-2 mg q4-6h

• *Child:* 0.03-0.08 mg/kg q4-6h, max 5 mg/dose

Antitussive

• *Adult:* **PO** 1 mg q3-4h prn

Available forms: Inj 1, 2, 3, 4, 10 mg/ml; tabs 1, 2, 3, 4, 8 mg; supp 3 mg; oral sol 5 mg/5 ml; syrup 1 mg/5 ml

---

Side effects/adverse reactions:
CNS: Drowsiness, dizziness, confusion, headache, sedation, euphoria, mood changes, ***seizures***
GI: Nausea, vomiting, anorexia, constipation, cramps, dry mouth
GU: Increased urinary output, dysuria, urinary retention
INTEG: Rash, urticaria, bruising, flushing, diaphoresis, pruritus
EENT: Tinnitus, blurred vision, miosis, diplopia
CV: Palpitations, bradycardia, change in B/P, hypotension, tachycardia
*RESP: **Respiratory depression***
Contraindications: Hypersensitivity, addiction (opiate)
Precautions: Addictive personality, pregnancy (C), lactation, increased intracranial pressure, MI (acute), severe heart disease, respiratory depression, hepatic disease, renal disease, child <18 yr
Do not confuse:
Dilaudid/Demerol
hydromorphone/meperidine
hydromorphone/morphine
Pharmacokinetics: Onset 15-30 min, peak ½-1 hr, duration 4-5 hr; metabolized by liver; excreted by kidneys; crosses placenta; excreted in breast milk, half-life 2-3 hr
Interactions:
• Effects may be increased with other CNS depressants: alcohol, opiates, sedative/hypnotics, antipsychotics, skeletal muscle relaxants
⧸ Increased action: kava
Lab test interferences:
Increase: Amylase
NURSING CONSIDERATIONS
Assess:
• I&O ratio; check for decreasing output; may indicate urinary retention
• CNS changes: dizziness, drowsiness, hallucinations, euphoria, LOC, pupil reaction
• Bowel function, constipation

• Allergic reactions: rash, urticaria
• Respiratory dysfunction: respiratory depression, character, rate, rhythm; notify prescriber if respirations are <10/min
• Need for pain medication, physical dependence
• Pain control, sedation by scoring on 0-10 scale, ATC dosing is best for pain control
Administer:
• With antiemetic if nausea, vomiting occur
• When pain is beginning to return; determine interval by response
• Rotate inj sites when giving SC
IV
• Direct, diluted with 5 ml sterile H$_2$O or NS; give through Y-connector or 3-way stopcock; give 2 mg or less/3-5 min
• IV INF: Dilute each 0.1-1 mg/ml NS (0.1-1 mg/ml), deliver by narcotic syringe infusor; may be diluted in D$_5$W, D$_5$/NaCl, 0.45% NaCl, or NS for larger amounts and delivery through an infusion pump
Additive compatibilities: Bupivacaine, fluorouracil, midazolam, ondansetron, promethazine, verapamil
Solution compatibilities: D$_5$W, D$_5$/0.45% NaCl, D$_5$/0.9% NaCl, D$_5$/LR, D$_5$/Ringer's sol, 0.45% NaCl, 0.9% NaCl, Ringer's and lactated Ringer's sol
Syringe compatibilities: Atropine, bupivacaine, ceftazidime, chlorpromazine, cimetidine, dimenhydrinate, diphenhydramine, fentanyl, glycopyrrolate, haloperidol, hydroxyzine, lorazepam, midazolam, pentazocine, pentobarbital, prochlorperazine, promethazine, ranitidine, scopolamine, tetracaine, thiethylperazine, trimethobenzamide
Y-site compatibilities: Acyclovir, allopurinol, amifostine, amikacin, amsacrine, aztreonam, cefamandole,

---

◆ = Nursing alert   ⧸ = Herb-drug interaction   ⊘ = Do not crush cefazolin, cefepime, cefmetazole, cefoperazone, cefotaxime, cefoxitin, ceftazidime, ceftizoxime, cefuroxime, cephalothin, cephapirin, chloramphenicol, cisatracurium, cisplatin, cladribine, clindamycin, cyclophosphamide, cytarabine, diltiazem, dobutamine, dopamine, doxorubicin, doxorubicin liposome, doxycycline, epinephrine, erythromycin lactobionate, famotidine, fentanyl, filgrastim, fludarabine, foscarnet, furosemide, gentamicin, granisetron, heparin, kanamycin, labetalol, lorazepam, magnesium sulfate, melphalan, methotrexate, metronidazole, mezlocillin, midazolam, milrinone, morphine, moxalactam, nafcillin, nicardipine, nitroglycerin, norepinephrine, ondansetron, oxacillin, paclitaxel, penicillin G potassium, piperacillin, piperacillin/tazobactam, propofol, ranitidine, remifentanil, teniposide, thiotepa, ticarcillin, tobramycin, trimethoprim-sulfamethoxazole, vancomycin, vecuronium, vinorelbine

Perform/provide:
• Storage in light-resistant area at room temperature
• Assistance with ambulation
• Safety measures: side rails, nightlight, call bell within easy reach

Evaluate:
• Therapeutic response: decrease in pain

Teach patient/family:
• To report any symptoms of CNS changes, allergic reactions
• That physical dependency may result when used for extended periods
• That withdrawal symptoms may occur: nausea, vomiting, cramps, fever, faintness, anorexia
• To avoid driving, other hazardous activities, drowsiness occurs

Treatment of overdose: Naloxone HCl (Narcan) 0.2-0.8 mg IV, O₂, IV fluids, vasopressors

hydromorphone/guaifenesin/alcohol (Rx)
(hye-droe-mor′fone)
Dilaudid Cough Syrup
Func. class.: Antitussive, opioid
Chem. class.: Phenanthrene derivative

Controlled Substance Schedule II
Action: Increases respiratory tract fluid by decreasing surface tension, adhesiveness, which increases removal of mucus; analgesic, antitussive suppresses the cough reflex by a direct central action
Uses: Cough
Dosage and routes:
• *Adult:* **PO** 1 mg q3-4h prn
Available forms: Syr 1 mg/5 ml
Side effects/adverse reactions:
CNS: Dizziness, drowsiness
GI: Nausea, constipation, vomiting, anorexia
CV: Hypotension
INTEG: Urticaria, rash
*RESP: **Respiratory depression***
Contraindications: Hypersensitivity, increased intracranial pressure, status asthmaticus
Precautions: Hypothyroidism, Addison's disease, CNS depression, brain tumor, asthma, hepatic disease, renal disease, COPD, psychosis, alcoholism, convulsive disorders, pregnancy (C), lactation
Pharmacokinetics: Metabolized by liver; half-life 2-4 hr
• Enhanced CNS depression: barbiturates, opioids, antipsychotics, antidepressants
⚫ Increased action: kava
NURSING CONSIDERATIONS
Assess:
• VS, cardiac status, including hypotension
• Respiratory rate, depth

• Cough: type, frequency, character, including sputum

Administer:
• Decreased dose to elderly patients; metabolism may be slowed

Perform/provide:
• Storage at room temperature
• Increased fluids, bulk, exercise to decrease constipation

Evaluate:
• Therapeutic response: absence of cough

Teach patient/family:
• To avoid driving, other hazardous activities until patient stabilized on medication if drowsiness occurs
• To avoid alcohol, other CNS depressants; will enhance sedating properties of this drug
• May be taken with food for GI upset
• Physical dependency may result when used for extended periods of time

---

RARELY USED

hydroquinone (R)
(hye-droh'quin-ohn)
Func. class.: Depigmentating agent

Uses: Bleaching skin, including age spots, freckles, lentigo, chloasma

Dosage and routes:
• *Adult and child:* **TOP** apply to affected area qd-bid

Contraindications: Hypersensitivity, inflamed skin, prickly heat, sunburn

hydroxocobalamin (vit B$_{12}$) (R)
(hye-drox'-o-ko-bal'a-min)
Acti-B$_{12}$*, Alphamin, Hydrobexan, Hydro-Cristi 12, Hydroxo-12, hydroxycobalamin, LA-12
Func. class.: Vitamin
Chem. class.: B$_{12}$—water-soluble vitamin

Action: Needed for adequate nerve functioning, protein and carbohydrate metabolism, normal growth, RBC development

Uses: Vit B$_{12}$ deficiency, pernicious anemia, vit B$_{12}$ malabsorption syndrome, Schilling test

Dosage and routes:
Vitamin B$_{12}$ deficiency
Adult: **IM** 30-100 µg qd × 5-10 days, maintenance 100-200 mg **IM** qmo
Child: **IM** 1-30 µg qd × 5-10 days, maintenance 60 µg **IM** qmo or more often
Pernicious anemia/malabsorption syndrome
• *Adult:* **IM** 100-1000 µg qd × 2 wk, then 100-1000 µg **IM** qmo
• *Child:* **IM** 1000-5000 µg × 2 wk or more given in 100-500 µg doses, then 60 µg **IM/SC** qmo
Schilling test
• *Adult and child:* **IM** 1000 µg in one dose
Available forms: Inj 1000 µg/ml
Side effects/adverse reactions:
CNS: Flushing, optic nerve atrophy
GI: Diarrhea
CV: **CHF,** peripheral vascular thrombosis, *pulmonary edema*
INTEG: Itching, rash
Contraindications: Hypersensitivity, optic nerve atrophy, cardiac disease
Precautions: Pregnancy (A), (C) if

◆ = Nursing alert   ✐ = Herb-drug interaction   ⊘ = Do not crush

used above RDA level, lactation, children

Pharmacokinetics: Stored in liver, kidneys, stomach; 50%-90% excreted in urine; crosses placenta, breast milk

Interactions:

• Decreased absorption of hydroxocobalamin: aminoglycosides, anticonvulsants, colchicine, chloramphenicol, antineoplastics, cimetidine, alcohol, vit C, K preparations

Lab test interferences:

False positive: Intrinsic factor

NURSING CONSIDERATIONS

Assess:

• K levels during beginning treatment

• CBC for increased reticulocyte count during first week of therapy, followed by increase in RBC and hemoglobin

• For pulmonary edema or worsening of CHF in cardiac patients

Administer:

• By IM inj for pernicious anemia unless contraindicated

Evaluate:

• Therapeutic response: decreased anorexia, dyspnea on excretion, palpitations, paresthesias, psychosis, visual disturbances

Teach patient/family:

• That treatment must continue for life in pernicious anemia

• The importance of a well-balanced diet

---

hydroxychloro-quine (℞)

(hye-drox-ee-klor'oh-kwin)

Plaquenil

Func. class.: Antimalarial

Chem. class.: 4-Aminoquinoline derivative

Action: Inhibits parasite replications, transcription of DNA to RNA by forming complexes with DNA in parasite

Uses: Malaria caused by *Plasmodium vivax, P. malariae, P. ovale, P. falciparum* (some strains): LE, rheumatoid arthritis

Dosage and routes:

Malaria

• *Adult:* **PO** suppression or prevention 200 mg qwk, begin 1-2 wk before travel, continue 4 wk after returning; treatment 400 mg, then 200 mg at 6, 24, 48 hr after 1st dose

• *Child:* **PO** suppression or prevention 5 mg/kg qwk, begin 1-2 wk before travel, continue 4 wk after returning; treatment 10 mg/kg, then 5 mg/kg at 6, 24, 48 hr after 1st dose

Lupus erythematosus

• *Adult:* **PO** 400 mg qd-bid; length depends on patient response; maintenance 200-400 mg qd

Rheumatoid arthritis

• *Adult:* **PO** 400-600 mg qd for 4-12 wk; then 200-300 mg qd after good response

• *Child:* **PO** 3-5 mg/kg/day max 400 mg/day

Available forms: Tabs 200 mg

Side effects/adverse reactions:

CV: Hypotension, heart block, *asystole with syncope*

INTEG: Pruritus, pigmentation changes, skin eruptions, lichen planus–like eruptions, eczema, *exfoliative dermatitis,* alopecia

CNS: Headache, stimulation, fatigue, irritability, *convulsions,* bad dreams, dizziness, confusion, psychosis, decreased reflexes

EENT: Blurred vision, corneal changes, retinal changes, difficulty focusing, tinnitus, vertigo, deafness, photophobia, corneal edema

GI: Nausea, vomiting, anorexia, diarrhea, cramps

*HEMA: **Thrombocytopenia, agranulocytosis, hemolytic anemia, leukopenia***

Contraindications: Hypersensitivity, retinal field changes, children (long-term)

Precautions: Blood dyscrasias, severe GI disease, neurologic disease, alcoholism, hepatic disease, G6PD deficiency, psoriasis, eczema, pregnancy (C), lactation

Pharmacokinetics:

PO: Peak 1-2 hr, half-life 3-5 days; metabolized in liver; excreted in urine, feces, breast milk; crosses placenta

Interactions:

• Decreased action of hydroxychloroquine: Mg or Al compounds
• Increased levels of digoxin
• Increased antibody titer: rabies vaccine

NURSING CONSIDERATIONS
Assess:

• Ophthalmic test baseline and q6mo if long-term treatment or drug dosage >150 mg/day
• Liver studies qwk: AST, ALT, bilirubin
• Blood studies: CBC, platelets; WBC, RBC, platelets may be decreased
• For decreased reflexes: knee, ankle
• ECG during therapy
• Watch for depression of T waves, widening of QRS complex

• Allergic reactions: pruritus, rash, urticaria
• Blood dyscrasias: malaise, fever, bruising, bleeding (rare)
• For ototoxicity (tinnitus, vertigo, change in hearing); audiometric testing should be done before, after treatment

◆ For toxicity: blurring vision, difficulty focusing, headache, dizziness, knee, ankle reflexes; drug should be discontinued immediately

Administer:
PO

• Before or after meals or with milk; at same time each day to maintain drug level

Perform/provide:

• Storage in tight, light-resistant container at room temperature; keep injection in cool environment

Evaluate:

• Therapeutic response: decreased symptoms of malaria, LE, rheumatoid arthritis

Teach patient/family:

• To use sunglasses in bright sunlight to decrease photophobia
• That urine may turn rust or brown
• To report hearing, visual problems, fever, fatigue, bruising, bleeding, which may indicate blood dyscrasias

Treatment of overdose: Induce vomiting; gastric lavage; administer barbiturate (ultrashort-acting), vasopressor, ammonium chloride; tracheostomy may be necessary

RARELY USED

hydroxyprogesterone (℞)
(hye-drox-ee-pro-jess'te-rone)
Func. class.: Progestin, hormone

Uses: Uterine carcinoma, menstrual disorders (abnormal uterine bleeding, amenorrhea)

Dosage and routes:

Menstrual disorders

• *Adult:* **IM** 125-375 mg q4wk; discontinue after 4 cycles

Uterine cancer:

• *Adult:* **IM** 1-5 g/wk

Contraindications: Breast cancer, hypersensitivity, thromboembolic disorders, genital bleeding (abnormal, undiagnosed), pregnancy (X)

hydroxyurea (℞)
(hye-drox'ee-yoo-ree-ah)
Droxia, Hydrea
Func. class.: Antineoplastic, antimetabolite
Chem. class.: Synthetic urea analog

Action: Acts by inhibiting DNA synthesis without interfering with RNA or protein synthesis; incorporates thymidine into DNA, causing direct damage to DNA strands; S phase specific of cell cycle

Uses: Melanoma, chronic myelocytic leukemia, recurrent or metastatic ovarian cancer, squamous cell carcinoma of the head and neck, sickle cell anemia, psoriasis

Dosage and routes:

Renal disease

• CrCl 10-50 ml/min dose 50%; CrCl <10 ml/min dose 20%

Solid tumors

• *Adult:* **PO** 80 mg/kg as a single dose q3d or 20-30 mg/kg as a single dose qd

In combination with radiation

• *Adult:* **PO** 80 mg/kg as a single dose q3d; should be started 7 days before irradiation

Resistant chronic myelocytic leukemia

• *Adult:* **PO** 20-30 mg/kg/day as a single daily dose

Sickle cell anemia

• *Adult:* **PO** 15 mg/kg/day, may increase by 5 mg/kg/day, max 35 mg/kg/day

Available forms: Caps 200, 300, 400, 500 mg

Side effects/adverse reactions:

HEMA: **Leukopenia, anemia, thrombocytopenia, megaloblastic erythropoiesis**

GI: Nausea, vomiting, anorexia, diarrhea, stomatitis, constipation

GU: Increased BUN, uric acid, creatinine, temporary renal function impairment

INTEG: Rash, urticaria, pruritus, dry skin, facial erythema

CV: Angina, ischemia

CNS: Headache, confusion, hallucinations, dizziness, **convulsions**

MISC: Fever, chills, malaise

Contraindications: Hypersensitivity, leukopenia (<2500/mm³), thrombocytopenia (<100,000/mm³), anemia (severe), pregnancy (D), lactation

Precautions: Renal disease (severe)

Pharmacokinetics: Readily absorbed when taken orally; peak level in 2 hr; degraded in liver; excreted in urine, almost totally eliminated in 24 hr; readily crosses blood-brain barrier, eliminated as CO_2

Interactions:

• Increased toxicity: radiation or other antineoplastics

Lab test interferences:

Increase: Renal function studies

NURSING CONSIDERATIONS
Assess:

• CBC, differential, platelet count qwk; withhold drug if WBC is <2500/mm^3 or platelet count is <100,000/mm^3; notify prescriber; drug should be discontinued

• Renal function studies: BUN, serum uric acid, urine CrCl, electrolytes before, during therapy

• I&O ratio; report fall in urine output to <30 ml/hr

• Monitor temp q4h; fever may indicate beginning infection

• Liver function tests before, during therapy: bilirubin, alk phosphatase, AST, ALT, LDH; prn or qmo

• B/P q3-4h; check for chest pain; angina, ischemia may occur

• Bleeding: hematuria, guaiac, bruising or petechiae, mucosa or orifices q8h

• Food preferences; list likes, dislikes

• Inflammation of mucosa, breaks in skin

• Buccal cavity q8h for dryness, sores or ulceration, white patches, oral pain, bleeding, dysphagia

• Symptoms indicating severe allergic reaction: rash, urticaria, itching, flushing

• Neurotoxicity: headaches, hallucinations, convulsions, dizziness

Administer:

• Allopurinol or NaHCO$_3$ concurrently to prevent high uric acid levels; extra fluids

• Antiemetic 30-60 min before giving drug and prn

• Antibiotics for prophylaxis of infection

• Transfusion for anemia

Perform/provide:

• Rinsing of mouth tid-qid with water, club soda; brushing of teeth bid-tid with soft brush or cotton-tipped applicators for stomatitis; use unwaxed dental floss

• Nutritious diet with iron, vitamin supplements as ordered

Evaluate:

• Therapeutic response: decreased tumor size, spread of malignancy

Teach patient/family:

🚫 Not to break, crush, or chew caps

• To report signs of infection: elevated temp, sore throat, flulike symptoms

• To report signs of anemia: fatigue, headache, faintness, shortness of breath, irritability

• To report bleeding: avoid use of razors, commercial mouthwash

• To avoid use of aspirin products, ibuprofen

• To avoid foods with citric acid, hot or rough texture if stomatitis is present

• To report stomatitis: any bleeding, white spots, ulcerations in the mouth; tell patient to examine mouth qd, report symptoms

• That contraceptive measures are recommended during therapy

• To notify prescriber of fever, chills, sore throat, nausea, vomiting, anorexia, diarrhea, bleeding, bruising; may indicate blood dyscrasias

---

◆ = Nursing alert   ∥ = Herb-drug interaction   🚫 = Do not crush

hydroxyzine (℞)

(hye-drox'i-zeen)
Apo-Hydroxyzine*, Atarax,
Atarax 100, hydroxyzine HCl,
hydroxyzine pamoate, Multi-
pax*, Novohydroxyzine*,
Vistaril, Vistazine 50

Func. class.: Antianxiety/anti-
histamine/sedative-hypnotic, antiemetic

Chem. class.: Piperazine derivative

Action: Depresses subcortical levels of CNS, including limbic system, reticular formation

Uses: Anxiety preoperatively, postoperatively to prevent nausea, vomiting, to potentiate narcotic analgesics; sedation; pruritus

Dosage and routes:
• *Adult:* **PO** 25-100 mg tid-qid, max
600 mg/day
• *Geriatric:* **PO** 10 mg tid-qid (pruritus)
• *Child >6 yr:* 50-100 mg/day in
divided doses
• *Child <6 yr:* 50 mg/day in divided
doses

Preoperatively/postoperatively
• *Adult:* **IM** 25-100 mg q4-6h
• *Child:* **IM** 0.5-1.1 mg/kg q4-6h

Pruritus
• *Adult:* **PO** 25 mg tid-qid

Antiemetic
• *Adult:* **IM** 25-100 mg/dose q4-6h
prn

Available forms: Tabs 10, 25, 50,
100 mg; caps 25, 50, 100 mg; syr 10
mg/5 ml; oral susp 25 mg/5 ml; inj
25, 50 mg/ml

Side effects/adverse reactions:
CV: Hypotension
CNS: Dizziness, drowsiness, confusion, headache, tremors, fatigue, depression, *seizures*

GI: Dry mouth, increased appetite,
nausea, diarrhea, weight gain

Contraindications: Hypersensitivity to this drug or cetirizine, early
pregnancy, lactation, acute asthma

Precautions: Elderly, debilitated,
hepatic disease, renal disease,
narrow-angle glaucoma, COPD,
prostatic hypertrophy, pregnancy (C)

Do not confuse:
Vistaril/Versed

Pharmacokinetics:
PO: Onset 15-30 min, duration 4-6
hr, half-life 3 hr, metabolized by
liver, excreted by kidneys

Interactions:
• Increased CNS depressant effect:
barbiturates, opioids, analgesics, alcohol
• Increased anticholinergic effects:
phenothiazines, quinidine, disopyramide, antihistamines, antidepressants, atropine, haloperidol
🍃 Increased anticholinergic effect:
henbane leaf
🍃 Increased action: kava

NURSING CONSIDERATIONS

Assess:
• B/P (lying, standing), pulse; if systolic B/P drops 20 mm Hg, hold
drug, notify prescriber
• Mental status: mood, sensorium,
affect
• Increased sedation

Administer:
PO
• With food or milk for GI symp-
toms (PO)
• Crushed if patient is unable to
swallow medication whole
• Gum, hard candy, frequent sips of
water for dry mouth
IM
• By Z-track inj in large muscle for
IM to decrease pain, chance of ne-
crosis, never give IV/SC

Additive compatibilities: Cisplatin,
cyclophosphamide, cytarabine, di-

H

menhydrinate, etoposide, lidocaine, mesna, methotrexate, nafcillin

Syringe compatibilities: Atropine, atropine/meperidine, benzquinamide, bupivacaine, butorphanol, chlorpromazine, cimetidine, codeine, diphenhydramine, doxapram, droperidol, fentanyl, fluphenazine, glycopyrrolate, hydromorphone, lidocaine, meperidine, meperidine/atropine, methotrimeprazine, metoclopramide, midazolam, morphine, nalbuphine, oxymorphone, pentazocine, perphenazine, procaine, prochlorperazine, promazine, promethazine, scopolamine, sufentanil, thiothixene

Perform/provide:

• Assistance with ambulation during beginning therapy, since drowsiness/dizziness occurs

• Safety measures, including side rails

• Checking to see if PO medication has been swallowed

Evaluate:

• Therapeutic response: decreased anxiety

Teach patient/family:

• That medication is not to be used for everyday stress or used longer than 4 mo

• To avoid OTC preparations (cold, cough, hay fever) unless approved by prescriber

• To avoid driving, activities that require alertness

• To avoid alcohol ingestion, other psychotropic medications

• Not to discontinue medication quickly after long-term use

• To rise slowly or fainting may occur

Treatment of overdose: Lavage if orally ingested; VS, supportive care; IV norepinephrine for hypotension

---

hyoscyamine (R̥)

(hye-oh-sye′a-meen)
Anaspaz, Cystospaz, Cystospaz-M, Gastrosed, Levsin, Levsin Drops, Levsinex Timecaps, Neoquess
Func. class.: Anticholinergic
Chem. class.: Belladonna alkaloid

Action: Inhibits muscarinic actions of acetylcholine at postganglionic parasympathetic neuroeffector sites

Uses: Treatment of peptic ulcer disease in combination with other drugs; other GI disorders, other spastic disorders, urinary incontinence

Dosage and routes:

• *Adult:* **PO/SL** 0.125-0.25 mg tid-qid ac, hs; **TIME REL** 0.375 q12h; **IM/SC/IV** 0.25-0.5 mg q6h

• *Child 2-10 yr:* ½ adult dose

• *Child <2 yr:* ¼ adult dose

Available forms: Tabs 0.125, 0.13, 0.15 mg; caps time rel 0.375 mg; sol 0.125 mg/ml; elix 0.125 mg/5 ml; inj 0.5 mg/ml

Side effects/adverse reactions:

CNS: Confusion, stimulation in elderly, headache, insomnia, dizziness, drowsiness, anxiety, weakness, hallucination

GI: Dry mouth, constipation, paralytic ileus, heartburn, nausea, vomiting, dysphagia, absence of taste

GU: Urinary hesitancy, retention, impotence

CV: Palpitations, tachycardia

EENT: Blurred vision, photophobia, mydriasis, cycloplegia, increased ocular tension

INTEG: Urticaria, rash, pruritus, anhidrosis, fever, allergic reactions

Contraindications: Hypersensitivity to anticholinergics, narrow-angle glaucoma, GI obstruction, myasthenia gravis, paralytic ileus,

---

◆ = Nursing alert   ∥ = Herb-drug interaction   ⊘ = Do not crush

GI atony, toxic megacolon, prostatic hypertrophy

Precautions: Hyperthyroidism, coronary artery disease, dysrhythmias, CHF, ulcerative colitis, hypertension, hiatal hernia, hepatic disease, renal disease, pregnancy (C), urinary retention, elderly

Pharmacokinetics:

PO: Duration 4-6 hr; metabolized by liver; excreted in urine; half-life 3.5 hr

Interactions:

• Decreased effect of hyoscyamine: antacids

• Increased anticholinergic effect: amantadine, tricyclics, MAOIs, H_1-antihistamines

• Decreased effect of phenothiazines, levodopa, ketoconazole

NURSING CONSIDERATIONS

Assess:

• VS, cardiac status: checking for dysrhythmias, increased rate, palpitations

• I&O ratio; check for urinary retention or hesitancy

• GI complaints: pain, bleeding (frank or occult), nausea, vomiting, anorexia

Administer:

• ½ hr ac for better absorption

• Decreased dose to elderly patients; metabolism may be slowed

• Gum, hard candy, frequent rinsing of mouth for dryness of oral cavity

Perform/provide:

• Storage in tight container protected from light

• Increased fluids, bulk, exercise to decrease constipation

Evaluate:

• Therapeutic response: absence of epigastric pain, bleeding, nausea, vomiting

Teach patient/family:

• To avoid driving, other hazardous activities until stabilized on medication

• To avoid alcohol or other CNS depressants; will enhance sedating properties of this drug

• To avoid hot environments; heat stroke may occur; drug suppresses perspiration

• To use sunglasses when outside to prevent photophobia; may cause blurred vision

🚫 Not to break, crush, or chew time rel caps

---

ibuprofen (OTC, R)

(eye-byoo-proe'fen)
Actiprofen*, Advil, Apo-Ibuprofen*, Bayer Select Ibuprofen Pain Relief, Children's Advil, Children's Motrin, Cramp End, Dolgesic, Excedrin IB, Genpril, Haltran, Ibuprin, ibuprofen, Ibren, Ibuprohm, IBU-Tab, Menadol, Medipren, Midol-200, Motrin, Motrin IB, Motrin Junior Strength, Novoprofen*, Nuprin, Pamprin-IB, PediaCare Children's Fever, Q-Profen, Rufen, Saleto-200, Saleto-400, Saleto-600, Saleto-800, Trendar

Func. class.: Nonsteroidal antiinflammatory, antipyretic

Chem. class.: Propionic acid derivative

Action: Inhibits prostaglandin synthesis by decreasing enzyme needed for biosynthesis; analgesic, antiinflammatory, antipyretic

Uses: Rheumatoid arthritis, osteoarthritis, primary dysmenorrhea, gout, dental pain, musculoskeletal disorders, fever

Dosage and routes:

Analgesic

• *Adult:* **PO** 200-400 mg q4-6h, not to exceed 3.2 g/day

• *Child:* **PO** 4-10 mg/kg/dose q6-8h

Antipyretic

• *Child 6 mo-12 yr:* **PO** 5 mg/kg (temp <102.5° F or 39.2° C), 10 mg/kg, (temp >102.5° F), may repeat q4-6h, max 40 mg/kg/day

Antiinflammatory

• *Adult:* **PO** 300-800 mg tid-qid, max 3.2 g/day

• *Child:* **PO** 30-40 mg/kg/day in 3-4 divided doses, max 50 mg/kg/day

Available forms: Tabs 100, 200, 300, 400, 600, 800 mg; cap, liq gels 200 mg; oral susp 100 mg/2.5 ml, 100 mg/5 ml; tabs, chew 50, 100 mg; drops 50 mg/1.25 ml

Side effects/adverse reactions:

CV: Tachycardia, peripheral edema, palpitations, dysrhythmias

CNS: Headache, dizziness, drowsiness, fatigue, tremors, confusion, insomnia, anxiety, depression

EENT: Tinnitus, hearing loss, blurred vision

GI: Nausea, anorexia, vomiting, diarrhea, jaundice, *hepatitis,* constipation, flatulence, cramps, dry mouth, peptic ulcer, *GI bleeding*

GU: Nephrotoxicity: dysuria, hematuria, oliguria, azotemia

HEMA: Blood dyscrasias, increased bleeding time

INTEG: Purpura, rash, pruritus, sweating

SYST: Anaphylaxis

Contraindications: Hypersensitivity, asthma, severe renal disease, severe hepatic disease

Precautions: Pregnancy (B) 1st trimester, lactation, children, bleeding disorders, GI disorders, cardiac disorders, hypersensitivity to other antiinflammatory agents, elderly, CHF, CrCl <25 ml/min

Do not confuse:

Nuprin/Lupron

Pharmacokinetics: Well absorbed (PO)

PO: Onset ½ hr; peak 1-2 hr, half-life 2-4 hr, metabolized in liver (inactive metabolites), excreted in urine (inactive metabolites), 90%-99% plasma protein binding, does not enter breast milk

Interactions:

• Decreased effect of: antihypertensives, thiazides, furosemide

• Decreased ibuprofen action: aspirin

• Increased risk of bleeding: cefamandole, cefotetan, cefoperazone, valproic acid, thrombolytics, antiplatelets, warfarin

• Increased possibility of blood dyscrasias: antineoplastics, radiation

• Increased toxicity: digoxin, lithium, oral anticoagulants, cyclosporine, probenecid

• Increased GI reactions: aspirin, corticosteroids, NSAIDs, alcohol

• Increased hypoglycemia: oral antidiabetics, insulin

NURSING CONSIDERATIONS

Assess:

• Renal, liver, blood studies: BUN, creatinine, AST, ALT, Hgb, before treatment, periodically thereafter

• Pain: note type, duration, location and intensity with ROM 1 hr after administration

• Audiometric, ophthalmic examination before, during, after treatment; for eye, ear problems: blurred vision, tinnitus; may indicate toxicity

• Fever: temp before and 1 hr after administration

• Cardiac status: edema (peripheral), tachycardia, palpitations; monitor B/P, pulse for character, quality, rhythm especially in patients with cardiac disease/elderly

---

◆ = Nursing alert   🖋 = Herb-drug interaction   🚫 = Do not crush

• For history of peptic ulcer disorder; asthma, aspirin, hypersensitivity, check closely for hypersensitivity reactions

Administer:

• With food, milk, or antacid to decrease GI symptoms; however, taking on empty stomach best facilitates absorption; if nausea and vomiting occur/persist, notify prescriber

Perform/provide:

• Storage at room temperature

Evaluate:

• Therapeutic response: decreased pain, stiffness in joints; decreased swelling in joints; ability to move more easily; reduction in fever or menstrual cramping

Teach patient/family:

• To report blurred vision, ringing, roaring in ears; may indicate toxicity; eye and hearing tests should be done during long-term therapy

• To avoid driving, other hazardous activities if dizziness or drowsiness occurs

◆ To report change in urinary pattern, increased weight, edema, increased pain in joints, fever, blood in urine; indicate nephrotoxicity

• That therapeutic inflammatory effects may take up to 1 mo

• To avoid alcohol, NSAIDs, salicylates; bleeding may occur

• To use sunscreen to prevent photosensitivity

---

ibutilide (℞)

(eye-byoo'tih-lide)

Corvert

Func. class.: Antidysrhythmic (Class III)

Action: Prolongs duration of action potential and effective refractory period, noncompetitive α- and β-adrenergic inhibition

Uses: Atrial fibrillation/flutter

Dosage and routes:

• *Adult:* **IV INF** (≥60 kg) 1 vial (1 mg) given over 10 min; **IV INF** (<60 kg) 0.01 mg/kg given over 10 min

Available forms: Inj 0.1 mg/ml

Side effects/adverse reactions:

CNS: Headache

GI: Nausea

CV: Hypotension, bradycardia, sinus arrest, CHF, dysrhythmias, hypertension, extrasystoles, ventricular tachycardia, bundle branch block, AV block

Contraindications: Hypersensitivity

Precautions: Sinus node dysfunction, 2nd- or 3rd-degree AV block, electrolyte imbalances, pregnancy (C), bradycardia, lactation, children <18 yr, renal/hepatic disease, elderly

Pharmacokinetics:

PO: Onset 1-3 wk, peak 2-10 hr; half-life 15-100 days; metabolized by liver, excreted by kidneys

Interactions:

• Prodysrhythmia: phenothiazines, tricyclics, tetracyclics, antidepressants, H$_2$-receptor antagonists, antihistamines

• Increased levels of digitalis, quinidine, procainamide, flecainide, disopyramide, phenytoin, amiodarone, sotalol

🌿 Increased action: aloe, buckthorn, cascara sagrada, senna

NURSING CONSIDERATIONS

Assess:

• I&O ratio; electrolytes: K, Na, Cl

• Liver function studies: AST, ALT, bilirubin, alk phosphatase

• ECG continuously to determine drug effectiveness, measure PR, QRS, QT intervals, check for PVCs, other dysrhythmias, discontinue if atrial fibrillation/flutter ceases

• For dehydration or hypovolemia

• For rebound hypertension after 1-2 hr
• Cardiac rate, respiration: rate, rhythm, character, chest pain

Administer:

IV

• Undiluted or diluted in 50 ml 0.9% NaCl, or D_5W (0.017 mg/ml) give over 10 min
• Solution is stable for 48 hr refrigerated or 24 hr, room temperature
• Do not admix with other solution, drugs
• Reduced dosage slowly with ECG monitoring

Evaluate:

• Therapeutic response: decrease in atrial fibrillation/flutter

Teach patient/family:

• To report side effects immediately
• Reason for medication

---

idarubicin (℞)

(eye-dah-roob'ih-sin)
Idamycin, Idamycin PFS

Func. class.: Antineoplastic, antibiotic

Chem. class.: Anthracycline glycoside

Action: Inhibits DNA synthesis by binding to DNA, a vesicant derived from daunorubicin by binding to DNA, which causes strand splitting; cell cycle specific (S phase)

Uses: Used in combination with other antineoplastics for acute myelocytic leukemia in adults

Investigational uses: Breast cancer, solid tumors

Dosage and routes:

• *Adult:* IV 12 mg/m²/day × 3 days in combination with cytosine (induction)

Available forms: Inj 1 mg/ml; pwd for inj, lyophilized 5, 10, 20 mg

Side effects/adverse reactions:

*HEMA: **Thrombocytopenia, leukopenia, anemia***

GI: Nausea, vomiting, abdominal pain, mucositis, diarrhea, ***hepatotoxicity***

INTEG: Rash, extravasation, dermatitis, reversible alopecia, urticaria, thrombophlebitis and tissue necrosis at injection site

*CV: **Dysrhythmias, CHF, pericarditis, myocarditis,** peripheral edema, angina, **MI***

CNS: Fever, chills, headache

*GU: **Nephrotoxicity***

Contraindications: Hypersensitivity, pregnancy (D), lactation, myelosuppression

Precautions: Renal and hepatic disease, gout, bone marrow depression, children

Do not confuse:

Idamycin/Adriamycin
idarubicin/doxorubicin

Pharmacokinetics: Half-life 22 hr; metabolized by liver; crosses placenta; excreted in bile, urine (primarily as metabolites)

Interactions:

• Increased toxicity: other antineoplastics or radiation
• Decreased antibody response: live virus vaccines

Lab test interferences:

Increase: Uric acid

NURSING CONSIDERATIONS

Assess:

• CBC, differential, platelet count weekly; withhold drug if WBC is <4000/mm³ or platelet count is <75,000/mm³; notify prescriber of these results
• Blood, urine, uric acid levels
• Renal function studies: BUN, serum uric acid, urine CrCl, electrolytes before, during therapy
• I&O ratio; report fall in urine output to <30 ml/hr

◆ = Nursing alert   ∅ = Herb-drug interaction   ⊘ = Do not crush

• Monitor temp q4h; fever may indicate beginning infection
• LFTs before, during therapy: bilirubin, AST, ALT, alk phosphatase prn or qmo; check for jaundice of skin, sclera, dark urine, clay-colored stools, itchy skin, abdominal pain, fever, diarrhea
• Cardiac toxicity: CHF, dysrhythmias, cardiomyopathy; cardiac studies should be done before and periodically during treatment: ECG, chest x-ray
• ECG: watch for ST-T wave changes, low QRS and T, possible dysrhythmias (sinus tachycardia, heart block, PVCs)
• Bleeding: hematuria, guaiac stools, bruising or petechiae, mucosa or orifices q8h
• Effects of alopecia on body image; discuss feelings about body changes
• Inflammation of mucosa, breaks in skin
• Buccal cavity q8h for dryness, sores, ulceration, white patches, oral pain, bleeding, dysphagia
• Local irritation, pain, burning at injection site
• GI symptoms: frequency of stools, cramping
• Acidosis, signs of dehydration: rapid respirations, poor skin turgor, decreased urine output, dry skin, restlessness, weakness

Administer:
• Allopurinol or sodium bicarbonate to reduce uric acid levels, alkalinization of urine
• Transfusion for anemia
• Hydrocortisone for extravasation; apply ice compress after stopping infusion
IV, direct
• After preparing in biologic cabinet wearing gown, gloves, mask

• Antiemetic 30-60 min before giving drug and 6-10 hr after treatment to prevent vomiting
• After reconstituting 5 mg vial with 5 ml 0.9% NaCl (1 mg/1 ml); give over 10-15 min through Y-tube or 3-way stopcock of inf of D_5 or NS; discard unused portion
Solution compatibilities: $D_{3.3}$/0.3% NaCl, D_5/0.9% NaCl, D_5W, LR, 0.9% NaCl
Y-site compatibilities: Amifostine, amikacin, aztreonam, cimetidine, cladribine, cyclophosphamide, cytarabine, diphenhydramine, droperidol, erythromycin, filgrastim, granisetron, imipenem/cisplatin, magnesium sulfate, mannitol, melphalan, metoclopramide, potassium chloride, ranitidine, sargramostim, thiotepa, vinorelbine
Perform/provide:
• Strict hand-washing technique, gloves, protective clothing
• Liquid diet: carbonated beverages, gelatin may be added if patient is not nauseated or vomiting
• Increase fluid intake to 2-3 L/day to prevent urate and calculi formation
• Diet low in purines: absence of organ meats (kidney, liver), dried beans, peas to reduce uric acid level
• Rinsing of mouth tid-qid with water, club soda; brushing of teeth tid-qid with soft brush or cotton-tipped applicators for stomatitis; use unwaxed dental floss
• Storage at room temperature for 3 days after reconstituting or 7 days refrigerated
Evaluate:
• Therapeutic response: decreased tumor size, spread of malignancy
Teach patient/family:
• To report any complaints, side effects to nurse or prescriber
• That hair may be lost during treatment and wig or hairpiece may make

patient feel better; tell patient that new hair may be different in color, texture

• To avoid foods with citric acid, hot or rough texture

• To report any bleeding, white spots, ulcerations in mouth; tell patient to examine mouth qd

• That urine may be red-orange for 48 hr

• To use contraception during treatment with this drug and for ≥4 mo after treatment

---

RARELY USED

idoxuridine-IDU (℞)
(eye-dox-yoor'i-deen)
Herplex, Stoxil
Func. class.: Antiviral

Uses: Herpes simplex keratitis, CMV, varicella-zoster alone or with corticosteroids
Dosage and routes:
• *Adult and child:* **INSTILL** 1 gtt q1h during day and 2 hr during night
Contraindications: Hypersensitivity

---

ifosfamide (℞)
(i-foss'fa-mide)
Ifex
Func. class.: Antineoplastic alkylating agent
Chem. class.: Nitrogen mustard
Action: Alkylates DNA, RNA, inhibits enzymes that allow synthesis of amino acids in proteins; also responsible for cross-linking DNA strands; activity is not cell cycle stage specific
Uses: Testicular cancer, soft tissue sarcoma, Ewing's sarcoma, non-

Hodgkin's lymphoma, lung, pancreatic sarcoma
Dosage and routes:
• *Adult:* **IV** 1.2 g/m^2/day × 5 days, repeat course q3wk, given with mesna
Available forms: Inj 1, 3 g
Side effects/adverse reactions:
CNS: Facial paresthesia, fever, malaise, somnolence, confusion, depression, hallucinations, dizziness, disorientation, *seizures, coma,* cranial nerve dysfunction
GI: Nausea, vomiting, anorexia, *hepatotoxicity,* stomatitis, constipation, diarrhea
INTEG: Dermatitis, alopecia, pain at injection site
GU: *Hematuria, nephrotoxicity, hemorrhagic cystitis,* dysuria, urinary frequency
HEMA: *Thrombocytopenia, leukopenia, anemia*
Contraindications: Hypersensitivity, bone marrow suppression, pregnancy (D)
Precautions: Renal disease, lactation, children
Pharmacokinetics: Metabolized by liver; saturation occurs at high doses; excreted in urine; half-life 7-15 hr
Interactions:
• Increased myelosuppression: other antineoplastics, radiation
• Decreased antibody response: live virus vaccines
• Increased toxicity: barbiturates, allopurinol
NURSING CONSIDERATIONS
Assess:
• Liver function studies before, during therapy (bilirubin, AST, ALT, LDH) as needed or monthly
• CBC, differential, platelet count weekly; withhold drug if WBC <2000 or platelet count <50,000; notify prescriber
• Monitor temp q4h (may indicate beginning of infection)

◆ = Nursing alert   ∅ = Herb-drug interaction   ⊘ = Do not crush

- Blood dyscrasias (anemia, granulocytopenia); bruising, fatigue, bleeding, poor healing
- Allergic reactions: dermatitis, exfoliative dermatitis, pruritus, urticaria
- I&O ratio; monitor for hematuria; hemorrhagic cystitis can occur; increase fluids to 3 L/day
- Neurologic symptoms: hallucinations, confusion, disorientation, drug should be discontinued
- Bleeding: hematuria, guaiac, bruising or petechiae, mucosa or orifices q8h
- Jaundice of skin, sclera, dark urine, clay-colored stools, itchy skin, abdominal pain, fever, diarrhea

Administer:
- Antiemetic 30-60 min before giving drug to prevent vomiting
- Antibiotics for prophylaxis of infection
- Always give with mesna to prevent ifosfamide-induced hemorrhagic cystitis

IV
- After diluting 1 g/20 ml sterile or bacteriostatic H_2O for inj with parabens or benzyl only; shake; may be diluted further with D_5W, LR, NS, sterile H_2O for inj; 1 g/20 ml = 50 mg/ml; 1 g/50ml = 20 mg/ml; 1 g/200 ml = 5 mg/ml; give over ≥30 min; may also give as cont inf over 72 hr

Additive compatibilities: Carboplatin, cisplatin, etoposide, fluorouracil, mesna

Syringe compatibilities: Mesna

Y-site compatibilities: Allopurinol, amifostine, amphotericin B cholesteryl, aztreonam, doxorubicin liposome, filgrastim, fludarabine, gallium, granisetron, melphalan, ondansetron, paclitaxel, piperacillin/tazobactam, propofol, sargramostim, sodium bicarbonate, teniposide, thiotepa, vinorelbine

Perform/provide:
- Storage of pwd at room temperature
- Increase fluid intake to 3 L/day to prevent hemorrhagic cystitis
- Warm compresses at inj site for inflammation

Evaluate:
- Therapeutic response: decrease in size and spread of tumor

Teach patient/family:
- To notify prescriber of sore throat, swollen lymph nodes, malaise, fever; other infections may occur
- Not to have vaccinations during treatment
- That hair may be lost during treatment; a wig or hairpiece may make the patient feel better; new hair may be different in color, texture
- To report signs of anemia: fatigue, headache, faintness, shortness of breath, irritability
- To report bleeding; avoid use of razors, commercial mouthwash
- To avoid use of aspirin products, NSAIDs, ibuprofen, hemorrhage can occur
- To use contraceptive measures during therapy
- To avoid crowds, those with infections

imatinib
See appendix a—selected new drugs

imipenem/cilastatin (℞)
(i-me-pen'em sye-la-stat'in)
Primaxin IM, Primaxin IV
Func. class.: Antiinfective, misc. penicillin
Chem. class.: Carbapenem

Action: Interferes with cell wall replication of susceptible organisms; osmotically unstable cell wall swells, bursts from osmotic pressure; addition of cilastatin prevents renal inactivation that occurs with high urinary concentrations of imipenem

Uses: Serious infections caused by gram-positive: *Streptococcus pneumoniae,* group A β-hemolytic streptococci, *Staphylococcus aureus,* enterococcus; gram-negative: *Klebsiella, Proteus, Escherichia coli, Acinetobacter, Serratia, Pseudomonas aeruginosa, Salmonella, Shigella*

Dosage and routes:
• *Adult:* IV 250-500 mg q8h; severe infections may require 1 g q8h; may give **IM** q12h (total daily **IM** dosage >1500 mg not recommended); mild to moderate infections
• *Child:* IV 600-100 mg/kg/day, max 4 g/day

Renal dose
• CrCl 30-70 ml/min give 50% dose q6-8h
• CrCl 20-30 ml/min give 40% dose q8-12h
• CrCl 5-20 ml/min give 25% dose q12h

Available forms: Inj 250, 500 mg (IV); inj 500, 750 mg (IM)

Side effects/adverse reactions:
CNS: Fever, somnolence, *seizures,* confusion, dizziness, weakness, myoclonia
GI: Diarrhea, nausea, vomiting, *pseudomembranous colitis, hepatitis,* glossitis
CV: Hypotension, palpitations
HEMA: Eosinophilia, neutropenia, decreased Hgb, Hct
INTEG: Rash, urticaria, pruritus, pain at injection site, phlebitis, erythema at injection site
SYST: Anaphylaxis
RESP: Chest discomfort, dyspnea, hyperventilation
Contraindications: Hypersensitiv-

ity, IM hypersensitivity to local anesthetics of the amide type

Precautions: Pregnancy (C), lactation, elderly, hypersensitivity to penicillins, seizure disorders, renal disease, children

Do not confuse:
imipenem/Omnipen
Primaxin/Premarin

Pharmacokinetics:
IV: Onset immediate, peak ½-1 hr, half-life 1 hr; 70%-80% excreted unchanged in urine

Interactions:
• Increased imipenem plasma levels: probenecid
• Increased toxicity: β-lactam antibiotics
• Increased risk of seizures: ganciclovir

Lab test interferences:
Increase: AST, ALT, LDH, BUN, alk phosphatase, bilirubin, creatinine
False-positive: Direct Coombs' test

NURSING CONSIDERATIONS
Assess:
• For infection: increased temp, WBC, characteristics of wounds, sputum, urine culture or stool culture
• Sensitivity to penicillin, other cephalosporins
• Renal disease: lower dose may be required
• Bowel pattern qd; if severe diarrhea occurs, drug should be discontinued; may indicate pseudomembranous colitis
◆ Allergic reactions, anaphylaxis: rash, urticaria, pruritus, wheezing, laryngeal edema; may occur few days after therapy begins; have epinephrine, antihistamine, emergency equipment available
• Overgrowth of infection: perineal itching, fever, malaise, redness, pain, swelling, drainage, rash, diarrhea, change in cough, sputum

◆ = Nursing alert   🌿 = Herb-drug interaction   🚫 = Do not crush

Administer:
• After C&S is taken
IV
• After reconstitution of 250 or 500 mg with 10 ml of diluent and shake; add to at least 100 ml of same inf sol
• 250-500 mg over 20-30 min; 1 g over 40-60 min; give through Y-tube or 3-way stopcock; do not give by IV bolus or if cloudy
Y-site compatibilities: Acyclovir, amifostine, aztreonam, cefepime, cisatracurium, diltiazem, famotidine, fludarabine, foscarnet, granisetron, idarubicin, insulin (regular), melphalan, methotrexate, ondansetron, propofol, remifentanil, tacrolimus, teniposide, thiotepa, vinorelbine, zidovudine
Evaluate:
• Therapeutic response: negative C&S; absence of signs and symptoms of infection
Teach patient/family:
• To report severe diarrhea; may indicate pseudomembranous colitis
• To report sore throat, bruising, bleeding, joint pain; may indicate blood dyscrasias (rare)
Treatment of anaphylaxis: Epinephrine, antihistamines; resuscitate if needed

---

imipramine (℞)

(im-ip′ra-meen)
Apo-Imipramine*, imipramine HCl*, Impril*, Novo Pramine*, Tofranil, Tofranil PM
Func. class.: Antidepressant, tricyclic
Chem. class.: Dibenzazepine, tertiary amine

Action: Blocks reuptake of norepinephrine, serotonin into nerve endings, increasing action of norepinephrine, serotonin in nerve cells

Uses: Depression, enuresis in children
Investigational uses: Chronic pain, migraine headaches, cluster headaches as adjunct, incontinence
Dosage and routes:
• *Adult:* **PO/IM** 75-100 mg/day in divided doses, may increase by 25-50 mg to 200 mg, not to exceed 300 mg/day; may give daily dose hs
• *Geriatric:* **PO** 25 mg hs, may increase to 100 mg/day in divided doses
• *Child:* **PO** 25-75 mg/day
Enuresis
• *Child:* **PO** 10 mg at hs, max 50 mg
Available forms: Tabs 10, 25, 50 mg; inj 25 mg/2 ml; caps 75, 100, 125, 150 mg
Side effects/adverse reactions:
HEMA: **Agranulocytosis, thrombocytopenia, eosinophilia, leukopenia**
CNS: Dizziness, drowsiness, confusion, **seizures,** headache, anxiety, tremors, stimulation, weakness, insomnia, nightmares, EPS (elderly), increased psychiatric symptoms, paresthesia
GI: Diarrhea, dry mouth, nausea, vomiting, **paralytic ileus;** increased appetite; cramps, epigastric distress, jaundice, **hepatitis,** stomatitis
GU: Retention, **acute renal failure**
INTEG: Rash, urticaria, sweating, pruritus, photosensitivity
CV: Orthostatic hypotension, ECG changes, tachycardia, hypertension, palpitations, **dysrhythmias**
EENT: Blurred vision, tinnitus, mydriasis
Contraindications: Hypersensitivity to tricyclics, recovery phase of MI, convulsive disorders, prostatic hypertrophy
Precautions: Suicidal patients, severe depression, increased intraocular pressure, narrow-angle glau-

coma, urinary retention, cardiac disease, hepatic disease, hyperthyroidism, electroshock therapy, elective surgery, elderly, pregnancy (C), lactation

Pharmacokinetics:

PO: Steady state 2-5 days; metabolized by liver; excreted in urine, breast milk, feces; crosses placenta; half-life 6-20 hr

Interactions:

• Decreased effects of guanethidine, clonidine, indirect-acting sympathomimetics (ephedrine)

• Increased effects of direct-acting sympathomimetics (epinephrine), alcohol, barbiturates, benzodiazepines, CNS depressants

◆ Increased toxicity: SSRIs, avoid concurrent use

◆ Hyperpyretic crisis, convulsions, hypertensive episode: MAOIs, clonidine

🌿 Increased anticholinergic effect: belladonna, henbane

🌿 Increased action of imipramine: scopolia, kava

Lab test interferences:

Increase: Serum bilirubin, alk phosphatase, blood glucose

Decrease: 5-HIAA, VMA, urinary catecholamines

NURSING CONSIDERATIONS

Assess:

• B/P (lying, standing), pulse q4h; if systolic B/P drops 20 mm Hg, hold drug, notify prescriber; take vital signs q4h in patients with cardiovascular disease

• Blood studies: CBC, leukocytes, differential, cardiac enzymes if patient is receiving long-term therapy

• Hepatic studies: AST, ALT, bilirubin

• Weight qwk; appetite may increase with drug

• ECG for flattening of T wave, bundle branch block, AV block, dysrhythmias in cardiac patients

• EPS primarily in elderly: rigidity, dystonia, akathisia

• Mental status: mood, sensorium, affect, suicidal tendencies, increase in psychiatric symptoms: depression, panic

• Urinary retention, constipation; constipation is more likely to occur in children, elderly

◆ Withdrawal symptoms: headache, nausea, vomiting, muscle pain, weakness; not usual unless drug discontinued abruptly

• Alcohol consumption; if alcohol is consumed, hold dose until morning

Administer:

• Increased fluids, bulk in diet for constipation, urinary retention

• With food or milk for GI symptoms

• Dosage hs if oversedation occurs during day; may take entire dose hs; elderly may not tolerate once/day dosing

• Gum, hard candy, or frequent sips of water for dry mouth

• In IM route after running warm water over ampule to dissolve crystals

Syringe compatibilities: Doxapram

Y-site compatibilities: Cladribine

Perform/provide:

• Storage in tight container at room temperature; do not freeze

• Assistance with ambulation during beginning therapy, since drowsiness/dizziness occurs

• Safety measures, primarily in elderly

• Checking to see if PO medication swallowed

Evaluate:

• Therapeutic response: decreased depression, enuresis, pain

Teach patient/family:

• That therapeutic effects may take 2-3 wk

• That drug is dispensed in small

◆ = Nursing alert   🌿 = Herb-drug interaction   🚫 = Do not crush

amounts because of suicide potential, especially in beginning of therapy
• To use caution in driving, other activities requiring alertness because of drowsiness, dizziness, blurred vision
• To avoid alcohol ingestion, other CNS depressants
• Not to discontinue medication quickly after long-term use; may cause nausea, headache, malaise
• To wear sunscreen or large hat, since photosensitivity occurs
🚫 Not to break, crush, or chew caps

Treatment of overdose: ECG monitoring; induce emesis; lavage, activated charcoal; administer anticonvulsant

---

immune globulin (℞)

Gamimune N, Gammagard S/D, gamma globulin, Gammar–P IV, Iveegam, Polygam, Polygam S/D, Sandoglobulin, Venoglobulin-I, Venoglobulin-S

Func. class.: Immune serum
Chem. class.: IgG

Action: Provides passive immunity to hepatitis A, measles, varicella, rubella, immune globulin deficiency; contains gamma globulin antibodies (IgG)

Uses: Immunodeficiency syndrome, B-cell chronic lymphocytic leukemia, Kawasaki syndrome, bone marrow transplantation, pediatric HIV infection, agammaglobulinemia, hepatitis A, B exposure, measles exposure, measles vaccine complications, purpura, rubella exposure, chickenpox exposure

Dosage and routes:
• *Adult:* IM 30-50 ml qmo; IV 100 mg/kg qmo, 0.01-0.02 ml/kg/min × ½ hr (Gamimune N); **IV** 200 mg/kg qmo, 0.05-1 ml/min × 15-30 min, then increase to 1.5-2.5 ml/min (Sandoglobulin)
• *Child:* IM 20-40 ml qmo

Hepatitis A exposure
• *Adult and child:* IM 0.02-0.04 ml/kg or 0.1 mg/kg if treatment is delayed

Hepatitis B exposure
• *Adult and child:* IM 0.06 ml/kg within 1 wk, qmo

Measles (postexposure)
• *Child:* IM 0.25 ml/kg within 6 days

Immunoglobulin deficiency
• *Adult and child:* IM 1.3 ml/kg, then 0.66 ml/kg after 2-4 wk and q2-4wk thereafter

Idiopathic thrombocytopenia, purpura
• *Adult and child:* IV 0.4 g/kg × 5 days or 1 g/kg/day × 1-2 days

Kawasaki syndrome
• *Child:* PO 2 g/kg as a single dose
Available forms: Inj 2, 10 ml/vial; 5% sol, 0.5, 1, 2.5, 3, 6, 10 g vials

Side effects/adverse reactions:
INTEG: Pain at injection site, rash, pruritus, chills, chest pain
MS: Arthralgia
SYST: Lymphadenopathy, **anaphylaxis**
CNS: Headache, fatigue, malaise
GI: Abdominal pain

Contraindications: Hypersensitivity

Precautions: Pregnancy (C)

Interactions:
• Do not administer live virus vaccines within 3 mo of this drug

NURSING CONSIDERATIONS
Assess:
• For exposure date: this drug should be given within 6 days of measles, 7 days of hepatitis B, 14 days of hepatitis A

• For anaphylaxis: diaphoresis, wheezing, chest tightness, hypotension

Administer:
• IM ≤3 ml in one site, use large muscle mass
• Only with epinephrine 1:1000, resuscitative equipment available
• Only within 2 wk of exposure to hepatitis A

IV
• Gamimune N: IV undiluted or dilute with D_5; give 0.01 ml/kg/min; may increase to 0.02-0.04 ml/kg/min
• Sandoglobulin: IV diluted with provided diluent; give 0.5-1 ml/min × 15-30 min; may increase to 1.5-2.5 ml/min
• Venoglobulin-I: (50 mg/ml sol) give 0.01-0.02 ml/kg/min; if no adverse reaction in ½ hr, increase to 0.04 ml/kg/min, store at room temperature
• Gammagard: reconstitute with sterile H_2O for inj (50 mg protein/ml); give 0.5 ml/kg/hr, may increase to 4 ml/kg/hr, use infusion set provided
• Gammar-IV: give 0.01 ml/kg/min (50 mg/ml sol) × 15-30 min, may increase to 0.02 ml/kg/min, may increase to 0.03-0.06 ml/kg/min

Y-site compatibilities: Fluconazole, sargramostim

Perform/provide:
• Storage at 36°-46° F (2°-8° C)

Evaluate:
• Prevention of infection, increased platelets

Teach patient/family:
• That passive immunity is temporary
• The treatment of anaphylaxis: epinephrine, diphenhydramine, O_2, vasopressors, corticosteroids

---

inamrinone (R)
(in-am'rih-nohn)

Func. class.: Cardiac inotropic agent

Chem. class.: Bipyrimidine derivative

Action: Positive inotropic agent with vasodilator properties; reduces preload and afterload by direct relaxation of vascular smooth muscle, increases cardiac output

Uses: Short-term management of CHF that has not responded to other medication; can be used with digitalis

Dosage and routes:
• *Adult and child:* **IV BOL** 0.75 mg/kg given over 2-3 min; start inf of 5-10 µg/kg/min; may give another bol 30 min after start of therapy, max 10 mg/kg total daily dose
• *Infant:* **IV** 3-4.5 mg/kg in divided doses, then give by infusion 10 µg/kg/min
• *Neonate:* **IV** 3-4.5 mg/kg in divided doses, then give by infusion 3-5 µg/kg/min

Available forms: Inj 5 mg/ml

Side effects/adverse reactions:
*HEMA: **Thrombocytopenia***
*CV: **Dysrhythmias,** hypotension,* headache, chest pain
GI: Nausea, vomiting, anorexia, abdominal pain, ***hepatotoxicity (rare), ascites,*** jaundice, hiccups
INTEG: Allergic reactions, burning at injection site
*HEMA: **Thrombocytopenia***
RESP: Pleuritis, ***pulmonary densities, hypoxemia***

Contraindications: Hypersensitivity to this drug or bisulfites, severe aortic disease, severe pulmonic valvular disease, acute MI

Precautions: Lactation, pregnancy (C), children, renal disease, hepatic

---

◆ = Nursing alert   ∥ = Herb-drug interaction   ⊘ = Do not crush

disease, atrial flutter/fibrillation, elderly

Do not confuse:
Inocor/Cordarone

Pharmacokinetics:
IV: Onset 2-5 min, peak 10 min, duration variable; half-life 4-6 hr, metabolized in liver, excreted in urine as drug and metabolites 60%-90%

Interactions:
• Excessive hypotension: antihypertensives, disopyramide
• Additive effect: cardiac glycosides

🌿 Possible increased action of amrinone: cascara sagrada bark, aloe, buckthorn bark/berry, ephedra, senna pod/leaf

Lab test interferences:
Decrease: Serum K
Increase: Hepatic enzymes

NURSING CONSIDERATIONS
Assess:
• B/P and pulse q5min during infusion; if B/P drops 30 mm Hg, stop infusion and call prescriber
• Electrolytes: K, S, Cl, Ca; renal function studies: BUN, creatinine; blood studies: platelet count; monitor fluid status (CVP) in elderly
• ALT, AST, bilirubin daily
• I&O ratio and weight qd; diuresis should increase with continuing therapy
◆ If platelets are <150,000/mm³, drug is usually discontinued and another drug started
• Extravasation; change site q48h

Administer:
• Do not mix directly with glucose solutions; chemical reaction occurs over 24 hr; precipitate forms if amrinone and furosemide come in contact
• Into running dextrose infusion through Y-connector or directly into tubing; may give undiluted over 2-3 min or dilute with 0.9%, 0.45% NaCl to 1-3 mg/ml, run at prescribed rate by continuous infusion
• By infusion pump for doses other than bolus
• K supplements if ordered for K levels <3.0, correct before using amrinone

Syringe compatibilities: Propranolol, verapamil

Y-site compatibilities: Aminophylline, atropine, bretylium, calcium chloride, cimetidine, cisatracurium, digoxin, dobutamine, dopamine, epinephrine, famotidine, hydrocortisone, isoproterenol, lidocaine, metaraminol, methylprednisolone, nitroglycerin, nitroprusside, norepinephrine, phenylephrine, potassium chloride, propofol, propranolol, remifentanil, verapamil

Evaluate:
• Therapeutic response: increased cardiac output, decreased PCWP, adequate CVP, decreased dyspnea, fatigue, edema, ECG

Teach patient/family:
• That burning may occur at IV site
• To report adverse reactions promptly

Treatment of overdose: Discontinue drug, support circulation

---

indapamide (℞)
(in-dap′a-mide)
indapamide, Lozide*, Lozol
Func. class.: Diuretic—thiazide-like, antihypertensive
Chem. class.: Indoline

Action: Acts on proximal section of distal renal tubule and thick ascending loop of Henle by inhibiting reabsorption of sodium; may act by direct vasodilation caused by blocking of calcium channel

Uses: Edema of CHF, hypertension, diuresis

Dosage and routes:

Edema

• *Adult:* **PO** 2.5 mg qd in AM; may be increased to 5 mg qd if needed

Antihypertensive

• *Adult:* 1.25-5 mg qd; may increase to 5 mg/day over 8 wk

Available forms: Tabs 1.25, 2.5 mg

Side effects/adverse reactions:

GU: Polyuria, nocturia, urinary frequency, impotence

ELECT: Hypochloremic alkalosis, hypomagnesemia, hyperuricemia, hypercalcemia, hyponatremia, hypokalemia, hyperglycemia

CNS: Headache, dizziness, fatigue, weakness, nervousness, agitation, extremity numbness, depression

GI: Nausea, diarrhea, dry mouth, vomiting, anorexia, cramps, constipation, abdominal pain

EENT: Blurred vision, nasal congestion, increased intraocular pressure

INTEG: Rash, pruritus

MS: Cramps

CV: Orthostatic hypotension, volume depletion, palpitations, dysrhythmias, PVCs

Contraindications: Hypersensitivity, anuria, hepatic coma

Precautions: Hypokalemia, dehydration, ascites, hepatic disease, severe renal disease, pregnancy (B), lactation, CrCl <25 ml/min (not effective)

Pharmacokinetics:

PO: Onset 1-2 hr, peak 2 hr, duration up to 36 hr; excreted in urine, feces; half-life 14-18 hr

Interactions:

• Hyperglycemia: diazoxide

• Increased toxicity of: muscle relaxants, steroids, lithium, digitalis

• Decreased K: steroids, amphotericin B, other diuretics

• Decreased effects: antidiabetics, antigout agents, anticoagulants

• Decreased absorption: cholestyramine, colestipol

• Decreased hypotensive effect: indomethacin, NSAIDs

🍂 Potassium deficiency: aloe, buckthorn, cascara sagrada, licorice, senna

Lab test interferences:

Increase: Ca, parathyroid test glucose, uric acid

NURSING CONSIDERATIONS

Assess:

• Weight daily, I&O daily to determine fluid loss; effect of drug may be decreased if used qd

• Rate, depth, rhythm of respiration, effect of exertion

• B/P lying, standing; postural hypotension may occur

• Electrolytes: K, Mg, Na, Cl: include BUN, CBC, serum creatinine, blood pH, ABGs, uric acid, Ca, glucose

• Signs of metabolic alkalosis, hypokalemia

• Rashes, fever qd

• Confusion, especially in elderly; take safety precautions if needed

• Hydration: skin turgor, thirst, dry mucous membranes

Administer:

• In AM to avoid interference with sleep

• With food; if nausea occurs, absorption may be decreased slightly

Evaluate:

• Therapeutic response: improvement in edema of feet, legs, sacral area daily, decreased B/P

Teach patient/family:

• Diet high in K; to rise slowly from lying or sitting position

• To recognize adverse reactions: muscle cramps, weakness, nausea, dizziness

• To take with food or milk for GI symptoms

• To use sunscreen for photosensitivity

◆ = Nursing alert   🍂 = Herb-drug interaction   🚫 = Do not crush

• To take early in day to prevent nocturia

Treatment of overdose: Lavage if taken orally; monitor electrolytes, administer IV fluids; monitor hydration, CV, renal status

---

RARELY USED

indecainide (R)

(in-de-kane′ide)
Func. class.: Antidysrhythmic (Class IC)

Uses: Life-threatening dysrhythmias, sustained ventricular tachycardia

Dosage and routes:
• *Adult:* PO 100-200 mg/day in divided dose q12h; 50 mg q12h initially, then increase dose by 25 mg increments q4d, max 400 mg/day

Contraindications: 2nd- or 3rd-degree AV block, right bundle branch block, cardiogenic shock, hypersensitivity

indinavir (R)

(en-den′a-veer)
Crixivan
Func. class.: Antiviral
Chem. class.: Synthetic peptide-like substrate analog

Action: Inhibits human immunodeficiency virus (HIV) protease; this prevents maturation of the infectious virus

Uses: HIV alone or in combination

Dosage and routes:
• Reduce dose in mild/moderate hepatic impairment and ketoconazole coadministration
• *Adult:* PO 800 mg q8h; if given

with ddI, give 1 hr apart on empty stomach

Available forms: Caps 200, 400 mg

Side effects/adverse reactions:

GU: Nephrolithiasis

GI: Diarrhea, abdominal pain, nausea, vomiting, anorexia, dry mouth

CNS: Headache, insomnia, dizziness, somnolence

INTEG: Rash

MS: Pain

OTHER: Asthenia, ***insulin-resistant hyperglycemia,*** hyperlipidemia, ***ketoacidosis***

Contraindications: Hypersensitivity

Precautions: Liver disease, pregnancy (C), lactation, children, renal disease, history of renal stones

Pharmacokinetics: Unknown

Interactions:
• Increased myopathy: cerivastatin, lovastatin, simvastatin
• Increase indinavir levels: ketoconazole, delavirdine, itraconazole
• Decreased indinavir levels: rifamycins, fluconazole, nevirapine, efavirenz
• Increased levels of both drugs: clarithromycin, zidovudine
• Increased levels of isoniazid, oral contraceptives
◆Life-threatening dysrhythmias: ergots, midazolam, rifampin, triazolam, cisapride
• Drug/food: decreased indinavir absorption: grapefruit juice, high-fat, high-protein foods
✎ Decreased indinavir levels: St. John's wort, avoid concurrent use

NURSING CONSIDERATIONS
Assess:
• Signs of infection, anemia
• Liver studies: ALT, AST
• The presence of other sexually transmitted diseases
• Bowel pattern before, during treatment; if severe abdominal pain

with bleeding occurs, drug should be discontinued; monitor hydration
• Skin eruptions; rash, urticaria, itching
• Allergies before treatment, reaction of each medication; place allergies on chart

Administer:
• With water, 1 hr ac or 2 hr pc

Teach patient/family:
• To take as prescribed; if dose is missed, take as soon as remembered up to 1 hr before next dose; do not double dose

🚫 Not to break, crush, or chew caps
• That drug must be taken in equal intervals around the clock to maintain blood levels for duration of therapy

◆ That hyperglycemia may occur; watch for increased thirst, weight loss, hunger, dry, itchy skin; notify prescriber
• To increase fluids to prevent kidney stones
• That drug does not cure AIDS, only controls symptoms

---

indomethacin (℞)

(in-doe-meth'a-sin)
Apo-Indomethacin*, Indameth*, Indocid*, Indocin, Indocin IV, Indocin PDA*, Indocin SR, indomethacin, Indochron E-R, Novomethacin*, Nu-Indo*

Func. class.: Nonsteroidal antiinflammatory (NSAID)

Chem. class.: Propionic acid derivative

Action: Inhibits prostaglandin synthesis by decreasing enzyme needed for biosynthesis; analgesic, antiinflammatory, antipyretic

Uses: Rheumatoid arthritis, ankylosing rheumatoid spondylitis, acute gouty arthritis, closure of patent ductus arteriosus in premature infants

Research note: Indomethacin reduces the antihypertensive effects of captopril and losartan; monitor carefully[18]

Dosage and routes:

Arthritis/antiinflammatory
• *Adult:* **PO/RECT** 25-50 mg bid; may increase by 25 mg/day qwk, not to exceed 200 mg/day; **SUS REL** 75 mg qd, may increase to 75 mg bid

Acute arthritis
• *Adult:* **PO/RECT** 50 mg tid; use only for acute attack, then reduce dose

Patent ductus arteriosus
Longer or repeated treatment courses may be necessary for very premature infants
• *Infant <2 days:* **IV** 0.2 mg/kg, then 0.1 mg/kg q12-24h
• *Infant 2-7 days:* **IV** 0.2 mg/kg, then 0.2 mg/kg × 2 doses after 12, 24 hr
• *Infant >7 days:* **IV** 0.2 mg/kg, then 0.25 mg/kg × 2 doses after 12, 24 hr

Available forms: Caps 25, 50 mg; caps ext rel 75 mg; susp 25 mg/5 ml; rec supp 50 mg; inj 1 mg vial

Side effects/adverse reactions:
GI: Nausea, anorexia, *vomiting,* diarrhea, jaundice, ***cholestatic hepatitis,*** constipation, flatulence, cramps, dry mouth, peptic ulcer, ***ulceration, perforation***, ***GI bleeding***
CNS: Dizziness, drowsiness, fatigue, tremors, confusion, insomnia, anxiety, depression, headache
CV: Tachycardia, peripheral edema, palpitations, dysrhythmias, hypertension
INTEG: Purpura, rash, pruritus, sweating

◆ = Nursing alert   ⫻ = Herb-drug interaction   🚫 = Do not crush

*GU: **Nephrotoxicity: dysuria, hematuria, oliguria, azotemia***

*HEMA: **Blood dyscrasias**,* prolonged bleeding

EENT: Tinnitus, hearing loss, blurred vision

Contraindications: Hypersensitivity, asthma, severe renal disease, severe hepatic disease, ulcer disease

Precautions: Pregnancy, lactation, children, bleeding disorders, GI disorders, cardiac disorders, hypersensitivity to other antiinflammatory agents, pregnancy (B) 1st trimester, lactation, depression

Pharmacokinetics:

PO: Onset 1-2 hr, peak 3 hr, duration 4-6 hr; metabolized in liver, kidneys; excreted in urine, bile, feces; crosses placenta; excreted in breast milk; 99% plasma protein binding

Interactions:

• Increased effect of: digoxin, penicillamine, phenytoin

• Decreased effect of antihypertensives

• Decreased levels of indomethacin: aspirin

• Toxicity: lithium, methotrexate, cyclosporine, aminoglycosides, aspirin, corticosteroids, triamterene, alcohol

• Increased risk of bleeding: anticoagulants

NURSING CONSIDERATIONS

Assess:

• Renal, liver, blood studies: BUN, creatinine, AST, ALT, Hgb, before treatment, periodically thereafter; if renal function has decreased, do not give subsequent doses

• Audiometric, ophthalmic exam before, during, after treatment

• For eye, ear problems: blurred vision, tinnitus; may indicate toxicity

• For confusion, mood changes, hallucinations, especially in elderly

Administer:

PO

• With food to decrease GI symptoms and prevent ulcerations; do not crush, chew, or break sus rel cap

IV

• After diluting 1 mg/ml or more NS or sterile H_2O for inj without preservative; give over 20-30 min to avoid dramatic shift in cerebral blood flow

Y-site compatibilities: Furosemide, insulin (regular), potassium chloride, sodium bicarbonate, sodium nitroprusside

Perform/provide:

• Storage at room temperature

Evaluate:

• Therapeutic response: decreased pain, stiffness in joints, decreased swelling in joints, ability to move more easily

Teach patient/family:

• To report blurred vision, ringing, roaring in ears; may indicate toxicity

• To avoid driving, other hazardous activities if dizziness, drowsiness occurs

• To report change in urine pattern, increased weight, edema, increased pain in joints, fever, blood in urine; indicate nephrotoxicity; to report mood changes: anxiety, depression

• That therapeutic antiinflammatory effects may take up to 1 mo

• To avoid alcohol, NSAIDs, salicylates; bleeding may occur

🚫 Not to break, crush, or chew sus rel or reg caps

• To use sunscreen to prevent photosensitivity

---

infliximab

(in-fliks′ih-mab)
Remicade
Func. class.: Monoclonal antibody

Action: Monoclonal antibody that neutralizes the activity of tumor necrosis factor alpha (TNF α) found in Crohn's disease; decreased infiltration of inflammatory cells

Uses: Crohn's disease, fistulizing (moderate-severe); rheumatoid arthritis given with methotrexate

Research note: An FDA adverse drug report showed a possibility of development of TB associated with infliximab administration[19]

Dosage and routes:

Crohn's disease (moderate-severe)

• *Adult:* **IV INF** 5 mg/kg × 1

Crohn's disease (fistulizing)

• *Adult:* **IV INF** 5 mg/kg initially, then repeat dose 2 wk, 6 wk after 1st dose

Rheumatoid arthritis

• *Adult:* **IV** 3 mg/kg initially and q2, 6, 8 wk thereafter given with methotrexate

Available forms: Pwd for inj 100 mg

Side effects/adverse reactions:

*SYST: **Anaphylaxis***

GI: Nausea, vomiting, abdominal pain, stomatitis, constipation, dyspepsia, flatulence

CNS: Headache, dizziness, depression, vertigo, fatigue, anxiety, fever

*HEMA: **Anemia***

INTEG: Rash, dermatitis, urticaria, dry skin, sweating, flushing, hematoma, pruritus

RESP: URI, pharyngitis, bronchitis, cough, dyspnea, sinusitis

MS: Myalgia, back pain, arthralgia

GU: Dysuria, urinary frequency

*CV: Chest pain, hyper- and hypotension, **tachycardia***

Contraindications: hypersensitivity to murines

Precautions: Pregnancy (C), lactation, children, elderly

Pharmacokinetics: Distributed to vascular compartment, half-life 9.5 days

NURSING CONSIDERATIONS

Assess:

• GI symptoms: nausea, vomiting, abdominal pain

• Periodic blood counts (CBC)

• CV status: B/P, pulse, chest pain

• Allergic reaction: rash, dermatitis, urticaria, dyspnea, hypotension, fever, chills; discontinue if severe, administer epinephrine, corticosteroids, antihistamines

Administer:

IV INF

• Immediately after reconstitution; reconstitute with 10 ml of sterile water for inj, further dilute total dose/250 ml of 0.9% NaCl inj to a total conc of 0.4-4 mg/ml; use 21G or smaller needle for reconstitution, direct sterile water at glass wall of vial, gently swirl

• Give over ≥2 hr, use polyethylene-lined infusion with in-line, sterile, low-protein-bind filter

Perform/provide:

• Refrigerated storage, do not freeze

Evaluate:

• Therapeutic response: absence of fever, mucus in stools

Teach patient/family:

• Not to breastfeed while taking this drug

• To notify prescriber of GI symptoms, hypersensitivity reactions

---

◆ = Nursing alert   ∥ = Herb-drug interaction   ⊘ = Do not crush

insulin, analog injection (lispro) (℞)

Humalog

insulin, isophane suspension (NPH) (℞)

Humulin N, Iletin NPH*, Iletin II NPH*, Novolin ge NPH*, Novolin N, Novolin N PenFill, Novolin N Prefilled, NPH Iletin I, NPH Iletin II, NPH-N

insulin, isophane suspension and regular insulin (℞)

Humulin 70/30, Humalin 30/70*, Novolin 70/30, Novolin 70/30 PenFill, Novolin 70/30 Prefilled, Novolin ge 30/70*

insulin, regular (℞)

Humulin R*, Iletin I*, Iletin II*, Novolin ge Toronto*, Novolin R, Novolin R Velosulin, Novolin R PenFill, Novolin R Prefilled, Regular Ilentin I, II, Regular Purified Pork Insulin, Velosulin Human BR

insulin, zinc suspension (Lente) (℞)

Humulin L, Iletin*, Iletin II*, Lente Iletin I, Lente Iletin II, Lente L, Novolin ge Lente*, Novolin L

insulin, zinc suspension extended (Ultralente) (℞)

Humulin U Ultralente, Humulin U*, Novolin ge Ultralente*

isophane insulin suspension and insulin injection (℞)

Humalin 50/50, Novolin 50/50*

Func. class.: Pancreatic hormone
Chem. class.: Exogenous unmodified insulin

Action: Decreases blood sugar; by transport of insulin into cells and the conversion of glucose to glycogen, indirectly increases blood pyruvate and lactate, decreases phosphate and potassium; insulin may be beef, pork, human (processed by recombinant DNA technologies)

Uses: Adult-onset diabetes, juvenile diabetes, ketoacidosis types I and II, type II (non–insulin-dependent) diabetes mellitus, type I (insulin-dependent) diabetes mellitus; insulin lispro may be used in combination with sulfonylureas in children >3 yr

Dosage and routes:

Insulin, isophane, suspension
• *Adult:* SC dosage individualized by blood, urine glucose; usual dose 7-26 U; may increase by 2-10 U/day if needed

Regular insulin (ketoacidosis)
• *Adult:* IV 5-10 U, then 5-10 U/hr until desired response, then switch to SC dose; IV/inf 2-12 U (50 U/500 ml of normal saline)
• *Child:* IV 0.1 U/kg

Replacement
• *Adult and child:* SC 0.5-1 U/kg/day qid given 30 min ac
• *Adolescent:* SC 0.8-1.2 mg/kg/day; this dosage is used during rapid growth

Available forms: NPH Inj 100 U/ml; regular inj 100 U/ml; zinc susp 100 U/ml; insulin analog inj 100 U/ml; insulin zinc susp, ext (Ultralente) 100 U/ml; isophane insulin/insulin inj 100 U/ml; insulin lispro 100 U/ml 1.5 ml cartridges

Side effects/adverse reactions:
EENT: Blurred vision, dry mouth
INTEG: Flushing, rash, urticaria, warmth, *lipodystrophy,* lipohypertrophy, swelling, redness
META: **Hypoglycemia,** rebound hy-

perglycemia (Somogyi effect 12-72 hr or longer)

SYST: **Anaphylaxis**

Contraindications: Hypersensitivity to protamine

Precautions: Pregnancy (B)

Do not confuse:
Novolin 70/30 Penfill
Novolin 70/30 Prefilled

Pharmacokinetics:

SC (lispro): Onset rapid, peak ½-1 hr, duration 3-4 hr

SC (NPH): Onset 1-2 hr, peak 4-12 hr, duration 18-24 hr

SC (regular susp): Onset ½ hr, peak 4-8 hr, duration 12-24 hr

SC (regular): Onset ½-1 hr, peak 2-4 hr, duration 5-7 hr

IV (regular): Onset 10-30 min, peak 10-30 min, duration ½-1 hr

SC (regular conc): Onset ½-1 hr, peak 2-5 hr, duration 5-7 hr

SC (zinc susp): Onset 1-2 ½ hr, peak 7-15 hr, duration 12-24 hr

SC (zinc susp conc): Onset 4-8 hr, peak 10-30 hr, duration, 7-36 hr

SC (zinc susp prompt): Onset 1-1 ½ hr, peak 5-10 hr, duration 12-16 hr

Metabolized by liver, muscle, kidneys; excreted in urine

Interactions:

• Increased hypoglycemia: salicylate, alcohol, β-blockers, anabolic steroids, fenfluramine, phenylbutazone, sulfinpyrazone, guanethidine, oral hypoglycemics, MAOIs, tetracycline

• Decreased hypoglycemia: thiazides, thyroid hormones, oral contraceptives, corticosteroids, estrogens, dobutamine, epinephrine

🌿 Decreased hypoglycemic effect: annato, cocoa seeds, coffee seeds, cola seeds, guarana, ma huang, maté, rosemary

🌿 Decreased or increased hypoglycemic effect: chromium

🌿 Increased glucose tolerance: karela

🌿 Increased hypoglycemics: aceitilla, adiantum agrimony, aloe gel, banana flowers/roots, banyan stembark, bilberry, bitter melon, broom, bugleweed, burdock, carob, cumin, damiana, dandelion, eucalyptus, fenugreek, fo-ti, garlic, goat's rue, guar gum, horse chestnut, jambue, juniper, konjac, maitake, onion, psyllium, reishi

Lab test interferences:

Increase: VMA

Decrease: K, Ca

Interference: Liver function studies, thyroid function studies

NURSING CONSIDERATIONS

Assess:

• Fasting blood glucose, 2 hr PP (80-150 mg/dl, normal fasting level; 70-130 mg/dl, normal 2 hr level); also glycosylated Hgb may be drawn to identify treatment effectiveness

• Urine ketones during illness; insulin requirements may increase during stress, illness, surgery

• For hypoglycemic reaction that can occur during peak time (sweating, weakness, dizziness, chills, confusion, headache, nausea, rapid weak pulse, fatigue, tachycardia, memory lapses, slurred speech, staggering gait, anxiety, tremors, hunger)

• For hyperglycemia: acetone breath, polyuria, fatigue, polydipsia, flushed, dry skin, lethargy

Administer:

SC

• After warming to room temperature by rotating in palms to prevent injecting cold insulin; use only insulin syringes with markings or syringe matching U/ml; rotate inj sites within one area: abdomen, upper back, thighs, upper arm, buttocks; keep record of sites

◆ = Nursing alert   🌿 = Herb-drug interaction   🚫 = Do not crush

• Increased dosages if tolerance occurs; give human insulin to those allergic to beef or pork
• Do not use if cloudy, thick, or discolored
• Lispro: 15 min ac

IV
• IV direct, undiluted via vein, Y-site, 3-way stopcock; give at 50 U/min or less
• By cont inf after diluting with IV sol and run at prescribed rate; use IV inf pump for correct dosing; give reduced dose at serum glucose level of 250 mg/100 ml

Additive compatibilities: Bretylium, cimetidine, lidocaine, meropenem, ranitidine, verapamil

Syringe compatibilities: Metoclopramide

Y-site compatibilities: Amiodarone, ampicillin, ampicillin/sulbactam, aztreonam, cefazolin, cefotetan, dobutamine, esmolol, famotidine, gentamicin, heparin, heparin/hydrocortisone, imipenem/cilastatin, indomethacin, magnesium sulfate, meperidine, meropenem, midazolam, morphine, nitroglycerin, oxytocin, pentobarbital, potassium chloride, propofol, ritodrine, sodium bicarbonate, sodium nitroprusside, tacrolimus, terbutaline, ticarcillin, ticarcillin/clavulanate, tobramycin, vancomycin, vit B/C

Perform/provide:
• Store at room temperature for <1 mo; keep away from heat and sunlight; refrigerate all other supply; do not use if discolored; do not freeze—IV route, regular only

Evaluate:
• Therapeutic response: decrease in polyuria, polydipsia, polyphagia, clear sensorium, absence of dizziness, stable gait

Teach patient/family:
• That blurred vision occurs; not to change corrective lens until vision is stabilized 1-2 mo
• To keep insulin, equipment available at all times
• That drug does not cure diabetes but controls symptoms
• To carry Medic Alert ID as diabetic
• To recognize hypoglycemia reaction: headache, tremors, fatigue, weakness
• The dosage, route, mixing instructions, if any diet restrictions, disease process
• To carry candy or lump sugar to treat hypoglycemia
• The symptoms of ketoacidosis: nausea, thirst, polyuria, dry mouth, decreased B/P, dry, flushed skin, acetone breath, drowsiness, Kussmaul respirations
• That a plan is necessary for diet, exercise; all food on diet should be eaten; exercise routine should not vary
• About blood glucose testing; make sure patient is able to determine glucose level
• To avoid OTC drugs unless directed by prescriber

Treatment of overdose: Glucose 25g IV, via dextrose 50% sol, 50 ml or glucagon 1 mg

---

insulin aspart (℞)
NovoLog
insulin glargine
Lantus
Func. class.: Pancreatic hormone

Action: Decreases blood sugar; by transport of insulin into cells and the conversion of glucose to glycogen, indirectly increases blood pyruvate and lactate, decreases phosphate and potassium; insulin may be beef, pork, human (processed by recombinant DNA technologies)

Uses: Adult-onset diabetes, juvenile diabetes, ketoacidosis types I and II, type II (non–insulin-dependent) diabetes mellitus, type I (insulin-dependent) diabetes mellitus

Dosage and routes:
Lantus
• *Adult and child ≥6 yr:* **SC** 10 IU qd HS, range 2-100 IU/day
NovoLog
• *Adult:* 0.5-1 U/kg/day; give close to meal

Available forms: Lantus (inj 100 IU); NovoLog (inj 100 U/ml human insulin aspart (rDNA)

Side effects/adverse reactions:
EENT: Blurred vision, dry mouth
INTEG: Flushing, rash, urticaria, warmth, *lipodystrophy,* lipohypertrophy, swelling, redness
META: Hypoglycemia, rebound hyperglycemia (Somogyi effect 12-72 hr or longer)
SYST: **Anaphylaxis**

Contraindications: Hypersensitivity to protamine

Precautions: Pregnancy (C)

Pharmacokinetics:
Aspart (NovoLog)
SC: Onset 0.25 hr, peak 1-3 hr, duration 3-5, half-life 1½ hr
Glargine (Lantus)
SC: Onset 1.1 hr, no peak, duration 24 hr

Metabolized by the liver, muscles, kidneys, excreted in urine, it is not known whether it is excreted in breast milk

Interactions:
• Increased hypoglycemia: salicylate, alcohol, β-blockers, anabolic steroids, fenfluramine, phenylbutazone, sulfinpyrazone, guanethidine, oral hypoglycemics, MAOIs, tetracycline

• Decreased hypoglycemia: thiazides, thyroid hormones, oral contraceptives, corticosteroids, estrogens, dobutamine, epinephrine

🖋 Decreased hypoglycemic effect: broom, buchu, dandelion, juniper

🖋 Decreased or increased hypoglycemic effect: chromium, fenugreek, ginseng

🖋 Increased glucose tolerance: karela

Lab test interferences:
Increase: VMA
Decrease: K, Ca
Interference: Liver function studies, thyroid function studies

NURSING CONSIDERATIONS
Assess:
• Fasting blood glucose, 2 hr PP (80-150 mg/dl, normal fasting level; 70-130 mg/dl, normal 2 hr level); also glycosylated Hgb may be drawn to identify treatment effectiveness
• Urine ketones during illness; insulin requirements may increase during stress, illness, surgery
• For hypoglycemic reaction that can occur during peak time (sweating, weakness, dizziness, chills, confusion, headache, nausea, rapid weak pulse, fatigue, tachycardia, memory lapses, slurred speech, staggering gait, anxiety, tremors, hunger)
• For hyperglycemia: acetone breath, polyuria, fatigue, polydipsia, flushed, dry skin, lethargy
Administer:
SC
• After warming to room temperature by rotating in palms to prevent injecting cold insulin; use only insulin syringes with markings or syringe matching U/ml; rotate inj sites within one area: abdomen, upper back, thighs, upper arm, buttocks; keep record of sites
• Increased dosages if tolerance occurs; give human insulin to those allergic to beef or pork

◆ = Nursing alert   🖋 = Herb-drug interaction   🚫 = Do not crush

• Do not mix or add insulin glargine to any other insulin or sol
• Do not mix insulin aspart with crystalline zinc insulin

Perform/provide:

• Store at room temperature for <1 mo; keep away from heat and sunlight; refrigerate all other supply; do not use if discolored

Evaluate:

• Therapeutic response: decrease in polyuria, polydipsia, polyphagia, clear sensorium, absence of dizziness, stable gait

Teach patient/family:

• That blurred vision occurs; not to change corrective lens until vision is stabilized 1-2 mo
• To keep insulin, equipment available at all times
• That drug does not cure diabetes but controls symptoms
• To carry Medic Alert ID as diabetic
• To recognize hypoglycemia reaction: headache, tremors, fatigue, weakness
• The dosage, route, mixing instructions, if any diet restrictions, disease process
• To carry candy or lump sugar to treat hypoglycemia
• The symptoms of ketoacidosis: nausea, thirst, polyuria, dry mouth, decreased B/P, dry, flushed skin, acetone breath, drowsiness, Kussmaul respirations
• That a plan is necessary for diet, exercise; all food on diet should be eaten; exercise routine should not vary
• About blood glucose testing; make sure patient is able to determine glucose level
• To avoid OTC drugs unless directed by prescriber

Treatment of overdose: Glucose 25 g IV, via dextrose 50% sol, 50 ml or glucagon 1 mg

interferon alfa-2a/ interferon alfa-2b ℞

(in-ter-feer′on)
Roferon-a/Intron-a
Func. class.: Misc. antineoplastic
Chem. class.: Protein product

Action: Antiviral action inhibits viral replication by reprogramming virus; antitumor action suppresses cell proliferation; immunomodulating action phagocytizes target cells; may also inhibit virus replication in virus-infested cells

Uses: Hairy cell leukemia in persons >18 yr, condylomata acuminata, malignant melanoma, AIDS (use phase II with zidovudine), chronic hepatitis B, C

Investigational uses: Bladder tumors, carcinoid tumors, non-Hodgkin's lymphoma, essential thrombocytopenia, cytomegaloviruses, herpes simplex, Kaposi's sarcoma, HPV-associated diseases

Dosage and routes:

alfa-2a

Hairy cell leukemia

• *Adult:* **SC/IM** 3 million IU/day × 16-24 wk, then 3 million IU 3×/wk maintenance

Condylomata acuminata

• 1 million IU/lesion 3×/wk × 3 wk

alfa-2b

Chronic hepatitis B

• 3 million IU/3×/wk × 18-24 mo **SC/IM** as 5 million IU/day or 10 million IU/3×/wk × 16 wk

Hairy cell leukemia

• 2 million IU/m^2 3×/wk; if severe adverse reactions occur, dose should be skipped or reduced by ½

Kaposi's sarcoma

• *Adult* **SC/IM:** 30 million IU/m^2 3×/wk

530 interferon alfa-2a/interferon alfa-2b

Available forms: alfa-2a inj 3, 6, 36 million IU/ml; alfa-2b inj 3, 5, 10, 18, 25 million U/vial, pwd for inj 5, 10, 18, 25, 50 million U/vial

Side effects/adverse reactions:

CNS: Dizziness, confusion, numbness, paresthesias, hallucinations, **seizures, coma,** amnesia, anxiety, mood changes, depression, somnolence, paranoia, irritability

CV: Edema, hypotension, hypertension, chest pain, palpitations, dysrhythmias, **CHF, MI, CVA,** tachycardia, syncope

INTEG: Rash, dry skin, itching, alopecia, flushing, photosensitivity

GI: Weight loss, taste changes, nausea, anorexia, diarrhea, xerostomia

GU: Impotence

*HEMA: **Neutropenia, thrombocytopenia***

MISC: Flulike syndrome; fever, fatigue, myalgias, headache, chills

Contraindications: Hypersensitivity

Precautions: Severe hypotension, dysrhythmia, tachycardia, pregnancy (C), lactation, children, severe renal or hepatic disease, convulsion disorder

Do not confuse:

Roferon-A/Imferon

Pharmacokinetics: Half-life (interferon alfa-2a) 3.7-8.5 hr, peak 3-4 hr; half-life (interferon alfa-2b) 2-7 hr, peak 6-8 hr

interferon alfa-2b

Interactions:

• Increased theophylline levels: aminophylline

• Increased neutropenia: zidovudine

Lab test interferences:

Interference: AST, ALT, LDH, alk phosphatase, WBC, platelets, granulocytes, creatinine

NURSING CONSIDERATIONS
Assess:

• For symptoms of infection; chills, fever, headache; may be masked by drug fever

• CNS reaction: LOC, mental status, dizziness, confusion, paresthesia, slurred speech

• Cardiac status: Lung sounds; ECG before and during treatment, especially in those with cardiac disease

• Bone marrow depression: bruising, bleeding, blood in stools, urine, sputum, emesis

• Mental status: depression, suicidal thoughts, hallucinations, amnesia

Administer:

alfa-2a

• SC/IM after reconstituting 18 million U/3 ml of diluent provided (6 million U/ml)

• 36 million U/ml is used for Kaposi's sarcoma only

alfa-2b

• IM/SC after reconstituting 3-5 million IU/1 ml, 10 million IU/2 ml, 25 million IU/5 ml, of diluent provided, mix gently

• Intralesional after reconstituting 10 million IU/1 ml bacteriostatic water for inj; no more than 5 lesions can safely be treated at a time

• At hs to minimize side effects

• Acetaminophen as ordered to alleviate fever and headache

Perform/provide:

• Reconstituted sol must be used within 30 days

• Increased fluid intake to 2-3 L/day

Evaluate:

• Therapeutic response: decrease in size, number of lesions

Teach patient/family:

• To take acetaminophen for fever

• To avoid hazardous tasks, since confusion, dizziness may occur;

◆ = Nursing alert   🖉 = Herb-drug interaction   🚫 = Do not crush

avoid prolonged sunlight, use sunscreen

• That brands of this drug should not be changed; each form is different, with different doses

• That fatigue is common; activity may have to be altered to take hs to minimize flulike symptoms

• Not to become pregnant while taking drug; possible mutagenic effects

• To report signs of infection: sore throat, fever, diarrhea, vomiting, sore or white patches in mouth

• That impotence may occur during treatment but is temporary

• That emotional lability is common; notify prescriber if severe or incapacitating

---

interferon alfacon-1 (℞)

(in-ter-feer'on al'fa-kon)

Infergen

Func. class.: Recombinant type I interferon

Action: Induces biologic responses and has antiviral, antiproliferative and immunomodulatory effects

Uses: Chronic hepatitis C infections

Investigational uses:

Hairy cell leukemia when used with G-CSF

Dosage and routes:

• *Adult:* **SC** 9 µg as a single inj 3×/wk × 24 wk

Available forms: Inj 9 µg/0.3 ml, 15 µg/0.5 ml

Side effects/adverse reactions:

CNS: Headache, fatigue, fever, rigors, insomnia, dizziness

GI: Abdominal pain, nausea, diarrhea, anorexia, dyspepsia, vomiting, constipation, flatulence, hemorrhoids, decreased salivation

MS: Back, limb, neck skeletal pain

GU: Dysmenorrhea, vaginitis, menstrual disorders

INTEG: Alopecia, pruritus, rash, erythema, dry skin

EENT: Tinnitus, earache, conjunctivitis, eye pain

HEMA: **Granulocytopenia, thrombocytopenia, leukopenia,** ecchymosis

CV: Hypertension, palpitation

PSYCH: Nervousness, depression, anxiety, lability, abnormal thinking

RESP: Pharyngitis, upper respiratory infection, cough, sinusitis, rhinitis, respiratory tract congestion, epistaxis, dyspnea, bronchitis

Contraindications: Hypersensitivity to alpha interferons, or products from *Escherichia coli*

Precautions: Thyroid disorders, myelosuppression, hepatic, cardiac disease, lactation, children <18 yr

Pharmacokinetics: Peak 24-36 hr

Interactions:

• None known

NURSING CONSIDERATIONS

Assess:

• Platelet counts, heme concentration, ANC, serum creatinine concentration, albumin, bilirubin, TSH, T_4

• For myelosuppression, hold dose if neutrophil count is $<500 \times 10^6$/L or if platelets are $<50 \times 10^9$/L

• For hypersensitivity: discontinue immediately if hypersensitivity occurs

Evaluate:

• Therapeutic response: decreased chronic hepatitis C signs/symptoms

Teach patient/family:

• Provide patient or family member with written, detailed information about drug

---

interferon alfa-n1 lymphoblastoid (℞)

(in-ter-feer′on al′fa n one lim-foh-blast′oid)

Wellferon

Func. class.: Recombinant type 1 interferon

Action: Induces biologic responses and has antiviral, antiproliferative and immunomodulatory effects; mixture of alpha interferons isolated from human cells after induction with parainfluenza virus

Uses: Chronic hepatitis C infections

Dosage and routes:
• *Adult:* **SC/IM** 3 MU × 3×/wk × 6-12 mo

Available forms: Solution 3 MU/ml

Side effects/adverse reactions:

CNS: Headache, fever, insomnia, dizziness, anxiety, hostility, lability, nervousness, depression, confusion, abnormal thinking, amnesia

GI: Abdominal pain, nausea, diarrhea, anorexia, vomiting

MS: Back pain

INTEG: Alopecia, pruritus, rash, erythema, dry skin

*HEMA: **Granulocytopenia, thrombocytopenia, leukopenia,** ecchymosis*

RESP: Pharyngitis, upper respiratory infection, cough, epistaxis, dyspnea, bronchitis

Contraindications: Hypersensitivity to alpha interferons, history of anaphylaxis to bovine or ovine immunoglobulins, egg protein, polymyxin B, neomycin sulfate

Precautions: Thyroid disorders, myelosuppression, hepatic, cardiac disease, lactation, children <18 yr, depression/suicide

Pharmacokinetics: Peak 24-36 hr

Interactions:
• Use caution when giving with theophylline, myelosuppressive agents

NURSING CONSIDERATIONS

Assess:
• ALT, HCV viral load; patients that show no reduction in ALT, HCV are unlikely to show benefit of treatment after 6 mo
• Platelet counts, heme concentration, ANC, serum creatinine concentration, albumin, bilirubin, TSH, T_4, AFP
• For myelosuppression, hold dose if neutrophil count is <500 × 10^6/L or if platelets are <50 × 10^9/L
• For hypersensitivity: discontinue immediately if hypersensitivity occurs

Administer:
• Same brand of product during course of treatment

Evaluate:
• Therapeutic response: decreased chronic hepatitis C signs/symptoms, undetectable viral load

Teach patient/family:
• Provide patient or family member with written, detailed information about drug
• Instructions for home use if appropriate
• Take in evening to reduce discomfort, sleep through some side effects

interferon alfa-n 3 (℞)

(in-ter-feer′on)

Alferon N

Func. class.: Antineoplastic

Chem. class.: Human interferon α-protein

Action: Binds interferon to membrane receptors on cell surface with high specificity; this produces protein synthesis, inhibition of virus replication, suppression

---

of cell proliferation, increased phagocytosis

Uses: Condylomata acuminata (venereal/genital warts)

Dosage and routes:
• *Adult:* 0.05 ml (250,000 IU) per wart, given 2×/wk × 8 wk; not to exceed 0.5 ml (2.5 million IU); inject into base of wart

Available forms: Inj 5 m IU/l ml vial with 3.3 mg/ml phenol and 1 mg/ml human albumin

Side effects/adverse reactions:

CNS: Fever, headache, sweating, vasovagal reaction, chills, fatigue, dizziness, insomnia, sleepiness, depression*

GI: Nausea, vomiting, heartburn, diarrhea, constipation, anorexia, stomatitis, dry mouth

MS: Myalgias, arthralgia, back pain, flulike symptoms

INTEG: Pain at injection site, pruritus

CV: Chest pain, hypotension

Contraindications: Hypersensitivity to this product, egg protein, IgG, neomycin

Precautions: Pregnancy (C), lactation, children, CHF, angina (unstable), COPD, diabetes mellitus with ketoacidosis, hemophilia, pulmonary embolism, thrombophlebitis, bone marrow depression, convulsive disorder

Pharmacokinetics: Unable to detect

Lab test interferences:

Interference: AST, ALT, LDH, alk phosphatase, WBC, platelets, granulocytes, creatinine

NURSING CONSIDERATIONS
Assess:
• For symptoms of infection; may be masked by drug fever
• CNS reaction: LOC, mental status, dizziness, confusion
• For body image disturbance

Administer:
• Acetaminophen to alleviate fever and headache

Perform/provide:
• Storage of reconstituted sol for 1 mo in refrigerator
• Increased fluid intake to 2-3 L/day

Evaluate:
• Therapeutic response: decrease in wart size

Teach patient/family:
• To avoid hazardous tasks, since confusion, dizziness may occur
• That brands of this drug should not be changed; each form is different, with different doses
• That fatigue is common; activity may have to be altered
• Not to become pregnant while taking drug; possible mutagenic effects
• To report signs of infection: sore throat, fever, diarrhea, vomiting
• To recognize the signs of hypersensitivity: liver, urticaria, wheezing, dyspnea; notify prescriber immediately

---

interferon beta-1a
(in-ter-feer′on)
Avonex
interferon beta-1b (℞)
Betaseron
Func. class.: Multiple sclerosis agent
Chem. class.: Escherichia coli derivative

Action: Antiviral, immunoregulatory; action not clearly understood; biologic response modifying properties mediated through specific receptors on cells, inducing expression of interferon-induced gene products

Uses: Ambulatory patients with relapsing-remitting multiple sclerosis

Investigational uses: May be useful in treatment of AIDS, AIDS-related Kaposi's sarcoma, malignant melanoma, metastatic renal cell carcinoma, cutaneous T cell lymphoma, acute non-A, non-B hepatitis

Dosage and routes:
interferon beta-1a
• *Adult:* IM 30 µg qwk
interferon beta-1b
Relapsing-remitting multiple sclerosis
• *Adult:* SC 0.25 mg (8 IU) qod
Available forms: beta-1a 33 µg (6.6 million IU/vial); beta-1b pwd for inj lyophilized 0.3 mg (9.6 mIU)

Side effects/adverse reactions:
CNS: Headache, fever, pain, chills, mental changes, hypertonia, **suicide attempts**
CV: Migraine, palpitations, hypertension, tachycardia, peripheral vascular disorders
EENT: Conjunctivitis, blurred vision
GI: Diarrhea, constipation, vomiting, abdominal pain
GU: Dysmenorrhea, irregular menses, metrorrhagia, cystitis, breast pain
*HEMA: **Decreased lymphocytes, ANC, WBC;** lymphadenopathy*
INTEG: Sweating, inj site reaction
*MS: Myalgia, **myasthenia***
RESP: Sinusitis, dyspnea

Contraindications: Hypersensitivity to natural or recombinant interferon-β or human albumin

Precautions: Pregnancy (C), lactation, child <18 yr, chronic progressive MS, depression, mental disorders

NURSING CONSIDERATIONS
Assess:
• Blood, renal, hepatic studies: CBC, differential, platelet counts, BUN, creatinine ALT, urinalysis; if abso-

lute neutrophil count < 750/mm^3, or if AST/ALT is 10 × normal, drug is discontinued
• CNS symptoms: headache, fatigue, depression
• GI status: diarrhea or constipation, vomiting, abdominal pain
• Cardiac status: increased B/P, tachycardia
• Mental status: depression, depersonalization, suicidal thoughts, insomnia
• For multiple sclerosis symptoms
Administer:
• Acetaminophen for fever, headache
• SC only
Interferon beta-1a
• Reconstitute with 1.1 ml diluent, swirl, give within 6 hr
Interferon beta-1b
• Reconstitute by injecting diluent provided (1.2 ml) into vial, swirl (8 mIU/ml), use 27G needle for inj
Perform/provide:
• Storage in refrigerator; do not freeze
Evaluate:
• Therapeutic response: decreased symptoms of multiple sclerosis
Teach patient/family:
• To provide patient or family member with written, detailed information about the drug
• That blurred vision, sweating may occur
• That female patients may experience irregular menses, dysmenorrhea, or metrorrhagia as well as breast pain
• To use sunscreen to prevent photosensitivity
• To notify prescriber if pregnancy is suspected
• Inj technique and care of equipment
• To notify prescriber of increased temp, chills, muscle soreness, fatigue

---

◆ = Nursing alert   ∥ = Herb-drug interaction   ⊘ = Do not crush

interferon gamma-1b (℞)

(in-ter-feer'on)

Actimmune

Func. class.: Biologic response modifier

Chem. class.: Lymphokine, interleukin type

Action: Species-specific protein synthesized in response to viruses, effects; can mediate killing of *Staphylococcus aureus, Toxoplasma gondii, Leishmania donovani, Listeria monocytogenes, Mycobacterium avium-intracellulare;* enhances oxidative metabolism of macrophages, enhances antibody-dependent cellular cytotoxicity

Uses: Serious infections associated with chronic granulomatous disease, osteoporosis

Dosage and routes:
• *Adult:* **SC** 50 µg/m² (1.5 million U/m²) for patients with surface area >0.5 m²; 1.5 µg/kg/dose for patient with surface area <0.5 m²; give Monday, Wednesday, Friday for 3×/wk dosing

Available forms: Inj 100 µg (3 million U)/single-dose vial

Side effects/adverse reactions:
GI: Nausea, anorexia, abdominal pain, weight loss, diarrhea, vomiting
CNS: Headache, fatigue, depression, fever, chills
INTEG: Rash, pain at inj site
MS: Myalgia, arthralgia

Contraindications: Hypersensitivity to interferon-γ, *Escherichia coli-*derived products

Precautions: Pregnancy (C), cardiac disease, seizure disorders, CNS disorders, myelosuppression, lactation, children

Pharmacokinetics:
SC: Dose absorbed 89%, elimination half-life 5.9 hr, peak 7 hr

Interactions:
• Increased myelosuppression: other myelosuppressive agents

NURSING CONSIDERATIONS
Assess:
• Blood, renal, hepatic studies: CBC, differential, platelet counts, BUN, creatinine, ALT, urinalysis
• CNS symptoms: headache, fatigue, depression

Administer:
• At hs to minimize adverse reactions; administer acetaminophen for fever, headache
• 50% of dose if severe reactions occur or discontinue treatment until reactions subside
• In right and left deltoid and anterior thigh
• Warm to room temperature before use; do not leave at room temperature over 12 hr (unopened vial)

Perform/provide:
• Storage in refrigerator upon receipt; do not freeze; do not shake

Evaluate:
• Therapeutic response: decreased serious infections, improvement in existing infections and inflammatory conditions

Teach patient/family:
• The method of administration if family members will be giving medication
• Provide patient or family member with written, detailed information about drug

---

RARELY USED

iodoquinol (℞)

(eye-oh-doh-kwin'ole)

Func. class.: Amebicide

Uses: Intestinal amebiasis
Dosage and routes:
• *Adult:* **PO** 630-650 mg tid × 20 days, not to exceed 2 g/day
• *Child:* **PO** 30-40 mg/kg/day in 2-3 divided doses × 20 days, not to exceed 1.95 g/24 hr × 20 days; do not repeat treatment before 2-3 wk
Contraindications: Hypersensitivity to this drug or iodine, renal disease, hepatic disease, severe thyroid disease, preexisting optic neuropathy

ipecac syrup (℞, OTC)

(ip'e-kak)

Func. class.: Emetic
Chem. class.: Cephaelis ipeca-cuanha derivative

Action: Acts on chemoreceptor trigger zone to induce vomiting; irritates gastric mucosa
Uses: In poisoning to induce vomiting
Dosage and routes:
• *Adult:* **PO** 15-30 ml, then 200-300 ml water; repeat 1×, if vomiting does not occur within 20 min
• *Child >1 yr:* **PO** 15 ml, then 200-300 ml water
• *Child 6-12 mo:* **PO** 5-10 ml, then 100-200 ml water; may repeat dose if needed
Available forms: Syr
Side effects/adverse reactions:
CNS: Depression, convulsions, coma
GI: Nausea, vomiting, bloody diarrhea
CV: Circulatory failure, atrial fi-brillation, fatal myocarditis, dysrhythmias
Contraindications: Hypersensitivity, unconscious/semiconscious, depressed gag reflex, poisoning with petroleum products or caustic substances, convulsions
Precautions: Lactation, pregnancy (C)
Pharmacokinetics:
PO: Onset 15-30 min
Interactions:
• Do not administer with activated charcoal, other antiemetics; effect will be decreased
• Drug/food: decreased effect: dairy products
• Increased abdominal distention: carbonated drinks
NURSING CONSIDERATIONS
Assess:
• VS, B/P; check patients with cardiac disease more often
• Type of poisoning; do not administer if petroleum products or caustic substances have been ingested: kerosene, gasoline, lye, Draño
• Respiratory status before, during, after administration; check rate, rhythm, character; respiratory depression can occur rapidly with elderly or debilitated patients
Administer:
◆ Ipecac syrup, not ipecac fluid, which is 14 times stronger; death may occur
• Activated charcoal after vomiting completed; may begin lavage after 10-15 min after 2 doses of ipecac syrup with no result
Evaluate:
• Therapeutic response: vomiting

◆ = Nursing alert   🌿 = Herb-drug interaction   🚫 = Do not crush

ipratropium (℞)

(i-pra-troe′pee-um)

Atrovent

Func. class.: Anticholinergic, bronchodilator

Chem. class.: Synthetic quaternary ammonium compound

Action: Inhibits interaction of acetylcholine at receptor sites on the bronchial smooth muscle, resulting in decreased cGMP and bronchodilation

Uses: Bronchodilation during bronchospasm in those with COPD; rhinorrhea in children 6-11 yr (nasal spray)

Dosage and routes:
• *Adult:* 2 **INH** 4 × day, not to exceed 12 **INH**/24 hr; sol 500 μg (1 unit dose) given 3-4 ×/day
• *Child 6-11 yr:* Nasal 1 spray in each nostril

Available forms: Aerosol 18 μg/actuation; nasal spray 0.03%, 0.06%; sol for inh 0.02%

Side effects/adverse reactions:

GI: Nausea, vomiting, cramps

EENT: Dry mouth, blurred vision

CNS: Anxiety, dizziness, headache, nervousness

RESP: Cough, worsening of symptoms, **bronchospasms**

INTEG: Rash

CV: Palpitation

Contraindications: Hypersensitivity to this drug, atropine, soya lecithin

Precautions: Pregnancy (B), lactation, children <12 yr, narrow-angle glaucoma, prostatic hypertrophy, bladder neck obstruction

Do not confuse:

Atrovent/Alupent

Pharmacokinetics: Half-life 2 hr; does not cross blood-brain barrier

NURSING CONSIDERATIONS

Assess:
• For palpitations; if severe, drug may have to be changed
• For tolerance over long-term therapy; dose may have to be increased or changed

Administer:

Nebulizer
• Use sol in nebulizer with a mouthpiece rather than a face mask

Nasal spray
• Priming pump initially requires 7 actuations of the pump, priming again is not necessary if used regularly

Perform/provide:
• Storage at room temperature
• Hard candy, frequent drinks, sugarless gum to relieve dry mouth

Evaluate:
• Therapeutic response: ability to breathe adequately

Teach patient/family:
• That compliance is necessary with number of inhalations/24 hr, or overdose may occur; spacer device in the elderly
• To shake before using
• The correct method of inhalation and cleaning of equipment daily

irbesartan (℞)

(er-be-sar′tan)

Avapro

Func. class.: Antihypertensive

Chem. class.: Angiotensin II receptor blocker (Type AT$_1$)

Action: Blocks the vasoconstrictor and aldosterone-secreting effects of angiotensin II; selectively blocks the binding of angiotensin II to the AT$_1$ receptor found in tissues

Uses: Hypertension, alone or in combination

Investigational uses: Heart failure, hypertensive patients with diabetic nephropathy caused by type II diabetes

Dosages and routes:
• *Adult:* **PO** 150 mg qd; may be increased to 300 mg qd
Available forms: 75, 150, 300 mg

Side effects/adverse reactions:
CNS: Dizziness, anxiety, headache, fatigue
GI: Diarrhea, dyspepsia
RESP: Cough, upper respiratory infection

Contraindications: Hypersensitivity, pregnancy (D) 2nd and 3rd trimester

Precautions: Hypersensitivity to ACE inhibitors; pregnancy (C) 1st trimester, lactation, children, elderly, renal disease

Pharmacokinetics: Extensively metabolized, half-life 11-15 hr, highly bound to plasma proteins, excreted in urine and feces

NURSING CONSIDERATIONS
Assess:
• B/P, pulse q4h; note rate, rhythm, quality
• Electrolytes: K, Na, Cl
• Baselines in renal, liver function tests before therapy begins
• Edema in feet, legs qd
• Skin turgor, dryness of mucous membranes for hydration status

Administer:
• Without regard to meals
• IV 0.9% NaCl and place supine for severe hypotension

Evaluate:
• Therapeutic response: decreased B/P

Teach patient/family:
• To comply with dosage schedule, even if feeling better
• That drug may cause dizziness, fainting; light-headedness may occur
• To rise slowly to sitting or standing position to minimize orthostatic hypotension
• To notify prescriber if pregnancy is suspected

---

irinotecan (℞)

(ear-een-oh-tee′kan)

Camptosar, Captothecan-11, CPT-11

Func. class.: Antineoplastic hormone

Chem. class.: Topoisomerase inhibitor

Action: Cytotoxic by producing damage to double-strand DNA during DNA synthesis

Uses: Metastatic carcinoma of the colon or rectum, or 1st-line treatment in combination with 5-FU and leucovorin for metastatic colon or rectal carcinomas

Dosage and routes:
• *Adult:* **IV** 125 mg/m^2 given over 1½ hr qwk × 4 wk, then 2 wk rest period, may be repeated; 4 wk or 2 wk off, dosage adjustments may be made to 150 mg/m^2 (high) or 50 mg/m^2 (low); adjustments should be made in increments of 25-50 mg/m^2 depending on patient's tolerance

Combination dosage schedules
• *Regimen 1:* irinotecan 75-125 mg/m^2, leucovorin 20 mg/m^2, 5-FU 300-500 mg/m^2 depending on dosing levels

Hepatic impairment
• *Adult:* **IV** 100 mg/m^2 qwk × 4 wk, then 2 wk rest, may repeat cycle or 300 mg/m^2 q3wk, dose may be adjusted up or down
Available forms: Inj 20 mg/ml

 = Nursing alert   🌿 = Herb-drug interaction   🚫 = Do not crush

Side effects/adverse reactions:
CNS: Fever, headache, chills, dizziness
GI: ***Severe diarrhea,*** nausea, vomiting, anorexia, constipation, cramps, flatus, stomatitis, dyspepsia, ***hepatotoxicity***
INTEG: Irritation at site, rash, sweating, alopecia
Leukopenia, anemia, neutropenia
RESP: Dyspnea, increased cough, rhinitis
CV: Vasodilation
MISC: Edema, asthenia, weight loss
Contraindications: Hypersensitivity, pregnancy (D)
Precautions: Lactation, children, elderly, myelosuppression, irradiation
Pharmacokinetics: Rapidly and completely absorbed; excreted in urine and bile as metabolites; half-life 10 hr, bound to plasma proteins 30%-68%
Interactions:
• Increased myelosuppression, diarrhea: other antineoplastics, radiation
• Increased lymphocytopenia: dexamethasone
• Increased akathisia: prochlorperazine
• Increased dehydration: diuretics
NURSING CONSIDERATIONS
Assess:
• For CNS symptoms: fever, headache, chills, dizziness
• CBC, differential, platelet count weekly; withhold drug if WBC is <2000/mm^3, or platelet count <100,000/mm^3, Hgb ≤9 g/dl, neutrophil ≤1000/mm^3; notify prescriber of these results; drug should be discontinued, and colony-stimulating factor given
• Buccal cavity q8h for dryness, sores, or ulceration, white patches, oral pain, bleeding, dysphagia
◆ GI symptoms: frequency of stools; cramping; severe life-threatening diarrhea may occur with fluid and electrolyte imbalances
• Signs of dehydration: rapid respirations, poor skin turgor, decreased urine output, dry skin, restlessness, weakness
• Bone marrow depression: bruising, bleeding, blood in stools, urine, sputum, emesis
Administer:
• Antiemetics and dexamethasone 10 mg at least ½ hr before antineoplastics
• After preparing in biologic cabinet using gloves, mask, gown
IV
• By intermittent inf after diluting with 0.9% NaCl or D$_5$ (0.12-1.1 mg/ml) give over 1½ hr
• Do not admix with other solutions or medications
• Stable for 24 hr at room temperature, 48 hr, refrigerated
Perform/provide:
• Increased fluid intake to 2-3 L/day to prevent dehydration, unless contraindicated
• Changing of IV site q48h
• Rinsing of mouth tid-qid with water, club soda; brushing of teeth bid-tid with soft brush or cotton-tipped applicator for stomatitis; use unwaxed dental floss
• Nutritious diet with iron, vitamin supplement, low fiber, few dairy products
Evaluate:
• Therapeutic response: decrease in tumor size, decrease in spread of cancer
Teach patient/family:
• To avoid foods with citric acid or hot or rough texture if stomatitis is present; to drink adequate fluids
• To report stomatitis; any bleeding, white spots, ulcerations in mouth; tell patient to examine mouth qd, report symptoms

• To report signs of anemia: fatigue, headache, faintness, shortness of breath, irritability

• To use contraception during therapy

• To avoid salicylates, NSAIDs, alcohol, bleeding may occur

• About alopecia, that when hair grows back, it will be different texture, thickness

• To avoid vaccinations while taking this drug

◆To report diarrhea that occurs 24 hr after administration, severe dehydration can occur rapidly

Treatment of overdose: Induce vomiting, provide supportive care, prevent dehydration

---

iron dextran (℞)
DexFerrum, Imferon, In Fed
Func. class.: Hematinic
Chem. class.: Ferric hydroxide complex with dextran

Action: Iron is carried by transferrin to the bone marrow, where it is incorporated into hemoglobin

Uses: Iron deficiency anemia

Dosage and routes:

• *Adult and child:* **IM** 0.5 ml as a test dose by Z-track, then no more than the following per day:

• *Adult <50 kg:* **IM** 100 mg

• *Adult >50 kg:* **IM** 250 mg

• *Infant <5 kg:* **IM** 25 mg

• *Child <5-9 kg:* **IM** 50 mg

• *Adult:* **IV** 0.5 ml (25 mg) test dose, then 100 mg qd after 2-3 days; give 25 mg test dose, wait 5 min, then infuse over 6-12 hr or use equation that follows:

$$\frac{0.3 \times \text{wt (lb)} \times \frac{100 - \text{Hgb (g/dl)} \times 100}{14.8}} = \text{mg iron}$$

<30 lb (66 kg) should be given 80% of above formula dose

Available forms: Inj 50 mg/ml

Side effects/adverse reactions:

CNS: Headache, paresthesia, dizziness, shivering, weakness, **seizures**

GI: Nausea, vomiting, metallic taste, abdominal pain

INTEG: Rash, pruritus, urticaria, fever, sweating, chills, brown skin discoloration, pain at inj site, necrosis, sterile abscesses, phlebitis

CV: Chest pain, **shock,** hypotension, tachycardia

RESP: Dyspnea

HEMA: **Leukocytosis**

OTHER: **Anaphylaxis**

Contraindications: Hypersensitivity, all anemias excluding iron deficiency anemia, hepatic disease

Precautions: Acute renal disease, children, asthma, lactation, rheumatoid arthritis (IV), infants <4 mo, pregnancy (C)

Do not confuse:
Imferon/Imuran
Imferon/Roferon-A

Pharmacokinetics:

IM: Excreted in feces, urine, bile, breast milk; crosses placenta; most absorbed through lymphatics; can be gradually absorbed over weeks/months from fixed locations

Interactions:

• Decreased reticulocyte response: chloramphenicol

• Increased toxicity: oral iron—do not use

• Decreased absorption of fluoroquinolones, penicillamine

Lab test interferences:

False increase: Serum bilirubin

False decrease: Serum Ca

False positive: ^{99m}Tc diphosphate bone scan, iron test (large doses >2 ml)

NURSING CONSIDERATIONS

Assess:

• Blood studies: Hct, Hgb, reticulocytes, transferrin, plasma iron concentrations, ferritin, total iron-

---

◆= Nursing alert   🌿= Herb-drug interaction   ⊘= Do not crush

binding, bilirubin before treatment, at least monthly
• Allergy: anaphylaxis, rash, pruritus, fever, chills, wheezing; notify prescriber immediately, keep emergency equipment available
• Cardiac status: anginal pain, hypotension, tachycardia
• Nutrition: amount of iron in diet (meat, dark green leafy vegetables, dried beans, dried fruits, eggs)
• Cause of iron loss or anemia, including use of salicylates, sulfonamides
• Toxicity: nausea, vomiting, diarrhea, fever, abdominal pain (early symptoms), cyanotic-looking lips, nailbeds, seizures, CV collapse (late symptoms)

Administer:
• D/C oral iron before parenteral; give only after test dose of 25 mg by preferred route; wait at least 1 hr before giving remaining portion
• IM deeply in large muscle mass; use Z-track method and a 19-20G 2-3-in needle; ensure needle is long enough to place drug deep in muscle, change needles after withdrawing drug and before injecting to prevent skin, tissue staining
◆ Only with epinephrine available in case of anaphylactic reaction during dose

IV
• IV after flushing with 10 ml 0.9% NaCl; give undiluted; may be diluted in 50-250 ml NS for infusion; give 1 ml (50 mg) or less over 1 min or more; flush line after use with 10 ml 0.9% NaCl; patient should remain recumbent for ½-1 hr
• IV injection requires single-dose vial without preservative; verify on label IV use is approved

Additive compatibilities: Netilmicin
Solution compatibility: TPN #211

Perform/provide:
• Storage at room temperature in cool environment
• Recumbent position 30 min after IV injection to prevent orthostatic hypotension
• Therapeutic response: increased serum iron levels, Hct, Hgb

Teach patient/family:
• That iron poisoning may occur if increased beyond recommended level; not to take oral iron preparation
• That delayed reaction may occur 1-2 days after administration and last 3-4 days (IV) 3-7 days (IM); report fever, chills, malaise, muscle, joint aches, nausea, vomiting, backache

Treatment of overdose: Discontinue drug, treat allergic reaction, give diphenhydramine or epinephrine as needed, give iron-chelating drug in acute poisoning

iron sucrose (℞)
Venofer
Func. class.: Hematinic
Chem. class.: Ferric hydroxide complex with dextran

Action: Iron is carried by transferrin to the bone marrow, where it is incorporated into hemoglobin
Uses: Iron deficiency anemia
Investigational uses: Dystrophic epidermolysis bullosa (DEB)
Dosage and routes:
• *Adult:* IV 5 ml (100 mg of elemental iron) given during dialysis, most will need 1000 mg of elemental iron over 10 dialysis sessions
Available forms: Inj 20 mg/ml
Side effects/adverse reactions:
CNS: Headache, dizziness
GI: Nausea, vomiting, abdominal pain

INTEG: Rash, pruritus, urticaria, fever, sweating, chills

CV: Chest pain, hypotension, hypertension, hypervolemia

RESP: Dyspnea, pneumonia, cough

OTHER: **Anaphylaxis**

Contraindications: Hypersensitivity, all anemias excluding iron deficiency anemia, iron overload

Precautions: Lactation, pregnancy (B), elderly, children

Pharmacokinetics: Excreted in urine, half-life 6 hr

Interactions:

• Increased toxicity: oral iron—do not use

NURSING CONSIDERATIONS

Assess:

• Blood studies: Hct, Hgb, reticulocytes, transferrin, plasma iron concentrations, ferritin, total iron-binding, bilirubin before teratment, at least monthly

• Allergy: anaphylaxis, rash, pruritus, fever, chills, wheezing; notify prescriber immediately, keep emergency equipment availble

• Cardiac status: hypotension, hypertension, hypervolemia

• Toxicity: nausea, vomiting, diarrhea, fever, abdominal pain (early symptoms), cyanotic-looking lips, nailbeds, seizures, CV collapse (late symptoms)

Administer:

◆Only with epinephrine available in case of anaphylactic reaction during dose

IV

• Give directly in dialysis line by slow inj or inf; give by slow inj at 1 ml/min (5 min/vial); inf dilute each vial exclusively in a maximum of 100 ml of 0.9% NaCl, give at rate of 100 mg of iron/15 min, discard unused portions

Perform/provide:

• Storage at room temperature in cool environment, do not freeze

• Therapeutic response: increased serum iron levels, Hct, Hgb

Teach patient/family:

• That iron poisoning may occur if increased beyond recommended level; not to take oral iron preparation

Treatment of overdose: Discontinue drug, treat allergic reaction, give diphenhydramine or epinephrine as needed, give iron-chelating drug in acute poisoning

---

isoniazid (℞)

(eye-soe-nye'a-zid)

INH, isoniazid, Isotamine*, Laniazid, Nydrazid, PMS-Isoniazid*

Func. class.: Antitubercular

Chem. class.: Isonicotinic acid hydrazide

Action: Bactericidal interference with lipid, nucleic acid biosynthesis

Uses: Treatment, prevention of TB

Dosage and routes:

Treatment

• *Adult:* **PO/IM** 300 mg/day or 15 mg/kg 2-3 ×/wk, max 900 mg 2-3 ×/wk

• *Child and infant:* **PO/IM** 10-20 mg/kg qd in 1-2 divided doses max 300 mg/day or 20-40 mg/kg, max 900 mg 2-3 ×/wk

Available forms: Tabs 50, 100, 300 mg; inj 100 mg/ml; pwd, syr 50 mg/5 ml

Side effects/adverse reactions:

Hypersensitivity: fever, skin eruptions, lymphadenopathy, vasculitis

CNS: Peripheral neuropathy, dizziness, memory impairment, **toxic encephalopathy, convulsions,** psychosis, slurred speech

EENT: Blurred vision, optic neuritis

HEMA: Agranulocytosis, hemolytic, aplastic anemia, thrombocytope-

---

◆ = Nursing alert   ∥ = Herb-drug interaction   Ⓢ = Do not crush

nia, eosinophilia, methemoglobin-emia

MISC: Dyspnea, B$_6$ deficiency, pellagra, hyperglycemia, metabolic acidosis, gynecomastia, rheumatic syndrome, SLE-like syndrome

GI: Nausea, vomiting, epigastric distress, ***jaundice, fatal hepatitis***

Contraindications: Hypersensitivity, acute liver disease

Precautions: Pregnancy (C), renal disease, diabetic retinopathy, cataracts, ocular defects, hepatic disease, child <13 yr

Pharmacokinetics:

PO: Peak 1-2 hr, duration 6-8 hr

IM: Peak 45-60 min

Metabolized in liver; excreted in urine (metabolites); crosses placenta; excreted in breast milk

Interactions:

• Increased toxicity: tyramine foods, alcohol, cycloserine, ethionamide, rifampin, carbamazepine, warfarin, phenytoin, benzodiazepines, meperidine

• Decreased absorption: aluminum antacids

• Decreased effectiveness of BCG vaccine, ketoconazole

NURSING CONSIDERATIONS
Assess:

• Liver studies qwk: ALT, AST, bilirubin; increased test results may indicate hepatitis

• Mental status often: affect, mood, behavioral changes; psychosis may occur

• Hepatic status: decreased appetite, jaundice, dark urine, fatigue

Administer:

• PO with meals to decrease GI symptoms; better to take on empty stomach 1 hr ac or 2 hr pc

• Antiemetic if vomiting occurs

• After C&S is completed; qmo to detect resistance

• IM deep in large muscle mass, massage, rotate inj site, warm inj to room temperature to dissolve crystals

Evaluate:

• Therapeutic response: decreased symptoms of TB

Teach patient/family:

• That compliance with dosage schedule, duration is necessary, not to skip or double dose

• That scheduled appointments must be kept or relapse may occur

◆To avoid alcohol while taking drug, may increase risk of hepatic injury

• That if diabetic, use blood glucose monitor to obtain correct result

◆To report weakness, fatigue, loss of appetite, nausea, vomiting, jaundice of skin or eyes, tingling/numbness of hands/feet

Treatment of overdose:
Pyridoxine

---

isoproterenol (Ƀ)
(eye-soe-proe-ter´e-nole)
Aerolone, Dispos-a-Medisoproterenol HCl, Isoproterenol HCl, Isuprel, Isuprel Glossets, Isuprel Mistometer, Medihaler-Iso, Vapo-Iso
Func. class.: β-Adrenergic agonist
Chem. class.: Catecholamine

Action: Has β$_1$ and β$_2$ action; relaxes bronchial smooth muscle and dilates the trachea and main bronchi by increasing levels of cAMP, which relaxes smooth muscles; causes increased contractility and heart rate by acting on β-receptors in heart

Uses: Bronchospasm, asthma, heart block, ventricular dysrhythmias, shock

Dosage and routes:
Asthma, bronchospasm
• *Adult:* **SL** 10-20 mg q6-8h; **INH** 1 puff, may repeat in 2-5 min, maintenance 1-2 puffs 4-6×/day; **IV** 10-20 μg during anesthesia
• *Child:* **SL** 5-10 mg q6-8h; **INH** 1 puff, may repeat in 2-5 min, maintenance 1-2 puffs 4-6×/day
Heart block/ventricular dysrhythmias
• *Adult:* **IV** 0.02-0.06, then 0.01-0.2 mg or 5 μg/min HCl; 0.2 mg, then 0.02-1 mg as needed HCl
Shock
• *Adult:* **IV INF** 0.5-5 μg/min 1 mg/500 ml D₅W, titrate to B/P, CVP, hourly urine output
Available forms: Sol for nebulization 1:400 (0.25%), 1:200 (0.5%), 1:100 (1%); aerosol 0.25%, 0.2%; pwd for inh 0.1 mg/cart; inj 1:5000 (0.2 mg/ml); glossets (SL) 10, 15 mg
Side effects/adverse reactions:
CNS: Tremors, anxiety, insomnia, headache, dizziness, stimulation
CV: Palpitations, tachycardia, hypertension, *cardiac arrest*
GI: Nausea, vomiting
RESP: Bronchial irritation, edema, dryness of oropharynx, *bronchospasms* (overuse)
META: Hyperglycemia
Contraindications: Hypersensitivity to sympathomimetics, narrow-angle glaucoma
Precautions: Pregnancy (C), cardiac disorders, hyperthyroidism, diabetes mellitus, prostatic hypertrophy, elderly
Pharmacokinetics:
IV: Onset rapid, duration 10 min
INH/SL: Onset 1-2 hr
RECT: Onset 2-4 hr
Metabolized in liver, lungs, GI tract
Interactions:
• Increased effects of both drugs: other sympathomimetics
• Decreased action when used with β-blockers

NURSING CONSIDERATIONS
Assess:
• Resp function: B/P, pulse, lung sounds
• Blood studies (CBC, WBC, differential), since blood dyscrasias may occur (rare)
• I&O ratio; check for urinary retention, frequency, hesitancy
• For paresthesias and coldness of extremities; peripheral blood flow may decrease
• Injection site: tissue sloughing; administer phentolamine mixed with 0.9% NaCl
Administer:
• With meals for GI symptoms
• SL ≤q3-4h or no more than tid
IV
• Direct dilute 0.2 mg/10 ml 0.9% NaCl (1:50,000 sol); give over 1 min; IV INF 2 mg (1:5000 sol)/500 ml of D₅W; run each 1 ml (1:250,000) sol/min; may be increased; use infusion pump, intracardiac, 1:5000 sol undiluted
Additive compatibilities: Atracurium, calcium chloride, calcium gluceptate, cephalothin, cimetidine, dobutamine, floxacillin, heparin, magnesium sulfate, multivitamins, netilmicin, potassium chloride, ranitidine, succinylchloride, verapamil, vit B/C
Syringe compatibilities: Ranitidine
Y-site compatibilities: Amiodarone, amrinone, atracurium, bretylium, cisatracurium, famotidine, heparin, hydrocortisone, pancuronium, potassium chloride, propofol, remifentanil, tacrolimus, vecuronium, vit B/C
Perform/provide:
• Storage at room temperature; do not use discolored sol

⬥ = Nursing alert 🌿 = Herb-drug interaction 🚫 = Do not crush

Evaluate:
• Therapeutic response: increased B/P with stabilization, ease of breathing

Teach patient/family:
• To rinse mouth after use
• Use of inhaler; review package insert with patient; to avoid getting aerosol in eyes; to wash inhaler in warm water and dry qd
• Use of spacer device in elderly
• About all aspects of drug; avoid smoking, smoke-filled rooms, persons with respiratory infections

Treatment of overdose: Administer a β-blocker

---

isosorbide dinitrate (℞)
(eye-soe-sor'bide)
Apo-ISDN*, Cedocard-SR*, Coronex*, Dilatrate-SR, ISDN, Iso-Bid, Isonate, Isorbid, Isordil, Isordil Tembids, Isordil Titradose, Isosorbide Dinitrate, Isotrate Timecelles, Novasorbide, Sorbitrate, Sorbitrate SA

isosorbide mononitrate
(eye-soe-sor'bide)
Imdur, Ismo, Isotrate ER, Monoket
Func. class.: Antianginal, vasodilator
Chem. class.: Nitrate

Action: Decreases preload, afterload, which is responsible for decreasing left ventricular end-diastolic pressure, systemic vascular resistance and reducing cardiac O_2 demand

Uses: Chronic stable angina pectoris, prophylaxis of angina pain, CHF

Dosage and routes:
Dinitrate
• *Adult:* PO 5-40 mg qid; SL 2.5-10 mg, may repeat q2-3h; CHEW TAB 5-10 mg prn or q2-3h as prophylaxis; SUS REL 40-80 mg q8-12h
Mononitrate
• *Adult:* PO Ismo, Monoket: 10-20 mg bid, 7 hr apart; Imdur: initiate at 30-60 mg/day as a single dose, increase q3d as needed, may increase to 120 mg qd, max 240 mg/day

Available forms:
Dinitrate: Caps sus rel 20, 40 mg; tabs 2.5, 5, 10, 20, 30, 40 mg; chew tabs 5, 10 mg; SL tabs 2.5, 5, 10 mg; ext rel tab 20, 40, 60 mg
Mononitrate: Tabs 10, 20 mg (Ismo, Monoket) 10, 20 mg; ext rel (Imdur) 30, 60, 120 mg

Side effects/adverse reactions:
MISC: Twitching, hemolytic anemia, ***methemoglobinemia***
CV: Postural hypotension, tachycardia, ***collapse,*** syncope
GI: Nausea, vomiting
INTEG: Pallor, sweating, rash
CNS: Vascular headache, flushing, dizziness, weakness, faintness

Contraindications: Hypersensitivity to this drug or nitrates, severe anemia, increased intracranial pressure, cerebral hemorrhage, acute MI
Precautions: Postural hypotension, pregnancy (C), lactation, children

Pharmacokinetics:
Mononitrate
Sus action: Duration 6-8 hr
Dinitrate
PO: Onset 15-30 min, duration 4-6 hr
SL: Onset 2-5 min, duration 1-4 hr
CHEW TAB: Onset 3 min, duration ½-3 hr
Metabolized by liver, excreted in urine as metabolites (80%-100%)

Interactions:
• Increased effects: β-blockers, di-

uretics, antihypertensives, alcohol, Ca channel blockers, phenothiazines

NURSING CONSIDERATIONS
Assess:
• Pain: duration, time started, activity being performed, character
• B/P, pulse, respirations during beginning therapy
• Tolerance if taken over long period
• Headache, light-headedness, decreased B/P; may indicate a need for decreased dosage
Administer:
• After checking expiration date
🚫Do not break, crush, or chew sus rel caps, SL tabs
• PO with 8 oz H_2O on empty stomach; do not crush SR or SL drug
• SL tabs should be placed under the tongue until dissolved
Evaluate:
• Therapeutic response: decrease or prevention of anginal pain
Teach patient/family:
• To leave tabs in original container
• To avoid alcohol products
• That drug may cause headache, but tolerance usually develops; taking with meals may reduce or eliminate headache
• That drug may be taken before stressful activity (exercise, sexual activity)
• That SL may sting when drug comes in contact with mucous membranes
• To avoid hazardous activities if dizziness occurs
• The importance of complying with complete medical regimen
• To make position changes slowly to prevent orthostatic hypotension
🚫Not to crush, chew sus rel caps, SL tabs

RARELY USED

isotretinoin (℞)
(eye-soe-tret'i-noyn)
Func. class.: Antiacne agent

Uses: Severe recalcitrant cystic acne
Dosage and routes:
• *Adult:* **PO** 0.5-2 mg/kg/day in 2 divided doses × 15-20 wk; if relapse occurs, repeat after 2 mo off drug
Contraindications: Hypersensitivity, inflamed skin, pregnancy (X)

RARELY USED

isoxsuprine (℞)
(eye-sox'syoo-preen)
Func. class.: Peripheral vasodilator

Uses: Symptoms of cerebrovascular insufficiency, peripheral vascular disease including arteriosclerosis obliterans, thromboangitis obliterans, Raynaud's disease
Dosage and routes:
• *Adult:* **PO** 10-20 mg tid or qid
Contraindications: Hypersensitivity, postpartum, arterial bleeding

isradipine (℞)
(is-ra'di-peen)
DynaCirc, DynaCirc CR
Func. class.: Antihypertensive, antianginal (calcium channel blocker)
Chem. class.: Dihydropyridine

Action: Inhibits calcium ion influx across cell membrane during cardiac depolarization; produces relaxation of coronary vascular smooth muscle, peripheral vascular smooth

---

muscle; dilates coronary vascular arteries; increases myocardial oxygen delivery in patients with vasospastic angina

Uses: Essential hypertension, angina pectoris, vasospastic angina

Dosage and routes:
• *Adult:* PO 2.5 mg bid; increase at 2-4 wk intervals up to 10 mg bid or 5 mg qd; cont rel may be increased q2-4wk, max 20 mg/day

Available forms: Caps 2.5, 5 mg, cont rel tabs 5, 10 mg

Side effects/adverse reactions:

*HEMA: **Thrombocytopenia, leukopenia, anemia***

CV: Peripheral edema, tachycardia, hypotension, chest pain, ***CHF, dysrhythmias***

GI: Nausea, vomiting, diarrhea, gastric upset, constipation, ***hepatitis***

GU: Nocturia, polyuria, ***acute renal failure***

INTEG: Rash, pruritus, urticaria, photosensitivity, hair loss

CNS: Headache, fatigue, dizziness, fainting, sleep disturbances

MISC: Flushing, ***Stevens-Johnson syndrome***

Contraindications: Sick sinus syndrome, 2nd- or 3rd-degree heart block, hypotension less than 90 mm Hg systolic, hypersensitivity

Precautions: CHF, hypotension, hepatic disease, pregnancy (C), lactation, children, renal disease, elderly

Pharmacokinetics: Metabolized in liver; metabolites excreted in urine, feces; secreted in breast milk, peak plasma levels at 2-3 hr

Interactions:
• Increased hypotension: nitrates, fentanyl, other antihypertensives, quinidine, alcohol
• Decreased antihypertensive effect: NSAIDs
• Bradycardia, conduction defects: digitalis, β-blockers, disopyramide, phenytoin

NURSING CONSIDERATIONS

Assess:
• I&O ratio, daily weight, watch for CHF: dyspnea, weight gain, rales, crackles, jugular vein distention
• Renal, hepatic, electrolytes prior to and during treatment
• Cardiac status: B/P, pulse, respiration, ECG; assess anginal pain, precipitating, ameliorating factors

Administer:
• Without regard to meals

Evaluate:
• Therapeutic response: decreased anginal pain, decreased B/P

Teach patient/family:

🚫 Not to break, crush, or chew cont rel tabs
• To avoid hazardous activities until stabilized on drug, dizziness is no longer a problem
• To limit caffeine consumption
• To avoid OTC drugs unless directed by prescriber
• The importance of compliance in all areas of medical regimen: diet, exercise, stress reduction, drug therapy
• To notify prescriber of irregular heartbeat, shortness of breath, swelling of feet and hands, pronounced dizziness, constipation, nausea, hypotension

Treatment of overdose: Defibrillation, β-agonists, IV Ca inotropic agents, diuretics, atropine for AV block, vasopressor for hypotension

---

itraconazole (℞)

(it-ra-con′a-zol)

Sporanox

Func. class.: Antifungal, systemic

Chem. class.: Triazole derivative

Action: Alters cell membranes and inhibits several fungal enzymes

Uses: Systemic candidiasis, chronic mucocandidiasis, oral thrush, candiduria, coccidioidomycosis, histoplasmosis, chromomycosis, paracoccidioidomycosis, blastomycosis (pulmonary and extrapulmonary), aspergillosis onychomycosis

Investigational uses: Dermatophytoses, pityriasis versicolor, sebopsoriasis, vaginal candidiasis, cryptococcus, subcutaneous mycoses, dimorphic infections, leishmaniasis, fungal keratitis, alternariosis, zygomycosis

Dosage and routes:
Dose varies with type of infection
• *Adult:* PO 200 mg qd with food; may increase to 400 mg qd if needed; life-threatening infections may require a loading dose of 200 mg tid × 3 days; IV 200 mg bid × 4 doses, then 200 mg qd, give each dose over 1 hr; maintenance **PO** 100 mg/day
• *Child:* PO 3-5 mg/kg/day
Available forms: Caps 100 mg; oral sol 10 mg/ml; inj 10 mg/ml

Side effects/adverse reactions:
CV: Hypertension
GU: Gynecomastia, impotence, decreased libido
INTEG: Pruritus, fever, *rash,*
CNS: Headache, dizziness, insomnia, somnolence, depression
GI: Nausea, vomiting, anorexia, diarrhea, cramps, abdominal pain, flatulence, **GI bleeding, hepatotoxicity**
MISC: Edema, fatigue, malaise, hypokalemia, tinnitus

Contraindications: Hypersensitivity, lactation, fungal meningitis, onychomycosis or dermatomycosis in cardiac dysfunction

Precautions: Hepatic disease, achlorhydria or hypochlorhydria (drug-induced), children, pregnancy (C)

Pharmacokinetics:
PO: Peak 3-5 hr, half-life 21 hr; metabolized in liver; excreted in bile, feces; requires acid pH for absorption; distributed poorly to CSF; highly protein bound

Interactions:
• Edema: calcium channel blockers
• Increased sedation: triazolam, oral midazolam
• Tinnitus, hearing loss: quinidine
• Increased levels, toxicity: busprione, busulfan, clarithromycin, cyclosporine, diazepam, digoxin, felodipine, indinavir, isradipine, nicardipine, nifedipine, nimoldipine, phenytoin, quinidine, ritonavir, saquinavir, tacrolimus, warfarin
• Hepatotoxicity: other hepatotoxic drugs
• Decreased action of itraconazole: antacids, H₂-receptor antagonists, rifamycins, didanosine
• Severe hypoglycemia: oral hypoglycemics
◆ Life-threatening CV reactions: pimozide, quinidine, cisapride, dofetilide

NURSING CONSIDERATIONS
Assess:
• For type of infection, may begin treatment prior to obtaining results
• For infection: temp, WBC, sputum, baseline and periodically
• I&O ratio, potassium levels
• Liver studies (ALT, AST, bilirubin) if on long-term therapy
• For allergic reaction: rash, photosensitivity, urticaria, dermatitis
◆ For hepatotoxicity: nausea, vomiting, jaundice, clay-colored stools, fatigue

Administer:
• In the presence of acid products only; do not use alkaline products or antacids within 2 hr of drug; may give coffee, tea, acidic fruit juices
• IV: after adding full contents 25-50 ml NaCl, mix gently, use flow

◆ = Nursing alert   🌿 = Herb-drug interaction   🚫 = Do not crush

control device, give over 1 hr; use separate line, flush after use
• Oral sol: patient should swish in mouth vigorously
• Oral sol and caps are not interchangeable on a mg/mg basis
• Give caps after full meal to ensure absorption, swallow whole

Perform/provide:
• Storage in tight container at room temperature

Evaluate:
• Therapeutic response: decreased fever, malaise, rash, negative C&S for infecting organism

Teach patient/family:
• That long-term therapy may be needed to clear infection (1 wk-6 mo depending on infection)
• To avoid hazardous activities if dizziness occurs
• To take 2 hr ac administration of other drugs that increase gastric pH (antacids, H_2-blockers, omeprazole, sucralfate, anticholinergics) to notify health-care provider of all medications taken; to take after a full meal (caps), on empty stomach (oral sol)
• The importance of compliance with drug regimen
• To notify prescriber of GI symptoms, signs of liver dysfunction (fatigue, nausea, anorexia, vomiting, dark urine, pale stools)
🚫 Not to break, crush, or chew caps; not to use oral sol, caps interchangeably

---

kanamycin (℞)

(kan-a-mye′sin)
kanamycin sulfate, Kantrex
Func. class.: Antiinfective
Chem. class.: Aminoglycoside

Action: Interferes with protein synthesis in bacterial cell by binding to the 30s ribosomal subunit, causing inaccurate peptide sequence to form in protein chain, causing bacterial death

Uses: Severe systemic infections of CNS, respiratory, GI, urinary tract, bone, skin, soft tissues caused by *Escherichia coli, Acinetobacter, Proteus, Klebsiella pneumoniae, Pseudomonas aeruginosa;* also used as adjunct in hepatic coma, peritonitis, preoperatively to sterilize bowel; decreases ammonia-producing bacteria in bowel and intraperitoneally after fecal spill during surgery

Dosage and routes:
Severe systemic infections
• *Adult and child:* **IV INF** 15 mg/kg/d in divided doses q8-12h; diluted 500 mg/200 ml of NS or D_5W given over 30-60 min, not to exceed 1.5 g/d; **IM** 15 mg/kg/d in divided doses q8-12h, not to exceed 1.5 g/d, irrigation not to exceed 1.5 g/d; **INH** 250 mg qid

Preoperative bowel sterilization
• *Adult:* **PO** 1 g qh × 4 doses, then q6h × 36-72 hr

Available forms: Inj 75, 500 mg/2 ml, 1 g/3 ml; cap 500 mg

Side effects/adverse reactions:
*GU: **Oliguria, hematuria, renal damage, azotemia, renal failure, nephrotoxicity***
CNS: Confusion, depression, numbness, tremors, ***convulsions,*** muscle twitching, ***neurotoxicity***
RESP: Respiratory depression
*EENT: **Ototoxicity,*** deafness, visual disturbances, dizziness, vertigo, tinnitus
*HEMA: **Agranulocytosis, thrombocytopenia, leukopenia, eosinophilia, anemia***
GI: Nausea, vomiting, anorexia, increased ALT, AST, bilirubin, hepatomegaly, ***hepatic necrosis,*** splenomegaly

---

CV: Hypotension

INTEG: Rash, burning, urticaria, dermatitis, alopecia

Contraindications: Bowel obstruction, severe renal disease, hypersensitivity, pregnancy (D)

Precautions: Neonates, myasthenia gravis, hearing deficits, mild renal disease, lactation, Parkinson's disease

Do not confuse:

kanamycin/Garamycin

Pharmacokinetics:

PO: Not absorbed

IM: Onset rapid, peak 1-2 hr

IV: Onset immediate, peak 1-2 hr
Plasma half-life 2-3 hr; not metabolized; excreted unchanged in urine; crosses placenta; poor penetration into CSF

Interactions:

• Increased ototoxicity, neurotoxicity, nephrotoxicity: other aminoglycosides, amphotericin B, polymyxin, vancomycin, ethacrynic acid, furosemide, mannitol, methoxyflurane, cisplatin, cephalosporins, bacitracin, penicillins

• Increased effects: nondepolarizing muscle relaxants, succinylcholine

• Decreased effects of oral anticoagulants

NURSING CONSIDERATIONS
Assess:

• Weight before treatment; dosage is usually calculated on ideal body weight, but may be calculated on actual body weight

• Renal impairment by CrCl, BUN, serum creatinine testing of urine; lower dosage should be given in renal impairment (CrCl <80 ml/min); I&O ratio, urinalysis daily for proteinuria, cells, casts; report sudden change in urine output; specific gravity

• VS during infusion; watch for hypotension, change in pulse

• IV site for thrombophlebitis, including pain, redness, swelling q30min; change site if needed; apply warm compresses to discontinued site

• Serum peak, drawn at 30-60 min after IV infusion or 60 min after IM injection; trough level drawn just before next dose; blood level should be 2-4 × bacteriostatic level; trough = 5-10 mEq/ml, peak = <30 mEq/ml

• Urine pH if drug is used for UTI; urine should be kept alkaline

• Deafness by audiometric testing, ringing, roaring in ears, vertigo; assess hearing before, during, after treatment

• Dehydration: high specific gravity, decrease in skin turgor, dry mucous membranes, dark urine

• Superinfection: fever, malaise, redness, pain, swelling, perineal itching, diarrhea, stomatitis, change in cough, sputum

• C&S before starting treatment to identify infecting organism

• Vestibular dysfunction: nausea, vomiting, dizziness, headache; drug should be discontinued if severe

• Inj sites for redness, swelling, abscesses; use warm compresses at site

Administer:

• IM inj in large muscle mass; rotate inj sites

• Penicillins at least 1 hr before or after this drug

• Drug in evenly spaced doses to maintain blood level

• Bicarbonate to alkalinize urine if ordered in treating UTI, as drug is most active in alkaline environment

IV

• After diluting 500 mg or less/100 ml of D_5W, D_5/NaCl, 0.9% NaCl, LR or more; give 3-4 ml/min or less; flush line after use

Additive compatibilities: Ascorbic acid, cefoxitin, chloramphenicol, clindamycin, dopamine, furo-

---

◆ = Nursing alert   ✎ = Herb-drug interaction   Ⓢ = Do not crush semide, penicillin G potassium, penicillin G sodium, polymyxin B, sodium bicarbonate, vit B/C; admixing is not recommended

Syringe compatibilities: Penicillin G sodium

Y-site compatibilities: Cyclophosphamide, furosemide, heparin with hydrocortisone, hydromorphone, magnesium sulfate, meperidine, morphine, perphenazine, potassium chloride, vit B/C

Perform/provide:
• Adequate fluids of 2-3 L/day unless contraindicated to prevent irritation of tubules
• Flush of IV line with NS or D_5W after infusion
• Supervised ambulation, other safety measures with vestibular dysfunction

Evaluate:
• Therapeutic effect: absence of fever, draining wounds, negative C&S after treatment

Teach patient/family:
• To report headache, dizziness, symptoms of overgrowth of infection, renal impairment
• To report loss of hearing, ringing, roaring in ears or feeling of fullness in head
• To continue full course of treatment

Treatment of overdose: Hemodialysis; monitor serum levels of drug

RARELY USED

ketamine (R)

(keet'a-meen)
Ketalar
Func. class.: General anesthetic

Uses: Short   anesthesia   for diagnostic/surgical procedures
Dosage and routes:
• *Adult and child:* IV 1-4.5 mg/kg over 1 min; IM 6.5-13 mg/kg; *Maintenance:* ½ to full induction dose may be repeated
Contraindications: Hypersensitivity, CVA, increased intracranial pressure, severe hypertension, cardiac decompensation, child <2 yr

---

ketoconazole (R)

(kee-toe-koe'na-zole)
Nizoral
Func. class.: Antifungal
Chem. class.: Imidazole derivative

Action: Alters cell membranes and inhibits several fungal enzymes
Uses: Systemic candidiasis, chronic mucocandidiasis, oral thrush, candiduria, coccidioidomycosis, histoplasmosis, chromomycosis, paracoccidioidomycosis, blastomycosis; tinea cruris, tinea corporis, tinea versicolor, *Pityrosporum ovale*
Investigational uses: Cushing's syndrome, advanced prostatic cancer, depression
Dosage and routes:
• *Adult:* PO 200-400 mg qd for 1-2 wk (candidiasis), 6 wk (other infections); 400 mg tid (prostate cancer—unlabeled); shampoo massage into scalp 1 min, reapply × 3 min, rinse, continue treatment 2×/wk × 1 mo, no more than q3d

• *Child >2 yr:* PO: 3.3-6.6 mg/kg/ day as single daily dose
• *Adult and child:* TOP 2% cream applied qd or bid
Depression
• *Adult:* PO 200 mg/day, increase by 200 mg q3-4d × 6 wk
Available forms: Tabs 200 mg; oral susp 100 mg/5 ml*, cream 2%, shampoo 2%
Side effects/adverse reactions:
GU: Gynecomastia, impotence
INTEG: Pruritus, fever, chills, photophobia, rash, dermatitis, purpura, urticaria
CNS: Headache, dizziness, somnolence
SYST: **Anaphylaxis**
GI: Nausea, vomiting, anorexia, diarrhea, abdominal pain, **hepatotoxicity**
HEMA: **Thrombocytopenia, leukopenia, hemolytic anemia**
Contraindications: Hypersensitivity, lactation, fungal meningitis; coadministration with terfenadine
Precautions: Renal disease, hepatic disease, achlorhydria (drug-induced), pregnancy (C), children <2 yr, other hepatotoxic agents including terfenadine
Pharmacokinetics:
PO: Peak 1-2 hr, half-life 2 hr, terminal 8 hr; metabolized in liver; excreted in bile, feces; requires acid pH for absorption; distributed poorly to CSF; highly protein bound
Interactions:
• Hepatotoxicity: other hepatotoxic drugs, alcohol
• Inhibition of CYP 450 3A4 pathway, toxicity: alfentanil, alprazolam, amprenavir, atorvastatin, calcium channel blockers, cerivastatin, cisapride, clarithromycin, corticosteroids, cyclophosphamide, cyclosporine, erythromycin, fentanyl, ifosfamide, indinavir, lovastatin, midazolam, nelfinavir, quinidine,

---

◆ = Nursing alert   ▮ = Herb-drug interaction   ⊘ = Do not crush

ritonavir, saquinavir, sildenafil, simvastatin, sufentanil, tamoxifen, triazolam, troleandomycin, vinblastine, vincristine

• Decreased action of ketoconazole: antacids, H_2-receptor antagonists, anticholinergics, isoniazid, rifampin, ddI, gastric acid pump inhibitors

• Increased anticoagulant effect: warfarin, anticoagulants

• Ketoconazole may decrease theophylline effect

• Inhibited metabolism: paclitaxel

🖉 Decreased ketoconazole action: Yew

NURSING CONSIDERATIONS
Assess:
• For infection symptoms before and after treatment

• Liver studies (ALT, AST, bilirubin) if on long-term therapy

• For allergic reaction: rash, photosensitivity, urticaria, dermatitis

◆ For hepatotoxicity: nausea, vomiting, jaundice, clay-colored stools, fatigue

Administer:
• In the presence of acid products only; do not use alkaline products, proton pump inhibitors, H_2-antagonists, antacids within 2 hr of drug; may give coffee, tea, acidic fruit juices, cola

• With food to decrease GI symptoms

• With HCl if achlorhydria is present; dissolve tab/4 ml of aqueous sol 0.2 NHCl, use straw to avoid contact, rinse with water afterward and swallow

Perform/provide:
• Storage in tight container at room temperature

Evaluate:
• Therapeutic response: decreased fever, malaise, rash, negative C&S for infecting organism, absence of scaling

Teach patient/family:
• That long-term therapy may be needed to clear infection (1 wk-6 mo depending on infection)

• To avoid hazardous activities if dizziness occurs

• To take 2 hr ac administration of other drugs that increase gastric pH (antacids, H_2-blockers, omeprazole, sucralfate, anticholinergics)

• The importance of compliance with drug regimen

◆ To notify prescriber of GI symptoms, signs of liver dysfunction (fatigue, nausea, anorexia, vomiting, dark urine, pale stools)

• Use sunglasses to prevent photophobia

K

---

ketoprofen (OTC, ℞)
(ke-toe-proe'fen)
Actron, Apo-Keto*, Apo-Keto-E*, ketoprofen, Orudis, Orudis-E*, Orudis-KT, Orudis-SR*, Oruvail, Rhodis*

Func. class.: Nonsteroidal antiinflammatory (NSAID)
Chem. class.: Propionic acid derivative

Action: Inhibits prostaglandin synthesis by decreasing enzyme needed for biosynthesis; analgesic, antiinflammatory, antipyretic

Uses: Mild to moderate pain, osteoarthritis, rheumatoid arthritis, dysmenorrhea

Dosage and routes:
Antiinflammatory
• *Adult:* PO 150-300 mg in divided doses tid-qid, not to exceed 300 mg/day or ext rel 150-200 mg qd
Analgesic
• *Adult:* PO 25-50 mg q6-8h
Available forms: Caps 12.5, 25, 50, 75 mg; ext rel cap 100, 150, 200 mg

---

Side effects/adverse reactions:

GI: Nausea, anorexia, vomiting, diarrhea, jaundice, ***hepatitis,*** constipation, flatulence, cramps, dry mouth, peptic ulcer, ***GI bleeding***

CNS: Dizziness, drowsiness, fatigue, tremors, confusion, insomnia, anxiety, depression, headache

CV: Tachycardia, peripheral edema, palpitations, dysrhythmias, hypertension

INTEG: Purpura, rash, pruritus, sweating

*GU: **Nephrotoxicity: dysuria, hematuria, oliguria, azotemia***

*HEMA: **Blood dyscrasias***

EENT: Tinnitus, hearing loss, blurred vision

*SYST: **Anaphylaxis***

Contraindications: Hypersensitivity, asthma, severe renal disease, severe hepatic disease, ulcer disease

Precautions: Pregnancy (B) 1st trimester, lactation, children, bleeding disorders, GI disorders, cardiac disorders, hypersensitivity to other antiinflammatory agents, elderly

Do not confuse:

Oruvail/Clinoril

Oruvail/Elavil

Pharmacokinetics:

PO: Peak 2 hr, half-life 2-4 hr; metabolized in liver; excreted in urine (metabolites); excreted in breast milk; 99% plasma protein binding

Interactions:

• Increased hypoglycemia: insulin, sulfonylureas

• Increased toxicity: cyclosporine, lithium, methotrexate, phenytoin, alcohol

• Increased risk of bleeding: cefamandole, cefoperazone, cefotetan, clopidogrel, eptifibatide, plicamycin, thrombolytics, ticlopidine, tirofiban, valproic acid, warfarin

• Increased levels of ketoprofen: aspirin, probenecid

• Decreased effect of: diuretics, antihypertensives

• Increased adverse GI reactions: aspirin, corticosteroids, NSAIDs, alcohol

NURSING CONSIDERATIONS
Assess:

• For pain: type, location, intensity, ROM before and 1-2 hr after treatment

• Renal, liver, blood studies: BUN, creatinine, AST, ALT, Hgb, before treatment, periodically thereafter

◆For aspirin sensitivity, asthma; these patients may be more likely to develop hypersensitivity to NSAIDs

• Audiometric, ophthalmic exam before, during, after treatment

• For eye, ear problems: blurred vision, tinnitus; may indicate toxicity

• For GI bleeding: blood in sputum, emesis, stools

Administer:

🚫Whole; do not crush, break, or chew ext rel caps

• With food to decrease GI symptoms; however, taking on empty stomach best facilitates absorption

Perform/provide:

• Storage at room temperature

Evaluate:

• Therapeutic response: decreased pain, stiffness in joints, decreased swelling in joints, ability to move more easily; decreased fever

Teach patient/family:

• To report blurred vision, ringing, roaring in ears; may indicate toxicity

• To avoid driving, other hazardous activities if dizziness, drowsiness occurs, especially elderly

• To report change in urine pattern, increased weight, edema, increased pain in joints, fever, blood in urine; indicate nephrotoxicity; rash, itching, blurred vision, ringing in the ears, flulike symptoms

• That therapeutic effects may take

◆= Nursing alert   🌿 = Herb-drug interaction   🚫= Do not crush up to 1 mo, to take with 8 oz of water and sit upright for ½ hr after administration to prevent GI irritation

• To avoid aspirin, alcohol, steroids, acetaminophen or other medications, supplements unless approved by prescriber

• To wear sunscreen to prevent photosensitivity

---

ketorolac (R̲)

(kee-toe′role-ak)
Acular, Toradol
Func. class.: Nonsteroidal antiinflammatory/nonopioid analgesic
Chem. class.: Pyrrolo-pyrrole

Action: Inhibits prostaglandin synthesis by decreasing an enzyme needed for biosynthesis; analgesic, antiinflammatory, antipyretic effects
Uses: Mild to moderate pain; seasonal allergic conjunctivitis (ophth)
Dosage and routes:
• *Adult <65 yr:* **PO** 20 mg then 10 mg q4-6h prn, max 40 mg/day
• *Adult >65 yr, renal disease, <50 kg:* **PO** 10 mg q4-6h prn, max 40 mg/day
• *Adult <65 yr:* **IM** (single dose) 60 mg **IV** 30 mg; **IM** (multiple dosing) 15 mg q6h, max 60 mg/day × 5 day combined either **PO/IM/IV**
• *Adult >65 yr, renal disease, <50 kg:* **IM** single dose 30 mg; **IV** 15 mg **IM/IV** (multiple dosing) 15 mg q6h, max 60 mg/day × 5 days combined either **PO/IM/IV**
• *Adult:* **OPHTH** 1 gtt qid
Available forms: Inj 15, 30 mg/ml (prefilled syringes); ophth 0.5% sol; tab 10 mg
Side effects/adverse reactions:
CV: Hypertension, flushing, syncope, pallor, edema, vasodilation

CNS: Dizziness, *drowsiness,* tremors
EENT: Tinnitus, hearing loss, blurred vision
GI: Nausea, anorexia, vomiting, diarrhea, constipation, flatulence, cramps, dry mouth, peptic ulcer, *GI bleeding, perforation,* taste change
GU: **Nephrotoxicity: dysuria, hematuria, oliguria, azotemia**
HEMA: **Blood dyscrasias,** prolonged bleeding
INTEG: Purpura, rash, pruritus, sweating
Contraindications: Hypersensitivity, asthma, severe renal disease, severe hepatic disease, peptic ulcer disease, L&D, lactation, CV bleeding
Precautions: Pregnancy (C), children, bleeding disorders, GI disorders, cardiac disorders, hypersensitivity to other antiinflammatory agents, elderly, CrCl <25 ml/min
Do not confuse:
Toradol/Tegretol
Toradol/Inderal
Toradol/Torecan
Toradol/tramadol
Pharmacokinetics:
PO: Peak 2-3 hr, duration 4-6 hr
IM: Peak 50 min, half-life 6 hr enters breast milk, <50% metabolized by liver, excreted by kidneys
Interactions:
• Increased toxicity: methotrexate, lithium, cyclosporine
• Increased risk of bleeding: anticoagulants, cefamandole, cefoperazone, cefotetan, clopidogrel, eptifibatide, plicamycin, salicylates, ticlopidine, tirofiban, thrombolytics, valproic acid
• Decreased effects: antihypertensives, diuretics
• Increased renal impairment: ACE inhibitors
• Increased levels of ketorolac: aspirin, probenecid

K

• Increased GI effects: steroids, alcohol, aspirin, NSAIDs, potassium products

• Compatible in 0.9% NaCl, D₅, Ringer's, LR, Plasmalate

NURSING CONSIDERATIONS

Assess:

• Patients with aspirin sensitivity, asthma; may be more likely to develop hypersensitivity to NSAIDs, monitor for hypersensitivity

• For pain: type, location, intensity, ROM before and 1 hr after treatment

• Eyes: redness, swelling, tearing, itching (ophth)

• Renal, liver, blood studies: BUN, creatinine, AST, ALT, Hgb before treatment, periodically thereafter; check for dehydration

• Bleeding times; check for bruising, bleeding; test for occult blood in urine

• For eye, ear problems: blurred vision, tinnitus (may indicate toxicity)

◆ Hepatic dysfunction: jaundice, yellow sclera and skin, clay-colored stools

• Audiometric, ophthalmic exam before, during, after treatment

• GI bleeding: blood in sputum, emesis, stools

Administer:

• IM/IV for 5 days or less; continue therapy with PO

IV

• Give undiluted over ≥15 sec

Solution compatibility: D₅W, 0.9% NaCl, LR

Syringe compatibilities: Sufentanil

Y-site compatibilities: Cisatracurium, remifentanil, sufentanil

Perform/provide:

• Storage at room temperature

Evaluate:

• Therapeutic response: decreased pain, stiffness, swelling in joints, ability to move more easily; decreased ocular itching (ophth)

Teach patient/family:

• To report blurred vision or ringing, roaring in ears (may indicate toxicity)

• To avoid driving, other hazardous activities if dizziness or drowsiness occurs

• To report change in urine pattern, weight increase, edema, pain increase in joints, fever, blood in urine (indicates nephrotoxicity)

• To avoid alcohol, salicylates, other NSAIDs, acetaminophen

• This drug may cause redness, burning if soft contact lenses are worn (ophth)

---

labetalol (℞)

(la-bet'a-lole)
Normodyne, Trandate
Func. class.: Antihypertensive, antianginal
Chem. class.: α/β-Blocker

Action: Produces decreases in B/P without reflex tachycardia or significant reduction in heart rate through mixture of α-blocking, β-blocking effects; elevated plasma renins are reduced

Uses: Mild to moderate hypertension; treatment of severe hypertension (IV)

Investigational uses: Angina pectoris (PO), hypotension during surgery (IV)

Dosage and routes:

Hypertension

• *Adult:* **PO** 100 mg bid; may be given with a diuretic; may increase to 200 mg bid after 2 days; may continue to increase q1-3 days; max 400 mg bid

Hypertensive crisis

• *Adult:* **IV INF** 200 mg/160 ml

◆ = Nursing alert   ⬧ = Herb-drug interaction   ⊘ = Do not crush

D_5W, run at 2 ml/min; stop inf at desired response, repeat q6-8h as needed; **IV BOL** 20 mg over 2 min, may repeat 40-80 mg q10min, not to exceed 300 mg

Available forms: Tabs 100, 200, 300 mg; inj 5 mg/ml in 20 ml amps

Side effects/adverse reactions:

*CV: Orthostatic hypotension, bradycardia, **CHF,** chest pain, **ventricular dysrhythmias,** AV block*

CNS: Dizziness, mental changes, drowsiness, fatigue, headache, catatonia, depression, anxiety, nightmares, paresthesias, lethargy

GI: Nausea, vomiting, diarrhea

INTEG: Rash, alopecia, urticaria, pruritus, fever

*HEMA: **Agranulocytosis, thrombocytopenia, purpura** (rare)*

EENT: Tinnitus, visual changes, sore throat, double vision, dry, burning eyes

GU: Impotence, dysuria, ejaculatory failure

*RESP: **Bronchospasm,** dyspnea, wheezing*

Contraindications: Hypersensitivity to β-blockers, cardiogenic shock, heart block (2nd or 3rd degree), sinus bradycardia, CHF, bronchial asthma

Precautions: Major surgery, pregnancy (C), lactation, diabetes mellitus, renal disease, thyroid disease, COPD, well-compensated heart failure, CAD, nonallergic bronchospasm, elderly, hepatic disease

Pharmacokinetics:

PO: Onset ½-2 hr, peak 2-4 hr, duration 8-12 hr

IV: Onset 5 min, peak 15 min, duration 2-4 hr

Half-life 6-8 hr; metabolized by liver (metabolites inactive); excreted in urine; crosses placenta; excreted in breast milk

Interactions:

• Do not use within 2 wk of MAOIs
• Decreased effects of labetalol: thyroid hormones
• Myocardial depression: hydantoins, general anesthetics, verapamil
• Increased hypotension: diuretics, other antihypertensives, cimetidine, nitroglycerin, alcohol, propranolol
• Decreased effects: sympathomimetics, lidocaine, indomethacin, theophylline, β-blockers, bronchodilators, xanthines
• Decreased antihypertensive effect: NSAIDs
• Increased bradycardia: cardiac glycosides
• Increased hypoglycemia: insulin, oral antidiabetics

Lab test interferences:

False increase: Urinary catecholamines

NURSING CONSIDERATIONS

Assess:

◆ I&O, weight daily; fluid overload: weight gain, jugular venous distention, edema, rales in lungs
• B/P during beginning treatment, periodically thereafter; pulse q4h; note rate, rhythm, quality
• Apical/radial pulse before administration; notify prescriber of any significant changes
• Baselines in renal tests, LFTs before therapy begins
• Edema in feet, legs daily
• Skin turgor, dryness of mucous membranes for hydration status

Administer:

• PO ac, hs; tab may be crushed or swallowed whole, give with meals to increase absorption
• Reduced dosage in renal dysfunction

IV

• Undiluted or diluted in LR, D_5W, D_5 in 0.2%, 0.9%, 0.33% NaCl or Ringer's inj, give undiluted 20 mg or less/2 min; inf is titrated to pa-

L

tient response; 200 mg of drug/160 ml sol = 1 mg/ml; 300 mg of drug/240 ml sol = 1 mg/ml; 200 mg of drug/250 ml sol = 2 mg/3 ml; use infusion pump

• Keeping patient recumbent during and for 3 hr after administration, monitor VS q5-15min

Solution compatibilities: D_5R, D_5LR, $D_{2½}/0.45\%$ NaCl, $D_5/0.2\%$ NaCl, $D_5/0.33\%$ NaCl, $D_50.9\%$ NaCl, D_5W, Ringer's, LR

Y-site compatibilities: Amikacin, aminophylline, amiodarone, ampicillin, butorphanol, calcium gluconate, cefazolin, ceftazidime, ceftizoxime, chloramphenicol, cimetidine, clindamycin, diltiazem, dobutamine, dopamine, enalaprilat, epinephrine, erythromycin, esmolol, famotidine, fentanyl, gentamicin, hydromorphone, lidocaine, lorazepam, magnesium sulfate, meperidine, metronidazole, midazolam, milrinone, morphine, nicardipine, nitroglycerin, norepinephrine, nitroprusside, oxacillin, penicillin G potassium, piperacillin, potassium chloride, potassium phosphate, propofol, ranitidine, sodium acetate, tobramycin, trimethoprim-sulfamethoxazole, vancomycin, vecuronium

Perform/provide:
• Storage in dry area at room temperature; do not freeze

Evaluate:
• Therapeutic response: decreased B/P after 1-2 wk

Teach patient/family:
• Not to discontinue drug abruptly; taper over 2 wk; may cause precipitate angina
• Not to use OTC products containing α-adrenergic stimulants (nasal decongestants, OTC cold preparations) unless directed by prescriber
• To report bradycardia, dizziness, confusion, depression, fever

• To take pulse at home, advise when to notify prescriber
• To avoid alcohol, smoking, Na intake
• To comply with weight control, dietary adjustments, modified exercise program
• To carry Medic Alert ID to identify drug, allergies
• To avoid hazardous activities if dizziness is present
• To report symptoms of CHF: difficulty breathing, especially on exertion or when lying down, night cough, swelling of extremities
• To take medication at bedtime to prevent effect of orthostatic hypotension
• To wear support hose to minimize effects of orthostatic hypotension

Treatment of overdose: Lavage, IV atropine for bradycardia, IV theophylline for bronchospasm, digitalis, O_2, diuretic for cardiac failure; hemodialysis is useful for removal, hypotension; administer vasopressor (norepinephrine)

---

lactulose (℞)

(lak'tyoo-lose)
Cephulac, Cholac, Chronulac, Constilac, Constulose, Duphalac, Enulose, Heptalac, Lactulax*, Lactulose PSE, Portalac

Func. class.: Laxative; ammonia detoxicant (hyperosmotic)

Chem. class.: Lactose synthetic derivative

Action: Prevents absorption of ammonia in colon; increases water in stool

Uses: Chronic constipation, portal-systemic encephalopathy in patients with hepatic disease

◆ = Nursing alert   ／ = Herb-drug interaction   ⊘ = Do not crush

Dosages and routes:

Constipation

• *Adult:* PO 15-60 ml qd

• *Child* (unlabeled): PO 7.5 ml qd

Encephalopathy

• *Adult:* PO 30-45 ml tid or qid until stools are soft; **RETENTION ENEMA** 300 ml diluted

• *Infant:* PO 2.5-10 ml/day in divided doses

• *Child:* PO 40-90 ml/day in divided doses given 2-4×/day

Available forms: Syr 10 g/15 ml

Side effects/adverse reactions:

GI: Nausea, vomiting, anorexia, abdominal cramps, diarrhea, flatulence, distention, belching

Contraindications: Hypersensitivity, low-galactose diet

Precautions: Pregnancy (B), lactation, diabetes mellitus, elderly, debilitated patients

Pharmacokinetics: Metabolized in intestine, excreted by kidneys; onset 1-2 days, peak unknown, duration unknown

Interactions:

• Decreased effects of lactulose: neomycin, other oral antiinfectives

NURSING CONSIDERATIONS

Assess:

• Stool: amount, color, consistency

• Blood ammonia level (30-70 mg/100 ml); may decrease ammonia level by 25%-50%

• Blood, urine electrolytes if drug is used often; may cause diarrhea, hypokalemia, hyponatremia

• I&O ratio to identify fluid loss

• Cause of constipation; determine whether fluids, bulk, or exercise is missing from lifestyle

• Cramping, rectal bleeding, nausea, vomiting; if these symptoms occur, drug should be discontinued

• Clearing of confusion, lethargy, restlessness, irritability if portal-systemic encephalopathy

Administer:

PO

• With 8 oz fruit juice, water, milk to increase palatability of oral form

RECT

• Retention enema by diluting 300 ml lactose/700 ml of water; administer by rectal balloon catheter

• Increased fluids to 2 L/day; do not give with other laxatives; if diarrhea occurs, reduce dosage

Evaluate:

• Therapeutic response: decreased constipation, decreased blood ammonia level, clearing of mental state

Teach patient/family:

• Not to use laxatives long-term

• To dilute with water or fruit juice to counteract sweet taste

• To store in cool environment; do not freeze

• To take on an empty stomach for rapid action

• To report diarrhea; may indicate overdose

lamivudine (℞)

(lam-i-voo'deen)

Epivir, Epivir-HBV, 3TC

Func. class.: Antiretroviral

Chem. class.: Nucleoside reverse transcriptase inhibitor

Action: Inhibits replication of HIV virus by incorporating into cellular DNA by viral reverse transcriptase, thereby terminating cellular DNA chain

Uses: HIV infection in combination with zidovudine (Epivir); chronic hepatitis B (Epivir-HBV)

Investigational uses: Prophylaxis of HIV—postexposure with indinavir and zidovudine

Dosage and routes:

HIV

• *Adult and child >12 yr:* PO 150 mg bid with zidovudine; <50 kg (110 lb): **PO** 2 mg/kg bid with zidovudine

• *Child 3 mo to 12 yr:* **PO** 4 mg/kg bid, may be given 150 mg bid with zidovudine

Renal dose

• *Adult:* **PO** CrCl 30-49 ml/min 150 mg qd; CrCl 15-29 ml/min 150 mg 1st dose, then 10 mg qd; CrCl 5-14 ml/min 150 mg qd, then 50 mg qd; CrCl <5 ml/min, 50 mg 1st dose, then 25 mg qd

Chronic hepatitis B

• *Adult:* **PO** 100 mg qd

Renal dose

• *Adult:* **PO** CrCl 30-49 ml/min 100 mg 1st dose, then 50 mg qd; CrCl 15-29 ml/min 100 mg 1st dose, then 25 mg qd; CrCl 5-14 ml/min 35 mg 1st dose, then 15 mg qd CrCl <5 ml/min 35 mg 1st dose, then 10 mg qd

Available forms: Tabs 100, 150 mg; oral sol 5, 10 mg/ml

Side effects/adverse reactions:

HEMA: **Neutropenia, anemia, thrombocytopenia**

CNS: Fever, headache, malaise, dizziness, insomnia, depression, fatigue, chills

GI: Nausea, vomiting, diarrhea, anorexia, cramps, dyspepsia, **pancreatitis (pediatrics)**

RESP: Cough

EENT: Taste change, hearing loss, photophobia

INTEG: Rash

MS: Myalgia, arthralgia, pain

Contraindications: Hypersensitivity

Precautions: Granulocyte count <1000/mm³ or Hgb <9.5 g/dl, pregnancy (C), lactation, children, renal disease, severe hepatic function, pancreatitis, elderly

Pharmacokinetics: Rapidly absorbed, distributed to extravascular space, excreted unchanged in urine

Interactions:

• Increased level of zidovudine when given with lamivudine

• Increased level of lamivudine: trimethoprim-sulfamethoxazole

NURSING CONSIDERATIONS
Assess:

• Blood counts q2wk; watch for neutropenia, thrombocytopenia, Hgb, CD4, viral load; if low, therapy may have to be discontinued and restarted after hematologic recovery; blood transfusions may be required

• Liver studies: AST, ALT, bilirubin; amylase, lipase, triglycerides, CD4, viral load periodically during treatment

• Children for pancreatitis

◆ Lactic acidosis, severe hepatomegaly with steatosis: obtain baseline LFTs, if elevated discontinue treatment; discontinue even if LFTs are normal if lactic acidosis, severe hepatomegaly develop

Administer:

• PO bid, without regard to meals

Perform/provide:

• With other antiretrovirals only

• Storage in cool environment; protect from light

Evaluate:

• Blood dyscrasias: bruising, fatigue, bleeding, poor healing

Teach patient/family:

• That GI complaints, insomnia resolve after 3-4 wk of treatment

• That drug is not a cure for HIV, but will control symptoms

• To notify prescriber of sore throat, swollen lymph nodes, malaise, fever; other infections may occur

• That patient is still infective, may pass HIV virus on to others

• That follow-up visits must be continued since serious toxicity may occur; blood counts must be done q2wk

• That drug must be taken twice a day, even if patient feels better

---

◆ = Nursing alert   🖉 = Herb-drug interaction   ⊘ = Do not crush

• That other drugs may be necessary to prevent other infections
• That drug may cause fainting or dizziness

---

lamotrigine (℞)

(la-mot′ri-geen)
Lamictal, Lamictal Chewable
Func. class.: Anticonvulsant, misc.
Chem. class.: Phenyltriazine

Action: Unknown, may inhibit voltage-sensitive sodium channels
Uses: Adjunct in the treatment of partial seizures; children with Lennox-Gastaut syndrome
Investigational uses: Generalized tonic-clonic, absence, atypical absence and myoclonic seizures; refractory bipolar disorder
Dosage and routes:

Monotherapy
• *Adult:* 50 mg/day for wk 1-2, then increase to 100 mg divided bid for wk 3-4; maintenance, 300-500 mg/day
• *Child:* 2 mg/kg/day in 2 divided doses × 2 wks, then 10 mg/kg/day, max 15 mg/kg/day or 400 mg/day
Multiple therapy
• *Adult:* 25 mg qod wk 1-4, then 150 mg/day in divided doses
• *Child:* 0.1-0.2 mg/kg/day initially, then increase q2wk as needed to 2 mg/kg/day or 150 mg/day
Available forms: Tabs 25, 100, 150, 200 mg; chew dispersible tabs 2, 5, 25 mg
Side effects/adverse reactions:
CNS: Dizziness, ataxia, *headache,* fever, insomnia, tremor, depression, anxiety
EENT: Nystagmus, *diplopia, blurred vision*
GI: Nausea, vomiting, anorexia, abdominal pain, **hepatotoxicity**
GU: Dysmenorrhea

INTEG: **Rash (potentially life-threatening),** alopecia, photosensitivity
SYST: **Stevens-Johnson syndrome**
Contraindications: Hypersensitivity
Precautions: Pregnancy (C), lactation, child <16 yr, renal, hepatic disease
Do not confuse:
Lamictal/Lomotil
Lamictal/Lamisil
Pharmacokinetics: Half-life varies depending on dose
Interactions:
• Increased metabolic clearance of lamotrigine: carbamazepine, phenobarbital, phenytoin, primidone
• Decreased metabolic clearance of lamotrigine: valproic acid
NURSING CONSIDERATIONS
Assess:
• For seizure activity: duration, type, intensity, halo before seizure
◆ For rash (Stevens-Johnson syndrome or toxic epidermal necrolysis) in pediatric patients, drug should be discontinued at first sign of rash
Administer:
• Chewable dispersible tabs
• Swallow whole, chew, or dispersed in water or diluted fruit juice; if chewed, drink a small amount of water
Evaluate:
• Therapeutic response: decrease in severity of seizures
Teach patient/family:
• To take PO doses divided with or after meals to decrease adverse effects, not to discontinue drug abruptly; seizures may occur
• To avoid hazardous activities until stabilized on drug
• To carry Medic Alert ID, to notify prescriber of skin rash or increased seizure activity, to use sunscreen and protective clothing if photosensitivity occurs

---

Side effects: *italics* = common; ***bold italics*** = life-threatening

hemolysis

• To notify prescriber if pregnant or intend to become pregnant

---

lansoprazole (℞)
(lan-so-prey′zole)
Prevacid
Func. class.: Antiulcer, proton pump inhibitor
Chem. class.: Benzimidazole

Action: Suppresses gastric secretion by inhibiting hydrogen/potassium ATPase enzyme system in gastric parietal cell; characterized as gastric acid pump inhibitor, since it blocks final step of acid production

Uses: Gastroesophageal reflux disease (GERD), severe erosive esophagitis, poorly responsive systemic GERD, pathologic hypersecretory conditions (Zollinger-Ellison syndrome, systemic mastocytosis, multiple endocrine adenomas); possibly effective for treatment of duodenal, gastric ulcers, maintenance of healed duodenal ulcers

Dosage and routes:
NG tube
• *Adult:* Use intact granules mixed in 40 ml of apple juice and injected through **NG** tube, then flush with apple juice
Duodenal ulcer
• *Adult:* **PO** 15 mg qd before eating for 4 wk, then 15 mg qd to maintain healing of ulcers; associated with *Helicobacter pylori*—30 mg lansoprazole, 500 mg clarithromycin, 1 g amoxicillin bid × 14 days or 30 mg lansoprazole, 1 g amoxicillin tid × 14 days
Erosive esophagitis
• *Adult:* **PO** 30 mg qd before eating for up to 8 wk, may use another 8 wk course if needed

Pathologic hypersecretory conditions
• *Adult:* **PO** 60 mg qd, may give up to 90 mg bid
Available forms: Caps, del rel 15, 30 mg
Side effects/adverse reactions:
CNS: Headache, dizziness, confusion, agitation, amnesia, depression
GI: Diarrhea, abdominal pain, vomiting, nausea, constipation, flatulence, acid regurgitation, anorexia, irritable colon
RESP: Upper respiratory infections, cough, epistaxis, asthma, bronchitis, dyspnea
INTEG: Rash, urticaria, pruritus, alopecia
META: Weight gain/loss, gout
EENT: Tinnitus, taste perversion, deafness, eye pain, otitis media
CV: Chest pain, angina, tachycardia, bradycardia, palpitations, **CVA,** hypertension/hypotension, **MI, shock,** vasodilation
GU: **Hematuria,** glycosuria, impotence, kidney calculus, breast enlargement
HEMA: **Hemolysis,** anemia
Contraindications: Hypersensitivity
Precautions: Pregnancy (B), lactation, children
Pharmacokinetics: Absorption after granules leave stomach—rapid; plasma half-life 1½ hr, protein binding 97%, extensively metabolized in liver, excreted in urine, feces; clearance decreased in the elderly, renal and hepatic impairment
Interactions:
• Delayed absorption of lansoprazole: sucralfate
• May be decreased absorption of ketoconazole, ampicillin, iron, digoxin

---

◆ = Nursing alert   ⫸ = Herb-drug interaction   ⊘ = Do not crush

NURSING CONSIDERATIONS
Assess:
• GI system: bowel sounds q8h, abdomen for pain, swelling, anorexia
• Hepatic enzymes: AST, ALT, alk phosphatase during treatment
Administer:
🚫 Before eating; swallow capsule whole; do not break, crush, or chew caps
Evaluate:
• Therapeutic response: absence of epigastric pain, swelling, fullness
Teach patient/family:
• To report severe diarrhea; drug may have to be discontinued
• That diabetic patient should know that hypoglycemia may occur
• To avoid hazardous activities; dizziness may occur
• To avoid alcohol, salicylates, ibuprofen; may cause GI irritation

---

leflunomide (℞)
(leh-floo'noh-mide)
Arava
Func. class.: Antirheumatic
Chem. class.: Pyrimidine synthesis inhibitor

Action: Inhibits an enzyme involved in pyrimidine synthesis and has antiproliferative, antiinflammatory effect

Uses: Rheumatoid arthritis, to reduce disease process and symptoms
Dosage and routes:
• *Adult:* **PO** loading dose 100 mg/day × 3 days, maintenance 20 mg/day, may be decreased to 10 mg/day if not well tolerated
Available forms: Tabs 10, 20, 100 mg
Side effects/adverse reactions:
GI: Nausea, anorexia, vomiting, constipation, flatulence, diarrhea, elevated LFTs
CNS: Headache, dizziness, insom-

nia, depression, paresthesia, anxiety, migraine, neuralgia
CV: Palpitations, hypertension, chest pain, angina pectoris, peripheral edema
INTEG: Rash, pruritus, alopecia, acne, hematoma, herpes infections
RESP: Pharyngitis, rhinitis, bronchitis, cough, respiratory infection, pneumonia, sinusitis
EENT: Pharyngitis, oral candidiasis, stomatitis, dry mouth, blurred vision
HEMA: Anemia, ecchymosis, hyperlipidemia
Contraindications: Hypersensitivity, pregnancy (X), lactation
Precautions: Hepatic, renal disorders
Pharmacokinetics:
PO: metabolized in liver to metabolite, excreted in urine
Interactions:
• Decreased antibody response: live virus vaccines
• Increased NSAIDs effect: NSAIDs
• Increased side effects of leflunomide: hepatotoxic agents, methotrexate
• Increased rifampin levels: rifampin
• Decreased effect of leflunomide: activated charcoal, cholestyramine
NURSING CONSIDERATIONS
Assess:
• Arthritic symptoms: ROM, mobility, swelling of joints baseline and during treatment
• Liver function studies: if ALT elevations are > twofold ULN, reduce dose to 10 mg/day
Administer:
PO
• With food for GI upset
• To eliminate drug: give cholestyramine 8 g tid × 11 days, check levels
Evaluate:
• Therapeutic response: decreased inflammation, pain in joints

---

Teach patient/family:

• That drug must be continued for prescribed time to be effective

• To take with food, milk, or antacids to avoid GI upset

• To use caution when driving; drowsiness, dizziness may occur

• To take with a full glass of water to enhance absorption

• To avoid pregnancy while taking this drug; not to breastfeed while taking this drug; men should also discontinue drug and begin leflunomide removal protocol if a pregnancy is planned

• That hair may be lost, review alternatives

• To avoid vaccinations during treatment (live virus)

---

lepirudin (℞)

(lep-ih-roo′din)
Refludan

Func. class.: Anticoagulant
Chem. class.: Hirudin

Action: Direct inhibitor of thrombin that is highly specific

Uses: Heparin-induced thrombocytopenia and other thromboembolic conditions

Dosage and routes:

• *Adult:* IV 0.4 mg/kg (≤110 kg) over 15-20 sec; then 0.15 mg/kg (≤110 kg/hr) as a cont inf for 2-10 days or longer

Available forms: Powder for inj 50 mg

Side effects/adverse reactions:

*CV: **Heart failure, pericardial effusion, ventricular fibrillation***
*SYST: **Multiorgan failure, sepsis***
CNS: Fever
GI: GI bleeding, abnormal LFTs
*GU: **Hematuria,** abnormal kidney function*

*HEMA: **Hemorrhage, thrombocytopenia***
RESP: Pneumonia
INTEG: Allergic skin reactions

Contraindications: Hypersensitivity to hirudins

Precautions: Intracranial bleeding, renal function impairment, lactation, children, hepatic disease, pregnancy (B)

Pharmacokinetics: May be metabolized by the release of amino acids during catabolism; 50% unchanged in urine

Interactions:

• Increased risk of bleeding: warfarin derivatives

• Increased action of lepirudin: thrombolytics

NURSING CONSIDERATIONS
Assess:

• Obtain baseline in APTT before treatment; do not start treatment if APTT ratio ≥2.5, then APTT 4 hr after initiation of treatment and at least qd thereafter, if APTT above target, stop inf for 2 hr, then restart at 50%, take APTT in 4 hr; if below target, increase inf rate by 20%, take APTT in 4 hr, do not exceed inf rate of 0.21 mg/kg/hr without checking for coagulation abnormalities

• APTT, which should be 1.5-2.5 × control

◆ Bleeding gums, petechiae, ecchymosis, black tarry stools, hematuria/epistaxis, B/P, vaginal bleeding and possible hemorrhage

• Fever, skin rash, urticaria

Administer:

• Avoiding all IM injections that may cause bleeding

• After reconstitution and further dilution under sterile conditions; use water for inj or 0.9% NaCl; for further dilution 0.9% NaCl or D₅; for rapid and complete reconstitution,

---

◆ = Nursing alert   ⫰ = Herb-drug interaction   ⊗ = Do not crush inject 1 ml of diluent into vial and shake gently, use immediately, warm to room temp before use

IV BOL

• Use sol with conc. of 5 mg/ml, reconstitute 5 mg (1 vial)/1 ml of water for inj or 0.9% NaCl, use body wt for correct calculation as to wt

IV INF

• Use sol with a conc. of 0.2 or 0.4 mg/ml; reconstitute 100 mg (2 vials) with 1 ml each (2 ml) water for inj or 0.9% NaCl, transfer to inf bag with either 500 or 250 ml of 0.9% NaCl or D_5

Evaluate:

• Therapeutic response

Teach patient/family:

• To use soft-bristle toothbrush to avoid bleeding gums, avoid contact sports, use electric razor, avoid IM injection

• To report any signs of bleeding: gums, under skin, urine, stools

---

letrozole (℞)

(let'tro-zohl)

Femara

Func. class.: Antineoplastic, nonsteroidal aromatase inhibitor

---

Action: Binds to the heme group of aromatase. Inhibits conversion of androgens to estrogens to reduce plasma estrogen levels. 30% of breast cancers decrease in size when deprived of estrogen

Uses: Metastatic breast cancer in postmenopausal women

Dosage and routes:

• *Adult:* **PO** 2.5 mg qd

Available forms: Tabs 2.5 mg

Side effects/adverse reactions:

RESP: Dyspnea, cough

*GI: Nausea, vomiting, anorexia, **he-** patotoxicity,* constipation, heartburn, diarrhea

INTEG: Rash, pruritus, alopecia, sweating, hot flashes

CV: Hypertension

CNS: Headache, lethargy, somnolence, dizziness, depression, anxiety

Contraindications: Hypersensitivity, pregnancy (D)

Precautions: Hepatic disease, respiratory disease

Pharmacokinetics: Metabolized in liver, excreted in urine

Interactions: Unknown

NURSING CONSIDERATIONS

Assess:

• Monitor temp q4h; may indicate beginning infection

• Liver function tests before, during therapy (bilirubin, AST, ALT, LDH) as needed or monthly

• Jaundiced skin, sclera, dark urine, clay-colored stools, itchy skin, abdominal pain, fever, diarrhea

Perform/provide:

• Liquid diet, including cola, Jell-O; dry toast or crackers as ordered may be added if patient is not nauseated or vomiting

• Nutritious diet with iron and vitamin supplements as ordered

Evaluate:

• Therapeutic response: decrease in size of tumor

Teach patient/family:

• To report any complaints, side effects to nurse or prescriber

• That drowsiness may occur and to avoid driving or operating heavy machinery

• May take without regard to meals

---

leucovorin (℞)
(loo-koe-vor'in)
citrovorum factor, folinic
acid, leucovorin calcium,
Wellcovorin

Func. class.: Vitamin, folic acid/
methotrexate antagonist antidote
Chem. class.: Tetrahydrofolic
acid derivative

Action: Needed for normal growth patterns; prevents toxicity during antineoplastic therapy by protecting normal cells

Uses: Megaloblastic or macrocytic anemia caused by folic acid deficiency, overdose of folic acid antagonist, methotrexate toxicity, toxicity caused by pyrimethamine or trimethoprim, pneumocystosis, toxoplasmosis

Dosage and routes:
Megaloblastic anemia caused by enzyme deficiency
• *Adult and child:* **PO/IV/IM** up to 6 mg/day

Megaloblastic anemia caused by deficiency of folate
• *Adult and child:* **IM** 1 mg or less qd until adequate response

Methotrexate toxicity
• *Adult and child:* **PO/IM/IV** normal elimination given 6 hr after dose of methotrexate (10 mg/m^2) until methotrexate is <10 M; CrCl is >50% above prior level or methotrexate level is 5×10 at 24 hr, or at 48 hr level is $>9 \times 10$ M, give leucovorin 100 mg/m^2 q3h until level drops to <10 M

Pyrimethamine toxicity
• *Adult and child:* **PO/IM** 5-15 mg qd

Trimethoprim toxicity
• *Adult and child:* **PO/IM** 400 mg qd

Advanced colorectal cancer
• *Adult:* **IV** 200 mg/m^2, then 5-FU 370 mg/m^2; or leucovorin 20 mg/m^2, then 5-FU 425 mg/m^2; give qd × 5 days q4-5wk

Available forms: Tabs 5, 10, 15, 25 mg; inj 3, 5 mg/ml; pwd for inj 10 mg/ml

Side effects/adverse reactions:
RESP: Wheezing
INTEG: Rash, pruritus, erythema, urticaria
HEMA: Thrombocytosis (intraarterial)

Contraindications: Hypersensitivity, anemias other than megaloblastic not associated with vit B$_{12}$ deficiency

Precautions: Pregnancy (C)

Do not confuse:
leucovorin/Leukeran
leucovorin/leukine

Interactions:
• Decreased folate levels: chloramphenicol
• Increased metabolism of phenobarbital, hydantoins

NURSING CONSIDERATIONS
Assess:
• CrCl before leucovorin rescue and qd to detect nephrotoxicity
• I&O; watch for nausea and vomiting
• Nutritional status: bran, yeast, dried beans, nuts, fruits, fresh vegetables, asparagus, which have high folic acid levels
• Other drugs taken: alcohol, hydantoins, trimethoprim may cause increased folic acid use by body

Administer:
• Within 1 hr of folic acid antagonist
IM
• No reconstitution needed
IV
• For IV reconstitute 50 mg/5 ml bacteriostatic or sterile H$_2$O for inj

◆ = Nursing alert   ▮ = Herb-drug interaction   ⊘ = Do not crush

(10 mg/ml) or (100 mg/10 ml); use immediately if sterile H_2O is used
• Give by direct IV over 160 mg/min or less (16 ml of 10 mg/ml sol/min)
• Give by intermittent inf after diluting in 100-500 ml of 0.9% NaCl, D_5W, $D_{10}W$, LR, Ringer's sol

Additive compatibilities: Cisplatin, cisplatin/floxuridine, floxuridine

Syringe compatibilities: Bleomycin, cisplatin, cyclophosphamide, doxorubicin, fluorouracil, furosemide, heparin, methotrexate, metoclopramide, mitomycin, vinblastine, vincristine

Y-site compatibilities: Amifostine, aztreonam, bleomycin, cefepime, cisplatin, cladribine, cyclophosphamide, doxorubicin, doxorubicin liposome, filgrastim, fluconazole, fluorouracil, furosemide, granisetron, heparin, methotrexate, metoclopramide, mitomycin, piperacillin/tazobactam, tacrolimus, teniposide, thiotepa, vinblastine, vincristine

Perform/provide:
• Increase fluid intake if used to treat folic acid inhibitor overdose
• Protection from light and heat

Evaluate:
• Therapeutic response: increased weight; improved orientation, well-being; absence of fatigue

Teach patient/family:
• For leucovorin rescue have patient drink 3 L fluid qd of rescue
• For folic acid deficiency eat folic acid rich foods: bran, yeast, dried beans, nuts, fresh, green leafy vegetables
• To take drug exactly as prescribed
• To notify prescriber of side effects
• To report signs of hyposensitivity reaction immediately

leuprolide (℞)
(loo-proe'lide)
Leupron Depo Ped, Lupron, Lupron Depot, Lupron Depot-3 month, Viadur

Func. class.: Antineoplastic hormone

Chem. class.: Gonadotropin-releasing hormone

Action: Causes initial increase in circulating levels of LH, FSH; continuous administration results in decreased LH, FSH; in men, testosterone is reduced to castrate levels; in premenopausal women, estrogen is reduced to menopausal levels

Uses: Metastatic prostate cancer, management of endometriosis, central precocious puberty

Dosage and routes:
Prostate cancer
• *Adult:* **SC** 1 mg/day; **IM:** 7.5 mg/dose qmo; Viadur implant qyr

Endometriosis/fibroids
• *Adult:* **IM** 3.75 mg qmo

Central precocious puberty
• *Child:* **SC** 50 mg/kg/day; may increase by 10 µg/kg/day as needed
• *Child >37.5 kg:* **IM** 15 mg q4wk
• *Child 25-37.5 kg:* **IM** 11.25 mg q4wk
• *Child ≤25 kg:* 7.5 mg q4wk

Available forms: Inj (depot) 3.75 mg, 7.5 mg single dose, multiple-dose vials (5 mg/ml), single-use kit 11.25 mg vial, pediatric depot 7.5, 11.25, 15 mg; 3 mo depot 22.5 mg single use; Viadur once a yr implant

Side effects/adverse reactions:
GU: Edema, hot flashes, impotence, decreased libido, amenorrhea, vaginal dryness, gynecomastia
CV: ***MI, pulmonary emboli, dysrhythmias***
GI: Anorexia, diarrhea, ***GI bleeding***

Contraindications: Hypersensitivity to GnRH or analogs, thromboembolic disorders, pregnancy (X), lactation, undiagnosed vaginal bleeding

Precautions: Edema, hepatic disease, CVA, MI, seizures, hypertension, diabetes mellitus

Do not confuse:

Lupron/Nuprin

Lupron/Lopurin

Pharmacokinetics:

SC: Onset 1-2 wk, peak 2-4 wk; absorbed rapidly (SC), slowly (IM depot); half-life 3 hr

NURSING CONSIDERATIONS

Assess:

• For symptoms of endometriosis (lower abdominal pain)/fibroids before, during, and after treatment

• Liver function tests before, during therapy (bilirubin, AST, ALT, LDH) as needed or monthly, PSA in prostate cancer

• Pituitary gonadotropic and gonadal function during therapy and 4-8 wk after therapy is decreased

• Worsening of signs and symptoms; normal during beginning therapy

• Fatigue, increased pulse, pallor, lethargy

• Edema in feet, joints; stomach pain; shaking

◆ Symptoms indicating severe allergic reaction: rash, pruritus, urticaria, purpuric skin lesions, itching, flushing

• For central precocious puberty (CPP) if treatment is for this condition; secondary S_4 characteristics to child <9 yr, estradiol/testosterone levels, GnRH test, tomography of head, adrenal steroids, chorionic gonadotropin, wrist x-ray, height, weight

Administer:

• IM/SC using syringe and drug packaged together, give deep in large muscle mass, rotate sites

• Use depot IM only

• Reconstitute vial (single dose)/1 ml of diluent, shake, use immediately

Perform/provide:

• Nutritious diet with iron, vitamin supplements as ordered

• Storage in tight container at room temperature

Evaluate:

• Therapeutic response: decreased tumor size and spread of malignancy

Teach patient/family:

• To notify prescriber if menstruation continues; menstruation should stop

• To use a nonhormonal method of contraception during therapy

• That bone pain will disappear after 1 wk

• To report any complaints, side effects to nurse or prescriber; hot flashes may occur; record weight, report gain of >2 lb/day

• How to prepare, give; to rotate sites for SC inj

• To keep accurate records of dose

• That tumor flare may occur: increase in size of tumor, increased bone pain, will subside rapidly; may take analgesics for pain; premenopausal women must use mechanical birth control; ovulation may be induced

---

levalbuterol (Ŗ)

(lev-al-byoo'ter-ole)

Xopenex

Func. class.: Bronchodilator, adrenergic β_2-agonist

Action: Causes bronchodilation by action on β_2 (pulmonary) receptors by increasing levels of cAMP, which relaxes smooth muscle; produces

---

◆ = Nursing alert   🥄 = Herb-drug interaction   🚫 = Do not crush bronchodilation, CNS, cardiac stimulation, as well as increased diuresis and gastric acid secretion; longer acting than isoproterenol

Uses: Treatment or prevention of bronchospasm (reversible obstructive airway disease)

Dosage and routes:
• *Adult and child ≥12 yr:* **INH** 0.63 mg tid, q6-8h by nebulization, may increase 1.25 mg q8h

Available forms: Sol, inh 0.63 mg, 1.25 mg/3 ml

Side effects/adverse reactions:
CNS: Tremors, anxiety, insomnia, headache, dizziness, stimulation, *restlessness,* hallucinations, flushing, irritability
EENT: Dry nose, irritation of nose and throat
CV: Palpitations, tachycardia, hypertension, angina, hypotension, dysrhythmias
GI: Heartburn, nausea, vomiting
MS: Muscle cramps

Contraindications: Hypersensitivity to sympathomimetics, tachydysrhythmias, severe cardiac disease

Precautions: Lactation, pregnancy (C), cardiac disorders, hyperthyroidism, diabetes mellitus, hypertension, prostatic hypertrophy, narrow-angle glaucoma, seizures

Pharmacokinetics: Metabolized in the liver and tissues, crosses placenta, breast milk, blood-brain barrier
INH: Onset 5-15 min, peak 1-1½ hr, duration 6-8 hr

Interactions:
• Increased action of aerosol bronchodilators
• Increased action of levalbuterol: tricyclics, MAOIs, other adrenergics
• May inhibit action of levalbuterol: other β-blockers

NURSING CONSIDERATIONS
Assess:
• Respiratory function: vital capacity, forced expiratory volume, ABGs, lung sounds, heart rate and rhythm (baseline)
• That patient has not received theophylline therapy before giving dose
• For evidence of allergic reactions

Administer:
• By nebulization q6-8h

Evaluate:
• Therapeutic response: absence of dyspnea, wheezing after 1 hr, improved airway exchange, improved ABGs

Teach patient/family:
• Not to use OTC medications; excess stimulation may occur
• To avoid getting aerosol in eyes; blurring may result
• To wash inhaler in warm water qd and dry
• To avoid smoking, smoke-filled rooms, persons with respiratory infections
⬦ That paradoxic bronchospasm may occur and to stop drug immediately, contact prescriber
• To limit caffeine products such as chocolate, coffee, tea, and colas

Treatment of overdose: Administer a $β_1$-adrenergic blocker

---

levetiracetam (Ŗ)
(lev-eh-teer-ass'eh-tam)
Keppra
Func. class.: Anticonvulsant

Action: Inhibits nerve impulses by limiting influx of sodium ions across cell membrane in motor cortex
Uses: Partial onset seizures
Dosage and routes:
• *Adult:* **PO** 500 mg bid
Available forms: Tabs 250, 500, 750 mg

Side effects/adverse reactions:
HEMA: Lowered Hct, Hgb, infection
CNS: Dizziness, somnolence, asthenia
Contraindications: Hypersensitivity
Precautions: Hepatic disease, renal disease, cardiac disease, psychosis, pregnancy (C), lactation, children
Pharmacokinetics: Rapidly absorbed, not protein bound, excreted via kidneys 66% unchanged; half-life 6-8 hr, longer in elderly
NURSING CONSIDERATIONS
Assess:
• Renal studies: urinalysis, BUN, urine creatinine q3mo
• Blood studies: RBC, Hct, Hgb
• Hepatic studies: ALT, AST, bilirubin
• Description of seizures
• Mental status: mood, sensorium, affect, behavioral changes; if mental status changes, notify prescriber
Administer:
• With food, milk to decrease GI symptoms
Perform/provide:
• Storage at room temperature
• Assistance with ambulation during early part of treatment; dizziness occurs
Evaluate:
• Therapeutic response: decreased seizure activity, document on patient's chart
Teach patient/family:
• To carry Medic Alert ID stating patient's name, drugs taken, condition, prescriber's name, phone number
• To avoid driving, other activities that require alertness
• Not to discontinue medication quickly after long-term use

RARELY USED

levobupivacaine (R)

(lee-voh-bu-piv′ah-kane)
Chirocaine
Func. class.: Local anesthetic

Uses: Local, regional anesthesia, surgical anesthesia, pain management, continuous epidural analgesia
Dosage and routes:
• Varies with route of anesthesia
Contraindications: Hypersensitivity, children <12 yr, elderly, severe liver disease

---

levodopa (R)

(lee′voe-doe-pa)
Dopar, Larodopa, L-Dopa
Func. class.: Antiparkinson agent
Chem. class.: Dopamine agonist

Action: Decarboxylation to dopamine, which increases dopamine levels in brain
Uses: Parkinsonism
Research note: Levodopa may be the cause of sleep attacks (daytime) in patients[20]
Dosage and routes:
• *Adult:* **PO** 0.5-1 g qd divided bid-qid with meals; may increase by up to 0.75 g q3-7d not to exceed 8 g/day unless closely supervised
Available forms: Caps 100, 250, 500 mg; tabs 100, 250, 500 mg
Side effects/adverse reactions:
*HEMA: **Hemolytic anemia, leukopenia, agranulocytosis***
CNS: Involuntary choreiform movements, hand tremors, fatigue, headache, anxiety, twitching, numbness, weakness, confusion, agitation, insomnia, nightmares, psychosis, hal-

---

◆ = Nursing alert   ∥ = Herb-drug interaction   Ⓢ = Do not crush

lucination, hypomania, severe depression, dizziness

GI: Nausea, vomiting, anorexia, abdominal distress, dry mouth, flatulence, dysphagia, bitter taste, diarrhea, constipation

INTEG: Rash, sweating, alopecia

CV: Orthostatic hypotension, tachycardia, hypertension, palpitation

EENT: Blurred vision, diplopia, dilated pupils

MISC: Urinary retention, incontinence, weight change, dark urine

Contraindications: Hypersensitivity, narrow-angle glaucoma, undiagnosed skin lesions

Precautions: Renal disease, cardiac disease, hepatic disease, respiratory disease, MI with dysrhythmias, convulsions, peptic ulcer, pregnancy (C), asthma, endocrine disease, affective disorders, psychosis, lactation, children <12 yr, peptic ulcer

Do not confuse:

L-dopa (levodopa)/methyldopa

Pharmacokinetics:

PO: Peak 1-3 hr, excreted in urine (metabolites)

Interactions:

◆ Hypertensive crisis: MAOIs, furazolidone

• Decreased effects of levodopa: anticholinergics, hydantoins, methionine, papaverine, pyridoxine, benzodiazepines

• Increased effects of levodopa: antacids, metoclopramide

• Drug/food: decreased levodopa absorption: high-protein foods

• Increased pyridoxine will decrease levodopa effect

✐ Decreased action of levodopa, increased EPS: Indian snakeroot

✐ Increased parkinsonian symptoms: kava

Lab test interferences:

False positive: Urine ketones, urine glucose, Coombs' test

False negative: Urine glucose (glucose oxidase)

False increase: Uric acid, urine protein

Decrease: VMA

NURSING CONSIDERATIONS

Assess:

• Liver, renal function studies: AST, ALT, alk phosphatase, LDH, bilirubin, CBC, BUN, protein-bound iodine

• Involuntary movements in parkinsonism: akinesia, tremors, staggering gait, muscle rigidity, drooling

◆ Levodopa toxicity: mental, personality changes, increased twitching, grimacing, tongue protrusion

• B/P, respiration during initial treatment; hypo/hypertension should be reported

• Mental status: affect, mood, behavioral changes, depression; complete suicide assessment

Administer:

• Drug until NPO before surgery

• Adjust dosage to patient response

• With meals; limit protein taken with drug

• Only after MAOIs have been discontinued for 2 wk

Perform/provide:

• Assistance with ambulation during beginning therapy

• Testing for diabetes mellitus, acromegaly if on long-term therapy

Evaluate:

• Therapeutic response: decrease in akathisia, increased mood

Teach patient/family:

• That therapeutic effects may take several wk to a few mo

• To change positions slowly to prevent orthostatic hypotension

• To report side effects: twitching, eye spasms; indicate overdose

• To use drug exactly as prescribed; if drug is discontinued abruptly, parkinsonian crisis may occur

• That urine, sweat may darken
• To avoid vit B_6 preparations, vitamin-fortified foods containing B_6; these foods can reverse effects of levodopa

---

levofloxacin (℞)

(lee-voh-floks'a-sin)
Levaquin
Func. class.: Antiinfective
Chem. class.: Fluoroquinolone

See Ophthalmic Appendix for Ophthalmic Product

Action: Interferes with conversion of intermediate DNA fragments into high-molecular-weight DNA in bacteria; DNA gyrase inhibitor

Uses: Acute sinusitis, acute chronic bronchitis, community-acquired pneumonia, uncomplicated skin infections, complicated UTI, acute pyelonephritis caused by *Streptococcus pneumoniae, Haemophilus influenzae, Haemophilis parainfluenzae, Moraxella catarrhalis*

Dosage and routes:
• *Adult:* **IV INF** 500 mg by slow inf over 1 hr q24h × 7-14 days depending on infection; **PO:** 500 mg q24h × 7-14 days depending on infection

Renal disease
• CrCl 20-49 ml/min initial 500 mg, then 250 mg, q24h; CrCl 10-19 ml/min 250 or 500 mg, depending on condition; then 250 mg q48h

Available forms: Single-use vials (500 mg); 25 mg/ml 20 ml vials; premixed flexible containers; tabs 250, 500, 750 mg

Side effects/adverse reactions:
MISC: Hypoglycemia, hypersensi-

tivity, *anaphylaxis, multisystem organ failure*
CNS: Headache, dizziness, *insomnia,* anxiety, *seizures,* encephalopathy, paresthesia
CV: Chest pain, palpitations, vasodilation
EENT: Dry mouth
HEMA: Eosinophilia, *hemolytic anemia,* lymphopenia
RESP: Pneumonitis
GI: Nausea, flatulence, *vomiting,* diarrhea, abdominal pain, *pseudomembranous colitis*
GU: Vaginitis, crystalluria
INTEG: Rash, pruritus, *photosensitivity, Stevens-Johnson syndrome*
Contraindications: Hypersensitivity to quinolones, photosensitivity
Precautions: Pregnancy (C), lactation, children
Pharmacokinetics: Metabolized in liver, excreted in urine unchanged, half-life 6-8 hr
Interactions:
• Nephrotoxicity: cyclosporine
• Decreased absorption of levofloxacin: antacids containing aluminum, magnesium; sucralfate, zinc, iron, calcium
• Altered blood glucose levels: antidiabetic agents
• Increased CNS stimulation, seizures: NSAIDs, foscarnet
• May decrease clearance of: theophylline, toxicity may result
• Increased risk of bleeding: warfarin
• Do not use with magnesium in the same IV line
• Increased toxicity/levels of digoxin, cimetidine
Lab test interferences:
Decrease: Glucose, lymphocytes
NURSING CONSIDERATIONS
Assess:
• For previous sensitivity reaction
• For signs and symptoms of infection: characteristics of sputum, WBC

◆ = Nursing alert   🖋 = Herb-drug interaction   🚫 = Do not crush

>10,000/mm^3, fever; obtain baseline information before and during treatment

• C&S before beginning drug therapy to identify if correct treatment has been initiated

⬥ For allergic reactions and anaphylaxis: rash, urticaria, pruritus, chills, fever, joint pain; may occur a few days after therapy begins; epinephrine and resuscitation equipment should be available for anaphylactic reaction

• Bowel pattern qd; if severe diarrhea occurs, drug should be discontinued

⬥ For overgrowth of infection: perineal itching, fever, malaise, redness, pain, swelling, drainage, rash, diarrhea, change in cough, sputum

Administer:

• PO 4 hr before or 2 hr after antacids, iron, calcium, zinc

IV

• Only by slow IV infusion over 1 hr

• Discard any unused sol in the single-dose vial

• Using premix, tear outer wrap at notch and remove sol container, check for leaks, close control clamps; remove cover from port at bottom of container, insert pin into port with a twist; suspend container from hanger, squeeze and release drip chamber to proper fluid level, open flow control to expel air, close clamp; regulate rate with flow control clamps

Solution compatibilities: 0.9% NaCl, D$_5$W, D$_5$/0.9% NaCl, D$_5$LR, D$_5$/0.45% NaCl, sodium lactate

Evaluate:

• Therapeutic response: absence of signs/symptoms of infection (WBC <10,000/mm^3, temp WNL)

Teach patient/family:

• To contact prescriber if vaginal itching, loose, foul-smelling stools,

furry tongue occur (may indicate superinfection); report itching, rash, pruritus, urticaria

• To notify prescriber of diarrhea with blood or pus

• To take 4 hr before or 2 hr after antacids, iron, calcium, zinc products

• To complete full course of therapy; to increase fluid intake to 2 L/day to prevent crystalluria

• To avoid hazardous activities until response is known

• To use frequent rinsing of mouth, sugarless candy or gum for dry mouth

• To avoid other medication unless approved by prescriber

• Not to use theophylline with this product, toxicity may result; contact prescriber if taking theophylline

• To prevent sun exposure or use sunscreen to prevent phototoxicity

levomethadyl (℞)

(lev-oh-meth'ah-dil)
ORLAMM
Func. class.: Opiate agonist analgesic

Action: Depresses pain impulse transmission at the spinal cord level by interacting with opioid receptors

Uses: Management of opiate dependency

Dosage and routes:

Opiate withdrawal

• Usually given 3×/wk (Monday, Wednesday, Friday or Tuesday, Thursday, Saturday)

• *Initial dose:* 20-40 mg each dose at 48 or 72 hr; may be adjusted in increments of 5-10 mg until steady state occurs (1-2 wk); patients dependent on methadone may require larger doses

• *Maintenance:* 60-90 mg 3×/wk
• *Transfer to methadone:* Initial treatment given after 48 hr; may give increased or decreased (5-10 mg) in the daily methadone dose (symptoms of withdrawal)

Available forms: Oral sol 10 mg/ml

Side effects/adverse reactions:

CNS: Drowsiness, dizziness, confusion, headache, sedation, euphoria
CV: Palpitations, bradycardia, change in B/P
EENT: Tinnitus, blurred vision, miosis, diplopia
GI: Nausea, vomiting, anorexia, constipation, cramps, biliary tract spasm
GU: Increased urinary output, dysuria, urinary retention
INTEG: Rash, urticaria, bruising, flushing, diaphoresis, pruritus
*RESP: **Respiratory depression***

Contraindications: Hypersensitivity

Precautions: Addictive personality, pregnancy (C), lactation, increased intracranial pressure, MI (acute), severe heart disease, respiratory depression, hepatic disease, renal disease, child <18 yr

Pharmacokinetics:
PO: Onset 30-60 min, duration 6-8 hr, cumulative 22-48 hr
Metabolized by liver, excreted by kidneys, crosses placenta, excreted in breast milk

Interactions:
• Increased effects with other CNS depressants: alcohol, opiates, sedative/hypnotics, antipsychotics, skeletal muscle relaxants, rifampin, phenytoin

NURSING CONSIDERATIONS
Assess:
• I&O ratio; check for decreasing output; may indicate urinary retention
Administer:
• With antiemetic for nausea, vomiting

Perform/provide:
• Storage in light-resistant container at room temperature
Evaluate:
• Therapeutic response: decreased dependence on opiate
• CNS changes: dizziness, drowsiness, hallucinations, euphoria, LOC, pupil reaction
• Allergic reactions: rash, urticaria
• Respiratory dysfunction: depression, character, rate, rhythm
Teach patient/family:
• To report any symptoms of CNS changes, allergic reactions
• That physical dependency may result after extended period of use
• That withdrawal symptoms may occur: nausea, vomiting, cramps, fever, faintness, anorexia
• To avoid pregnancy; if suspected, notify prescriber
• To use contraception during treatment

---

levonorgestrel implant (℞)
(lee-voe-nor-jess'trel)
Norplant System
Func. class.: Contraceptive system
Chem. class.: Synthetic progestin

Action: As a progestin, transforms proliferative endometrium into secretory endometrium; inhibits secretion of pituitary gonadotropins, which prevents follicular maturation and ovulation

Uses: Prevention of pregnancy for 5 yr

Dosage and routes:
• *Adult:* 6 caps subdermally implanted in the upper arm during first

---

7 days after onset of menses, replace q5yr

Available forms: Kit of 6 caps, 36 mg/cap

Side effects/adverse reactions:

CV: ***Cerebral hemorrhage, coronary thrombosis, pulmonary embolism, cerebral thrombosis***

CNS: Dizziness, headache, nervousness

GU: Amenorrhea, cervical erosion, breakthrough bleeding, dysmenorrhea, vaginal candidiasis, breast changes, vaginitis

GI: Nausea, abdominal discomfort

INTEG: Alopecia, dermatitis, hirsutism, acne, hypertrichosis, infection at site, pain/itching at site

OTHER: Change in appetite, weight gain

Contraindications: Hypersensitivity, pregnancy (X), thrombophlebitis, undiagnosed genital bleeding, liver tumors, breast carcinoma, liver disease

Precautions: Depression, psychosis, lactation, fluid retention, contact lens wearers

Pharmacokinetics: Onset 1 mo, peak 1 mo, duration 5 yr

Interactions:
• Decreased contraception: phenytoin, carbamazepine

NURSING CONSIDERATIONS
Assess:
• Blood studies: cholesterol, triglycerides; may be increased or decreased; sex hormone—binding globulin, thyroxine, T_3 uptake, LDL, HDL
• Menstrual irregularities: spotting, prolonged bleeding, amenorrhea; usually diminish
• For jaundice, thrombophlebitis; implants should be removed, hepatic studies
• For acne, dermatitis, hirsutism, alopecia

Administer:
• 8 cm (3 in) above the crease of the elbow; implantation should be during first 7 days after onset of menses; implantation should be fanlike, 15 degrees apart

Evaluate:
• Therapeutic response: absence of pregnancy

Teach patient/family:
• To notify prescriber if pregnancy is suspected
• To use sunscreen or stay out of the sun
• That this product only prevents pregnancy, does not protect against HIV or other STDs
• That if vision problems occur, an ophthalmologist should be seen
• That physical examinations are necessary
◆To report fluid retention: weight gain, edema; hepatic symptoms: yellowing skin or eyes, clay-colored stools, dark urine; thrombosis: blurred vision, headache, tenderness in extremities

---

RARELY USED

levorphanol (℞)

(lee-vor'fa-nole)

Levo-Dromoran, Levorphan

Func. class.: Opioid analgesic (agonist)

Controlled Substance Schedule II

Uses: Moderate to severe pain

Dosage and routes:
• *Adult:* **PO/SC/IV** 2-3 mg q4-5h prn; **PCA** 0.1 mg/ml

Contraindications: Hypersensitivity, addiction (narcotic)

---

levothyroxine (T$_4$) (Ɍ)

(lee-voe-thye-rox'een)
Eltroxin*, Levo-T, Levoxyl,
Levothroid, levothyroxine
sodium, Levoxyl, PMS-
Levothyroxine Sodium*,
Synthroid, T$_4$

Func. class.: Thyroid hormone
Chem. class.: Levoisomer of thyroxine

Action: Increases metabolic rate, controls protein synthesis, increases cardiac output, renal blood flow, O$_2$ consumption, body temp, blood volume, growth, development at cellular level

Uses: Hypothyroidism, myxedema coma, thyroid hormone replacement, congenital hypothyroidism, thyrotoxicosis, congenital hypothyroidism, some types of thyroid cancer

Dosage and routes:

Severe hypothyroidism
• *Adult:* PO 50 µg qd, increased by 50-100 µg q1-4 wk until desired response, maintenance dose 75-125 µg qd; **IM/IV** 50-100 µg/day as a single dose
• *Child >12 yr:* PO 2-3 µg/kg/day as a single dose AM
• *Child 6-12 yr:* PO 4-5 µg/kg/day as a single dose AM
• *Child 1-5 yr:* PO 5-6 µg/kg/day as a single dose AM
• *Child 6-12 mo:* PO 6-8 µg/kg/day as a single dose AM
• *Child to 6 mo:* PO 8-10 µg/kg/day as a single dose AM

Myxedema coma
• *Adult:* IV 200-500 µg, may increase by 100-300 µg after 24 hr; place on oral medication as soon as possible

Available forms: Pwd for inj 50, 200, 500 µg/vial; tabs 0.025, 0.05, 0.075, 0.088, 0.1, 0.112, 0.125, 0.137, 0.15, 0.175, 0.2, 0.3 mg

Side effects/adverse reactions:

CNS: Anxiety, insomnia, tremors, headache, **thyroid storm**
CV: Tachycardia, palpitations, angina, dysrhythmias, hypertension, **cardiac arrest**
GI: Nausea, diarrhea, increased or decreased appetite, cramps
MISC: Menstrual irregularities, weight loss, sweating, heat intolerance, fever

Contraindications: Adrenal insufficiency, myocardial infarction, thyrotoxicosis, hypersensitivity to beef, alcohol intolerance (inj only)

Precautions: Elderly, angina pectoris, hypertension, ischemia, cardiac disease, pregnancy (A), lactation

Do not confuse:
Synthroid/Symmetrel

Pharmacokinetics:
PO: Onset unknown, peak 1-3 wk, duration 1-3 wk
IV: Onset 6-8 hr, peak 24 hr, duration unknown
Half-life 6-7 days; distributed throughout body tissues

Interactions:
• Increased risk of cardiac insufficiency when used with epinephrine products
• Decreased absorption of levothyroxine: cholestyramine, colestipol
• Increased effects of anticoagulants, sympathomimetics, tricyclics
• Decreased effects of digitalis drugs, insulin, hypoglycemics
• Decreased effects of levothyroxine: estrogens
• Considered to be incompatible in syringe with all other drugs
🍃 Do not give with bugleweed

Lab test interferences:
Increase: CPK, LDH, AST, PBI, blood glucose
Decrease: Thyroid function tests

◆ = Nursing alert   🍃 = Herb-drug interaction   🚫 = Do not crush

NURSING CONSIDERATIONS
Assess:
• B/P, pulse periodically during treatment
• Weight qd in same clothing, using same scale, at same time of day
• Height, growth rate of a child
• T_3, T_4, FTIs, which are decreased; radioimmunoassay of TSH, which is increased; radio uptake, which is increased if patient is on too low a dose of medication
• PT may require decreased anticoagulant; check for bleeding, bruising
• Increased nervousness, excitability, irritability, which may indicate too high dose of medication, usually after 1-3 wk of treatment
• Cardiac status: angina, palpitation, chest pain, change in VS

Administer:
• IV after diluting with provided diluent 0.5 mg/5 ml; shake; give through Y-tube or 3-way stopcock; give 0.1 mg or less over 1 min; do not add to IV inf; 0.1 mg = 1 ml
• In AM if possible as a single dose to decrease sleeplessness
• At same time each day to maintain drug level
• Only for hormone imbalances; not to be used for obesity, male infertility, menstrual conditions, lethargy
• Lowest dose that relieves symptoms; lower dose to the elderly and in cardiac diseases
• Crushed and mixed with water, nonsoy formula, or breast milk for infants/children

Perform/provide:
• Storage in tight, light-resistant container; sol should be discarded if not used immediately
• Withdrawal of medication 4 wk before RAIU test

Evaluate:
• Therapeutic response: absence of depression; increased weight loss, diuresis, pulse, appetite; absence of constipation, peripheral edema, cold intolerance; pale, cool, dry skin; brittle nails, alopecia, coarse hair, menorrhagia, night blindness, paresthesias, syncope, stupor, coma, rosy cheeks

Teach patient/family:
• That hair loss will occur in child, is temporary
• To report excitability, irritability, anxiety, which indicate overdose
• Not to switch brands unless approved by prescriber
• That drug may be discontinued after giving birth, thyroid panel evaluated after 1-2 mo
• That hypothyroid child will show almost immediate behavior/personality change
• That drug is not to be taken to reduce weight
• To avoid OTC preparations with iodine; read labels
• To avoid iodine food, iodized salt, soybeans, tofu, turnips, some seafood, some bread
• That drug is not a cure but controls symptoms and treatment is life-long

lidocaine (parenteral) (℞)
(lye′doe-kane)
LidoPen Auto-Injector,
Xylocard*

Func. class.: Antidysrhythmic (Class Ib)

Chem. class.: Aminoacyl amide

Action: Increases electrical stimulation threshold of ventricle, His-Purkinje system, which stabilizes

L

cardiac membrane, decreases automaticity

Uses: Ventricular tachycardia, ventricular dysrhythmias during cardiac surgery, myocardial infarction, digitalis toxicity, cardiac catheterization

Dosage and routes:

• *Adult:* **IV BOL** 50-100 mg (1 mg/kg) over 2-3 min, repeat q3-5min, not to exceed 300 mg in 1 hr; begin **IV INF; IV INF** 20-50 µg/kg/min; **IM** 200-300 mg (4.3 mg/kg) in deltoid muscle, may repeat in 1-1½ hr if needed

• *Elderly, CHF, reduced liver function:* **IV BOL** give ½ adult dose

• *Child:* **IV BOL** 1 mg/kg, then **IV INF** 30 µg/kg/min

Available forms: IV INF 0.2% (2 mg/ml), 0.4% (4 mg/ml), 0.8% (8 mg/ml); IV ad 4% (40 mg/ml), 10% (100 mg/ml), 20% (200 mg/ml); IV dir 1% (10 mg/ml), 2% (20 mg/ml); IM 10% 300 mg/ml

Side effects/adverse reactions:

CNS: Headache, dizziness, involuntary movement, confusion, tremor, drowsiness, euphoria, ***convulsions***

EENT: Tinnitus, blurred vision

GI: Nausea, vomiting, anorexia

*CV: Hypotension, bradycardia, **heart block, cardiovascular collapse, arrest***

RESP: Dyspnea, ***respiratory depression***

INTEG: Rash, urticaria, edema, swelling

MISC: Febrile response, phlebitis at injection site

Contraindications: Hypersensitivity to amides, severe heart block, supraventricular dysrhythmias, Adams-Stokes syndrome, Wolff-Parkinson-White syndrome

Precautions: Pregnancy (B), lactation, children, renal disease, liver disease, CHF, respiratory depression, malignant hyperthermia

Pharmacokinetics:

IV: Onset 2 min, duration 20 min

IM: Onset 5-15 min, duration 1½ hr; half-life 8 min, 1-2 hr (terminal); metabolized in liver; excreted in urine; crosses placenta

Interactions:

• Increased neuromuscular blockade of neuromuscular blockers, tubocurarine

• Increased effects of lidocaine: cimetidine, phenytoin, propranolol, metoprolol

• Decreased effects of lidocaine: barbiturates

🌿 Increased action of lidocaine: aloe, buckthorn, cascara sagrada, senna

Lab test interferences:

Increase: CPK

NURSING CONSIDERATIONS

Assess:

◆ ECG continuously to determine increased PR or QRS segments; if these develop, discontinue or reduce rate; watch for increased ventricular ectopic beats; may have to rebolus, B/P

• IV infusion rate using infusion pump; run at less than 4 mg/min

• Blood levels (therapeutic level: 1.5-5 µg/ml)

• I&O ratio, electrolytes (K, Na, Cl)

◆ Malignant hyperthermia: tachypnea, tachycardia, changes in B/P, increased temp

• Respiratory status: rate, rhythm, lung fields for rales, watch for respiratory depression; lung fields, bilateral rales may occur in CHF patient; increased respiration, increased pulse; drug should be discontinued

• CNS effects: dizziness, confusion, psychosis, paresthesias, convulsions; drug should be discontinued

Administer:

• IM injection in deltoid; aspirate to

◆ = Nursing alert   🌿 = Herb-drug interaction   🚫 = Do not crush

avoid intravascular administration; check site daily for infiltration or extravasation

IV

• Bolus undiluted (1%, 2% only) give 50 mg or less over 1 min or dilute 1 g/250-500 ml of D₅W; titrate to patient response; use infusion pump; pediatric inf is 120 mg of lidocaine/100 ml D₅W; 1-2.5 ml/kg/hr = 20-50 μg/kg/min; use only 1%, 2% sol for IV bol

Additive compatibilities: Alteplase, aminophylline, amiodarone, atracurium, bretylium, calcium chloride, calcium gluceptate, calcium gluconate, chloramphenicol, chlorothiazide, cimetidine, dexamethasone, digoxin, diphenhydramine, dobutamine, dopamine, ephedrine, erythromycin lactobionate, floxacillin, flumazenil, furosemide, heparin, hydrocortisone, hydroxyzine, insulin (regular), mephentermine, metaraminol, nafcillin, nitroglycerin, penicillin G potassium, pentobarbital, phenylephrine, potassium chloride, procainamide, prochlorperazine, promazine, ranitidine, sodium bicarbonate, sodium lactate, theophylline, verapamil, vit B/C

Solution compatibilities: D₅W, D₅/0.9% NaCl, D₅/0.45% NaCl, D₅/LR, LR, 0.9% NaCl, 0.45% NaCl

Syringe compatibilities: Cloxacillin, glycopyrrolate, heparin, hydroxyzine, methicillin, metoclopramide, milrinone, moxalactam, nalbuphine

Y-site compatibilities: Alteplase, amiodarone, amrinone, cefazolin, ciprofloxacin, cisatracurium, diltiazem, dobutamine, dopamine, enalaprilat, etomidate, famotidine, haloperidol, heparin, heparin/hydrocortisone, labetalol, meperidine, morphine, nitroglycerin, nitroprusside, potassium chloride, propofol, remifentanil, streptokinase, theophylline, vit B/C, warfarin

Evaluate:

• Therapeutic response: decreased dysrhythmias

Teach patient/family:

• The use of automatic lidocaine injection device if ordered for personal use

Treatment of overdose: O₂, artificial ventilation, ECG; administer dopamine for circulatory depression, diazepam or thiopental for convulsions; decrease drug if needed

RARELY USED

lincomycin (℞)
(lin-koe-mye′sin)
Func. class.: Antibacterial

Uses: Infections caused by group A β-hemolytic streptococci, pneumococci, staphylococci (respiratory tract, skin, soft tissue, urinary tract infections, osteomyelitis, septicemia)

Dosage and routes:

• *Adult:* PO 500 mg q6-8h, not to exceed 8 g/day; IM 600 mg/day or q12h; IV 600 mg-1 g q8-12h; dilute in 100 ml IV sol; infuse over 1 hr, not to exceed 8 g/day

• *Child >1 mo:* PO 30-60 mg/kg/day in divided doses q6-8h; IM 10 mg/kg/day q12h; IV 10-20 mg/kg/day in divided doses q8-12h; dilute to 100 ml IV sol; infuse over 1 hr

Contraindications: Hypersensitivity, ulcerative colitis/enteritis, infants <1 mo

lindane (R)

(lin'dane)

Bio-Well, GBH*, G-Well*, Hexit*, Kwell, Kwellada*, Kwildane, lindane, PMS-Lindane*, Scabene, Thionex

Func. class.: Scabicide, pediculicide

Chem. class.: Chlorinated hydrocarbon (synthetic)

Action: Stimulates nervous system of arthropods, resulting in seizures, death of organism

Uses: Scabies, lice (head/pubic/body), nits

Dosage and routes:

Lice

• *Adult and child:* **CREAM/LOTION** wash area with soap, water; remove visible crusts; apply to skin surfaces; remove with soap, water in 8-12 hr; may reapply in 1 wk if needed; shampoo using 30 ml: work into lather, rub for 5 min, rinse, dry with towel; comb with fine-toothed comb to remove nits

Scabies

• *Adult and child:* **TOP** apply 1% cream/lotion to skin, neck to bottom of feet, toes; repeat in 1 wk prn

Available forms: Lotion, shampoo, cream (1%)

Side effects/adverse reactions:

INTEG: Pruritus, rash, irritation, contact dermatitis

GI: Nausea, vomiting, diarrhea, liver damage (inhalation of vapors)

HEMA: **Aplastic anemia** (chronic inhalation of vapors)

CV: **Ventricular fibrillation** (chronic inhalation of vapors)

GU: **Kidney damage** (chronic inhalation of vapors)

CNS: Tremors, **convulsions,** stimulation, dizziness (chronic inhalation of vapors)

Contraindications: Hypersensitivity; premature neonate; patients with known seizure disorders; inflammation of skin, abrasions, or skin breaks

Precautions: Pregnancy (B); avoid contact with eyes; children <10 yr, infants, lactation

Interactions:

• Oils may enhance absorption; if an oil-based hair dressing is used, shampoo, rinse, dry hair before applying lindane shampoo

NURSING CONSIDERATIONS

Assess:

• Head, hair for lice and nits before and after treatment; if scabies are present check all skin surfaces

• Identify source of infection: school, family, sexual contacts

Administer:

• To body areas, scalp only; do not apply to face, lips, mouth, eyes, any mucous membrane, anus, or meatus

• Topical corticosteroids as ordered to decrease contact dermatitis

• Antihistamines

• Lotions of menthol or phenol to control itching

• Topical antibiotics for infection

Perform/provide:

• Isolation until areas on skin, scalp have cleared and treatment is completed

• Removal of nits by using a fine-toothed comb rinsed in vinegar after treatment; use gloves

Evaluate:

• Therapeutic response: decreased crusts, nits, brownish trails on skin, itching papules in skin folds, decreased itching after several wk

Teach patient/family:

• To wash all inhabitants' clothing, using insecticide; preventive treatment may be required of all persons living in same house, using lotion or shampoo to decrease spread of infection; use rubber gloves when applying drug

⬥ = Nursing alert   🌿 = Herb-drug interaction   🚫 = Do not crush

• That itching may continue for 4-6 wk

• That drug must be reapplied if accidently washed off, or treatment will be ineffective

• Not to apply to face; if accidental contact with eyes occurs, flush with water

• Instruct patient to remove after specified time to prevent toxicity

• To treat sexual contacts simultaneously

Treatment of ingestion: Gastric lavage, saline laxatives, IV diazepam (Valium) for convulsions

---

linezolid (℞)

(line-zoe'lide)

Zyvox

Func. class.: Broad-spectrum antiinfective

Chem. class.: Oxalodinone

Action: Binds to bacterial 23S ribosomal RNA of the 50S subunit preventing formation of the bacterial translation process

Uses: Vancomycin-resistant *Enterococcus faecium* infections, nosocomial pneumonia, uncomplicated or complicated skin and skin structure infections, community-acquired pneumonia

Research note: One case of myelosuppression occurring with linezolid led researchers to suggest monitoring of hematologic parameters[21]

Dosage and routes:

Vancomycin-resistant **Enterococcus faecium** *infections*

• *Adult:* **IV/PO** 600 mg q12h × 14-28 days

Nosocomial pneumonia/ complicated skin infections/ community-acquired pneumonia/ concurrent bacterial infection

• *Adult:* **IV/PO** 600 mg q12h × 10-14 days

Uncomplicated skin infections

• *Adult:* **IV/PO** 400 mg q10-14 days

Available forms: Tab 400, 600 mg; powder for reconstitution 100 mg/5 ml; inj 2 mg/ml

Side effects/adverse reactions:

CNS: Headache, dizziness

GI: Nausea, diarrhea, increased ALT, AST, *vomiting,* taste change, tongue color change

MISC: Vaginal moniliasis, fungal infection, oral moniliasis

*HEMA: **Myelosuppression***

Contraindications: Hypersensitivity

Precautions: Pregnancy (C), lactation, children, thrombocytopenia

Do not confuse:

Zyvox/Vioxx

Pharmacokinetics: Rapidly and extensively absorbed, protein binding 31%, metabolized by oxidation of the morpholine ring

Interactions:

• May decrease the effects of MAOIs

• Increased effects of adrenergic agents, serotonergic agents

NURSING CONSIDERATIONS

Assess:

• CBC weekly, assess for myelosuppression (anemias, leukopenia, pancytopenia, thrombocytopenia)

• CNS symptoms: headache, dizziness

• Liver function studies: AST, ALT

• Allergic reactions: fever, flushing, rash, urticaria, pruritus

• For pseudomembranous colitis

Administer:

PO

• Store reconstituted oral suspension at room temperature, use within 3 wk

IV

• 30-120 min; do not use IV infusion bag in series connections, do not use with additives in sol, do not use with another drug, administer separately

---

Side effects: *italics* = common; ***bold italics*** = life-threatening

Solution compatibilities:
D₅, 0.9% NaCl, LR
Evaluate:
• Therapeutic response: decreased symptoms of infection, blood cultures negative
Teach patient/family:
• If dizziness occurs, to ambulate, perform activities with assistance
• To complete full course of drug therapy
• To contact prescriber if adverse reaction occurs
• To avoid large amounts of high-tyramine foods (provide list)

---

liothyronine (T₃) (R̟)
(lye-oh-thye′roe-neen)
Cytomel, *l*-triiodothyronine, T₃, liothyronine sodium, Triostat
Func. class.: Thyroid hormone
Chem. class.: Synthetic T₃

Action: Increases metabolic rates, cardiac output, O₂ consumption, body temp, blood volume, growth, development at cellular level
Uses: Hypothyroidism, myxedema coma, thyroid hormone replacement, congenital hypothyroidism, nontoxic goiter, T₃ suppression test
Dosage and routes:
• *Adult:* **PO** 25 µg qd, increased by 12.5-25 µg q1-2wk until desired response, maintenance dose 25-75 µg qd
• *Geriatric:* **PO** 5 µg/day, increase by 5 µg/day q1-2wk
Congenital hypothyroidism
• *Child >3 yr:* **PO** 50-100 µg qd
• *Child <3 yr:* **PO** 5 µg qd, increased by 5 µg q3-4d titrated to response
Myxedema, severe hypothyroidism
• *Adult:* **PO** 25-50 µg then may increase by 5-10 µg q1-2wk; maintenance dose 50-100 µg qd
Nontoxic goiter
• *Adult:* **PO** 5 µg qd, increased by 12.5-25 µg q1-2wk; maintenance dose 75 µg qd
Suppression test
• *Adult:* **PO** 75-100 µg qd × 1 wk; radioactive ¹³¹I is given before and after 1 wk dose
Available forms: Tabs 5, 25, 50 µg; inj 10 µg/ml
Side effects/adverse reactions:
CNS: Insomnia, tremors, headache, ***thyroid storm***
CV: Tachycardia, palpitations, angina, dysrhythmias, hypertension, ***cardiac arrest***
GI: Nausea, diarrhea, increased or decreased appetite, cramps
MISC: Menstrual irregularities, weight loss, sweating, heat intolerance, fever
Contraindications: Adrenal insufficiency, myocardial infarction, thyrotoxicosis
Precautions: Elderly, angina pectoris, hypertension, ischemia, cardiac disease, pregnancy (A), lactation
Pharmacokinetics:
PO/IV: Peak 12-48 hr, duration 72 hr, half-life 1-2 days
Interactions:
• Decreased absorption of liothyronine: cholestyramine
• Increased effects of anticoagulants, sympathomimetics, tricyclics
• Decreased effects of digitalis drugs, insulin, hypoglycemics
• Decreased effects of liothyronine: estrogens
🍃 Do not use with bugleweed
Lab test interferences:
Increase: CPK, LDH, AST, PBI, blood glucose
Decrease: Thyroid function tests

◆ = Nursing alert   🍃 = Herb-drug interaction   🚫 = Do not crush

NURSING CONSIDERATIONS
Assess:

• B/P, pulse, periodically during treatment
• Weight qd in same clothing, using same scale, at same time of day
• Height, growth rate of child
• T_3, T_4, which are decreased; radioimmunoassay of TSH, which is increased; radio uptake, which is increased if patient is on too low a dose of medication
• PT may require decreased anticoagulant; check for bleeding, bruising
• Increased nervousness, excitability, irritability, which may indicate too high dose of medication, usually after 1-3 wk of treatment
• Cardiac status: angina, palpitation, chest pain, change in VS

Administer:

• In AM if possible as a single dose to decrease sleeplessness
• At same time each day to maintain drug level
• Only for hormone imbalances; not to be used for obesity, male infertility, menstrual conditions, lethargy
• Lowest dose that relieves symptoms
• Liothyronine after discontinuing other thyroid preparation

Perform/provide:

• Removal of medication 4 wk before RAIU test

Evaluate:

• Therapeutic response: absence of depression; increased weight loss, diuresis, pulse, appetite; absence of constipation, peripheral edema, cold intolerance; pale, cool, dry skin; brittle nails, alopecia, coarse hair, menorrhagia, night blindness, paresthesia, syncope, stupor, coma, rosy cheeks

Teach patient/family:

• That hair loss will occur in child but is temporary
• To report excitability, irritability, anxiety, which indicates overdose
• Not to switch brands unless approved by prescriber
• That hypothyroid child will show almost immediate behavior/personality change
• That drug is not to be taken to reduce weight
• To avoid OTC preparations with iodine; read labels
• To avoid iodine food, iodized salt, soybeans, tofu, turnips, some seafood, some bread
• That drug controls symptoms but does not cure; treatment is lifelong

---

liotrix (R)
(lye'oh-trix)
Thyrolar, T_3/T_4
Func. class.: Thyroid hormone
Chem. class.: Levothyroxine/liothyronine (synthetic T_4, T_3)

Action: Increases metabolic rates, cardiac output, O_2 consumption, body temp, blood volume, growth, development at cellular level

Uses: Hypothyroidism, thyroid hormone replacement

Dosage and routes:

• *Adult and child:* **PO** 50 µg levothyroxine mg qd, increased by 12.5 µg liothyronine mg qmo until desired response
• *Elderly:* **PO** 12.5-25 µg levothyroxine/3.1-6.2 µg liothyronine, may increase by 12.5-25 µg levothyroxine/3.1-6.2 µg liothyronine q6-8wk until adequate response

Available forms: Tabs: 12.5 µg levothyroxine/3.1 µg liothyronine, 25 µg levothyroxine/6.25 µg liothyronine, 50 µg levothyroxine/12.5 µg liothyronine, 100 µg levothyroxine/25 µg liothyronine, 150 μg levothyroxine/ 37.5 μg liothyronine

Side effects/adverse reactions:

CNS: Insomnia, tremors, headache, ***thyroid storm***

CV: Tachycardia, palpitations, angina, dysrhythmias, hypertension, ***cardiac arrest***

GI: Nausea, diarrhea, increased or decreased appetite, cramps

MISC: Menstrual irregularities, weight loss, sweating, heat intolerance, fever

Contraindications: Adrenal insufficiency, myocardial infarction, thyrotoxicosis

Precautions: Elderly, angina pectoris, hypertension, ischemia, cardiac disease, pregnancy (A), lactation

Do not confuse:

Thyrolar/Thyrar

Pharmacokinetics:

PO (T₄): Onset unknown, peak 1-3 wk, duration 1-3 wk

PO (T₃): Onset unknown, peak 24-72 hr, duration 72 hr, half-life 1 wk

Interactions:

• Decreased absorption of liotrix: cholestyramine, colestipol

• Increased effects of anticoagulants, sympathomimetics, tricyclics, catecholamines

• Decreased effects of digitalis, insulin, hypoglycemics

• Decreased effects of liotrix: estrogens

🍃 Do not use with bugleweed

Lab test interferences:

Increase: CPK, LDH, AST, PBI, blood glucose

Decrease: Thyroid function tests

NURSING CONSIDERATIONS

Assess:

• B/P, pulse periodically during treatment

• Weight qd in same clothing, using same scale, at same time of day

• Height, growth rate of child

• T₃, T₄, FTIs, which are decreased; radioimmunoassay of TSH, which is increased; radio uptake, which is increased if patient is on too low a dose of medication

• PT may require decreased anticoagulant; check for bleeding, bruising

• Increased nervousness, excitability, irritability, which may indicate too high dose of medication, usually after 1-3 wk of treatment

• Cardiac status: angina, palpitation, chest pain, change in VS

Administer:

• In AM if possible as a single dose to decrease sleeplessness

• At same time each day to maintain drug level

• Only for hormone imbalances; not to be used for obesity, male infertility, menstrual conditions, lethargy

• Lowest dose that relieves symptoms

Perform/provide:

• Withdrawal of medication 4 wk before RAIU test

• Storage in airtight, light-resistant container

Evaluate:

• Therapeutic response: absence of depression; increased weight loss, diuresis, pulse, appetite; absence of constipation, peripheral edema, cold intolerance; pale, cool, dry skin; brittle nails, coarse hair, menorrhagia, night blindness, paresthesias, syncope, stupor, coma, rosy cheeks

Teach patient/family:

• That hair loss will occur in child, is temporary

• To report excitability, irritability, anxiety, which indicate overdose

• Not to switch brands unless approved by prescriber

• That hypothyroid child will show almost immediate behavior/personality change

⬥ = Nursing alert   🍃 = Herb-drug interaction   🚫 = Do not crush

- That drug is not to be taken to reduce weight
- To avoid OTC preparations with iodine; read labels
- To avoid iodine food, iodized salt, soybeans, tofu, turnips, some seafood, some bread
- That drug does not cure, but controls symptoms, treatment is lifelong

---

lisinopril (℞)

(lyse-in'oh-pril)
Prinivil, Zestril

Func. class.: Antihypertensive, angiotensin converting enzyme inhibitor (ACE)

Chem. class.: Enalaprilat lysine analog

Action: Selectively suppresses renin-angiotensin-aldosterone system; inhibits ACE, preventing conversion of angiotensin I to angiotensin II

Uses: Mild to moderate hypertension, adjunctive therapy of systolic CHF

Research note: Rofecoxib may decrease the effects of lisinopril, dosage adjustment may be required[22]

Dosage and routes:

Hypertension

- *Adult:* PO 10-40 mg qd; may increase to 80 mg qd if required
- *Geriatric:* PO 2.5-5 mg/day, increase q7 days

CHF

- *Adult:* PO 5 mg initially with diuretics/digitalis

Available forms: Tabs 2.5, 5, 10, 20, 40 mg

Side effects/adverse reactions:

GI: Nausea, vomiting, anorexia, constipation, flatulence, GI irritation

GU: **Proteinuria, renal insufficiency,** sexual dysfunction, impotence

HEMA: **Agranulocytopenia,** neutropenia

INTEG: Rash, pruritus

CNS: Vertigo, depression, **stroke,** insomnia, paresthesias, headache, *fatigue,* asthenia

EENT: Blurred vision, nasal congestion

SYST: **Angioedema**

RESP: Dry cough, dyspnea

Contraindications: Hypersensitivity, pregnancy (D) 2nd/3rd trimesters

Precautions: Pregnancy (C) 1st trimester, lactation, renal disease, hyperkalemia, renal artery stenosis

Do not confuse:

Prinivil/Plendil
Prinivil/Proventil
Prinivil/Prilosec

Pharmacokinetics: Onset 1 hr, peak 6-8 hr, duration 24 hr; excreted unchanged in urine

Interactions:

- Increased hypotensive effect: diuretics, other hypertensives, probenecid, phenothiazines, nitrates, acute alcohol ingestion
- Decreased effects of lisinopril: aspirin, indomethacin
- Increased K levels: K salt substitutes, K-sparing diuretics, K supplements
- Possible toxicity: lithium, digoxin
- Increased hypersensitivity reactions: allopurinol
- Drug/food: high-K diet (bananas, orange juice, avocados, nuts, spinach) should be avoided; hyperkalemia may occur

Lab test interferences:

Interference: Glucose/insulin tolerance tests, ANA titer

NURSING CONSIDERATIONS

Assess:

◆ Blood studies, platelets; WBC with diff baseline and periodically q3mo; if neutrophils <1000/mm³, discontinue treatment

---

• B/P, pulse q4h; note rate, rhythm, quality
• Electrolytes: K, Na, Cl
• Apical/pedal pulse before administration; notify prescriber of any significant changes
• Baselines in renal tests, LFTs before therapy begins and periodically increased LFTs, uric acid and glucose may be increased
• Edema in feet, legs qd, weight qd in CHF
• Skin turgor, dryness of mucous membranes for hydration status
• Symptoms of CHF: edema, dyspnea, wet rales

Evaluate:
• Therapeutic response: decreased B/P, CHF symptoms

Teach patient/family:
• Not to discontinue drug abruptly
• To rise slowly to sitting or standing position to minimize orthostatic hypotension
• To avoid increasing K in the diet
Treatment of overdose: Lavage, IV atropine for bradycardia, IV theophylline for bronchospasm, digitalis, O_2, diuretic for cardiac failure

---

lithium (R)

(li'thee-um)
Carbolith*, Cibalith-S, Duralith*, Eskalith, Eskalith-CR, Lithane, lithium carbonate, Lithizine*, Lithonate, Lithotabs

Func. class.: Antimanic, antipsychotic

Chem. class.: Alkali metal ion salt

Action: May alter sodium, potassium ion transport across cell membrane in nerve, muscle cells; may balance biogenic amines of norepinephrine, serotonin in CNS areas involved in emotional responses

Uses: Bipolar disorders (manic phase), prevention of bipolar manic-depressive psychosis

Dosage and routes:
• *Adult:* **PO** 300-600 mg tid, maintenance 300 mg tid or qid; slow rel tabs 300 mg bid; dose should be individualized to maintain blood levels at 0.5-1.5 mEq/L
• *Geriatric:* **PO** 300 mg bid, increase q7 days by 300 mg to desired dose

Renal dose
• **PO** CrCl 10-50 ml/min 50%-75% of dose; CrCl <10 ml/min 25%-50% of dose
• *Child:* **PO** 15-20 mg (0.4-0.5 mEq)/kg/day in 2-3 divided doses, increase as needed, do not exceed adult doses

Available forms: Caps 150, 300, 600 mg; tabs 300 mg; tabs ext rel 300, 450 mg; syr 300 mg/5 ml (8 mEq/5 ml); cap slow rel 150, 300 mg*

Side effects/adverse reactions:
CNS: Headache, drowsiness, dizziness, tremors, twitching, ataxia, ***seizure,*** slurred speech, restlessness, confusion, stupor, memory loss, clonic movements, fatigue
GI: Dry mouth, anorexia, nausea, vomiting, diarrhea, incontinence, abdominal pain, metallic taste
*GU: **Polyuria, glycosuria, proteinuria, albuminuria,*** urinary incontinence, polydipsia, edema
CV: Hypotension, ECG changes, ***dysrhythmias, circulatory collapse,*** edema
INTEG: Drying of hair, alopecia, rash, pruritus, hyperkeratosis, acneiform lesions, folliculitis
*HEMA: **Leukocytosis***
EENT: Tinnitus, blurred vision
ENDO: Hyponatremia, hypothyroid-

---

ism, goiter, hyperglycemia, hyperthyroidism
MS: Muscle weakness
Contraindications: Hepatic disease, brain trauma, OBS, pregnancy
(D), lactation, children <12 yr,
schizophrenia, severe cardiac disease, severe renal disease, severe
dehydration
Precautions: Elderly, thyroid disease, seizure disorders, diabetes mellitus, systemic infection, urinary retention
Pharmacokinetics:
PO: Onset rapid, peak ½-4 hr, half-
life 18-36 hr depending on age;
crosses blood-brain barrier; 80% of
filtered lithium is reabsorbed by the
renal tubules, excreted in urine;
crosses placenta; enters breast milk;
well absorbed by oral method
Interactions:
• Increased hypothyroid effects: antithyroid agents, calcium iodide, potassium iodide, iodinated glycerol
• Neurotoxicity: haloperidol, thioridazine
• Increased effects of neuromuscular blocking agents, phenothiazines
• Increased renal clearance: sodium
bicarbonate, acetazolamide, mannitol, aminophylline
• Increased toxicity: indomethacin,
diuretics, nonsteroidal antiinflammatories, losartan
• Decreased effects of lithium: theophyllines, urea, urinary alkalinizers
• Increased lithium effect/toxicity:
carbamazepine, fluoxetine, methyldopa, NSAIDs, thiazide diuretics,
probenecid
• Drug/food: significant changes in
sodium intake will alter lithium excretion
🖋 Increased effects of lithium, increased toxicity: broom, buchu, dandelion, juniper

Lab test interferences:
Increase: K excretion, urine glucose, blood glucose, protein, BUN
Decrease: VMA, T_3, T_4, PBI, ^{131}I
NURSING CONSIDERATIONS
Assess:
• Weight qd; check for and report
edema in legs, ankles, wrists
• Na intake; decreased Na intake
with decreased fluid intake may lead
to lithium retention; increased Na
and fluids may decrease lithium re-
tention
• Skin turgor at least qd
• Urine for albuminuria, glycosuria,
uric acid during beginning treat-
ment, q2mo thereafter
• Neurologic status: LOC, gait, mo-
tor reflexes, hand tremors
• Serum lithium levels qwk initially,
then q2mo (therapeutic level: 0.5-
1.5 mEq/L)
Administer:
• Reduced dose to elderly
• With meals to avoid GI upset
• Adequate fluids (2-3 L/day) to prevent dehydration during initial treatment, 1-2 L/day during maintenance
Evaluate:
• Therapeutic response: decrease in
excitement, manic phase
Teach patient/family:
• The symptoms of minor toxicity:
vomiting, diarrhea, poor coordination, fine motor tremors, weakness,
lassitude; major toxicity: coarse
tremors, severe thirst, tinnitus, diluted urine
• To monitor urine specific gravity,
emphasize need for follow-up care
to determine lithium levels
• That contraception is necessary,
since lithium may harm fetus
• Not to operate machinery until
lithium levels are stable
• That beneficial effects may take
1-3 wk
• About drugs that interact with lithium (provide list) and discuss need

for adequate stable intake of salt and fluids

🚫 Not to break, crush, or chew caps, ext rel tabs

Treatment of overdose: Induce emesis or lavage, maintain airway, respiratory function; dialysis for severe intoxication

---

lomefloxacin (℞)

(lo-meh-flox′a-sin)
Maxaquin
Func. class.: Antiinfective
Chem. class.: Fluoroquinolone

Action: Interferes with conversion of intermediate DNA fragments into high-molecular-weight DNA in bacteria; DNA gyrase inhibitor

Uses: Treatment of lower respiratory tract infections (pneumonia, bronchitis), genitourinary infections (prostatitis, UTIs), preoperatively to reduce UTIs in transurethral surgical procedures; gram-negative bacteria: *Aeromonas, Citrobacter, Enterobacter, Escherichia coli, Haemophilus influenzae, Klebsiella, Legionella, Moraxella catarrhalis, Morganella morganii, Proteus vulgaris, Proteus mirabillis, Providencia alcalifaciens, Providencia rettgeri, Pseudomonas aeruginosa, Serratia;* gram-positive bacteria: *Staphylococcus aureus, Staphylococcus epidermidis, Staphylococcus saprophyticus*

Dosage and routes:
• *Adult:* **PO** 400 mg/day × 7-14 days depending on type of infection
In renal impairment
• *Adult:* **PO** 200 mg/day
Surgical prophylaxis
• *Adult:* **PO** 400 mg 2-6 hr before surgery
Available forms: Tabs 400 mg

Side effects/adverse reactions:
CNS: Dizziness, headache, somnolence, depression, insomnia, nervousness, confusion, agitation
GI: Diarrhea, *nausea,* vomiting, anorexia, flatulence, heartburn, dry mouth; increased AST, ALT; constipation, abdominal pain, oral thrush, glossitis, stomatitis
INTEG: Rash, pruritus, urticaria, *photosensitivity*
EENT: Visual disturbances
Contraindications: Hypersensitivity to quinolones
Precautions: Pregnancy (C), lactation, children, elderly, renal disease, seizure disorders, excessive exposure to sunlight
Pharmacokinetics:
PO: Peak 1-2 hr, half-life 6-8 hr; excreted in urine as active drug, metabolites
Interactions:
• Decreased absorption: antacids containing aluminum, magnesium, sucralfate, zinc, iron, give 4 hr ac or 2 hr pc
• May increase CNS stimulation, seizures: NSAIDs
• May increase toxicity of lomefloxacin: cimetidine, probenecid
• Increased levels: cyclosporine, warfarin, watch for toxicity
• May decrease clearance of theophylline, toxicity may result
NURSING CONSIDERATIONS
Assess:
• Kidney, liver function studies: BUN, creatinine, AST, ALT
• I&O ratio; urine pH, <5.5 is ideal
• CNS symptoms: insomnia, vertigo, headache, agitation, confusion
◆ Allergic reactions and anaphylaxis: rash, flushing, urticaria, pruritus, chills, fever, joint pain; may occur a few days after therapy begins; epinephrine and resuscitation equipment should be available for anaphylactic reaction

---

◆ = Nursing alert　　🌿 = Herb-drug interaction　　🚫 = Do not crush

• Bowel pattern qd, if severe diarrhea occurs, drug should be discontinued
• For overgrowth of infection: perineal itching, fever, malaise, redness, pain, swelling, drainage, rash, diarrhea, change in cough, sputum
Administer:
• After clean-catch urine for C&S
• 4 hr before or 2 hrs after antacids, iron, calcium, zinc products
Evaluate:
• Therapeutic response: negative C&S, absence of signs/symptoms of infection
Teach patient/family:
• That fluids must be increased to 2 L/day to avoid crystallization in kidneys
• That if dizziness or light-headedness occurs, to ambulate, perform activities with assistance
• To complete full course of drug therapy
• To contact prescriber if adverse reactions occur
• To avoid iron- or mineral-containing supplements or antacids within 4 hr before and after dosing
• That photosensitivity may occur and sunscreen should be used
• To use frequent rinsing of mouth, sugarless candy or gum for dry mouth
• To avoid other medication unless approved by prescriber
• Not to use theophylline with this product, toxicity may result; contact prescriber if taking theophylline

lomustine (℞)
(loe-mus'teen)
CCNU, CeeNU
Func. class.: Antineoplastic alkylating agent
Chem. class.: Nitrosourea

Action: Responsible for crosslinking DNA strands, which leads to cell death; activity is not cell cycle phase specific
Uses: Hodgkin's disease, lymphomas, melanomas, multiple myeloma; brain, lung, bladder, kidney, colon cancer
Investigational uses: Brain, breast, renal, GI tract, bronchogenic carcinoma; melanomas
Dosage and routes:
• *Adult:* **PO** 130 mg/m^2 as a single dose q6wk; titrate dose to WBC; do not give repeat dose unless WBC >4000/mm^3, platelet count >100,000/mm^3
Available forms: Caps 10, 40, 100 mg
Side effects/adverse reactions:
*HEMA: **Thrombocytopenia, leukopenia, myelosuppression, anemia***
*GI: Nausea, vomiting, anorexia, stomatitis, **hepatotoxicity***
*GU: **Azotemia, renal failure***
INTEG: Burning at injection site
*RESP: **Fibrosis, pulmonary infiltrate***
Contraindications: Hypersensitivity, leukopenia, thrombocytopenia, pregnancy (D), lactation, "blastic" phase of CML
Precautions: Radiation therapy
Pharmacokinetics: Metabolized in liver, excreted in urine; half-life 16-48 hr; 50% protein bound; crosses blood-brain barrier; appears in breast milk

Interactions:
• Increased toxicity: barbiturates, phenytoin, chloral hydrate
• Increased metabolism of lomustine: phenobarbital
• Potentiation of lomustine: succinylcholine
• Increased bone marrow depression: allopurinol

NURSING CONSIDERATIONS
Assess:
• CBC, differential, platelet count qwk; withhold drug if WBC <4000/mm^3 or platelet count <100,000/mm^3; notify prescriber
• Pulmonary function tests, chest x-ray films before, during therapy; chest film should be obtained q2wk during treatment
• Renal function studies: BUN, serum uric acid, urine CrCl before, during therapy
• I&O ratio; report fall in urine output of 30 ml/hr
• Monitor temp q4h (may indicate beginning infection); no rectal temps
• LFTs before, during therapy (bilirubin, AST, ALT, LDH) as needed or monthly
• Bleeding: hematuria, guaiac, bruising or petechiae, mucosa or orifices q8h
• Dyspnea, rales, unproductive cough, chest pain, tachypnea
• Food preferences; list likes, dislikes
• Jaundiced skin and sclera, dark urine, clay-colored stools, itchy skin, abdominal pain, fever, diarrhea
• Inflammation of mucosa, breaks in skin
• Buccal cavity q8h for dryness, sores or ulceration, white patches, oral pain, bleeding, dysphagia
• Local irritation, pain, burning, discoloration at inj site
◆ Symptoms indicating severe allergic reaction: rash, pruritus, urticaria, purpuric skin lesions, itching, flushing

Administer:
• Antiemetic 30-60 min before giving drug to prevent vomiting
• Antibiotics for prophylaxis of infection

Perform/provide:
• Storage in tight container at room temperature
• Strict medical asepsis, protective isolation if WBC levels are low
• Deep-breathing exercises with patient tid-qid; place in semi-Fowler's position
• Increase fluid intake to 2-3 L/day to prevent urate deposits, calculi formation
• Rinsing of mouth tid-qid with water, club soda; brushing of teeth bid-tid with soft brush or cotton-tipped applicators for stomatitis; use unwaxed dental floss

Evaluate:
• Therapeutic response: decreased tumor size, spread of malignancy

Teach patient/family:
• About protective isolation
• To report any changes in breathing or coughing
• To avoid foods with citric acid, hot or rough texture if buccal inflammation is present
• To report any bleeding, white spots, or ulcerations in mouth to prescriber; tell patient to examine mouth qd
• To report signs of infection: fever, sore throat, flulike symptoms
• To report signs of anemia: fatigue, headache, faintness, shortness of breath, irritability
• To avoid use of razors, commercial mouthwash
• To avoid use of aspirin products or ibuprofen

◆ = Nursing alert   ▮▮ = Herb-drug interaction   Ⓝ = Do not crush

loperamide (OTC, ℞)

(loe-per'a-mide)
A-D Kaopectate II Caplets, loperamide solution, Imodium, Imodium A-D, Imodium A-D Caplet, loperamide, Maalox Antidiarrheal Caplets, Pepto Diarrhea Control
Func. class.: Antidiarrheal
Chem. class.: Piperidine derivative

Action: Direct action on intestinal muscles to decrease GI peristalsis; reduces volume, increases bulk, electrolytes not lost

Uses: Diarrhea (cause undetermined), chronic diarrhea, ileostomy discharge

Dosage and routes:
• *Adult:* **PO** 4 mg, then 2 mg after each loose stool, max 16 mg/day
• *Child 9-11 yr:* **PO** 2 mg, then 1 mg after each loose stool, max 6 mg/24 hr
• *Child 2-5 yr:* **PO** 1 mg then 0.1 mg/kg after each loose stool, max 4 mg/24 hr
Available forms: Caps 2 mg; liq 1 mg/5 ml; tabs 2 mg
Side effects/adverse reactions:
CNS: Dizziness, drowsiness, fatigue, fever
GI: Nausea, dry mouth, vomiting, constipation, abdominal pain, anorexia, **toxic megacolon**
INTEG: Rash
Contraindications: Hypersensitivity, severe ulcerative colitis, pseudomembranous colitis, acute diarrhea associated with *Escherichia coli*
Precautions: Pregnancy (B), lactation, children <2 yr, liver disease, dehydration, bacterial disease
Pharmacokinetics:
PO: Onset ½-1 hr, duration 4-5 hr, half-life 7-14 hr; metabolized in liver; excreted in feces as unchanged drug; small amount in urine
Interactions:
• Do not mix oral sol with other sols

NURSING CONSIDERATIONS
Assess:
• Stools: volume, color, characteristics
• Electrolytes (K, Na, Cl) if on long-term therapy
• Skin turgor q8h if dehydration is suspected
• Bowel pattern before; for rebound constipation
• Response after 48 hr; if no response, drug should be discontinued
• Dehydration, CNS problems in children
• Abdominal distention, toxic megacolon; may occur in ulcerative colitis
Administer:
• For 48 hr only
Perform/provide:
• Storage in tight container
Evaluate:
• Therapeutic response: decreased diarrhea
Teach patient/family:
• To avoid OTC products unless directed by prescriber
• That ostomy patient may take this drug for extended time
• That if drowsiness occurs, not to operate machinery
• To use hard candy, sips of water for dry mouth
🚫 Not to break, crush, or chew caps

loracarbef

See cephalosporins—2nd generation

loratadine (R)

(lor-a'ti-deen)
Claritin, Claritin Reditabs

Func. class.: Antihistamine, 2nd generation

Chem. class.: Selective histamine (H_1)-receptor antagonist

Action: Binds to peripheral histamine receptors, providing antihistamine action without sedation

Uses: Seasonal rhinitis

Dosage and routes:

• *Adult and child ≥12 yr:* **PO** 10 mg qd

• *Child 2-12 yr:* **PO** 5 mg qd

Available forms: Tabs 10 mg; tabs rapid-disintegrating 10 mg; syr 5 mg/5 ml

Side effects/adverse reactions:

CNS: Sedation (more common with increased doses), headache

Contraindications: Hypersensitivity, acute asthma attacks, lower respiratory tract disease

Precautions: Pregnancy (B), increased intraocular pressure, bronchial asthma

Pharmacokinetics: Peak 1½ hr, elimination half-life 8½-28 hr; metabolized in liver to active metabolites, excreted in urine

Interactions:

• Additive CNS depressant effects: alcohol, other CNS depressants

🔗 Increased anticholinergic effect: henbane leaf

NURSING CONSIDERATIONS

Assess:

• Allergy: hives, rash, rhinitis; monitor respiratory status

Administer:

• Rapid-disintegrating tabs by placing on tongue, then swallow after disintegrated with or without water

• On empty stomach

Perform/provide:

• Storage in tight container at room temperature

Evaluate:

• Therapeutic response: absence of running or congested nose, other allergy symptoms

Teach patient/family:

• To avoid driving, other hazardous activities if drowsiness occurs

• To use sunscreen or stay out of the sun to prevent photosensitivity

• To avoid use of other CNS depressants

lorazepam (R)

(lor-a'ze-pam)
Apo-Lorazepam*, Ativan, lorazepam, Novolorazem*, Nu-Loraz*

Func. class.: Sedative, hypnotic; antianxiety

Chem. class.: Benzodiazepine

Controlled Substance Schedule IV

Action: Potentiates the actions of GABA, especially in system and reticular formation

Uses: Anxiety, irritability in psychiatric or organic disorders, preoperatively, insomnia, adjunct in endoscopic procedures

Investigational uses: Antiemetic prior to chemotherapy, status epilepticus, rectal use

Dosage and routes:

Anxiety

• *Adult:* **PO** 2-6 mg/day in divided doses, not to exceed 10 mg/day

• *Geriatric:* **PO** 0.5-1 mg/day in divided doses; or 0.5-1 mg hs

• *Child:* **PO** 0.05 mg/kg/dose, q4-8h

Insomnia

• *Adult:* **PO** 2-4 mg hs; only minimally effective after 2 wk continuous therapy

---

⬦ = Nursing alert   🔗 = Herb-drug interaction   🚫 = Do not crush

Preoperatively
• *Adult:* **IM** 50 µg/kg 2 hr prior to surgery; **IV** 44 µg/kg 15-20 min prior to surgery
• *Child:* **IV** 0.05 mg/kg
Status epilepticus
• *Neonate:* **IV** 0.05 mg/kg
• *Child:* **IV** 0.1 mg/kg up to 4 mg/dose; rectal (off label) 0.05-0.1 mg ×2; wait 7 min before giving 2nd dose

Available forms: Tabs 0.5, 1, 2 mg; inj 2, 4 mg/ml; conc sol 2 mg/ml

Side effects/adverse reactions:
CNS: Dizziness, drowsiness, confusion, headache, anxiety, tremors, stimulation, fatigue, depression, insomnia, hallucinations, weakness, unsteadiness
GI: Constipation, dry mouth, nausea, vomiting, anorexia, diarrhea
INTEG: Rash, dermatitis, itching
*CV: Orthostatic hypotension, **ECG changes, tachycardia,** hypotension; **apnea, cardiac arrest (IV, rapid)***
EENT: Blurred vision, tinnitus, mydriasis

Contraindications: Hypersensitivity to benzodiazepines, narrow-angle glaucoma, psychosis, pregnancy (D), lactation, child <12 yr, history of drug abuse, COPD

Precautions: Elderly, debilitated, hepatic disease, renal disease

Do not confuse:
lorazepam/alprazolam

Pharmacokinetics:
PO: Onset ½ hr, peak 1-6 hr, duration 24-48 hr
IM: Onset 15-30 min, peak 1-1½ hr, duration 24-48 hr
IV: Onset 5-15 min, peak unknown, duration 24-48 hr
Metabolized by liver; excreted by kidneys; crosses placenta, breast milk; half-life 14 hr

Interactions:
• Decreased effects of lorazepam: oral contraceptives, valproic acid
• Increased effects of lorazepam: CNS depressants, alcohol, disulfiram, oral contraceptives
🌿 Increased action: kava

Lab test interferences:
Increase: AST, ALT, serum bilirubin
Decrease: RAIU
False increase: 17-OHCS

NURSING CONSIDERATIONS
Assess:
• B/P (lying, standing), pulse; if systolic B/P drops 20 mm Hg, hold drug, notify prescriber; respirations q5-15min if given IV
• Blood studies: CBC during long-term therapy; blood dyscrasias have occurred rarely
• Hepatic studies: AST, ALT, bilirubin, creatinine, LDH, alk phosphatase
• Mental status: mood, sensorium, affect, sleeping pattern, drowsiness, dizziness
• Physical dependency, withdrawal symptoms: headache, nausea, vomiting, muscle pain, weakness, tremors, convulsions, after long-term, excessive use
◆ Suicidal tendencies

Administer:
• With food or milk for GI symptoms
• Crushed if patient is unable to swallow medication whole
• Sugarless gum, hard candy, frequent sips of water for dry mouth
• Deep into large muscle mass (IM inj)
IV
• IV after diluting in equal vol sterile H_2O, 5% dextrose or 0.9% NaCl for inj; give through Y-tube or 3-way stopcock; give at 2 mg or less over 1 min

L

Syringe compatibilities: Cimetidine, hydromorphone

Y-site compatibilities: Acyclovir, albumin, allopurinol, amifostine, amikacin, amoxicillin, amoxicillin/clavulanate, amphotericin B cholesteryl, amsacrine, atracurium, bumetanide, cefepime, cefmetazole, cefotaxime, ciprofloxacin, cisatracurium, cisplatin, cladribine, clonidine, cyclophosphamide, cytarabine, dexamethasone, diltiazem, dobutamine, dopamine, doxorubicin, doxorubicin liposome, epinephrine, erythromycin, etomidate, famotidine, fentanyl, filgrastim, fluconazole, fludarabine, furosemide, gentamicin, granisetron, haloperidol, heparin, hydrocortisone, hydromorphone, ketanserin, labetalol, melphalan, methotrexate, metronidazole, midazolam, milrinone, morphine, nicardipine, nitroglycerin, norepinephrine, paclitaxel, pancuronium, piperacillin, piperacillin/tazobactam, potassium chloride, propofol, ranitidine, remifentanil, tacrolimus, teniposide, thiotepa, trimethoprim-sulfamethoxazole, vancomycin, vecuronium, vinorelbine, zidovudine

Perform/provide:

• Assistance with ambulation during beginning therapy, since drowsiness/dizziness occurs
• Check to see if PO medication has been swallowed
• Refrigerate parenteral form

Evaluate:

• Therapeutic response: decreased anxiety, restlessness, insomnia

Teach patient/family:

• That drug may be taken with food
• Not to use drug for everyday stress or used longer than 4 mo unless directed by prescriber
• Not to take more than prescribed amount; may be habit forming
• To avoid OTC preparations (cough, cold, hay fever) unless approved by prescriber
• To avoid driving, activities that require alertness, since drowsiness may occur
• To avoid alcohol ingestion, other psychotropic medications, unless directed by prescriber
• Not to discontinue medication abruptly after long-term use
• To rise slowly or fainting may occur, especially elderly
• That drowsiness may worsen at beginning of treatment
• To use birth control if child-bearing age

Treatment of overdose: Lavage, VS, supportive care, flumazenil

---

losartan (R)

(lo-zar′tan)
Cozaar
Func. class.: Antihypertensive
Chem. class.: Angiotensin II receptor (type AT_1)

Action: Blocks the vasoconstrictor and aldosterone-secreting effects of angiotensin II; selectively blocks the binding of angiotensin II to the AT_1 receptor found in tissues

Uses: Hypertension, alone or in combination

Research note: Indomethacin reduces the antihypertensive effects of captopril and losartan; monitor carefully[23]

Dosage and routes:

• *Adult:* **PO** 50 mg qd alone or 25 mg qd when used in combination
Hepatic dose
• *Adult:* **PO** 25 mg qd

Available forms: Tabs 25, 50 mg

Side effects/adverse reactions:

CNS: Dizziness, insomnia, anxiety, confusion, abnormal dreams, migraine, tremor, vertigo

---

CV: Angina pectoris, 2nd-degree AV block, ***cerebrovascular accident,*** hypotension, ***myocardial infarction, dysrhythmias***

EENT: Blurred vision, burning eyes, conjunctivitis

GI: Diarrhea, dyspepsia, anorexia, constipation, dry mouth, flatulence, gastritis, vomiting

GU: Impotence, nocturia, urinary frequency, UTI

HEMA: Anemia

INTEG: Alopecia, dermatitis, dry skin, flushing, photosensitivity, rash, pruritus, sweating

META: Gout

MS: Cramps, myalgia, pain, stiffness

RESP: Cough, upper respiratory infection, congestion, dyspnea, bronchitis

Contraindications: Hypersensitivity, pregnancy (D) 2nd/3rd trimesters

Precautions: Hypersensitivity to ACE inhibitors; pregnancy (C) 1st trimester; lactation, children, elderly

Do not confuse:
Cozaar/Zocor

Pharmacokinetics: Extensively metabolized, half-life 2 hr, metabolite 6-9 hr, highly bound to plasma proteins, excreted in urine and feces

Interactions:
• Increased lithium toxicity: lithium

NURSING CONSIDERATIONS

Assess:
• B/P with position changes, pulse q4h; note rate, rhythm, quality
• Electrolytes: K, Na, Cl
• Baselines in renal tests, LFTs before therapy begins
• Edema in feet, legs qd
• Skin turgor, dryness of mucous membranes for hydration status

Administer:
• Without regard to meals

Evaluate:
• Therapeutic response: decreased B/P

Teach patient/family:
• To avoid sunlight or wear sunscreen if in sunlight; photosensitivity may occur
• To comply with dosage schedule, even if feeling better
• To notify prescriber of mouth sores, fever, swelling of hands or feet, irregular heartbeat, chest pain
• That excessive perspiration, dehydration, vomiting, diarrhea may lead to fall in blood pressure; consult prescriber if these occur
• That drug may cause dizziness, fainting; light-headedness may occur
• To rise slowly to sitting or standing position to minimize orthostatic hypotension
• To use contraception while taking this product

---

lovastatin (℞)

(loh-vah-stat′in)
Mevacor
Func. class.: Antilipemic
Chem. class.: Aspergillus terreus strain derivative

Action: Inhibits HMG-CoA reductase enzyme, which reduces cholesterol synthesis

Uses: As an adjunct in primary hypercholesterolemia (types IIa, IIb), mixed hyperlipidemia, atherosclerosis

Dosage and routes:
(Patient should first be placed on a cholesterol–lowering diet)
• *Adult:* **PO** 20 mg qd with evening meal; may increase to 20-80 mg/day in single or divided doses, not to exceed 80 mg/day; dosage ad-

---

justments should be made qmo, reduce dose in renal disease

Available forms: Tabs 10, 20, 40 mg

Side effects/adverse reactions:

*GI: Flatus, nausea, constipation, diarrhea, dyspepsia, abdominal pain, heartburn, **liver dysfunction***

*MS: Muscle cramps, myalgia, **myositis, rhabdomyolysis***

CNS: Dizziness, headache, tremor

INTEG: Rash, pruritus, photosensitivity

*HEMA: **Thrombocytopenia, hemolytic anemia, leukopenia***

EENT: Blurred vision, dysgeusia, lens opacities

Contraindications: Hypersensitivity, pregnancy (X), lactation, active liver disease

Precautions: Past liver disease, alcoholism, severe acute infections, trauma, hypotension, uncontrolled seizure disorders, severe metabolic disorders, electrolyte imbalances, visual disorder, children

Pharmacokinetics:

PO: Peak 2-4 hr, metabolized in liver (metabolites), highly protein bound; excreted in urine, feces; crosses placenta, excreted in breast milk; half-life 3-4 hr

Interactions:

• Increased effects: bile acid sequestrants, warfarin

• Increased myalgia, myositis: cyclosporine, gemfibrozil, niacin, erythromycin, clofibrate

• Decreased antihyperlipidemic effect: propranolol

• Increased bleeding: warfarin

• Drug/food: increased levels of lovastatin with food

Lab test interferences:

Increase: CPK, LFTs

NURSING CONSIDERATIONS

Assess:

• Diet, obtain diet history including fat, cholesterol in diet

• Fasting cholesterol, LDL, HDL, triglycerides periodically during treatment

• Liver function studies q1-2mo during the first 1½ yr of treatment; AST, ALT, LFTs may increase

• Renal function in patients with compromised renal system: BUN, creatinine, I&O ratio

• Ophthalmic exam before, 1 mo after treatment begins, annually; lens opacities may occur

• For muscle pain, tenderness, obtain CPK; if these occur, drug may need to be discontinued

Administer:

• In evening with meal; if dose is increased, take with breakfast and evening meal

Perform/provide:

• Storage in cool environment in airtight, light-resistant container

Evaluate:

• Therapeutic response: cholesterol at desired level after 8 wk

Teach patient/family:

• To report suspected pregnancy

• That blood work and eye exam will be necessary during treatment

• To report blurred vision, severe GI symptoms, dizziness, headache, muscle pain, weakness

• To use sunscreen or stay out of the sun to prevent photosensitivity

• That previously prescribed regimen will continue: low-cholesterol diet, exercise program, smoking cessation

loxapine (R)

(lox'a-peen)
Loxapac*, loxapine succinate*, Loxitane, Loxitane IM, Loxitane-C
Func. class.: Antipsychotic, neuroleptic
Chem. class.: Dibenzoxazepine

Action: Depresses cerebral cortex, hypothalamus, limbic system, which control activity and aggression; blocks neurotransmission produced by dopamine at synapse; exhibits strong α-adrenergic, anticholinergic blocking action; mechanism for antipsychotic effects is unclear

Uses: Psychotic disorders, nonpsychotic symptoms associated with dementia

Investigational uses: Depression, anxiety

Dosage and routes:
• *Adult:* PO 10 mg bid-qid initially, may be rapidly increased depending on severity of condition, maintenance 60-100 mg/day; **IM** 12.5-50 mg q4-6h or more until desired response, then start **PO** form
• *Geriatric:* PO 5-10 mg qd-bid, increase q4-7 days by 5-10 mg, max 125 mg

Available forms: Caps 5, 10, 25, 50 mg; tabs 5, 10, 25, 50 mg; conc 25 mg/ml; inj 50 mg/ml

Side effects/adverse reactions:
*RESP: **Laryngospasm**, dyspnea, **respiratory depression***
*CNS: EPS: pseudoparkinsonism, akathisia, dystonia, tardive dyskinesia, drowsiness, headache, **seizures**, confusion*
*HEMA: **Anemia, leukopenia, leukocytosis, agranulocytosis***
INTEG: Rash, photosensitivity, dermatitis
EENT: Blurred vision, glaucoma

GI: Dry mouth, nausea, vomiting, anorexia, constipation, diarrhea, jaundice, weight gain
GU: Urinary retention, urinary frequency, enuresis, impotence, amenorrhea, gynecomastia
*CV: Orthostatic hypotension, **cardiac arrest**, ECG changes, tachycardia*

Contraindications: Hypersensitivity, blood dyscrasias, coma, brain damage, bone marrow depression, alcohol and barbiturate withdrawal states, severe CNS depression

Precautions: Pregnancy (C), lactation, seizure disorders, hepatic disease, cardiac disease, prostatic hypertrophy, cardiac conditions, child <16 yr, elderly

Pharmacokinetics:
PO: Onset 20-30 min, peak 2-4 hr, duration 12 hr
IM: Onset 15-30 min, peak 15-20 min, duration 12 hr
Metabolized by liver; excreted in urine; crosses placenta; enters breast milk; initial half-life 5 hr; terminal half-life 19 hr

Interactions:
• Toxicity: epinephrine
• Increased EPS: other antipsychotics
• Decreased effects: guanadrel, guanethidine
• Increased CNS depression: MAOIs, antidepressants, alcohol
🍃 Increased action: kava

NURSING CONSIDERATIONS
Assess:
• Mental status before initial administration
• Swallowing of PO medication; check for hoarding or giving of medication to other patients
• I&O ratio; palpate bladder if low urinary output occurs
• Bilirubin, CBC, liver function studies qmo

• Urinalysis is recommended before and during prolonged therapy

• Affect, orientation, LOC, reflexes, gait, coordination, sleep pattern disturbances

• B/P standing and lying; take pulse and respirations q4h during initial treatment; establish baseline before starting treatment; report drops of 30 mm Hg

• Dizziness, faintness, palpitations, tachycardia on rising

• EPS including akathisia (inability to sit still, no pattern to movements), tardive dyskinesia (bizarre movements of the jaw, mouth, tongue, extremities), pseudoparkinsonism (rigidity, tremors, pill rolling, shuffling gait)

◆ For neuroleptic malignant syndrome: muscle rigidity, increased CPK, altered mental status, hyperthermia

• Constipation, urinary retention qd; if these occur, increase bulk, water in diet

Administer:

• Reduced dose to elderly

• Antiparkinsonian agent if EPS symptoms occur

IM

• IM injection into large muscle mass

PO

• Concentrate mixed in orange or grapefruit juice

Perform/provide:

• Decreased sensory input by dimming lights, avoiding loud noises

• Supervised ambulation until stabilized on medication; do not involve in strenuous exercise program because fainting is possible; patient should not stand still for long periods

• Increased fluids to prevent constipation

• Sips of water, candy, gum for dry mouth

• Storage in airtight, light-resistant container

Evaluate:

• Therapeutic response: decrease in emotional excitement, hallucinations, delusions, paranoia; reorganization of patterns of thought, speech

Teach patient/family:

• That orthostatic hypotension may occur and to rise from sitting or lying position gradually

• To remain lying down after IM injection for at least 30 min

• To avoid hot tubs, hot showers, tub baths, as hypotension may occur; that in hot weather heat stroke may occur; take extra precautions to stay cool

• To avoid abrupt withdrawal of this drug, or EPS may result; drug should be withdrawn slowly

• To avoid OTC preparations (cough, hay fever, cold) unless approved by prescriber; serious drug interactions may occur; avoid use with alcohol, CNS depressants; increased drowsiness may occur

• To avoid hazardous activities until stabilized on medication

• To use a sunscreen during sun exposure to prevent burns

• About necessity for meticulous oral hygiene, since oral candidiasis may occur

• To report impaired vision, jaundice, tremors, muscle twitching

Treatment of overdose: Lavage if orally ingested; provide an airway

---

◆ = Nursing alert   ∥ = Herb-drug interaction   ⊘ = Do not crush

lymphocyte immune globulin (antithymocyte) (℞)
Atgam
Func. class.: Immune globulins—immunosuppressant

Action: Produces immunosuppression by inhibiting the function of lymphocytes (T)

Uses: Organ transplants to prevent rejection, aplastic anemia

Investigational uses: MS; myasthenia gravis; immunosuppressant in liver, bone marrow, heart, and other organ transplants; pure red-cell aplasia; scleroderma

Dosage and routes:

Renal allograft
• *Adult:* IV 10-30 mg/kg/day
• *Child:* IV 5-25 mg/kg/day

Delay of renal allograft rejection
• *Adult:* IV 15 mg/kg/day × 14 days, then qod × 14 days for a total of 21 doses in 28 days

Aplastic anemia
• *Adult:* IV 10-20 mg/kg/day × 8-14 days

Available forms: Inj 50 mg horse gamma globulin/ml

Side effects/adverse reactions:

Renal transplant
CNS: Fever, chills, headache, dizziness, weakness, faintness, *seizures*
INTEG: Rash, pruritus, urticaria, wheal
GI: Diarrhea, nausea, vomiting, epigastric pain
CV: Chest pain, hypertension, tachycardia
SYST: **Anaphylaxis**

Aplastic anemia
CNS: Fever, chills, headache, *seizures,* lightheadedness, encephalitis, postviral encephalopathy

CV: Bradycardia, myocarditis, irregularity
GI: Nausea, LFTs abnormality

Contraindications: Hypersensitivity

Precautions: Severe renal disease, severe hepatic disease, pregnancy (C), lactation, children

Pharmacokinetics: Onset rapid, half-life 5.7 days

Interactions: None known

NURSING CONSIDERATIONS

Assess:
• For infection; if infection occurs, evaluation will be needed to continue therapy
• Renal studies: BUN, creatinine at least monthly during treatment, 3 mo after treatment
• Liver function studies: alk phosphatase, AST, ALT, bilirubin

Administer:
• Do not infuse <4 hr

Aplastic anemia
• Skin testing must be completed prior to treatment; use intradermal inj of 0.1 ml of a 1:1000 dilution (5 μg horse IgG) in 0.9% NaCl, if a wheal or rash >10 mm or both, use caution during inf
• Dilute in saline sol before inf, invert IV bag, so undiluted drug does not contact the air inside, concentration should not be >1 mg/ml
• Keep emergency equipment nearby for severe allergic reaction

Evaluate:
• Therapeutic response: absence of rejection; hematologic recovery (aplastic anemia)

Teach patient/family:
• To report fever, chills, sore throat, fatigue, since serious infections may occur
• To use contraceptive measures during treatment, for 12 wk after ending therapy

L

magaldrate (OTC)

(mag'al-drate)
Losapan*, Lowsium, Riopan,
Riopan Extra Strength*
Func. class.: Antacid
Chem. class.: Aluminum/magnesium hydroxide

Action: Neutralizes gastric acidity; drug is dissolved in gastric contents; combination of aluminum, magnesium

Uses: Antacid, peptic ulcer disease (adjunct), duodenal, gastric ulcers, reflux esophagitis, hyperacidity, indigestion, heartburn

Dosage and routes:
• *Adult:* **SUSP** 5-10 ml (400-800 mg) with H_2O between meals, hs, not to exceed 100 ml/day

Available forms: Susp 540 mg/5 ml, liquid 540 mg/5 ml

Side effects/adverse reactions:
GI: Constipation, diarrhea
META: Hypermagnesemia, hypophosphatemia

Contraindications: Hypersensitivity to this drug or aluminum

Precautions: Elderly, fluid restriction, decreased GI motility, GI obstruction, dehydration, renal disease, Na-restricted diets, pregnancy (C)

Pharmacokinetics:
PO: Duration 60 min

Interactions:
• Decreased effectiveness of tetracyclines, ketoconazole
• Decreased absorption of anticholinergics, chlordiazepoxide, cimetidine, corticosteroids, iron salts, phenothiazines, phenytoin, salicylates

NURSING CONSIDERATIONS
Assess:
• GI status: location of pain, intensity, characteristics, heartburn, hematemesis
• Serum magnesium levels with impaired renal function; Ca, phosphate, K if using long term
• Constipation: increase bulk in diet if needed

Administer:
• Laxatives or stool softeners if constipation occurs
• After shaking; give between meals and hs

Evaluate:
• Therapeutic response: absence of pain, decreased acidity

Teach patient/family:
• To separate enteric-coated drugs and antacid by 2 hr
• To notify prescriber immediately of coffee-ground emesis, emesis with frank blood, black tarry stools

magnesium salicylate (OTC, ℞)

Doan's Pills, Magan, Mobidin
Func. class.: Nonopioid analgesic, nonsteroidal antiinflammatory
Chem. class.: Salicylate

Action: Blocks pain impulses in CNS that occur in response to inhibition of prostaglandin synthesis; antipyretic action results from inhibition of hypothalamic heat-regulating center to produce vasodilation to allow heat dissipation

Uses: Mild to moderate pain or fever including arthritis, juvenile rheumatoid arthritis

Dosage and routes:
Arthritis
• *Adult:* **PO** not to exceed 4.8 g/day in divided doses

◆ = Nursing alert   ▟ = Herb-drug interaction   ⊘ = Do not crush

Pain/fever

• *Adult:* **PO** 600 mg tid or qid

Available forms: Tabs 325, 500, 545, 600 mg

Side effects/adverse reactions:

*HEMA: **Thrombocytopenia, agranulocytosis, leukopenia, neutropenia, hemolytic anemia,*** increased pro-time

CNS: Stimulation, drowsiness, dizziness, confusion, ***seizures,*** headache, flushing, hallucinations, ***coma***

GI: Nausea, vomiting, ***GI bleeding,*** *diarrhea, heartburn,* anorexia, ***hepatitis***

INTEG: Rash, urticaria, bruising

EENT: Tinnitus, hearing loss

CV: Rapid pulse, ***pulmonary edema***

RESP: Wheezing, hyperpnea

ENDO: Hypoglycemia, hyponatremia, hypokalemia

*SYST: **Anaphylaxis***

Contraindications: Hypersensitivity to salicylates, GI bleeding, bleeding disorders, children <12 yr, vit K deficiency, pregnancy (D) 1st trimester

Precautions: Anemia, hepatic disease, renal disease, Hodgkin's disease, lactation

Pharmacokinetics:

PO: Onset 15-30 min, peak 1-2 hr, duration 4-6 hr; metabolized by liver; excreted by kidneys; crosses placenta; excreted in breast milk; half-life 1-3½ hr

Interactions:

• Decreased effects of magnesium-salicylate: antacids, steroids, urinary alkalizers

• Increased effects of anticoagulants, insulin, methotrexate, penicillins, valproic acid, phenytoin, sulfonamides

• Decreased effects of probenecid, spironolactone, sulfinpyrazone, some NSAIDs, diuretics, antihypertensives

• Decreased blood sugar levels: salicylates

Lab test interferences:

Increase: Coagulation studies, liver function studies, serum uric acid, amylase, CO_2, urinary protein

Decrease: Serum K, cholesterol, blood glucose

Interference: Urine catecholamines, pregnancy test

NURSING CONSIDERATIONS

Assess:

• Liver function studies: AST, ALT, bilirubin, creatinine (long-term therapy)

• Renal function studies: BUN, urine creatinine (long-term therapy)

• Blood studies: CBC, Hct, Hgb, PT (long-term therapy); monitor salicylate levels

• I&O ratio; decreasing output may indicate renal failure (long-term therapy)

◆ Hepatotoxicity: dark urine, clay-colored stools, jaundiced skin and sclera, itching, abdominal pain, fever, diarrhea (long-term therapy)

◆ Allergic reactions, anaphylaxis: rash, urticaria; if these occur, drug may have to be discontinued; those with asthma or nasal polyp are more prone to reactions

• Renal dysfunction: decreased urine output

• Ototoxicity: tinnitus, ringing, roaring in ears; audiometric testing is needed before, after long-term therapy

• Visual changes: blurring, halos, corneal and retinal damage

• Edema in feet, ankles, legs

• Prior drug history; there are many drug interactions

Administer:

• To patient crushed or whole; chewable tablets may be chewed

• With food or milk to decrease gas-

M

tric symptoms; give 30 min before or 2 hr after antacids
• With full glass of water
Evaluate:
• Therapeutic response: decreased pain, fever
Teach patient/family:
• To report any symptoms of hepatotoxicity, renal toxicity, visual changes, ototoxicity, allergic reactions, bleeding (long-term therapy)
• Not to exceed recommended dosage; acute poisoning may result
• To read label on other OTC drugs; many contain aspirin
• That therapeutic response takes 2 wk (arthritis)
• To avoid alcohol ingestion; GI bleeding may occur
• That if anticoagulants are given with this drug, both should be discontinued 2 wk before surgery
Treatment of overdose: Lavage, activated charcoal, monitor electrolytes, VS

magnesium salts (OTC)
(mag-nee'zee-um)
magnesium chloride, Chloromag, Slo-Mag
magnesium citrate (OTC)
citrate of magnesia, Citroma, CitroMag*, Evac-Q-Mag
magnesium hydroxide (OTC)
Phillips' Magnesium Tablets, Phillips' Milk of Magnesia, MOM
magnesium oxide (OTC)
Mag-Ox 400, Maox, Uro-Mag
magnesium sulfate (OTC)
epsom salts
Func. class.: Electrolyte; anticonvulsant; laxative, saline; antacid

Action: Increases osmotic pressure, draws fluid into colon, neutralizes HCl
Uses: Constipation, bowel preparation before surgery or exam
Dosage and routes:
Laxative
• *Adult:* **PO** 30-60 ml hs (Milk of Magnesia), 300 mg
• *Adult and child >6 yr:* **PO** 15 g in 8 oz H₂O (magnesium sulfate); **PO** 10-20 ml (Concentrated Milk of Magnesia); **PO** 5-10 oz hs (magnesium citrate)
• *Child 2-6 yr:* 5-15 ml (Milk of Magnesia)
Prevention of magnesium deficiency
• *Adult and child ≥10 yr:* **PO** male: 270-400 mg/day; female: 280-300 mg/day; lactation: 335-350 mg/day; pregnancy 320 mg/day
• *Child 8-10 yr:* **PO** 170 mg/day

• *Child 4-7 yr:* **PO** 120 mg/day
• *Child infant to 4 yr:* 40-80 mg/day
Magnesium sulfate
Deficiency
• *Adult:* **PO** 200-400 mg in divided doses tid-qid; **IM** 1 g q6h × 4 doses; **IV** 5 g (severe)
• *Child 6-12 yr:* 3-6 mg/kg/day in divided doses tid-qid
Pre-eclampsia/eclampsia
magnesium sulfate
• *Adult:* **IM/IV** 4-5 g **IV inf;** with 5 g **IM** in each gluteus, then 5 g q4h or 4 g **IV inf,** then 1-2 g/hr **cont inf**
Available forms:
• Chloride: sus rel tabs 535 mg (64 mg Mg) enteric tabs 833 mg (100 mg Mg)
• Hydroxide: Liq 400 mg/5 ml; conc liquid 800 mg/5 ml; chew tabs 300, 600 mg
• Oxide: Tabs 400 mg; caps 140 mg
• Sulfate: Powder for oral; bulk packages; epsom salts, bulk packages; inj 10%, 12.5%, 25%, 50%
Side effects/adverse reactions:
CNS: Muscle weakness, flushing, sweating, confusion, sedation, depressed reflexes, *flaccidity, paralysis,* hypothermia
GI: Nausea, vomiting, anorexia, cramps
CV: Hypotension, heart block, *circulatory collapse*
META: Electrolyte, fluid imbalances
Contraindications: Hypersensitivity, renal diseases, abdominal pain, nausea/vomiting, obstruction, acute surgical abdomen, rectal bleeding
Precautions: Pregnancy (A)
Pharmacokinetics:
PO: Onset 3-6 hr
IM: Onset 1 hr, duration 4 hr
IV: Duration ½ hr
Interactions:
• Increased effect of neuromuscular blockers

• Decreased absorption of tetracyclines, other antiinfectives, nitrofurantoin
NURSING CONSIDERATIONS
Assess:
• I&O ratio; check for decrease in urinary output
• Cause of constipation; lack of fluids, bulk, exercise
• Cramping, rectal bleeding, nausea, vomiting; drug should be discontinued
◆ Mg toxicity: thirst, confusion, decrease in reflexes
Administer:
• With 8 oz H_2O
• Refrigerate magnesium citrate before giving
• Shake susp before using as antacid at least 2 hr pc
IV
• Only when calcium gluconate available for magnesium toxicity
• IV undiluted 1.5 ml of 10% sol over 1 min; may dilute to 20% sol, infuse over 3 hr
• IV at less than 150 mg/min; circulatory collapse may occur
Additive compatibilities: Calcium gluconate, cephalothin, chloramphenicol, cisplatin, heparin, hydrocortisone, isoproterenol, meropenem, methyldopa, norepinephrine, penicillin G potassium, potassium phosphate, verapamil
Y-site compatibilities: Acyclovir, aldesleukin, amifostine, amikacin, ampicillin, aztreonam, cefamandole, cefazolin, cefmetazole, cefoperazone, cefotaxime, cefoxitin, cephalothin, cephapirin, chloramphenicol, cisatracurium, clindamycin, dobutamine, doxycycline, doxorubicin liposome, enalaprilat, erythromycin, esmolol, famotidine, fludarabine, gallium, gentamicin, granisetron, heparin, hydrocortisone, hydromorphone, idarubicin, insulin, kanamycin, labetalol, meperi-

M

dine, metronidazole, minocycline, morphine, moxalactam, nafcillin, ondansetron, oxacillin, paclitaxel, penicillin G potassium, piperacillin, piperacillin/tazobactam, potassium chloride, propofol, remifentanil, sargramostim, thiotepa, ticarcillin, tobramycin, trimethoprim-sulfamethoxazole, vancomycin, vit B complex/C

Evaluate:

• Therapeutic response: decreased constipation

Teach patient/family:

• Not to use laxatives for long-term therapy; bowel tone will be lost

• That chilling helps the taste of magnesium citrate

• To shake suspension well

• To not give at hs as a laxative; may interfere with sleep

• To give citrus fruit after administering to counteract unpleasant taste

---

mannitol (℞)

(man'i-tole)

mannitol, Osmitrol, Resectisol

Func. class.: Osmotic diuretic

Chem. class.: Hexahydric alcohol

Action: Acts by increasing osmolarity of glomerular filtrate, which raises osmotic pressure of fluid in renal tubules; decrease in reabsorption of water, electrolytes; increase in urinary output, sodium, chloride excretion

Uses: Edema, promote systemic diuresis in cerebral edema, decrease intraocular pressure, improve renal function in acute renal failure, chemical poisoning

Dosage and routes:

Oliguria, prevention

• *Adult:* IV 50-100 g 5%-25% sol, may use test dose 0.2 g/kg over 3-5 min

Oliguria, treatment

• *Adult:* IV 300-400 mg/kg 20%-25% sol up to 100 g 15%-20% sol

• *Child:* IV 0.25-2 g/kg as 15%-20% sol run over 2-6 hr

Intraocular pressure/intracranial pressure

• *Adult:* IV 1½-2 g/kg 15%-25% sol over ½-1 hr

• *Child:* IV 1-2 g/kg (30-60 g/m^2) as 15%-20% sol run over ½-1 hr

Renal failure

• *Adult:* IV 50-200 g/24 hr, adjusted to maintain output of 30-50 mg/hr

Diuresis in drug intoxication

• *Adult and child >12 yr:* 5%-10% sol continuously up to 200 g **IV,** while maintaining 100-500 ml urine output/hr

Available forms: Inj 5%, 10%, 15%, 20%, 25%; GU irrigation: 5%

Side effects/adverse reactions:

GU: Marked diuresis, urinary retention, thirst

CNS: Dizziness, headache, ***convulsions, rebound increased ICP,*** confusion

GI: Nausea, *vomiting,* dry mouth, diarrhea

CV: Edema, thrombophlebitis, hypotension, hypertension, ***tachycardia,*** angina-like chest pains, fever, chills

RESP: Pulmonary congestion

ELECT: Fluid, electrolyte imbalances, *acidosis,* electrolyte loss, dehydration

EENT: Loss of hearing, blurred vision, nasal congestion, decreased intraocular pressure

Contraindications: Active intracranial bleeding, hypersensitivity, anuria, severe pulmonary congestion, edema, severe dehydration, progressive heart, renal failure

Precautions: Dehydration, pregnancy (C), severe renal disease, CHF, lactation

---

⬥ = Nursing alert   🖋 = Herb-drug interaction   🚫 = Do not crush

Pharmacokinetics:

IV: Onset 30-60 min for diuresis, ½-1 hr for intraocular pressure, 25 min for cerebrospinal fluid; duration 4-6 hr for intraocular pressure, 3-8 hr for cerebrospinal fluid; excreted in urine, half-life 100 min

Interactions:

• Decreased effect: lithium

• Drug/food: potassium foods: increased hyperkalemia

Lab test interferences:

Interference: Inorganic phosphorus, ethylene glycol

NURSING CONSIDERATIONS
Assess:

• Weight, I&O qd to determine fluid loss; effect of drug may be decreased if used qd; output qh prn

• Rate, depth, rhythm of respiration, effect of exertion

• B/P lying, standing; postural hypotension may occur

• Electrolytes: K, Na, Cl; include BUN, CBC, serum creatinine, blood pH, ABGs, CVP, PAP

• Signs of metabolic acidosis: drowsiness, restlessness

• Signs of hypokalemia: postural hypotension, malaise, fatigue, tachycardia, leg cramps, weakness

• Rashes, temp qd

• Confusion, especially in elderly; take safety precautions if needed

• Hydration including skin turgor, thirst, dry mucous membranes

• For blurred vision, pain in eyes, before and during treatment (increased intraocular pressure); neurologic checks, intracranial pressure during treatment (increased intracranial pressure)

Administer:
IV

• In 15%-25% sol with filter; give over ½-1½ hr; rapid infusion may worsen CHF; warm in hot water and shake to dissolve crystals

• Test dose in severe oliguria, 0.2 g/kg over 3-5 min; if no urine increase, give second test dose; if no response, reassess patient

Irrigation:

• 100 ml of 25%/900 ml of sterile water for inj (2.5% sol)

Additive compatibilities: Amikacin, bretylium, cefamandole, cefoxitin, cimetidine, cisplatin, dopamine, fosphenytoin, furosemide, gentamicin, metoclopramide, netilmicin, nizatidine, ofloxacin, ondansetron, sodium bicarbonate, tobramycin, verapamil

Y-site compatibilities: Allopurinol, amifostine, amphotericin B cholesteryl, aztreonam, cisatracurium, cladribine, fludarabine, fluorouracil, gallium, idarubicin, melphalan, ondansetron, paclitaxel, piperacillin, propofol, remifentanil, sargramostim, teniposide, thiotepa, vinorelbine

Evaluate:

• Therapeutic response: improvement in edema of feet, legs, sacral area daily if medication is being used in CHF; decreased intraocular pressure, prevention of hypokalemia, increased excretion of toxic substances; decreased ICP

Teach patient/family:

• To rise slowly from lying or sitting position

• The reason for and method of treatment

Treatment of overdose: Discontinue infusion; correct fluid, electrolyte imbalances; hemodialysis; monitor hydration, CV, renal function

M

masoprocol (℞)
(mas-o-proe′cole)
Func. class.: Miscellaneous topical product

Uses: Actinic keratoses
Dosage and routes:
• *Adult:* **TOP** apply to lesion bid × 2-4 wk
Contraindications: Hypersensitivity, children

mazindol (℞)
(may′zin-dole)
Func. class.: Anorexiant

Uses: Exogenous obesity
Dosage and routes:
• *Adult:* **PO** 1 mg 1 hr ac, or 2 mg 1 hr ac lunch, or 1 mg tid 1 hr ac
Contraindications: Hypersensitivity to sympathomimetic amine, glaucoma, drug abuse, cardiovascular disease, children <12 yr, hypertension, severe arteriosclerosis, agitated states, hyperthyroidism, concurrent MAOI use or use within 14 days

mebendazole (℞)
(me-ben′da-zole)
Vermox
Func. class.: Anthelmintic
Chem. class.: Carbamate

Action: Inhibits glucose uptake, degeneration of cytoplasmic microtubules in the cell; interferes with absorption, secretory function
Uses: Pinworms, roundworms, hookworms, whipworms, threadworms, pork tapeworms, dwarf tapeworms, beef tapeworms, hydatid cyst
Dosage and routes:
• *Adult and child >2 yr:* **PO** 100 mg as a single dose (pinworms) or bid × 3 days (whipworms, roundworms, or hookworms); course may be repeated in 3 wk if needed
Available forms: Tabs, chew 100 mg
Side effects/adverse reactions:
CNS: Dizziness, fever, headache
GI: Transient diarrhea, abdominal pain, nausea, vomiting
Contraindications: Hypersensitivity
Precautions: Child <2 yr, lactation, pregnancy (C) (1st trimester)
Pharmacokinetics:
PO: Peak ½-7 hr; excreted in feces primarily (metabolites), small amount in urine (unchanged); highly bound to plasma proteins 95%
Interactions:
• Decreased effect of mebendazole: carbamazepine, hydantoins
• Drug/food: increased absorption: high-fat meal
NURSING CONSIDERATIONS
Assess:
• Stools during entire treatment; specimens must be sent to lab while still warm, also 1-3 wk after treatment is completed
• For allergic reaction: rash (rare)
• For diarrhea during expulsion of worms; avoid self-contamination with patient's feces
• For infection in other family members, since infection from person to person is common
• Blood studies: AST, ALT, alk phosphatase, BUN, CBC during treatment
Administer:
• May be crushed, chewed, swallowed whole, mixed with food

- PO after meals to avoid GI symptoms, since absorption is not altered by food
- Second course after 3 wk if needed; usually recommended

Perform/provide:
- Storage in tight container

Evaluate:
- Therapeutic response: expulsion of worms and 3 negative stool cultures after completion of treatment

Teach patient/family:
- Proper hygiene after BM, including hand-washing technique; tell patient to avoid putting fingers in mouth; clean fingernails
- That infected person should sleep alone; do not shake bed linen, change bed linen qd, wash in hot water, change and wash undergarments daily
- To clean toilet qd with disinfectant (green soap solution)
- The need for compliance with dosage schedule, duration of treatment
- To wear shoes, wash all fruits and vegetables well before eating; use commercial fruit/vegetable cleaner
- That all members of the family should be treated (pinworms)

---

mechlorethamine (R)

(me-klor-eth'a-meen)
Mustargen, nitrogen mustard
Func. class.: Antineoplastic alkylating agent
Chem. class.: Nitrogen mustard

Action: Responsible for crosslinking DNA strands leading to cell death; rapidly degraded, a vesicant; activity is not cell cycle phase-specific

Uses: Hodgkin's disease, leukemias, lymphomas, lymphosarcoma; ovarian, breast, lung carcinoma; neoplastic effusions

Dosage and routes:
- *Adult:* **IV** 0.4 mg/kg or 10 mg/m² as 1 dose or 2-4 divided doses over 2-4 days; second course after 3 wk depending on blood cell count

Neoplastic effusions
- *Adult:* **INTRACAVITARY** 0.4 mg/kg, may be 200-400 µg/kg

Available forms: Inj 10 mg

Side effects/adverse reactions:
EENT: Tinnitus, hearing loss
HEMA: ***Thrombocytopenia, leukopenia, agranulocytosis,*** anemia
GI: Nausea, vomiting, diarrhea, stomatitis, weight loss, colitis, ***hepatotoxicity***
CNS: Headache, dizziness, drowsiness, paresthesia, peripheral neuropathy, ***coma***
INTEG: Alopecia, pruritus, herpes zoster, extravasation

Contraindications: Lactation, pregnancy (D), myelosuppression, acute herpes zoster

Precautions: Radiation therapy, chronic lymphocytic leukopenia

Pharmacokinetics: Metabolized in liver, excreted in urine

Interactions:
- Increased toxicity: antineoplastics, radiation
- Blood dyscrasias: amphotericin B
- Decreased antibody reaction: live virus vaccines

NURSING CONSIDERATIONS
Assess:
- CBC, differential, platelet count qwk; withhold drug if WBC is <1000/mm³ or platelet count is <75,000/mm³; notify prescriber, recovery of WBCs, platelets within 20 days
- Renal function studies: BUN, serum uric acid, urine CrCl before, during therapy
- I&O ratio; report fall in urine output of 30 ml/hr
- Monitor temp q4h (may indicate beginning infection); no rectal temps

---

• LFTs before, during therapy (bilirubin, AST, ALT, LDH) as needed or monthly
• Bleeding: hematuria, guaiac, bruising or petechiae, mucosa or orifices q8h
• Jaundiced skin and sclera, dark urine, clay-colored stools, itchy skin, abdominal pain, fever, diarrhea
• Effects of alopecia on body image; discuss feelings about body changes
• Buccal cavity q8h for dryness, sores, ulceration, white patches, oral pain, bleeding, dysphagia
• Local irritation, pain, burning, discoloration at injection site
⬥ Symptoms indicating severe allergic reaction: rash, pruritus, urticaria, purpuric skin lesions, itching, flushing

Administer:
• After using guidelines for preparation of cytotoxic drugs
• Antiemetic 30-60 min before giving drug and prn
• IV after diluting 10 mg/10 ml sterile H_2O or NaCl; leave needle in vial, shake, withdraw dose, give through Y-tube or 3-way stopcock or directly over 3-5 min
• Watch for infiltration; infiltrate area with isotonic sodium thiosulfate or 1% lidocaine; apply ice for 6-12 hr
• Topical or systemic analgesics for pain
• Local or systemic drugs for infection

Y-site compatibilities: Amifostine, aztreonam, filgrastim, fludarabine, granisetron, melphalan, ondansetron, sargramostim, teniposide, vinorelbine

Perform/provide:
• Storage at room temperature in dry form
• Increase fluid intake to 2-3 L/day to prevent urate deposits, calculi formation
• Diet low in purines: organ meats (kidney, liver), dried beans, peas to maintain alkaline urine
• Preparation under hood using gloves and mask
• Rinsing of mouth tid-qid with water, club soda; brushing of teeth bid-tid with soft brush or cotton-tipped applicators for stomatitis; use unwaxed dental floss
• Warm compresses at injection site for inflammation

Evaluate:
• Therapeutic response: decreased tumor size, spread of malignancy

Teach patient/family:
• The rationale for and techniques of protective isolation
• That sterility, amenorrhea can occur; reversible after discontinuing treatment
• That hair may be lost during treatment; a wig or hairpiece may make patient feel better; new hair may be different in color, texture
• To avoid foods with citric acid, hot or rough texture
• To report any bleeding, white spots, or ulcerations in mouth to prescriber; tell patient to examine mouth qd
• To report signs of infection: fever, sore throat, flulike symptoms
• To report signs of anemia: fatigue, headache, faintness, shortness of breath, irritability
• To avoid use of razors, commercial mouthwash
• To avoid use of aspirin products, NSAIDs
• To notify prescriber if pregnancy is suspected; to use contraception during treatment

---

⬥ = Nursing alert   🍃 = Herb-drug interaction   🚫 = Do not crush

meclizine (OTC, R̥)

(mek'li-zeen)
Antivert, Antivert/25,
Antivert/25 Chewable,
Antivert-50, Antrizine,
Bonamine*, Bonine, Dizmiss,
Dramamine II, meclizine HCl,
Meni-D, Vergan

Func. class.: Antiemetic, antihistamine, anticholinergic
Chem. class.: H₁-Receptor antagonist, piperazine derivative

Action: Acts centrally by blocking chemoreceptor trigger zone, which in turn acts on vomiting center
Uses: Vertigo, motion sickness
Dosage and routes:
• *Adult:* PO 25-100 mg qd in divided doses or 1 hr before traveling
Available forms: Tabs 12.5, 25, 50 mg; chew tabs 25 mg; caps 15, 25, 30 mg
Side effects/adverse reactions:
CNS: Drowsiness, fatigue, restlessness, headache, insomnia
CV: Hypotension
GU: Urinary retention
GI: Nausea, anorexia
EENT: Dry mouth, blurred vision
Contraindications: Hypersensitivity to cyclizines, shock
Precautions: Children, narrowangle glaucoma, glaucoma, urinary retention, lactation, prostatic hypertrophy, elderly, pregnancy (B), CV disease, hypertension, seizure disease
Pharmacokinetics:
PO: Duration 8-24 hr, half-life 6 hr
Interactions:
• Increased effect of alcohol, opioids, other CNS depressants
⬥ Increased anticholinergic effect: henbane leaf
Lab test interferences:
False negative: Allergy skin testing

NURSING CONSIDERATIONS
Assess:
• VS, B/P
⬥ Signs of toxicity of other drugs or masking of symptoms of disease: brain tumor, intestinal obstruction
• Observe for drowsiness, dizziness, level of consciousness
Administer:
PO
• Tablets may be swallowed whole, chewed, or allowed to dissolve; give with food to decrease GI upset
• Lowest possible dose in elderly, anticholinergic effects
Evaluate:
• Therapeutic response: absence of dizziness, vomiting
Teach patient/family:
• That a false-negative result may occur with skin testing for allergies; these procedures should not be scheduled for 4 days after discontinuing use
• To avoid hazardous activities, activities requiring alertness; dizziness may occur; instruct patient to request assistance with ambulation
• To avoid alcohol, other depressants

M

medroxyprogesterone (R̥)

(me-drox'ee-proe-jess'te-rone)
Amen, Curretab, Cycrin,
Depo-Provera, medroxyprogesterone, Provera
Func. class.: Antineoplastic, hormone, contraceptive
Chem. class.: Progesterone derivative

Action: Inhibits secretion of pituitary gonadotropins, which prevents follicular maturation and ovulation; stimulates growth of mammary tissue; antineoplastic action against endometrial cancer

Uses: Uterine bleeding (abnormal), secondary amenorrhea, endometrial cancer, renal cancer, contraceptive, prevent endometrial changes associated with estrogen replacement therapy (ERT)

Investigational uses: Pickwickian syndrome, sleep apnea, hypersomnolence

Dosage and routes:

Secondary amenorrhea

• *Adult:* **PO** 5-10 mg qd × 5-10 days

Endometrial/renal cancer

• *Adult:* **IM** 400-1000 mg/wk may repeat qwk, dose may be decreased after adequate response

Uterine bleeding

• *Adult:* **PO** 5-10 mg qd × 5-10 days starting on 16th or 21st day of menstrual cycle

Contraceptive

• *Adult:* **INJ** q3mo

With ERT

• *Adult:* **PO** monophasic 2.5 mg qd; Biphasic 5 mg days 15-28 of cycle

Available forms: Tabs 2.5, 5, 10, 100 mg; inj susp 50, 100, 150, 400 mg/ml

Side effects/adverse reactions:

CNS: Dizziness, headache, migraines, depression, fatigue

CV: Hypotension, thrombophlebitis, edema, ***thromboembolism, stroke, pulmonary embolism, MI***

GI: Nausea, vomiting, anorexia, cramps, increased weight, ***cholestatic jaundice***

EENT: Diplopia

GU: Amenorrhea, cervical erosion, breakthrough bleeding, dysmenorrhea, vaginal candidiasis, breast changes, *gynecomastia, testicular atrophy, impotence,* endometriosis, ***spontaneous abortion***

INTEG: Rash, urticaria, acne, hirsutism, alopecia, oily skin, seborrhea, purpura, melasma, photosensitivity

META: Hyperglycemia

SYST: ***Angioedema, anaphylaxis***

Contraindications: Breast cancer, hypersensitivity, thromboembolic disorders, reproductive cancer, genital bleeding (abnormal, undiagnosed), pregnancy (D)

Precautions: Lactation, hypertension, asthma, blood dyscrasias, gallbladder disease, CHF, diabetes mellitus, bone disease, depression, migraine headache, convulsive disorders, hepatic disease, renal disease, family history of cancer of breast or reproductive tract

Do not confuse:

Amen/Ambien

medroxyprogesterone/
methylprednisolone

Provera/Premarin

Pharmacokinetics:

PO: Duration 24 hr, excreted in urine and feces, metabolized in liver

Lab test interferences:

Increase: Alk phosphatase, N (urine), pregnanediol, amino acids

Decrease: GTT, HDL

NURSING CONSIDERATIONS

Assess:

◆ Symptoms indicating severe allergic reaction, angioedema, have epinephrine and rescusiative equipment available

• Weight qd; notify prescriber of weekly weight gain >5 lb

• B/P at beginning of treatment and periodically

• I&O ratio; be alert for decreasing urinary output, increasing edema

• Liver function studies: ALT, AST, bilirubin, periodically during long-term therapy

• Edema, hypertension, cardiac symptoms, jaundice

• Mental status: affect, mood, behavioral changes, depression

Administer:

• Titrated dose; use lowest effective dose

• 150 mg/ml for contraception

◆ = Nursing alert   🌿 = Herb-drug interaction   🚫 = Do not crush

• Oil solution deep in large muscle mass (IM), rotate sites
• With food or milk to decrease GI symptoms (PO)
Perform/provide:
• Storage in dark area
Evaluate:
• Therapeutic response: decreased abnormal uterine bleeding, absence of amenorrhea, decrease in size and growth of tumor
Teach patient/family:
• To avoid sunlight or use sunscreen; photosensitivity can occur
• About cushingoid symptoms
◆ To report breast lumps, vaginal bleeding, edema, jaundice, dark urine, clay-colored stools, dyspnea, headache, blurred vision, abdominal pain, numbness or stiffness in legs, chest pain; male to report impotence or gynecomastia
• To report suspected pregnancy

RARELY USED

mefenamic acid (R)
(me-fe-nam'ik)
Func. class.: Nonsteroidal antiinflammatory

Uses: Mild to moderate pain, dysmenorrhea, inflammatory disease
Dosage and routes:
• *Adult and child >14 yr:* **PO** 500 mg, then 250 mg q6h, use not to exceed 1 wk
Contraindications: Hypersensitivity, asthma, severe renal disease, severe hepatic disease, ulcer disease

---

RARELY USED

mefloquine (R)
(meh'floh-quin)
Func. class.: Antimalarial

Uses: Treatment and prevention of *Plasmodium falciparum, P. vivax,* malaria
Dosage and routes:
• *Adult:* **PO** 1250 mg as a single dose (treatment); 250 mg 1 wk prior to trip, then for 4 wk after returning, then 250 mg q2wk (prevention)
Contraindications: Hypersensitivity

---

megestrol (R)
(me-jess'trole)
Megace, megestrol
Func. class.: Antineoplastic, contraceptive
Chem. class.: Hormone, progestin

Action: Affects endometrium by antiluteinizing effect; this is thought to bring about cell death
Uses: Breast, endometrial cancer, renal cell cancer, cachexia
Investigational uses: Hot flashes
Dosage and routes:
Endometrial/ovarian carcinoma
• *Adult:* **PO** 40-320 mg/day in divided doses
Breast carcinoma
• *Adult:* **PO** 40 mg qid or 160 mg qd
Anorexia (AIDS)
• *Adult:* **PO** 800 mg qd (oral susp)
Hot flashes (off label)
• *Adult:* **PO** 20 mg qd
Available forms: Tabs 20, 40 mg; oral susp 200 mg/5 ml
Side effects/adverse reactions:
GI: Nausea, vomiting, diarrhea, abdominal cramps, weight gain

M

GU: Gynecomastia, fluid retention, **hypercalcemia**, vaginal bleeding, discharge, impotence, decreased libido

CV: **Thrombophlebitis, thromboembolism**

INTEG: Alopecia, rash, pruritus, purpura, itching

CNS: Mood swings

Contraindications: Hypersensitivity, pregnancy D (tabs); X (susp)

Do not confuse:

Megace/Reglan

Pharmacokinetics:

PO: Duration 1-3 days, half-life 60 min; metabolized in liver; excreted in feces, breast milk

Lab test interferences:

Increase: Alk phosphatase, urinary N, urinary pregnanediol, plasma amino acids

False positive: Urine glucose

Decrease: HDL, glucose tolerance test

NURSING CONSIDERATIONS
Assess:

• I&O ratio; weights

• Effects of alopecia on body image; discuss feelings about body changes

◆ Symptoms indicating severe allergic reaction: rash, pruritus, urticaria, purpuric skin lesions, itching, flushing

• Frequency of stools, characteristics: cramping, acidosis, signs of dehydration (rapid respirations, poor skin turgor, decreased urine output, dry skin, restlessness, weakness)

• Anorexia, nausea, vomiting, constipation, weakness, loss of muscle tone

• Thrombophlebitis: Homans' sign, edema, pain in calf, thigh, notify prescriber

Administer:

• Oral susp for AIDS patients

Perform/provide:

• Nutritious diet with iron, vitamin supplements as ordered

• Storage in tight container at room temperature

Evaluate:

• Therapeutic response: decreased tumor size, spread of malignancy; weight gain in AIDS patients

Teach patient/family:

• To report vaginal bleeding

• That nonhormonal contraception should be used during and 4 mo after treatment

• That gynecomastia can occur; reversible after discontinuing treatment

• To recognize and report signs of fluid retention, thromboemboli

---

meloxicam (℞)

(mel-ox′i-kam)

Mobic

Func. class.: Nonsteroidal antiinflammatory/nonopioid analgesic

Chem. class.: Oxicam

Action: Inhibits prostaglandin synthesis by decreasing an enzyme needed for biosynthesis; analgesic, antiinflammatory, antipyretic effects

Uses: Osteoarthritis

Dosage and routes:

• *Adult:* **PO** 7.5 mg qd, may increase to 15 mg qd

Available forms: Tabs 7.5 mg

Side effects/adverse reactions:

CV: Hypertension, angina, **cardiac failure, MI,** hypotension, palpitations, **dysrhythmias,** tachycardia

CNS: Dizziness, drowsiness, tremors, headache, nervousness, malaise, fatigue, insomnia, depression, **seizures**

EENT: Tinnitus, hearing loss

◆ = Nursing alert   🌿 = Herb-drug interaction   🚫 = Do not crush

GI: Pancreatitis, nausea, colitis, GERD, vomiting, diarrhea, constipation, flatulence, cramps, dry mouth, peptic ulcer, *__GI bleeding, perforation__*
GU: __Nephrotoxicity: dysuria, hematuria, oliguria, azotemia__
HEMA: __Blood dyscrasias,__ anemia, prolonged bleeding
INTEG: Rash, urticaria, photosensitivity
SYST: __Angioedema, anaphylaxis__
Contraindications: Hypersensitivity, asthma, severe renal disease, severe hepatic disease, peptic ulcer disease, L&D, lactation, CV bleeding
Precautions: Pregnancy (C), children, bleeding disorders, GI disorders, cardiac disorders, hypersensitivity to other antiinflammatory agents, elderly, CrCl <25 ml/min
Pharmacokinetics:
PO: Peak 4-5 hr
IM: Peak 50 min, half-life 6 hr, enters breast milk, <50% metabolized by liver, excreted by kidneys
Interactions:
• Increased action of meloxicam: phenytoin, sulfonamides
• Decreased action of meloxicam: cholestyramine, salicylates
• Increased action of: aminoglycosides, hydantoins, diuretics, anticoagulants
• Decreased action of: β-blockers
• Nephrotoxicity: cyclosporine
NURSING CONSIDERATIONS
Assess:
• Renal, liver, blood studies: BUN, creatinine, AST, ALT, Hgb before treatment, periodically thereafter
• Bleeding times; check for bruising, bleeding; test for occult blood in urine
◆ For anaphylaxis and angioedema; emergency equipment should be nearby

◆ Hepatic dysfunction: jaundice, yellow sclera and skin, clay-colored stools
• Audiometric, ophthalmic exam before, during, after teratment
• GI condition, hypertension, cardiac conditions
Administer:
• May take without regard to meals, to take with food for GI upset
Perform/provide:
• Storage at room temperature
Evaluate:
• Therapeutic response: decreased pain, stiffness, swelling in joints, ability to move more easily
Teach patient/family:
• To report blurred vision or ringing, roaring in ears (may indicate toxicity)
• To avoid driving, other hazardous activities if dizziness or drowsiness occurs
• To report change in urine pattern, weight increase, edema, pain increase in joints, fever, blood in urine (indicates nephrotoxicity); to report rash, black stools, or continuing headache
• To avoid alcohol, ASA

M

---

melphalan (℞)

(mel'fa-lan)
Alkeran, Alkeran IV, L-PAM, phenylalanine mustard
Func. class.: Antineoplastic, alkylating agent
Chem. class.: Nitrogen mustard
Action: Responsible for cross-linking DNA strands leading to cell death; activity is not cell cycle phase specific
Uses: Multiple myeloma, malignant melanoma, advanced ovarian cancer
Investigational uses: Breast, testicular, prostate carcinoma; osteo-

genic sarcoma, chronic myelogenous leukemia

Dosage and routes:

Multiple myeloma

• *Adult:* **PO** 150 μg/kg/day × 1 wk, then 21 days after, then 50 μg/kg/day or 100-150 μg/kg/day or 250 μg/kg/day × 4 days for 2-3 wk, then 2-4 wk after, then 2-4 mg/day or 7 mg/m² × 5 day q5-6wk

Ovarian carcinoma

• *Adult:* **IV INF** 16 mg/m², reduce in renal insufficiency, give over 15-20 min, give at 2 wk intervals × 4 doses, then at 4 wk intervals

Available forms: Tabs 2 mg, pwd for inj 50 mg

Side effects/adverse reactions:

*HEMA: **Thrombocytopenia, neutropenia, leukopenia,** anemia*

GI: Nausea, vomiting, stomatitis, diarrhea

GU: Amenorrhea, hyperuricemia, gonadal suppression

INTEG: Rash, urticaria, alopecia, pruritus

*RESP: **Fibrosis, dysplasia***

*SYST: **Anaphylaxis,** allergic reactions*

Contraindications: Lactation, pregnancy (D), hypersensitivity to this drug or other nitrogen mustards

Precautions: Radiation therapy, bone marrow depression, infections, renal disease, children

Pharmacokinetics: Metabolized in liver, excreted in urine, half-life 1½ hr

Interactions:

• Increased toxicity: antineoplastics, radiation

• Decreased antibody response: live virus vaccines

• Increased pulmonary toxicity: carmustine

NURSING CONSIDERATIONS

Assess:

• CBC, differential, platelet count qwk; withhold drug if WBC is <3000/mm³ or platelet count is <100,000/mm³; notify prescriber

Renal function studies: BUN, serum uric acid, urine CrCl before, during therapy

I&O ratio; report fall in urine output to 30 ml/hr

For infection: fever, cough, temp, sore throat, notify prescriber

For bleeding: bruising, blood in urine, stools, emesis

LFTs before, during therapy (bilirubin, AST, ALT, LDH) as needed or monthly

Bleeding: hematuria, guaiac, bruising or petechiae, mucosa or orifices q8h

Jaundiced skin and sclera, dark urine, clay-colored stools, itchy skin, abdominal pain, fever, diarrhea

Buccal cavity q8h for dryness, sores, ulceration, white patches, oral pain, bleeding, dysphagia

Local irritation, pain, burning, discoloration at injection site

◆ Symptoms indicating severe allergic reaction: rash, pruritus, urticaria, purpuric skin lesions, itching, flushing

Administer:

• Antiemetic 30-60 min before giving drug to prevent vomiting

Y-site compatibilities: Acyclovir, amikacin, aminophylline, ampicillin, aztreonam, bleomycin, bumetanide, buprenorphine, butorphanol, calcium gluconate, carboplatin, carmustine, cefazolin, cefepime, cefoperazone, cefotaxime, cefotetan, ceftazidime, ceftizoxime, ceftriaxone, cefuroxime, cimetidine, cisplatin, clindamycin, cyclophosphamide, cytarabine, dacarbazine, dactinomycin, daunorubicin, dexamethasone, diphenhydramine, doxorubicin, doxycycline, droperidol, enalaprilat, etoposide, famotidine, floxuridine, fluconazole, fludarabine, fluorouracil, furosemide, gallium, ganciclovir, gentamicin, granisetron, haloperidol, heparin, hydrocortisone, hydrocortisone sodium phosphate, hydromorphone, hydroxyzine, idarubicin, ifosfamide, imipenem-cilastatin, lorazepam, mannitol, mechlorethamine, meperidine, mesna, methotrexate, methylprednisolone, metoclopramide, metronidazole, miconazole, minocycline, mitomycin, mitoxantrone, morphine, nalbuphine, netilmicin, ondansetron, pentostatin, piperacillin, plicamycin, potassium chloride, prochlorperazine, promethazine, ranitidine, sodium bicarbonate, streptozocin, teniposide, thiotepa, ticarcillin, ticarcillin/clavulanate, tobramycin, trimethoprim-sulfamethoxazole, vancomycin, vinblastine, vincristine, vinorelbine, zidovudine

Perform/provide:

• Storage in airtight, light-resistant container

• Strict medical asepsis, protective isolation if WBC levels are low

• Increase fluid intake to 2-3 L/day to prevent urate deposits, calculi formation

• Diet low in purines: organ meats (kidney, liver), dried beans, peas to maintain alkaline urine

• Rinsing of mouth tid-qid with water, club soda; brushing of teeth bid-tid with soft brush or cotton-tipped applicators for stomatitis; use unwaxed dental floss

• Warm compresses at injection site for inflammation

Evaluate:

• Therapeutic response: decreased tumor size, spread of malignancy

Teach patient/family:

• That sterility, amenorrhea can occur; reversible after discontinuing treatment

• To avoid foods with citric acid, hot or rough texture

• To report any bleeding, white spots, or ulcerations in mouth to prescriber; tell patient to examine mouth qd

• To report signs of infection: fever, sore throat, flulike symptoms

• To report suspected pregnancy; to use contraception during treatment

• To report signs of anemia: fatigue, headache, faintness, shortness of breath, irritability

• To avoid use of razors, commercial mouthwash

• To avoid use of aspirin products, NSAIDs, alcohol

---

menotropins (℞)

(men-oh-troe′pins)
Humegon, Pergonal, Repronex
Func. class.: Gonadotropin
Chem. class.: Exogenous gonadotropin

M

Action: In women, increases follicular growth, maturation; in men, when given with HCG, stimulates spermatogenesis

Uses: Infertility, anovulation in women, stimulates spermatogenesis in men

Dosage and routes:

Infertility

• *Men:* **IM** 1 ampule 3 × wk with HCG 2000 U 2 × wk × 4 mo

• *Women:* **IM** 75 IU FSH, LH qd × 9-12 days, then 10,000 U HCG 1 day after these drugs; repeat × 2 menstrual cycles, then increase to 150 IU FSH, LH qd × 9-12 days, then 10,000 U HCG 1 day after these drugs × 2 menstrual cycles

Anovulation

• *Women:* **IM** 75 IU FSH, LH qd × 9-12 days, then 10,000 U HCG 1 day after last dose of these drugs; repeat × 1-3 menstrual cycles

Available forms: Pwd for inj lyoph-

---

ilized 75 IU FSH, LH activity 150 IU FSH, LH activity

Side effects/adverse reactions:
CNS: Fever
CV: **Hypovolemia**
RESP: **ARDS, pulmonary embolism, pulmonary infarction**
SYST: **Anaphylaxis**
GI: Nausea, vomiting, diarrhea, anorexia
GU: Ovarian enlargement, abdominal distention/pain, multiple births, ovarian hyperstimulation: sudden ovarian enlargement, ascites with or without pain, pleural effusion; gynecomastia in men
HEMA: **Hemoperitoneum, arterial thromboembolism**

Contraindications: Primary ovarian failure, abnormal bleeding, thyroid/adrenal dysfunction, organic intracranial lesion, ovarian cysts, primary testicular failure, pregnancy (X)

NURSING CONSIDERATIONS
Assess:
• Weight qd; notify prescriber if weight increases rapidly
• Estrogen excretion level; if >100 μg/24 hr, drug is withheld; hyperstimulation syndrome may occur
• I&O ratio; be alert for decreasing urinary output
• Ovarian enlargement, abdominal distention/pain; report symptoms immediately
Administer:
IM
• After reconstituting with 1-2 ml sterile saline inj; use immediately
Evaluate:
• Therapeutic response: ovulation, pregnancy
Teach patient/family:
• That multiple births are possible; if pregnancy occurs, usually 4-6 wk after start of treatment

• To keep appointment during treatment qd × 2 wk

RARELY USED

mepenzolate (℞)
(me-pen'zoe-late)
Func. class.: GI anticholinergic

Uses: Treatment of peptic ulcer disease, irritable bowel syndrome in combination with other drugs; for other GI disorders
Dosage and routes:
• *Adult:* **PO** 25-50 mg qid with meals, hs; titrate to patient response
Contraindications: Hypersensitivity to anticholinergics, narrow-angle glaucoma, GI obstruction, myasthenia gravis, paralytic ileus, GI atony, toxic megacolon

---

meperidine (℞)
(me-per'i-deen)
Demerol, meperidine, Pethidine
Func. class.: Opiate analgesic
Chem. class.: Phenylpiperidine derivative
Controlled Substance Schedule II
Action: Depresses pain impulse transmission at the spinal cord level by interacting with opioid receptors
Uses: Moderate to severe pain, preoperatively, postoperatively
Dosage and routes:
Pain
• *Adult:* **PO/SC/IM** 50-150 mg q3-4h prn; dose should be decreased if given **IV**
• *Child:* **PO/SC/IM** 1 mg/kg q3-4h prn, not to exceed 100 mg q4h
Labor analgesia
• *Adult:* **SC/IM** 50-100 mg given

◆ = Nursing alert   �િ = Herb-drug interaction   ⊘ = Do not crush when contractions are regularly spaced, repeat q1-3h prn

Preoperatively
• *Adult:* **IM/SC** 50-100 mg q30-90 min before surgery; dose should be reduced if given **IV**
• *Child:* **IM/SC** 1-2.2 mg/kg 30-90 min before surgery

Renal disease
• CrCl 10-50 ml/min 75% of dose; CrCl <10 ml/min 50% of dose

Available forms include: Inj 10, 25, 50, 75, 100 mg/ml; tabs 50, 100 mg; syr 50 mg/5 ml

Side effects/adverse reactions:
CNS: Drowsiness, dizziness, confusion, headache, sedation, euphoria, increased intracranial pressure, seizures

CV: Palpitations, bradycardia, change in B/P, tachycardia (IV)

EENT: Tinnitus, blurred vision, miosis, diplopia, depressed corneal reflex

GI: Nausea, vomiting, anorexia, constipation, cramps

GU: Urinary retention, dysuria

INTEG: Rash, urticaria, bruising, flushing, diaphoresis, pruritus

RESP: Respiratory depression

Contraindications: Hypersensitivity, addiction (narcotic)

Precautions: Addictive personality, pregnancy (B), lactation, increased intracranial pressure, MI (acute), severe heart disease, respiratory depression, hepatic disease, renal disease, child <18 yr, elderly

Do not confuse:
Demerol/Dilaudid
meperidine/hydromorphone

Pharmacokinetics: Absorption 50% (PO), well absorbed IM, SC
PO: Onset 15 min, peak ½-1 hr, duration 2-4 hr
SC/IM: Onset 10 min, peak ½-1 hr, duration 2-4 hr
IV: Onset 5 min, duration 2 hr
Metabolized by liver (to active/

inactive metabolites), excreted by kidneys; crosses placenta, excreted in breast milk; half-life 3-4 hr; toxic by-product can result from regular use

Interactions:
• Increased effects with: other CNS depressants, alcohol, opioids, sedative/hypnotics, antipsychotics, skeletal muscle relaxants
• Increased adverse reactions: protease inhibitor antiretrovirals, chlorpromazine
• Decreased meperidine effect: phenytoin
◆ May cause fatal reaction: MAOIs, procarbazine

Lab test interferences:
Increase: Amylase, lipase

NURSING CONSIDERATIONS
Assess:
• Pain: location, type, character; give before pain becomes extreme
• Renal function prior to initiating therapy; poor renal function can lead to accumulation of toxic metabolite and seizures
• I&O ratio; check for decreasing output; may indicate urinary retention
• For constipation; increase fluids, bulk in diet
• CNS changes: dizziness, drowsiness, hallucinations, euphoria, LOC, pupil reactions; at chronic or high-dose use
• Allergic reactions: rash, urticaria
• Respiratory dysfunction: depression, character, rate, rhythm; notify prescriber if respirations are <12/min

Administer:
• Patient should remain recumbent for 1 hr after IM/SC route
• With antiemetic for nausea, vomiting
• When pain is beginning to return; determine dosage interval by patient response

M

• In gradually decreasing dose after long-term use; withdrawal symptoms may occur

IV

• After diluting with 5 ml or more sterile H_2O or NS; give directly over 4-5 min; may be further diluted in sol to 1 mg/ml during anesthesia in D_5W or NS; if diluted in NS, may be given through patient-controlled inf device

Additive compatibilities: Cefazolin, dobutamine, ondansetron, scopolamine, succinylcholine, triflupromazine, verapamil

Syringe compatibilities: Atropine, benzquinamide, butorphanol, chlorpromazine, cimetidine, dimenhydrinate, diphenhydramine, droperidol, fentanyl, glycopyrrolate, hydroxyzine, ketamine, metoclopramide, midazolam, pentazocine, perphenazine, prochlorperazine, promazine, promethazine, ranitidine, scopolamine

Y-site compatibilities: Amifostine, amikacin, ampicillin, atenolol, aztreonam, bumetanide, cefamandole, cefazolin, cefmetazole, cefotaxime, cefotetan, cefoxitin, ceftazidime, ceftizoxime, ceftriaxone, cefuroxime, cephalothin, cephapirin, chloramphenicol, cisatracurium, cladribine, clindamycin, dexamethasone, diltiazem, diphenhydramine, dobutamine, dopamine, doxorubicin liposome, doxycycline, droperidol, erythromycin, famotidine, filgrastim, fluconazole, fludarabine, gallium, gentamicin, granisetron, heparin, hydrocortisone, insulin (regular), kanamycin, labetalol, lidocaine, methyldopate, magnesium sulfate, melphalan, methylprednisolone, metoclopramide, metoprolol, metronidazole, moxalactam, ondansetron, oxacillin, oxytocin, paclitaxel, penicillin G potassium, piperacillin, potassium chloride, propofol, propranolol, ranitidine, remifentanil, sargramostim, teniposide, thiotepa, ticarcillin, ticarcillin/clavulanate, tobramycin, trimethoprim-sulfamethoxazole, vancomycin, verapamil, vinorelbine

Perform/provide:

• Storage in light-resistant container at room temperature

• Assistance with ambulation

• Safety measures: night-light, call bell within easy reach

Evaluate:

• Therapeutic response: decrease in pain

Teach patient/family:

• To report any symptoms of CNS changes, allergic reactions

• That physical dependency may result from extended use

• That drowsiness, dizziness may occur; to call for assistance

• That withdrawal symptoms may occur: nausea, vomiting, cramps, fever, faintness, anorexia

• To make position changes slowly; orthostatic hypotension can occur

• To avoid OTC medications, alcohol unless directed by prescriber

Treatment of overdose: Naloxone (Narcan) 0.2-0.8 mg IV, O_2, IV fluids, vasopressors

---

mercaptopurine (R)

(mer-kap-toe-pyoor′een)
Purinethol, 6-MP
Func. class.: Antineoplastic-antimetabolite
Chem. class.: Purine analog

Action: Inhibits purine metabolism at multiple sites, which inhibits DNA and RNA synthesis, S phase of cell cycle specific

Uses: Chronic myelocytic or acute lymphoblastic leukemia in children, acute myelogenous leukemia

---

Investigational uses: Polycythemia vera, psoriatic arthritis, colitis, lymphoma

Dosage and routes:
• *Adult:* **PO** 80-100 mg/m^2 qd max 5 mg/kg/day; maintenance 1.5-2.5 mg/kg/day
• *Child:* 75 mg/m^2/day; maintenance 1.5-2.5 mg/kg/day

Available forms: Tabs 50 mg

Side effects/adverse reactions:
CNS: Fever, headache, weakness
HEMA: ***Thrombocytopenia, leukopenia, myelosuppression, anemia***
GI: *Nausea, vomiting, anorexia, diarrhea, stomatitis,* ***hepatotoxicity*** (high doses), *jaundice, gastritis*
GU: ***Renal failure,*** *hyperuricemia,* ***oliguria,*** *crystalluria,* ***hematuria***
INTEG: *Rash,* dry skin, urticaria

Contraindications: Patients with prior drug resistance, leukopenia (<2500/mm^3), thrombocytopenia (<100,000/mm^3), anemia, pregnancy (D)

Precautions: Renal disease

Pharmacokinetics: Incompletely absorbed when taken orally; metabolized in liver, excreted in urine

Interactions:
• Increased toxicity: radiation or other antineoplastics
• Increased bone marrow depression: allopurinol, co-trimoxazole
• Reversal of neuromuscular blockade: nondepolarizing muscle relaxants
• Increased or decreased anticoagulant action: warfarin

NURSING CONSIDERATIONS
Assess:
• CBC, differential, platelet count qwk; withhold drug if WBC is <3500 or platelet count is <100,000; notify prescriber; drug should be discontinued
• Renal function studies: BUN, serum uric acid, urine CrCl, electrolytes before, during therapy

• I&O ratio; report fall in urine output to <30 ml/hr
• Monitor temp q4h; fever may indicate beginning infection; no rectal temps
• Liver function tests before, during therapy: bilirubin, alk phosphatase, AST, ALT, qwk during beginning therapy
• Bleeding: hematuria, guaiac, bruising, petechiae; mucosa or orifices q8h
• Buccal cavity q8h for dryness, sores, ulceration, white patches, oral pain, bleeding, dysphagia
◆ Symptoms indicating severe allergic reaction: rash, urticaria, itching, flushing

Administer:
• Antacid before oral agent; give drug after evening meal before bedtime
• Allopurinol or sodium bicarbonate to maintain uric acid levels, alkalinization of urine

Perform/provide:
• Strict medical asepsis, protective isolation if WBC levels are low
• Increase fluid intake to 2-3 L/day to prevent urate deposits, calculi formation, unless contraindicated
• Diet low in purines: absence of organ meats (kidney, liver), dried beans, peas to maintain alkaline urine
• Rinsing of mouth tid-qid with water, club soda; brushing of teeth bid-tid with soft brush or cotton-tipped applicators for stomatitis; use unwaxed dental floss
• Nutritious diet with iron, vitamin supplements as ordered
• Storage in tightly closed container in cool environment

Evaluate:
• Therapeutic response: decreased size of tumor, spread of malignancy

Teach patient/family:
• To avoid foods with citric acid, hot or rough texture for stomatitis

• To report stomatitis: any bleeding, white spots, ulcerations in mouth; tell patient to examine mouth qd, report symptoms

• That contraceptive measures are recommended during therapy; to avoid breastfeeding

• To drink 10-12 (8 oz) glasses of fluid/day

• To notify prescriber of fever, chills, sore throat, nausea, vomiting, anorexia, diarrhea, bleeding, bruising, which may indicate blood dyscrasias

• To report signs of infection: fever, sore throat, flulike symptoms

• To report signs of anemia: fatigue, headache, faintness, shortness of breath, irritability

• To report bleeding: avoid use of razors, commercial mouthwash

• To avoid use of aspirin products, NSAIDs

---

meropenem (℞)

(mer-oh-pen′em)
Merrem IV
Func. class.: Antiinfective-misc.
Chem. class.: Carbapenem

Action: Interferes with cell wall replication of susceptible organisms; osmotically unstable cell wall swells, bursts from osmotic pressure

Uses: Serious infections caused by gram-positive bacteria: *Streptococcus pneumoniae,* group A β-hemolytic streptococci, enterococcus; gram-negative: *Klebsiella, Proteus, Escherichia coli, Pseudomonas aeruginosa;* appendicitis, peritonitis caused by *viridans* group streptococci; *Bacteroides fragilis, Bacterioides thetaiotamicron,* bacterial meningitis (≥3 mo)

Dosage and routes:
• *Adult:* IV 1 g q8h, given over 15-30 min or as an **IV BOL** 5-20 ml given over 3-5 min

• *Child ≥3 mo:* IV 20-40 mg/kg q8h (max 2g q8h meningitis)

• *Child >50 kg:* IV 1 g q8h (intraabdominal infection) or 2 g q8h (meningitis) given over 15-30 min or as an **IV BOL** 5-20 ml over 3-5 min

Renal disease
• *Adult:* IV CrCl 26-50 ml/min 1 g q12h; CrCl 10-25 ml/min 500 mg q12h; CrCl <10 ml/min 500 mg q24h
Available forms: Inj 500 mg, 1 g
Side effects/adverse reactions:
CNS: Fever, somnolence, *seizures,* dizziness, weakness, myoclonia, *headache*
GI: Diarrhea, nausea, vomiting, *pseudomembranous colitis, hepatitis,* glossitis
CV: Hypotension, palpitations
*HEMA: **Eosinophilia, neutropenia,*** decreased Hgb, Hct
INTEG: Rash, urticaria, *pruritus,* pain at injection site, phlebitis, erythema at inj site
*SYST: **Anaphylaxis***
RESP: Chest discomfort, dyspnea, hyperventilation
Contraindications: Hypersensitivity to meropenem or imipenem
Precautions: Pregnancy (B), lactation, elderly, renal disease
Pharmacokinetics:
IV: Onset immediate, peak dose dependent, half-life 1 hr, hepatic metabolism
Interactions:
• Increased meropenem plasma levels: probenecid
Lab test interferences:
Increase: AST, ALT, LDH, BUN, alk phosphatase, bilirubin, creatinine
False positive: Direct Coombs' test

◆ = Nursing alert   ⫸ = Herb-drug interaction   ⊗ = Do not crush

NURSING CONSIDERATIONS
Assess:
• Sensitivity to carbapenem antibiotics, penicillins
• Renal disease: lower dose may be required
• Bowel pattern qd; if severe diarrhea occurs, drug should be discontinued; may indicate pseudomembranous colitis
• For infection: temp, sputum, characteristics of wound, before, during, and after treatment
◆ Allergic reactions, anaphylaxis: rash, urticaria, pruritus; may occur few days after therapy begins
• Overgrowth of infection: perineal itching, fever, malaise, redness, pain, swelling, drainage, rash, diarrhea, change in cough, sputum
Administer:
• By IV INF or IV BOL
• After C&S is taken
• Reconstitute with 0.9% NaCl, D_5W, LR, dilute in 5-20 ml comp sol, give by direct IV over 3-5 min; give by intermittent inf, dilute in 5-20 ml of comp sol, give over 15-30 min
Additive compatibilities: Aminophylline, atropine, cimetidine, dexamethasone, dobutamine, dopamine, enalaprilat, fluconazole, furosemide, gentamicin, heparin, insulin (regular), magnesium sulfate, metoclopramide, morphine, norepinephrine, phenobarbital, ranitidine, vancomycin
Y-site compatibilities: Aminophylline, atenolol, atropine, cimetidine, dexamethasone, digoxin, diphenhydramine, enalaprilat, fluconazole, furosemide, gentamicin, heparin, insulin (regular), metoclopramide, morphine, norepinephrine, phenobarbital, vancomycin

Evaluate:
• Therapeutic response: negative C&S; absence of symptoms and signs of infection
Teach patient/family:
• To report severe diarrhea; may indicate pseudomembranous colitis
• To report sore throat, bruising, bleeding, joint pain; may indicate blood dyscrasias (rare)
• To report overgrowth of infection: black, furry tongue; vaginal itching; foul-smelling stools
• To avoid breastfeeding; drug is excreted in breast milk
Treatment of overdose: Epinephrine, antihistamines; resuscitate if needed (anaphylaxis)

---

mesalamine (R_x)
(mez-al'a-meen)
Asacol, Mesasal, Pentasa, Rowasa Salofalk*
Func. class.: GI antiinflammatory
Chem. class.: 5-Aminosalicylic acid

M

Action: May diminish inflammation by blocking cyclooxygenase, inhibiting prostaglandin production in colon; local action only
Uses: Mild to moderate active distal ulcerative colitis, proctosigmoiditis, proctitis
Dosage and routes:
• *Adult:* **RECT** 60 ml (4 g) hs, retained for 8 hr × 3-6 wk; **PO** 800 mg tid × 6 wk; **SUPP** 500 mg bid × 3-6 wk
Available forms: Rect susp 4 g/60 ml; supp 500 mg; tab del rel 400 mg; con rel cap 250 mg (Pentasa)
Side effects/adverse reactions:
CV: Pericarditis, myocarditis
GI: Cramps, gas, nausea, diarrhea, rectal pain, constipation

CNS: Headache, fever, dizziness, insomnia, asthenia, weakness, fatigue
INTEG: Rash, itching, acne
SYST: Flulike symptoms, malaise, back pain, peripheral edema, leg and joint pain, arthralgia, dysmenorrhea
EENT: Sore throat, cough, pharyngitis, rhinitis
Contraindications: Hypersensitivity to this drug or salicylates
Precautions: Renal disease, pregnancy (B), lactation, children, sulfite sensitivity
Do not confuse:
Asacol/Ansaid
Pharmacokinetics:
RECT: Primarily excreted in feces but some in urine as metabolite; half-life 1 hr, metabolite half-life 5-10 hr
Interactions:
• Increased mesalamine absorption: omeprazole
NURSING CONSIDERATIONS
Assess:
• GI symptoms: cramps, gas, nausea, diarrhea, rectal pain; if severe, drug should be discontinued
• Renal function prior to treatment
Administer:
• May give orally; tabs should be swallowed whole
• Rectally; drug should be given hs, retained until morning
Perform/provide:
• Storage at room temperature
Evaluate:
• Therapeutic response: absence of pain, bleeding from GI tract, decrease in number of diarrhea stools
Teach patient/family:
• That usual course of therapy is 3-6 wk
• To shake bottle well (rectal susp)
• Method of rectal administration
• To inform prescriber of GI symptoms
🚫 Not to break, crush, or chew tabs

• To report abdominal cramping, pain, diarrhea with blood, headache, fever, rash, chest pain; drug should be discontinued

---

mesoridazine (℞)
(mez-oh-rid′a-zeen)
Serentil, Serentil Concentrate
Func. class.: Antipsychotic, neuroleptic
Chem. class.: Phenothiazine, piperidine

Action: Depresses cerebral cortex, hypothalamus, limbic system, which control activity, aggression; blocks neurotransmission produced by dopamine at synapse; exhibits strong α-adrenergic, anticholinergic blocking action; mechanism for antipsychotic effects is unclear
Uses: Psychotic disorders, schizophrenia, anxiety, alcoholism, behavioral problems in mental deficiency, chronic brain syndrome
Dosage and routes:
Schizophrenia
• *Adult:* PO 50 mg tid, optimum dose 100-400 mg/day; **IM** 25 mg may repeat ½-1 hr; dosage range 25-200 mg/day
Behavior problems
• *Adult:* PO 25 mg tid; optimum dose 75-300 mg/day
• *Geriatric:* PO 10 mg qd-bid, increase q3-7days by 10-25 mg to desired dose
Alcoholism
• *Adult:* PO 25 mg bid; optimum dose 50-200 mg/day
Psychoneurotic disorders
• *Adult:* PO 10 mg tid; optimum dose 30-150 mg/day
Available forms: Tabs 10, 25, 50, 100 mg; conc 25 mg/ml; inj 25 mg/ml

---

 ◆ = Nursing alert   🖋 = Herb-drug interaction   🚫 = Do not crush

Side effects/adverse reactions:

*RESP: **Laryngospasm,** dyspnea, **respiratory depression***

CNS: EPS: pseudoparkinsonism, akathisia, dystonia, tardive dyskinesia, drowsiness, headache

*HEMA: **Anemia, leukopenia, leukocytosis, agranulocytosis***

INTEG: Rash, photosensitivity, dermatitis

EENT: Blurred vision, glaucoma

GI: Dry mouth, nausea, vomiting, anorexia, constipation, diarrhea, jaundice, weight gain

GU: Urinary retention, urinary frequency, enuresis, impotence, amenorrhea, gynecomastia

CV: Orthostatic hypotension, hypertension, **cardiac arrest,** ECG changes, tachycardia

Contraindications: Hypersensitivity, severe CNS depression, circulatory collapse, liver damage, cerebral arteriosclerosis, coronary disease, severe hypertension/hypotension, blood dyscrasias, coma, brain damage, bone marrow depression, narrow-angle glaucoma

Precautions: Pregnancy (C), lactation, seizure disorders, hypertension, hepatic disease, cardiac disease, prostatic hypertrophy, intestinal obstruction, respiratory conditions

Do not confuse:

Serentil/Sinequan

Pharmacokinetics:

PO: Onset erratic, peak 2 hr, duration 4-6 hr

IM: Onset 15-30 min, peak 30 min, duration 6-8 hr

Metabolized by liver, excreted in urine, crosses placenta, enters breast milk

Interactions:

• Oversedation: other CNS depressants, alcohol, barbiturate anesthetics

• Decreased absorption: aluminum hydroxide, magnesium hydroxide antacids

• Increased anticholinergic effects: anticholinergics

🍃 Increased anticholinergic effect: henbane

Lab test interferences:

Increase: LFTs, cardiac enzymes, cholesterol, blood glucose, prolactin, bilirubin, PBI, cholinesterase, [131]I

Decrease: Hormones (blood, urine)

False-positive: Pregnancy tests, PKU

False-negative: Urinary steroids, 17-OHCS

NURSING CONSIDERATIONS
Assess:

• Mental status before initial administration

• Swallowing of PO medication; check for hoarding or giving to other patients

• I&O ratio; palpate bladder if low urinary output occurs

• Bilirubin, CBC, liver function studies monthly

• Urinalysis is recommended before, during prolonged therapy

• Affect, orientation, LOC, reflexes, gait, coordination, sleep pattern disturbances

• B/P standing and lying, pulse, respirations q4h during initial treatment; establish baseline before starting treatment; report drops of 30 mm Hg

• Dizziness, faintness, palpitations, tachycardia on rising

• EPS including akathisia (inability to sit still, no pattern to movements), tardive dyskinesia (bizarre movements of jaw, mouth, tongue, extremities), pseudoparkinsonism (rigidity, tremors, pill rolling, shuffling gait)

◆ For neuroleptic malignant syndrome: hyperthermia, altered men-

M

tal status, muscle rigidity, increased CPK

• Constipation, urinary retention daily; if these occur, increase bulk, water in diet

Administer:

• Antiparkinsonian agent after securing order from prescriber for extrapyramidal symptoms

• Concentrate mixed in distilled water, orange, grape juice; do not prepare, store bulk dilutions

• Use gloves when preparing sol, prevent contact with skin and clothes

• IM inj into large muscle mass; do not use if precipitate present

• Lowest possible dose to elderly to minimize side effects

Perform/provide:

• Decreased sensory input by dimming lights, avoiding loud noises

• Supervised ambulation until stabilized on medication; do not involve in strenuous exercise program because fainting is possible; patient should not stand still for long periods

• Dose reduction in patients treated for behavior problems

• Increased fluids to prevent constipation

• Sips of water, candy, gum for dry mouth

• Storage in airtight, light-resistant container

Evaluate:

• Therapeutic response: decrease in emotional excitement, hallucinations, delusions, paranoia, and reorganization of patterns of thought, speech

Teach patient/family:

• That orthostatic hypotension is common and to rise from sitting or lying position gradually; to avoid hazardous activities until stabilized on medication

• To remain lying down for at least 30 min after IM injection

• To avoid hot tubs, hot showers, tub baths; hypotension may occur

• To avoid abrupt withdrawal of mesoridazine, or EPS may result; drug should be withdrawn slowly

• To avoid OTC preparations (cough, hay fever, cold) unless approved by prescriber; serious drug interactions may occur; to avoid use with alcohol, CNS depressants; increased drowsiness may occur

• To use sunscreen during sun exposure to prevent burns

• Regarding compliance with drug regimen

• About necessity for meticulous oral hygiene, since oral candidiasis may occur

• To report sore throat, malaise, fever, bleeding, mouth sores; if these occur, a CBC should be drawn and drug discontinued

• That in hot weather heat stroke may occur; take extra precautions to stay cool

Treatment of overdose: Lavage if orally ingested; provide an airway; *do not induce vomiting*

---

metaproterenol (℞)
(met-a-proe-ter´e-nole)
Alupent, Arm-A-Med,
Dey-Lute Metaproterenol
**metaproterenol
sulfate** (℞)
Metaprel
Func. class.: Bronchodilator-selective β₂-agonist

Action: Relaxes bronchial smooth muscle by direct action on β₂-adrenergic receptors with increased levels of cAMP with increased bronchodilation, diuresis, cardiac CNS stimulation

Uses: Bronchial asthma, bronchospasm

 = Nursing alert   = Herb-drug interaction   = Do not crush

Dosage and routes:
• *Adult and child >12 yr:* **INH** 2-3 inhalations; may repeat q3-4h, not to exceed 12 inhalations/day
• *Adult:* **PO** 20 mg q6-8h
• *Geriatric:* **PO** 10 mg tid-qid, initially
• *Child >9 yr or >27 kg:* **PO** 20 mg q6-8h or 0.4-0.9 mg/kg tid
• *Child 6-9 yr or <27 kg:* **PO** 10 mg q6-8h or 0.4-0.9 mg/kg tid
• *Child 2-6 yr:* **PO** 1.3-2.6 mg/kg divided q6-8h

Available forms: Tabs 10, 20 mg; aerosol 0.65 mg/dose; syr 10 mg/5 ml; sol for inh 0.4%, 0.6%, 5%

Side effects/adverse reactions:
CNS: Tremors, anxiety, insomnia, headache, dizziness, stimulation
CV: Palpitations, tachycardia, hypertension, dysrhythmias, ***cardiac arrest*** (high dose)
GI: Nausea, vomiting
*RESP: **Paradoxical bronchospasm***

Contraindications: Hypersensitivity to sympathomimetics, narrow-angle glaucoma

Precautions: Pregnancy (C), cardiac disorders, hyperthyroidism, diabetes mellitus, prostatic hypertrophy

Do not confuse:
Alupent/Atrovent

Pharmacokinetics: Well absorbed (PO)
PO: Onset 15-30 min, peak 1 hr, duration 4 hr, excreted in urine as metabolites
INH: Onset 5 min, peak 1 hr, duration 4 hr

Interactions:
• Increased effects of both drugs: other sympathomimetics
• Decreased action of β-blockers, oral hypoglycemics
• Hypertensive crisis: MAOIs
• Increased effect: ephedra

Lab test interferences:
Decrease: Potassium

NURSING CONSIDERATIONS
Assess:
• Respiratory function: vital capacity, forced expiratory volume, ABGs; also B/P; lung sounds, secretions before and after treatment
• Tolerance over long-term therapy; dose may have to be changed; check for rebound bronchospasm

Administer:
• 2 hr before hs to avoid sleeplessness
• PO with food for GI upset

Perform/provide:
• Storage at room temperature; do not use discolored sol
• Spacer device for elderly

Evaluate:
• Therapeutic response: absence of dyspnea, wheezing; improved ABGs

Teach patient/family:
• To increase fluid intake (2-3 L/day) to liquefy secretions
• Not to use OTC medications; excess stimulation may occur
• To notify prescriber of headaches, chest pain, weakness, dizziness, anxiety
• Use of inhaler; review package insert with patient
• To avoid getting aerosol in eyes
• To wash inhaler in warm water and dry qd
• All aspects of drug; avoid smoking, smoke-filled rooms, persons with respiratory infections

M

metformin (℞)
(met-for′min)
Glucophage, Glucophage XR
Func. class.: Antidiabetic, oral
Chem. class.: Biguanide

Action: Inhibits hepatic glucose production and increases sensitivity of peripheral tissue to insulin
Uses: Stable adult-onset diabetes mellitus (type II) (NIDDM)

Dosage and routes:
• *Adult:* **PO** 500 mg bid initially, then increase to desired response 1-3 g; dosage adjustment q2-3wk or 850 mg qd with morning meal with dosage increased every other wk, max 2500 mg/day
• *Geriatric:* **PO,** use lowest effective dose
Available forms: Tabs 500, 850 mg
Side effects/adverse reactions:
CNS: Headache, weakness, dizziness, drowsiness, tinnitus, fatigue, vertigo, *agitation*
GI: Nausea, vomiting, diarrhea, heartburn, anorexia, metallic taste
HEMA: **Thrombocytopenia,** decreased vit B_{12} concentration
INTEG: Rash
ENDO: Lactic acidosis, hypoglycemia
Contraindications: Hypersensitivity, hepatic, renal disease, alcoholism, cardiopulmonary disease, history of lactic acidosis
Precautions: Previous hypersensitivity, pregnancy (B), elderly, thyroid disease, CHF, renal disease
Pharmacokinetics: Excreted by the kidneys unchanged 35%-50%, half-life 1½-5 hr, terminal 6-20 hr, peak 1-3 hr
Interactions:
• Increased metformin level: cimetidine, digoxin, morphine, procainamide, quinidine, ranitidine, triamterene, vancomycin
• Increased hypoglycemia: cimetidine, calcium channel blockers, corticosteroids, estrogens, oral contraceptives, phenothiazines, sympathomimetics, diuretics, thyroid replacement, isoniazid, phenytoin
• Do not give with radiologic contrast media; may cause renal failure
🌿 Quinine: increased metformin level

NURSING CONSIDERATIONS
Assess:
• For hypoglycemic reactions (sweating, weakness, dizziness, anxiety, tremors, hunger), hyperglycemic reactions soon after meals
• CBC (baseline, q3mo) during treatment; check LFTs periodically AST, LDH, renal studies: BUN, creatinine during treatment
🔷 For lactic acidosis: malaise, myalgia, abdominal distress; risk increases with age, poor renal function
Administer:
PO
• Twice a day given with meals to decrease GI upset and provide best absorption, may also be taken as a single dose
• Tabs crushed and mixed with meal or fluids for patients with difficulty swallowing
Perform/provide:
• Conversion from other oral hypoglycemic agents; change may be made without gradual dosage change; monitor serum or urine glucose and ketones tid during conversion
• Storage in tight container in cool environment
Evaluate:
• Therapeutic response: decrease in polyuria, polydipsia, polyphagia; clear sensorium; absence of dizziness; stable gait, blood glucose at normal level
Teach patient/family:
🔷 Lactic acidosis symptoms: hyperventilation, fatigue, malaise, myalgia, somnolence; to notify prescriber immediately
• To use capillary blood glucose test or Chemstrip tid
• The symptoms of hypo/hyperglycemia, what to do about each
• That drug must be continued on

🔷 = Nursing alert   🌿 = Herb-drug interaction   🚫 = Do not crush daily basis; explain consequence of discontinuing drug abruptly

• To avoid OTC medications unless approved by prescriber

• That diabetes is a lifelong illness; that this drug is not a cure; only controls symptoms

• That all food included in diet plan must be eaten to prevent hypoglycemia

• To carry emergency ID and glucagon emergency kit for emergencies

Treatment of overdose: Glucose 25 g IV via dextrose 50% sol, 50 ml or 1 mg glucagon

methadone (℞)

(meth'a-done)

Dolophine, methadone, Methadose

Func. class.: Opiate analgesic

Chem. class.: Synthetic diphenylheptane derivative

Controlled Substance Schedule II

Action: Depresses pain impulse transmission at the spinal cord level by interacting with opioid receptors, produce CNS depression

Uses: Severe pain, opiate withdrawal

Dosage and routes:

Severe pain

• *Adult:* **PO/SC/IM** 2.5-10 mg q3-4h prn

Opiate withdrawal

• *Adult:* **PO** 15-40 mg/day individualized initially, then 20-120 mg/day titrated to patient response

• *Child:* 0.05-0.1 mg/kg/dose q6-12h

Renal disease

• CrCl 10-50 ml/min dose q8h; CrCl <10 ml/min dose q8-12h

Available forms: Inj 10 mg/ml; tabs 5, 10 mg; oral sol 5, 10 mg/5 ml; dispersible tabs 40 mg; oral conc 10 mg/ml; oral sol 5 mg/5 ml, 10 mg/5 ml, 10 mg/10 ml

Side effects/adverse reactions:

*CNS: Drowsiness, dizziness, confusion, headache, sedation, euphoria, **seizures***

GI: Nausea, vomiting, anorexia, constipation, cramps, biliary tract spasm

GU: Increased urinary output, dysuria, urinary retention

INTEG: Rash, urticaria, bruising, flushing, diaphoresis, pruritus

EENT: Tinnitus, blurred vision, miosis, diplopia

CV: Palpitations, bradycardia, change in B/P, **cardiac arrest, shock**

*RESP: **Respiratory depression, respiratory arrest***

Contraindications: Hypersensitivity to this drug or chlorobutanol (inj), addiction (opiate)

Precautions: Addictive personality, pregnancy (C), lactation, increased intracranial pressure, MI (acute), severe heart disease, respiratory depression, hepatic disease, renal disease, children <18 yr, elderly

Do not confuse:

methadone/methylphenidate

Pharmacokinetics:

PO: Onset 30-60 min, peak 1½-2 hr, duration 6-8 hr, cumulative 22-48 hr

SC/IM: Onset 10-20 min, peak 1½-2 hr, duration 4-6 hr, cumulative 22-48 hr

Metabolized by liver; excreted by kidneys; crosses placenta; excreted in breast milk; half-life 15-30 hr, extended interval with continued dosing; 90% bound to plasma proteins

Interactions:

• Increased effects with other CNS depressants: alcohol, opiates, sedative/hypnotics, antipsychotics, skeletal muscle relaxants, rifampin, phenytoin

M

• Unpredictable reactions: MAOIs, do not use together

Lab test interferences:

Increase: Amylase

NURSING CONSIDERATIONS

Assess:

• For pain: type, location, intensity, grimacing before and 1½-2 hr after administration; use pain scoring

• I&O ratio; check for decreasing output; may indicate urinary retention

• CNS changes: dizziness, drowsiness, hallucinations, euphoria, LOC, pupil reaction

• Allergic reactions: rash, urticaria

• Respiratory dysfunction: respiratory depression, character, rate, rhythm; notify prescriber if respirations are <10/min

Administer:

• With antiemetic if nausea/vomiting occurs

• When pain is beginning to return; determine dosage interval by patient response

• Rotating inj sites, give deep in large muscle mass (IM)

Perform/provide:

• Storage in light-resistant container at room temperature

• Assistance with ambulation

• Safety measures: night-light, call bell within easy reach

Evaluate:

• Therapeutic response: decrease in pain, successful opiate withdrawal

Teach patient/family:

• To report any symptoms of CNS changes, allergic reactions

• That physical dependency may result from extended use

⬥ Withdrawal symptoms may occur: nausea, vomiting, cramps, fever, faintness, anorexia

Treatment of overdose: Naloxone (Narcan) 0.2-0.8 mg IV, O_2, IV fluids, vasopressors

---

methamphetamine (℞)

(meth-am-fet′a-meen)

Desoxyn, Desoxyn Gradumet

Func. class.: CNS stimulant

Chem. class.: Amphetamine

Controlled Substance Schedule II

Action: Increases release of norepinephrine and dopamine in cerebral cortex to reticular activating system

Uses: Short-term adjunct in exogenous obesity, attention deficit disorder with hyperactivity

Dosage and routes:

Attention deficit disorder

• *Child ≥6 yr:* **PO** 2.5-5 mg qd or bid increasing by 5 mg/wk

Obesity

• *Adult:* **PO** 2.5-5 mg, 30 min ac or 10-15 mg long-acting tab qd in AM

Available forms: Tabs 5 mg; tabs long-acting 5, 10, 15 mg

Side effects/adverse reactions:

CNS: Hyperactivity, insomnia, restlessness, talkativeness, dizziness, headache, chills, stimulation, dysphoria, irritability, aggressiveness, tremor

GI: Anorexia, dry mouth, diarrhea, constipation, weight loss, metallic taste, cramps

GU: Impotence, change in libido

*CV: Palpitations, **tachycardia**,* hypertension, decreased heart rate, ***dysrhythmia***

INTEG: Urticaria

Contraindications: Hypersensitivity to sympathomimetic amines, hyperthyroidism, hypertension, glaucoma hypertrophy, severe arteriosclerosis, drug abuse, cardiovascular disease, anxiety

---

⬥ = Nursing alert   🌿 = Herb-drug interaction   🚫 = Do not crush

Alendronate Sodium

Fosamax
5mg: Merck

Fosamax
10mg: Merck

Fosamax
40mg: Merck

Amlodipine

Norvasc
2.5mg: Pfizer

Norvasc
5mg: Pfizer

Norvasc
10mg: Pfizer

Amoxicillin

Amoxil
125mg: SmithKline Beecham

Amoxil
250mg: SmithKline Beecham

Amoxil
250mg: SmithKline Beecham

Amoxil
500mg: SmithKline Beecham

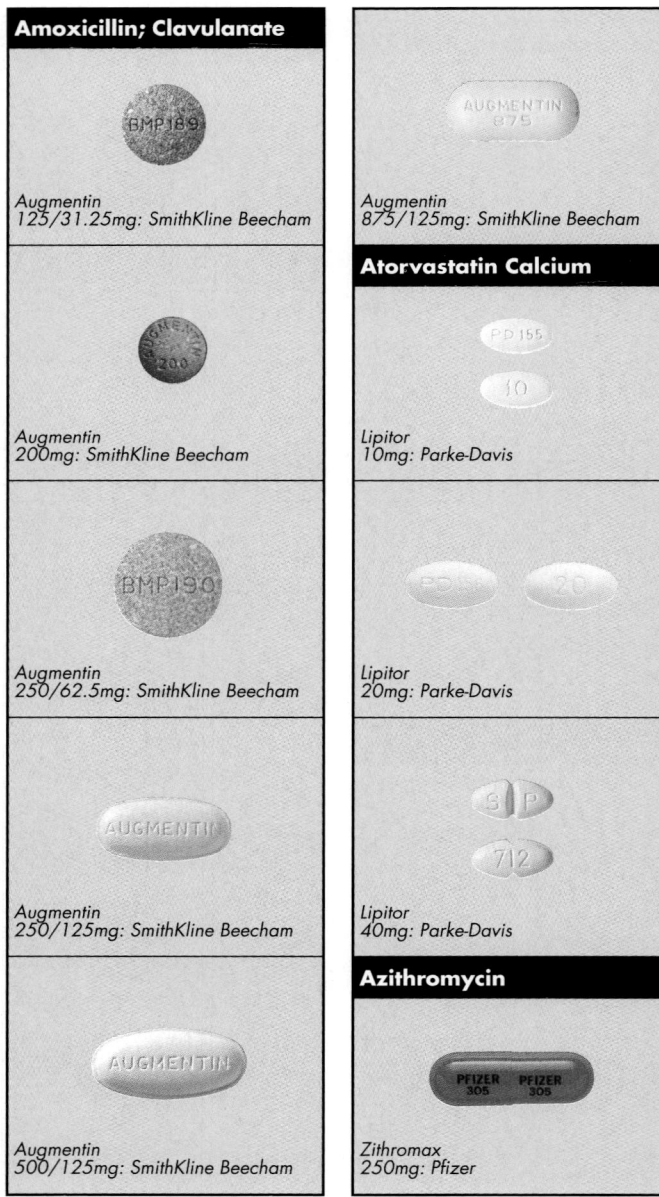

Amoxicillin; Clavulanate

Augmentin
125/31.25mg: SmithKline Beecham

Augmentin
200mg: SmithKline Beecham

Augmentin
250/62.5mg: SmithKline Beecham

Augmentin
250/125mg: SmithKline Beecham

Augmentin
500/125mg: SmithKline Beecham

Augmentin
875/125mg: SmithKline Beecham

Atorvastatin Calcium

Lipitor
10mg: Parke-Davis

Lipitor
20mg: Parke-Davis

Lipitor
40mg: Parke-Davis

Azithromycin

Zithromax
250mg: Pfizer

Zithromax
250mg: Pfizer

Benazepril HCl

Lotensin
5mg: Novartis

Lotensin
10mg: Novartis

Lotensin
20mg: Novartis

Lotensin
40mg: Novartis

Bupropion HCl

Wellbutrin SR
100mg: Glaxo Wellcome

Wellbutrin SR
150mg: Glaxo Wellcome

Cefprozil

Cefzil
250mg: Bristol-Myers Squibb

Cefzil
500mg: Bristol-Myers Squibb

Cefuroxime Axetil

Ceftin
125mg: Glaxo Wellcome

Ciprofloxacin HCl

Ceftin
250mg: Glaxo Wellcome

Cipro
250mg: Miles

Ceftin
500mg: Glaxo Wellcome

Cipro
500mg: Miles

Celecoxib

Cipro
750mg: Miles

Celebrex
100mg: Searle

Clarithromycin

Celebrex
200mg: Searle

Biaxin
250mg: Abbott

Cetirizine

Zyrtec
10mg: Pfizer

Biaxin
500mg: Abbott

Biaxin XL
500mg: Abbott

Digoxin

Lanoxicaps
0.1mg: Glaxo Wellcome

Diltiazem HCl

Cardizem CD
120mg: Hoechst Marion Roussel

Cardizem CD
180mg: Hoechst Marion Roussel

Cardizem CD
240mg: Hoechst Marion Roussel

Cardizem CD
300mg: Hoechst Marion Roussel

Divalproex

Depakote
125mg: Abbott

Depakote
250mg: Abbott

Depakote
500mg: Abbott

Doxazosin

Cardura
1mg: Roerig

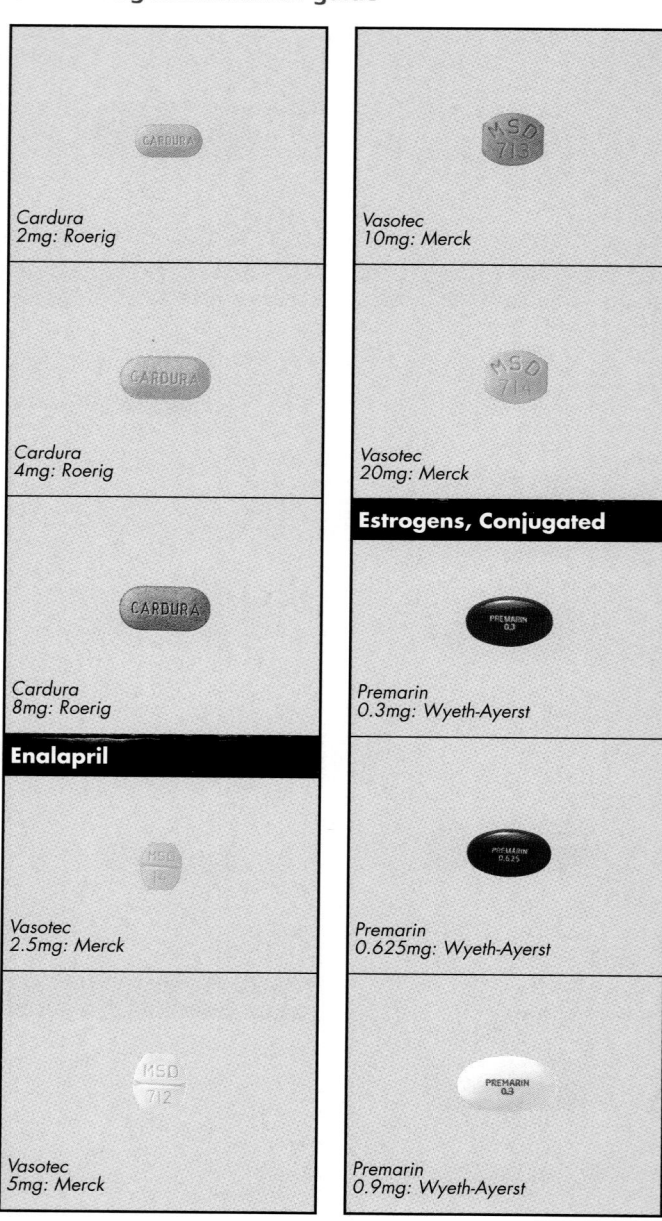

Cardura
2mg: Roerig

Vasotec
10mg: Merck

Cardura
4mg: Roerig

Vasotec
20mg: Merck

Estrogens, Conjugated

Cardura
8mg: Roerig

Premarin
0.3mg: Wyeth-Ayerst

Enalapril

Vasotec
2.5mg: Merck

Premarin
0.625mg: Wyeth-Ayerst

Vasotec
5mg: Merck

Premarin
0.9mg: Wyeth-Ayerst

Premarin
1.25mg: Wyeth-Ayerst

Premarin
2.5mg: Wyeth-Ayerst

Estrogens, Conjugated, Medroxyprogesterone

Prempro
0.625/2.5mg: Wyeth-Ayerst

Premphase
0.625/5mg: Wyeth-Ayerst

Ethinyl Estradiol; Levonorgestrel

Triphasil Inert/ 0.03/0.125/0.03/
0.05/0.04/0.075mg: Wyeth-Ayerst

Famotidine

Pepcid
20mg: Merck

Pepcid
40mg: Merck

Fexofenadine HCl

Allegra
180mg: Aventis

Allegra
60mg: Hoechst Marion Roussel

Fluconazole

Diflucan
50mg: Roerig

Diflucan
100mg: Roerig

Diflucan
200mg: Roerig

Fluoxetine HCl

Prozac
10mg: Dista

Prozac
20mg: Dista

Prozac
10mg: Lilly

Gabapentin

Neurontin
100mg: Parke-Davis

Neurontin
300mg: Parke-Davis

Neurontin
400mg: Parke-Davis

Glipizide

Glucotrol XL
5mg: Pfizer

Glucotrol XL
10mg: Pfizer

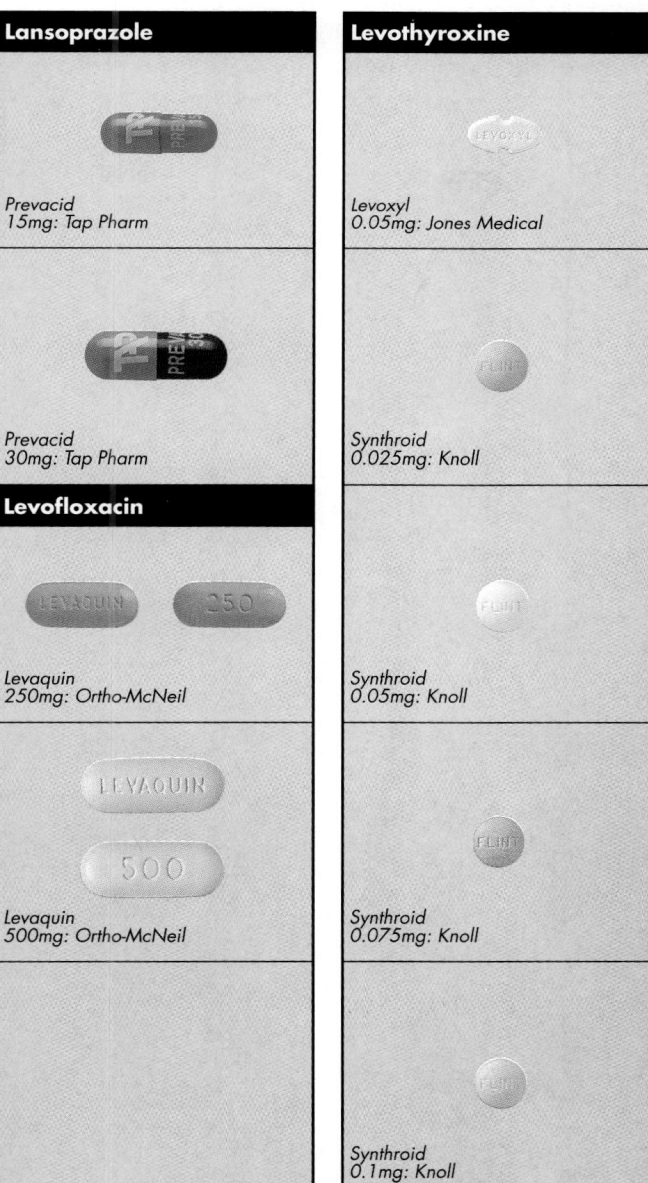

Lansoprazole

Prevacid
15mg: Tap Pharm

Prevacid
30mg: Tap Pharm

Levofloxacin

Levaquin
250mg: Ortho-McNeil

Levaquin
500mg: Ortho-McNeil

Levothyroxine

Levoxyl
0.05mg: Jones Medical

Synthroid
0.025mg: Knoll

Synthroid
0.05mg: Knoll

Synthroid
0.075mg: Knoll

Synthroid
0.1mg: Knoll

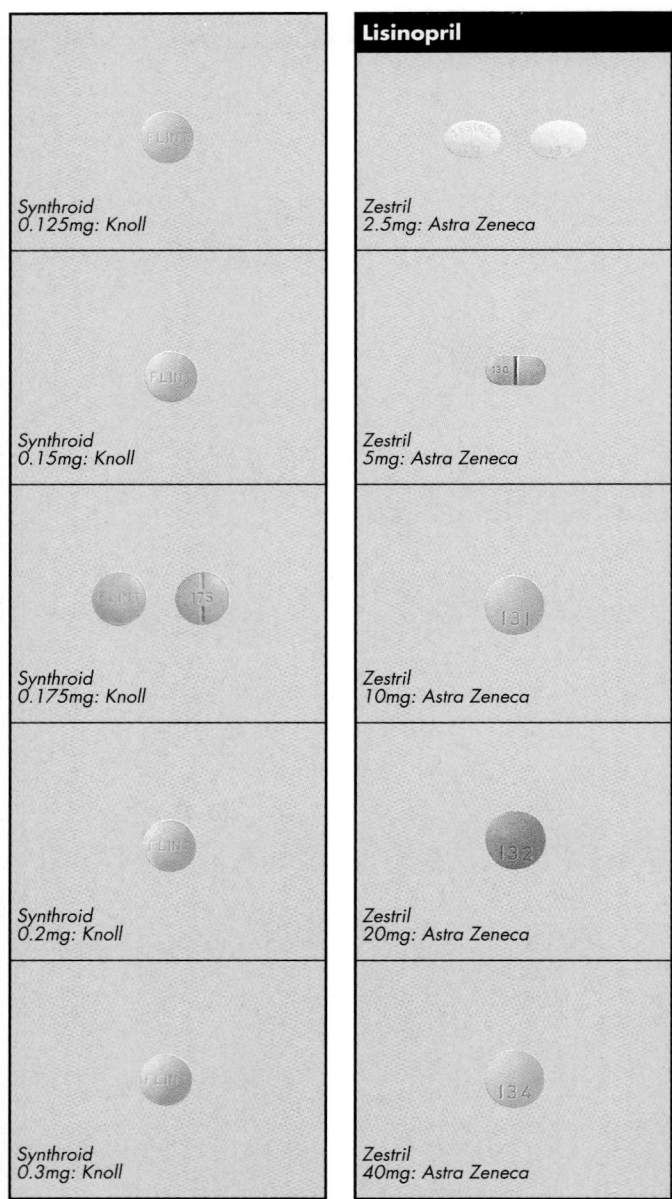

Lisinopril

Synthroid
0.125mg: Knoll

Zestril
2.5mg: Astra Zeneca

Synthroid
0.15mg: Knoll

Zestril
5mg: Astra Zeneca

Synthroid
0.175mg: Knoll

Zestril
10mg: Astra Zeneca

Synthroid
0.2mg: Knoll

Zestril
20mg: Astra Zeneca

Synthroid
0.3mg: Knoll

Zestril
40mg: Astra Zeneca

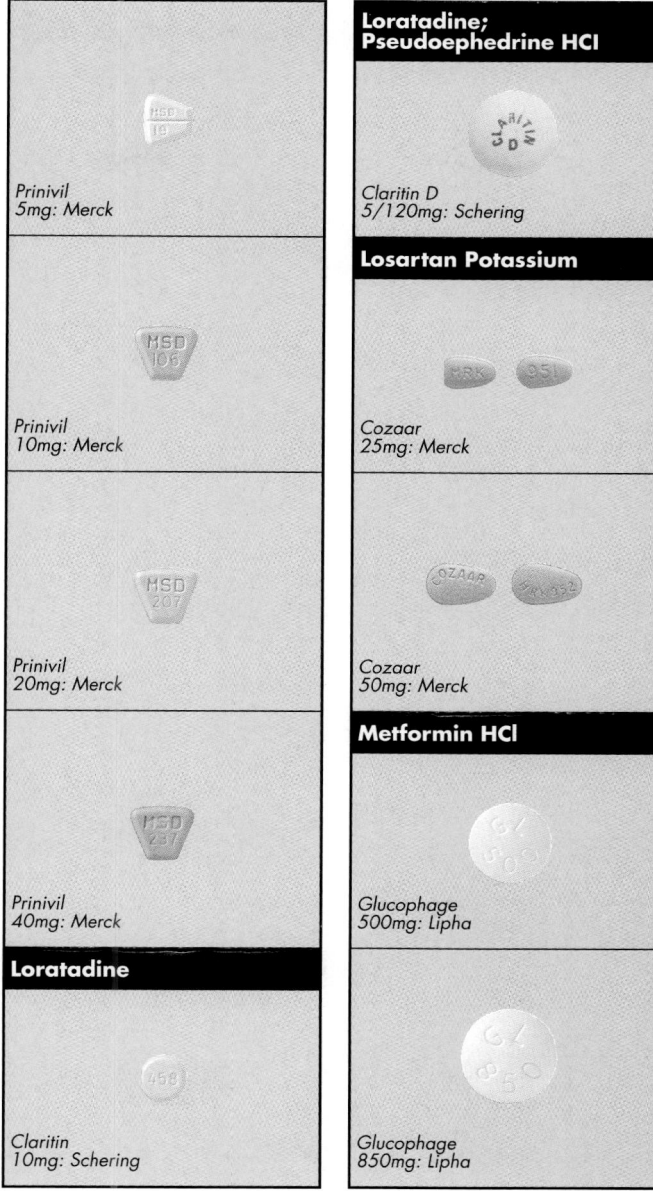

Prinivil
5mg: Merck

Prinivil
10mg: Merck

Prinivil
20mg: Merck

Prinivil
40mg: Merck

Loratadine

Claritin
10mg: Schering

**Loratadine;
Pseudoephedrine HCl**

Claritin D
5/120mg: Schering

Losartan Potassium

Cozaar
25mg: Merck

Cozaar
50mg: Merck

Metformin HCl

Glucophage
500mg: Lipha

Glucophage
850mg: Lipha

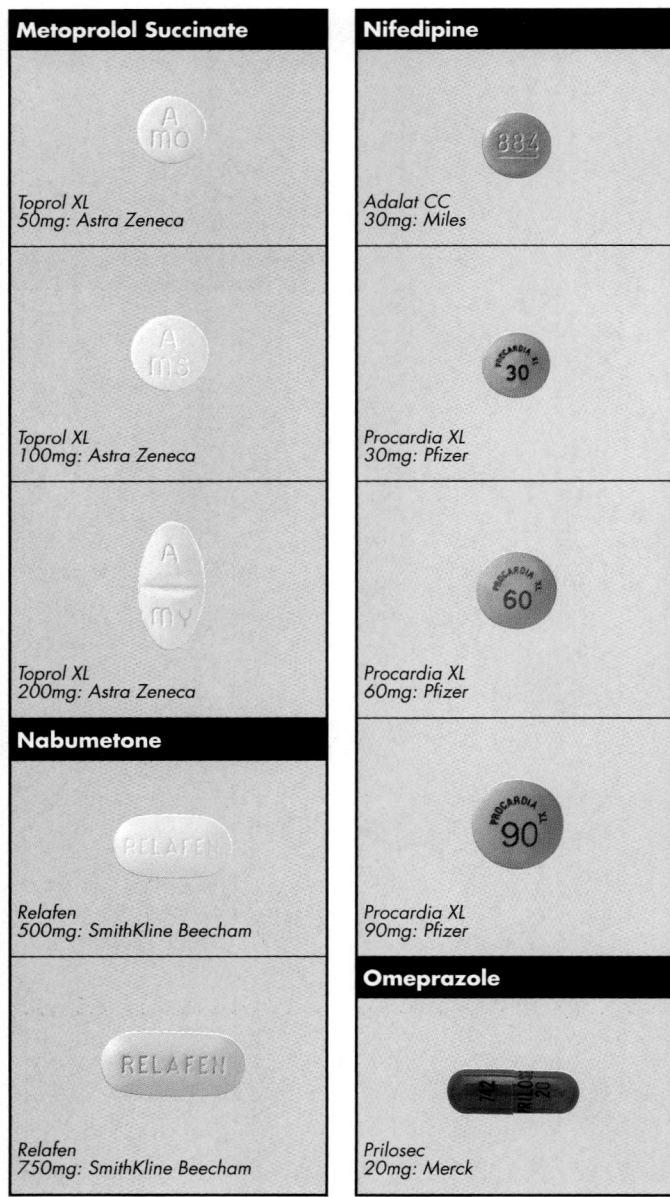

Metoprolol Succinate

Toprol XL
50mg: Astra Zeneca

Toprol XL
100mg: Astra Zeneca

Toprol XL
200mg: Astra Zeneca

Nabumetone

Relafen
500mg: SmithKline Beecham

Relafen
750mg: SmithKline Beecham

Nifedipine

Adalat CC
30mg: Miles

Procardia XL
30mg: Pfizer

Procardia XL
60mg: Pfizer

Procardia XL
90mg: Pfizer

Omeprazole

Prilosec
20mg: Merck

Paroxetine HCl

Paxil
10mg: SmithKline Beecham

Paxil
20mg: SmithKline Beecham

Paxil
30mg: SmithKline Beecham

Paxil
40mg: SmithKline Beecham

Penicillin V Potassium

Veetids
250mg: Bristol-Myers Squibb

Veetids
500mg: Bristol-Myers Squibb

Potassium Chloride

K-Dur
750mg: Schering

K-Dur
1500mg: Schering

Pravastatin

Pravachol
10mg: Bristol-Myers Squibb

Pravachol
20mg: Bristol-Myers Squibb

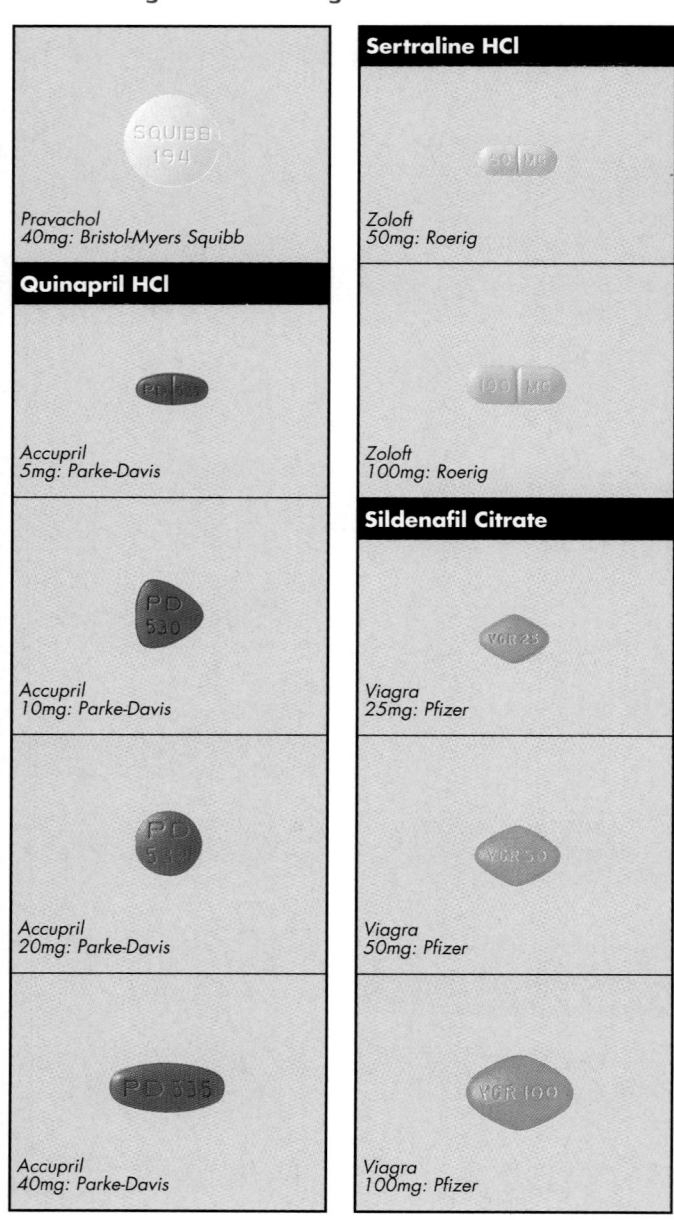

Pravachol
40mg: Bristol-Myers Squibb

Quinapril HCl

Accupril
5mg: Parke-Davis

Accupril
10mg: Parke-Davis

Accupril
20mg: Parke-Davis

Accupril
40mg: Parke-Davis

Sertraline HCl

Zoloft
50mg: Roerig

Zoloft
100mg: Roerig

Sildenafil Citrate

Viagra
25mg: Pfizer

Viagra
50mg: Pfizer

Viagra
100mg: Pfizer

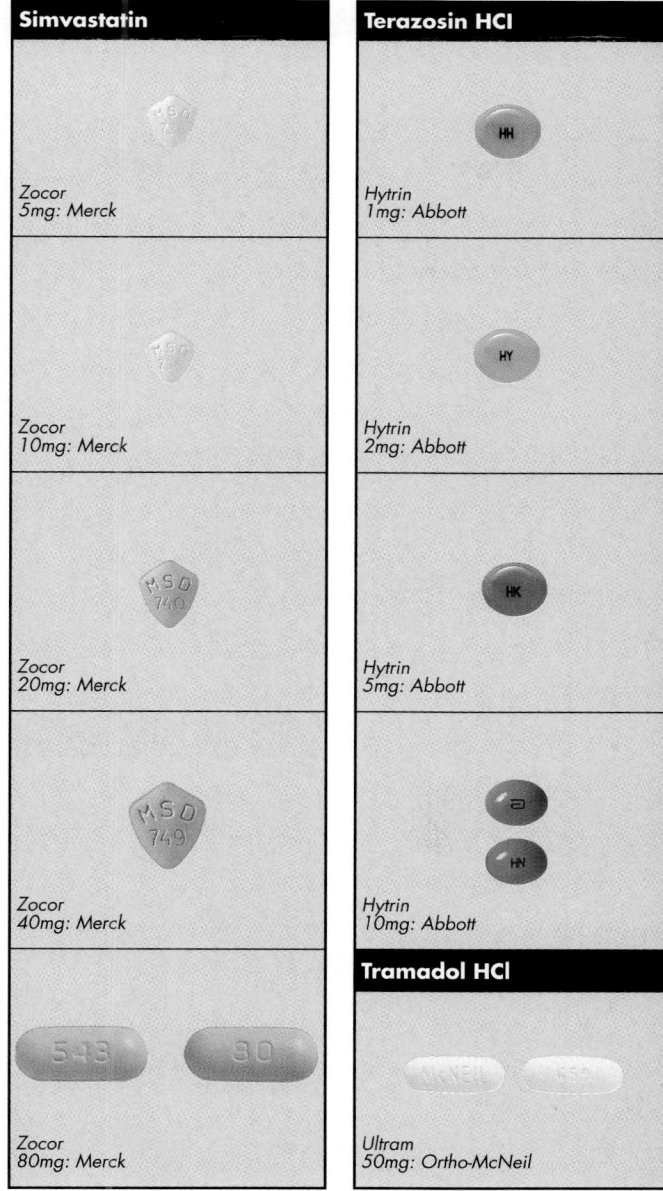

Simvastatin

Zocor
5mg: Merck

Zocor
10mg: Merck

Zocor
20mg: Merck

Zocor
40mg: Merck

Zocor
80mg: Merck

Terazosin HCl

Hytrin
1mg: Abbott

Hytrin
2mg: Abbott

Hytrin
5mg: Abbott

Hytrin
10mg: Abbott

Tramadol HCl

Ultram
50mg: Ortho-McNeil

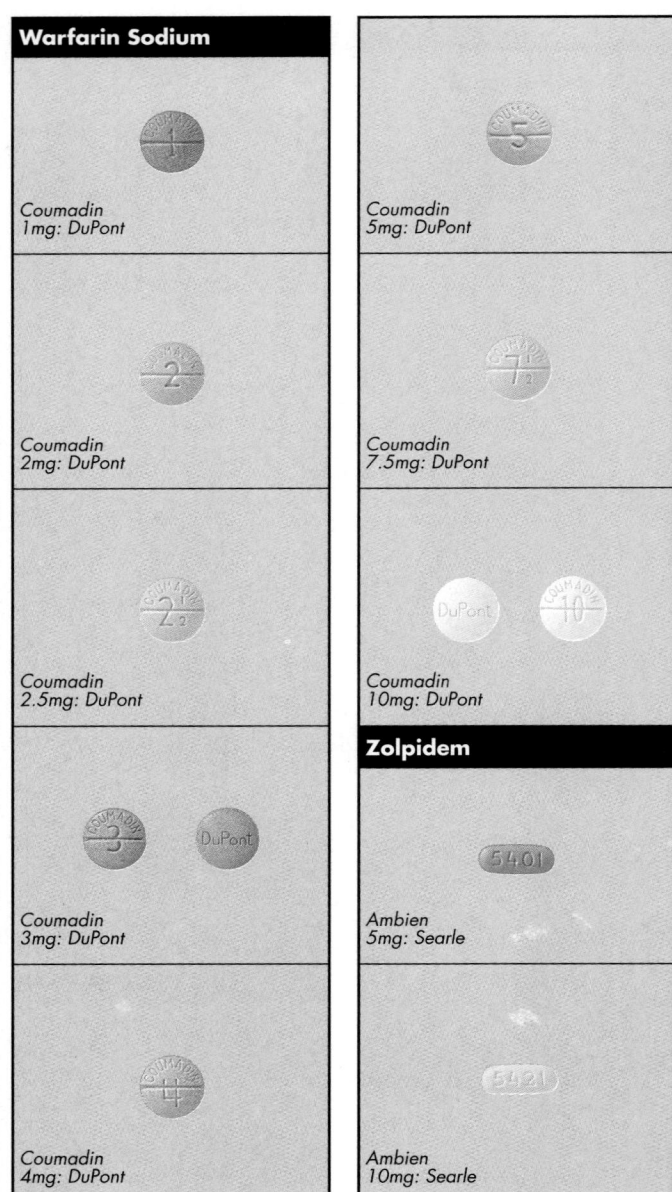

Warfarin Sodium

Coumadin
1mg: DuPont

Coumadin
2mg: DuPont

Coumadin
2.5mg: DuPont

Coumadin
3mg: DuPont

Coumadin
4mg: DuPont

Coumadin
5mg: DuPont

Coumadin
7.5mg: DuPont

Coumadin
10mg: DuPont

Zolpidem

Ambien
5mg: Searle

Ambien
10mg: Searle

Precautions: Gilles de la Tourette's disorder, pregnancy (C), lactation, child <3 yr

Pharmacokinetics:

PO: Duration 3-6 hr, metabolized by liver, excreted by kidneys, crosses blood-brain barrier

Interactions:

• Hypertensive crisis: MAOIs or within 14 days of MAOIs

• Increased effect of methamphetamine: acetazolamide, antacids, sodium bicarbonate

• Decreased effects of methamphetamine: barbiturates, tricyclics, ascorbic acid, ammonium chloride

• Drug/food: increased amine effects: caffeine products

🖉 May increase effects of methamphetamine, increased insomnia: melatonin

NURSING CONSIDERATIONS
Assess:

• VS, B/P; may reverse antihypertensives; check patients with cardiac disease more often

• CBC, urinalysis, in diabetes: blood sugar, urine sugar; insulin changes may have to be made, since eating will decrease

• Height, growth rate in children; growth rate may be decreased

• Mental status: mood, sensorium, affect, stimulation, insomnia, aggressiveness

• Physical dependency: should not be used for extended time; dose should be discontinued gradually; tolerance will occur (long-term use)

◆ Withdrawal symptoms: headache, nausea, vomiting, muscle pain, weakness

• Weight per regimen protocol

Administer:

• At least 6 hr before hs to avoid sleeplessness

• For obesity only if patient is on program including dietary changes, exercise; patient will develop tolerance; loss of weight won't occur without additional methods; give 2 hr before meals

• Gum, hard candy, or frequent sips of water for dry mouth

Evaluate:

• Therapeutic response: decreased weight, decreased hyperactivity

Teach patient/family:

• To decrease caffeine consumption (coffee, tea, cola, chocolate), which may increase irritability, stimulation

• To avoid OTC preparations unless approved by prescriber

• To taper off drug over several wk, or depression, increased sleeping, lethargy may ensue

• To avoid alcohol ingestion

• To avoid hazardous activities until patient is stabilized on medication

• To get needed rest; patients will feel more tired at end of day

🚫 Not to break, crush, or chew sus rel forms

Treatment of overdose: Administer fluids, hemodialysis or peritoneal dialysis; antihypertensive for increased B/P; ammonium Cl for increased excretion

M

---

methimazole (℞)

(meth-im'a-zole)

Tapazole

Func. class.: Thyroid hormone antagonist (antithyroid)

Chem. class.: Thioamide

Action: Inhibits synthesis of thyroid hormones by decreasing iodine use in manufacture of thyroglobin and iodothyronine; does not affect already formed hormones

Uses: Hyperthyroidism, preparation for thyroidectomy, thyrotoxic crisis, thyroid storm

---

Dosage and routes:
Hyperthyroidism
• *Adult:* PO 5-20 mg tid depending on severity of condition; continue until euthyroid; maintenance dose 5-10 mg qd-tid, maximal dose 150 mg qd
• *Child:* PO 0.4 mg/kg/day in divided doses q8h; continue until euthyroid; maintenance dose 0.2 mg/kg/day in divided doses q8h
Preparation and thyroidectomy
• *Adult and child:* PO same as above; iodine may be added × 10 days before surgery
Thyrotoxic crisis
• *Adult and child:* PO same as hyperthyroidism with iodine and propranolol
Available forms: Tabs 5, 10 mg
Side effects/adverse reactions:
ENDO: Enlarged thyroid
INTEG: Rash, urticaria, pruritus, alopecia, hyperpigmentation, lupus-like syndrome
GU: Nephritis
CNS: Drowsiness, headache, vertigo, fever, paresthesias, neuritis
*HEMA: **Agranulocytosis, leukopenia, thrombocytopenia, hypothrombinemia, lymphadenopathy,** bleeding,* vasculitis
*GI: Nausea, diarrhea, vomiting, **jaundice, hepatitis,** loss of taste*
MS: Myalgia, arthralgia, nocturnal muscle cramps
Contraindications: Hypersensitivity, pregnancy (D), lactation
Precautions: Infection, bone marrow depression, hepatic disease
Pharmacokinetics:
PO: Onset 1 wk, duration is up to 10 wk, half-life 1-2 hr; excreted in urine, breast milk; crosses placenta
Interactions:
• Increased bone marrow depression: radiation, antineoplastic agents
• Decreased effectiveness: amiodarone, potassium iodide

• Agranulocytosis: phenothiazines
• Altered response to digitalis, warfarin
Lab test interferences:
Increase: PT, AST, ALT, alk phosphatase
NURSING CONSIDERATIONS
Assess:
• Pulse, B/P, temp
• I&O ratio; check for edema: puffy hands, feet, periorbits; indicate hypothyroidism
• Weight qd; same clothing, scale, time of day
• T_3, T_4, which are increased; serum TSH, which is decreased; free thyroxine index, which is increased if dosage is too low; discontinue drug 3-4 wk before RAIU
• Blood work: CBC for blood dyscrasias: leukopenia, thrombocytopenia, agranulocytosis; LFTs
⬥ Overdose: peripheral edema, heat intolerance, diaphoresis, palpitations, dysrhythmias, severe tachycardia, fever, delirium, CNS irritability
• Hypersensitivity: rash, enlarged cervical lymph nodes; drug may have to be discontinued
• Hypoprothrombinemia: bleeding, petechiae, ecchymosis
• Clinical response: after 3 wk should include increased weight, pulse; decreased T_4
• Bone marrow depression: sore throat, fever, fatigue
Administer:
• With meals to decrease GI upset
• At same time each day to maintain drug level
• Lowest dose that relieves symptoms; discontinue before RAIU
Perform/provide:
• Storage in light-resistant container
• Fluids to 3-4 L/day, unless contraindicated

⬥ = Nursing alert   🖊 = Herb-drug interaction   🚫 = Do not crush

Evaluate:

• Therapeutic response: weight gain, decreased pulse, decreased T_4, B/P

Teach patient/family:

• Not to breastfeed

• To take pulse daily

• To report redness, swelling, sore throat, mouth lesions, fever, which indicate blood dyscrasias

• To keep graph of weight, pulse, mood

• To avoid OTC products that contain iodine

• That seafood, other iodine products may be restricted

• Not to discontinue this medication abruptly; thyroid crisis may occur; stress patient response

• That response may take several mo if thyroid is large

• The symptoms and signs of overdose: periorbital edema, cold intolerance, mental depression

• The symptoms of inadequate dose: tachycardia, diarrhea, fever, irritability

---

methocarbamol (℞)

(meth-oh-kar′ba-mole)
Carbacot, methocarbamol, Robaxin, Robaxin-750, Skelex
Func. class.: Skeletal muscle relaxant, central acting
Chem. class.: Carbamate derivative

Action: Depresses multisynaptic pathways in the spinal cord, causing skeletal muscle relaxation

Uses: Adjunct for relief of spasm and pain in musculoskeletal conditions, tetanus management

Dosage and routes:

Pain

• *Adult:* **PO** 1.5 g × 2-3 days, then 1 g qid; **IM** 500 mg in each gluteal region, may repeat q8h; **IV BOL** 1-3 g/day at 3 ml/min; **IV INF** 1 g/ 250 ml D_5W or NS, not to exceed 3 g/day

• *Geriatric:* **PO** 500 mg qid, titrate to needed dose

Tetanus

• *Adult:* **IV INF** 1-3 g/L of solution q6h; **IV BOL** 1-2 g injected into running **IV**

• *Child:* **IV** 15 mg/kg q6h

Available forms: Tabs 500, 750 mg; inj 100 mg/ml

Side effects/adverse reactions:

CNS: Dizziness, weakness, drowsiness, headache, tremor, depression, insomnia; *seizures* (IV use)

HEMA: Hemolysis, increased hemoglobin (IV only)

EENT: Diplopia, temporary loss of vision, blurred vision, nystagmus

CV: Postural hypotension, ***bradycardia***

GI: Nausea, vomiting, hiccups, anorexia, metallic taste

GU: Brown, black, green urine

INTEG: Rash, pruritus, fever, facial flushing, urticaria

SYST: **Anaphylaxis** (IM, IV)

Contraindications: Hypersensitivity, child <12 yr, intermittent porphyria

Precautions: Renal disease, hepatic disease, addictive personalities, pregnancy (C), myasthenia gravis, epilepsy

Pharmacokinetics:

IM/IV: Onset rapid

PO: Onset ½ hr, peak 1-2 hr, half-life 1-2 hr

Metabolized in liver, excreted in urine unchanged, crosses placenta

Interactions:

• Increased CNS depression: alcohol, tricyclics, opiates, barbiturates, sedatives, hypnotics

• Considered incompatible with any drug in sol or syringe

M

Lab test interferences:

False increase: VMA, urinary 5-HIAA

NURSING CONSIDERATIONS

Assess:

• Blood studies: CBC, WBC, differential; blood dyscrasias may occur

• During and after injection: CNS effects, rash, conjunctivitis, nasal congestion may occur

• Liver function studies: AST, ALT, alk phosphatase; hepatitis may occur

• ECG in epileptic patients; poor seizure control has occurred

• Allergic reactions: rash, fever, respiratory distress

• Severe weakness, numbness in extremities

• Tolerance: increased need for medication, more frequent requests for medication, increased pain

• CNS depression: dizziness, drowsiness, psychiatric symptoms

Administer:

PO

• With meals for GI symptoms

IV

• IV undiluted over 1 min or more, give 300 mg or less/1 min or longer; may be diluted in 250 ml or less D_5 or isotonic NaCl sol

• By slow IV to prevent phlebitis; keep recumbent for 15 min to prevent orthostatic hypotension; check for extravasation

IM

• IM deep in large muscle mass; rotate sites

Perform/provide:

• Storage in tight container at room temperature

• Assistance with ambulation if dizziness/drowsiness occurs

• Recumbent position after IV administration

Evaluate:

• Therapeutic response: decreased pain, spasticity

Teach patient/family:

• Not to discontinue medication quickly; insomnia, nausea, headache, spasticity, tachycardia will occur; drug should be tapered off over 1-2 wk

• That urine may turn green, black, or brown

• Not to take with alcohol, other CNS depressants

• To avoid altering activities while taking this drug

• To avoid hazardous activities if drowsiness, dizziness occurs

• To avoid using OTC medication: cough preparations, antihistamines, unless directed by prescriber

Treatment of overdose: Induce emesis of conscious patient, lavage, dialysis; have epinephrine, antihistamines, and corticosteroids available

---

RARELY USED

methohexital (℞)

(meth-oh-hex′i-tal)

Brevital Sodium, Brietal Sodium*

Func. class.: General anesthetic

Uses: General anesthesia for electroshock therapy, reduction of fractures, adjunct with other anesthetics, balanced anesthesia

Dosage and routes:

• *Adult and child:* **IV** 50-120 mg given 1 ml/5 sec

Maintenance:

• *Adult and child:* **IV** 20-40 mg q4-7min 0.1% sol; **CONT IV** 3 ml/min (6 mg/min) 0.2% sol

 = Nursing alert   ℱ = Herb-drug interaction   🚫 = Do not crush

Contraindications: Hypersensitivity, status asthmaticus, hepatic/intermittent porphyrias, pregnancy (D)

---

methotrexate (amethopterin, MTX) (℞)

(meth-oh-trex'ate)
Folex, Folex PFS, methotrexate, Methotrexate LPF, Rheumatrex, Trexall

Func. class.: Antineoplastic-antimetabolite

Chem. class.: Folic acid antagonist

Action: Inhibits an enzyme that reduces folic acid, which is needed for nucleic acid synthesis in all cells; S phase of cell cycle specific; immunosuppressive

Uses: Acute lymphocytic leukemia, in combination for breast, lung, head, neck carcinoma; lymphosarcoma, gestational choriocarcinoma, hydatidiform mole, psoriasis, rheumatoid arthritis, mycosis fungoides

Investigational uses: Used investigationally to produce abortion

Dosage and routes:

Acute lymphocytic leukemia
• *Adult and child:* **PO** 3.3 mg/m²/day with prednisone **IT** 12 mg/m², maintenance 30 mg/m²/day 2 ×/wk; **IV** 2.5 mg/kg q2wk

Choriocarcinoma
• *Adult and child:* **PO** 15-30 mg/m² qd × 5 days, then off 1 wk; may repeat

Meningeal leukemia
• *Adult and child:* 12 mg/m² **INTRATHECALLY** q2-5 days until CSF is normal, then 1 additional dose, max 15 mg

Burkitt's lymphoma (stages I, II, III)
• *Adult:* **PO** 10-25 mg qd × 4-8 days with 7-day rest period

Lymphosarcoma (stage III)
• *Adult:* **PO/IM/IV** 0.625-2.5 mg/kg/day

Osteosarcoma
• *Adult and child:* **IV** 12 g/m² given over 4 hr, then leucovorin rescue

Mycosis fungoides
• *Adult:* **PO** 2.5-10 mg/day until cleared (may be many months); **IM** 50 mg qwk or 25 mg 2 ×/wk

Psoriasis
• *Adult:* **PO/IM/IV** 10 mg qwk, may increase to 25 mg qwk

Breast cancer
• *Adult:* **IV** 40 mg/m² on days 1 and 8 with other antineoplastics

Rheumatoid arthritis
• *Adults:* **PO** 7.5 mg/wk; max 20 mg/wk

Available forms: Tabs 2.5, 5, 7.5, 10, 15 mg; inj 25 mg/ml; pwd for inj 20, 25, 50, 100, 250 mg, 1 g; sodium inj 2.5, 25 mg/ml

Side effects/adverse reactions:

HEMA: ***Leukopenia, thrombocytopenia, myelosuppression, anemia***

GI: Nausea, vomiting, anorexia, diarrhea, stomatitis, ***hepatotoxicity,*** cramps, ulcer, gastritis, ***GI hemorrhage,*** abdominal pain, hematemesis

GU: Urinary retention, ***renal failure,*** menstrual irregularities, defective spermatogenesis, ***hematuria, azotemia, uric acid nephropathy***

INTEG: Rash, alopecia, dry skin, urticaria, photosensitivity, folliculitis, vasculitis, petechiae, ecchymosis, acne, alopecia

CNS: Dizziness, ***seizures, leukencephalopathy,*** headache, confusion, hemiparesis, malaise, fatigue, chills, fever; arachnoiditis (intrathecal)

Contraindications: Hypersensitivity, leukopenia (<3500/mm³), thrombocytopenia (<100,000/mm^3), anemia, psoriatic patients with severe renal/hepatic disease, pregnancy (X), alcoholism, HIV

Do not confuse:
methotrexate/metolazone

Precautions: Renal disease, lactation

Pharmacokinetics:
PO: Readily absorbed
PO/IM/IV: Onset 4-7 days; peak 1-2 wk; duration 3 wk
IT: Onset, peak, duration unknown
Not metabolized; excreted in urine (unchanged); crosses placenta, blood-brain barrier; 50% plasma protein bound

Interactions:
• Increased toxicity: aspirin, sulfa drugs, other antineoplastics, radiation, alcohol, probenecid, phenytoin, phenylbutazone, theophylline, penicillins
• Decreased effect of oral digoxin, vaccines
• Increased hypoprothrombinemia: oral anticoagulants
• Decreased effect of methotrexate: folic acid supplements

◆ Possible fatal interactions: NSAIDs

NURSING CONSIDERATIONS
Assess:
• CBC, differential, platelet count weekly; withhold drug if WBC is <3500/mm^3 or platelet count is <100,000/mm^3; notify prescriber; drug should be discontinued
• Renal function studies: BUN, serum uric acid, urine CrCl, electrolytes before, during therapy
• I&O ratio; report fall in urine output to <30 ml/hr
• Monitor temp q4h; fever may indicate beginning infection; no rectal temps
• LFTs before and during therapy: bilirubin, alk phosphatase, AST, ALT; liver biopsy should be done before start of therapy (psoriasis patients)
Bleeding time, coagulation time during treatment; bleeding: hematuria, guaiac, bruising or petechiae, mucosa or orifices q8h
Effects of alopecia on body image; discuss feelings about body changes
◆ Hepatotoxicity: jaundiced skin and sclera, dark urine, clay-colored stools, pruritus, abdominal pain, fever, diarrhea
• Buccal cavity q8h for dryness, sores, ulceration, white patches, oral pain, bleeding, dysphagia
• Symptoms indicating severe allergic reaction: rash, urticaria, itching, flushing

Administer:
• Antacid before oral agent; give drug after evening meal before bedtime
• Antiemetic 30-60 min before giving drug
• Allopurinol or sodium bicarbonate to maintain uric acid levels, alkalinization of urine (pH >6.5), adequate fluids

IV
• After diluting 5 mg/2 ml of sterile H$_2$O for inj; give through Y-tube or 3-way stopcock at 10 mg or less/min
◆ Leucovorin Ca within 12 hr of this drug to prevent tissue damage; check agency policy

Additive compatibilities: Cephalothin, cyclophosphamide, cytarabine, fluorouracil, hydroxyzine, mercaptopurine, ondansetron, sodium bicarbonate, vincristine

Solution compatibilities: Amino acids, 4.25%/D$_{25}$, D$_5$W, sodium bicarbonate 0.05 mol/L, sodium chloride 0.9%

Syringe compatibilities: Bleomycin, cisplatin, cyclophosphamide, doxapram, doxorubicin, fluorouracil, furosemide, heparin, leucovorin, mitomycin, vinblastine, vincristine

Y-site compatibilities: Allopurinol, amifostine, amphotericin B cholesteryl, asparaginase, aztreonam, bleomycin, cefepime, ceftriaxone, cimetidine, cisplatin, cyclophosphamide, cytarabine, daunorubicin, dexchlorpheniramine, diphenhydramine, doxorubicin, doxorubicin liposome, etoposide, famotidine, filgrastim, fludarabine, fluorouracil, furosemide, gallium, ganciclovir, granisetron, heparin, hydromorphone, imipenem/cilastatin, leucovorin, lorazepam, melphalan, mesna, methylprednisolone, metoclopramide, mitomycin, morphine, ondansetron, oxacillin, paclitaxel, piperacillin/tazobactam, prochlorperazine, ranitidine, sargramostim, teniposide, thiotepa, vinblastine, vincristine, vinorelbine

Perform/provide:
• Strict medical asepsis and protective isolation if WBC levels are low
• Liquid diet: carbonated beverage, Jell-O; dry toast, crackers may be added when patient is not nauseated or vomiting
• Increased fluid intake to 2-3 L/day to prevent urate deposits, calculi formation, unless contraindicated
• Diet low in purines: absence of organ meats (kidney, liver), dried beans, peas to maintain alkaline urine
• Rinsing of mouth tid-qid with water, club soda; brushing of teeth bid-tid with soft brush or cotton-tipped applicators for stomatitis; use unwaxed dental floss
• Nutritious diet with iron, vitamin supplements
• Storage in tightly closed container in cool environment; store injection, pwd for inj in dark, dry area

Evaluate:
• Therapeutic response: decreased tumor size, spread of malignancy

Teach patient/family:
• To report any complaints, side effects to nurse or prescriber: black tarry stools, chills, fever, sore throat, bleeding, bruising, cough, shortness of breath, dark or bloody urine
• That hair may be lost during treatment; wig or hairpiece may make patient feel better; tell patient that new hair may be different in color, texture (alopecia is rare)
• To avoid foods with citric acid, hot or rough texture if stomatitis is present
• To report stomatitis: any bleeding, white spots, ulcerations in mouth to prescriber; tell patient to examine mouth qd, report symptoms to nurse
• That contraceptive measures are recommended during therapy and for at least 8 wk following cessation of therapy
• To drink 10-12 glasses of fluid/day
• To avoid alcohol, salicylates, live vaccines
• To avoid use of razors, commercial mouthwash
• To use sunblock to prevent burns

RARELY USED

methoxsalen (℞)

(meth-ox′a-len)

Func. class.: Pigmenting agent

Uses: Vitiligo, psoriasis

Dosage and routes:

Vitiligo
• *Adult and child >12 yr:* **PO** 20 mg qd 2-4 hr before exposure to therapeutic ultraviolet rays; administer on alternate days; **TOP** apply 1-2 hr before exposure to UVA light; treat-

ment intervals regulated by erythema response

Psoriasis

• *Adult:* **PO** dosage individualized to weight; taken 2 hr before exposure to therapeutic ultraviolet rays

Contraindications: Hypersensitivity, melanoma, LE, albinism, sunburn, cataracts, squamous cell cancer, child ≤12 yr, diseases associated with photosensitivity

---

RARELY USED

methscopolamine (℞)
(meth-skoe-pol'a-meen)
Func. class.: GI anticholinergic

Uses: Peptic ulcer disease, preoperatively
Dosage and routes:
• *Adult:* **PO** 2.5-5 mg 1/2 hr ac, hs
Contraindications: Hypersensitivity to anticholinergics, narrow-angle glaucoma, GI obstruction, myasthenia gravis, paralytic ileus, GI atony, toxic megacolon

---

RARELY USED

methsuximide (℞)
(meth-sux'i-mide)
Func. class.: Anticonvulsant

Uses: Refractory absence seizures (petit mal)
Dosage and routes:
• *Adult and child:* **PO** 300 mg/day; may increase by 300 mg/wk, not to exceed 1.2 g/day in divided doses
Contraindications: Hypersensitivity to succinimide derivatives

methylcellulose (OTC)
(meth-ill-sell'yoo-lose)
Citrucel
Func. class.: Laxative, bulk
Chem. class.: Hydrophilic semi-synthetic cellulose derivative

---

Action: Attracts water, expands in intestine to increase peristalsis; also absorbs excess water in stool; decreases diarrhea
Uses: Constipation
Dosage and routes:
• *Adult:* **PO** 1-3 tbs heaping in 1 cup cold water qd-tid
• *Child 6-12 yr:* **PO** 1-1½ tsps-level in ½ cup cold water qd-tid
Available forms: Pwd 2 g/tbs (heaping)
Side effects/adverse reactions:
*GI: **Obstruction,*** abdominal distention
Contraindications: Hypersensitivity, GI obstruction, hepatitis
Pharmacokinetics:
PO: Onset 12-24 hr, peak 1-3 days
Interactions:
• Decreased absorption: antibiotics, digitalis, nitrofurantoin, salicylates, tetracyclines, oral anticoagulants
NURSING CONSIDERATIONS
Assess:
• Blood, urine electrolytes if used often
• I&O ratio to identify fluid loss
• Cause of constipation; lack of fluids, bulk, exercise
• Cramping, rectal bleeding, nausea, vomiting; drug should be discontinued
Administer:
PO
• Alone for better absorption; do not take within 1 hr of other drugs
• In morning or evening (oral dose)

◆ = Nursing alert   ✦ = Herb-drug interaction   ⃠ = Do not crush

Evaluate:
• Therapeutic response: decrease in constipation

Teach patient/family:

🚫 To swallow tabs whole; do not break, crush, or chew

• To increase fluid intake

• That normal bowel movements do not always occur daily

• Not to use in presence of abdominal pain, nausea, vomiting

• To notify prescriber if constipation unrelieved or if symptoms of electrolyte imbalance occur: muscle cramps, pain, weakness, dizziness, excessive thirst

---

methyldopa/methyldopate (Ⴑ)

(meth-ill-doe′pa)
Aldomet, Apo-Methyldopa*, Dopamet*, methyldopa/methyldopate, Novamedopa*, Nu-Medopa*

Func. class.: Antihypertensive
Chem. class.: Centrally acting α-adrenergic inhibitor

Action: Stimulates central inhibitory α-adrenergic receptors or acts as false transmitter, resulting in reduction of arterial pressure

Uses: Hypertension

Dosage and routes:
• *Adult:* **PO** 250-500 mg bid or tid, then adjusted q2d as needed, 0.5-2 g qd in 2-4 divided doses (maintenance), not to exceed 3 g/day; **IV** 250-500 mg in 100 ml D_5W q6h, run over 30-60 min, not to exceed 1 g q6h, switch to oral as soon as possible

• *Geriatric:* **PO** 125 mg bid-tid, increase q2d as needed, max 3 g/day

• *Child:* **PO** 10 mg/kg/day in 2-4 divided doses, not to exceed 65 mg/kg or 3 g/day, whichever is less;

IV 20-40 mg/kg/day in 4 divided doses, not to exceed 65 mg/kg or 3g, whichever is less

Available forms: Methyldopa: tabs 125, 250, 500 mg; oral susp 50 mg/ml; methyldopate: inj 50 mg/ml

Side effects/adverse reactions:

ENDO: Breast enlargement, gynecomastia, lactation, amenorrhea

GI: Nausea, vomiting, diarrhea, constipation, ***hepatic dysfunction,*** sore or "black" tongue, ***pancreatitis***

CV: Bradycardia, ***myocarditis,*** orthostatic hypotension, angina, edema, weight gain, ***CHF***

CNS: Drowsiness, weakness, dizziness, sedation, headache, depression, psychosis paresthesias, parkinsonism, Bell's palsy, nightmares

EENT: Nasal congestion

HEMA: ***Leukopenia, thrombocytopenia, hemolytic anemia, granulocytopenia,*** positive Coombs' test

INTEG: Rash, ***toxic epidermal necrolysis,*** lupuslike syndrome, eczema

GU: Impotence, failure to ejaculate

Contraindications: Active hepatic disease, hypersensitivity, blood dyscrasias

Precautions: Pregnancy (B) (PO); (C) (IV), liver disease, eclampsia, severe cardiac disease

Do not confuse:
methyldopa/ʟ-dopa (levodopa)

Pharmacokinetics:
PO: Peak 2-4 hr, duration 12-24 hr
IV: Peak 2 hr, duration 10-16 hr
Metabolized by liver, excreted in urine

Interactions:
• Increased pressor effect: sympathomimetic amines (norepinephrine, phenylpropanolamine), MAOIs
• Increased hypotension: levodopa
• Increased psychosis: haloperidol
• Lithium toxicity: lithium

M

• Increased B/P: phenothiazines, β-blockers, amphetamines, NSAIDs, tricyclics, barbiturates

🍃 Decreased effect: capsicum, Indian snakeroot

Lab test interferences:

Interference: Urinary uric acid, serum creatinine, AST

False increase: Urinary catecholamines

NURSING CONSIDERATIONS
Assess:

• Blood studies: neutrophils, decreased platelets

• Baselines in renal tests, LFTs before therapy begins

• B/P when beginning treatment, periodically thereafter

• Allergic reaction: rash, fever, pruritus, urticaria; drug should be discontinued if antihistamines fail to help

• CNS symptoms, especially in the elderly

• Symptoms of CHF: edema, dyspnea, wet rales, B/P

• Renal symptoms: polyuria, oliguria, urinary frequency; I&O ratio, weight

Administer:
IV route

• After diluting with 100-200 ml D₅W; run over ½-1 hr

Additive compatibilities: Aminophylline, ascorbic acid, chloramphenicol, diphenhydramine, heparin, magnesium sulfate, multivitamins, netilmicin, potassium chloride, promazine, sodium bicarbonate, succinylcholine, verapamil, vit B/C

Solution compatibilities: D_5W, D_5/0.9% NaCl, Ringer's, sodium bicarbonate 5%, 0.9% NaCl, amino acids 4.25%/D_{25}, Dextran₆/0.9% NaCl, Normosol R, Normosol M/D_5W

Y-site compatibilities: Esmolol, heparin, meperidine, morphine, theophylline

Perform/provide:

• Storage of tabs in tight container

Evaluate:

• Therapeutic response: decrease in B/P in hypertension

Teach patient/family:

• To avoid hazardous activities

• To administer 1 hr before meals

• Not to discontinue drug abruptly, or withdrawal symptoms may occur: anxiety, increased B/P, headache, insomnia, increased pulse, tremors, nausea, sweating

• Not to use OTC (cough, cold, allergy) products unless directed by prescriber

• To avoid sunlight or wear sunscreen; photosensitivity may occur

• To comply with dosage schedule even if feeling better

• To rise slowly to sitting or standing position to minimize orthostatic hypotension

• To notify prescriber of mouth sores, sore throat, fever, swelling of hands or feet, irregular heartbeat, chest pain, signs of angioedema

• That excessive perspiration, dehydration, vomiting, diarrhea may lead to fall in blood pressure; consult prescriber

• That dizziness, fainting, lightheadedness may occur during first few days of therapy

• That compliance is necessary; not to skip or stop drug unless directed by prescriber

• That drug may cause skin rash or impaired perspiration

Treatment of overdose: Gastric evacuation, sympathomimetics may be indicated; if severe, hemodialysis

---

◆ = Nursing alert   🍃 = Herb-drug interaction   🚫 = Do not crush

methylergonovine (℞)

(meth-ill-er-goe-noe'veen)
Methergine,
methylergonovine
Func. class.: Oxytocic
Chem. class.: Ergot alkaloid

Action: Stimulates uterine, vascular, smooth muscle, causing contractions; decreases bleeding

Uses: Treatment of hemorrhage postpartum or postabortion, uterine contractions

Dosage and routes:
• *Adult:* **IM** 0.2 mg q2-5h, not to exceed 5 doses; **IV** 0.2 mg given over 1 min; **PO** 0.2-0.4 mg q6-12h × 2-7 days after initial **IM** or **IV** dose

Available forms: Inj 0.2 mg/ml; tabs 0.2 mg

Side effects/adverse reactions:
RESP: Dyspnea
GU: Cramping
*CNS: Headache, dizziness, **seizures***
GI: Nausea, vomiting
CV: Chest pain, palpitation, *hypertension, dysrhythmias; **CVA (IV)***
EENT: Tinnitus
INTEG: Sweating, rash, allergic reactions

Contraindications: Hypersensitivity to ergot preparations, indication of labor, before delivery of placenta, hypertension, pelvic inflammatory disease, respiratory disease, cardiac disease, peripheral vascular disease

Precautions: Pregnancy (C), severe hepatic disease, severe renal disease, jaundice, diabetes mellitus, convulsive disorders, sepsis

Pharmacokinetics:
PO: Onset 5-25 min, duration 3 hr
IM: Onset 2-5 min, duration 3 hr
IV: Onset immediate, duration 45 min

Metabolized in liver, excreted in urine

Interactions:
• Increase vasoconstriction: vasopressors, nicotine

NURSING CONSIDERATIONS
Assess:
• B/P, pulse, character and amount of vaginal bleeding; watch for indications of hemorrhage
• Respiratory rate, rhythm, depth; notify prescriber of abnormalities
• For uterine relaxation; observe for severe cramping
◆ Ergot toxicity: tinnitus, hypertension, palpitations, chest pain, nausea, vomiting, weakness; cold, numb extremities

Administer:
• Only during fourth stage of labor; not to be used to augment labor
• IM in deep muscle mass; rotate injection sites of additional doses

IV
• Undiluted through Y-tube or 3-way stopcock; give 0.2 mg or less/min or diluted in 5 ml 0.9% NaCl given through Y-site
• With crash cart available on unit; IV route used only in emergencies

Y-site compatibilities: Heparin, hydrocortisone sodium succinate, potassium chloride, vit B/C

Evaluate:
• Therapeutic response: absence of hemorrhage

Teach patient/family:
• To report increased blood loss, severe abdominal cramps, fever or foul-smelling lochia
• To avoid smoking

Side effects: *italics* = common; ***bold italics*** = life-threatening

methylphenidate (R)

(meth-ill-fen'i-date)
Concerta, Metadate CD,
Metadate ER, Methylin,
Methylin ER, PMS-
methylphenidate, Methidate,
Ritalin, Ritalin SR
Func. class.: Cerebral stimulant
Chem. class.: Piperidine deriv-
ative

Controlled Substance Schedule II
Action: Increases release of norepinephrine, dopamine in cerebral cortex to reticular activating system;
exact action not known
Uses: Attention deficit hyperactivity disorder, narcolepsy
Investigational uses: Depression in
the elderly; cancer, post-stroke patients, HIV, brain injury, anesthesia-
related hiccups
Dosage and routes:
*Attention deficit hyperactivity dis-
order*
• *Child >6 yr:* **PO** 5 mg before
breakfast and lunch, increasing by
5-10 mg/wk, not to exceed 60 mg/
day; sus rel 20 mg qd-tid
Narcolepsy
• *Adult:* **PO** 10 mg bid-tid, 30-45
min before meals, may increase up
to 40-60 mg/day
Depression (elderly)
• *Geriatric:* **PO** 2.5 mg qAM, increase q 3rd day by 2.5 mg to desired dose, max 20 mg/day
Available forms: Tabs 5, 10, 20 mg;
tabs ext rel 10, 18, 20, 36, 54 mg;
tabs, sus rel 20 mg; cap, ext rel 20
mg
Side effects/adverse reactions:
MISC: Fever, arthralgia, scalp hair
loss
*CNS: Hyperactivity, insomnia, rest-
lessness, talkativeness,* dizziness,
drowsiness, toxic psychosis, head-

ache, akathisia, dyskinesia, mask-
ing or worsening of Gilles de la
Tourette's syndrome, *seizures*
GI: Nausea, anorexia, dry mouth,
weight loss, abdominal pain
CV: Palpitations, tachycardia, B/P
changes, angina, *dysrhythmias,* palpitations
INTEG: Exfoliative dermatitis, urticaria, rash, erythema multiforme
ENDO: Growth retardation
*HEMA: Leukopenia, anemia, throm-
bocytopenic purpura*
Contraindications: Hypersensitivity, anxiety, history of Gilles de la
Tourette's syndrome; children <6 yr,
glaucoma
Precautions: Hypertension, depres-
sion, pregnancy (C), seizures, lac-
tation, drug abuse
Do not confuse:
methylphenidate/methadone
Pharmacokinetics:
PO: Onset ½-1 hr, duration 4-6 hr,
metabolized by liver, excreted by
kidneys
Interactions:
• Hypertensive crisis: MAOIs or
within 14 days of MAOIs, vasopressors
• Decreased effect of: guanethidine
• Increased effects of: tricyclics, anticonvulsants, SSRIs
• Drug/food: increased stimulation:
caffeine
NURSING CONSIDERATIONS
Assess:
• VS, B/P; may reverse antihypertensives; check patients with cardiac disease more often for increased B/P
• CBC, urinalysis, in diabetes: blood
sugar, urine sugar; insulin changes
may have to be made, since eating
will decrease
• Height, growth rate q3mo in children; growth rate may be decreased

◆ = Nursing alert   ✐ = Herb-drug interaction   ⊘ = Do not crush

• Mental status: mood, sensorium, affect, stimulation, insomnia, aggressiveness

◆ Withdrawal symptoms: headache, nausea, vomiting, muscle pain, weakness

• Appetite, sleep, speech patterns
• For attention span, decreased hyperactivity in ADHD persons

Administer:
• At least 6 hr before hs to avoid sleeplessness (regular release); at least 10 hr (SR, ER)
• Gum, hard candy, frequent sips of water for dry mouth

Evaluate:
• Therapeutic response: decreased hyperactivity (ADHD) or ability to stay awake (narcolepsy)

Teach patient/family:
• To decrease caffeine consumption (coffee, tea, cola, chocolate); may increase irritability, stimulation
🚫 Not to break, crush, or chew time-released medication
• To avoid OTC preparations unless approved by prescriber
• To taper off drug over several wk, or depression, increased sleeping, lethargy will occur
• To avoid alcohol ingestion
• To avoid hazardous activities until stabilized on medication
• To get needed rest; patients will feel more tired at end of day

Treatment of overdose: Administer fluids; hemodialysis or peritoneal dialysis; antihypertensive for increased B/P; administer short-acting barbiturate before lavage

---

methylprednisolone (℞)

(meth-il-pred-niss′oh-lone)

A-methaPred, depMedalone, Depoject, Depo-Medrol, Depopred, Depo-Predate, Medrol, Duralone, Medralone, Rep-Pred, Solu-Medrol

Func. class.: Corticosteroid

Chem. class.: Glucocorticoid, immediate acting

Action: Decreases inflammation by suppression of migration of polymorphonuclear leukocytes, fibroblasts; reversal of increased capillary permeability and lysosomal stabilization

Uses: Severe inflammation, shock, adrenal insufficiency, collagen disorders

Dosage and routes:

Adrenal insufficiency/inflammation
• *Adult:* **PO** 2-60 mg in 4 divided doses; **IM** 10-80 mg (acetate); **IM/IV** 10-250 mg (succinate); intraarticular 4-30 mg (acetate)
• *Child:* **IV** 117 µg-1.66 mg/kg in 3-4 divided doses (succinate)

Shock
• *Adult:* **IV** 100-250 mg q2-6h or 30 mg/kg, then q4-6h prn, for 2-3 days (succinate)

Multiple sclerosis
• *Adult:* **PO** 160 mg/day × 1 wk, then 64 mg qod × 30 days

Available forms: Tabs 2, 4, 6, 8, 16, 24, 32 mg; inj 20, 40, 80 mg/ml acetate; inj 40, 125, 500, 1000 mg/ vial succinate; dose pack 4 mg tabs; enema 40 mg

Side effects/adverse reactions:
CNS: Depression, flushing, sweating, headache, mood changes
CV: Hypertension, *circulatory col-*

---

lapse, thrombophlebitis, embolism, tachycardia

EENT: Fungal infections, increased intraocular pressure, blurred vision, cataracts

GI: Diarrhea, nausea, abdominal distention, **GI hemorrhage,** increased appetite, pancreatitis

HEMA: **Thrombocytopenia**

INTEG: Acne, poor wound healing, ecchymosis, petechiae

MS: Fractures, osteoporosis, weakness

Contraindications: Psychosis, hypersensitivity, idiopathic thrombocytopenia, acute glomerulonephritis, amebiasis, fungal infections, nonasthmatic bronchial disease, child <2 yr, AIDS, TB

Precautions: Pregnancy (C), lactation, diabetes mellitus, glaucoma, osteoporosis, seizure disorders, ulcerative colitis, CHF, myasthenia gravis, renal disease, esophagitis, peptic ulcer

Do not confuse:
methylprednisolone/prednisone
methylprednisolone/medroxyprogesterone

Pharmacokinetics: Well absorbed PO, IM

PO: Peak 1-2 hr, duration 1½ days
IM: Peak 4-8 days, duration 1-4 wk
Intraarticular: Peak 1 wk

Half-life >3½ hr; crosses placenta, enters breast milk in small amounts; metabolized in liver, excreted by kidneys (unchanged)

Interactions:

• Decreased action of methylprednisolone: cholestyramine, colestipol, barbiturates, rifampin, ephedrine, phenytoin, theophylline

• Decreased effects of anticoagulants, anticonvulsants, antidiabetics, ambenonium, neostigmine, isoniazid, toxoids, vaccines, anticholinesterases, salicylates, somatrem

• Increased side effects: alcohol, salicylates, indomethacin, amphotericin B, digitalis, cyclosporine, diuretics

• Increased action of methylprednisolone: salicylates, estrogens, indomethacin, oral contraceptives, ketoconazole, macrolide antibiotics

🍂 Potassium deficiency: aloe, cascara sagrada, buckthorn, rhubarb root, senna

Lab test interferences:

Increase: Cholesterol, Na, blood glucose, uric acid, Ca, urine glucose
Decrease: Ca, K, T_4, T_3, thyroid ^{131}I uptake test, urine 17-OHCS, 17-KS

False negative: Skin allergy tests

NURSING CONSIDERATIONS
Assess:

• Potassium depletion: parethesias, fatigue, nausea, vomiting, depression, polyuria, dysrhythmias, weakness

• Edema, hypertension, cardiac symptoms

• Mental status: affect, mood, behavioral changes, aggression

• Potassium, blood sugar, urine glucose while on long-term therapy; hypokalemia and hyperglycemia

• Joint mobility, pain, edema if given intraarticularly

• Weight daily; notify prescriber of weekly gain >5 lb

• B/P q4h, pulse; notify prescriber of chest pain, rales

• I&O ratio; be alert for decreasing urinary output, increasing edema

• Adrenal insufficiency: weight loss, nausea, vomiting, confusion, anxiety, hypotension, weakness

• Plasma cortisol levels during long-term therapy (normal level: 138-635 nmol/L SI units when drawn at 8 AM)

• Growth in children on long-term treatment

Administer:
• Titrated dose; use lowest effective dose
• IM inj deep in large muscle mass; rotate sites; avoid deltoid; use 21G needle; after shaking suspension (parenteral)
• In one dose in AM to prevent adrenal suppression; avoid SC administration; may damage tissue
• With food or milk to decrease GI symptoms (PO)
◆ Do not give Solu-Medrol intrathecally
IV
• After diluting with diluent provided; agitate slowly; give 500 mg or less/1 min or longer; may be given as IV infusion in its own diluent over 10-20 min
Additive compatibilities: Chloramphenicol, cimetidine, clindamycin, dopamine, granisetron, heparin, norepinephrine, penicillin G potassium, ranitidine, theophylline, verapamil
Syringe compatibilities: Granisetron, metoclopramide
Y-site compatibilities: Acyclovir, amifostine, amphotericin B cholesteryl, amrinone, aztreonam, cefepime, cisplatin, cladribine, cyclophosphamide, cytarabine, dopamine, doxorubicin, enalaprilat, famotidine, fludarabine, granisetron, heparin, melphalan, meperidine, methotrexate, metronidazole, midazolam, morphine, piperacillin/tazobactam, remifentanil, sodium bicarbonate, tacrolimus, teniposide, theophylline, thiotepa
Perform/provide:
• Assistance with ambulation in patient with bone tissue disease to prevent fractures
Evaluate:
• Therapeutic response: ease of respirations, decreased inflammation; decreased symptoms of adrenal insufficiency
• Infection: increased temp, WBC, even after withdrawal of medication; drug masks infection
Teach patient/family:
• To increase intake of K, Ca, protein
• To carry ID (steroid user)
• To notify prescriber if therapeutic response decreases; dosage adjustment may be needed
• Not to discontinue abruptly, or adrenal crisis can result
• To avoid OTC products: salicylates, alcohol in cough products, cold preparations unless directed by prescriber; to avoid vaccinations, since immunosuppression occurs
• About cushingoid symptoms
• To recognize the symptoms of adrenal insufficiency: nausea, anorexia, fatigue, dizziness, dyspnea, weakness, joint pain

methysergide (℞)
(meth-i-ser'jide)
Sansert
Func. class.: Adrenergic blocker, serotonin antagonist
Chem. class.: Ergot derivative

Action: Competitively blocks serotonin HT receptors in CNS and periphery; potent vasoconstrictor
Uses: Prophylaxis for migraine and other vascular headaches. If no improvement is noted in 3 wk, drug is unlikely to be beneficial
Dosage and routes:
• *Adult:* **PO** 2 mg bid with meals; 3-4 wk rest period after each 6 mo treatment
Available forms: Tabs 2 mg
Side effects/adverse reactions:
CNS: Tremors, anxiety, insomnia, headache, dizziness, euphoria,

confusion, depersonalization, hallucination, paresthesias, drowsiness

*CV: **Retroperitoneal fibrosis,*** valvular thickening, palpitations, tachycardia, postural hypertension, angina, ***thrombophlebitis,*** ECG changes, ***cardiac fibrosis***

GI: Nausea, vomiting, weight gain

MS: Arthralgia, myalgia

INTEG: Flushing, rash, alopecia

*HEMA: **Blood dyscrasias***

Contraindications: Hypersensitivity to ergot, tartrazine, occlusion (peripheral, vascular), CAD, hepatic disease, renal disease, peptic ulcer, hypertension, connective tissue disease, fibrotic pulmonary disease, pregnancy (X)

Precautions: Lactation, children

Pharmacokinetics:

PO: Half-life 10 hr, metabolized by liver, excreted in urine (metabolites/unchanged drug)

Interactions:

• Increased vasoconstriction: β-blockers

NURSING CONSIDERATIONS

Assess:

• Weight daily; check for peripheral edema in feet, legs; B/P

• For stress, activity, recreation, coping mechanisms

• Neurologic status: LOC, blurring vision, nausea, vomiting, tingling in extremities that precedes headache

• Ingestion of tyramine foods (pickled products, beer, wine, aged cheese), food additives, preservatives, colorings, artificial sweeteners, chocolate, caffeine may precipitate these types of headaches

Administer:

PO

• Give with or after meals to avoid GI symptoms

• Only to women who are not pregnant; harm to fetus may occur

• For less than 6 mo continuously, a 3-4 wk drug-free period must follow each 6 mo period

Perform/provide:

• Storage in dark area

• Quiet, calm environment with decreased stimulation such as noise, bright light, or excessive talking

Evaluate:

• Therapeutic response: decrease in frequency, severity of headache

Teach patient/family:

• Not to use OTC medications; serious interactions may occur

• To maintain dose at approved level, not to increase even if drug does not relieve headache

• To report side effects: increased vasoconstriction starting with cold extremities, then paresthesia, weakness

• That headaches may increase when drug discontinued after long-term use

◆ To keep drug out of reach of children; death may occur

• To report at once: dyspnea, paresthesias, urinary problems, pain in abdomen, chest, back, legs

• To use drug for less than 6 mo unless a 3-4 wk rest period has been taken

• That drug may cause drowsiness

---

metoclopramide (℞)

(met-oh-kloe-pra′mide)

Apo-Metoclop*, Clopra, Emex*, Maxeran*, Maxolon, metoclopramide, Octamide PFS, Reclomide, Reglan

Func. class.: Cholinergic, antiemetic

Chem. class.: Central dopamine receptor antagonist

Action: Enhances response to acetylcholine of tissue in upper GI tract, which causes contraction of gastric

---

◆ = Nursing alert   🍃 = Herb-drug interaction   🚫 = Do not crush

muscle; relaxes pyloric, duodenal segments; increases peristalsis without stimulating secretions, blocks dopamine in chemoreceptor trigger zone of CNS

Uses: Prevention of nausea, vomiting induced by chemotherapy, radiation, delayed gastric emptying, gastroesophageal reflux

Investigational uses: Hiccups, migraines

Dosage and routes:
Renal dose
• CrCl <40 ml/min 50% of dose
Nausea/vomiting
• *Adult:* IV 1-2 mg/kg 30 min before administration of chemotherapy, then q2h × 2 doses, then q3h × 3 doses
• *Child:* IV 0.1-0.2 mg/kg/dose
Facilitate small bowel intubation, in radiologic exams
• *Adult and child >14 yr:* IV 10 mg over 1-2 min
• *Child <6 yr:* IV 0.1 mg/kg
• *Child 6-14 yr:* IV 2.5-5 mg
Delayed gastric emptying
• *Adult:* PO 10 mg 30 min ac, hs × 2-8 wk
• *Geriatric:* PO 5 mg ½ hr ac hs, increase to 10 mg if needed
Gastroesophageal reflux
• *Adult:* PO 10-15 mg qid 30 min ac
Available forms: Tabs 5, 10 mg; syr 5 mg/5 ml; inj 5 mg/ml
Side effects/adverse reactions:
CNS: Sedation, fatigue, restlessness, headache, sleeplessness, dystonia, dizziness, drowsiness, ***suicide ideation, seizures***
GI: Dry mouth, constipation, nausea, anorexia, vomiting, diarrhea
GU: Decreased libido, prolactin secretion, amenorrhea, galactorrhea
CV: Hypotension, supraventricular tachycardia

INTEG: Urticaria, rash
*HEMA: **Neutropenia, leukopenia, agranulocytosis***

Contraindications: Hypersensitivity to this drug or procaine or procainamide, seizure disorder, pheochromocytoma, breast cancer (prolactin dependent), GI obstruction

Precautions: Pregnancy (B), lactation, GI hemorrhage, CHF, Parkinson's disease

Do not confuse:
metoclopramide/metolazone
Reglan/Megace

Pharmacokinetics:
IV: Onset 1-3 min, duration 1-2 hr
PO: Onset ½-1 hr, duration 1-2 hr
IM: Onset 10-15 min, duration 1-2 hr
Metabolized by liver, excreted in urine, half-life 4 hr

Interactions:
• Decreased action of metoclopramide: anticholinergics, opiates
• Increased sedation: alcohol, other CNS depressants
• Increased risk of EPS: haloperidol, phenothiazines
• Avoid use with MAOIs

Lab test interferences:
Increase: Prolactin, aldosterone, thyrotropin

NURSING CONSIDERATIONS
Assess:
• For EPS and tardive dyskinesia, more likely to occur in elderly patient
• Mental status: depression, anxiety, irritability
• GI complaints: nausea, vomiting, anorexia, constipation
Administer:
• ½-1 hr before meals for better absorption
• Gum, hard candy, frequent rinsing of mouth for dry oral cavity

M

IV

• Diphenhydramine IV for EPS

• Undiluted if dose is ≤10 mg; give over 2 min; more than 10 mg may be diluted in 50 ml or more D₅W, NaCl, Ringer's, LR and given over 15 min or more

Additive compatibilities: Clindamycin, meropenem, morphine, multivitamins, potassium acetate, potassium chloride, potassium phosphate, verapamil

Syringe compatibilities: Aminophylline, ascorbic acid, atropine, benztropine, bleomycin, butorphanol, chlorpromazine, cisplatin, cyclophosphamide, cytarabine, dexamethasone, dimenhydrinate, diphenhydramine, doxorubicin, droperidol, fentanyl, fluorouracil, heparin, hydrocortisone, hydroxyzine, insulin (regular), leucovorin, lidocaine, magnesium sulfate, meperidine, methotrimeprazine, methylprednisolone, midazolam, mitomycin, morphine, pentazocine, perphenazine, prochlorperazine, promazine, promethazine, ranitidine, scopolamine, sufentanil, vinblastine, vincristine, vit B/C

Y-site compatibilities: Acyclovir, aldesleukin, amifostine, aztreonam, bleomycin, ciprofloxacin, cisatracurium, cisplatin, cladribine, cyclophosphamide, cytarabine, diltiazem, doxorubicin, droperidol, famotidine, filgrastim, fluconazole, fludarabine, fluorouracil, foscarnet, gallium, granisetron, heparin, idarubicin, leucovorin, melphalan, meperidine, meropenum, methotrexate, mitomycin, morphine, ondansetron, paclitaxel, piperacillin/tazobactam, propofol, remifentanil, sargramostim, sufentanil, tacrolimus, teniposide, thiotepa, vinblastine, vincristine, vinorelbine, zidovudine

Perform/provide:

• Protect from light with aluminum foil during infusion

• Discard open ampules

Evaluate:

• Therapeutic response: absence of nausea, vomiting, anorexia, fullness

Teach patient/family:

• To avoid driving, other hazardous activities until patient is stabilized on this medication

• To avoid alcohol, other CNS depressants that will enhance sedating properties of this drug

---

metolazone (℞)

(me-tole′a-zone)

Mykrox, Zaroxolyn

Func. class.: Diuretic

Chem. class.: Thiazide-like quinazoline derivative

Action: Acts on distal tubule and cortical thick ascending limb of the loop of Henle by increasing excretion of water, sodium, chloride, potassium, magnesium, bicarbonate

Uses: Edema, hypertension, CHF

Dosage and routes:

Edema

• *Adult:* **PO** 5-20 mg/day

Hypertension

• *Adult:* **PO** 2.5-5 mg/day (Zaroxolyn)

• *Child:* **PO** 0.2-0.4 mg/kg/day divided q12-24h

• *Adult:* **PO** 0.5 mg (Mykrox) qd in AM, may increase to 1 mg

Available forms: Tabs 0.5 (Mykrox), 2.5, 5, 10 mg

Side effects/adverse reactions:

GU: Urinary frequency, polyuria, *uremia, glucosuria*

CNS: Drowsiness, paresthesia, anxiety, depression, headache, *dizziness, fatigue, weakness*

GI: Nausea, vomiting, anorexia, con-

♦ = Nursing alert   🌿 = Herb-drug interaction   🚫 = Do not crush stipation, diarrhea, cramps, pancreatitis, GI irritation, *__hepatitis__*

EENT: Blurred vision

INTEG: Rash, urticaria, purpura, photosensitivity, fever

META: Hyperglycemia, increased creatinine, BUN

HEMA: __Aplastic anemia, hemolytic anemia, leukopenia, agranulocytosis, neutropenia__

CV: Irregular pulse, orthostatic hypotension, palpitations, volume depletion

ELECT: Hypokalemia, hypomagnesemia, hypercalcemia, hyponatremia, hypochloremia, hypophosphatemia

Contraindications: Hypersensitivity to thiazides or sulfonamides, anuria, lactation

Precautions: Hypokalemia, renal disease, hepatic disease, gout, COPD, lupus erythematosus, diabetes mellitus, pregnancy (B)

Do not confuse:

metolazone/methotrexate

metolazone/metoclopramide

Pharmacokinetics:

PO: Onset 1 hr, peak 2 hr, duration 12-24 hr; excreted unchanged by kidneys; crosses placenta; enters breast milk; half-life 8 hr

Interactions:

• Decreased action of metolazone: NSAIDs, salicylates

• Increased hypokalemia: mezlocillin, piperacillin, amphotericin B, glucocorticoids, digoxin

• Increased hypotension: alcohol (large amounts), nitrates, antihypertensives, barbiturates, opioids

• Increased toxicity: lithium

🌿 Potassium deficiency: aloe, cascara sagrada, buckthorn, rhubarb root, senna

Lab test interferences:

Increase: BSP retention, Ca, amylase, parathyroid test

Decrease: PBI, PSP

NURSING CONSIDERATIONS

Assess:

• Weight, I&O daily to determine fluid loss; effect of drug may be decreased if used qd

• Rate, depth, rhythm of respiration, effect of exertion

• B/P lying, standing; postural hypotension may occur

• Electrolytes: K, Mg, Na, Cl; include BUN, blood sugar, CBC, serum creatinine, blood pH, ABGs, uric acid, Ca

• Improvement in edema of feet, legs, sacral area daily if medication is being used in CHF

• Improvement in CVP q8h

• Signs of metabolic alkalosis: drowsiness, restlessness

• Signs of hypokalemia: postural hypotension, malaise, fatigue, tachycardia, leg cramps, weakness

• Rashes, fever qd

• Confusion, especially in elderly; take safety precautions if needed

Administer:

• In AM to avoid interference with sleep if using drug as a diuretic

• K replacement if K <3 mg/dl

• With food, if nausea occurs; absorption may be decreased slightly

• Extended product is Zaroxolyn; prompt product is Mykrox

Evaluate:

• Therapeutic response: decreased edema, B/P

Teach patient/family:

• To increase fluid intake to 2-3 L/day unless contraindicated, to rise slowly from lying or sitting position

• To notify prescriber of muscle weakness, cramps, nausea, dizziness

• That drug may be taken with food or milk

• To use sunscreen for photosensitivity

• That blood sugar may be increased in diabetics

M

• To take early in day to avoid nocturia

Treatment of overdose: Lavage if taken orally; monitor electrolytes; administer dextrose in saline; monitor hydration, CV, renal status

---

metoprolol (℞)

(meh-toe'proe-lole)
Apo-Metoprolol*, Betaloc*, Betaloc Durules*, Lopresor*, Lopressor, Lopressor SR*, Novometoprol*, Toprol-XL
Func. class.: Antihypertensive, antianginal
Chem. class.: β₁-Blocker

Action: Lowers B/P by β-blocking effects; reduces elevated renin plasma levels; blocks β₂-adrenergic receptors in bronchial, vascular smooth muscle only at high doses
Uses: Mild to moderate hypertension, acute MI to reduce cardiovascular mortality, angina pectoris, NYHA class II, III heart failure
Investigational uses: Dysrhythmias, hypertrophic cardiomyopathy, mitral valve prolapse, pheochromocytoma, tremors, prevention of vascular headaches, aggression
Dosage and routes:
Hypertension
• *Adult:* PO 50 mg bid, or 100 mg qd; may give up to 200-450 mg in divided doses; **EXT REL** give qd
• *Geriatric:* PO 25 mg/day initially, increase weekly as needed
Myocardial infarction
• *Adult:* (early treatment) **IV BOL** 5 mg q2min × 3, then 50 mg **PO** 15 min after last dose and q6h × 48 hr; (late treatment) **PO** maintenance 100 mg bid for 3 mo
Angina
• *Adult:* PO 100 mg qd, increase qwk prn or 100 mg ext rel qd

Available forms: Tabs 50, 100 mg; inj 1 mg/ml; ext rel tab 25, 50, 100, 200 mg
Side effects/adverse reactions:
CV: Hypotension, *bradycardia, CHF, palpitations,* dysrhythmias, *cardiac arrest, AV block*
CNS: Insomnia, dizziness, mental changes, hallucinations, *depression,* anxiety, headaches, nightmares, confusion, fatigue
GI: Nausea, vomiting, colitis, cramps, *diarrhea,* constipation, flatulence, dry mouth, *hiccups*
INTEG: Rash, purpura, alopecia, dry skin, urticaria, pruritus
HEMA: **Agranulocytosis, eosinophilia, thrombocytopenia, purpura**
EENT: Sore throat; dry, burning eyes
GU: Impotence
Uses: Refractory absence seizures (petit mal) RESP:
Bronchospasm, dyspnea, wheezing
Contraindications: Hypersensitivity to β-blockers, cardiogenic shock, heart block (2nd, 3rd degree), sinus bradycardia, bronchial asthma
Precautions: Major surgery, pregnancy (C), lactation, diabetes mellitus, renal disease, thyroid disease, COPD, heart failure, CAD, nonallergic bronchospasm, hepatic disease, CHF
Do not confuse:
metoprolol/misoprostol
Pharmacokinetics:
PO: Peak 2-4 hr, duration 13-19 hr; half-life 3-4 hr; metabolized in liver (metabolites); excreted in urine; crosses placenta; enters breast milk
Interactions:
• Increased hypotension, bradycardia: reserpine, hydralazine, methyldopa, prazosin, amphetamines, ephedrine, epinephrine, norepinephrine, H₂-antagonists
• Increased hypoglycemic effects: insulin oral antidiabetics

◆ = Nursing alert   ▮ = Herb-drug interaction   🚫 = Do not crush

- Do not use with MAOIs
- Decreased antihypertensive effect: indomethacin
- Decreased effects of dopamine, dobutamine, xanthines
- Drug/food: increased absorption with food

Lab test interferences:
Increase: LFTs, renal function tests

NURSING CONSIDERATIONS
Assess:
- ECG directly when giving IV during initial treatment
- I&O, weight daily
- B/P during initial treatment, periodically thereafter; pulse q4h; note rate, rhythm, quality
- Apical/radial pulse before administration; notify prescriber of any significant changes or pulse <50 bpm
- Baselines in renal, liver function tests before therapy begins
- Edema in feet, legs daily
- Skin turgor, dryness of mucous membranes for hydration status

Administer:
- PO ac, hs, tab may be crushed or swallowed whole, except for sus rel tab

IV
- IV, undiluted, give over 1 min, keep patient recumbent for 3 hr

Y-site compatibilities: Alteplase, meperidine, morphine

Perform/provide:
- Storage in dry area at room temperature, do not freeze

Evaluate:
- Therapeutic response: decreased B/P after 1-2 wk

Teach patient/family:
- To take with or immediately after meals
- Not to discontinue drug abruptly; taper over 2 wk; may cause precipitate angina
- Not to use OTC products containing α-adrenergic stimulants (nasal decongestants, OTC cold preparations) unless directed by prescriber
- To report bradycardia, dizziness, confusion, depression, fever, sore throat, shortness of breath to prescriber
- To take pulse at home; advise when to notify prescriber
- To avoid alcohol, smoking, Na intake
- To comply with weight control, dietary adjustments, modified exercise program
- To carry Medic Alert ID to identify drug, allergies
- To avoid hazardous activities if dizziness is present
- To report symptoms of CHF: difficult breathing, especially on exertion or when lying down, night cough, swelling of extremities
- To take medication hs to prevent effect of orthostatic hypotension
- To wear support hose to minimize effects of orthostatic hypotension

Treatment of overdose: Lavage, IV atropine for bradycardia, IV theophylline for bronchospasm, digitalis, O_2, diuretic for cardiac failure, hemodialysis, hypotension administer vasopressor (norepinephrine)

M

---

metronidazole (R)

(me-troe-ni'da-zole)
Apo-Metronidazole*, Flagyl,
Flagyl ER, Flagyl IV, Flagyl IV
RTU, metronidazole,
Novonidazole*, Protostat,
Trikacide*

Func. class.: Antiinfective, misc
Chem. class.: Nitroimidazole derivative

Action: Direct-acting amebicide/trichomonacide binds, degrades DNA in organism
Uses: Intestinal amebiasis, amebic

Side effects: *italics* = common; ***bold italics*** = life-threatening

abscess, trichomoniasis, refractory trichomoniasis, bacterial anaerobic infections, giardiasis, septicemia, endocarditis, bone, joint infections, lower respiratory tract infections

Dosage and routes:

Trichomoniasis

• *Adult:* PO 250 mg tid × 7 days or 2 g in single dose; do not repeat treatment for 4-6 wk

• *Child:* PO 5 mg/kg tid × 7 days

Refractory trichomoniasis

• *Adult:* PO 250 mg bid × 10 days

Amebic hepatic abscess

• *Adult:* PO 500-750 mg tid × 5-10 days

• *Child:* PO 35-50 mg/kg/day in 3 divided doses × 10 days

Intestinal amebiasis

• *Adult:* PO 750 mg tid × 5-10 days

• *Child:* PO 35-50 mg/kg/day in 3 divided doses × 10 days; then oral iodoquinol

Anaerobic bacterial infections

• *Adult:* IV INF 15 mg/kg over 1 hr, then 7.5 mg/kg IV or PO q6h, not to exceed 4 g/day; first maintenance dose should be administered 6 hr following loading dose

Giardiasis

• *Adult:* PO 250 mg tid × 5 days

• *Child:* PO 5 mg/kg tid × 5 days

Antibiotic-associated pseudomembranous colitis

• *Adult:* PO 250-500 mg 3-4 ×/day × 10-14 days

• *Child:* PO 20 mg/kg/day (max 2 g) divided q6h

Available forms: Tabs 250, 375, 500 mg; tab, ext rel 750 mg; inj 500 mg/100 ml; pwd for inj 500 mg single dose

Side effects/adverse reactions:

CV: Flat T waves

CNS: Headache, dizziness, confusion, irritability, restlessness, ataxia, depression, fatigue, drowsiness, insomnia, paresthesia, peripheral neuropathy, *seizures,* incoordination, depression

EENT: Blurred vision, sore throat, retinal edema, dry mouth, metallic taste, furry tongue, glossitis, stomatitis

GI: Nausea, vomiting, diarrhea, epigastric distress, *anorexia,* constipation, *abdominal cramps,* metallic taste, *pseudomembranous colitis*

GU: Darkened urine, vaginal dryness, polyuria, *albuminuria,* dysuria, cystitis, decreased libido, *neurotoxicity,* incontinence, dyspareunia

HEMA: Leukopenia, bone marrow, depression, aplasia

INTEG: Rash, pruritus, urticaria, flushing

Contraindications: Hypersensitivity to this drug, renal disease, hepatic disease, contracted visual or color fields, blood dyscrasias, pregnancy (1st trimester), lactation, CNS disorders

Precautions: *Candida* infections, pregnancy (B) (2nd, 3rd trimesters)

Pharmacokinetics:

IV: Onset immediate, peak end of inf

PO: Peak 1-2 hr, half-life 6-11 hr

Crosses placenta, enters breast milk, excreted in feces; absorbed PO (80%-85%)

Interactions:

• Disulfiram reaction: alcohol

• May increase action of: anticoagulants

• Decreased action of metronidazole: phenobarbital, phenytoin

• Toxicity: cimetidine, lithium

Lab test interferences:

Decrease: AST, ALT

NURSING CONSIDERATIONS

Assess:

• For infection: WBC, wound symptoms, fever, skin or vaginal secretions; start treatment after C&S

◆ = Nursing alert   ◢ = Herb-drug interaction   ⊘ = Do not crush

• Stools during entire treatment; should be clear at end of therapy; stools should be free of parasites for 1 yr before patient is considered cured (amebiasis)

• Vision by ophthalmic exam during, after therapy; vision problems often occur

• I&O; weight daily; stools for number, frequency, character

◆ Neurotoxicity: peripheral neuropathy, seizures, dizziness, uncoordination, pruritus, joint pains; drug may be discontinued

• Allergic reaction: fever, rash, itching, chills; drug should be discontinued if these symptoms occur

• Superinfection: fever, monilial growth, fatigue, malaise

• Renal and reproductive dysfunction: dysuria, polyuria, impotence, dyspareunia, decreased libido

Administer:

• PO with or after meals to avoid GI symptoms, metallic taste; crush tabs if needed

IV

• Prediluted; metronidazole IV, dilute with 4.4 ml sterile H_2O or 0.9% NaCl; must be diluted further with 8 mg/ml or more 0.9% NaCl, D_5W, or LR; must neutralize with 5 mEq Na_2CO_3/500 mg; CO_2 gas will be generated and may require venting; run over 1 hr or more; primary IV must be discontinued; may be given as continuous infusion; do not use aluminum products; IV may require venting

Additive compatibilities: Amikacin, aminophylline, cefazolin, cefotaxime, cefotiam, ceftazidime, ceftizoxime, ceftriaxone, cefuroxime, chloramphenicol, ciprofloxacin, clindamycin, disopyramide, floxacillin, fluconazole, gentamicin, heparin, moxalactam, multielectrolyte concentrate, multivitamins,

netilmicin, penicillin G potassium, tobramycin

Y-site compatibilities: Acyclovir, allopurinol, amifostine, amiodarone, cefepime, cisatracurium, cyclophosphamide, diltiazem, dopamine, doxorubicin liposome, enalaprilat, esmolol, fluconazole, foscarnet, granisetron, heparin, hydromorphone, labetalol, lorazepam, magnesium sulfate, melphalan, meperidine, methylprednisolone, midazolam, morphine, perphenazine, piperacillin/tazobactam, remifentanil, sargramostim, tacrolimus, teniposide, theophylline, thiotepa, vinorelbine

Perform/provide:

• Storage in light-resistant container; do not refrigerate

Evaluate:

• Therapeutic response: decreased symptoms of infection

Teach patient/family:

• That urine may turn dark-reddish brown, drug may cause metallic taste

• Proper hygiene after BM; handwashing technique

• To notify physician for numbness or tingling of extremities

• To avoid hazardous activities, since dizziness can occur

• Need for compliance with dosage schedule, duration of treatment

• To use condoms if treatment for trichomoniasis, or cross-contamination may occur

• To use frequent sips of water, sugarless gum for dry mouth

• That treatment of both partners is necessary in trichomoniasis

• Not to drink alcohol or use preparations containing alcohol for 24 hr after use of drug; disulfiram-like reaction can occur

M

mexiletine (R)

(mex-il′e-teen)
Mexitil
Func. class.: Antidysrhythmic
(Class IB)
Chem. class.: Lidocaine analog

Action: Increases electrical stimulation threshold of ventricle, His-Purkinje system, which stabilizes cardiac membrane

Uses: Ventricular tachycardia, ventricular dysrhythmias during cardiac surgery, MI

Investigational uses: Diabetic neuropathy

Research note: Fluvoxamine given with mexiletine resulted in an increase of AUC and peak concentration of mexiletine[24]

Dosage and routes:
• *Adult:* **PO** 200-400 mg (loading dose), then 200 mg q8h, then 200-400 mg q8h

Diabetic neuropathy (off-label)
• *Adult:* **PO** 75 mg tid with gradual titration to 450-675 mg/day; maintenance dose 150-675 mg/day in 3 divided doses

Available forms: Caps 100*, 150, 200, 250 mg

Side effects/adverse reactions:
CNS: Headache, dizziness, confusion, *seizures,* tremors, psychosis, nervousness, paresthesias, weakness, fatigue, coordination difficulties, change in sleep habits
EENT: Blurred vision, hearing loss, tinnitus
GI: Nausea, vomiting, anorexia, diarrhea, abdominal pain, *hepatitis,* dry mouth, peptic ulcer, altered taste, *GI bleeding*
CV: Hypotension, bradycardia, angina, PVCs, *heart block, cardiovascular collapse or arrest,* sinus node slowing, *left ventricular failure,* syncope, *cardiogenic shock*
RESP: Dyspnea, *fibrosis, embolism, pneumonia*
INTEG: Rash, alopecia, dry skin
HEMA: Thrombocytopenia, leukopenia, agranulocytosis, hypoplastic anemia, systemic lupus erythematosus syndrome
GU: Urinary hesitancy, decreased libido
MISC: Edema, arthralgia, fever

Contraindications: Hypersensitivity to amides, cardiogenic shock, blood dyscrasias, severe heart block

Precautions: Pregnancy (C), lactation, children, renal disease, liver disease, CHF, respiratory depression, myasthenia gravis

Pharmacokinetics:
PO: Peak 2-3 hr; half-life 12 hr, metabolized by liver, excreted unchanged by kidneys (10%), excreted in breast milk

Interactions:
• Decreased or increased effects of mexiletine: cimetidine, lidocaine
• Decreased levels of mexiletine: phenytoin, phenobarbital, rifampin, urinary acidifiers, aluminum/magnesium hydroxide, atropine, opiates
• Increased effects of mexiletine: metoclopramide, urinary alkalinizers
• Increased levels of: caffeine, theophylline
• Drug/smoking: decreased drug effect
🗲 Increased potassium loss, increased antidysrhythmic action: aloe, cascara sagrada, buckthorn, rhubarb, senna

Lab test interferences:
Increase: CPK

NURSING CONSIDERATIONS
Assess:
• ECG continuously for increased PR or QRS segments; discontinue

◆ = Nursing alert   🗲 = Herb-drug interaction   🚫 = Do not crush or reduce rate; watch for increased ventricular ectopic beats; may have to rebolus

• Blood levels (therapeutic level 0.5-2 μg/ml)

• B/P continuously for fluctuations in cardiac rate

• I&O ratio, electrolytes (K, Na, Cl), liver enzymes

◆ Malignant hyperthermia: tachypnea, tachycardia, changes in B/P, fever

• Respiratory status: rate, rhythm, lung fields for rales, watch for respiratory depression

• CNS effects: dizziness, confusion, psychosis, paresthesias, convulsions; drug should be discontinued

• Lung fields, bilateral rales may occur in CHF patient

• Increased respiration, increased pulse; drug should be discontinued

Administer:

• With food for GI upset

Evaluate:

• Therapeutic response: decreased dysrhythmias

Treatment of overdose: O$_2$, artificial ventilation, ECG; administer dopamine for circulatory depression, diazepam or thiopental for convulsions, to acidify urine

---

mezlocillin (R)

(mez-loe-sill'in)
Mezlin

Func. class.: Antiinfective, broad-spectrum

Chem. class.: Extended-spectrum penicillin

Action: Interferes with cell wall replication of susceptible organisms; osmotically unstable cell wall swells, bursts from osmotic pressure

Uses: Effective for gram-positive cocci *(Staphylococcus aureus, Streptococcus viridans, Streptococcus faecalis, Streptococcus pneumoniae),* gram-negative cocci *(Neisseria gonorrhoeae),* gram-positive bacilli *(Clostridium perfringens, Clostridium tetani),* gram-negative bacilli *(Bacteroides, Escherichia coli, Haemophilus influenzae, Klebsiella, Proteus mirabilis, Proteus vulgaris, Providencia rettgeri, Peptococcus, Peptostreptococcus, Morganella morganii, Enterobacter, Serratia, Pseudomonas, Shigella, Citrobacter, Veillonella)*

Dosage and routes:

• *Adult:* **IM/IV** 200-300 mg/kg/day (serious infections) q4-6h or **IV** 500 mg q8h, may give up to 24 g/day for severe infections

• *Child:* **IM/IV** 50 mg/kg q4-6h

• *Infant >8 days (>2000 g):* 75 mg/kg q6h; *<2000 g:* 75 mg/kg q8h

• *Infant <8 days:* 75 mg/kg q12h

Renal dose

• Dose reduction indicated in renal impairment (CrCl <30 ml/min)

Hepatic dose

• Hepatic dose give 50% of dose

Available forms: Pwd for inj 1, 2, 3, 4, 20 g

Side effects/adverse reactions:

HEMA: Anemia, increased bleeding time, ***bone marrow depression, granulocytopenia***

GI: Nausea, vomiting, diarrhea; increased AST, ALT; abdominal pain, glossitis, colitis, abnormal taste

GU: Oliguria, proteinuria, hematuria, (vaginitis, moniliasis), ***glomerulonephritis,*** increased BUN, creatinine

CNS: Lethargy, hallucinations, anxiety, depression, twitching, ***coma, seizures***

META: Hyperkalemia, hypokalemia, alkalosis, hypernatremia

Contraindications: Hypersensitivity to penicillins

Precautions: Pregnancy (B), lactation, hypersensitivity to cephalosporins, neonates, renal disease

Pharmacokinetics:

IM: Peak 45 min

IV: Peak 5 min

Half-life 50-55 min; partially metabolized in liver; excreted in urine, bile, breast milk (small amount); crosses placenta

Interactions:

• Decreased excretion of lithium

• Increased hypokalemia: diuretics, digoxin

• Increased mezlocillin concentrations: aspirin, probenecid

🍃 Delayed/reduced absorption: khat, separate by ≥2 hr

Lab test interferences:

False positive: Urine glucose, urine protein

NURSING CONSIDERATIONS

Assess:

• I&O ratio; report hematuria, oliguria, since penicillin in high doses is nephrotoxic

• Any patient with compromised renal system, since drug is excreted slowly in poor renal system function; toxicity may occur rapidly

• Liver studies: AST, ALT

• Blood studies: WBC, RBC, Hct, Hgb, bleeding time

• Renal studies: urinalysis, protein, blood, BUN, creatinine

• C&S before drug therapy; drug may be given as soon as culture is taken

• Bowel pattern before and during treatment

• Skin eruptions after administration of penicillin to 1 wk after discontinuing drug

• Respiratory status: rate, character, wheezing, and tightness in chest

• Check IV site for thrombophlebitis

• For possible seizures; seizure precautions in those on high doses

• WBC, differential, liver, renal studies periodically for patients on long-term therapy

• Allergies before initiation of treatment, and reaction of each medication; highlight allergies on chart

Administer:

• Drug after C&S completed

IV

• After diluting 1 g or less/10 ml of sterile H_2O, D_5, or 0.9% NaCl for inj; shake, dilute further with D_5W or 0.45 NaCl, and give over 3-5 min; may be given by intermittent inf over ½ hr, change site q48h

Solution compatibilities: $D_{10}W$, D_5W, 0.9% NaCl

Syringe compatibilities: Heparin

Y-site compatibilities: Amifostine, aztreonam, cyclophosphamide, doxorubicin liposome, famotidine, fludarabine, granisetron, hydromorphone, morphine, perphenazine, propofol, remifentanil, sargramostim, tacrolimus, teniposide, thiotepa

Perform/provide:

• Adrenaline, suction, tracheostomy set, endotracheal intubation equipment

• Adequate fluid intake (2 L) during diarrhea episodes

• Scratch test to assess allergy after securing order from prescriber; usually done when penicillin is only drug of choice

• Storage at room temperature; reconstituted sol is stable for 24 hr refrigerated

Evaluate:

• Therapeutic response: absence of fever, draining wounds

Teach patient/family:

• That culture may be taken after completed course of medication

• To report sore throat, fever, fatigue (may indicate superinfection)

• To wear or carry Medic Alert ID if allergic to penicillins

◆ = Nursing alert   🍃 = Herb-drug interaction   🚫 = Do not crush

• To report diarrhea, symptoms of *Candida* vaginitis

Treatment of anaphylaxis: Withdraw drug, maintain airway, administer epinephrine, aminophylline, O_2, IV corticosteroids

---

midazolam (R)

(mid′ay-zoe-lam)

Versed

Func. class.: Sedative, hypnotic, antianxiety

Chem. class.: Benzodiazepine, short-acting

Controlled Substance Schedule IV

Action: Depresses subcortical levels in CNS; may act on limbic system, reticular formation; may potentiate γ-aminobutyric acid (GABA) by binding to specific benzodiazepine receptors

Uses: Preoperative sedation, general anesthesia induction, sedation for diagnostic endoscopic procedures, intubation

Investigational uses: Epileptic seizures, refractory status epilepticus

Dosage and routes:

Preoperative sedation

• *Adult:* **IM** 0.07-0.08 mg/kg ½-1 hr before general anesthesia

• *Child:* **IM** 0.1-0.15 mg/kg, may give up to 0.5 mg/kg if needed

Induction of general anesthesia

• *Adult and child 12-16 yr:* **IV** (unpremedicated patients) 0.3-0.35 mg/kg over 30 sec, wait 2 min, follow with 25% of initial dose if needed; (premedicated patients) 0.15-0.35 mg/kg over 20-30 sec, allow 2 min for effect

• *Child 6-12 yr:* **IV** 0.025-0.05 mg/kg, total dose up to 0.4 mg/kg may be needed

• *Child 6 mo-5 yr:* **IV** 0.05-0.1 mg/

kg, total dose up to 0.6 mg/kg may be needed

• *Child <6 mo:* Titrate with small increments

Available forms: Inj 1, 5 mg/ml, syr 2 mg/ml

Side effects/adverse reactions:

CNS: Retrograde amnesia, euphoria, confusion, headache, anxiety, insomnia, slurred speech, paresthesia, tremors, weakness, chills

RESP: Coughing, **apnea, bronchospasm, laryngospasm,** dyspnea, **respiratory depression**

CV: Hypotension, PVCs, tachycardia, bigeminy, nodal rhythm, **cardiac arrest**

EENT: Blurred vision, nystagmus, diplopia, blocked ears, loss of balance

GI: Nausea, vomiting, increased salivation, hiccups

INTEG: Urticaria, pain, swelling at inj site, rash, pruritus

Contraindications: Pregnancy (D), hypersensitivity to benzodiazepines, shock, coma, alcohol intoxication, acute narrow-angle glaucoma

Precautions: COPD, CHF, chronic renal failure, chills, elderly, debilitated, children, lactation

Do not confuse:

Versed/Vepesid

Versed/Vistaril

Pharmacokinetics:

IM: Onset 15 min, peak ½-1 hr

IV: Onset 3-5 min, onset of anesthesia 1½-2½ min; protein binding 97%; half-life 1.2-12.3 hr

Metabolized in liver; metabolites excreted in urine; crosses placenta, blood-brain barrier

Interactions:

• Prolonged respiratory depression: other CNS depressants, alcohol, barbiturates, opiate analgesics, verapamil, ritonavir, indinavir, fluvoxamine

M

• May alter midazolam metabolism: erythromycin, theophylline

• Extended half-life: oral contraceptives

NURSING CONSIDERATIONS
Assess:

• Injection site for redness, pain, swelling

• Degree of amnesia in elderly; may be increased

• Anterograde amnesia

• Vital signs for recovery period in obese patient, since half-life may be extended

• Apnea, respiratory depression that may be increased in the elderly

Administer:

• IM deep into large muscle mass

IV

• After diluting with D_5W or 0.9% NaCl to 0.25 mg/ml; give over 2 min (conscious sedation) or over 30 sec (anesthesia induction)

Additive compatibility: Hydromorphone

Syringe compatibilities: Atracurium, atropine, benzquinamide, buprenorphine, butorphanol, chlorpromazine, cimetidine, cisatracurium, diphenhydramine, droperidol, fentanyl, glycopyrrolate, hydromorphone, hydroxyzine, meperidine, metoclopramide, morphine, nalbuphine, promazine, promethazine, remifentanil, scopolamine, sufentanil, thiethylperazine, trimethobenzamide

Y-site compatibilities: Amikacin, amiodarone, atracurium, calcium gluconate, cefazolin, cefmetazole, cefotaxime, cimetidine, ciprofloxacin, clindamycin, digoxin, diltiazem, dopamine, epinephrine, erythromycin, esmolol, etomidate, famotidine, fentanyl, fluconazole, gentamicin, haloperidol, heparin, hydromorphone, insulin (regular), labetalol, lorazepam, methylprednisolone, metronidazole, milrinone, morphine, nicardipine, nitroglycerin, norepinephrine, pancuronium, piperacillin, potassium chloride, ranitidine, sodium nitroprusside, sufentanil, theophylline, tobramycin, vancomycin, vecuronium

Perform/provide:

• Assistance with ambulation until drowsy period relieved

• Storage at room temperature

• Immediate availability of resuscitation equipment, O_2 to support airway; do not give by rapid bolus

Evaluate:

• Therapeutic response: induction of sedation, general anesthesia

Teach patient/family:

• That amnesia occurs; events may not be remembered

Treatment of overdose: O_2, vasopressors, physostigmine, resuscitation

---

midodrine (℞)
(mye'doh-dreen)
ProAmatine
Func. class.: Vasopressor

Action: Activates α-adrenergic receptors of arteriolar venous vasculature by increasing vascular tone

Uses: Orthostatic hypotension

Dosage and routes:

• *Adult:* **PO** 10 mg tid

Renal dose

• *Adult:* **PO** 2.5 mg tid

Available forms: Tabs 2.5, 5 mg

Side effects/adverse reactions:

CNS: Drowsiness, restlessness, headache, *paresthesia, pain,* chills

GI: Nausea, anorexia

EENT: Dry mouth, blurred vision

INTEG: Pruritus, piloerection, rash

GU: Urinary urgency

*CV: **Supine hypertension***

Contraindications: Hypersensitivity, severe organic heart disease, acute renal disease, urinary reten-

◆ = Nursing alert   ∅ = Herb-drug interaction   ⊘ = Do not crush

tion, pheochromocytoma, thyrotoxicosis, persistent/excessive supine hypertension

Precautions: Children, urinary retention, lactation, prostatic hypertrophy, pregnancy (C)

Pharmacokinetics:

PO: Peak 1-2 hr, half-life 3-4 hr

Interactions:

• Increased bradycardia: β-blockers, psychotropics, cardiac glycosides

• Increased pressor effects: α-agonist

• Increased supine hypertension: fludrocortisone

NURSING CONSIDERATIONS
Assess:

• VS, B/P (standing, supine); notify prescriber if B/P supine is increased

• Observe for drowsiness, dizziness, LOC

Administer:

• Tablets may be swallowed whole, chewed, or allowed to dissolve

• Upon arising, midday, and late afternoon (no later than 6 PM)

• Avoid administering if patient is to be supine during day

Evaluate:

• Therapeutic response: decreased orthostatic hypotension

Teach patient/family:

• To avoid hazardous activities, activities requiring alertness; dizziness may occur; instruct patient to request assistance with ambulation

• To avoid alcohol, other depressants

---

mifepristone (℞)

(mif-ee-press'tone)

Mifeprex

Func. class.: Abortifacient

Action: Stimulates uterine contractions, causing complete abortion

Uses: Abortion through 49 days' gestation

Investigational uses: Postcoital contraception/contragestation, intrauterine fetal death, endometriosis, Cushing's syndrome, unresectable meningioma

Dosage and routes:

• *Adult:* **PO** 600 mg day 1, 400 μg misoprostol day 3

Available forms: Tabs 200 mg

Side effects/adverse reactions:

MISC: Fatigue, back pain, fever, viral infections, chills, sinusitis

CNS: Dizziness, insomnia, anxiety, syncope, fainting, headache

GI: Nausea, vomiting, diarrhea, dyspepsia

GU: Uterine cramping, uterine hemorrhage, vaginitis, pelvic pain

Contraindications: Hypersensitivity, severe hepatic disease, severe renal disease, PID, respiratory disease, cardiac disease

Precautions: Asthma, anemia, jaundice, diabetes mellitus, convulsive disorders, past uterine surgery, pregnancy (C)

Pharmacokinetics: Rapidly absorbed, peak 90 min, 98% bound to plasma proteins, albumin, glycoprotein, excretion via feces, urine

Interactions:

• May inhibit metabolism of: erythromycin, ketoconazole, itraconazole, grapefruit juice

NURSING CONSIDERATIONS
Assess:

• B/P, pulse; watch for change that may indicate hemorrhage

• Respiratory rate, rhythm, depth; notify prescriber of abnormalities

• For length, duration of contraction; notify prescriber of contractions lasting over 1 min or absence of contractions

• For incomplete abortion, pregnancy must be terminated by another method; drug is teratogenic

M

Perform/provide:
• Emotional support before and after abortion
Evaluate:
• Therapeutic response: expulsion of fetus
Teach patient/family:
• To report increased blood loss, abdominal cramps, increased temp, foul-smelling lochia
• Some methods of comfort control and pain control
• Must continue with follow-up
• That cramping and vaginal bleeding will occur

---

miglitol (Ⓡ)
(mig′lih-tol)
Glyset
Func. class.: Oral hypoglycemic
Chem. class.: α-Glucosidase inhibitor

Action: Delays digestion of ingested carbohydrates, results in smaller rise in blood glucose after meals; does not increase insulin production
Uses: Non–insulin-dependent diabetes mellitus (NIDDM) type II
Dosage and routes:
• *Adult:* PO 25 mg tid initially, with first bite of meal; maintenance dose may be increased to 50 mg tid; may be increased to 100 mg tid if needed (only in patients >60 kg) with dosage adjustment at 4-8 wk intervals
Available forms: Tabs 25, 50, 100 mg
Side effects/adverse reactions:
GI: Abdominal pain, diarrhea, flatulence, **hepatotoxicity**
HEMA: Low iron
INTEG: Rash
Contraindications: Hypersensitivity, diabetic ketoacidosis, cirrhosis, inflammatory bowel disease, co-

lonic ulceration, partial intestinal obstruction, chronic intestinal disease
Precautions: Pregnancy (B), renal disease, lactation, children, hepatic disease
Pharmacokinetics: Peak 2-3 hr, not metabolized, excreted in urine as unchanged drug, half-life 2 hr
Interactions:
• Decreased levels of: digoxin, propranolol, ranitidine
• Decreased levels of miglitol: digestive enzymes, intestinal adsorbents; do not use together
🔥 Decreased hypoglycemic effect: broom, buchu, dandelion, juniper
🔥 Increased or decreased hypoglycemic effect: chromium, fenugreek, ginseng
🔥 Improved glucose tolerance: karela
NURSING CONSIDERATIONS
Assess:
• Hypoglycemia, hyperglycemia; even though drug does not cause hypoglycemia, if patient is on sulfonylureas or insulin, hypoglycemia may be additive
• Blood glucose levels, glycosylated hemoglobin, LFTs
Administer:
• Tid with first bite of each meal
Perform/provide:
• Storage in tight container in cool environment
Evaluate:
• Therapeutic response: decreased signs/symptoms of diabetes mellitus (polyuria, polydipsia, polyphagia, clear sensorium, absence of dizziness, stable gait)
Teach patient/family:
• The symptoms of hypo/hyperglycemia, what to do about each, that during periods of stress, infection, surgery, insulin may be required
• That medication must be taken as prescribed; explain consequences of discontinuing medication abruptly

---

◆ = Nursing alert   🔥 = Herb-drug interaction   🚫 = Do not crush

- To avoid OTC medications unless approved by health-care provider
- That diabetes is lifelong illness; that this drug is not a cure
- To carry a Medic Alert ID for emergency purposes
- That diet and exercise regimen must be followed

---

milrinone (℞)

(mill'rih-nohn)
Primacor

Func. class.: Inotropic/vasodilator agent with phosphodiesterase activity

Chem. class.: Bipyridine derivative

Action: Positive inotropic agent, increases contractility of cardiac muscle with vasodilator properties; reduces preload and afterload by direct relaxation on vascular smooth muscle

Uses: Short-term management of advanced CHF that has not responded to other medication; can be used with digitalis

Dosage and routes:
- *Adult:* IV BOL 50 μg/kg given over 10 min; start infusion of 0.375-0.75 μg/kg/min; reduce dose in renal impairment

Available forms: Inj 1 mg/ml; premixed inj 200 μg/ml in D_5W

Side effects/adverse reactions:

*HEMA: **Thrombocytopenia***

MISC: Headache, hypokalemia, tremor

*CV: **Dysrhythmias,*** hypotension, chest pain

GI: Nausea, vomiting, anorexia, abdominal pain, ***hepatotoxicity, jaundice***

Contraindications: Hypersensitivity to this drug, severe aortic disease, severe pulmonic valvular disease, acute myocardial infarction

Precautions: Lactation, pregnancy (C), children, renal disease, hepatic disease, atrial flutter/fibrillation, elderly

Pharmacokinetics:
IV: Onset 2-5 min, peak 10 min, duration variable; half-life 4-6 hr; metabolized in liver; excreted in urine as drug and metabolites 60%-90%

NURSING CONSIDERATIONS
Assess:
- B/P and pulse q5min during infusion; if B/P drops 30 mm Hg, stop infusion and call prescriber
- Electrolytes: K, Na, Cl, Ca; renal function studies: BUN, creatinine; blood studies: platelet count
- ALT, AST, bilirubin qd
- I&O ratio and weight qd; diuresis should increase with continuing therapy
- If platelets are <150,000/mm³, drug is usually discontinued and another drug started
- Extravasation; change site q48h

Administer:
- Potassium supplements if ordered for K levels <3 mg/dl

IV
- Into running dextrose infusion through Y-connector or directly into tubing; dilute with 0.9% NaCl to 1-3 mg/ml; do not mix with glucose for long-term infusion
- By infusion pump for doses other than bolus

Additive compatibilities: Quinidine

Syringe compatibilities: Atropine, calcium chloride, digoxin, epinephrine, lidocaine, morphine, propranolol, sodium bicarbonate, verapamil

Y-site compatibilities: Digoxin, diltiazem, dobutamine, dopamine, epinephrine, fentanyl, heparin, hydro-

M

---

morphone, labetalol, lorazepam, midazolam, morphine, nicardipine, nitroglycerin, norepinephrine, propranolol, quinidine, ranitidine, thiopental, vecuronium

Evaluate:

• Therapeutic response: increased cardiac output, decreased PCWP, adequate CVP, decreased dyspnea, fatigue, edema, ECG

Treatment of overdose: Discontinue drug, support circulation

---

mineral oil (OTC)

Agoral Plain, Fleet Mineral Oil Enema, Kondremul*, Kondremul Plain, Liqui-doss, Lansoyl*, Milkinol, Neo-Cultol, Nujol, Petrogalar Plain, Zymenol

Func. class.: Laxative-lubricant
Chem. class.: Petroleum hydrocarbon

Action: Eases passage of stool by increasing water retention in feces; acts as lubricant

Uses: Constipation, preparation for bowel surgery or exam

Dosage and routes:

• *Adult:* **PO** 15-30 ml hs; **ENEMA** 4 oz

• *Child 6-12 yr:* **PO** 5-15 ml hs; **ENEMA** 1-2 oz

• *Child 2-11 yr:* **ENEMA** 1-2 oz

Available forms: Oil, enema; jelly 55%; susp 1.4, 2.5, 2.75 mg/5 ml

Side effects/adverse reactions:

CNS: Muscle weakness

GI: Nausea, vomiting, anorexia, diarrhea, pruritus ani, hepatic infiltration

*META: **Hypoprothrombinemia***

*RESP: **Lipid pneumonia***

Contraindications: Hypersensitivity, intestinal obstruction, abdominal pain, nausea/vomiting

Precautions: Pregnancy (UK), swallowing difficulty

Pharmacokinetics: Excreted in feces

Interactions:

• Increased effect of oral anticoagulants

• Decreased absorption: fat-soluble vitamins (A, D, E, K) if used for prolonged time

NURSING CONSIDERATIONS

Assess:

• Stool for color, consistency, amount

• Blood, urine electrolytes if drug is used often by patient

• I&O ratio to identify fluid loss

• Cause of constipation; lack of fluids, bulk, exercise

• Cramping, rectal bleeding, nausea, vomiting; drug should be discontinued

Administer:

• Alone for better absorption

• In morning or evening (oral dose)

• Cautiously in elderly to prevent aspiration

Evaluate:

• Therapeutic response: decrease in constipation

Teach patient/family:

• Not to use laxatives for long-term therapy; bowel tone will be lost

• That normal bowel movements do not always occur daily

• Not to use in presence of abdominal pain, nausea, vomiting

• To notify prescriber if constipation unrelieved or if symptoms of electrolyte imbalance occur: muscle cramps, pain, weakness, dizziness, excessive thirst

• Not to use with food or vitamin preparations; delays digestion and absorption of fat-soluble vitamins

---

◆ = Nursing alert   🌿 = Herb-drug interaction   🚫 = Do not crush

minocycline (R)

(min-oh-sye'kleen)

Apo-Minocycline*, Arestin, Dynacin, Minocin, Minocin IV, Vectrin

Func. class.: Broad-spectrum antiinfective

Chem. class.: Tetracycline

Action: Inhibits protein synthesis, phosphorylation in microorganisms by binding to 30S ribosomal subunits, reversibly binding to 50S ribosomal subunits; bacteriostatic

Uses: Syphilis, *Chlamydia trachomatis,* gonorrhea, lymphogranuloma venereum, rickettsial infections, inflammatory acne, *Neisseria meningitidis, Neisseria gonorrheae, Treponema pallidum, Chlamydia trachomatis, Ureaplasma urealyticum, Mycoplasma pneumoniae, Nocardia,* periodontitis

Investigational uses: Rheumatoid arthritis

Dosage and routes:

• *Adult:* **PO/IV** 200 mg, then 100 mg q12h or 50 mg q6h, not to exceed 400 mg/24 hr **IV**

• *Child >8 yr:* **PO/IV** 4 mg/kg then 4 mg/kg/day **PO** in divided doses q12h

Gonorrhea

• *Adult:* **PO** 200 mg, then 100 mg q12h × 4 days

Chlamydia trachomatis

• *Adult:* **PO** 100 mg bid × 7 days

Syphilis

• *Adult:* **PO** 200 mg, then 100 mg q12h × 10-15 days

Uncomplicated gonococcal urethritis in men

• *Adult:* **PO** 100 mg bid × 5 days

Rheumatoid arthritis (off-label)

• *Adult:* **PO** 100 mg bid for ≤48 wk

Available forms: Tabs 50, 100 mg; caps 50, 100 mg; oral susp 50 mg/5 ml; inj 100 mg; microspheres

Side effects/adverse reactions:

CNS: Dizziness, fever, light-headedness, vertigo

*HEMA: **Eosinophilia, neutropenia, thrombocytopenia, hemolytic anemia***

EENT: Dysphagia, glossitis, decreased calcification of deciduous teeth, permanent discoloration of teeth, oral candidiasis

GI: Nausea, abdominal pain, *vomiting, diarrhea,* anorexia, enterocolitis, ***hepatotoxicity,*** flatulence, abdominal cramps, epigastric burning, stomatitis

CV: Pericarditis

GU: Increased BUN, polyuria, polydipsia, ***renal failure, nephrotoxicity***

INTEG: Rash, urticaria, photosensitivity, increased pigmentation, ***exfoliative dermatitis,*** pruritus, angioedema, blue-gray color of skin, mucous membranes

Contraindications: Hypersensitivity to tetracyclines, children <8 yr, pregnancy (D)

Precautions: Hepatic disease, lactation

Pharmacokinetics:

PO: Peak 2-3 hr, half-life 11-17 hr; excreted in urine, feces, breast milk; crosses placenta; 70%-75% protein bound

Interactions:

• Decreased effect of minocycline: antacids, sodium bicarbonate, alkali products, iron, kaolin/pectin, cimetidine

• Increased effect: warfarin

• Decreased effect of barbiturates, carbamazepine, phenytoin, penicillins, oral contraceptives

• Nephrotoxicity: methoxyflurane

Lab test interferences:

False negative: Urine glucose with Clinistix or Tes-Tape

M

Side effects: *italics* = common; ***bold italics*** = life-threatening

NURSING CONSIDERATIONS
Assess:
• I&O ratio
• Blood studies: PT, CBC, AST, ALT, BUN, creatinine
• Signs of anemia: Hct, Hgb, fatigue
• Allergic reactions: rash, itching, pruritus, angioedema
• Nausea, vomiting, diarrhea; administer antiemetic, antacids as ordered
• Overgrowth of infection: fever, malaise, redness, pain, swelling, drainage, perineal itching, diarrhea, changes in cough or sputum, black, furry tongue
Administer:
• After C&S obtained
• 2 hr before or after laxative or ferrous products; 3 hr after antacid or kaolin-pectin product (PO)
IV
• After diluting 100 mg/5 ml sterile H_2O for inj; further dilute in 500-1000 ml of NaCl, dextrose sol, LR, Ringer's sol; run 100 mg/6 hr
Y-site compatibilities: Aztreonam, cisatracurium, cyclophosphamide, filgrastim, fludarabine, granisetron, heparin, hydrocortisone, magnesium sulfate, melphalan, perphenazine, potassium chloride, remifentanil, sargramostim, teniposide, vinorelbine, vit B/C
Perform/provide:
• Storage in airtight, light-resistant container at room temperature
Evaluate:
• Therapeutic response: decreased temp, absence of lesions, negative C&S
Teach patient/family:
• To avoid sunlight; sunscreen does not seem to decrease photosensitivity
• That all prescribed medication must be taken to prevent superinfection; not to use outdated product, Fanconi's syndrome may occur
• To take with a full glass of water; take with food for GI symptoms

---

minoxidil (℞)

(mi-nox′i-dill)
Loniten, minoxidil, Rogaine (top)
Func. class.: Antihypertensive
Chem. class.: Vasodilator, peripheral

Action: Directly relaxes arteriolar smooth muscle, causing vasodilation
Uses: Severe hypertension unresponsive to other therapy (use with diuretic); topically to treat alopecia
Dosage and routes:
Severe hypertension
• *Adult:* **PO** 2.5-5 mg/day not to exceed 100 mg daily, usual range 10-40 mg/day in single doses
• *Geriatric:* **PO** 2.5 mg qd, may be increased gradually
• *Child <12 yr:* **PO** (initial) 0.2 mg/kg/day; (effective range) 0.25-1 mg/kg/day; (max) 50 mg/day
Alopecia
• *Adult:* Apply topically, rub into scalp daily
Available forms: Tabs 2.5, 10 mg; top 20, 50 mg/ml
Side effects/adverse reactions:
Systemic
CV: Severe rebound hypertension, tachycardia, angina, increased T wave, *CHF, pulmonary edema, pericardial effusion,* edema, sodium, water retention
CNS: Drowsiness, dizziness, sedation, headache, depression, fatigue
GI: Nausea, vomiting
GU: Gynecomastia, breast tenderness
INTEG: Pruritus, Stevens-Johnson syndrome, rash, hirsutism

◆ = Nursing alert   ∅ = Herb-drug interaction   ⊘ = Do not crush

HEMA: Hct, Hgb, erythrocyte count may decrease initially

Contraindications: Acute MI, dissecting aortic aneurysm, hypersensitivity, pheochromocytoma

Precautions: Pregnancy (C), lactation, children, renal disease, CAD, CHF

Do not confuse:
Loniten/Lotensin
minoxidil/Monopril

Pharmacokinetics:
PO: Onset 30 min, peak 2-3 hr, duration 75 hr; half-life 4.2 hr; metabolized in liver; metabolites excreted in urine, feces

Interactions:
• Orthostatic hypotension: antihypertensives

Lab test interferences:
Increase: Renal function studies
Decrease: Hgb/Hct/RBC

NURSING CONSIDERATIONS
Assess:
• Nausea, edema in feet, legs daily
• Skin turgor, dryness of mucous membranes for hydration status
• Rales, dyspnea, orthopnea
• Electrolytes: K, Na, Cl, CO_2
• Renal function studies: catecholamines, BUN, creatinine
• Hepatic function studies: AST, ALT, alk phosphatase
• B/P, pulse
• Weight daily, I&O

Administer:
TOP
• 1 ml no matter how much balding has occurred; increasing dosage does not speed growth

PO
• With meals for better absorption, to decrease GI symptoms
• With β-blocker and/or diuretic for hypertension

Perform/provide:
• Storage protected from light and heat

Evaluate:
• Therapeutic response: decreased B/P or increased hair growth

Teach patient/family:
• That body hair will increase but is reversible after discontinuing treatment
• Not to discontinue drug abruptly
• To report pitting edema, dizziness, weight gain >5 lb, shortness of breath, bruising or bleeding, heart rate >20 beats/min over normal, severe indigestion, dizziness, lightheadedness, panting, new or aggravated symptoms of angina
• To take drug exactly as prescribed, or serious side effects may occur

Topical
• That for topical use, treatment must continue long-term or new hair will be lost
• Not to use except on scalp

Treatment of overdose: Administer normal saline IV, vasopressors

M

---

mirtazapine (℞)
(mer-ta′za-peen)
Remeron, Remeron SolTab
Func. class.: Antidepressant
Chem. class.: Tetracyclic

Action: Blocks reuptake of norepinephrine, serotonin into nerve endings, increasing action of norepinephrine, serotonin in nerve cells

Uses: Depression, dysthymic disorder, bipolar disorder—depressed, agitated depression

Dosage and routes:
• *Adult:* PO 15 mg/day at hs, maintenance to continue for 6 mo; orally disintegrating tabs: open blister pack, place tab on tongue, allow to disintegrate, swallow
• *Geriatric:* PO 7.5 mg q hs, increase by 7.5 mg q1-2wk to desired dose, max 45 mg/day

Available forms: Tabs 15, 30 mg; orally disintegrating tab 15, 30, 45 mg

Side effects/adverse reactions:

HEMA: **Agranulocytosis, thrombocytopenia, eosinophilia, leukopenia**

CNS: *Dizziness, drowsiness,* confusion, headache, anxiety, tremors, stimulation, weakness, insomnia, nightmares, EPS (elderly), increased psychiatric symptoms, *seizures*

GI: *Diarrhea, dry mouth,* nausea, vomiting, *paralytic ileus,* increased appetite, cramps, epigastric distress, *jaundice, hepatitis,* stomatitis

GU: *Urinary retention,* ***acute renal failure***

INTEG: Rash, urticaria, sweating, pruritus, photosensitivity

CV: *Orthostatic hypotension, ECG changes, tachycardia,* ***hypertension,*** palpitations

EENT: *Blurred vision,* tinnitus, mydriasis

Contraindications: Hypersensitivity to tricyclics, recovery phase of MI, convulsive disorders, prostatic hypertrophy

Precautions: Suicidal patients, severe depression, increased intraocular pressure, narrow-angle glaucoma, urinary retention, cardiac disease, hepatic disease, hypothyroidism, hyperthyroidism, electroshock therapy, elective surgery, elderly, pregnancy (C)

Pharmacokinetics:

PO: Peak 12 hr, metabolized by liver; excreted in urine, feces; crosses placenta; half-life 20-40 hr

Interactions:

• Decreased effects of clonidine, indirect-acting sympathomimetics (ephedrine)

• Increased CNS depression, alcohol, barbiturates, benzodiazepines, CNS depressants

 Hyperpyretic crisis, seizures, hypertensive episode: MAOIs

 Increased anticholinergic effect: belladonna, henbane

 Increased antidepressant action: scopolia

Lab test interferences:

Increase: Serum bilirubin, blood glucose, alk phosphatase

False increase: Urinary catecholamines

Decrease: VMA, 5-HIAA

NURSING CONSIDERATIONS

Assess:

• B/P (lying, standing), pulse q4h; if systolic B/P drops 20 mm Hg, hold drug, notify prescriber; take vital signs q4h in patients with cardiovascular disease

• Blood studies: CBC, leukocytes, differential, cardiac enzymes if patient is receiving long-term therapy

• Hepatic studies: AST, ALT, bilirubin, creatinine

• Weight qwk; appetite may increase with drug

• ECG for flattening of T wave, bundle branch block, AV block, dysrhythmias in cardiac patients

• EPS primarily in elderly: rigidity, dystonia, akathisia

• Mental status: mood, sensorium, affect, suicidal tendencies, increase in psychiatric symptoms: depression, panic

• Alcohol consumption; if alcohol is consumed, hold dose until morning

Administer:

• Increased fluids, bulk in diet for constipation, especially elderly

• With food, milk for GI symptoms

• Dosage hs if oversedation occurs during day; may take entire dose hs; elderly may not tolerate once/day dosing

• Gum, hard candy, or frequent sips of water for dry mouth

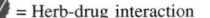 = Nursing alert   = Herb-drug interaction   = Do not crush

• Orally disintegrating tab: no water needed; allow to dissolve on tongue

Perform/provide:

• Storage in tight container at room temperature; do not freeze

• Assistance with ambulation during beginning therapy, since drowsiness/dizziness occurs

• Safety measures, including side rails, primarily in elderly

• Checking to see PO medication swallowed

Evaluate:

• Therapeutic response: decreased depression

Teach patient/family:

• That therapeutic effects may take 2-3 wk

• To use caution in driving, other activities requiring alertness, because of drowsiness, dizziness, blurred vision

• To avoid alcohol ingestion, other CNS depressants

Treatment of overdose: ECG monitoring, induce emesis; lavage, activated charcoal; administer anticonvulsant

misoprostol (℞)

(mye-soe-prost′ole)

Cytotec

Func. class.: Gastric mucosa protectant

Chem. class.: Prostaglandin E_1-analog

Action: Inhibits gastric acid secretion; may protect gastric mucosa; can increase bicarbonate, mucus production

Uses: Prevention of nonsteroidal antiinflammatory drug-induced gastric ulcers

Investigational uses: Used investigationally with methotrexate to produce abortion

Dosage and routes:

• *Adult:* PO 200 µg qid with food for duration of nonsteroidal antiinflammatory therapy; if 200 µg is not tolerated, 100 µg may be given

Available forms: Tabs 100, 200 µg

Side effects/adverse reactions:

GI: Diarrhea, nausea, vomiting, flatulence, constipation, dyspepsia, abdominal pain

GU: Spotting, cramps, hypermenorrhea, menstrual disorders

Contraindications: Hypersensitivity, pregnancy (X)

Precautions: Lactation, children, elderly, renal disease

Do not confuse:

cytotec/Cytoxan

misoprostol/metoprolol

Pharmacokinetics:

PO: Peak 12 min, plasma steady state achieved within 2 days, excreted in urine

Interactions:

• Drug/food: decreased absorption when taken with food

NURSING CONSIDERATIONS

Assess:

• GI symptoms: hematemesis, occult or frank blood in stools, gastric aspirate, cramping, severe diarrhea

• Obtain a negative pregnancy test; miscarriages are common

• Gastric pH (>5 should be maintained)

Administer:

• PO with meals for prolonged drug effect; avoid use of magnesium antacids

Perform/provide:

• Storage at room temperature

Evaluate:

• Therapeutic response: absence of pain or GI complaints; prevention of ulcers

Teach patient/family:

• To take only as directed

• Not to take if pregnant (can cause miscarriage) and not to become pregnant while taking this medication; if pregnancy occurs during therapy, discontinue drug, notify prescriber; not to administer to nursing mothers

• Not to give drug to anyone else or take for more than 4 wk unless directed by prescriber

• To avoid OTC preparations: aspirin, cough, cold products; condition may worsen

---

mitomycin (R)

(mye-toe-mye′sin)
mitomycin, Mutamycin
Func. class.: Antineoplastic, antiinfective

Action: Inhibits DNA synthesis, primarily; derived from *Streptomyces caespitosus;* appears to cause cross-linking of DNA, a vesicant

Uses: Pancreas, stomach cancer, head and neck or breast cancer

Investigational uses: Palliative treatment of head, neck, colon, breast, biliary, cervical, lung malignancies

Dosage and routes:
• *Adult:* **IV** 10-20 mg/m^2 q6-8wk
Available forms: Inj 5, 20, 40 mg/vial

Side effects/adverse reactions:
HEMA: **Thrombocytopenia, leukopenia, anemia**
GI: Nausea, vomiting, anorexia, stomatitis, hepatotoxicity, diarrhea
GU: Urinary retention, **renal failure,** edema
INTEG: Rash, alopecia, **extravasation**
RESP: **Fibrosis, pulmonary infiltrate,** dyspnea
CNS: Fever, headache, confusion, drowsiness, syncope, fatigue
EENT: Blurred vision, drowsiness, syncope

Contraindications: Hypersensitivity, pregnancy (D) (1st trimester), as a single agent, thrombocytopenia, coagulation disorders, lactation

Precautions: Renal disease, bone marrow depression

Pharmacokinetics: Half-life 1 hr, metabolized in liver, 10% excreted in urine (unchanged)

Interactions:
• Increased toxicity: other antineoplastics (vinca alkaloids), radiation

NURSING CONSIDERATIONS
Assess:
• CBC, differential, platelet count weekly; withhold drug if WBC is <2000/mm^3, granulocyte count <1000/mm^3, or platelet count is <100,000/mm^3; notify prescriber

• Pulmonary function tests, chest x-ray before, during therapy; chest x-ray should be obtained q2wk during treatment

• Renal function studies: BUN, serum uric acid, urine CrCl, electrolytes before, during therapy

• I&O ratio; report fall in urine output to <30 ml/hr

• Monitor temp q4h; fever may indicate beginning infection

• LFTs before, during therapy: bilirubin, AST, ALT, alk phosphatase as needed or monthly; check for jaundiced skin and sclera, dark urine, clay-colored stools, itchy skin, abdominal pain, fever, diarrhea

• Alkalosis if severe vomiting is present

• Bleeding: hematuria, guaiac, bruising, petechiae, mucosa or orifices q8h

• Dyspnea, rales, unproductive cough, chest pain, tachypnea, fatigue, increased pulse, pallor, lethargy

• Effects of alopecia on body image; discuss feelings about body changes

---

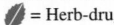

• Inflammation of mucosa, breaks in skin
• Buccal cavity q8h for dryness, sores, ulceration, white patches, oral pain, bleeding, dysphagia
• Local irritation, pain, burning at injection site
• GI symptoms: frequency of stools, cramping
• Acidosis, signs of dehydration: rapid respirations, poor skin turgor, decreased urine output, dry skin, restlessness, weakness

Administer:
• Apply ice compress for extravasation; stop infusion
• Antiemetic 30-60 min before giving drug to prevent vomiting
• IV after diluting 5 mg/10 ml sterile H_2O for inj; allow to stand, give through Y-tube or 3-way stopcock; give over 5-10 min
• Transfusion for anemia
• Antispasmodic for GI symptoms

Additive compatibilities: Dexamethasone, hydrocortisone
Solution compatibilities: LR, 0.3% NaCl, 0.5% NaCl
Syringe compatibilities: Bleomycin, cisplatin, cyclophosphamide, doxorubicin, droperidol, fluorouracil, furosemide, heparin, leucovorin, methotrexate, metoclopramide, vinblastine, vincristine
Y-site compatibilities: Allopurinol, amifostine, bleomycin, cisplatin, cyclophosphamide, doxorubicin, droperidol, fluorouracil, furosemide, granisetron, heparin, leucovorin, melphalan, methotrexate, metoclopramide, ondansetron, teniposide, thiotepa, vinblastine, vincristine

Perform/provide:
• Liquid diet: carbonated beverages, gelatin may be added if patient is not nauseated or vomiting
• Rinsing of mouth tid-qid with water; brushing of teeth with baking soda bid-tid with soft brush or cotton-tipped applicators for stomatitis; use unwaxed dental floss
Storage at room temperature 1 wk after reconstituting or 2 wk refrigerated

Evaluate:
• Therapeutic response: decreased tumor size, spread of malignancy

Teach patient/family:
• To report any complaints, side effects to nurse or prescriber
• That hair may be lost during treatment and wig or hairpiece may make the patient feel better; tell patient that new hair may be different in color, texture
• To avoid foods with citric acid, hot or rough texture
• To report any bleeding, white spots, ulcerations in mouth; tell patient to examine mouth qd
• To avoid crowds, people with infections if granulocyte count is low

M

RARELY USED

mitotane (R)
(mye′toe-tane)
Lysodren, p′-DDD
Func. class.: Antineoplastic

Uses: Adrenocortical carcinoma
Dosage and routes:
• *Adult:* **PO** 9-10 g/day in divided doses tid or qid; may have to decrease dose for severe reaction
Contraindications: Hypersensitivity

---

mitoxantrone (R)

(mye-toe-zan'trone)
Novantrone

Func. class.: Antineoplastic, antiinfective, immunomodulator

Chem. class.: Synthetic anthraquinone

Action: DNA reactive agent, cytocidal effect on both proliferating and nonproliferating cells, suggesting lack of cell cycle phase specificity (vesicant)

Uses: Acute nonlymphocytic leukemia (adult), relapsed leukemia, breast cancer; used with steroids to treat bone pain (advanced prostate cancer), MS

Investigational uses: Breast and liver malignancies, non-Hodgkin's lymphoma

Dosage and routes:
• *Adult:* **IV INF** 12 mg/m^2/day on days 1-3, and 100 mg/m^2 cytosine arabinoside × 7 days as a continuous 24 hr infusion
• *Adult:* **IV** 12 mg/m^2 given as a short 5-15 min inf

Available forms: Inj 2 mg/ml

Side effects/adverse reactions:

*GI: Nausea, vomiting, diarrhea, anorexia, mucositis, **hepatotoxicity***

*HEMA: **Thrombocytopenia, leukopenia, myelosuppression, anemia***

INTEG: Rash, necrosis at injection site, dermatitis, thrombophlebitis at injection site, alopecia

*CV: **CHF, cardiopathy, dysrhythmias***

MISC: Fever

RESP: Cough, dyspnea

Contraindications: Hypersensitivity, pregnancy (D)

Precautions: Myelosuppression, lactation, cardiac disease, children; renal, hepatic disease; gout

Pharmacokinetics: Highly bound to plasma proteins, metabolized in liver, excreted via renal, hepatobiliary systems; half-life 24-72 hr

Interactions:
• Do not mix with heparin; precipitate will form
• Do not mix with any other drug

NURSING CONSIDERATIONS

Assess:
• CBC, differential, platelet count qwk; withhold drug if WBC is <4000/mm^3 or platelet count is <75,000/mm^3; notify prescriber of these results
• LFTs before, during therapy: bilirubin, AST, ALT, alk phosphatase prn or qmo
• Renal function studies: BUN, serum uric acid, urine CrCl, electrolytes before, during therapy
• Bleeding, hematuria, guaiac, bruising or petechiae, mucosa or orifices q8h
• Jaundiced skin and sclera, dark urine, clay-colored stools, itchy skin, abdominal pain, fever, diarrhea
• Acidosis, signs of dehydration: rapid respirations, poor skin turgor, decreased urine output, dry skin, restlessness, weakness
• For MS: obtain MUGA, LVEF baselines; repeat LVEF if symptoms of CHF occur or if cumulative dose is >100 mg/m^2; do not administer to patients who have received a lifetime dose of ≥140 mg/m^2 or if LVEF <50% or significant L LVEF
• Do not administer to patients with MS if neutrophils <1500 cells/mm^3
• Obtain pregnancy test in all women of childbearing age, even if birth control is used

Administer:
• Medications by oral route if possible; avoid IM, SC, IV routes to prevent infections

◆ = Nursing alert   🖋 = Herb-drug interaction   ⊘ = Do not crush

• Antiemetic 30-60 min before giving drug to prevent vomiting
• IV after diluting with 50 ml or more NS or D$_5$W; give over 3-5 min, running IV of D$_5$W or NS; may be diluted further in D$_5$W, NS and run over 15-30 min; check for extravasation

Additive compatibilities: Cyclophosphamide, cytarabine, fluorouracil, hydrocortisone, potassium chloride
Solution compatibilities: D$_5$/0.9 NaCl, D$_5$W, 0.9% NaCl
Y-site compatibilities: Allopurinol, amifostine, cladribine, filgrastim, fludarabine, granisetron, melphalan, ondansetron, sargramostim, teniposide, thiotepa, vinorelbine
Perform/provide:
• Liquid diet: carbonated beverages, Jell-O; dry toast, crackers may be added if patient is not nauseated or vomiting
• Rinsing of mouth tid-qid with water, club soda; brushing of teeth bid-qid with soft brush or cotton-tipped applicators for stomatitis; use unwaxed dental floss
Evaluate:
• Therapeutic response: decreased tumor size, spread of malignancy
Teach patient/family:
• To report side effects to nurse or physician
• To avoid foods with citric acid, rough texture, or hot
• To report any bleeding, white spots, ulcerations in mouth; tell patient to examine mouth qd
• That sclera, urine may turn blue or green
• To notify prescriber if pregnancy is suspected or planned

mivacurium (℞)
(miv-a-kure′ee-um)
Mivacron
Func. class.: Nondepolarizing neuromuscular blocker

Action: Inhibits transmission of nerve impulses by binding competitively with cholinergic receptor sites, antagonizing action of acetylcholine
Uses: Facilitation of endotracheal intubation, skeletal muscle relaxation during mechanical ventilation, surgery, or general anesthesia
Dosage and routes:
• *Adult:* **IV** 0.15 mg/kg; maintenance q15min
• *Child 2-12 yr:* **IV** 0.2 mg/kg for a 10 min block
Available forms: 5, 10 ml single-use vial (2 mg/ml); premixed infusion in D$_5$W 50-ml flex container
Side effects/adverse reactions:
CV: Decreased B/P, bradycardia, tachycardia
*RESP: **Prolonged apnea, bronchospasm, wheezing, respiratory depression***
EENT: Diplopia
MS: Weakness, prolonged skeletal muscle relaxation, ***paralysis***
INTEG: Rash, urticaria
Contraindications: Hypersensitivity
Precautions: Pregnancy (C), renal or hepatic disease, lactation, children <3 mo, fluid and electrolyte imbalances, neuromuscular disease, respiratory disease, obesity, elderly
Do not confuse:
Mivacron/Mazicon
Pharmacokinetics: Rapidly hydrolyzed by plasma cholinesterases, peak 2-3 min, reversal within 15-30 min

Interactions:
• Increased neuromuscular blockade: aminoglycosides, quinidine, local anesthetics, polymyxin antibiotics, enflurane, isoflurane, tetracyclines, halothane, Mg, colistin, procainamide, bacitracin, lincomycin, clindamycin, lithium

NURSING CONSIDERATIONS
Assess:
• For electrolyte imbalances (K, Mg); may lead to increased action of this drug
• Vital signs (B/P, pulse, respirations, airway) until fully recovered; rate, depth, pattern of respirations, strength of hand grip
• I&O ratio; check for urinary retention, frequency, hesitancy
• Recovery: decreased paralysis of face, diaphragm, leg, arm, rest of body
• Allergic reactions: rash, fever, respiratory distress, pruritus; drug should be discontinued

Administer:
• Using nerve stimulator by anesthesiologist to determine neuromuscular blockade
• Anticholinesterase to reverse neuromuscular blockade
• By slow IV over 1-2 min (only by qualified persons, usually an anesthesiologist)
• Only fresh sol
Y-site compatibilities: Etomidate, thiopental
Perform/provide:
• Storage at room temperature; do not freeze
• Reassurance if communication is difficult during recovery from neuromuscular blockade
• Frequent (q2h) instillation of artificial tears and covering eyes to prevent drying of cornea
Evaluate:
• Therapeutic response: paralysis of jaw, eyelid, head, neck, rest of body

Treatment of overdose: Neostigmine, monitor VS; may require mechanical ventilation

---

modafinil (R)
(moh-daf'ih-nil)
Provigil
Func. class.: Cerebral stimulant

Controlled Substance Schedule IV
Action: Promotes wakefulness, exact mechanism is unknown
Uses: Narcolepsy
Dosage and routes:
• *Adult:* **PO** 200 mg qd in the AM, may increase to 400 mg qd if needed
Hepatic dose
• Reduce dose by 50%
Available forms: Tabs 100, 200 mg
Side effects/adverse reactions:
META: Hyperglycemia, albuminuria
RESP: Rhinitis, pharyngitis, lung disorder, dyspnea, asthma, epistaxis
EENT: Abnormal vision, amblyopia
CNS: Hyperactivity, insomnia, restlessness, dizziness, headache, chills, stimulation
GI: Anorexia, dry mouth, diarrhea, nausea, vomiting, mouth ulcer, gingivitis, thirst
GU: Urinary retention, abnormal ejaculation
CV: Palpitations, tachycardia, hypertension, *dysrhythmias*
INTEG: Herpes simplex, dry skin
Contraindications: Hypersensitivity, hyperthyroidism, hypertension, glaucoma, severe arteriosclerosis, drug abuse, cardiovascular disease, anxiety
Precautions: Gilles de la Tourette's disorder, pregnancy (C), elderly, lactation, children <16 yr
Pharmacokinetics: Absorbed rapidly, well distributed, protein bind-

---

⬥ = Nursing alert   🌿 = Herb-drug interaction   🚫 = Do not crush

ing 60%, metabolized extensively, half-life 15 hr with multiple dosing, peak 2-4 hr

Interactions:

• Increased levels of drugs metabolized by CYP-2C19, CYP-2C9: clomipramine, phenytoin, warfarin, diazepam, propranolol

• Decreased levels of: cyclosporine, oral contraceptives, theophylline

• Decreased modafinil absorption: methylphenidate

• Use cautiously with MAOIs

• Altered levels of drugs metabolized by CYP-3A4: carbamazepine, phenobarbital, rifampin, itraconazole, ketoconazole

• Increased levels of: tricyclics

• Decreased absorption of: methylphenidate

NURSING CONSIDERATIONS

Assess:

• For improvement in narcolepsy

Administer:

• Gum, hard candy, frequent sips of water for dry mouth

Evaluate:

• Therapeutic response: increased CNS stimulation, decreased drowsiness

Teach patient/family:

• To decrease caffeine consumption (coffee, tea, cola, chocolate); may increase irritability, stimulation

• To avoid OTC preparations unless approved by prescriber

• To notify prescriber if rash or other symptoms of allergy occur

• To notify prescriber if pregnancy is suspected, or if breast-feeding; another form of contraception is needed if using hormonal contraception while on this drug and for a month afterwards

• To avoid hazardous activities until stabilized on medication

---

moexipril (℞)

(moe-ex′ih-prill)
Univasc
Func. class.: Antihypertensive
Chem. class.: Angiotensin-converting enzyme inhibitor

Action: Selectively suppresses renin-angiotensin-aldosterone system; inhibits ACE; prevents conversion of angiotensin I to angiotensin II; results in dilation of arterial, venous vessels

Uses: Hypertension, alone or in combination with thiazide diuretics

Dosage and routes:

• *Adult:* **PO** 7.5 mg 1 hr ac initially, may be increased or divided depending on B/P response; maintenance dosage; 7.5-30 mg qd in 1-2 divided doses 1 hr ac

Renal dose

• CrCl <40 ml/min 3.75 mg/day titrate to desired dose

Available forms: Tabs 7.5, 15 mg

Side effects/adverse reactions:

CV: Hypotension, postural hypotension

GU: Impotence, dysuria, nocturia, proteinuria, nephrotic syndrome, acute reversible renal failure, polyuria, oliguria, frequency

HEMA: **Neutropenia**

INTEG: Rash

RESP: **Bronchospasm,** dyspnea, dry cough

META: Hypokalemia

GI: Loss of taste

CNS: Fever, chills

SYST: **Angioedema, anaphylaxis**

Contraindications: Hypersensitivity, children, lactation, heart block, bilateral renal stenosis, K-sparing diuretics, pregnancy (D) 2nd/3rd trimester

Precautions: Dialysis patients, hypovolemia, leukemia, scleroderma,

M

---

lupus erythematosus, blood dyscrasias, CHF, diabetes mellitus, renal disease, thyroid disease, COPD, asthma, pregnancy (C) (1st trimester)

Pharmacokinetics: Metabolized by liver (metabolites), excreted in urine; crosses placenta; excreted in breast milk

Interactions:
• Increased hypotension: diuretics, other antihypertensives, ganglionic blockers, adrenergic blockers
• Do not use with potassium-sparing diuretics, sympathomimetics, potassium supplements

Lab test interferences:
False positive: Urine acetone

NURSING CONSIDERATIONS
Assess:
• Blood studies: neutrophils, decreased platelets
• B/P
• Renal studies: protein, BUN, creatinine; watch for increased levels that may indicate nephrotic syndrome
• Baselines in renal, liver function tests before therapy begins
• K levels, although hyperkalemia rarely occurs
• Edema in feet, legs daily
• Allergic reaction: rash, fever, pruritus, urticaria; drug should be discontinued if antihistamines fail to help
• Symptoms of CHF; edema, dyspnea, wet rales, B/P
• Renal symptoms: polyuria, oliguria, frequency

Administer:
• PO 1 hr before meals

Perform/provide:
• Storage in tight container at 86° F (30° C) or less

Evaluate:
• Therapeutic response: decrease in B/P in hypertension

Teach patient/family:
• To take 1 hr ac
• Not to discontinue drug abruptly
• Not to use OTC (cough, cold, or allergy) products unless directed by prescriber
• To comply with dosage schedule, even if feeling better
• To rise slowly to sitting or standing position to minimize orthostatic hypotension
• To notify prescriber of mouth sores, sore throat, fever, swelling of hands and feet, irregular heartbeat, chest pain, signs of angioedema
• That excessive perspiration, dehydration, vomiting, diarrhea may lead to fall in blood pressure; consult prescriber if these occur
• That dizziness, fainting, lightheadedness may occur during first few days of therapy
• That skin rash or impaired perspiration may occur
• How to take B/P

Treatment of overdose: 0.9% NaCl IV inf, hemodialysis

RARELY USED

molindone (℞)
(moe-lin'done)
Func. class.: Antipsychotic/neuroleptic

Uses: Psychotic disorders

Dosage and routes:
• *Adult:* **PO** 50-75 mg/day increasing to 225 mg/day if needed

Contraindications: Hypersensitivity, coma, child

---

montelukast (R)

(mon-teh-loo'kast)
Singulair
Func. class.: Bronchodilator
Chem. class.: Leukotriene receptor, cysteinyl

Action: Inhibits leukotriene (LTD_4) formation; leukotrienes exert their effects by increasing neutrophil, eosinophil migration; aggregation of neutrophils, monocytes; smooth muscle contraction, capillary permeability; these actions further lead to bronchoconstriction, inflammation, edema

Uses: Chronic asthma in adults and children

Dosage and routes:
Asthma
• *Adult and child ≥15 yr:* **PO** 10 mg qd PM
• *Child 6-14 yr:* **PO** 5 mg chew tab qd PM
• *Child 2-5 yr:* **PO** chew tab 4 mg qd
Available forms: Tabs 10 mg; tabs, chew 4, 5 mg

Side effects/adverse reactions:
CNS: Dizziness, fatigue, headache
GI: Abdominal pain, dyspepsia
INTEG: Rash
MS: Asthenia
RESP: Influenza, cough, nasal congestion

Contraindications: Hypersensitivity

Precautions: Acute attacks of asthma, alcohol consumption, pregnancy (B), lactation, child <6 yr, aspirin sensitivity

Pharmacokinetics: Rapidly absorbed, peak 3-4 hr, half-life 2.7-5.5 hr; protein binding 99%; metabolized by liver, excreted via bile

Interactions:
• Decreased montelukast levels: phenobarbital, rifampin
• Increased stimulation: ephedrine

NURSING CONSIDERATIONS
Assess:
◆Adult patients carefully for symptoms of Churg-Strauss syndrome (rare), including eosinophilia, vasculitic rash, worsening pulmonary symptoms, cardiac complications, and/or neuropathy
• CBC, blood chemistry, during treatment
• Respiratory rate, rhythm, depth; auscultate lung fields bilaterally; notify prescriber of abnormalities
• Allergic reactions: rash, urticaria; drug should be discontinued

Administer:
PO
• In PM qd

Evaluate:
• Therapeutic response: ability to breathe more easily

Teach patient/family:
• To check OTC medications, current prescription medications for ephedrine, which will increase stimulation; to avoid alcohol
• To avoid hazardous activities; dizziness may occur
• That drug is not to be used for acute asthma attacks

moricizine (R)

(more-i'siz-een)
Ethmozine
Func. class.: Antidysrhythmic, group I
Chem. class.: Phenothiazine

Action: Decreased rate of rise of action potential, prolonging refractory period and shortening the action potential duration; depression of inward influx if sodium mediates the effects; drug may slow atrial and AV nodal conduction

Uses: Life-threatening ventricular dysrhythmias

Dosage and routes:
• *Adult:* **PO** 10-15 mg/kg/day or 600-900 mg/day in 2-3 divided doses
Hepatic dose
• *Adult:* **PO** 600 mg or less qd
Available forms: Film-coated tabs 200, 250, 300 mg

Side effects/adverse reactions:
GI: Nausea, abdominal pain, vomiting, diarrhea
CNS: Dizziness, headache, fatigue, perioral numbness, euphoria, nervousness, sleep disorders, depression, tinnitus, fatigue
RESP: Dyspnea, hyperventilation, *apnea,* asthma, pharyngitis, cough
GU: Sexual dysfunction, difficult urination, dysuria, incontinence
CV: Palpitations, chest pain, *CHF,* hypertension, syncope, dysrhythmias, bradycardia, *MI, thrombophlebitis*
MISC: Sweating, musculoskeletal pain

Contraindications: 2nd/3rd degree AV block, right bundle branch block, cardiogenic shock, hypersensitivity

Precautions: CHF, hypokalemia, hyperkalemia, sick sinus syndrome, pregnancy (B), lactation, children, impaired hepatic and renal function, cardiac dysfunction

Pharmacokinetics: Half-life 1.5-3.5 hr; peak 0.5-2.2 hr; metabolized by the liver; metabolites excreted in feces and urine, protein binding >90%

Interactions:
• Increased plasma levels of moricizine: cimetidine
• Digoxin or propranolol may enhance some cardiac effects of moricizine; moricizine may decrease effects of theophylline

💉 Increased anticholinergic effect: henbane

💉 Increased potassium loss, increased antidysrhythmic action: aloe, cascara sagrada, buckthorn, rhubarb, senna

Lab test interferences:
Increase: CPK

NURSING CONSIDERATIONS
Assess:
• GI status: bowel pattern, number of stools
• Cardiac status: rate, rhythm, quality
• Chest x-ray, pulmonary function test during treatment
• I&O ratio; check for decreasing output
• B/P for fluctuations
• Lung fields: bilateral rales may occur in CHF patient
• Increased respirations, increased pulse; drug should be discontinued
◆➤ Toxicity: fine tremors, dizziness
• Cardiac status: respiration, rate, rhythm, character continuously
Evaluate:
• Therapeutic response: absence of dysrhythmias
Teach patient/family:
• To report side effects to prescriber

Treatment of overdose: O_2 artificial ventilation, ECG; administer dopamine for circulatory depression, diazepam or thiopental for convulsions

---

◆ = Nursing alert   💉 = Herb-drug interaction   🚫 = Do not crush

morphine (℞)

(mor′feen)

Astramorph PF, Duramorph, Epimorph*, Kadian, Infumorph 200, Infumorph 500, morphine sulfate, Morphitec*, M.O.S.*, M.O.S.-S.R.*, MS Contin, MSIR, OMS Concentrate, Oramorph SR, RMS, Roxanol, Roxanol 100, Roxanol Rescudose, Roxanol SR, UltraJect

Func. class.: Opiate analgesic
Controlled Substance Schedule II
Action: Depresses pain impulse transmission at the spinal cord level by interacting with opioid receptors
Uses: Severe pain
Dosage and routes:
• *Adult:* **SC/IM** 4-15 mg q4h prn; **PO** 10-30 mg q4h prn; **EXT REL** q8-12h; **RECT** 10-20 mg q4h prn; **IV** 4-10 mg diluted in 4-5 ml H₂O for injection, over 5 min
• *Child:* **SC/IV** 0.1-0.2 mg/kg, not to exceed 15 mg; **PO** 0.2-0.5 mg/kg q4-6h (reg rel), q12h (sus rel)
Available forms: Inj 0.5, 1, 2, 3, 4, 5, 8, 10, 15, 25, 50 mg/ml; sol tabs 10, 15, 30 mg; oral sol 10, 20 mg/5 ml, 20 mg/10 ml, 20 mg/ml; oral tabs 15, 30 mg; rect supp 5, 10, 20, 30 mg; ext rel tabs 15, 30, 60, 100, 200 mg; caps 15, 30 mg; syr 1, 5 mg/ml
Side effects/adverse reactions:
*HEMA: **Thrombocytopenia***
CNS: Drowsiness, dizziness, confusion, headache, sedation, euphoria
CV: Palpitations, ***bradycardia***, change in B/P, ***shock, cardiac arrest***
EENT: Tinnitus, blurred vision, miosis, diplopia
GI: Nausea, vomiting, anorexia, constipation, cramps, biliary tract pressure
GU: Urinary retention
INTEG: Rash, urticaria, bruising, flushing, diaphoresis, pruritus
*RESP: **Respiratory depression, respiratory arrest, apnea***
Contraindications: Hypersensitivity, addiction (narcotic), hemorrhage, bronchial asthma, increased intracranial pressure
Precautions: Addictive personality, pregnancy (C), lactation, acute MI, severe heart disease, elderly, respiratory depression, hepatic disease, renal disease, child <18 yr
Do not confuse:
morphine/hydromorphone
Roxanol/Roxicet
Pharmacokinetics:
PO: Onset variable, peak variable, duration variable
IM: Onset ½ hr, peak ½-1 hr, duration 3-7 hr
SC: Onset 15-20 min, peak 50-90 min, duration 3-5 hr
IV: Peak 20 min
RECT: Peak ½-1 hr, duration 4-5 hr
Intrathecal: Onset rapid, duration up to 24 hr
Metabolized by liver, crosses placenta; excreted in urine, breast milk; half-life 1½-2 hr
Interactions:
• Unpredictable reaction, avoid use: MAOIs
• Increased effects with other CNS depressants: alcohol, opiates, sedative/hypnotics, antipsychotics, skeletal muscle relaxants
• Decreased morphine action: rifampin
Lab test interferences:
Increase: Amylase
NURSING CONSIDERATIONS
Assess:
• Pain: location, type, character; give dose before pain becomes severe

M

• Bowel status; constipation common

• I&O ratio; check for decreasing output; may indicate urinary retention

• B/P, pulse, respirations (character, depth, rate)

• CNS changes: dizziness, drowsiness, hallucinations, euphoria, LOC, pupil reaction

• Allergic reactions: rash, urticaria

• Respiratory dysfunction: depression, character, rate, rhythm; notify prescriber if respirations are <12/min

Administer:

• With antiemetic for nausea, vomiting

• When pain is beginning to return; determine dosage interval by response; continuous dosing is more effective than prn

• May be given by patient: controlled analgesia

• Epidural cautiously in the elderly

IV

• After diluting with 5 ml or more sterile H_2O or NS; give 15 mg or less over 4-5 min; give through Y-tube or 3-way stopcock; may be added to IV sol, each 0.1-1 mg diluted in 1 ml D_5W, $D_{10}W$, 0.9% NaCl, 0.45% NaCl, Ringer's, LR, given with inf pump titrated to patient response

Additive compatibilities: Alteplase, atracurium, baclofen, bupivacaine, dobutamine, fluconazole, furosemide, meropenem, metoclopramide, ondansetron, succinylcholine, verapamil

Syringe compatibilities: Atropine, benzquinamide, bupivacaine, butorphanol, cimetidine, dimenhydrinate, diphenhydramine, droperidol, fentanyl, glycopyrrolate, hydroxyzine, ketamine, metoclopramide, midazolam, milrinone, pentazocine, per-

phenazine, promazine, ranitidine, scopolamine

Y-site compatibilities: Allopurinol, amifostine, amikacin, aminophylline, amiodarone, ampicillin, ampicillin/sulbactam, amsacrine, atenolol, atracurium, aztreonam, bumetanide, calcium chloride, cefamandole, cefazolin, cefmetazole, cefoperazone, cefotaxime, cefotetan, cefoxitin, ceftazidime, ceftizoxime, ceftriaxone, cefuroxime, cephalothin, cephapirin, chloramphenicol, cisatracurium, cisplatin, cladribine, clindamycin, cyclophosphamide, cytarabine, dexamethasone, digoxin, diltiazem, dobutamine, dopamine, doxycycline, enalaprilat, epinephrine, erythromycin, esmolol, etomidate, famotidine, fentanyl, filgrastim, fluconazole, fludarabine, foscarnet, gentamicin, granisetron, heparin, hydrocortisone, hydromorphone, IL-2, insulin (regular), kanamycin, labetalol, lidocaine, lorazepam, magnesium sulfate, melphalan, meropenem, methotrexate, methyldopa, methylprednisolone, metoclopramide, metoprolol, metronidazole, mezlocillin, midazolam, milrinone, moxalactam, nafcillin, nicardipine, nitroglycerin, norepinephrine, ondansetron, oxacillin, oxytocin, paclitaxel, pancuronium, penicillin G potassium, piperacillin, piperacillin/tazobactam, potassium chloride, propofol, propranolol, ranitidine, remifentanil, sodium bicarbonate, sodium nitroprusside, teniposide, thiotepa, ticarcillin, ticarcillin/clavulanate, tobramycin, trimethoprim-sulfamethoxazole, vancomycin, vecuronium, vinorelbine, vit B/C, warfarin, zidovudine

Perform/provide:

• Storage in light-resistant container at room temperature

• Assistance with ambulation

◆ = Nursing alert   ∅ = Herb-drug interaction   ⊘ = Do not crush

- Safety measures: side rails, night-light, call bell within easy reach
- Gradual withdrawal after long-term use

Evaluate:
- Therapeutic response; decrease in pain intensity

Teach patient/family:
- To change position slowly; orthostatic hypotension may occur
- To report any symptoms of CNS changes, allergic reactions
- That physical dependency may result from long-term use
- To avoid use of alcohol, CNS depressants
- That withdrawal symptoms may occur: nausea, vomiting, cramps, fever, faintness, anorexia

Treatment of overdose: Naloxone (Narcan) 0.2-0.8 mg IV, O_2, IV fluids, vasopressors

---

moxalactam
See cephalosporins—3rd generation

---

moxifloxacin
Avelox
Func. class.: Antiinfective
Chem. class.: Fluoroquinolone

Action: Interferes with conversion of intermediate DNA fragments into high-molecular-weight DNA in bacteria; DNA gyrase inhibitor

Uses: Acute bacterial sinusitis: *Streptococcus pneumoniae, Haemophilus influenzae, Moraxella catarrhalis;* acute bacterial exacerbation of chronic bronchitis: *S. pneumoniae, H. influenzae, Haemophilus parainfluenzae, Klebsiella pneumoniae, Staphylococcus aureus, M. catarrhalis;* community-acquired pneumonia: *S. pneumoniae, H. influenzae, Mycoplasma pneumoniae, Chlamydia pneumoniae, M. catarrhalis;* uncomplicated skin/skin structure infections: *S. aureus, Streptococcus pyogenes*

Dosage and routes:
Urinary tract infections
- *Adult:* 400 mg qd × 5-10 days depending on condition

Available forms: Tabs 400 mg

Side effects/adverse reactions:
CV: Prolonged QT interval, ***dysrhythmias***
CNS: Headache, dizziness, fatigue, insomnia, depression, *restlessness, seizures,* confusion
GI: Nausea, diarrhea, increased ALT, AST, flatulence, heartburn, *vomiting,* oral candidiasis, dysphagia
INTEG: Rash, pruritus, urticaria, photosensitivity, flushing, fever, chills
MS: Tremor, arthralgia, tendon rupture
*SYST: **Anaphylaxis, Stevens-Johnson syndrome***

Contraindications: Hypersensitivity to quinolones

Precautions: Pregnancy (C), lactation, children, renal disease, epilepsy, uncorrected hypokalemia, prolonged QT interval, patients receiving class IA, III antidysrhythmics

Pharmacokinetics: Excreted in urine as active drug, metabolites

Interactions:
- Decreased absorption of moxifloxacin: magnesium antacids, aluminum hydroxide, zinc, iron, sucralfate, calcium, enteral feeding, didanosine
- Increased serum levels of moxifloxacin: probenecid
- Increased toxicity: caffeine, theophylline, cyclosporine
- Increased warfarin, cyclosporine effect

M

• Prolonged QT: antidysrhythmics class IA, III

NURSING CONSIDERATIONS
Assess:

• CNS symptoms: headache, dizziness, fatigue, insomnia, depression

• Kidney, liver function studies: BUN, creatinine, AST, ALT

• I&O ratio, urine pH <5.5 is ideal

◆ Allergic reactions and anaphylaxis: fever, flushing, rash, urticaria, pruritus; keep epinephrine, emergency equipment nearby for anaphylaxis

Administer:

• 2 hr before or 2 hr after antacids, zinc, iron, calcium

Perform/provide:

• Limited intake of alkaline foods, drugs: milk, dairy products, alkaline antacids, sodium bicarbonate

Evaluate:

• Therapeutic response: decreased pain, C&S; absence of infection

Teach patient/family:

• Not to take any products containing magnesium or calcium (such as antacids), iron, or aluminum with this drug or within 2 hr of drug

• That photosensitivity may occur; patient should avoid sunlight or use sunscreen to prevent burns

• To use frequent rinsing of mouth, sugarless candy or gum for dry mouth

• To take as prescribed, not to double or miss doses

• Not to use theophylline with this product, may cause toxicity; contact prescriber if taking theophylline

• That fluids must be increased to 3 L/day to avoid crystallization in kidneys

• If dizziness occurs, to ambulate, perform activities with assistance

• To complete full course of drug therapy

• To contact prescriber if adverse reaction occurs or if inflammation or pain in tendon occurs

---

multivitamins (OTC, R)
Adavite, Dayalets, LKV Drops, Multi-75, Multiday, One-A-Day, Optilets, Poly-Visol, Quin tabs, Ru-Lets, Sesame Street Vitamins, Tab-A-Vite, Therabid, Theragram, Unicaps, Vita-Bob, Vita-Kid, many other brands
Func. class.: Vitamins, multiple

Action: Needed for adequate metabolism

Uses: Prevention and treatment of vitamin deficiencies

Dosage and routes:

• *Adult and child:* **PO/IV**—depends on brand

Available forms: Many

Side effects/adverse reactions:
None known at recommended dosage

Precautions: Pregnancy (A)

Do not confuse:
Theragran/Phenergan

NURSING CONSIDERATIONS
Assess:

• Vitamin deficiency: usually more than one vitamin is deficient

Administer:

• Liquid multivitamins diluted or dropped into patient's mouth using dropper provided with some brands

• Chew tabs should be chewed, not swallowed whole

• Give by cont IV inf only after diluting 5-10 ml multivitamins/500-1000 ml of D_5W, $D_{10}W$, $D_{20}W$, LR, D_5/LR, D_5/0.9% NaCl, 0.9% NaCl, 3% NaCl

• Do not use sol with crystals, precipate, or color other than bright yellow

---

◆ = Nursing alert   ⬤ = Herb-drug interaction   ⊘ = Do not crush

Additive compatibilities: Cefoxitin, isoproterenol, methyldopa, metoclopramide, metronidazole, netilmicin, norepinephrine, sodium bicarbonate, verapamil

Y-site compatibilities: Acyclovir, ampicillin, cefazolin, cephalothin, cephapirin, diltiazem, erythromycin, fludarabine, gentamicin, tacrolimus

Evaluate:

• Therapeutic response: check each individual vitamin for guidelines

Teach patient/family:

• That adequate nutrition must be maintained to prevent further deficiencies

• The drug interactions that should be avoided

• To comply with regimen

• To avoid presenting flavored multivitamins as candy; child may overdose

• To store out of children's reach

---

muromonab-CD3 (℞)
(mur-oo-mone'ab)
Orthoclone OKT3
Func. class.: Immunosuppressant
Chem. class.: Murine monoclonal antibody

Action: Reverses graft rejection by blocking T-cell function

Uses: Acute allograft rejection in renal, cardiac/hepatic transplant patients

Dosage and routes:

• *Adult:* **IV BOL** 5 mg/day × 10-14 days

• *Child:* **IV** 100 µg/kg/day × 10-14 days

Cardiac/hepatic allograft rejection, steroid resistant

• *Adult:* **IV BOL** 5 mg/day × 10-14 days; begin when it is known that rejection has not been reversed by steroids

Available forms: Inj 5 mg/5 ml

Side effects/adverse reactions:

*CNS: Pyrexia, chills, tremors, **aseptic meningitis***

*RESP: Dyspnea, wheezing, **pulmonary edema***

CV: Chest pain

GI: Vomiting, nausea, diarrhea

*MISC: **Infection, cytokine release syndrome, anaphylaxis***

Contraindications: Hypersensitivity to murine origin, fluid overload

Precautions: Pregnancy (C), child <2 yr, fever

Pharmacokinetics: Trough level steady state 3-14 days

Interactions:

• Increased immunosuppression: immunosuppressants

• Increased risk of infection: cyclosporine, corticosteroids, azathioprine

• Increased CNS symptoms: indomethacin

• Decreased immune response: vaccines

NURSING CONSIDERATIONS
Assess:

◆ For cytokine release syndrome (CRS): nausea, vomiting, chills, fever, joint pain, weakness, dizziness, diarrhea, tremors, abdominal pain

◆ For hypersensitivity, **anaphylaxis:** dyspnea, bronchospasm, urticaria, tachycardia, angioedema; emergency equipment must be available

• Blood studies: Hgb, WBC, platelets during treatment qmo; if leukocytes are <3000/mm³, drug should be discontinued; CD3, CD4, CD8, CD3 ≤25 cells/mm³

• Liver function studies: alk phosphatase, AST, ALT, bilirubin

◆ Hepatotoxicity: dark urine, jaundice, itching, light-colored stools; drug should be discontinued

---

• For infection: sore throat, fever, chills, temp, notify prescriber immediately

🔷 For aseptic meningitis: fever, headache, photophobia

🔷 For fluid overload: increased weight, I&O, edema, rales

Administer:
• For several days before transplant surgery
• All medications PO if possible; avoid IM injection, since infection may occur

IV
• IV undiluted; withdraw with a 0.2-0.22 low protein-binding μm filter, discard and use new needle for administration; give over 1 min
• Incompatible with any drug in syringe or sol

Evaluate:
• Therapeutic response: absence of graft rejection

Teach patient/family:
• To report fever, chills, sore throat, fatigue, since serious infection may occur; rash, dyspnea, fast heartbeat
• To use contraceptive measures during treatment
• To report cytokine release syndrome, give symptoms
• To avoid vaccinations during treatment
• To avoid persons with infections, crowds; infections may occur

---

mycophenolate (℞)
(mye-koe-phen'oh-late)
CellCept
Func. class.: Immunosuppressant

Action: Inhibits inflammatory responses that are mediated by the immune system; prolongs the survival of allogenic transplants

Uses: Organ transplants (to prevent rejection); prophylaxis of organ rejection in allogenic cardiac, hepatic, renal transplants

Investigational uses: Refractory uveitis, second-line therapy for Churg-Strauss syndrome, diffuse proliferative lupus nephritis (in combination)

Research note: When iron was administered with mycophenolate, a decreased absorption of mycophenolate resulted[25]

Dosage and routes:
Renal transplant
• *Adult:* **PO/IV** give initial dose 72 hr prior to transplantation; 1 g bid given to renal transplant patients in combination with corticosteroids, cyclosporine

Renal dose
• *Adult:* **PO/IV** GFR <25 ml/min, max 2 g/day

Cardiac transplant
• *Adult:* **PO/IV** 1.5 g bid, IV can be started ≤24 hr after transplant, switch to **PO** when able

Hepatic transplant
• *Adult:* **PO/IV** 1.5 gm bid; give IV over ≥2 hr

Available forms: Caps 250 mg; tabs 500 mg; inj (pwd) 500 mg/20 ml vial; pwd for oral susp 200 mg/ml

Side effects/adverse reactions:
GI: Diarrhea, constipation, nausea, vomiting, stomatitis, ***GI bleeding***
*HEMA: **Leukopenia, thrombocytopenia, anemia, pancytopenia***
INTEG: Rash
MS: Arthralgia, muscle wasting
RESP: Dyspnea, respiratory infection, increased cough, pharyngitis, bronchitis, pneumonia
CNS: Tremor, dizziness, insomnia, headache, fever
META: Peripheral edema, hypercholesterolemia, hypophosphatemia, edema, hyperkalemia, hypokalemia, hyperglycemia
*GU: UTI, hematuria, **renal tubular necrosis***

🔷 = Nursing alert   🌿 = Herb-drug interaction   🚫 = Do not crush

CV: Hypertension, chest pain
*SYST: **Lymphoma**, nonmelanoma skin carcinoma*

Contraindications: Hypersensitivity to this drug or mycophenolic acid
Precautions: Lymphomas, malignancies, neutropenia, renal disease, pregnancy (C), lactation
Pharmacokinetics: Rapidly and completely absorbed, metabolized to active metabolite (MPA), excreted in urine, feces
Interactions:
• Increased concentration of both drugs: acyclovir, ganciclovir
• Increased levels of mycophenolate: probenecid, salicylate
• Decreased levels of mycophenolate: antacids, cholestyramine
• Decreased protein binding of phenytoin, theophylline
• Avoid administration with azathioprine
• Drug/food: decreased absorption if taken with food
NURSING CONSIDERATIONS
Assess:
• Blood studies: CBC during treatment monthly
• Liver function studies: alk phosphatase, AST, ALT, bilirubin
Administer:
• 72 hr prior to transplantation; may be given in combination with corticosteroids, cyclosporine
• Give alone for better absorption (PO)
IV
• Do not give by rapid or bolus inj; reconstitute and dilute to 6 mg/ml with D₅W, give over ≥2 hr
• Do not admix with mycophenolate IV in infusion catheter or with other IV drugs or infusion admixtures
Evaluate:
• Therapeutic response: absence of graft rejection

Teach patient/family:
• To report fever, rash, severe diarrhea, chills, sore throat, fatigue, since serious infections may occur
• To reduce risk of infection by avoiding crowds
🚫 Not to break, crush, or chew tabs, do not open caps
• The need for repeated lab tests
• To limit exposure to sunlight/UV light
• To use contraception before, during, and 6 wk after therapy

nabumetone (Ⓡ)
(na-byoo'me-tone)
Relafen
Func. class.: Nonsteroidal antiinflammatory
Chem. class.: Acetic acid derivative

Action: Inhibits prostaglandin synthesis by decreasing enzyme needed for biosynthesis; analgesic, antiinflammatory
Uses: Osteoarthritis, rheumatoid arthritis, acute or chronic treatment
Dosage and routes:
• *Adult:* **PO** 1 g as a single dose; may increase to 2 g/day if needed; may give qd or bid as a divided dose
Available forms: Tabs 500, 750 mg
Side effects/adverse reactions:
CNS: Dizziness, headache, drowsiness, fatigue, tremors, confusion, insomnia, anxiety, depression, nervousness
*GU: **Nephrotoxicity, dysuria, hematuria, oliguria, azotemia,** cystitis*
GI: Nausea, anorexia, vomiting, diarrhea, jaundice, ***cholestatic hepatitis,*** constipation, flatulence, cramps, dry mouth, peptic ulcer, gastritis, ***ulceration, perforation***
CV: Tachycardia, peripheral edema, palpitations, dysrhythmias, ***CHF***

INTEG: Purpura, rash, pruritus, sweating, photosensitivity

HEMA: **Blood dyscrasias**

EENT: Tinnitus, hearing loss, blurred vision

RESP: Dyspnea, pharyngitis, **bronchospasm**

SYST: **Anaphylaxis, angioneurotic edema**

Contraindications: Hypersensitivity to this drug or aspirin, iodides, NSAIDs, asthma, severe renal disease, severe hepatic disease

Precautions: Pregnancy (B) 2nd trimester, (C) 1st trimester; lactation, children, bleeding disorders, GI disorders, cardiac disorders, renal disorders, hepatic dysfunction, elderly

Pharmacokinetics:

PO: Peak 2½-4 hr, plasma protein binding >90%, half-life 22-30 hr; metabolized in liver to active metabolite; excreted in urine (metabolites), breast milk

Interactions:

• Decreased effect of: diuretics, antihypertensives

• Increased risk of bleeding: anticoagulants, thrombolytics, valproic acid, cefamandole, cefotetan, cefoperazone, plicamycin, clopidogrel, eptifibatide, ticlopidine

• Increased risk of hematologic reactions: antineoplastics, radiation

• Increased GI reactions: salicylates, NSAIDs, alcohol, potassium, corticosteroids

NURSING CONSIDERATIONS

Assess:

• Pain: frequency, intensity, characteristics; relief of pain after med

• Asthma, aspirin sensitivity or nasal polyps; increased hypersensitivity reactions

• Renal, liver, blood studies: BUN, creatinine, AST, ALT, Hgb, LDH, blood glucose, WBC, platelets, CrCl before treatment, periodically thereafter

• Audiometric, ophthalmic exam before, during, after treatment

• For eye, ear problems: blurred vision, tinnitus; may indicate toxicity

Administer:

• With food for GI symptoms

Perform/provide:

• Storage at room temperature

Evaluate:

• Therapeutic response: decreased pain and stiffness in joints

Teach patient/family:

• To avoid alcoholic beverages and aspirin

• To report blurred vision, ringing, roaring in ears; may indicate toxicity

• To avoid driving, other hazardous activities if dizziness, drowsiness occur

• To report change in urine pattern, increased weight, edema, increased pain in joints, fever, blood in urine; indicates nephrotoxicity

• That therapeutic effects may take up to 1 mo

• To take with a full glass of water to enhance absorption and sit upright

• To report dark stools; may indicate GI bleeding

---

nadolol (℞)

(nay-doe′lole)

Corgard, Syn-Nadolol*

Func. class.: Antihypertensive, antianginal

Chem. class.: β-Adrenergic receptor blocker

Action: Long-acting, nonselective β-adrenergic receptor blocking agent; mechanism is similar to that of propranolol

Uses: Chronic stable angina pectoris, mild to moderate hypertension, prophylaxis of migraine headaches

---

◆ = Nursing alert   ✐ = Herb-drug interaction   ⊘ = Do not crush

Investigational uses: Tachydysrhythmias, aggression, anxiety, tremors, esophageal varices (rebleeding only), hyperthyroidism adjunctive therapy

Dosage and routes:
• *Adult:* **PO** 40 mg qd, increase by 40-80 mg q3-7d; maintenance 40-240 mg/day for angina, 40-320 mg/day for hypertension
• *Geriatric:* **PO** 20 mg/day, may increase by 20 mg until desired dose
Renal dose
• CrCl 31-50 ml/min give q24-36h; CrCl 10-30 ml/min give q24-48h
Available forms: Tabs 20, 40, 80, 120, 160 mg

Side effects/adverse reactions:
RESP: Dyspnea, respiratory dysfunction, ***bronchospasm,*** cough, wheezing, nasal stuffiness, pharyngitis, ***laryngospasm***
CV: ***Bradycardia,*** hypotension, ***CHF,*** palpitations, ***AV block,*** chest pain, peripheral ischemia, flushing, edema, vasodilation, conduction disturbances, ***pulmonary edema***
HEMA: ***Agranulocytosis, thrombocytopenia***
GI: Nausea, vomiting, diarrhea, colitis, constipation, cramps, dry mouth, flatulence, hepatomegaly, ***pancreatitis,*** taste distortion
INTEG: Rash, pruritus, fever
CNS: Depression, hallucinations, dizziness, fatigue, lethargy, paresthesias, headache
EENT: Sore throat
GU: Impotence

Contraindications: Hypersensitivity to this drug, cardiac failure, cardiogenic shock, 2nd/3rd degree heart block, bronchospastic disease, sinus bradycardia, CHF, COPD
Precautions: Diabetes mellitus, pregnancy (C), renal disease, lactation, hyperthyroidism, peripheral vascular disease, myasthenia gravis

Do not confuse:
Corgard/Cognex
Pharmacokinetics:
PO: Onset variable, peak 3-4 hr, duration 17-24 hr; half-life 20-24 hr; not metabolized; excreted in urine (unchanged), bile, breast milk; protein binding 30%
Interactions:
• Decreased antihypertensive effect: NSAIDs
• Increased bradycardia: digoxin
• Increased hypotension, bradycardia: amphetamines, clonidine, ephedrine, epinephrine, norepinephrine, phenylephrine, pseudoephedrine
• Do not use with MAOIs, hypertension may occur
• Increased hypotensive effects: other hypotensive agents, diuretics, phenothiazines
• Decreased effects of xanthines, thyroid
Lab test interferences:
Increase: Serum K, serum uric acid, ALT, AST, alk phosphatase, LDH, blood glucose, cholesterol

NURSING CONSIDERATIONS
Assess:
• B/P, pulse, respirations during beginning therapy, orthostatic hypotension
• Weight qd; report gain of 5 lb
• I&O ratio, CrCl if kidney damage is diagnosed
• qd, note need to be administered more often
• Pain: duration, time started, activity being performed, character
• Headache, light-headedness, decreased B/P; may indicate a need for decreased dosage
Administer:
PO
• With 8 oz water
Evaluate:
• Therapeutic response: decreased B/P, symptoms of angina

N

Teach patient/family:
• That drug may mask signs of hypoglycemia or alter blood glucose in diabetics

⬦ Not to discontinue abruptly, serious dysrhythmias may occur
• To avoid OTC drugs unless prescriber approves
• To avoid hazardous activities if dizziness occurs
• To comply with complete medical regimen
• To rise slowly to prevent orthostatic hypotension
• How and when to check B/P and pulse; to hold dose if pulse ≤50 bpm

---

nafarelin (℞)
(naf-ah-rell'in)
Synarel
Func. class.: Gonadotropin
Chem. class.: Analog of gonadotropin-releasing hormone

Action: Stimulates the release of LH and FSH, which increases ovarian steroid production; repeated dosing prevents stimulation of the pituitary gland

Uses: Endometriosis, gonadotropin-dependent precocious puberty

Dosage and routes:
• *Adult:* **NASAL** 400 µg/day as one spray (200 µg) into one nostril in morning and one spray into other nostril in evening; start treatment between days 2 and 4 of menstrual cycle; may increase to 800 µg/day (one spray into each nostril twice a day); recommended duration of treatment is 6 mo
• *Child:* **NASAL** 2 sprays in each nostril AM and PM, may increase to 3 sprays alternating nostril tid
Available forms: Nasal spray 2 mg/ml (200 µg/spray)

Side effects/adverse reactions:
GU: Decreased libido, vaginal dryness, breast tenderness, increased pubic hair
CNS: Headache, flushing, depression, insomnia, emotional lability, hot flashes
INTEG: Nasal irritation, acne
MISC: Body odor, seborrhea, rhinitis
SENSITIVITY: Shortness of breath, chest pain, urticaria, pruritus
Contraindications: Hypersensitivity, pregnancy (X), lactation, undiagnosed abnormal vaginal bleeding
Precautions: Children
Pharmacokinetics: Rapidly absorbed, peak 10-40 min, half-life 3 hr; 80% bound to plasma proteins
Interactions:
• Decrease nafarelin absorption: nasal decongestants (nasal sprays)
NURSING CONSIDERATIONS
Assess:
• Pain in endometriosis during treatment
• Endocrine studies, bone age, sex steroids, RHCG, GnRH, baseline q8wk
• For precocious puberty including secondary sex characteristics
• Test results: pituitary/hypothalamus dysfunction (decreased LH); postmenopausal (increased LH)
Administer:
NASAL
• Repeated doses may be necessary to elevate pituitary gonadotropin reserve
Perform/provide:
• Storage at room temperature; protect from light
Evaluate:
• Therapeutic response: decreased symptoms of endometriosis; adequate resolution of central precocious puberty

---

⬦ = Nursing alert　　🖋 = Herb-drug interaction　　🚫 = Do not crush

Teach patient/family:

• To use nonhormonal contraception

• About correct nasal use, one spray in right nostril AM, one in left nostril PM

• That medication may cause hot flashes, decreased libido, vaginal dryness

---

nafcillin (R)

(naf-sill'in)
Nafcil, nafcillin sodium, Nallpen, Unipen
Func. class.: Antiinfective, broad-spectrum
Chem. class.: Penicillinase-resistant penicillin

Action: Interferes with cell wall replication of susceptible organisms; osmotically unstable cell wall swells, bursts from osmotic pressure

Uses: Effective for gram-positive cocci *(Staphylococcus aureus, Streptococcus viridans, Streptococcus pneumoniae),* infections caused by penicillinase-producing *Staphylococcus*

Dosage and routes:

• *Adult:* PO 250-1000 mg q4-6h; **IM** 500 mg q4-6h; **IV** 500-1500 mg q4-6h

• *Child and infants, most infections:* **PO** 6.25-12.5 mg/kg q6h; pharyngitis **PO** 250 mg q8h; **IM** 25 mg/kg q12h; **IV** most infections 10-20 mg/kg q4h or 20-40 mg/kg q8h, max 200 mg/kg/day

• *Neonates:* **PO** 10 mg/kg q6-8h; **IM** 10 mg/kg q12h; **IV:** most infections 10-20 mg/kg q4h or 20-40 mg/kg q8h, max 200 mg/kg/day
Meningitis

• *Neonates ≥2 kg:* 50 mg/kg q8h × 1 wk of life, then 50 mg/kg q6h

• *Neonates <2 kg:* 25-50 mg/kg q12h × 1 wk of life, then 50 mg/kg q8h
Available forms: Caps 250 mg; tabs 500 mg; pwd for inj 1, 2, 10 g
Side effects/adverse reactions:

HEMA: Anemia, increased bleeding time, ***bone marrow depression, granulocytopenia***

GI: Nausea, vomiting, diarrhea, increased AST, ALT, abdominal pain, glossitis, ***pseudomembranous colitis***

GU: Oliguria, ***proteinuria, hematuria,*** vaginitis, moniliasis, ***glomerulonephritis,*** interstitial nephritis

CNS: Lethargy, hallucinations, anxiety, depression, twitching, ***coma, seizures***

Contraindications: Hypersensitivity to penicillins

Precautions: Pregnancy (B), hypersensitivity to cephalosporins, neonates

Pharmacokinetics:

IM/PO: Peak 30-60 min, duration 4-6 hr, half-life 1 hr, metabolized by liver, excreted in bile, urine

Interactions:

• Increased risk of bleeding: anticoagulants

• Decreased effect of oral contraceptives

• Increased nafcillin concentrations: aspirin, probenecid, disulfiram

• Drug/food: decreased absorption: food, carbonated drinks, citrus juice

Delayed/reduced absorption: khat, separate by ≥2 hr

Lab test interferences:

False-positive: Urine glucose, urine protein

NURSING CONSIDERATIONS
Assess:

• I&O ratio; report hematuria, oliguria, since penicillin in high doses is nephrotoxic

◆ Any patient with compromised renal system, since drug is excreted

slowly in poor renal system function; toxicity may occur rapidly
• Liver studies: AST, ALT
• Blood studies: WBC, RBC, H&H, bleeding time
• Renal studies: urinalysis, protein, blood, BUN, creatinine
• C&S before drug therapy; drug may be given as soon as culture is taken
• Bowel pattern before and during treatment
• Respiratory status: rate, character, wheezing, and tightness in chest
• Allergies before initiation of treatment; monitor for anaphylaxis, dyspnea, rash, laryngeal edema; stop drug; keep emergency equipment nearby; skin eruptions after administration of penicillin to 1 wk after discontinuing drug
• Differential WBC in patients on long-term therapy
Administer:
• IM deep in gluteal muscle
• Drug after C&S has been completed
• Divided oral doses on empty stomach before meals; oral absorption is erratic
IV
• After diluting 1 g/3.4 ml or 2 g/6.8 ml to 250 mg/ml sterile H_2O for inj; further dilute 15-30 ml sterile H_2O or NS sol; give through Y-tube or 3-way stopcock; 500 mg or less/5-10 min; may be further diluted and run over 24 hr
Additive compatibilities: Chloramphenicol, chlorothiazide, dexamethasone, diphenhydramine, ephedrine, heparin, hydroxyzine, lidocaine, potassium chloride, prochlorperazine, sodium bicarbonate, sodium lactate
Syringe compatibilities: Cimetidine, heparin
Y-site compatibilities: Acyclovir, atropine, cyclophosphamide, diazepam, enalaprilat, esmolol, famotidine, fentanyl, fluconazole, foscarnet, hydromorphone, magnesium sulfate, morphine, perphenazine, propofol, theophylline, zidovudine
Perform/provide:
• Adrenalin, suction, tracheostomy set, endotracheal intubation equipment
• Adequate fluid intake (2 L) during diarrhea episodes
• Scratch test to assess allergy after securing order from prescriber; usually done when penicillin is only drug of choice
• Storage in tight container; refrigerate reconstituted sol
Evaluate:
• Therapeutic response: absence of fever, draining wounds
Teach patient/family:
• All aspects of drug therapy, including need to complete course of medication to ensure organism death (10-14 days); culture may be taken after completed course
• To report sore throat, fever, fatigue (may indicate superinfection)
• To wear or carry Medic Alert ID if allergic to penicillins
• To notify nurse of diarrhea
🚫 Not to break, crush, or chew caps
Treatment of anaphylaxis: Withdraw drug; maintain airway; administer epinephrine, aminophylline, O_2, IV corticosteroids

nalbuphine (℞)
(nal'byoo-feen)
Nubain, nalbuphine HCl
Func. class.: Opioid analgesic
Chem. class.: Synthetic opioid agonist, antagonist
Action: Depresses pain impulse transmission at the spinal cord level by interacting with opioid receptors

◆ = Nursing alert　　🖊 = Herb-drug interaction　　🚫 = Do not crush

Uses: Moderate to severe pain
Dosage and routes:
Analgesic
• *Adult:* **SC/IM/IV** 10-20 mg q3-6h prn, not to exceed 160 mg/day
Balanced anesthesia supplement
• *Adult:* **IV** 0.3-3 mg/kg given over 10-15 min, may give 0.25-0.5 mg/kg as needed for maintenance
Available forms: Inj 10, 20 mg/ml
Side effects/adverse reactions:
CNS: Drowsiness, dizziness, confusion, headache, sedation, euphoria, dysphoria (high doses), hallucinations, dreaming, tolerance, physical, psychological dependency
GI: Nausea, vomiting, anorexia, constipation, cramps
GU: Increased urinary output, dysuria, urinary retention, urgency
INTEG: Rash, urticaria, bruising, flushing, diaphoresis, pruritus
EENT: Tinnitus, blurred vision, miosis, diplopia
CV: Palpitations, bradycardia, change in B/P, orthostatic hypotension
*RESP: **Respiratory depression***
Contraindications: Hypersensitivity, addiction (opiate)
Precautions: Addictive personality, pregnancy (C), lactation, increased intracranial pressure, MI (acute), severe heart disease, respiratory depression, hepatic disease, renal disease
Pharmacokinetics:
SC/IM/IV: Duration 3-6 hr; metabolized by liver, excreted by kidneys, half-life 5 hr
Interactions:
• Increased effects with other CNS depressants: alcohol, opiates, sedative/hypnotics, antipsychotics, skeletal muscle relaxants
◆ Avoid use with MAOIs, unpredictable reactions may occur
Lab test interferences:
Increase: Amylase

NURSING CONSIDERATIONS
Assess:
• I&O ratio; check for decreasing output; may indicate urinary retention
◆ For withdrawal reactions in opiate-dependent individuals: pulmonary embolus, vascular occlusion; abscesses, ulcerations, nausea, vomiting, seizures; however, there is a low potential for dependence
• CNS changes: dizziness, drowsiness, hallucinations, euphoria, LOC, pupil reaction
• Allergic reactions: rash, urticaria
• Respiratory dysfunction: respiratory depression, character, rate, rhythm; notify prescriber if respirations are <10/min
• Need for pain medication by pain sedation scoring, physical dependency
Administer:
• With antiemetic if nausea, vomiting occur
• When pain is beginning to return; determine dosage interval by response
• IM deep in large muscle mass, rotate inj sites
IV
• Undiluted 10 mg or less over 3-5 min
Syringe compatibilities: Atropine, cimetidine, diphenhydramine, droperidol, glycopyrrolate, hydroxyzine, lidocaine, midazolam, prochlorperazine, ranitidine, scopolamine, trimethobenzamide
Y-site compatibilities: Amifostine, aztreonam, cefmetazole, cisatracurium, cladribine, filgrastim, fludarabine, granisetron, melphalan, paclitaxel, propofol, remifentanil, teniposide, thiotepa, vinorelbine
Perform/provide:
• Storage in light-resistant area at room temperature

• Assistance with ambulation
• Safety measures: night-light, call bell within easy reach
Evaluate:
• Therapeutic response: decrease in pain
Teach patient/family:
• To report any symptoms of CNS changes, allergic reactions
• That physical dependency may result from long-term use
• That withdrawal symptoms may occur: nausea, vomiting, cramps, fever, faintness, anorexia
Treatment of overdose: Naloxone (Narcan) 0.2-0.8 mg IV, O₂, IV fluids, vasopressors

---

nalidixic acid (℞)

(nal-i-dix'ik)
NegGram
Func. class.: Urinary tract anti-infective
Chem. class.: Fluoroquinolone

Action: Appears to inhibit DNA polymerization, primary target is single-stranded DNA precursors in late-stage chromosomal replication
Uses: UTIs (acute/chronic) caused by *Escherichia coli, Klebsiella, Enterobacter, Proteus mirabilis, Proteus vulgaris, Proteus morganii*
Dosage and routes:
• *Adult:* PO 1 g qid × 1-2 wk, 2 g/day for long-term treatment
• *Child >3 mo:* PO 55 mg/kg/day in 4 divided doses for 1-2 wk; 33 mg/kg/day in 4 divided doses for long-term treatment
Renal dose
• CrCl <50 ml/min avoid use
Available forms: Tabs 250, 500 mg, 1 g; susp 250 mg/5 ml
Side effects/adverse reactions:
INTEG: Pruritus, rash, urticaria, photosensitivity

CNS: Dizziness, headache, drowsiness, insomnia, ***seizures***
GI: Nausea, vomiting, abdominal pain, diarrhea
EENT: Sensitivity to light, blurred vision, change in color perception
Contraindications: Hypersensitivity, CNS damage, liver failure, infants <3 mo
Precautions: Elderly, renal disease, hepatic disease, pregnancy (B), lactation
Pharmacokinetics:
PO: Peak 1-2 hr, metabolized in liver, excreted in urine (unchanged/conjugates), crosses placenta, enters breast milk
Interactions:
• Increased effects of oral coagulants, check for bleeding
• Decreased effect: nitrofurantoin
Lab test interferences:
False positive: Urinary glucose
False increase: 17-OHCS, VMA
NURSING CONSIDERATIONS
Assess:
• Blood count for patients on chronic therapy
• I&O ratio; urine pH <5.5 is ideal
• Renal, hepatic function
• Photosensitivity: drug should be discontinued
• CNS symptoms: insomnia, vertigo, headache, drowsiness, convulsions
• Allergy: fever, flushing, rash, urticaria, pruritus
Administer:
PO
• After clean-catch urine for C&S
• Two daily doses if urine output is high or if patient has diabetes
• 2 hr before or 2 hr after antacids
Perform/provide:
• Protection from freezing
Evaluate:
• Therapeutic response: decreased dysuria, negative culture

⬥ = Nursing alert   ⁄⁄ = Herb-drug interaction   ⃠ = Do not crush

Teach patient/family:

• That photosensitivity occurs; that patient should avoid sunlight or use sunscreen to prevent burns

• To take medication with food or milk to decrease GI irritation; take 2 hr before or 2 hr after antacids

• To protect suspension from freezing, shake well before taking

• That drug may cause drowsiness; instruct client to seek aid in walking, other activities; advise client not to drive or operate machinery while on medication

• That diabetics should monitor blood glucose

---

naloxone (R)

(nal-oks'one)
naloxone HCl, Narcan
Func. class.: Opioid antagonist, antidote
Chem. class.: Thebaine derivative

Action: Competes with opioids at opiate receptor sites

Uses: Respiratory depression induced by opioids, pentazocine, propoxyphene; refractory circulatory shock, asphyxia neonatorum

Dosage and routes:

Opioid-induced respiratory depression

• *Adult:* **IV/SC/IM** 0.4-2 mg; repeat q2-3min if needed

• *Child:* **IV/SC/IM** 0.5-2 µg/kg as small frequent, q/min **BOL** or as **INF** titrated to response

Postoperative respiratory depression

• *Adult:* **IV** 0.1-0.2 mg q2-3min prn

• *Child:* **IV/IM/SC** 0.01 mg/kg q2-3min prn

Asphyxia neonatorum

• *Neonate:* **IV** 0.01 mg/kg given into umbilical vein after delivery; may repeat q2-3min × 3 doses

Available forms: Inj 0.02, 0.4, 1 mg/ml

Side effects/adverse reactions:

CNS: Drowsiness, nervousness

CV: Rapid pulse, increased systolic B/P (high doses), ***ventricular tachycardia, fibrillation***

GI: Nausea, vomiting

RESP: Hyperpnea

Contraindications: Hypersensitivity, respiratory depression

Precautions: Pregnancy (B), children, cardiovascular disease, opioid dependency, lactation

Do not confuse:

Narcan/Norcuron

Pharmacokinetics: Well absorbed IM, SC; metabolized by liver, crosses placenta; excreted in urine, breast milk; half-life 1 hr

IV: Onset 1 min, duration 45 min

IM/SC: Onset 2-5 min, duration 45-60 min

Interactions:

• Decreased effect of opioid analgesics

Lab test interferences:

Interference: Urine VMA, 5-HIAA, urine glucose

NURSING CONSIDERATIONS

Assess:

• Withdrawal: cramping, hypertension, anxiety, vomiting, signs of withdrawal in drug-dependent individuals may occur up to 2 hr after administration

• VS q3-5min

• ABGs including Po_2, Pco_2

• Cardiac status: tachycardia, hypertension; monitor ECG

• Respiratory dysfunction: respiratory depression, character, rate, rhythm; if respirations are <10/min, administer naloxone; probably due to opioid overdose; monitor LOC

N

Side effects: *italics* = common; ***bold italics*** = life-threatening

• For pain: duration, intensity, location, before and after administration; may be used for respiratory depression

Administer:
• Only with resuscitative equipment, O₂ nearby
• Only sol prepared within 24 hr

IV
• Undiluted with sterile H_2O for inj; may be further diluted with NS or D_5 and given as an inf; give 0.4 mg or less over 15 sec or titrate inf to response

Additive compatibilities: Verapamil

Syringe compatibilities: Benzquinamide, heparin

Y-site compatibilities: Propofol

Perform/provide:
• Dark storage at room temperature

Evaluate:
• Therapeutic response: reversal of respiratory depression; LOC-alert

---

naltrexone (R)

(nal-trex'one)
Depade, ReVia, Trexan
Func. class.: Opioid antagonist
Chem. class.: Thebaine derivative

Action: Competes with narcotics at narcotic receptor sites

Uses: Blockage of opioid analgesics, used in treatment of opiate addiction

Investigational uses: Pruritus, alcohol dependence

Dosage and routes:
• *Adult:* PO 25 mg, may give 25 mg after 1 hr if no withdrawal symptoms; 50-150 mg may be given qd depending on need, maintenance 50 mg q24h; 100-150 mg may be given on alternate days or 3 days per wk

Pruritus (off-label)
• *Adult:* PO 50 mg qd

Available forms: Tabs 50 mg

Side effects/adverse reactions:

MISC: Increased thirst, chills, fever

MS: Joint and muscle pain

GU: Delayed ejaculation, decreased potency

CNS: Stimulation, drowsiness, dizziness, confusion, *seizures,* headache, flushing, hallucinations, nervousness, irritability

GI: Nausea, vomiting, diarrhea, heartburn, anorexia, *hepatitis,* constipation

INTEG: Rash, urticaria, bruising, oily skin, acne, pruritus

EENT: Tinnitus, hearing loss, blurred vision

CV: Rapid pulse, *pulmonary edema,* hypertension

RESP: Wheezing, hyperpnea, nasal congestion, rhinorrhea, sneezing, sore throat

Contraindications: Hypersensitivity, opioid dependence, hepatic failure, hepatitis

Precautions: Pregnancy (C), hepatic disease, lactation, children

Pharmacokinetics:

PO: Onset 15-30 min, peak 1-2 hr, duration is dose dependent

Metabolized by liver, excreted by kidneys; crosses placenta, excreted in breast milk; half-life 4 hr; extensive first-pass metabolism

NURSING CONSIDERATIONS
Assess:
• VS q3-5min
• ABGs including Po_2, Pco_2
• Signs of withdrawal in drug-dependent individuals
• Cardiac status: tachycardia, hypertension
• Respiratory dysfunction: respiratory depression, character, rate, rhythm; if respirations are <10/min, respiratory stimulant should be administered

◆ = Nursing alert   ✦ = Herb-drug interaction   ⊘ = Do not crush

Administer:

• Only if resuscitative equipment is nearby

Perform/provide:

• Storage in tight container

Evaluate:

• Therapeutic response: blocking opiate ingestion

Teach patient/family:

• That they must be drug-free to start treatment

• That using opioid while taking this drug could prove fatal because high dose is needed to overcome this antagonist

• To carry MedicAlert ID stating med used

• If surgery is needed, all involved should be aware of this drug

---

nandrolone (℞)

(nan'droe-lone)
Deca-Durabolin, Hybolin
Decanoate, Kabolin

Func. class.: Androgenic anabolic steroid, antianemic

Chem. class.: Halogenated testosterone derivative

Action: Increases weight by building body tissue, increases potassium, phosphorus, chloride, nitrogen levels, increases bone development

Uses: Tissue building, severe disease, refractory anemias, metastatic breast cancer

Dosage and routes:

Tissue building (possibly effective)

• *Adult:* **IM** 50-100 mg q3-4wk (decanoate)

• *Child 2-13 yr:* **IM** 25-50 mg q3-4wk (decanoate)

Severe disease/refractory anemias

• *Adult:* **IM** 100-200 mg qwk (decanoate)

Breast cancer

• *Adult:* **IM** 50-100 mg qwk (phen-propionate)

Available forms: Inj 100, 200 mg/ml

Side effects/adverse reactions:

INTEG: Rash, acneiform lesions, oily hair, skin, flushing, sweating, acne vulgaris, alopecia, hirsutism

CNS: Dizziness, headache, fatigue, tremors, paresthesias, flushing, sweating, anxiety, lability, insomnia, carpal tunnel syndrome, chills

MS: Cramps, spasms

CV: Increased B/P

GU: **Hematuria,** amenorrhea, vaginitis, decreased libido, decreased breast size, clitoral hypertrophy, testicular atrophy, priapism

GI: Nausea, vomiting, constipation, weight gain, *cholestatic jaundice*

EENT: Conjunctival edema, nasal congestion

ENDO: Abnormal GTT

Contraindications: Severe renal, severe cardiac, severe hepatic disease, hypersensitivity, pregnancy (X), lactation, abnormal genital bleeding, males with cancer of breast, prostate

Precautions: Diabetes mellitus, CV disease, MI

Pharmacokinetics:

IM: Metabolized in liver, crosses placenta, excreted in breast milk, urine

Interactions:

• Increased effects of oral antidiabetics, oxyphenbutazone

• Increased PT: anticoagulants

• Edema: ACTH, adrenal steroids

• Decreased effects of insulin

Lab test interferences:

Increase: Serum cholesterol, blood glucose, urine glucose

Decrease: Serum Ca, serum K, T_4, T_3, thyroid ^{131}I uptake test, urine 17-OHCS, 17-KS, PBI, BSP

N

NURSING CONSIDERATIONS
Assess:
• Weight daily; notify prescriber if weekly weight gain is >5 lb
• B/P q4h
• I&O ratio; be alert for decreasing urinary output, increasing edema
• Growth rate in children, since growth rate may be uneven (linear/bone growth) with extended use
• Electrolytes: K, Na, Cl, Ca; cholesterol
• Liver function studies: ALT, AST, bilirubin
• Edema, hypertension, cardiac symptoms, jaundice
• Mental status: affect, mood, behavioral changes, aggression
• Signs of masculinization in female: increased libido, deepening of voice, decreased breast tissue, enlarged clitoris, menstrual irregularities; male: gynecomastia, impotence, testicular atrophy
• Hypercalcemia: lethargy, polyuria, polydipsia, nausea, vomiting, constipation, drug may have to be decreased
• Hypoglycemia in diabetics, since oral antidiabetic action is increased
Administer:
• Titrated dose; use lowest effective dose
Perform/provide:
• Diet with increased calories, protein; decrease Na if edema occurs
Evaluate:
• Therapeutic response: increased appetite, increased stamina
Teach patient/family:
• That drug must be combined with complete health plan: diet, rest, exercise
• To notify prescriber if therapeutic response decreases
• Not to discontinue abruptly
• About changes in sex characteristics
• That females should report menstrual irregularities
• That 1-3 mo course is necessary for response in breast cancer

---

naproxen (OTC, ℞)
(na-prox′en)
Apo-Naproxen*, EC-Naprosyn, Naprelan, Napron X, Naprosyn, Naprosyn-E*, Naprosyn-SR*, Naxen*, Novo-Naprox*, Nu-Naprox*
naproxen sodium
Aleve, Anaprox, Anaprox DS, Apo-Napro-Na*, Apo-Napro-Na DS, Naprelan, Novo-Naprox Sodium*, Novo-Naprox Sodium DS*, Synflex*, Synflex DS*
Func. class.: Nonsteroidal antiinflammatory, nonopioid analgesic
Chem. class.: Propionic acid derivative

Action: Inhibits prostaglandin synthesis by decreasing an enzyme needed for biosynthesis; analgesic, antiinflammatory, antipyretic
Uses: Mild to moderate pain, osteoarthritis, rheumatoid, gouty arthritis, juvenile arthritis, primary dysmenorrhea
Dosage and routes:
• *Adult:* **PO** 250-500 mg bid, not to exceed 1 g/day (base); 525 mg, then 275 mg q6-8h prn, not to exceed 1475 mg (sodium)
• *Child:* **PO** 10 mg/kg in 2 divided doses
Available forms: Tabs, naproxen: 250, 375, 500 mg; tabs, del rel 375, 500 mg; tabs, ext rel 750, 1000 mg; oral susp 125 mg/5 ml; naproxen sodium tabs, cont rel 421.5, 550 mg; tabs 220, 275, 550 mg
Side effects/adverse reactions:
GI: Nausea, anorexia, vomiting, di-

◆ = Nursing alert   ∥ = Herb-drug interaction   ⊘ = Do not crush

arrhea, jaundice, ***cholestatic hepatitis,*** constipation, flatulence, cramps, dry mouth, peptic ulcer, ***GI ulceration, bleeding, perforation***

CNS: Dizziness, drowsiness, fatigue, tremors, confusion, insomnia, anxiety, depression

CV: Tachycardia, peripheral edema, palpitations, dysrhythmias

INTEG: Purpura, rash, pruritus, sweating

GU: ***Nephrotoxicity: dysuria, hematuria, oliguria, azotemia***

HEMA: ***Blood dyscrasias***

EENT: Tinnitus, hearing loss, blurred vision

Contraindications: Hypersensitivity, asthma, severe renal disease, severe hepatic disease, ulcer disease

Precautions: Pregnancy (B) 1st trimester, lactation, children <2 yr, bleeding disorders, GI disorders, cardiac disorders, hypersensitivity to other antiinflammatory agents, elderly, CrCl <25 ml/min

Pharmacokinetics:

PO: Peak 2-4 hr, half-life 3-3½ hr; metabolized in liver; excreted in urine (metabolites), breast milk; 99% protein binding

Interactions:

• Increased toxicity: methotrexate, oral anticoagulants, sulfonylureas, probenecid

• Decreased effect of: antihypertensives, diuretics

• Increased risk of GI side effects: aspirin, corticosteroids, alcohol

• Possible renal impairment: ACE inhibitors

Lab test interferences:

Increase: BUN, alk phosphatase
False increase: 5-HIAA, 17KGS

NURSING CONSIDERATIONS

Assess:

• Pain: frequency, characteristics, intensity; relief prior to and 1-2 hr after med

• Asthma, aspirin hypersensitivity

or nasal polyps, increased risk of hypersensitivity

• Renal, liver, blood studies: BUN, creatinine, AST, ALT, Hgb, LDH, blood glucose, Hct, WBC, platelets CrCl before treatment, periodically thereafter

• Audiometric, ophthalmic exam before, during, after treatment

• For eye, ear problems: blurred vision, tinnitus (may indicate toxicity)

Administer:

• With food to decrease GI symptoms; take on empty stomach to facilitate absorption

Perform/provide:

• Storage at room temperature

Evaluate:

• Therapeutic response: decreased pain, stiffness, swelling in joints, ability to move more easily

Teach patient/family:

• To use sunscreen to prevent photosensitivity

• To report blurred vision, ringing, roaring in ears (may indicate toxicity)

• To avoid driving, other hazardous activities if dizziness or drowsiness occurs

• To report change in urine pattern, weight increase, edema (face, lower extremities), pain increase in joints, fever, blood in urine (indicates nephrotoxicity); black stools, flulike symptoms

• That therapeutic effects may take up to 1 mo

• To avoid ASA, alcohol, steroids

naratriptan (R)

(nair'ah-trip-tan)

Amerge

Func. class.: Antimigraine agent
Chem. class.: 5-HT$_1$ receptor agonist

Action: Binds selectively to the vascular 5-HT$_1$ receptor subtype, exerts antimigraine effect; causes vasoconstriction in cranial arteries

Uses: Acute treatment of migraine with or without aura

Dosage and routes:

• *Adult:* PO 1 or 2.5 mg with fluids, if headache returns, repeat once after 4 hr, max 5 mg/24 hr

Hepatic/renal dose

Max 2.5 mg/24 hr

Available forms: Tab 1, 2.5 mg

Side effects/adverse reactions:

GI: Nausea, vomiting

MS: Weakness, neck stiffness, myalgia

CNS: Dizziness, sedation, fatigue

CV: Increased B/P, palpitations, *tachydysrhythmias, PR, QTc prolongation, ST/T wave changes, PVCs, atrial flutter/fibrillation, coronary vasospasm*

EENT: EENT infections, photophobia

MISC: Temperature change sensations; tightness, pressure sensations

Contraindications: Angina pectoris, history of MI, documented silent ischemia, ischemic heart disease, concurrent ergotamine-containing preparations, uncontrolled hypertension, CV syndromes, hemiplegic or basilar migraines, hypersensitivity, severe renal disease (CrCl <15 ml/min); severe hepatic disease (Child-Pugh grade C)

Precautions: Postmenopausal women, men >40 yr, risk factors for CAD, hypercholesterolemia, obesity, diabetes, impaired hepatic or renal function, pregnancy (C), lactation, children, elderly, peripheral vascular disease

Pharmacokinetics: Peak 2-3 hr, 28%-31% plasma protein binding, half-life 6 hr, metabolized in the liver (metabolite), excreted in urine, feces; may be excreted in breast milk

Interactions:

• Extended vasospastic effects: ergot, ergot derivatives, other 5-HT$_1$ agonists

• Weakness, hyperreflexia, incoordination: SSRIs (fluoxetine, fluvoxamine, paroxetine, sertraline)

NURSING CONSIDERATIONS

Assess:

• For stress level, activity, recreation, coping mechanisms

• Neurologic status: LOC blurred vision, nausea, vomiting, tingling in extremities preceding headache

Administer:

• With fluids as soon as symptoms appear, may take another dose after 4 hr; do not take >5 mg in any 24-hr period

Perform/provide:

• Quiet, calm environment with decreased stimulation for noise, bright light, excessive talking

Evaluate:

• Therapeutic response: decrease in frequency, severity of headache

Teach patient/family:

• To report pain, tightness in chest, neck, throat, or jaw; notify prescriber immediately if sudden, severe abdominal pain occurs

• Not to use if another 5-HT$_1$ agonist or an ergot preparation has been used in the past 24 hr

• Advise patient to notify prescriber if pregnancy is planned or suspected

---

◆ = Nursing alert   🖊 = Herb-drug interaction   🚫 = Do not crush

nedocromil (R)

(ned-o-kroe′mill)
Tilade
Func. class.: Antiasthmatic
Chem. class.: Mast cell stabilizer

Action: Stabilizes the membrane of the sensitized mast cell, preventing release of chemical mediators after an antigen-IgE interaction

Uses: Severe perennial bronchial asthma, exercise-induced bronchospasm (prevention), prevention of acute bronchospasm induced by environmental pollutants; *not* for treatment of acute asthma attacks

Dosage and routes:
• *Adult and child >12 yr:* **INH** 2 inhalations 2-4 ×/day at regular intervals to provide 14 g/day

Available forms: 1.75 mg nedocromil Na per activation in 16.2 g canisters providing at least 112 metered inhalations

Side effects/adverse reactions:
EENT: Throat irritation, cough, nasal congestion, burning eyes, rhinitis
CNS: Headache, dizziness, neuritis, dysphonia
GI: Nausea, vomiting, anorexia, dry mouth, bitter taste

Contraindications: Hypersensitivity to this drug or lactose, status asthmaticus

Precautions: Pregnancy (B), lactation, children

Pharmacokinetics:
INH: Peak 15 min, duration 4-6 hr; excreted unchanged in urine; half-life 80 min

NURSING CONSIDERATIONS
Assess:
• Pulmonary function testing baseline (asthma)

• Respiratory status: rate, rhythm, characteristics, cough, wheezing, dyspnea

Administer:
• By inhalation only, with spacer device if needed
• Gargle, sip of water to decrease irritation in throat

Evaluate:
• Therapeutic response: decrease in asthmatic symptoms, congested, runny nose

Teach patient/family:
• To clear mucus before using
• The proper technique: exhale; using inhaler, inhale deeply with head tipped back to open airway; remove, hold breath, exhale; use Halermatic or Spinhaler with Intal caps
• That therapeutic effect may take up to 4 wk
• That drug is preventive only, not restorative

nefazodone (R)

(ne-faz′o-done)
Serzone
Func. class.: Antidepressant—misc
Chem. class.: Phenylpiperazine

Action: Selectively inhibits serotonin uptake by brain, potentiates behavioral changes, occupies central S-H$_2$ receptors

Uses: Major depression

Research note: Clozapine given with nefazodone resulted in an increase of clozapine[26]

Dosage and routes:
• *Adult:* **PO** 200 mg/day (100 mg bid); dose may be increased to 300 mg/day (150 mg bid), max 600 mg/day
• *Elderly:* 100 mg/day (50 mg bid); increase to 100 mg bid after 2 wk to desired dose

N

Available forms: Tabs 50, 100, 150, 200, 250 mg

Side effects/adverse reactions:

CNS: Somnolence, dizziness, *headache, insomnia*

GI: Nausea, constipation, dry mouth

GU: Urinary frequency, retention, UTI

CV: Postural hypotension

RESP: Pharyngitis, cough

EENT: Blurred vision, abnormal vision

Contraindications: Hypersensitivity to this drug or phenylpiperazines

Precautions: Pregnancy (C), lactation, children, elderly, cardiovascular disease, seizure disorder

Pharmacokinetics: Metabolized in liver extensively to metabolites; excreted in urine, breast milk; peak 1-3 hr; half-life triphasic 2-4 hr

Interactions:

• Increased effect: CNS depressants, alcohol

 Fatal reaction: antihistamines, nonsedating

• Increased plasma concentrations: benzodiazepines

 Hypertensive crisis: MAOIs

• Increased toxicity: triazolam, alprazolam, midazolam, phenytoin, MAOI

NURSING CONSIDERATIONS

Assess:

• B/P (lying, standing), pulse q4h; if systolic B/P drops 20 mm Hg, hold drug, notify prescriber; take vital signs q4h in patients with cardiovascular disease

• Blood studies: CBC, leukocytes, differential, cardiac enzymes (long-term therapy)

• Hepatic studies: AST, ALT, bilirubin

• Mental status: mood, sensorium, affect, suicidal tendencies; increase in psychiatric symptoms: depression, panic

• Urinary retention, constipation; constipation is more likely in children, elderly

• Alcohol consumption; hold dose until morning

Administer:

• With food, milk for GI symptoms

• Crushed if patient cannot swallow whole

Perform/provide:

• Storage at room temperature; do not freeze

Evaluate:

• Therapeutic response: decrease in depression; absence of suicidal thoughts

Teach patient/family:

• That therapeutic effects may take 3-4 wk

• To use caution in driving, other activities requiring alertness because of drowsiness, dizziness; to avoid rising quickly from sitting to standing, especially elderly

• To avoid alcohol ingestion, other CNS depressants, benzodiazepines

• To increase bulk in diet for constipation, especially elderly

• To take gum, hard sugarless candy, frequents sips of water for dry mouth

Treatment of overdose: ECG monitoring; induce emesis; lavage, activated charcoal; administer anticonvulsant

---

nelfinavir (R)

(nell-fin'a-ver)
Viracept

Func. class.: Antiretroviral
Chem. class.: HIV protease inhibitor

Action: Inhibits human immunodeficiency virus (HIV) protease, which prevents maturation of the infectious virus

Uses: HIV alone or in combination

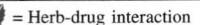

Dosage and routes:
• *Adult:* **PO** 750 mg tid
• *Child 2-13 yr:* **PO** 20-30 mg/kg tid

Available forms: Tabs 250 mg; powder, oral 50 mg/g

Side effects/adverse reactions:
*HEMA: **Anemia, leukopenia, thrombocytopenia, Hgb abnormalities***
GI: Diarrhea, anorexia, dyspepsia, *nausea, flatulence*
CNS: Headache, asthenia, poor concentration, *seizures*
INTEG: Rash, dermatitis
MS: Pain, arthralgia, myalgia, myopathy
CV: Bleeding
ENDO: Hypoglycemia, hyperlipidemia

Contraindications: Hypersensitivity to protease inhibitors

Precautions: Liver disease, pregnancy (B), lactation, renal disease, hemophilia, PKU

Pharmacokinetics: Half-life 3½-5 hr

Interactions:
◆Serious dysrhythmias: ergots, midazolam, triazolam, amiodarone, cisapride, quinidine
• Decreased effect of: oral contraceptives
• Increased effect: rifabutin
• Increased nelfinavir levels: ketoconazole, indinavir, ritonavir
• Decreased nelfinavir levels: rifamycins, nevirapine, phenobarbital, phenytoin, carbamazepine
• Drug/food: increased absorption with food

NURSING CONSIDERATIONS
Assess:
• Signs of infection, anemia
• Liver function studies: ALT, AST
• C&S before drug therapy; drug may be taken as soon as culture is taken; repeat C&S after treatment; determine the presence of other sexually transmitted diseases

• Bowel pattern before, during treatment; if severe abdominal pain with bleeding occurs, drug should be discontinued; monitor hydration
• Skin eruptions, rash, urticaria, itching
• Allergies before treatment, reaction of each medication; place allergies on chart
• Viral load, CD4 cell counts baseline and throughout treatment

Administer:
• With food
• Oral powder mixed with fluids if desired, do not mix with juice or acidic fluids, stable mixed for 6 hr

Teach patient/family:
• To avoid taking with other medications unless directed by prescriber
• That drug does not cure, but does manage symptoms, and does not prevent transmission of HIV to others
• To use a nonhormonal form of birth control while taking this drug
• If dose is missed, to take as soon as remembered up to 1 hr before next dose; do not double dose
• To take with food

neomycin (℞)
(nee-oh-mye'sin)
Mycifradin, Myciguent
Func. class.: Antiinfective
Chem. class.: Aminoglycoside

Action: Interferes with protein synthesis in bacterial cell by binding to 30S ribosomal subunit, causing inaccurate peptide sequence to form in protein chain, causing bacterial death

Uses: Severe systemic infections of CNS, respiratory, GI, urinary tract, eye, bone, skin, soft tissues caused by *Pseudomonas aeruginosa, Escherichia coli, Enterobacter, Klebsiella pneumoniae, Proteus vulgaris;*

also used for hepatic coma, preoperatively to sterilize bowel, infectious diarrhea caused by enteropathogenic *E. coli*

Dosage and routes:

Hepatic encephalopathy

• *Adult:* **PO** 4-12 g/day in divided doses × 5-6 days

• *Child:* **PO** 50-100 mg/kg/day in divided doses

Preoperative intestinal antisepsis

• *Adult:* **PO** on 3rd day of a 3-day regimen, give 1 g early PM, repeat in 1 hr, repeat at hs (given with erythromycin); give saline cathartic before giving this drug

• *Child:* **PO** 14.7 mg/kg or 4.7 mg/m^2 q4h × 3 days

Available forms: Tabs 500 mg; oral sol 125 mg/5 ml

Side effects/adverse reactions:

*GU: **Oliguria, hematuria, renal damage, azotemia, renal failure, nephrotoxicity***

CNS: Confusion, depression, numbness, tremors, ***seizures,*** muscle twitching, ***neurotoxicity,*** dizziness, vertigo

*EENT: **Ototoxicity,*** deafness, visual disturbances, tinnitus

*HEMA: **Agranulocytosis, thrombocytopenia,*** leukopenia, eosinophilia, anemia

GI: Nausea, vomiting, anorexia; increased ALT, AST, bilirubin; hepatomegaly, ***hepatic necrosis,*** splenomegaly

CV: Hypotension, hypertension, palpitation

INTEG: Rash, burning, urticaria, photosensitivity, dermatitis, alopecia

Contraindications: Bowel obstruction (oral use), severe renal disease, hypersensitivity, infants, children

Precautions: Mild renal disease, pregnancy (C), hearing deficits, lactation, myasthenia gravis, Parkinson's disease

Pharmacokinetics:

PO: Onset rapid, peak 1-2 hr Plasma half-life 2-3 hr; not metabolized, excreted unchanged in feces, crosses placenta

Interactions:

• Increased ototoxicity, neurotoxicity, nephrotoxicity: other aminoglycosides, amphotericin B, polymyxin, vancomycin, ethacrynic acid, furosemide, mannitol, methoxyflurane, cisplatin, cephalosporins, bacitracin

• Increased effects: nondepolarizing muscle relaxants, succinylcholine, oral anticoagulants when given with oral neomycin

• Decreased effects of digoxin, penicillin V when given with oral neomycin

NURSING CONSIDERATIONS

Assess:

• Weight before treatment; calculation of dosage is usually based on ideal body weight, but may be calculated on actual body weight

• I&O ratio, urinalysis qd for proteinuria, cells, casts; report sudden change in urine output

• Urine pH if drug is used for UTI; urine should be kept alkaline

• Renal impairment by securing urine for CrCl testing, BUN, serum creatinine; lower dosage should be given in renal impairment

• Deafness by audiometric testing, ringing, roaring in ears, vertigo; assess hearing before, during, after treatment

• Dehydration: high specific gravity, decrease in skin turgor, dry mucous membranes, dark urine

• Overgrowth of infection: fever, malaise, redness, pain, swelling, perineal itching, diarrhea, stomatitis, change in cough, sputum

• C&S before starting treatment to identify infecting organism

---

◆ = Nursing alert   ✦ = Herb-drug interaction   ⃠ = Do not crush

• Vestibular dysfunction: nausea, vomiting, dizziness, headache; drug should be discontinued if severe

• Injection sites for redness, swelling, abscesses; use warm compresses at site

Administer:

• Drug in evenly spaced doses to maintain blood level

• Bicarbonate to alkalinize urine if ordered in treating UTI, as drug is most active in alkaline environment

Perform/provide:

• Adequate fluids of 2 L/day unless contraindicated to prevent irritation of tubules

• Supervised ambulation, other safety measures, with vestibular dysfunction

Evaluate:

• Therapeutic response: absence of fever, draining wounds, negative C&S after treatment

Teach patient/family:

• To report headache, dizziness, symptoms of overgrowth of infection, renal impairment

• To report loss of hearing, ringing, roaring in ears or a feeling of fullness in head

• To take all of medication, to take a missed dose as soon as remembered, do not double doses

Treatment of overdose: Hemodialysis; monitor serum levels of drug

---

neostigmine (℞)

(nee-oh-stig′meen)

neostigmine, Prostigmin

Func. class.: Cholinergic stimulant; anticholinesterase

Chem. class.: Quaternary compound

Action: Inhibits destruction of acetylcholine, which increases concentration at sites where acetylcholine is released; this facilitates transmission of impulses across myoneural junction

Uses: Myasthenia gravis, nondepolarizing neuromuscular blocker antagonist, bladder distention, postoperative ileus

Dosage and routes:

Renal dose

• CrCl 10-50 ml/min 50% of dose; CrCl <10 ml/min 25% of dose

Myasthenia gravis

• *Adult:* **PO** 15 q3-4h, may increase to 375 mg/day; **IM/IV** 0.5-2 mg q1-3h

• *Child:* **PO** 2 mg/kg/day q3-4h

Nondepolarizing neuromuscular blocker antagonist

• *Adult:* **IV** 0.5-2 mg slowly, may repeat if needed (give 0.6-1.2 mg atropine before this drug)

• *Infant/child:* **IV** 0.025-0.1 mg/kg/dose

Abdominal distention/postoperative ileus

• *Adult:* **IM/SC** 0.25-1 mg (1:4000) q4-6h depending on condition × 2-3 days

Available forms: Tabs 15 mg; inj 1:1000, 1:2000, 1:4000

Side effects/adverse reactions:

INTEG: Rash, urticaria, flushing

CNS: Dizziness, headache, sweating, weakness, *convulsions,* incoordination, *paralysis,* drowsiness, loss of consciousness

GI: Nausea, diarrhea, vomiting, cramps, increased peristalsis, salivary and gastric secretions

CV: Tachycardia, dysrhythmias, bradycardia, hypotension, AV block, ECG changes, *cardiac arrest,* syncope

GU: Urinary frequency, incontinence, urgency

RESP: Respiratory depression, bronchospasm, constriction, laryngospasm, respiratory arrest, dyspnea

N

EENT: Miosis, blurred vision, lacrimation, visual changes

Contraindications: Obstruction of intestine, renal system, bromide sensitivity, peritonitis

Precautions: Bradycardia, pregnancy (C), hypotension, seizure disorders, bronchial asthma, coronary occlusion, hyperthyroidism, dysrhythmias, peptic ulcer, megacolon, poor GI motility, lactation, children

Pharmacokinetics:

PO: Onset 45-75 min, duration 2½-4 hr

IM/SC: Onset 10-30 min, duration 2½-4 hr

IV: Onset 4-8 min; duration 2-4 hr; metabolized in liver, excreted in urine

Interactions:

• Decreased action of gallamine, metocurine, pancuronium, tubocurarine, atropine

• Increased action of decamethonium, succinylcholine

• Decreased action of neostigmine: aminoglycosides, anesthetics, procainamide, quinidine, mecamylamine, polymyxin, magnesium

NURSING CONSIDERATIONS

Assess:

• VS, respiration q8h

• I&O ratio; check for urinary retention or incontinence

◆ For bradycardia, hypotension, bronchospasm, headache, dizziness, convulsions, respiratory depression; drug should be discontinued if toxicity occurs

Administer:

• Only with atropine sulfate available for cholinergic crisis

• Only after all other cholinergics have been discontinued

• Increased doses, as ordered if tolerance occurs

• Larger doses after exercise or fatigue, as ordered

PO

• On empty stomach for better absorption

IV

• Undiluted, give through Y-tube or 3-way stopcock; give 0.5 mg or less over 1 min

Additive compatibilities: Netilmicin

Syringe compatibilities: Glycopyrrolate, heparin, pentobarbital, thiopental

Y-site compatibilities: Heparin, hydrocortisone, potassium chloride, vit B/C

Perform/provide:

• Storage at room temperature

Evaluate:

• Therapeutic response: increased muscle strength, hand grasp, improved gait, absence of labored breathing (if severe)

Teach patient/family:

• That drug is not a cure; it only relieves symptoms

• To wear Medic Alert ID specifying myasthenia gravis, drugs taken

Treatment of overdose: Respiratory support, atropine 1-4 mg (IV)

---

nesiritide

See appendix a—selected new drugs

---

nevirapine

(ne-veer′a-peen)

Viramune

Func. class.: Antiretroviral

Chem. class.: Non-nucleoside reverse transcriptase inhibitor (NNRTI)

Action: Binds directly to reverse transcriptase and blocks RNA, DNA,

---

 = Nursing alert   ✻ = Herb-drug interaction   ⊘ = Do not crush

causing a disruption of the enzyme's site

Uses: HIV-1 in combination with nucleoside analogs in those experiencing deterioration

Research note: Nevirapine given with warfarin resulted in decreased warfarin action[27]

Dosage and routes:
• *Adult:* **PO** 200 mg qd × 2 wk, then 200 mg bid in combination with nucleoside analogs
• *Child ≥8 yr:* **PO** 4 mg/kg/qd × 2 wk, then 4 mg/kg/bid
• *Child 2 mo-8 yr:* **PO** 4 mg/kg qd × 2 wk, then 7 mg/kg bid

Available forms: Tabs 200 mg; oral susp 50 mg/5 ml

Side effects/adverse reactions:

GI: Diarrhea, abdominal pain, *nausea, stomatitis,* **hepatotoxicity**

CNS: Paresthesia, headache, fever, peripheral neuropathy

INTEG: Rash, toxic epidermal necrolysis

MS: Pain, myalgia

HEMA: **Neutropenia, anemia, thrombocytopenia**

MISC: **Stevens-Johnson syndrome**

Contraindications: Hypersensitivity

Precautions: Liver disease, pregnancy (C), lactation, children, renal disease

Pharmacokinetics: Rapidly absorbed, 60% bound to plasma proteins, metabolized by liver

Interactions:
• Decreased nevirapine levels: rifamycins
• Decreased effects of protease inhibitors, oral contraceptives

NURSING CONSIDERATIONS
Assess:
• Signs of infection, anemia
• Liver, blood studies during treatment: ALT, AST, viral load, CD4; renal studies

• C&S before drug therapy; drug may be taken as soon as culture is taken; repeat C&S after treatment; determine the presence of other sexually transmitted disease
• Bowel pattern before, during treatment; if severe abdominal pain with bleeding occurs, drug should be discontinued; monitor hydration
• Skin eruptions; rash, urticaria, itching
• Allergies before treatment, reaction to each medication; place allergies on chart

Administer:
• Without regard to meals

Teach patient/family:
• To report any right quadrant pain, jaundice, rash immediately
• That drug may be taken with food, antacids, didanosine
• To take as prescribed; if dose is missed, take as soon as remembered up to 1 hr before next dose; do not double dose
• That drug is not a cure, controls symptoms of HIV
• To avoid OTC agents unless approved by prescriber
• To use a nonhormonal form of contraception during treatment
• That drug must be taken in equal intervals around the clock to maintain blood levels for duration of therapy

niacin (OTC, ℞)
(nye′a-sin)
Edur-Acin, Nia-Bid, Niac,
Niacels, Niacor, Niaspan,
Nicobid, Nico-400, Nicolar,
Nicotinex
nicotinic acid (OTC, ℞)
Novo-Niacin*, Slo-Niacin,
vitamin B
niacinamide (OTC, ℞)
nicotinamide (OTC, ℞)
Func. class.: Vit B$_3$, antihyperlipidemic
Chem. class.: Water-soluble vitamin

Action: Needed for conversion of
fats, protein, carbohydrates, by oxidation reduction; acts directly on
vascular smooth muscle, causing vasodilation; high doses decrease serum lipids

Uses: Pellagra, hyperlipidemias, peripheral vascular disease

Research note: Extended release
niacin may cause less flushing and
does not cause increased hepatotoxicity[28]

Dosage and routes:
Adjunct in hyperlipidemia
• *Adult:* **PO** 100-500 mg qd in 3
divided doses after meals, may be
increased to 4 g/day
Pellagra
• *Adult:* **PO** 300-500 mg qd in divided doses
• *Child:* **PO** 100-300 mg qd in divided doses
Peripheral vascular disease
• *Adult:* **PO** 250-800 mg qd in divided doses
Available forms: Niacin tabs 25, 50,
100, 125, 250, 500 mg; caps, time
rel 125, 250, 300, 400, 500 mg; tabs,
ext rel 125, 250, 400, 500, 750, 1000
mg; cap, ext rel 125, 250, 300, 400,
500 mg; elix 50 mg/5 ml;

nicotinamide—tabs 50, 100, 125,
250, 500 mg
Side effects/adverse reactions:
CNS: Paresthesias, headache, dizziness, anxiety
GI: Nausea, vomiting, anorexia, flatulence, xerostomia, *jaundice,*
diarrhea, peptic ulcer
GU: Hyperuricemia, *glycosuria, hypoalbuminemia*
CV: Postural hypotension, vasovagal attacks, dysrhythmias, vasodilation
EENT: Blurred vision, ptosis
INTEG: Flushing, dry skin, rash, pruritus
RESP: Wheezing

Contraindications: Hypersensitivity, peptic ulcer, hepatic disease, lactation, hemorrhage, severe hypotension

Precautions: Glaucoma, cardiovascular disease, CAD, diabetes
mellitus, gout, schizophrenia, pregnancy (C)

Do not confuse:
Nicobid/Nitro-Bid

Pharmacokinetics:
PO: Peak 30-70 min, half-life 45
min; metabolized in liver; 30% excreted unchanged in urine

Interactions:
• Increased action of ganglionic
blockers

Lab test interferences:
Increase: Bilirubin, alk phospha-
tase, liver enzymes, LDH, uric acid
Decrease: Cholesterol
False increase: Urinary catechol-
amines
False-positive: Urine glucose

NURSING CONSIDERATIONS
Assess:
• Liver function studies: AST, ALT,
bilirubin, uric acid, alk phosphatase; blood glucose before and during treatment

---

◆ = Nursing alert   ∥ = Herb-drug interaction   ⊘ = Do not crush

• Cardiac status: rate, rhythm, quality; postural hypotension, dysrhythmias

• Nutritional status: liver, yeast, legumes, organ meat, lean poultry; fat in diet

• Liver dysfunction: clay-colored stools, itching, dark urine, jaundice

• CNS symptoms: headache, paresthesias, blurred vision

• For symptoms of niacin deficiency: nausea, vomiting, anemia, poor memory, confusion, dermatitis

• For lipid, triglyceride, cholesterol level, if using for hyperlipidemia

Administer:

• With meals for GI symptoms, and 325 mg aspirin ½ hr before dose to decrease flushing

Evaluate:

• Therapeutic response: decreased lipids, warm extremities, absence of numbness in extremities

Teach patient/family:

• That flushing and increase in feelings of warmth will occur several hr after taking drug (PO); after 2 wk of therapy, these side effects diminish

• To remain recumbent if postural hypotension occurs; to rise slowly to prevent orthostatic hypotension

• To abstain from alcohol if drug is prescribed for hyperlipidemia

• To avoid sunlight if skin lesions are present

🚫 Not to break, crush, or chew ext rel tabs, caps

---

nicardipine (℞)

(nye-card′i-peen)
Cardene, Cardene IV,
Cardene SR
Func. class.: Calcium channel blocker, antianginal, antihypertensive
Chem. class.: Dihydropyridine

Action: Inhibits calcium ion influx across cell membrane during cardiac depolarization; produces relaxation of coronary vascular smooth muscle, peripheral vascular smooth muscle; dilates coronary vascular arteries; increases myocardial oxygen delivery in patients with vasospastic angina

Uses: Chronic stable angina pectoris, hypertension

Research note: Grapefruit juice given with nicardipine resulted in increased nicardipine levels[29]

Dosage and routes:

• *Adult:* **PO** 20 mg tid initially, may increase after 3 days (range 20-40 mg tid); **IV** 0.5-2.2 mg/hr

Available forms: Caps 20, 30 mg; caps sus rel 30, 45, 60 mg; inj 2.5 mg/ml

Side effects/adverse reactions:

CV: Dysrhythmia, edema, *CHF,* bradycardia, hypotension, palpitations, *MI, pulmonary edema*

GI: Nausea, vomiting, diarrhea, gastric upset, constipation, *hepatitis,* abdominal cramps

GU: Nocturia, polyuria, *acute renal failure*

INTEG: Rash, pruritus, urticaria, photosensitivity, hair loss

CNS: Headache, fatigue, drowsiness, dizziness, anxiety, depression, weakness, insomnia, confusion, paresthesia, somnolence

OTHER: Blurred vision, flushing, nasal congestion, sweating, shortness

---

of breath, gynecomastia, hyperglycemia, sexual difficulties, ***Stevens-Johnson syndrome***

Contraindications: Sick sinus syndrome, 2nd-/3rd-degree heart block, hypotension <90 mm Hg systolic, hypersensitivity

Precautions: CHF, hypotension, hepatic injury, pregnancy (C), lactation, children, renal disease, elderly

Do not confuse:

Cardene/Cardizem

Cardene SR/Cardizem SR

Pharmacokinetics:

PO: Onset 30 min, peak 1-2 hr, duration 8 hr

PO-SR: Onset unknown, peak 2-6 hr, duration 10-12 hr, half-life 2-5 hr
Metabolized by liver, excreted in urine (98% as metabolites)

Interactions:

• Increased effects of digitalis, neuromuscular blocking agents, theophylline, other antihypertensives, nitrates, alcohol, quinidine

• Increased effects of nicardipine: cimetidine

• Decreased antihypertensive effect: NSAIDs

• Increased risk of toxicity: cyclosporine, prazosin, carbamazepine, quinidine, cimetidine, propranolol

• Food/drug: increased hypotensive effect: grapefruit juice

NURSING CONSIDERATIONS

Assess:

• Cardiac status: B/P, pulse, respiration, ECG

• Anginal pain: intensity, location, duration, alleviating factors

• K, LFTs, renal studies, periodically

• CHF: weight gain, rales, jugular venous distention, dyspnea

Administer:

• Without regard to meals

IV

• Dilute each 25 mg/240 ml of compatible sol (0.1 mg/ml), give slowly

• Stable at room temperature 24 hr

Y-site compatibilities: Diltiazem, dobutamine, dopamine, epinephrine, fentanyl, hydromorphone, labetalol, lorazepam, midazolam, milrinone, morphine, nitroglycerin, norepinephrine, ranitidine, vecuronium

Evaluate:

• Therapeutic response: decreased anginal pain, decreased B/P

Teach patient/family:

• To avoid hazardous activities until stabilized on drug, dizziness is no longer a problem

• To limit caffeine consumption, take no alcohol products

• To avoid OTC drugs unless directed by prescriber

• To comply in all areas of medical regimen: diet, exercise, stress reduction, drug therapy

• To notify prescriber of irregular heartbeat, shortness of breath, swelling of feet and hands, pronounced dizziness, constipation, nausea, hypotension

Treatment of overdose: Defibrillation, β-agonists, IV Ca, diuretics, atropine for AV block, vasopressor for hypotension

nicotine (OTC, R)
(nik'o-teen)
nicotine chewing gum (OTC, R)
Nicorette, Nicotine gum
nicotine inhaler (OTC, R)
Nicotrol Inhaler
nicotine nasal spray (R)
Nicotrol NS Nasal Spray
nicotine transdermal (R)
Habitrol, Nicoderm CQ, Nicotine Transdermal System, Nicotrol

Func. class.: Smoking deterrent
Chem. class.: Ganglionic cholinergic agonist

Action: Agonist at nicotinic receptors in peripheral, central nervous systems; acts at sympathetic ganglia, on chemoreceptors of aorta, carotid bodies; also affects adrenalin-releasing catecholamines

Uses: Deter cigarette smoking

Investigational uses: Gilles de la Tourette's syndrome

Dosage and routes:
Nicotine chewing gum
• *Adult:* Gum 1 piece chewed × ½ hr as needed to abstain from smoking, not to exceed 30/day
Nicotine inhaler
• *Adult:* INH 6 cartridges/day for first 3-6 wk, max 16/day × 12 wk
Nicotine nasal spray
• *Adults:* 1 spray in each nostril 1-2 ×/hr, max 5 ×/hr or 40 ×/day, max 3 mo
Nicotine transdermal/inhaler system
• *Habitrol, Nicoderm:* 21 mg/day × 4-8 wk; 14 mg/day × 2-4 wk; 7 mg/day × 2-4 wk

• *Nicotrol:* 15 mg/day × 12 wk; 10 mg/day × 2 wk; 5 mg/day × 2 wk
• *Nicotrol Inhaler:* delivers 30% of what a smoker receives from an actual cigarette
Gilles de la Tourette's syndrome (off-label)
• *Adult/child:* Chewing gum: 2 mg chewed × ½ hr bid for 1-6 mo; TD: 7 or 10 mg patch qd × 2 days
Available forms: Transdermal patch delivering 7, 14, 21 mg/day (Habitrol, Nicoderm, Nicotine transdermal system); 5, 10, 15 mg/day (Nicoderm); nicotine inhaler: 4 mg delivered; nasal spray: 0.5 mg nicotine/actuation; Gum: 2 mg/piece
Side effects/adverse reactions:
RESP: Breathing difficulty, cough, hoarseness, sneezing, wheezing
EENT: Jaw ache, irritation in buccal cavity
CNS: Dizziness, vertigo, insomnia, headache, confusion, convulsions, depression, euphoria, numbness, tinnitus, strange dreams
GI: Nausea, vomiting, anorexia, indigestion, diarrhea, abdominal pain, constipation, eructation
CV: Dysrhythmias, tachycardia, palpitations, edema, flushing, hypertension
Contraindications: Hypersensitivity, immediate post MI recovery period, severe angina pectoris, pregnancy (D)
Precautions: Vasospastic disease, dysrhythmias, diabetes mellitus, hyperthyroidism, pheochromocytoma, coronary disease, esophagitis, peptic ulcer, lactation, hepatic/renal disease
Pharmacokinetics: Onset 15-30 min, metabolized in liver, excreted in urine, half-life 2-3 hr, 30-120 hr (terminal)
Interactions:
• Decreased absorption: glutethimide

N

• Increased absorption: SC insulin
• Decreased metabolism of propoxyphene
• Smoking cessation increases diuretic effects of furosemide
• Increased blood levels with cessation of smoking: caffeine, theophylline, pentazocine, imipramine, oxazepam, propranolol, acetaminophen

NURSING CONSIDERATIONS
Assess:
• Adverse reaction: irritation of buccal cavity, dislike of taste, jaw ache
Evaluate:
• Therapeutic response: decrease in urge to smoke, decreased need for gum after 3-6 mo
Teach patient/family:
• To chew gum slowly for 30 min to promote buccal absorption of the drug; do not chew over 45 min
• To begin drug withdrawal after 3 mo use; not to exceed 6 mo
• All aspects of drug use; give package insert to patient and explain
• That gum will not stick to dentures, dental appliances
• That gum is as toxic as cigarette; to be used only to deter smoking
• Not to use during pregnancy; birth defects may occur

Transdermal patch
• That patch is as toxic as cigarettes; to be used only to deter smoking
• Not to use during pregnancy; birth defects may occur
• To keep used and unused system out of reach of children and pets
• To apply once a day to a nonhairy, clean, dry area of skin on upper body or upper outer arm; to rotate sites to prevent skin irritation
• To stop smoking immediately when beginning patch treatment
• To apply promptly after removing from protective patch; system may lose strength

Inhaler
• That puffing on mouthpiece delivers nicotine through the mouth lining

---

nifedipine (Ŗ)
(nye-fed'i-peen)
Adalat, Adalat CC, Apo-Nifed*, nifedipine, Novo-Nifedin*, Nu-Nifedin*, Procardia, Procardia XL
Func. class.: Calcium-channel blocker, antianginal, antihypertensive
Chem. class.: Dihydropyridine

Action: Inhibits calcium ion influx across cell membrane during cardiac depolarization; relaxes coronary vascular smooth muscle; dilates coronary arteries; increases myocardial oxygen delivery in patients with vasospastic angina; dilates peripheral arteries
Uses: Chronic stable angina pectoris, vasospastic angina, hypertension
Investigational uses: Migraines, CHF, Raynaud's disease, anal fissures
Dosage and routes:
• *Adult:* **PO** immediate release 10 mg tid, increase in 10 mg increments q4-6h, not to exceed 180 mg/24 hr or single dose of 30 mg; sus rel 30-60 mg/qd, may increase q7-14d, doses >120 mg not recommended
• *Child:* **PO** 0.25-0.5 mg/kg/dose q4-6h, max 1-2 mg/kg/day
Anal fissures (off-label)
• *Adult:* **TOP** 0.2% gel q12h × 21 days
Available forms: Caps 5, 10, 20 mg; tabs, ext rel 10, 20, 30, 60, 90 mg; tabs 10 mg

---

⬙ = Nursing alert   🌿 = Herb-drug interaction   🚫 = Do not crush

Side effects/adverse reactions:

CNS: Headache, fatigue, drowsiness, dizziness, anxiety, depression, weakness, insomnia, light-headedness, paresthesia, tinnitus, blurred vision, nervousness

CV: ***Dysrhythmias,*** edema, ***CHF,*** hypotension, palpitations, ***MI, pulmonary edema,*** tachycardia

GI: Nausea, vomiting, diarrhea, gastric upset, constipation, increased liver function studies, dry mouth

GU: Nocturia, polyuria

INTEG: Rash, pruritus, flushing, photosensitivity, hair loss

MISC: Flushing, sexual difficulties, cough, fever, chills

Contraindications: Hypersensitivity

Precautions: CHF, hypotension, sick sinus syndrome, 2nd-/3rd-degree heart block, hypotension less than 90 mm Hg systolic, hepatic injury, pregnancy (C), lactation, children, renal disease

Pharmacokinetics:

Well absorbed PO

PO-ER: Duration 24 hr

PO: Onset 20 min, peak 0.5-6 hr, duration 6-8 hr, half-life 2-5 hr

Metabolized by liver, excreted in urine (98% as metabolites)

Interactions:

• Decreased antihypertensive effect: NSAIDs

• Increased risk of toxicity: cimetidine, propranolol, cyclosporine, prazosin, carbamazepine, quinidine, digoxin

• Increased effects of theophylline, β-blockers, antihypertensives

• Food/drug: increased nifedipine level: grapefruit juice

• Decreased effects: quinidine

Lab test interferences:

Positive: ANA, direct Coombs' test

NURSING CONSIDERATIONS

Assess:

• Anginal pain: location, intensity, duration, character, alleviating, aggravating factors

• Cardiac status: B/P, pulse, respiration, ECG

• Potassium, LFTs, renal studies periodically during treatment

Administer:

• Without regard to meals

• SL: may puncture cap and squeeze drug into buccal pouch

Evaluate:

• Therapeutic response: decreased anginal pain, B/P, activity tolerance

Teach patient/family:

• To avoid hazardous activities until stabilized on drug, dizziness is no longer a problem

• To limit caffeine consumption; take no alcohol products

• To avoid OTC drugs unless directed by a prescriber

• That ext rel nonabsorbable shell may appear in stools

• To comply with all areas of medical regimen: diet, exercise, stress reduction, drug therapy

• To change position slowly; orthostatic hypotension is common

🚫 Not to break, crush, or chew ext rel tabs

• To notify prescriber of dyspnea, edema of extremities, nausea, vomiting, severe ataxia

Treatment of overdose: Defibrillation, atropine for AV block, vasopressor for hypotension

N

---

nilutamide
(nye-loo'ta-mide)
Anandron*, Nilandron
Func. class.: Antineoplastic-hormone
Chem. class.: Antiandrogen

Action: Interferes with testosterone uptake in the nucleus or testosterone activity in target tissues; arrests tumor growth in androgen-sensitive tissue (e.g., prostate gland); prostatic carcinoma is androgen-sensitive, so tumor growth is arrested

Uses: Metastatic prostatic carcinoma, stage D2 in combination with surgical castration

Dosage and routes:
• *Adult:* **PO** 300 mg qd × 30 days, then 150 mg qd
Available forms: Tabs 50, 100*, 150 mg

Side effects/adverse reactions:
CNS: Hot flashes, drowsiness, insomnia, dizziness, hyperthesia, depression
GU: Decreased libido, impotence, testicular atrophy, UTI, hematuria, nocturia, gynecomastia
GI: Diarrhea, nausea, vomiting, increased liver function studies, constipation, dyspepsia, ***hepatotoxicity***
INTEG: Rash, sweating, alopecia, dry skin
RESP: Dyspnea, URI, pneumonia, ***interstitial pneumonitis***
HEMA: Anemia
EENT: Delay in adaptation to dark
MISC: Edema

Contraindications: Hypersensitivity, severe hepatic impairment, severe respiratory disease, women
Precautions: Pregnancy (C)
Pharmacokinetics: Rapidly and completely absorbed; excreted in urine and feces as metabolites

Interactions:
• Increased toxicity of vit K, phenytoin, theophylline

NURSING CONSIDERATIONS
Assess:
• Liver function studies: AST, ALT, alk phosphatase, which may be elevated
• For CNS symptoms: drowsiness, insomnia, dizziness
• Chest x-rays, routinely, baseline pulmonary function studies, dyspnea, cough, which may indicate interstitial pneumonitis; discontinue treatment if this condition is suspected

Administer:
• Without regard to meals
Perform/provide:
• Storage at room temperature
Evaluate:
• Therapeutic response: decrease in prostatic tumor size, decrease in spread of cancer

Teach patient/family:
• To report side effects: decreased libido, impotence, breast enlargement, hot flashes, diarrhea, dyspnea, cough, shortness of breath; if SOB occurs notify prescriber immediately
• To report signs of hepatotoxicity
• To wear tinted lens to alleviate delay in adapting to the dark
• That drug is started on day of or day after surgical castration
• To avoid alcohol consumption

Treatment of overdose: Induce vomiting, provide supportive care

◆ = Nursing alert   ∅ = Herb-drug interaction   ⊘ = Do not crush

nisoldipine
(nye-sole′dih-peen)
Sular
Func. class.: Antihypertensive, calcium channel blocker
Chem. class.: Dihydropyridine

Action: Inhibits calcium ion influx across cell membrane, resulting in dilation of peripheral arteries

Uses: Essential hypertension, alone or with other antihypertensives

Dosage and routes:
• *Adult:* **PO** 20 mg qd initially, may increase by 10 mg/wk, usual dose 20-40 mg qd
• *Geriatric:* **PO** 10 mg/day, increase by 10 mg/wk

Available forms: Tabs, ext rel 10, 20, 30, 40 mg

Side effects/adverse reactions:
CV: Dysrhythmia, edema, CHF, hypotension, palpitations, *MI, pulmonary edema,* tachycardia, syncope, AV block, angina
GI: Nausea, vomiting, diarrhea, gastric upset, constipation, increased liver function studies, dry mouth
GU: Nocturia, polyuria
INTEG: Rash, pruritus
MISC: Flushing, sexual difficulties, cough, nasal congestion, SOB, wheezing, epistaxis, respiratory infection, chest pain
CNS: Headache, fatigue, drowsiness, dizziness, anxiety, depression, nervousness, insomnia, lightheadedness, paresthesia, tinnitus, psychosis, somnolence
HEMA: Anemia

Contraindications: Hypersensitivity, sick sinus syndrome, 2nd-/3rd-degree heart block

Precautions: CHF, hypotension <90 mm Hg systolic, hepatic injury, pregnancy (C), lactation, children, renal disease, elderly

Pharmacokinetics: Metabolized by liver, excreted in urine

Interactions:
• Increased effects of β-blockers, antihypertensives, digitalis
• Increased felodipine level: cimetidine, ranitidine
• Drug/food: increased nisoldipine level: high-fat foods; increased hypotensive effect: grapefruit juice

NURSING CONSIDERATIONS
Assess:
• Cardiac status: B/P, pulse, respiration, ECG
• I&O ratios, weight qd
• For CHF: weight gain, jugular vein distention, edema, rales

Administer:
• Once daily as whole tablet; avoid high-fat foods, grapefruit juice

Evaluate:
• Therapeutic response: decreased B/P

Teach patient/family:
🚫 To swallow whole; not to break, crush, or chew
• To avoid hazardous activities until stabilized on drug, dizziness is no longer a problem
• To report nausea, dizziness, edema, shortness of breath, palpitations
• To limit caffeine consumption
• To avoid OTC drugs unless directed by a prescriber
• The importance of complying with all areas of medical regimen: diet, exercise, stress reduction, drug therapy
• To rise slowly to prevent orthostatic hypotension

Treatment of overdose: Defibrillation, atropine for AV block, vasopressor for hypotension

nitric oxide (Ⴆ)

(nye'trik ok'side)

INOmax

Func. class.: Respiratory inhalant

Action: Increases partial pressure of arterial oxygen (Pao_2) by dilating pulmonary vessels

Uses: Treatment of term and near-term (>34 wk) neonates with hypoxic respiratory failure associated with pulmonary hypertension; used with other agents and ventilatory support

Dosage and routes:

• *Neonate:* **INH** 20 ppm × up to 2 wk until O_2 desaturation has been resolved and neonate is ready to be weaned from therapy

Available forms: Gas 100, 800 ppm

Side effects/adverse reactions:

RESP: **Pulmonary hemorrhage,** atelectasis

SYST: **Intracranial hemorrhage,** hematuria, hyperglycemia, **sepsis,** cellulitis, **stridor,** withdrawal syndrome, **methemoglobinemia, seizures, cerebral infarction, posttreatment infection,** hypotension

Contraindications: Dependence on right to left shunting of blood, hypersensitivity

Precautions: Bradycardia, rales, infections, pregnancy (C)

Pharmacokinetics: Unknown

NURSING CONSIDERATIONS

Assess:

• Respiratory rate, rhythm, character, chest expansion, color, transcutaneous saturation, ABGs, methemoglobinemia

Administer:

• Only by persons trained in neonatal ventilation, inhalation

• Only in neonates; not indicated for other populations

Perform/provide:

• Weaning off therapy; do not discontinue abruptly

Evaluate:

• Therapeutic response: significant improvement in respiratory status and pulmonary hypertension

nitrofurantoin (Ⴆ)

(nye-troe-fyoor'an-toyn)

Apo-Nitrofurantoin*, Furadantin, Furalan, Furatoin, Macrobid, Macrodantin, Nitrofuracot, nitrofurantoin

Func. class.: Urinary tract anti-infective

Chem. class.: Synthetic nitrofuran derivative

Action: Appears to inhibit bacterial enzymes

Uses: Urinary tract infections caused by *Escherichia coli, Klebsiella, Pseudomonas, Proteus vulgaris, Proteus morganii, Serratia, Citrobacter, Staphylococcus aureus, Staphylococcus epidermidis, Enterococcus, Salmonella, Shigella*

Dosage and routes:

Active infections

• *Adult and child >12 yr:* **PO** 50-100 mg qid pc or 50-100 mg hs for long-term treatment

• *Child 1 mo-3 yr:* **PO** 5-7 mg/kg/day in 4 divided doses; 1-3 mg/kg/day for long-term treatment

Chronic suppression

• *Adult:* **PO** 50-100 mg qPM

• *Child:* **PO** 1 mg/kg/day qPM

Available forms: Caps 25, 50, 100 mg; tabs 50, 100 mg; susp 25 mg/5 ml; ext rel caps 100 mg; macrocrystal caps (Macrodantin) 25, 50, 100 mg

Side effects/adverse reactions:

INTEG: Pruritus, rash, urticaria, angioedema, alopecia, tooth staining

---

◆ = Nursing alert   ∥ = Herb-drug interaction   ⊘ = Do not crush

CNS: Dizziness, headache, drowsiness, peripheral neuropathy, chills
*GI: Nausea, vomiting, abdominal pain, diarrhea, **cholestatic jaundice,*** loss of appetite
Contraindications: Hypersensitivity, anuria, severe renal disease, infants <1 mo
Precautions: Pregnancy (B), lactation, G-6-PD deficiency, elderly, CrCl <40
Pharmacokinetics:

PO: Half-life 20-60 min; crosses blood-brain barrier, placenta; enters breast milk; excreted as inactive metabolites in liver, unchanged in urine
Interactions:
• Increased levels of nitrofurantoin: probenecid
• Antagonistic effect: norfloxacin
• Decreased absorption of Mg trisilicate antacid
NURSING CONSIDERATIONS
Assess:
• Blood count during chronic therapy
• I&O ratio; urine pH <5.5 is ideal; C&S before treatment, after completion; symptoms of UTI
• CNS symptoms: insomnia, vertigo, headache, drowsiness, convulsions
• Allergy: fever, flushing, rash, urticaria, pruritus
Administer:

PO
• After clean-catch urine for C&S
• Two daily doses if urine output is high or if patient has diabetes
Evaluate:
• Therapeutic response: decreased dysuria, fever; neg C&S
Teach patient/family:
• To take with food or milk; avoid alcohol
• To protect susp from freezing and shake well before taking
• That drug may cause drowsiness; instruct client to seek aid in walking

and other activities; advise client not to drive or operate machinery while on medication
• That diabetics should monitor blood glucose level
🚫 Not to crush tabs, open caps
• That drug may turn urine rust-yellow to brown

---

nitroglycerin (℞)
(nye-troe-gli'ser-in)
extended-release buccal tablets (℞)
Nitrogard, Nitrogard SR
extended-release capsules (℞)
Nitrocap T.D., Nitroglyn, Nitrolin, Nitrospan, Nitro-Time
extended-release tablets (℞)
Nitrong
IV (℞)
Nitro-Bid I.V., Tridil
ointment (℞)
Nitro-Bid, Nitrol
SL (℞)
Nitrostat, NitroQuick
spray (℞)
Nitrolingual Translingual Spray
transdermal (℞)
Deponit, Minitran, Nitrek, Nitrocine, Nitrodisc, Nitro-Dur, Transderm-Nitro
Func. class.: Coronary vasodilator, antianginal
Chem. class.: Nitrate

Action: Decreases preload, afterload, which is responsible for decreasing left ventricular end-diastolic pressure, systemic vascular resistance; dilates coronary arteries, improves blood flow through coronary vasculature

N

Uses: Chronic stable angina pectoris, prophylaxis of angina pain, CHF associated with acute MI, controlled hypotension in surgical procedures

Dosage and routes:
• *Adult:* **SL** dissolve tab under tongue when pain begins; may repeat q5min until relief occurs; take no more than 3 tabs/15 min; use 1 tab prophylactically 5-10 min before activities; **SUS CAP** q6-12h on empty stomach; **TOP** 1-2 in q8h, increase to 4 in q4h as needed; **IV** 5 µg/min, then increase by 5 µg/min q3-5min; if no response after 20 µg/min, increase by 10-20 µg/min until desired response; **TRANS** apply a pad qd to a site free of hair; remove patch hs to provide 10-12h nitrate-free interval to avoid tolerance
• *Child:* **IV** initial: 0.25-0.5 µg/kg/min, titrate to patient response, usual dose 1-3 µg/kg/min

Available forms: Buccal tabs 1, 2, 3 mg; aero 0.4 mg/metered spray; sus rel caps 2.5, 6.5, 9, 13 mg; tabs, sus rel 2.6, 6.5, 9 mg; inj 0.5, 5, mg/ml; SL tabs 0.15, 0.3, 0.4, 0.6 mg; trans oint 2%; trans syst 0.1, 0.2, 0.3, 0.4, 0.6 mg/24 hr; inj sol 25 mg/250 ml, 50 mg/250 ml, 50 mg/500 ml, 100 mg/500 ml, 200 mg/500 ml; patch 22.4, 44.8, 67.2 mg

Side effects/adverse reactions:
CV: Postural hypotension, tachycardia, *collapse,* syncope
GI: Nausea, vomiting
INTEG: Pallor, sweating, rash
CNS: Headache, flushing, dizziness

Contraindications: Hypersensitivity to this drug or nitrites, severe anemia, increased intracranial pressure, cerebral hemorrhage

Precautions: Postural hypotension, pregnancy (C), lactation

Do not confuse:
Nitro-Bid/Nicobid

Pharmacokinetics:
SUS REL: Onset 20-45 min, duration 3-8 hr
SL: Onset 1-3 min, duration 30 min
TRANS: Onset ½-1 hr, duration 12-24 hr
IV: Onset 1-2 min, duration 3-5 min
TRANSMUC: Onset 3 min, duration 3-5 hr
AEROSOL: Onset 2 min, duration 30-60 min
TOP OINT: Onset 30-60 min, duration 2-12 hr
Metabolized by liver, excreted in urine, half-life 1-4 min

Interactions:
• Increased effects: β-blockers, diuretics, antihypertensives, anticoagulants, alcohol
• Decreased heparin: IV nitroglycerin

NURSING CONSIDERATIONS
Assess:
• Orthostatic B/P, pulse
• Pain: duration, time started, activity being performed, character
• Tolerance if taken over long period
• Headache, light-headedness, decreased B/P; may indicate a need for decreased dosage

Administer:
• With 8 oz H_2O on empty stomach (oral tablet) 1 hr before or 2 hr after meals
• Trans tab should be placed between cheek and gum line
• Topical ointment should be measured on papers supplied
• Apply a new TD patch qd and remove after 12-14 hr to prevent tolerance
IV
• Diluted in amount specified D_5, D_5W, 0.9% NaCl for infusion; use glass infusion bottles, non–polyvinyl chloride infusion tubing; titrate to patient response; do not use filters

---

◆ = Nursing alert   ⫽ = Herb-drug interaction   ⊘ = Do not crush

Additive compatibilities: Alteplase, aminophylline, dobutamine, dopamine, enalaprilat, furosemide, lidocaine, verapamil

Syringe compatibilities: Heparin

Y-site compatibilities: Amiodarone, amphotericin B cholesteryl, amrinone, atracurium, cefmetazole, cisatracurium, diltiazem, dobutamine, dopamine, epinephrine, esmolol, famotidine, fentanyl, fluconazole, furosemide, haloperidol, heparin, hydromorphone, insulin (regular), labetalol, lidocaine, lorazepam, midazolam, milrinone, morphine, nicardipine, norepinephrine, pancuronium, propofol, ranitidine, remifentanil, sodium nitroprusside, streptokinase, tacrolimus, theophylline, thiopental, vecuronium, warfarin

Evaluate:

• Therapeutic response: decrease, prevention of anginal pain

Teach patient/family:

• To place buccal tab between lip and gum above incisors or between cheek and gum

🚫 That sus rel must be swallowed whole, not chewed

• That SL should be dissolved under tongue, not swallowed

• That aerosol should be sprayed under tongue, not inhaled

• To use inhaler only when lying down

• Not to inhale spray

• To keep tabs in original container

• If 3 SL tabs in 15 min do not relieve pain, to seek immediate medical attention

• To avoid alcohol

• That drug may cause headache; tolerance usually develops; use nonnarcotic analgesic

• That drug may be taken before stressful activity: exercise, sexual activity

• That SL may sting when drug comes in contact with mucous membranes

• To avoid hazardous activities if dizziness occurs

• To comply with complete medical regimen

• To make position changes slowly to prevent fainting

---

nitroprusside (℞)

(nye-troe-pruss'ide)

Nitropress, sodium nitroprusside

Func. class.: Antihypertensive, vasodilator

Action: Directly relaxes arteriolar, venous smooth muscle, resulting in reduction in cardiac preload, afterload

Uses: Hypertensive crisis, to decrease bleeding by creating hypotension during surgery, acute CHF, cardiogenic shock

Dosage and routes:

• *Adult:* IV INF dissolve 50 mg in 2-3 ml of D_5W, then dilute in 250-1000 ml of D_5W; run at 0.5-8 µg/kg/min

• *Child:* IV 0.3-0.5 µg/kg/min, titrate to response

Available forms: Inj 50 mg

Side effects/adverse reactions:

GI: Nausea, vomiting, abdominal pain

CNS: Dizziness, headache, agitation, twitching, decreased reflexes, *LOC,* restlessness

EENT: Tinnitus, blurred vision

GU: Impotence

INTEG: Pain, irritation at injection site, sweating

CV: Palpitation, severe hypotension, dyspnea

MISC: Cyanide, thiocyanate toxicity

Contraindications: Hypersensitivity, hypertension (compensatory)

N

Precautions: Pregnancy (C), lactation, children, fluid, electrolyte imbalances, hepatic disease, renal disease, hypothyroidism, elderly

Pharmacokinetics:

IV: Onset 1-2 min, duration 1-10 min, half-life 4 days in patients with abnormal renal function; metabolized in liver, excreted in urine

Interactions:

• Severe hypotension: ganglionic blockers, volatile liquid anesthetics, halothane, enflurane, circulatory depressants

NURSING CONSIDERATIONS
Assess:

• Electrolytes: K, Na, Cl, CO_2, CBC, serum glucose, serum methemoglobin if pulmonary O_2 levels are decreased

• Renal function studies: catecholamines, BUN, creatinine

• Hepatic function studies: AST, ALT, alk phosphatase

• B/P by direct means if possible; check ECG continuously; pulse, jugular vein distention; PCWP

• Weight qd, I&O

• Thiocyanate, lactate, cyanide levels if on long-term treatment

• Nausea, vomiting, diarrhea

• Edema in feet, legs daily; skin turgor, dryness of mucous membranes for hydration status

• Rales, dyspnea, orthopnea q30min

• For decrease in bicarbonate, P_{CO_2} blood pH, acidosis

Administer:

IV

• Depending on B/P reading q15min

• IV after diluting 50 mg/2-3 ml of D_5W, further dilute in 250 ml of D_5W; use an infusion pump only; wrap bottle with aluminum foil to protect from light; observe for color change in the infusion; discard if highly discolored (blue, green, dark red); titrate to patient response

Syringe compatibilities: Heparin

Y-site compatibilities: Amrinone, atracurium, diltiazem, dobutamine, dopamine, enalaprilat, famotidine, lidocaine, nitroglycerin, pancuronium, tacrolimus, theophylline, vecuronium

Evaluate:

• Therapeutic response: decreased B/P, absence of bleeding

Teach patient/family:

• To report headache, dizziness, loss of hearing, blurred vision, dyspnea, faintness

Treatment of overdose: Administer amyl nitrite inhalation until 3% sodium nitrate solution can be prepared for IV administration, then inject sodium thiosulfate IV, correct drop in B/P with vasopressor

---

nizatidine (OTC, ℞)

(ni-za'ti-deen)

Axid, Axid AR

Func. class.: H$_2$-Receptor antagonist

Chem. class.: Substituted thiazole

Action: Blocks H$_2$-receptors, thereby reducing gastric acid output

Uses: Benign gastric and duodenal ulceration, prevention of duodenal ulcer recurrence, symptomatic relief of gastroesophageal reflux, heartburn prevention

Dosage and routes:

Renal dose

• CrCl 20-50 ml/min give 150 mg/day; CrCl <20 ml/min give 150 mg qod

Gastric and duodenal ulcer

• *Adult:* **PO** 300 mg at night or 150 mg bid for 4-8 wk; maintenance 150 mg at night

---

Prophylaxis of duodenal ulcer
• *Adult:* **PO** 150 mg qd hs
Gastroesophageal reflux
• *Adult:* **PO** 150 mg bid
Heartburn prevention
• *Adult:* **PO** 75 mg before eating
Available forms: Caps 150, 300 mg; tabs 75 mg
Side effects/adverse reactions:
CNS: Headache, somnolence, confusion, abnormal dreams, dizziness
ENDO: Gynecomastia
HEMA: **Thrombocytopenia**
INTEG: Pruritus, sweating, urticaria, **exfoliative dermatitis**
MS: Myalgia
RESP: **Bronchospasm, laryngeal edema**
METAB: Hyperuricemia
GI: Elevated liver enzymes, **hepatitis,** jaundice, nausea
CV: Cardiac dysrhythmias, **cardiac arrest**
Contraindications: Hypersensitivity
Precautions: Renal or hepatic impairment (reduce dose in renal impairment), pregnancy (C), lactation
Pharmacokinetics: Partially metabolized by liver, excreted by kidneys, plasma half-life 1½ hr, 70% absorbed orally, small amount (0.1% of plasma concentration) enters breast milk, 35% bound to plasma proteins
NURSING CONSIDERATIONS
Assess:
• Gastric pH (>5 should be maintained)
• Fluid balance, I&O
Administer:
PO
• With meals for prolonged drug effect; antacids 1 hr before or 1 hr after drug
Evaluate:
• Mental status, confusion, dizziness, depression, anxiety, weakness, tremors, psychosis, diarrhea, jaundice, report immediately
• For GI symptoms: nausea, vomiting, diarrhea, cramps
Teach patient/family:
• That gynecomastia, impotence may occur, are reversible
• To avoid driving or other hazardous activities until patient is stabilized on this medication; dizziness may occur
• To avoid black pepper, caffeine, alcohol, harsh spices, extremes in temp of food
• To avoid OTC preparations: aspirin, cough, cold preparations
Treatment of overdose: Symptomatic and supportive therapy is recommended; activated charcoal, emesis or lavage may reduce absorption

N

norepinephrine (℞)
(nor-ep-i-nef'rin)
Levophed
Func. class.: Adrenergic
Chem. class.: Catecholamine
Action: Causes increased contractility and heart rate by acting on β-receptors in heart; also acts on α-receptors, causing vasoconstriction in blood vessels; B/P is elevated, coronary blood flow improves, cardiac output increases
Uses: Acute hypotension, shock
Dosage and routes:
• *Adult:* **IV INF** 8-12 µg/min titrated to B/P
• *Child:* **IV INF** 0.05-0.1 µg/kg/min titrated to B/P
Available forms: Inj 1 mg/ml
Side effects/adverse reactions:
CNS: Headache, anxiety, dizziness, insomnia, restlessness, tremor
CV: Palpitations, tachycardia, hypertension, ectopic beats, angina

GI: Nausea, vomiting
INTEG: Necrosis, tissue sloughing with extravasation, ***gangrene***
RESP: Dyspnea
GU: Decreased urine output
Contraindications: Hypersensitivity, ventricular fibrillation, tachydysrhythmias, pheochromocytoma
Precautions: Lactation, arterial embolism, peripheral vascular disease, hypertension, hyperthyroidism, elderly, heart disease, pregnancy (C)
Pharmacokinetics:
IV: Onset 1-2 min; metabolized in liver; excreted in urine (inactive metabolites); crosses placenta
Interactions:
• Severe hypertension: guanethidine
◆Do not use within 2 wk of MAOIs, or hypertensive crisis may result
• Dysrhythmias: general anesthetics, bretylium
• Decreased action of norepinephrine: α-blockers
• Increased B/P: oxytocics
• Increased pressor effect: tricyclics, MAOIs
• Incompatible with alkaline solutions: Na, HCO_3^-
NURSING CONSIDERATIONS
Assess:
• I&O ratio; notify prescriber if output <30 ml/hr
• ECG during administration continuously; if B/P increases, drug is decreased
• B/P and pulse q2-3min after parenteral route
• CVP or PWP during infusion if possible
• For paresthesias and coldness of extremities; peripheral blood flow may decrease
• Injection site: tissue sloughing; administer phentolamine mixed with 0.9% NaCl
• Sulfite sensitivity, which may be life-threatening

Administer:
• Plasma expanders for hypovolemia
• IV after diluting with 500-1000 ml D_5W or D_5/0.9% NaCl; average dilution is 4 mg/1000 ml diluent (4 μg base/ml); give as infusion 2-3 ml/min; titrate to response
• Using 2-bottle setup so drug may be discontinued while IV is still running; use infusion pump
Additive compatibilities: Amikacin, calcium chloride, calcium gluconate, cimetidine, corticotropin, dimenhydrinate, dobutamine, heparin, hydrocortisone, magnesium sulfate, meropenem, methylprednisolone, multivitamins, netilmicin, potassium chloride, succinylcholine, verapamil, vit B/C
Syringe compatibilities: Heparin
Y-site compatibilities: Amiodarone, amrinone, cisatracurium, diltiazem, dobutamine, dopamine, epinephrine, esmolol, famotidine, fentanyl, furosemide, haloperidol, heparin, hydrocortisone, hydromorphone, labetalol, lorazepam, meropenem, midazolam, milrinone, morphine, nicardipine, nitroglycerin, potassium chloride, propofol, ranitidine, remifentanil, vecuronium, vit B/C
Perform/provide:
• Storage of reconstituted sol if refrigerated no longer than 24 hr
• Do not use discolored sol
Evaluate:
• Therapeutic response: increased B/P with stabilization
Teach patient/family:
• The reason for drug administration and to report dyspnea, dizziness, chest pain
Treatment of overdose: Administer fluids, electrolyte replacement

---

◆ = Nursing alert   ▮ = Herb-drug interaction   ⊘ = Do not crush

norethindrone (℞)

(nor-eth-in'drone)

Micronor, Nor-QD

Func. class.: Progestogen

Chem. class.: Progesterone derivative

Action: Inhibits secretion of pituitary gonadotropins, which prevents follicular maturation, ovulation; stimulates growth of mammary tissue; antineoplastic action against endometrial cancer

Uses: Uterine bleeding (abnormal), amenorrhea, endometriosis

Dosage and routes:

• *Adult:* **PO** 5-20 mg qd days 5-25 of menstrual cycle

Endometriosis

• *Adult:* **PO** 10 mg qd × 2 wk, then increased by 5 mg qd × 2 wk, up to 30 mg qd

Available forms: Tabs 5 mg

Side effects/adverse reactions:

CNS: Dizziness, headache, migraines, depression, fatigue

CV: Hypotension, ***thrombophlebitis,*** edema, ***thromboembolism, stroke, pulmonary embolism, MI***

GI: Nausea, vomiting, anorexia, cramps, increased weight, ***cholestatic jaundice***

EENT: Diplopia

GU: Amenorrhea, cervical erosion, breakthrough bleeding, dysmenorrhea, vaginal candidiasis, breast changes, (gynecomastia, testicular atrophy, impotence), endometriosis, ***spontaneous abortion***

INTEG: Rash, urticaria, acne, hirsutism, alopecia, oily skin, seborrhea, purpura, melasma

META: Hyperglycemia

Contraindications: Breast cancer, hypersensitivity, thromboembolic disorders, reproductive cancer, genital bleeding (abnormal, undiagnosed), pregnancy (X)

Precautions: Lactation, hypertension, asthma, blood dyscrasias, gallbladder disease, CHF, diabetes mellitus, bone disease, depression, migraine headache, convulsive disorders, hepatic disease, renal disease, family history of breast or reproductive tract cancer

Pharmacokinetics:

PO: Duration 24 hr, excreted in urine, feces, metabolized in liver

Lab test interferences:

Increase: Alk phosphatase, nitrogen (urine), pregnanediol, amino acids, factors VII, VIII, IX, X

Decrease: GTT, HDL

NURSING CONSIDERATIONS

Assess:

• Weight qd: notify prescriber of weekly weight gain >5 lb

• B/P at beginning of treatment and periodically

• I&O ratio; be alert for decreasing urinary output, increasing edema

• Liver function studies: ALT, AST, bilirubin, periodically during long-term therapy

• Edema, hypertension, cardiac symptoms, jaundice

• Mental status: affect, mood, behavioral changes, depression

• Hypercalcemia

Administer:

• Titrated dose; use lowest effective dose

• In one dose in AM

• With food or milk to decrease GI symptoms

Perform/provide:

• Storage in dark area

Evaluate:

• Therapeutic response: decreased abnormal uterine bleeding, absence of amenorrhea

Teach patient/family:

• About cushingoid symptoms

• To report breast lumps, vaginal

N

Side effects: *italics* = common; ***bold italics*** = life-threatening

bleeding, edema, jaundice, dark urine, clay-colored stools, dyspnea, headache, blurred vision, abdominal pain, numbness or stiffness in legs, chest pain; male to report impotence or gynecomastia
• To report suspected pregnancy

---

norfloxacin (℞)
(nor-flox'-a-sin)
Noroxin
Func. class.: Urinary antiinfective
Chem. class.: Fluoroquinolone

Action: Interferes with conversion of intermediate DNA fragments into high-molecular-weight DNA in bacteria, inhibits DNA gyrase
Uses: Adult urinary tract infections (including complicated) caused by *Escherichia coli, Enterobacter cloacae, Proteus mirabilis, Klebsiella pneumoniae,* group D strep, indole-positive *Proteus, Citrobacter freundii, Staphylococcus aureus;* uncomplicated gonorrhea, ocular infection
Dosage and routes:
Renal dose
• CrCl ≤30 ml/min 400 mg **PO** qd
Uncomplicated infections
• *Adult:* **PO** 400 mg bid × 3-10 days 1 hr before or 2 hr after meals
Complicated infections
• *Adult:* **PO** 400 mg bid × 10-21 days; 400 mg qd × 7-10 days in impaired renal function
Uncomplicated gonorrhea
• *Adult:* **PO** 800 mg as a single dose
Ocular infection
• *Adult and child:* **OPHTH** 1 gtt qid, may increase to 1 gtt q2h for severe infections
Prostatitis
• *Adult:* **PO** 400 mg bid × 4 wk
Available forms: Tabs 400 mg

Side effects/adverse reactions:
CNS: Headache, dizziness, fatigue, somnolence, depression, insomnia
GI: Nausea, constipation, increased ALT, AST, flatulence, heartburn, vomiting, diarrhea, dry mouth
INTEG: Rash
EENT: Visual disturbances
Contraindications: Hypersensitivity to quinolones
Precautions: Pregnancy (C), lactation, children, renal disease, seizure disorders
Pharmacokinetics: Peak 1 hr, half-life 3-4 hr; steady state 2 days; excreted in urine as active drug, metabolites
Interactions:
• Decreased effect of norfloxacin: antacids, iron products, sucralfate; give 2 hr apart
• Increased serum concentrations of: cyclosporine, probenecid
• Antagonizes effects of norfloxacin: nitrofurantoin, monitor closely
• Increased anticoagulation: oral anticoagulants
• Possible increased levels, toxicity: theophylline
Lab test interferences:
Increase: AST, ALT, BUN, creatinine, alk phosphatase
NURSING CONSIDERATIONS
Assess:
• Kidney, liver function studies: BUN, creatinine, AST, ALT
• I&O ratio; urine pH, <5.5 is ideal
• CNS symptoms: insomnia, vertigo, headache, agitation, confusion
• Allergic reactions: fever, flushing, rash, urticaria, pruritus
Administer:
PO
• After clean-catch urine for C&S
• Two daily doses if urine output is high or if patient has diabetes

---

◆ = Nursing alert   🖊 = Herb-drug interaction   🚫 = Do not crush

Evaluate:
• Therapeutic response: decreased pain, frequency, urgency, C&S, absence of infection

Teach patient/family:
• That fluid intake must be 3 L/day to avoid crystallization in kidneys
• That if dizziness occurs, to walk, perform activities with assistance
• To complete full course of drug therapy
• To contact prescriber if adverse reaction occurs
• To take 1 hr before or 2 hr after meals; not to take antacids with or within 2 hr of this drug; to sip water or use hard candy for dry mouth

---

norgestrel (℞)

(nor-jess'trel)
Ovrette
Func. class.: Progestogen
Chem. class.: Progesterone derivative

Action: Inhibits secretion of pituitary gonadotropins, which prevents follicular maturation, ovulation, stimulates growth of mammary tissue, antineoplastic action against endometrial cancer

Uses: Female contraception

Dosage and routes:
• *Adult:* **PO** 1 tab qd
Available forms: Tabs 0.075 mg

Side effects/adverse reactions:
CNS: Dizziness, headache, migraines, depression, fatigue
CV: Hypotension, ***thrombophlebitis,*** edema, ***thromboembolism, stroke, pulmonary embolism, myocardial infarction***
GI: Nausea, vomiting, anorexia, cramps, increased weight, ***cholestatic jaundice***
EENT: Diplopia
GU: Amenorrhea, cervical erosion, breakthrough bleeding, dysmenorrhea, vaginal candidiasis, breast changes, *gynecomastia, testicular atrophy, impotence,* endometriosis, ***spontaneous abortion***
INTEG: Rash, urticaria, acne, hirsutism, alopecia, oily skin, seborrhea, purpura, melasma
META: Hyperglycemia

Contraindications: Breast cancer, hypersensitivity, thromboembolic disorders, reproductive cancer, genital bleeding (abnormal, undiagnosed), cerebral hemorrhage, pregnancy (X)

Precautions: Lactation, hypertension, asthma, blood dyscrasias, gallbladder disease, CHF, diabetes mellitus, bone disease, depression, migraine headache, convulsive disorders, hepatic disease, renal disease, family history of breast or reproductive tract cancer

Pharmacokinetics:
PO: Duration 24 hr; excreted in urine, feces; metabolized in liver

Lab test interferences:
Increase: Alk phosphatase, nitrogen (urine), pregnanediol, amino acids, factors VII, VIII, IX, X
Decrease: GTT, HDL

NURSING CONSIDERATIONS
Assess:
• Weight qd; notify prescriber of weekly weight gain >5 lb
• B/P at beginning of treatment and periodically
• I&O ratio; be alert for decreasing urinary output, increasing edema
• Liver function studies: ALT, AST, bilirubin, periodically during long-term therapy
• Edema, hypertension, cardiac symptoms, jaundice
• Mental status: affect, mood, behavioral changes, depression
• Hypercalcemia

Administer:
- Titrated dose; use lowest effective dose
- In one dose in AM
- With food or milk to decrease GI symptoms
- After warming to dissolve crystals

Perform/provide:
- Storage in dark area

Evaluate:
- Therapeutic response: absence of pregnancy

Teach patient/family:
- About cushingoid symptoms
- To report breast lumps, vaginal-bleeding, edema, jaundice, dark urine, clay-colored stools, dyspnea, headache, blurred vision, abdominal pain, numbness or stiffness in legs, chest pain
- To report suspected pregnancy
- To monitor blood sugar if diabetic

---

nortriptyline (℞)

(nor-trip'ti-leen)
Aventyl, Pamelor

Func. class.: Antidepressant, tricyclic

Chem. class.: Dibenzocycloheptene—secondary amine

Action: Blocks reuptake of norepinephrine, serotonin into nerve endings, increasing action of norepinephrine, serotonin in nerve cells

Uses: Major depression

Investigational uses: Chronic pain management

Dosage and routes:
- *Adult:* **PO** 25 mg tid or qid; may increase to 150 mg/day; may give daily dose hs
- *Geriatric:* **PO** 10-25 mg q hs, increase by 10-25 mg at weekly intervals to desired dose; usual maintenance 30-50 mg

Available forms: Caps 10, 25, 50, 75 mg; sol 10 mg/5 ml

Side effects/adverse reactions:

HEMA: **Agranulocytosis, thrombocytopenia, eosinophilia, leukopenia**

CNS: *Dizziness, drowsiness,* confusion, headache, anxiety, tremors, stimulation, weakness, insomnia, nightmares, EPS (elderly), increased psychiatric symptoms

GI: *Constipation, dry mouth,* nausea, vomiting, ***paralytic ileus,*** increased appetite, cramps, epigastric distress, jaundice, ***hepatitis,*** stomatitis

GU: Urinary retention, **acute renal failure**

INTEG: Rash, urticaria, sweating, pruritus, photosensitivity

CV: *Orthostatic hypotension, ECG changes, tachycardia,* **hypertension,** palpitations

EENT: *Blurred vision,* tinnitus, mydriasis

Contraindications: Hypersensitivity to tricyclics, recovery phase of MI, convulsive disorders, prostatic hypertrophy

Precautions: Suicidal patients, severe depression, increased intraocular pressure, narrow-angle glaucoma, urinary retention, cardiac disease, hepatic disease, hyperthyroidism, electroshock therapy, elective surgery, pregnancy (C), lactation

Do not confuse:
nortriptyline/amitriptyline

Pharmacokinetics:
PO: Steady state 4-19 days; metabolized by liver; excreted by kidneys; crosses placenta; excreted in breast milk; half-life 18-28 hr

Interactions:
- Decreased effects of guanethidine, clonidine, indirect-acting sympathomimetics (ephedrine)

◆ = Nursing alert   ∥ = Herb-drug interaction   ⊘ = Do not crush

• Increased effects of direct-acting sympathomimetics (epinephrine), alcohol, barbiturates, benzodiazepines, CNS depressants

◆ Hyperpyretic crisis, convulsions, hypertensive episode: MAOI

🖊 Increased anticholinergic effect: belladonna, henbane

🖊 Increased antidepressant action: scopolia

Lab test interferences:

Increase: Serum bilirubin, blood glucose, alk phosphatase

False increase: Urinary catecholamines

Decrease: VMA, 5-HIAA

NURSING CONSIDERATIONS

Assess:

• B/P (lying, standing), pulse q4h; if systolic B/P drops 20 mm Hg, hold drug, notify prescriber; take vital signs q4h in patients with cardiovascular disease

• Blood studies: CBC, leukocytes, differential, cardiac enzymes if patient is receiving long-term therapy

• Hepatic studies: AST, ALT, bilirubin

• Weight qwk; appetite may increase with drug

• ECG for flattening of T wave, bundle branch block, AV block, dysrhythmias in cardiac patients

• EPS primarily in elderly: rigidity, dystonia, akathisia

• Mental status changes: mood, sensorium, affect, suicidal tendencies, increase in psychiatric symptoms, depression, panic

• Urinary retention, constipation; constipation is more likely to occur in children

◆ Withdrawal symptoms: headache, nausea, vomiting, muscle pain, weakness; do not usually occur unless drug was discontinued abruptly

• Alcohol intake; if alcohol is consumed, hold dose until AM

Administer:

• Increased fluids, bulk in diet if constipation occurs

• With food, milk for GI symptoms

• Dosage hs for oversedation during day; may take entire dose hs; elderly may not tolerate once/day dosing

• Gum, hard candy, frequent sips of water for dry mouth

• Concentrate with fruit juice, water, or milk to disguise taste

Perform/provide:

• Storage in tight, light-resistant container at room temperature

• Assistance with ambulation during beginning therapy, since drowsiness/dizziness occurs

• Safety measures including side rails, primarily for elderly

• Checking to see if PO medication swallowed

Evaluate:

• Therapeutic response: decreased depression

Teach patient/family:

• That therapeutic effects may take 2-3 wk

• To use caution in driving, other activities requiring alertness because of drowsiness, dizziness, blurred vision

• To avoid alcohol ingestion, other CNS depressants

• Not to discontinue medication quickly after long-term use; may cause nausea, headache, malaise

• To wear sunscreen or large hat, since photosensitivity occurs

Treatment of overdose: ECG monitoring; induce emesis; lavage, activated charcoal; administer anticonvulsant

nystatin (R)

(nye-stat′in)
Mycostatin, Nadostine*, Nilstat, Nystex, PMS-Nystatin*, Pastilles, Nadostine*, nystatin
Func. class.: Antifungal
Chem. class.: Amphoteric polyene

Action: Interferes with fungal DNA replication; binds sterols in fungal cell membrane, which increases permeability, leaking of cell nutrients

Uses: *Candida* species causing oral, vaginal, intestinal infections

Dosage and routes:
Oral infection
• *Adult:* **SUSP** 400,000-600,000 U qid, use ½ dose in each side of mouth, swish and swallow
Infants: 200,000 U qid (100,000 U in each side of mouth)
• *Newborn and premature infant:* **SUSP** 100,000 U qid
• *Adult and child:* Troches 200,000-400,000 U qid × up to 2 wk
GI infection
• *Adult:* **PO** 500,000-1,000,000 U tid

Available forms: Tabs 500,000 U; powder 50 million, 150 million, 500 million, 1 billion, 2 billion, 5 billion U; susp 100,000 U per ml; troches 200,000 U

Side effects/adverse reactions:
INTEG: Rash, urticaria (rare)
GI: Nausea, vomiting, anorexia, diarrhea, cramps

Contraindications: Hypersensitivity

Precautions: Pregnancy (B)

Pharmacokinetics:
PO: Little absorption, excreted in feces

NURSING CONSIDERATIONS
Assess:
• For allergic reaction: rash, urticaria; drug may have to be discontinued
• For predisposing factors: antibiotic therapy, pregnancy, diabetes mellitus, sexual partner infection (vaginal infections)

Administer:
• Oral susp dose by placing ½ in each cheek, then swallow
• Topical dose after cleansing area; mouth may be swabbed

Perform/provide:
• Storage in refrigerator for oral susp; tabs in tight, light-resistant containers at room temperature

Evaluate:
• Therapeutic response: culture negative for *Candida*

Teach patient/family:
• That long-term therapy may be needed to clear infection; to complete entire course of medication
• Proper hygiene: changing socks if feet are infected; using no commercial mouthwashes for mouth infection
• Shake susp before measuring each dose
• To avoid getting preparation on hands
• To wear light-day pad for vaginal preparations
• To avoid tight shoes, bandages when using on feet
• To avoid sexual contact during treatment to minimize reinfection
• To notify prescriber of irritation; drug may have to be discontinued
• That relief from itching may occur after 24-72 hr

◆ = Nursing alert 🖊 = Herb-drug interaction 🚫 = Do not crush

octreotide (℞)

(ok-tree′oh-tide)

Sandostatin, Sandostatin LAR Depot

Func. class.: Hormone, antidiarrheal

Chem. class.: Octapeptide

Action: A potent growth hormone similar to somatostatin

Uses: Sandostatin: acromegaly, carcinoid tumors, vasoactive intestinal peptide tumors (VIPomas); LAR Depot: long-term maintenance of acromegaly, carcinoid tumors, VIPomas

Investigational uses: GI fistula, variceal bleeding, diarrheal conditions, pancreatic fistula, irritable bowel syndrome, dumping syndrome

Dosage and routes:

Initial dose

• *Adult:* **IV/SC** 50 µg bid-tid CSI (continuous SC inf) has been used but is not approved

Acromegaly

• *Adult:* **SC** 50 µg tid, adjust q2wk based on somatomedin C

VIPomas

• *Adult:* **SC** 0.2-0.3 mg qd in 2-4 doses for 2 wk, not to exceed 0.45 mg qd

Carcinoid tumors

• *Adult:* **SC** 0.1-0.6 mg qd in 2-4 doses for 2 wk, titrated to patient response

GI fistula

• *Adult:* **SC** 50-200 µg q8h

Irritable bowel syndrome

• *Adult:* **SC** 100 µg single dose to 125 µg bid

Dumping syndrome

• *Adult:* **SC** 50-150 µg/day

Variceal bleeding

• *Adult:* **IV** 25-50 µg/hr cont **IV** inf for 18 hr-5 days

Available forms: Sandostatin: inj 0.05, 0.1, 0.2 0.5, 1 mg/ml; LAR Depot: inj 10, 20, 30 mg/5 ml

Side effects/adverse reactions:

CNS: Headache, dizziness, fatigue, weakness, depression, anxiety, tremors, **seizure,** paranoia

*CV: Sinus bradycardia, conduction abnormalities, **dysrhythmias,** chest pain, SOB, thrombophlebitis, ischemia, **CHF,** hypertension, palpitations*

ENDO: Hyperglycemia, ketosis, hypothyroidism, hypoglycemia, galactorrhea, diabetes insipidus

*GI: Diarrhea, nausea, abdominal pain, vomiting, flatulence, distention, constipation, **hepatitis,** increased LFTs, **GI bleeding, pancreatitis***

GU: UTI, pollakiuria

HEMA: Hematoma of inj site, bruise

INTEG: Rash, urticaria, pain; inflammation at injection site

MS: Joint and muscle pain

Contraindications: Hypersensitivity

Precautions: Diabetes mellitus, hypothyroidism, pregnancy (B), elderly, lactation, children, renal disease

Pharmacokinetics: Absorbed rapidly, completely, peak ½ hr, half-life 1.7 hr, duration 12 hr, excreted unchanged in urine

Interactions:

• Cyclosporine: Possible increased rejection

• Drug/food: decreased absorption of dietary fat, decreased vit B_{12} levels

NURSING CONSIDERATIONS

Assess:

• Growth hormone antibodies, IGF-1, 1-4 hr intervals for 8-12 hr post dose in acromegaly; 5-HIAA, plasma serotonin, plasma substance P in carcinoid; VIP in VIPomas

• Thyroid function tests: T_3, T_4, T_7, TSH to identify hypothyroidism
• Fecal fat, serum carotene
• Allergic reaction: rash, itching, fever, nausea, wheezing
• For cardiac status: bradycardia, conduction abnormalities, dysrhythmias; monitor ECG for QT prolongation, low voltage, axis shifts, early repolarization, R/S transition, early wave progression

Administer:
SC
• Rotate inj site
Perform/provide:
• Storage in refrigerator for unopened amps, vials; or room temperature for 2 wk, protect from light; do not use discolored or cloudy sol
Evaluate:
• Therapeutic response: growth in children
Teach patient/family:
• Regular assessments are required
• Regarding SC injection if patient or other persons will be giving injection

---

ofloxacin (℞)

(o-flox'a-sin)
Floxin, Occuflox
Func. class.: Antiinfective
Chem. class.: Fluoroquinolone

Action: Interferes with conversion of intermediate DNA fragments into high-molecular-weight DNA in bacteria, inhibits DNA gyrase

Uses: Treatment of lower respiratory tract infections (pneumonia, bronchitis), genitourinary infections (prostatitis, UTIs) caused by *Escherichia coli, Klebsiella pneumoniae, Chlamydia trachomatis, Neisseria gonorrhoeae;* skin and skin structure infections; conjunctivitis (ophth)

Dosage and routes:
Renal dose
• CrCl 10-50 ml/min give q24h; CrCl <10 ml/min give ½ of dose q24h
Lower respiratory tract infections/ skin and skin structure infections
• *Adult:* **PO, IV** 400 mg q12h × 10 days
Cervicitis, urethritis
• *Adult:* **PO, IV** 300 mg q12h × 7 days
Prostatitis
• *Adult:* **PO, IV** 300 mg q12h × 6 wk
Acute, uncomplicated gonorrhea
• *Adult:* **PO, IV** 400 mg as a single dose
Conjunctivitis
• *Adult and child:* **OPHTH** 1-2 gtt q2-4h × 2 days, then qid × 5 days
Urinary tract infection
• *Adult:* **PO, IV** 200-400 mg q12h × 3-10 days
Available forms: Tabs 200, 300, 400 mg; 200, 400 mg; ophth sol 0.3%

Side effects/adverse reactions:

CNS: Dizziness, headache, fatigue, somnolence, depression, insomnia, lethargy, malaise
GI: Diarrhea, nausea, vomiting, anorexia, flatulence, heartburn, dry mouth, increased AST, ALT, abdominal pain, constipation
INTEG: Rash, pruritus
EENT: Visual disturbances

Contraindications: Hypersensitivity to quinolones
Precautions: Pregnancy (C), lactation, children, elderly, renal disease, seizure disorders, excessive sunlight
Do not confuse:
Ocuflox/Ocufen

Pharmacokinetics:
PO: Peak 1-2 hr, half-life 9 hr, steady state 2 days; excreted in urine as active drug, metabolites; 90%-95% bioavailability

---

◆ = Nursing alert   ⫰ = Herb-drug interaction   ⊘ = Do not crush

Interactions:

• May decrease absorption: antacids with aluminum, magnesium, iron products, sucralfate, zinc products; separate by 2 hr

• May alter blood glucose levels: antidiabetics

• May increase CNS stimulation, seizures: NSAIDs

• Increased anticoagulation: oral anticoagulants

• Possible theophylline toxicity: theophylline

• Drug/food: decreased absorption

NURSING CONSIDERATIONS
Assess:

• Kidney, liver function studies: BUN, creatinine, AST, ALT

• I&O ratio; urine pH <5.5 is ideal

• CNS symptoms: insomnia, vertigo, headache, agitation, confusion

• Allergic reactions: rash, flushing, urticaria, pruritus

Administer:

PO

• 2 hr before or 2 hr after antacids, calcium, iron, zinc products

• After clean-catch urine for C&S

IV

• Over 1 hr or more

Additive compatibilities: Amoxicillin, ceftazidime, clindamycin, gentamicin, piperacillin, tobramycin, vancomycin

Syringe compatibilities: Cefotaxime

Y-site compatibilities: Ampicillin, cisatracurium, granisetron, propofol, remifentanil, thiotepa

Perform/provide:

• Storage for 2 wk refrigerated or 6 mo frozen after reconstitution

Evaluate:

• Therapeutic response: negative C&S; absence of redness, swelling (ophth)

Teach patient/family:

• That fluid intake must be 3 L/day to avoid crystallization in kidneys

• That if dizziness or lightheadedness occurs, ambulate, perform activities with assistance

• To complete full course of therapy

• To notify prescriber of adverse reactions or tendon pain

• To avoid iron- or mineral-containing supplements within 2 hr before or after dose

• To prevent sun exposure, photosensitivity can occur

---

olanzapine

(oh-lanz′a-peen)

Zyprexa, Zyprexa Zydis

Func. class.: Antipsychotic, neuroleptic

Chem. class.: Thienbenzodiazepine

Action: Unknown; may mediate antipsychotic activity by both dopamine and serotonin type 2 (5-HT2) antagonist; also, may antagonize muscarinic receptors, histaminic (H_1)- and α-adrenergic receptors

Uses: Schizophrenia, acute manic episodes in bipolar disorder

Investigational uses: Dementia related to Alzheimer's disease

Research note: One case of writer's cramp has been attributed to olanzapine use[30]

Dosage and routes:

Schizophrenia

• *Adult:* **PO** 5-10 mg initially qd, may increase dosage by 5 mg at 1 wk or more intervals; orally disintegrating tabs: open blister pack, place tab on tongue, let disintegrate, swallow

• *Elderly:* **PO** 5 mg, may increase cautiously at 1 wk intervals

Bipolar mania

• *Adult:* **PO** 10-15 mg qd, may increase dose >24 hr, by 5 mg

Available forms: Tab 2.5, 5, 7.5, 10,

15, 20 mg; orally disintegrating tabs 5, 10 mg

Side effects/adverse reactions:

CV: Orthostatic hypotension, tachycardia, chest pain

EENT: Blurred vision

GI: Dry mouth, nausea, vomiting, anorexia, constipation, abdominal pain, weight gain

GU: Urinary retention, urinary frequency, enuresis, impotence, amenorrhea, gynecomastia, breast engorgement, premenstrual syndrome

INTEG: Rash

RESP: Dyspnea, rhinitis, cough, pharyngitis

CNS: EPS: pseudoparkinsonism, akathisia, dystonia, tardive dyskinesia, seizures, headache, ***neuroleptic malignant syndrome (rare),*** fever, insomnia, somnolence, agitation, nervousness, hostility, dizziness, hypertonia, tremor, euphoria

MS: Joint pain, twitching

Contraindications: Hypersensitivity

Precautions: Pregnancy (C), lactation, hypertension, hepatic disease, cardiac disease, elderly

Pharmacokinetics: Well absorbed, peak 6 hr, metabolized by liver, excreted in urine, 93% bound to plasma proteins

Interactions:

• Oversedation: other CNS depressants, alcohol, barbiturate anesthetics, antihistamines, sedatives/hypnotics, antidepressants

• Decreased levels of olanzapine: carbamazepine, omeprazole, rifampin

• Increased hypotension: antihypertensives, alcohol, diazepam

• Decreased antiparkinson activity: levodopa, bromocriptine, other dopamine agonists

• Increased anticholinergic effects: anticholinergics

Lab test interferences:

Increase: LFTs, prolactin, CPK

NURSING CONSIDERATIONS

Assess:

• Mental status: orientation, mood, behavior, presence of hallucinations and type before initial administration and monthly

• Swallowing of PO medication: check for hoarding or giving of medication to other patients

• I&O ratio; palpate bladder if low urinary output occurs, especially in elderly

• Bilirubin, CBC

• Urinalysis recommended before, during prolonged therapy

• Affect, orientation, LOC, reflexes, gait, coordination, sleep pattern disturbances

• B/P sitting, standing, lying: take pulse and respirations q4h during initial treatment; establish baseline before starting treatment; report drops of 30 mm Hg; obtain baseline ECG

• Dizziness, faintness, palpitations, tachycardia on rising

⬥ For neuroleptic malignant syndrome: hyperpyrexia, muscle rigidity, increased CPK, altered mental status, for acute dystonia (check chewing, swallowing, eyes, pill rolling)

• EPS, including akathisia (inability to sit still, no pattern to movements), tardive dyskinesia (bizarre movements of the jaw, mouth, tongue, extremities), pseudoparkinsonism (rigidity, tremors, pill rolling, shuffling gait)

• Skin turgor daily

• Constipation, urinary retention daily; increase bulk, H_2O in diet

Administer:

• Antiparkinsonian agent for EPS

• Decreased dose in elderly

⬥ = Nursing alert   🖊 = Herb-drug interaction   🚫 = Do not crush

• PO with full glass of water, milk; or with food to decrease GI upset
• Orally disintegrating tabs: open blister pack, place tab on tongue until dissolved, swallow; no water needed

Perform/provide:
• Decreased stimuli by dimming light, avoiding loud noises
• Supervised ambulation until stabilized on medication; do not involve in strenuous exercise program because fainting is possible; patient should not stand still for long periods
• Increased fluids to prevent constipation
• Sips of water, candy, gum for dry mouth
• Storage in tight, light-resistant container

Evaluate:
• Therapeutic response: decrease in emotional excitement, hallucinations, delusion, paranoia, reorganization of patterns of thought, speech

Teach patient/family:
• To use good oral hygiene; frequent rinsing of mouth, sugarless gum for dry mouth
• To avoid hazardous activities until drug response is determined
• That orthostatic hypotension occurs often and to rise from sitting or lying position gradually
• To avoid hot tubs, hot showers, tub baths, since hypotension may occur
• To avoid abrupt withdrawal of this drug, or EPS may result; drug should be withdrawn slowly
• To avoid OTC preparations (cough, hay fever, cold) unless approved by prescriber, since serious drug interactions may occur; avoid use with alcohol, CNS depressants; increased drowsiness may occur
• That in hot weather, heat stroke

may occur; take extra precautions to stay cool

Treatment of overdose: Lavage if orally ingested; provide airway; do not induce vomiting or use epinephrine

---

olsalazine (℞)

(ohl-sal′ah-zeen)
Dipentum
Func. class.: Antiinflammatory
Chem. class.: Salicylate derivative

Action: Bioconverted to 5-aminosalicylic acid, which decreases inflammation
Uses: Maintenance of remission of ulcerative colitis in patients intolerant to sulfasalazine
Dosage and routes:
• *Adult:* **PO** 500 mg bid
Available forms: Caps 250 mg
Side effects/adverse reactions:
EENT: Dry mouth, dry eyes, watery eyes, blurred vision
SYST: **Anaphylaxis**
GI: Nausea, vomiting, abdominal pain, stomatitis, ***hepatitis,*** pancreatitis, diarrhea, bloating
CNS: Headache, insomnia, hallucinations, depression, vertigo, fatigue, ***drug fever,*** chills, dizziness, drowsiness, tremors
HEMA: **Leukopenia, neutropenia, thrombocytopenia, agranulocytosis, anemia**
INTEG: Rash, dermatitis, urticaria, **Stevens-Johnson syndrome,** erythema, photosensitivity, alopecia
GU: Urinary frequency, dysuria, hematuria, impotence
CV: **Allergic myocarditis,** 2nd-degree heart block, hypertension, peripheral edema, chest pain, palpitations
RESP: **Bronchospasm,** shortness of breath

Contraindications: Hypersensitivity to salicylates

Precautions: Pregnancy (C), child <14 yr, lactation; impaired hepatic, renal function, severe allergy, bronchial asthma

Pharmacokinetics:

PO: Partially absorbed, peak 1½ hr, half-life 5-10 hr, excreted in urine as 5-aminosalicylic acid and metabolites, crosses placenta

Lab test interferences:

False positive: Urinary glucose test

NURSING CONSIDERATIONS

Assess:

• I&O ratio: note color, character, pH of urine in treatment for UTIs; output should be 800 ml less than intake; if urine is highly acidic, alkalization may be needed

• Kidney function studies: BUN, creatinine, urinalysis (long-term therapy)

• Blood dyscrasias: skin rash, fever, sore throat, bruising, bleeding, fatigue, joint pain

• Allergic reaction: rash, dermatitis, urticaria, pruritus, dyspnea, bronchospasm

Administer:

• Medication after C&S; repeat C&S after full course of medication

• With resuscitative equipment available; severe allergic reactions may occur

• Total daily dose evenly spaced to minimize GI intolerance, with food

Perform/provide:

• Storage in tight, light-resistant container at room temperature

Evaluate:

• Therapeutic response: absence of fever, mucus in stools

---

omeprazole (℞)

(oh-mep′ray-zole)
Losec*, Prilosec
Func. class.: Antiulcer, proton pump inhibitor
Chem. class.: Benzimidazole

Action: Suppresses gastric secretion by inhibiting hydrogen/potassium ATPase enzyme system in gastric parietal cell; characterized as gastric acid pump inhibitor, since it blocks final step of acid production

Uses: Gastroesophageal reflux disease (GERD), severe erosive esophagitis, poorly responsive systemic GERD, pathologic hypersecretory conditions (Zollinger-Ellison syndrome, systemic mastocytosis, multiple endocrine adenomas); treatment of active duodenal ulcers with or without antiinfectives for *Helicobacter pylori*

Investigational uses: Posterior laryngitis, enhancing pancreatin

Dosage and routes:

Active duodenal ulcers

• *Adult:* **PO** 20 mg qd × 4-8 wk; associated with *H. pylori* 40 mg q AM and clarithromycin 500 mg tid on day 1-14, then 20 mg qd on day 15-28

Severe erosive esophagitis/poorly responsive GERD

• *Adult:* **PO** 20 mg qd × 4-8 wk

Pathologic hypersecretory conditions

• *Adult:* **PO** 60 mg/day; may increase to 120 mg tid; daily doses >80 mg should be divided

Gastric ulcer

• *Adult:* **PO** 40 mg qd 4-8 wk
• *Elderly:* ≤20 mg/day

Laryngitis (off-label)

• *Adult:* **PO** 20-40 mg qhs × 6-24 wk or 20 mg bid × 4-12 wk

---

◆ = Nursing alert   ∅ = Herb-drug interaction   ⊘ = Do not crush

Available forms: Caps, delayed rel 10, 20, 40 mg

Side effects/adverse reactions:

CNS: Headache, dizziness, asthenia

GI: Diarrhea, abdominal pain, vomiting, nausea, constipation, flatulence, acid regurgitation, abdominal swelling, anorexia, irritable colon, esophageal candidiasis, dry mouth

RESP: Upper respiratory infections, cough, epistaxis

INTEG: Rash, dry skin, urticaria, pruritus, alopecia

META: Hypoglycemia, increased hepatic enzymes, weight gain

EENT: Tinnitus, taste perversion

CV: Chest pain, angina, tachycardia, bradycardia, palpitations, peripheral edema

GU: UTI, urinary frequency, increased creatinine, *proteinuria, hematuria,* testicular pain, glycosuria

HEMA: Pancytopenia, thrombocytopenia, neutropenia, leukocytosis, anemia

MISC: Back pain, fever, fatigue, malaise

Contraindications: Hypersensitivity

Precautions: Pregnancy (C), lactation, children

Do not confuse:

Prilosec/Prinivil

Prilosec/Prozac

Prilosec/prednisone

Pharmacokinetics: Peak ½-3½ hr, half-life ½-1 hr, protein binding 95%, eliminated in urine as metabolites and in feces; in elderly elimination rate decreased, bioavailability increased

Interactions:

• Increased serum levels of omeprazole: diazepam, phenytoin, flurazepam, triazolam, clarithromycin

• Possible increased bleeding: warfarin

• Delayed absorption: sucralfate

NURSING CONSIDERATIONS

Assess:

• GI system: bowel sounds q8h, abdomen for pain, swelling, anorexia

• Hepatic enzymes: AST, ALT, alk phosphatase during treatment

Administer:

🚫 Before eating; swallow capsule whole; do not break, crush, or chew

Evaluate:

• Therapeutic response: absence of epigastric pain, swelling, fullness

Teach patient/family:

• To report severe diarrhea; drug may have to be discontinued

• That diabetic patient should know hypoglycemia may occur

• To avoid hazardous activities; dizziness may occur

• To avoid alcohol, salicylates, ibuprofen; may cause GI irritation

---

ondansetron (℞)

(on-dan-seh′tron)

Zofran

Func. class.: Antiemetic

Chem. class.: 5-HT3 receptor antagonist

o

Action: Prevents nausea, vomiting by blocking serotonin peripherally, centrally, and in the small intestine

Uses: Prevention of nausea, vomiting associated with cancer chemotherapy, radiotherapy, and prevention of postoperative nausea, vomiting

Investigational uses: Bulimia, pruritus, rectal use

Dosage and routes:

Hepatic dose

• Max dose 8 mg qd

Prevention of nausea/vomiting of cancer chemotherapy

• *Adult and child 4-18 yr:* IV 0.15 mg/kg infused over 15 min, 30 min before start of cancer chemother-

---

apy; 0.15 mg/kg given 4 hr and 8 hr after first dose or 32 mg as a single dose; dilute in 50 ml of D$_5$ or 0.9% NaCl before giving; rectal use (off-label) 16 mg qd 2 hr prior to chemotherapy

Prevention of nausea/vomiting of radiotherapy
• *Adult:* **PO** 8 mg tid

Prevention of postoperative nausea/vomiting
• *Adult:* **IV** 4 mg undiluted over >30 sec
• *Child 2-12 yr:* **IV** 0.1 mg/kg (≤40 kg); **IV** 4 mg (≥40 kg) give ≥30 sec

Bulimia (off-label)
• *Adult:* **PO** 4 mg tid (base dose); prn during bingeing/purging

Pruritus (off-label)
• *Adult:* **PO** 4 mg bid

Available forms: Inj 2 mg/ml, 32 mg/50 ml (premixed); tabs 4, 8 mg; oral sol 4 mg/5 ml; oral disintegrating tabs 4, 8 mg

Side effects/adverse reactions:
GI: Diarrhea, constipation, abdominal pain
CNS: Headache, dizziness, drowsiness, fatigue, extrapyramidal syndrome
*MISC: Rash, **bronchospasm** (rare), MS pain, wound problems, shivering, fever, hypoxia, urinary retention*

Contraindications: Hypersensitivity

Precautions: Pregnancy (B), lactation, children, elderly

Do not confuse:
Zofran/Zantac

Pharmacokinetics:
IV: Mean elimination half-life 3.5-4.7 hr, plasma protein binding 70%-76%; extensively metabolized in the liver

NURSING CONSIDERATIONS
Assess:
• For absence of nausea, vomiting during chemotherapy

• Hypersensitivity reaction: rash, bronchospasm
• For EPS: shuffling gait, tremors, grimacing, rigidity

Administer:
IV
• After diluting a single dose in 50 ml NS or D$_5$W, 0.45% NaCl or NS and given over 15 min

Additive compatibilities: Cisplatin, cyclophosphamide, cytarabine, dacarbazine, dexamethasone, doxorubicin, etoposide, fluconazole, hydromorphone, meperidine, methotrexate, morphine

Solution compatibilities: May also be diluted with D$_5$W, lactated Ringer's, D$_5$/0.9% NaCl, D$_5$/0.45% NaCl

Y-site compatibilities: Aldesleukin, amifostine, amikacin, aztreonam, bleomycin, carboplatin, carmustine, cefazolin, cefmetazole, cefotaxime, cefoxitin, ceftazidime, ceftizoxime, cefuroxime, chlorpromazine, cimetidine, cisatracurium, cisplatin, cladribine, clindamycin, cyclophosphamide, cytarabine, dacarbazine, dactinomycin, daunorubicin, dexamethasone, diphenhydramine, dopamine, doxorubicin, doxorubicin liposome, doxycycline, droperidol, etoposide, famotidine, filgrastim, floxuridine, fluconazole, fludarabine, gallium, gentamicin, haloperidol, heparin, hydrocortisone, hydromorphone, hydroxyzine, ifosfamide, imipenem/cilastatin, magnesium sulfate, mannitol, mechlorethamine, melphalan, meperidine, mesna, methotrexate, metoclopramide, miconazole, mitomycin, mitoxantrone, morphine, paclitaxel, pentostatin, piperacillin/tazobactam, potassium chloride, prochlorperazine, promethazine, ranitidine, remifentanil, streptozocin, teniposide, thiotepa, ticarcillin, ticarcillin/clavulanate, vancomycin, vinblastine, vincristine, vinorelbine, zidovudine

Perform/provide:

• Storage at room temperature 48 hr after dilution

Evaluate:

• Therapeutic response: absence of nausea, vomiting during cancer chemotherapy

Teach patient/family:

• To report diarrhea, constipation, rash, or changes in respirations or discomfort at insertion site

---

opium tincture/ camphorated opium tincture (paregoric) (℞)
(oh'pee-um)

Func. class.: Antidiarrheal
Chem. class.: Opium, opium and morphine

Controlled Substance Schedule III/II (depending on amount of opium)

Action: Antiperistaltic activity

Uses: Diarrhea (cause undetermined); withdrawal symptoms in infants born to addicted mothers

Dosage and routes:

• *Adult:* **PO** 0.3-1 ml qid, not to exceed 6 ml/day (tincture) or 5-10 ml qd-qid (camphorated)

• *Child:* **PO** 0.25-0.5 ml/kg qd-qid (camphorated)

Withdrawal

• *Neonate:* **PO** 1:25 dilution, 3-6 gtt q3-6h (tincture), dosage adjustment to control symptoms

Available forms: Liquid 2 mg morphine equivalent per 5 ml

Side effects/adverse reactions:

CNS: Dizziness, drowsiness, fainting, flushing, physical dependency, **CNS depression**

GI: Nausea, vomiting, constipation, abdominal pain

Contraindications: Hypersensitivity, severe ulcerative colitis, pseudomembranous colitis

Precautions: Liver disease, addiction proneness, prostatic hypertrophy (severe), pregnancy (B)

Pharmacokinetics:

PO: Duration 4 hr, half-life 2-3 hr; metabolized in liver; excreted in urine

Interactions:

• Increased action of both drugs: other CNS depressants

• Increased CNS toxicity: cimetidine

NURSING CONSIDERATIONS

Assess:

• Electrolytes (K, Na, Cl) if on long-term therapy

• Skin turgor q8h if dehydration is suspected

• Bowel pattern before; for rebound constipation

• Response after 48 hr; if no response, drug should be discontinued

• Dehydration in children

• Abdominal distention; toxic megacolon may occur in ulcerative colitis

Administer:

• Undiluted with water

• For 48 hr only

Evaluate:

• Therapeutic response: decreased diarrhea

Teach patient/family:

• To avoid OTC products (cough, cold, hay fever preparations) unless directed by prescriber

• Not to exceed recommended dose

• That drug may be habit-forming

• To avoid hazardous activities; drowsiness may occur

---

oral contraceptives (R)

Func. class.: Hormone
Chem. class.: Estrogen, progestin combinations

Action: Prevents ovulation by suppressing FSH, LH; *monophasic:* estrogen/progestin (fixed dose) used during a 21-day cycle; ovulation is inhibited by suppression of FSH and LH; thickness of cervical mucus and endometrial lining prevents pregnancy; *biphasic:* ovulation is inhibited by suppression of FSH and LH; alteration of cervical mucus, endometrial lining prevents pregnancy; *triphasic:* ovulation is inhibited by suppression of FSH and LH; change of cervical mucus, endometrial lining prevents pregnancy; variable doses of estrogen/progestin combinations may be similar to natural hormonal fluctuations; *progestin-only pill and implant:* change of cervical mucus and endometrial lining prevents pregnancy; ovulation may be suppressed
Uses: To prevent pregnancy, endometriosis, hypermenorrhea
Dosage and routes:
• *Adult:* PO 1 qd starting on day 5 of menstrual cycle; day 1 is 1st day of period
21 tablet packs
• *Adult:* PO 1 qd starting on day 7 of menstrual cycle; day 1 is 1st day of period, then on 20 or 21 days, off 7 days
28 tablet packs
• *Adult:* PO 1 qd continuously
Biphasic
• *Adult:* 1 qd × 10 days, then next color 1 qd × 11 days
Triphasic
• *Adult:* 1 qd; check package insert

Endometriosis
• *Adult:* PO 1 qd × 20 days from day 5 to 24 of cycle
Available forms: Check specific brand
Side effects/adverse reactions:
GI: Nausea, vomiting, cramps, diarrhea, bloating, constipation, change in appetite, ***cholestatic jaundice***
INTEG: Chloasma, melasma, acne, rash, urticaria, erythema, pruritus, hirsutism, alopecia, photosensitivity
CV: Increased B/P, ***cerebral hemorrhage, thrombosis, pulmonary embolism,*** fluid retention, edema
ENDO: Decreased glucose tolerance, increased TBG, PBI, T_4, T_3
GU: Breakthrough bleeding, amenorrhea, spotting, dysmenorrhea, galactorrhea, endocervical hyperplasia, vaginitis, cystitis-like syndrome, breast change
CNS: Depression, fatigue, dizziness, nervousness, anxiety, headache
EENT: Optic neuritis, retinal thrombosis, cataracts
HEMA: Increased fibrinogen, clotting factor
Contraindications: Pregnancy (X), lactation, reproductive cancer, thrombophlebitis, MI, hepatic tumors, hepatic disease, CAD, women 40 and over, CVA
Precautions: Depression, hypertension, renal disease, seizure disorders, lupus erythematosus, rheumatic disease, migraine headache, amenorrhea, irregular menses, breast cancer (fibrocystic), gallbladder disease, diabetes mellitus, heavy smoking, acute mononucleosis, sickle cell disease
Pharmacokinetics: Excreted in breast milk
Interactions:
• Decreased effectiveness of oral contraceptives: anticonvulsants, ri-

---

◆ = Nursing alert   ∥ = Herb-drug interaction   ⊘ = Do not crush

fampin, analgesics, antibiotics, antihistamines, chenodiol, griseofulvin

• Decreased action of oral anticoagulants

• Increased clotting: aminocaproic acid

• Drug/food: increased peak level: grapefruit juice

🖉 Decreased effect of oral contraceptives: St. John's wort

Lab test interferences:

Increase: Pro-time; clotting factors VII, VIII, IX, X; TBG, PBI, T_4, platelet aggregability, BSP, triglycerides, bilirubin, AST, ALT

Decrease: T_3, antithrombin III, folate, metyrapone test, GTT, 17-OHCS

NURSING CONSIDERATIONS
Assess:

• Glucose, thyroid function, LFTs

• Reproductive changes: change in breasts, tumors, positive Pap smear; drug should be discontinued

Administer:

• PO with food for GI symptoms; give at same time each day

• Subdermal implant of 6 caps effective for 5 yr; then should be removed

• IM inj deep in large muscle mass after shaking suspension; ensure patient not pregnant if injections are 2 wk or more apart

Evaluate:

• Therapeutic response: absence of pregnancy, endometriosis, hypermenorrhea

Teach patient/family:

• About detection of clots using Homan's sign

• To use sunscreen or avoid sunlight; photosensitivity can occur

• To take at same time each day to ensure equal drug level

• To report GI symptoms that occur after 4 mo

• To use another birth control method during 1st week of oral contraceptive use

• To take another tablet as soon as possible if one is missed

• That after drug is discontinued, pregnancy may not occur for several months

• To report abdominal pain, change in vision, shortness of breath, change in menstrual flow, spotting, breakthrough bleeding, breast lumps, swelling, headache, severe leg pain

• That continuing medical care is needed: Pap smear and gynecologic examinations q6mo

• To notify health care providers and dentists of oral contraceptive

---

orlistat (℞)
(or′lih-stat)
Xenical
Func. class.: Lipase inhibitor

Action: Inhibits the absorption of dietary fats

Uses: Obesity management

Dosage and routes:

• *Adult:* **PO** 120 mg tid with each main meal containing fat

Available forms: Caps 120 mg

Side effects/adverse reactions:

MS: Back pain, arthritis, myalgia, tendinitis

CNS: Insomnia, depression, anxiety, dizziness, headache, fatigue

GI: Oily spotting, flatus with discharge, fecal urgency, fatty/oily stool, oily evacuation, fecal incontinence, nausea, vomiting, abdominal pain, infectious diarrhea, rectal pain, tooth disorder

GU: UTI, vaginitis, menstrual irregularity

RESP: Influenza, URI, LRI, EENT symptoms

INTEG: Dry skin, rash

Contraindications: Hypersensitivity, malabsorption syndrome, cholestasis

Precautions: Hypothyroidism, other organic causes of obesity, lactation, children, pregnancy (B)

Pharmacokinetics: Minimal absorption, peak 8 hr, 99% protein binding, excretion in feces, half-life 1-2 hr

Interactions:
• Decreased absorption: fat-soluble vitamins, cyclosporine
• Increased lipid-lowering effect: pravastatin

NURSING CONSIDERATIONS
Assess:
• Weight weekly, diabetic patients may need reduction in oral hypoglycemics
• For misuse in certain population (anorexia nervosa, bulimia)

Administer:
• For obesity only if patient is on weight-reduction program that includes dietary changes, exercise; patient should be on a diet with 30% of calories from fat, omit dose of orlistat if a meal contains no fat

Evaluate:
• Therapeutic response: decrease in weight

Teach patient/family:
• Safety and effectiveness beyond 2 yr have not been determined
• By instructing patient to read patient's information sheet
• To take a multivitamin containing fat-soluble vitamins 2 hr before or after orlistat
• To avoid hazardous activities until PT is stabilized on medication, discuss unpleasant side effects

---

oseltamivir (℞)

(oss-el-tam'ih-veer)
Tamiflu
Func. class.: Antiviral
Chem. class.: Ethyl ester prodrug

Action: Inhibits influenza virus neuraminidase with possible alteration of virus particle aggregation and release

Uses: Prevention/treatment of influenza type A

Dosage and routes:
Treatment
• *Adult:* **PO** 75 mg bid × 5 days, begin treatment within 2 days of onset of symptoms
Prevention
• *Adult:* **PO** 75 mg qd × ≥7 days
Available forms: Caps 75 mg; pwd for oral susp 12 mg/ml after reconstitution

Side effects/adverse reactions:
CNS: Headache, dizziness, fatigue, *insomnia*
GI: Nausea, vomiting, diarrhea, abdominal pain
RESP: Cough

Contraindications: Hypersensitivity

Precautions: Hepatic disease, renal disease, elderly, pregnancy (C)

Pharmacokinetics: Rapidly absorbed, protein binding low, converted to oseltamivir carboxylate, half-life 1-3 hr

NURSING CONSIDERATIONS
Assess:
• Bowel pattern before, during treatment
• Signs of infection

Administer:
• Within 2 days of symptoms of influenza; continue for 5 days
• At least 4 hr before hs to prevent insomnia

◆ = Nursing alert   ∥ = Herb-drug interaction   ⊘ = Do not crush

Perform/provide:
• Storage in tight, dry container
Evaluate:
• Therapeutic response: absence of fever, malaise, cough, dyspnea in infection
Teach patient/family:
• About aspects of drug therapy
• To avoid hazardous activities if dizziness occurs
• To take missed dose as soon as remembered within 2 hr of next dose

---

oxacillin (Ŗ)

(ox-a-sill'in)
Bactocill, oxacillin sodium
Func. class.: Broad-spectrum antiinfective
Chem. class.: Penicillinase-resistant penicillin

Action: Interferes with cell wall replication of susceptible organisms; osmotically unstable cell wall swells, bursts from osmotic pressure
Uses: Effective for gram-positive cocci *(Staphylococcus aureus, Streptococcus pneumoniae),* infections caused by penicillinase-producing *Staphylococcus*
Dosage and routes:
• *Adult:* **PO** 2-6 g/day in divided doses q4-6h; **IM/IV** 2-12 g/day in divided doses q4-6h
• *Child:* **PO** 50-100 mg/kg/day in divided doses q6h; **IM/IV** 50-100 mg/kg/day in divided doses q4-6h
Available forms: Caps 250, 500 mg; pwd for oral susp 250 mg/5 ml; pwd for inj 250, 500 mg, 1, 2, 4, 10 g
Side effects/adverse reactions:
HEMA: Anemia, increased bleeding time, *bone marrow depression, granulocytopenia*
GI: Nausea, vomiting, diarrhea, increased AST, ALT, abdominal pain, glossitis, colitis

GU: **Oliguria, proteinuria, hematuria,** *vaginitis, moniliasis,* **glomerulonephritis**
CNS: Lethargy, hallucinations, anxiety, depression, twitching, **coma, convulsions**
Contraindications: Hypersensitivity to penicillins
Precautions: Pregnancy (B), hypersensitivity to cephalosporins, neonates
Do not confuse:
Bactocill/Pathocil
Pharmacokinetics:
PO/IM: Peak 30-60 min, duration 4-6 hr
IV: Peak 5 min, duration 4-6 hr, half-life 30-60 min
Metabolized in the liver; excreted in urine, bile, breast milk; crosses placenta
Interactions:
• Decreased antimicrobial effectiveness of oxacillin: tetracyclines
• Decreased effect of oral contraceptives
• Increased oxacillin concentrations: aspirin, probenecid, disulfiram
🌠 Delayed/reduced absorption: khat, separate by ≥2 hr
Lab test interferences:
False positive: Urine glucose, urine protein
NURSING CONSIDERATIONS
Assess:
• I&O ratio; report hematuria, oliguria, since penicillin in high doses is nephrotoxic
◆ Any patient with compromised renal system, since drug is excreted slowly in poor renal system function; toxicity may occur rapidly
• Liver studies: AST, ALT
• Blood studies: WBC, RBC, Hct/ Hgb, bleeding time
• Renal studies: urinalysis, protein
• C&S before therapy; drug may be given as soon as culture is taken

• Bowel pattern before and during treatment
• Skin eruptions after administration of penicillin to 1 wk after discontinuing drug
• Respiratory status: rate, character, wheezing, tightness in chest
• Allergies before initiation of treatment, and reaction of each medication; highlight allergies on chart

Administer:
• Drug after C&S completed
• PO with full glass of water 1 hr before or 2 hr after meals
• IM inj deep in gluteal muscle

IV
• After diluting 500 mg or less/5 ml sterile H_2O or NaCl for inj; may dilute further in D_5W, NS, LR and give 1 g over 10 min; may be given as infusion over 6 hr

Additive compatibilities: Cephapirin, chloramphenicol, dopamine, potassium chloride, sodium bicarbonate

Y-site compatibilities: Acyclovir, cyclophosphamide, diltiazem, famotidine, fluconazole, foscarnet, heparin, hydrocortisone, hydromorphone, labetalol, magnesium sulfate, meperidine, methotrexate, morphine, perphenazine, potassium chloride, tacrolimus, vit B/C, zidovudine

Perform/provide:
• Adrenalin, suction, tracheostomy set, endotracheal intubation equipment
• Scratch test to assess allergy, after securing order from prescriber; usually done when penicillin is only drug of choice
• Storage in airtight container; refrigerate reconstituted sol up to 2 wk

Evaluate:
• Therapeutic response: absence of fever, draining wounds

Teach patient/family:
• All aspects of drug therapy, including need to complete course of medication to ensure organism death (10-14 days); culture may be taken after completed course
• To report sore throat, fever, fatigue (may indicate superinfection); persistent diarrhea
• To wear or carry Medic Alert ID if allergic to penicillins
• To take on empty stomach with a full glass of water

Treatment of anaphylaxis: Withdraw drug, maintain airway, administer epinephrine, aminophylline, O_2, IV corticosteroids

---

oxaprozin (℞)

(ox-a-proe′zin)
Daypro
Func. class.: Nonsteroidal antiinflammatory
Chem. class.: Propionic acid derivative

Action: May inhibit prostaglandin synthesis by decreasing enzyme needed for biosynthesis; analgesic, antiinflammatory

Uses: Acute and long-term management of osteoarthritis, rheumatoid arthritis

Dosage and routes:
• *Adult:* **PO** 1200 mg qd; maximum dose 1800 mg/day or 26 mg/kg, whichever is lower

Available forms: Tabs 600 mg

Side effects/adverse reactions:
MISC: **Anaphylaxis, angioneurotic edema**
GI: Nausea, anorexia, vomiting, diarrhea, jaundice, ***cholestatic hepatitis,*** constipation, flatulence, cramps, dry mouth, peptic ulcer, ***GI bleeding***

◆ = Nursing alert   ✦ = Herb-drug interaction   ⊘ = Do not crush

CNS: Dizziness, headache, drowsiness, fatigue, tremors, confusion, insomnia, anxiety, depression

CV: Tachycardia, peripheral edema, palpitations, dysrhythmias

INTEG: Purpura, rash, pruritus, sweating

*GU: **Nephrotoxicity: dysuria, hematuria, oliguria, azotemia***

*HEMA: **Increased bleeding time***

EENT: Tinnitus, hearing loss, blurred vision

Contraindications: Hypersensitivity, asthma, patients in whom aspirin and iodides have induced symptoms of allergic reactions or asthma

Precautions: Pregnancy (C), lactation, children, bleeding disorders, GI disorders, cardiac disorders, hypersensitivity to other antiinflammatory agents, severe renal and hepatic disease, elderly, CHF

Do not confuse:

Daypro/Diupres

Pharmacokinetics:

PO: Onset 1 wk, peak unknown, duration unknown, half-life 40-50 hr; metabolized in liver; excreted in urine (metabolites), breast milk; 99% plasma protein binding

Interactions:

• Increased toxicity: aspirin, cyclosporine, methotrexate

• Possible risk of bleeding: oral anticoagulants

• Increased levels of phenytoin, lithium, avoid concomitant use

• Decreased effect: antihypertensives, diuretics

• Increased GI side effects: aspirin, corticosteroids

NURSING CONSIDERATIONS

Assess:

• Pain: frequency, intensity, characteristics; relief of pain after med

• Asthma, aspirin hypersensitivity, oronasal polyps; increased hypersensitivity reactions

• Renal, liver, blood studies: BUN, creatinine, AST, ALT, Hgb, before treatment, periodically thereafter

• Audiometric, ophthalmic exam before, during, after treatment

• For eye, ear problems: blurred vision, tinnitus; may indicate toxicity

Administer:

• With food to decrease GI symptoms

Perform/provide:

• Storage at room temperature

Evaluate:

• Therapeutic response: decreased pain, stiffness in joints, decreased swelling in joints, ability to move more easily

Teach patient/family:

• To report blurred vision, ringing, roaring in ears; may indicate toxicity

• To avoid driving, other hazardous activities if dizziness/drowsiness occurs

• To report change in urine pattern, increased weight, edema, increased pain in joints, fever, blood in urine; indicates nephrotoxicity

• That therapeutic effects may take up to 1 mo

• To take with a full glass of water to enhance absorption

---

oxazepam (℞)

(ox-ay′ze-pam)

Apo-Oxazepam*, Novoxapam*, oxazepam, Serax

Func. class.: Sedative/hypnotic; antianxiety

Chem. class.: Benzodiazepine

Controlled Substance Schedule IV

Action: Potentiates the actions of GABA, especially in limbic system and reticular formation

Uses: Anxiety, alcohol withdrawal

Dosage and routes:

Anxiety

• *Adult:* **PO** 10-30 mg tid-qid

Alcohol withdrawal
• *Adult:* PO 15-30 mg tid-qid
Available forms: Caps 10, 15, 30 mg; tabs 10, 15, 30 mg
Side effects/adverse reactions:
CNS: Dizziness, drowsiness, confusion, headache, anxiety, tremors, fatigue, depression, insomnia, hallucinations, paradoxical excitement, transient amnesia
GI: Nausea, vomiting, anorexia
INTEG: Rash, dermatitis, itching
*CV: Orthostatic hypotension, **ECG changes, tachycardia,*** hypotension
EENT: Blurred vision, tinnitus, mydriasis
Contraindications: Hypersensitivity to benzodiazepines, narrow-angle glaucoma, psychosis, pregnancy (D), lactation, child <12 yr
Precautions: Elderly, debilitated, hepatic disease, renal disease
Pharmacokinetics:
PO: Peak 2-4 hr, metabolized by liver, excreted by kidneys, half-life 5-15 hr
Interactions:
• Decreased effects of oxazepam: oral contraceptives, valproic acid
• Increased effects of oxazepam: CNS depressants, alcohol, disulfiram, oral contraceptives
Lab test interferences:
Increase: AST, ALT, serum bilirubin
Decrease: RAIU
False increase: 17-OHCS
NURSING CONSIDERATIONS
Assess:
• B/P (lying, standing), pulse; if systolic B/P drops 20 mm Hg, hold drug, notify prescriber
• Blood studies: CBC during long-term therapy; blood dyscrasias have occurred rarely
• Hepatic studies: AST, ALT, bilirubin, creatinine, LDH, alk phosphatase if taking long term

• Mental status: mood, sensorium, affect, sleeping pattern, drowsiness, dizziness
◆ Physical dependency, withdrawal symptoms: headache, nausea, vomiting, muscle pain, weakness, tremors, convulsions (long-term use)
• Suicidal tendencies
Administer:
PO
• With food, milk for GI symptoms
• Sugarless gum, hard candy, frequent sips of water for dry mouth
Perform/provide:
• Assistance with ambulation during beginning therapy; drowsiness/dizziness occurs
• Safety measures, including side rails
• Check to see if PO medication has been swallowed
Evaluate:
• Therapeutic response: decreased anxiety, restlessness, insomnia
Teach patient/family:
• That drug may be taken with food
• That medication is not to be used for everyday stress or used longer than 4 mo unless directed by prescriber; not to take more than prescribed dose; may be habit forming
• To avoid OTC preparations (cough, cold, hay fever) unless approved by prescriber
• To avoid driving, activities that require alertness, since drowsiness may occur
• To avoid alcohol ingestion, other psychotropic medications unless directed by prescriber
• Not to discontinue medication abruptly after long-term use
• To rise slowly, or fainting may occur, especially elderly
• That drowsiness may worsen at beginning of treatment
Treatment of overdose: Lavage, VS, supportive care, flumazenil

---

◆ = Nursing alert   🖊 = Herb-drug interaction   🚫 = Do not crush

oxcarbazepine (℞)
(ox'kar-baz'uh-peen)
Trileptal
Func. class.: Anticonvulsant

Action: May inhibit nerve impulses by limiting influx of sodium ions across cell membrane in motor cortex

Uses: Partial seizures

Dosage and routes:
Seizures
• *Adult:* **PO** 300 mg bid, may be increased to 600 mg/day in divided doses bid; maintenance 1200 mg/day
• *Child:* **PO** 8-10 mg/kg/day divided bid, max 600 mg/day; dose is determined by weight

Conversion to monotherapy in partial seizures
• *Adult:* **PO** 300 mg bid with reduction in other anticonvulsants, increase oxcarbazepine to max 600 mg/day q1wk over 2-4 wk; withdraw other anticonvulsants over 3-6 wk

Initiation of monotherapy in partial seizures
• *Adult:* **PO** 300 mg bid, increase by 300 mg/day q3days to 1200 mg divided bid

Renal dose
• CrCl <30 ml/min 150 mg bid and increase slowly

Available forms: Tabs, film-coated, 150, 300, 600 mg

Side effects/adverse reactions:
CNS: Dizziness, confusion, fatigue, feeling abnormal, ataxia, abnormal gait, tremors, anxiety, agitation, headache, ***worsening of seizures***
CV: Hypotension, chest pain, edema
EENT: Blurred vision, diplopia, nystagmus, rhinitis, sinusitis
GI: Nausea, constipation, diarrhea, anorexia, vomiting, abdominal pain, gastritis, dry mouth, thirst, ***rectal hemorrhage***
GU: Frequency, UTI, vaginitis
INTEG: Purpura, rash, acne, bruising, sweating

Contraindications: Hypersensitivity

Precautions: Hypersensitivity to carbamazepine, pregnancy (C), lactation, child <4 yr

Pharmacokinetics:
PO: Onset unknown, peak unknown, metabolized by liver

Interactions:
• Decreased oxcarbazepine levels: phenobarbital, phenytoin
• Increased CNS depression: alcohol
• Decreased effects of felodipine

NURSING CONSIDERATIONS
Assess:
• Description of seizures: frequency, duration, aura
• Mental status: mood, sensorium, affect, behavioral changes; if mental status changes, notify prescriber
• Eye problems: need for ophthalmic examinations before, during, after treatment (slit lamp, funduscopy, tonometry)
• Allergic reaction: purpura or red, raised rash; if these occur, drug should be discontinued

Administer:
PO
• With food, milk to decrease GI symptoms

Perform/provide:
• Storage at room temperature
• Hard candy, gum, frequent rinsing for dry mouth
• Assistance with ambulation during early part of treatment; dizziness occurs

Evaluate:
• Therapeutic response: decreased seizure activity

Teach patient/family:
• To carry ID stating patient's name, drugs taken, condition, prescriber's name and phone number
• To avoid driving, other activities that require alertness
• Not to discontinue medication quickly after long-term use
• To inform prescriber if hypersensitive to carbamazepine
• To avoid use of alcohol while taking this medication
• To use alternative contraception if using hormonal method

---

oxtriphylline (℞)
(ox-trye'fi-lin)
Choledyl SA
Func. class.: Bronchodilator, spasmolytic
Chem. class.: Choline salt of theophylline

Action: Relaxes smooth muscle of respiratory system by blocking phosphodiesterase, which increases cAMP; 64% theophylline
Uses: Acute bronchial asthma, reversible bronchospasm in chronic bronchitis and COPD
Dosage and routes:
• *Adult and child >12 yr:* **PO** 4.7 mg/kg q8h or sus action q12h
• *Child 9-16 yr and smokers (adult):* 4.7 mg/kg q6h
• *Child 1-9 yr:* 6.2 mg/kg q6h
Available forms: Elix 100 mg/5 ml*; syr 50 mg/5 ml; tabs 100, 200 mg; sus rel tabs 400, 600 mg
Side effects/adverse reactions:
CNS: Anxiety, restlessness, insomnia, dizziness, **convulsions,** headache, light-headedness
CV: Palpitations, **sinus tachycardia,** hypotension
GI: Nausea, vomiting, anorexia, diarrhea, bitter taste, dyspepsia

RESP: Increased rate, ***respiratory arrest***
INTEG: Flushing, urticaria, alopecia
Contraindications: Hypersensitivity to xanthines, tachydysrhythmias
Precautions: Elderly, CHF, cor pulmonale, hepatic disease, active peptic ulcer disease, diabetes mellitus, hyperthyroidism, hypertension, children, pregnancy (C), glaucoma, prostatic hypertrophy
Pharmacokinetics:
ELIXIR: Peak 1 hr
PO-ER: Peak 4-7 hr, duration 8-12 hr
Metabolized in liver; excreted in urine, breast milk; crosses placenta
Interactions:
• Increased action, toxicity: fluoroquinolones, β- blockers, cimetidine, oral contraceptives, corticosteroids, fluvoxamine, disulfiram, mexiletine
• May increase effects of: ephedrine, anticoagulants, coffee (caffeine items)
• Decreased effect of lithium
• Decreased theophylline level: rifampin, phenytoin, barbiturates, ketoconazole, nicotine products
• Drug/food: caffeine: increased effect
• Decreased effect: charbroiled foods
⌀ Increased action of both: ephedra, cola tree
NURSING CONSIDERATIONS
Assess:
• Therapeutic blood levels; toxicity may occur with small increase above therapeutic level; therapeutic theophylline levels: 11-20 μg/ml; watch for toxicity: nausea, vomiting, diarrhea, restlessness, tachycardia
• Smoking: reduces effects of theophyllines, requiring larger doses
• Respiratory rate, rhythm, depth; auscultate lung fields bilaterally; notify prescriber of abnormalities

---

◆ = Nursing alert   ⌀ = Herb-drug interaction   🚫 = Do not crush

- Allergic reactions: rash, urticaria; drug should be discontinued
- I&O ratios, increase in weight
- Pulmonary function studies baseline and during treatment

Administer:
- PO after meals to decrease GI symptoms; absorption may be affected

Perform/provide:
- Storage in closed container away from heat; protect elixir from light

Evaluate:
- Therapeutic response: absence of dyspnea, wheezing

Teach patient/family:
- Not to break, crush, or chew tab
- To check OTC medications, prescription medications for ephedrine, which will increase stimulation
- To avoid hazardous activities; dizziness may occur
- If GI upset occurs, to take drug with 8 oz water; avoid food; absorption may be decreased
- To notify prescriber of toxicity: nausea, vomiting, anxiety, convulsions, insomnia, rapid pulse
- To notify prescriber of change in smoking habit; may need to change dose; encourage not to smoke

---

oxybutynin (R)

(ox-i-byoo'ti-nin)
Ditropan, Ditropan XL, oxybutynin
Func. class.: Anticholinergic
Chem. class.: Synthetic tertiary amine

Action: Relaxes smooth muscles in urinary tract by inhibiting acetylcholine at postganglionic sites

Uses: Antispasmodic for neurogenic bladder

Dosage and routes:
- *Adult:* **PO** 5 mg bid-tid, not to exceed 5 mg qid; ER 5 mg qd, may increase by 5 mg, max 30 mg/day
- *Geriatric:* **PO** 2.5-5 mg tid, increase by 2.5 mg q several days
- *Child >5 yr:* **PO** 5 mg bid, not to exceed 5 mg tid
- *Child 1-5 yr:* **PO** 0.2 mg/kg/dose 2-4 ×/day

Available forms: Syr 5 mg/5 ml; tabs 5 mg; tabs, ext rel 5, 10, 15 mg

Side effects/adverse reactions:
*CNS: Anxiety, restlessness, dizziness, **convulsions,** headache, drowsiness, confusion*
CV: Palpitations, sinus tachycardia, hypotension
GI: Nausea, vomiting, anorexia, abdominal pain, constipation
GU: Dysuria, urinary retention, hesitancy
EENT: Blurred vision, increased intraocular tension, dry mouth, throat

Contraindications: Hypersensitivity, GI obstruction, GI hemorrhage, GU obstruction, glaucoma, severe colitis, myasthenia gravis, unstable CV status in acute hemorrhage

Precautions: Pregnancy (B), lactation, suspected glaucoma, children <12 yr, elderly

Do not confuse:
Ditropan/diazepam

Pharmacokinetics: Onset ½-1 hr, peak 3-4 hr, duration 6-10 hr; metabolized by liver, excreted in urine

Interactions:
- Increased levels of atenolol, digoxin, nitrofurantoin, oxybutynin
- Decreased levels of acetaminophen, haloperidol, levodopa
- Increased or decreased levels of phenothiazines

NURSING CONSIDERATIONS
Assess:
- Urinary patterns: distention, nocturia, frequency, urgency, incontinence

• Allergic reactions: rash, urticaria; if these occur, drug should be discontinued
• CNS effects: confusion, anxiety; anticholinergic effects in the elderly

Administer:
• Without regard to meals

Evaluate:
• Urinary status: dysuria, frequency, nocturia, incontinence

Teach patient/family:
• To avoid hazardous activities; dizziness, blurred vision may occur
• To avoid OTC medications with alcohol, other CNS depressants
• To prevent photophobia by wearing sunglasses
• Avoid hot weather, strenuous activity, drug decreases perspiration

---

oxycodone (℞)
(ox-i-koe′done)
Endocodone, M-oxy, Oxy Contin, OxyFAST, OxyIR, Roxicodone, Roxicodone Supeudol*
oxycodone/aspirin
Endodan*, Oxycodan*, Percodan, Percodan-Demi, Roxiprin
oxycodone/ acetaminophen
Endocet*, Oxycocet*, Percocet, Roxicet, Roxilox, Tylox
Func. class.: Opiate analgesic
Chem. class.: Semisynthetic derivative

Controlled Substance Schedule II
Action: Inhibits ascending pain pathways in CNS, increases pain threshold, alters pain perception
Uses: Moderate to severe pain
Investigational uses: Postherpetic neuralgic (cont rel)
Dosage and routes:
• *Adult:* **PO** 10-30 mg q4hr (5 mg

q6h for OxyIR, OxyFast) **OxyFast Conc. Sol is extremely concentrated; do not use interchangeably**
• *Child:* **PO** 0.05-0.15 mg/kg/dose up to 5 mg/dose q4-6h; not recommended in children

Available forms: Oxycodone tabs, cont rel 10, 20, 40, 80, 160 mg; tabs, immediate rel 15, 30 mg; tabs 5 mg; caps, immediate rel 5 mg; oral sol 5 mg/5 ml, 20 mg/ml; oxycodone with acetaminophen tabs 5 mg/325 mg; cap 5 mg/500 mg; oral sol 5 mg/325 mg/5 ml; oxycodone with aspirin 2.44 mg/325 mg, 4.88/325 mg

Side effects/adverse reactions:
CNS: Drowsiness, dizziness, confusion, headache, sedation, euphoria
GI: Nausea, vomiting, anorexia, constipation, cramps
GU: Increased urinary output, dysuria, urinary retention
INTEG: Rash, urticaria, bruising, flushing, diaphoresis, pruritus
EENT: Tinnitus, blurred vision, miosis, diplopia
CV: Palpitations, bradycardia, change in B/P
RESP: Respiratory depression

Contraindications: Hypersensitivity, addiction (opiate)
Precautions: Addictive personality, pregnancy (B), lactation, increased intracranial pressure, MI (acute), severe heart disease, respiratory depression, hepatic disease, renal disease, child <18 yr

Do not confuse:
Percodan/Decadron
Roxicet/Roxanol
Tylox/Xanax
Tylox/Trimox
Tylox/Wymox

Pharmacokinetics:
PO: Onset 15-30 min, peak 1 hr, duration 4-6 hr; detoxified by liver, excreted in urine, crosses placenta, excreted in breast milk

---

⬥ = Nursing alert   ⫻ = Herb-drug interaction   ⃠ = Do not crush

Interactions:
• Increased effects with other CNS depressants: alcohol, narcotics, sedative/hypnotics, antipsychotics, skeletal muscle relaxants
Lab test interferences:
Increase: Amylase
NURSING CONSIDERATIONS
Assess:
• I&O ratio; check for decreasing output; may indicate urinary retention
• CNS changes: dizziness, drowsiness, hallucinations, euphoria, LOC, pupil reaction
• Allergic reactions: rash, urticaria
• Respiratory dysfunction: respiratory depression, character, rate, rhythm; notify prescriber if respirations are <10/min
• Need for pain medication by pain, sedation scoring; physical dependence
Administer:
• 80, 160 mg cont rel tabs only in opioid-tolerant patients
• With antiemetic if nausea, vomiting occur
• When pain is beginning to return; determine dosage interval by response
🚫 Do not break, crush, or chew controlled release tabs
Perform/provide:
• Storage in light-resistant area at room temperature
• Assistance with ambulation
• Safety measures: night-light, call bell within easy reach
Evaluate:
• Therapeutic response: decrease in pain
Teach patient/family:
• To report any symptoms of CNS changes, allergic reactions
• That physical dependency may result from extended use

• That withdrawal symptoms may occur: nausea, vomiting, cramps, fever, faintness, anorexia
Treatment of overdose: Naloxone (Narcan) 0.2-0.8 mg IV, O_2, IV fluids, vasopressors

---

oxymorphone (℞)

(ox-i-mor'fone)
Numorphan
Func. class.: Opiate analgesic
Chem. class.: Semisynthetic phenanthrene derivative

Controlled Substance Schedule II
Action: Inhibits ascending pain pathways in CNS, increases pain threshold, alters pain perception
Uses: Moderate to severe pain
Dosage and routes:
• *Adult:* **IM/SC** 1-1.5 mg q4-6h prn; **IV** 0.5 mg q4-6h prn; **RECT** 5 mg q4-6h prn
Labor analgesia
• *Adult:* **IM:** 0.5-1 mg
Available forms: Inj 1, 1.5 mg/ml; supp 5 mg
Side effects/adverse reactions:
CNS: Drowsiness, dizziness, confusion, headache, sedation, seizures, euphoria (elderly)
GI: Nausea, vomiting, anorexia, constipation, cramps
GU: Increased urinary output, dysuria, urinary retention
INTEG: Rash, urticaria, bruising, flushing, diaphoresis, pruritus
EENT: Tinnitus, blurred vision, miosis, diplopia
CV: Palpitations, ***bradycardia,*** change in B/P
*RESP: **Respiratory depression***
Contraindications: Hypersensitivity, addiction (opiate)
Precautions: Addictive personality, pregnancy (B) (short-term), lactation, increased intracranial pres-

O

sure, MI (acute), severe heart disease, respiratory depression, hepatic disease, renal disease, child <18 yr
Pharmacokinetics:
SC/IM: Onset 10-15 min, peak 1½ hr, duration, 3-6 hr
IV: Onset 5-10 min, peak 15-30 min, duration 3-6 hr
RECT: Onset 15-30 min, duration 3-6 hr
Metabolized by liver, excreted in urine, crosses placenta
Interactions:
• Increased effects with other CNS depressants: alcohol, opiates, sedative/hypnotics, antipsychotics, skeletal muscle relaxants
Lab test interferences:
Increase: Amylase
NURSING CONSIDERATIONS
Assess:
• I&O ratio for decreasing output; may indicate urinary retention
• CNS changes: dizziness, drowsiness, hallucinations, euphoria, LOC, pupil reaction
• Allergic reactions: rash, urticaria
• Respiratory dysfunction: respiratory depression, character, rate, rhythm; notify prescriber if respirations are <10/min
• Need for pain medication, physical dependence
Administer:
• With antiemetic for nausea, vomiting
• When pain is beginning to return; determine interval by response
IV
• After diluting with 5 ml sterile H_2O or NS for inj; give over 2-5 min through Y-tube or 3-way stopcock
Syringe compatibilities: Glycopyrrolate, hydroxyzine, ranitidine
Perform/provide:
• Storage in light-resistant area at room temperature

• Assistance with ambulation
• Safety measures: night-light, call bell within easy reach
Evaluate:
• Therapeutic response: decrease in pain
Teach patient/family:
• To report any symptoms of CNS changes, allergic reactions
• That physical dependency may result from extended use
• That withdrawal symptoms may occur: nausea, vomiting, cramps, fever, faintness, anorexia
Treatment of overdose: Naloxone (Narcan) 0.2-0.8 mg IV, O_2, IV fluids, vasopressors

---

oxytocin (℞)

(ox-i-toe'sin)
Pitocin, Syntocinon
Func. class.: Oxytocic
Chem. class.: Hormone

Action: Acts directly on myofibrils, producing uterine contraction; stimulates milk ejection by the breast
Uses: Stimulation, induction of labor; missed or incomplete abortion; postpartum bleeding
Dosage and routes:
Postpartum hemorrhage
• *Adult:* IV 10 U infused at 20-40 mU/min
• *Adult:* IM 10 U after delivery of placenta
Fetal stress test
• *Adult:* IV 0.5 mU/min, increase q20min until 3 contractions within 10 min
Stimulation of labor
• *Adult:* IV 1-2 mU/min, increase by 1-2 mU q15-60 min until contractions occur; then decrease dose
Incomplete abortion
• *Adult:* IV INF 10 U/500 ml D_5W or 0.9% NaCl at 20-40 mU/min

---

◆ = Nursing alert   ⫽ = Herb-drug interaction   🚫 = Do not crush

Available forms: Inj 10 U/ml

Side effects/adverse reactions:

*CNS: **Convulsions, tetanic contractions***

CV: Hypotension, hypertension, dysrhythmias, increased pulse, bradycardia, tachycardia, PVC

FETUS: Dysrhythmias, jaundice, hypoxia, ***intracranial hemorrhage***

GI: Anorexia, nausea, vomiting, constipation

*GU: **Abruptio placentae, decreased uterine blood flow***

HEMA: Increased hyperbilirubinemia

INTEG: Rash

*RESP: **Asphyxia***

Contraindications: Hypersensitivity, serum toxemia, cephalopelvic disproportion, fetal distress, hypertonic uterus

Precautions: Cervical/uterine surgery, uterine sepsis, primipara >35 yr, 1st, 2nd stage of labor

Pharmacokinetics:

IM: Onset 3-7 min, duration 1 hr, half-life 12-17 min

IV: Onset 1 min, duration 30 min, half-life 12-17 min

Interactions:

• Hypertension: vasopressors

• Hypertension: ephedra

NURSING CONSIDERATIONS

Assess:

• I&O ratio

• Respiration

• B/P, pulse; watch for changes that may indicate hemorrhage

• Respiratory rate, rhythm, depth; notify prescriber of abnormalities

• Length, intensity, duration of contraction; notify prescriber of contractions lasting over 1 min or absence of contractions; turn patient on her side

• FHTs, fetal distress; watch for acceleration, deceleration; notify prescriber if problems occur; fetal presentation, pelvic dimensions; turn patient on left side if FHT change in rate

◆ For signs and symptoms of water intoxication; confusion, anuria, drowsiness, headache

Administer:

Labor induction

• After diluting 10 U/L of 0.9% NS or D₅ NS run at 1-2 mU/min at 15-30 min intervals to begin normal labor; dilute 10-40 mU/min, titrate to control postpartum bleeding; dilute 10 U/500 ml sol; run 10 U-20 mU/ml; administer by only 1 route at a time; use inf pump; rotate inf to provide mixing; do not shake

Control of postpartum bleeding

• Dilute 10-40 U/1 L of sol, run at 10-20 mU/min; adjust rate as needed

• With crash cart available on unit (Mg⁺SO₄ at bedside)

Additive compatibilities: Chloramphenicol, metaraminol, netilmicin, sodium bicarbonate, thiopental, verapamil

Y-site compatibilities: Heparin, hydrocortisone, insulin (regular), meperidine, morphine, potassium chloride, vit B/C, warfarin

Evaluate:

• Therapeutic response: stimulation of labor, control of postpartum bleeding

Teach patient/family:

• To report increased blood loss, abdominal cramps, fever, foul-smelling lochia

• That contractions will be similar to menstrual cramps, gradually increasing in intensity

paclitaxel (℞)

(pa-kli-tax'el)

Onxol, Taxol

Func. class.: Misc. antineoplastic

Chem. class.: Antimicrotubule, natural diterpene

Action: Inhibits reorganization of microtubule network needed for interphase and mitotic cellular functions; also causes abnormal bundles of microtubules during cell cycle and multiple esters of microtubules during mitosis

Uses: Taxol: Metastatic carcinoma of the ovary, breast; AIDS-related Kaposi's sarcoma (2nd-line), non–small cell lung cancer (1st-line), adjuvant treatment for node-positive breast cancer; Onxol: failure of other treatment in breast cancer, advanced carcinoma in ovarian cancer

Investigational uses: Advanced head, neck, small cell lung cancer; non-Hodgkin's lymphoma, adenocarcinoma of the upper GI tract, hormone-refractory prostate cancer

Dosage and routes:

Ovarian cancer

• *Adult:* **IV INF** 135 mg/m² given over 24 hr q3wk then cisplatin 75 mg/m²; or 175 mg/m² over 3 hr q3wk; or 175 mg/m² over 3 hr

Advanced ovarian carcinoma

• *Adult:* **IV/INF** 175 mg/m² with cisplatin 75 mg/m² using a 3-hr regimen q3wk

Breast carcinoma

• *Adult:* **IV INF** 175 mg/m² over 3 hr q3wk × 4 courses

AIDS-related Kaposi's sarcoma

• *Adult:* **IV INF** 135 mg/m² over 3 hr q3wk or 100 mg/m² over 3 hr q2wk

1st-line non–small cell lung cancer

• *Adult:* **IV INF** 135 mg/m²/24 hr inf with cisplatin 75 mg/m² × 3 wk

Available forms: Inj 30 mg/5 ml vial (6 mg/ml)

Side effects/adverse reactions:

HEMA: **Neutropenia, leukopenia, thrombocytopenia, anemia,** bleeding, infections

SYST: **Hypersensitivity reactions, anaphylaxis**

CV: Bradycardia, *hypotension,* abnormal ECG

NEURO: Peripheral neuropathy

MS: Arthralgia, myalgia

GI: Nausea, vomiting, diarrhea, mucositis, increased bilirubin, alk phosphatase, AST

INTEG: Alopecia

Contraindications: Hypersensitivity to paclitaxel or other drugs with polyoxyethylated castor oil, neutropenia of <1500/mm³, pregnancy (D)

Precautions: Children, lactation; hepatic, cardiovascular disease; CNS disorder

Do not confuse:

paclitaxel/paroxetine

paclitaxel/Paxil

Taxol/Paxil

Taxol/Taxotera

Pharmacokinetics: 89%-98% of drug is serum protein bound, metabolized in liver, excreted in bile and urine; terminal half-life 5.3-17.4 hr

Interactions:

• Increased myelosuppression: other antineoplastics, radiation

• Decreased metabolism of paclitaxel: ketoconazole, verapamil, diazepam, cyclosporine, teniposide, etoposide, quinidine, dexamethasone, vincristine, testosterone

• Increased doxorubicin levels: doxorubicin

• Decreased immune response: live virus vaccines

 = Nursing alert   = Herb-drug interaction   ⃠ = Do not crush

NURSING CONSIDERATIONS
Assess:

• CBC, differential, platelet count prior to and qwk; withhold drug if WBC is <1500/mm³ or platelet count is <100,000/mm³, notify prescriber
• Monitor temp q4h (may indicate beginning infection)
• Liver function tests before, during therapy (bilirubin, AST, ALT, LDH, bilirubin) prn or qmo, check for jaundiced skin and sclera, dark urine, clay-colored stool, itchy skin, abdominal pain, fever, diarrhea
• VS during 1st hr of infusion, check IV site for signs of infiltration
◆ Hypersensitive reactions, anaphylaxis including hypotension, dyspnea, angioedema, generalized urticaria; discontinue infusion immediately
• Bleeding: hematuria, guaiac, bruising or petechiae, mucosa or orifices q8h; obtain prescription for viscous lidocaine (Xylocaine)
• Effects of alopecia on body image; discuss feelings about body changes

Administer:

• Antiemetic 30-60 min before giving drug and prn
IV
• After diluting in 0.9% NaCl, D₅, D₅ and 0.9% NaCl, D₅LR to a concentration of 0.3-1.2 mg/ml
• Using an in-line filter ≤0.22 μm
• After premedicating with dexamethasone 20 mg PO 12 hr and 6 hr before paclitaxel, diphenhydramine 50 mg IV ½-1 hr before paclitaxel and cimetidine 300 mg or ranitidine 50 mg IV ½-1 hr before paclitaxel
• Using only glass bottles, polypropylene, polyolefin bags and administration sets; do not use PVC infusion bags or sets
• Using gloves and cytotoxic handling precautions

Y-site compatibilities: Acyclovir, amikacin, aminophylline, ampicillin/sulbactam, bleomycin, butorphanol, calcium chloride, carboplatin, cefepime, cefotetan, ceftazidime, ceftriaxone, cimetidine, cisplatin, cladribine, cyclophosphamide, cytarabine, dacarbazine, dexamethasone, diphenhydramine, doxorubicin, droperidol, etoposide, famotidine, floxuridine, fluconazole, fluorouracil, furosemide, ganciclovir, gentamicin, granisetron, haloperidol, heparin, hydrocortisone, hydromorphone, ifosfamide, lorazepam, magnesium sulfate, mannitol, meperidine, mesna, methotrexate, metoclopramide, morphine, nalbuphine, ondansetron, pentostatin, potassium chloride, prochlorperazine, propofol, ranitidine, sodium bicarbonate, thiotepa, vancomycin, vinblastine, vincristine, zidovudine

Perform/provide:

• Confirmation that dexamethasone was given 12 hr and 6 hr before infusion begins
• Storage of prepared sol up to 27 hr in refrigeration

Evaluate:

• Therapeutic response: decreased tumor size, spread of malignancy

Teach patient/family:

• To report signs of infection: fever, sore throat, flulike symptoms
• To report signs of anemia: fatigue, headache, faintness, shortness of breath, irritability
• To report bleeding; avoid use of razors, commercial mouthwash
• To avoid use of aspirin, ibuprofen
• To report any complaints or side effects to nurse or prescriber
• That hair may be lost during treatment; a wig or hairpiece may make patient feel better; new hair may be different in color, texture
• That pain in muscles and joints 2-5 days after infusion is common

P

Side effects: *italics* = common; ***bold italics*** = life-threatening

• To use nonhormonal type of contraception
• To avoid receiving vaccinations while on this drug

---

palivizumab (R)
(pal-ih-viz′uh-mab)
Synagis
Func. class.: Monoclonal antibody

Action: A humanized monoclonal antibody that exhibits neutralizing and fusion-inhibitory activity against respiratory syncytial virus (RSV)
Uses: Prevention of serious lower respiratory tract disease caused by RSV in pediatric patients
Dosage and routes:
• *Child:* **IM** 15 mg/kg, those patient who develop RSV should receive monthly doses during RSV season
Available forms: Lyophilized inj 100 mg
Side effects/adverse reactions:
GI: Nausea, vomiting, diarrhea, increased AST
RESP: URI, *apnea*
EENT: Otitis media, rhinitis, pharyngitis
INTEG: Rash, inj site reaction
Contraindications: Hypersensitivity, adults, cyanotic congenital heart disease
Precautions: Thrombocytopenia, coagulation disorders, established RSV, congenital heart disease, chronic lung disease, systemic allergic reactions, pregnancy (C)
Pharmacokinetics: Mean half-life 20 days
NURSING CONSIDERATIONS
Assess:
• For presence of RSV infection, drug is given to prevent infection For side effects; report if allergic reaction is evident

Administer:
• IM only
• After adding 1 ml of sterile water for inj per 100 mg vial, gently swirl, let stand at room temperature for 20 min until sol clarifies; given within 6 hr of reconstitution
Teach patient/family:
• To report upper respiratory infections, earaches, rash, sore throat

---

pamidronate (R)
(pam-i-drone′ate)
Aredia
Func. class.: Bone-resorption inhibitor, electrolyte modifier
Chem. class.: Bisphosphonate

Action: Absorbs calcium phosphate crystals in bone and may directly block dissolution of hydroxyapatite crystals of bone; inhibits bone resorption, apparently without inhibiting bone formation and mineralization
Uses: Moderate to severe hypercalcemia associated with malignancy with or without bone metastases, osteolytic lesions in breast cancer patients
Dosage and routes:
• *Adult:* **IV INF** 60-90 mg in moderate hypercalcemia, 90 mg in severe hypercalcemia over 24 hr
Paget's disease
• *Adult:* **IV** 90-180 mg/treatment, may use 30 mg qd × 3 days up to 30 mg/wk × 6 wk
Available forms: Inj 30, 60, 90 mg/vial
Side effects/adverse reactions:
INTEG: Redness, swelling, induration, pain on palpation at site of catheter insertion
META: Anemia, hypokalemia, hypomagnesemia, hypophosphatemia
GI: Abdominal pain, anorexia, constipation, nausea, vomiting

◆ = Nursing alert　　 ∥ = Herb-drug interaction　　 ⊘ = Do not crush

MS: Bone pain
CV: Hypertension
GU: UTI, fluid overload
Contraindications: Hypersensitivity to bisphosphonates
Precautions: Children, nursing mothers, pregnancy (C), renal dysfunction
Do not confuse:
Aredia/Adriamycin
Pharmacokinetics: Rapidly cleared from circulation and taken up mainly by bones, eliminated primarily by kidneys
Interactions:
• Hypomagnesemia, hypokalemia: digoxin
• Decreased effect of pamidronate: calcium, vit D
• Do not mix with Ca-containing infusion sol such as Ringer's sol
NURSING CONSIDERATIONS
Assess:
• Renal studies and Ca, P, Mg, K
• For hypercalcemia: paresthesia, twitching, laryngospasm, Chvostek's, Trousseau's signs
Administer:
IV
• After reconstituting by adding 10 ml of sterile water for inj to each vial (30 mg/10 ml, or 60 mg/10 ml, or 90 mg/10 ml depending on vial used), then add to 1000 ml of sterile 0.45%, 0.9% NaCl, D₅W, run over 24 hr for hypercalcemia or 60 mg ≥4 hr, 90 mg over 24 hr; dilute reconstituted sol in 500 ml of 0.9% NaCl, 0.45% NaCl, or D₅W, give over 4 hr (multiple myeloma, Paget's disease)
Perform/provide:
• Storage of infusion sol up to 24 hr at room temperature
• Reconstituted sol with sterile water may be stored under refrigeration for up to 24 hr

Evaluate:
• Therapeutic response: decreased Ca levels
Teach patient/family
• To report hypercalcemic relapse: nausea, vomiting, bone pain, thirst
• To continue with dietary recommendations including calcium and vit D

---

pancreatin (℞)
(pan'kree-a-tin)
Creon, Donnazyme, Hi-Vegi-Lip, 4× Pancreatin 600 mg, 8× Pancreatin 900 mg, Pancrezyme 4×
Func. class.: Digestant
Chem. class.: Pancreatic enzyme concentrate—bovine/porcine

Action: Pancreatic enzyme needed for breakdown of substances released from the pancreas
Uses: Exocrine pancreatic secretion insufficiency, cystic fibrosis (digestive aid)
Dosage and routes:
• *Adult:* **PO** 8000-24,000 USP U with meals
Available forms: Tabs 650, 2000, 12,000 U, others in combination
Side effects/adverse reactions:
GI: Anorexia, nausea, vomiting, diarrhea, glossitis, anal soreness
GU: Hyperuricuria, hyperuricemia
INTEG: Rash, hypersensitivity
EENT: Buccal soreness
Contraindications: Hypersensitivity to pork, chronic pancreatic disease
Precautions: Pregnancy (C), lactation
• Decreased absorption: cimetidine, antacids, oral iron
NURSING CONSIDERATIONS
Assess:
• I&O ratio; watch for increasing urinary output

P

• Fecal fat, nitrogen, PT, Ca during treatment
• For polyuria, polydipsia, polyphagia (may indicate diabetes mellitus)
• For allergy to pork
Administer:
PO
• After antacid or H₂-blockers; decreased pH inactivates drug

$\bigcirc$ Whole; do not break, crush, or chew (enteric coated)
• Low-fat diet for GI symptoms
Perform/provide:
• Storage in tight container at room temperature
Evaluate:
• Therapeutic response: relief of GI symptoms

---

pancrelipase (Ŗ)

(pan-kre-li'pase)
Cotazym, Cotazym Capsules, Cotazym-S Capsules, Creon Capsules, Festal II Tablets, Ilozyme, Ku-Zyme HP Capsules, Pancrease Capsules, Pancrease MT 4, Pancrease MT 10, Pancrease MT 16, Ultrase MT 12, Ultrase MT 20, Ultrase MT 24, Viokase Powder, Viokase Tablets, Zymase
Func. class.: Digestant
Chem. class.: Pancreatic enzyme—bovine/porcine

Action: Pancreatic enzyme needed for breakdown of substances released from the pancreas
Uses: Exocrine pancreatic secretion insufficiency, cystic fibrosis (digestive aid), steatorrhea, pancreatic enzyme deficiency
Dosage and routes:
• *Adult and child:* **PO** 1-3 caps/tabs ac or with meals, or 1 cap/tab with snack or 1-2 pwd pkt ac
Available forms: Pwd: 16,800 U lipase/70,000 U protease and amylase; caps: 8000 U lipase/30,000 U protease and amylase; cap, delayed rel 4000 U lipase/12,000 U protease and amylase, 4000 U lipase/25,000 U protease/ 20,000 U amylase, 5000 U lipase/20,000 U protease and amylase, 10,000 U lipase/30,000 U protease and amylase, 12,000 U lipase/24,000 U protease and amylase, 12,000 U lipase/39,000 U protease and amylase, 16,000 U lipase/48,000 U protease and amylase, 20,000 U lipase/65,000 U protease and amylase, 24,000 U lipase/78,000 U protease and amylase
Side effects/adverse reactions:
GI: Anorexia, nausea, vomiting, diarrhea
GU: Hyperuricuria, hyperuricemia
Contraindications: Allergy to pork
Precautions: Pregnancy (C)
Interactions:
• Decreased absorption: cimetidine, antacids, oral iron
NURSING CONSIDERATIONS
Assess:
• For appropriate height, weight development; may be delayed
• I&O ratio; watch for increasing urinary output
• Fecal fat, nitrogen, PT during treatment
• For polyuria, polydipsia, polyphagia (may indicate diabetes mellitus)
• For pork sensitivity, cross-sensitivity may occur
Administer:
• After antacid or cimetidine; decreased pH inactivates drug
• Powder mixed in prepared fruit juice for infants, children
• Low-fat diet for GI symptoms

$\Leftrightarrow$ = Nursing alert   �ില = Herb-drug interaction $\bigcirc$ = Do not crush

Perform/provide:
• Storage in tight container at room temperature

Evaluate:
• Therapeutic response: improved digestion of carbohydrates, protein, fat; absence of steatorrhea

Teach patient/family:
• Not to inhale powder; may be very irritating to mucous membranes; some powder may irritate skin
• To take with 8 oz water or more, not to allow to sit in mouth, have patient sit up during administration
• To notify prescriber of allergic reactions, abdominal pain, cramping, or blood in the urine

---

pancuronium (℞)

(pan-kyoo-roe'nee-um)
pancuronium bromide,
Pavulon

Func. class.: Neuromuscular blocker (nondepolarizing)
Chem. class.: Synthetic curariform

Action: Inhibits transmission of nerve impulses by binding with cholinergic receptor sites, antagonizing action of acetylcholine

Uses: Facilitation of endotracheal intubation, skeletal muscle relaxation during mechanical ventilation, surgery, or general anesthesia

Dosage and routes:
• *Adult:* IV 0.04-0.1 mg/kg, then 0.01 mg/kg q½-1h
• *Child >10 yr:* IV 0.04-0.1 mg/kg, then ⅕ initial dose q½-1h

Available forms: Inj 1, 2 mg/ml

Side effects/adverse reactions:
CV: Bradycardia; tachycardia; increased, decreased B/P; ventricular extrasystoles

RESP: **Prolonged apnea, bronchospasm, cyanosis, respiratory depression**
EENT: Increased secretions
MS: Weakness to prolonged skeletal muscle relaxation
INTEG: Rash, flushing, pruritus, urticaria, sweating, salivation

Contraindications: Hypersensitivity to bromide ion

Precautions: Pregnancy (C), renal disease, cardiac disease, lactation, children <2 yr, electrolyte imbalances, dehydration, neuromuscular disease, respiratory disease

Pharmacokinetics:
IV: Onset 30-45 sec, peak 3-5 min; metabolized (small amounts), excreted in urine (unchanged), crosses placenta

Interactions:
• Increased neuromuscular blockade: aminoglycosides, clindamycin, enflurane, isoflurane, lincomycin, lithium, local anesthetics, narcotic analgesics, polymyxin antiinfectives, quinidine, thiazides
• Dysrhythmias: theophylline

Lab test interferences:
Decrease: Cholinesterase

NURSING CONSIDERATIONS
Assess:
• For electrolyte imbalances (K, Mg); may lead to increased action of this drug
• Vital signs (B/P, pulse, respirations, airway) until fully recovered; rate, depth, pattern of respirations, strength of hand grip
• I&O ratio; check for urinary retention, frequency, hesitancy
• Recovery: decreased paralysis of face, diaphragm, leg, arm, rest of body; allow to recover fully before neuro assessment
• Allergic reactions: rash, fever, respiratory distress, pruritus; drug should be discontinued

P

Administer:

IV, direct

• With diazepam or morphine when used for therapeutic paralysis; this drug provides no sedation

• Using nerve stimulator by anesthesiologist to determine neuromuscular blockade

• Atropine to counteract muscarinic effects

• After succinylcholine effects subside

• Anticholinesterase to reverse neuromuscular blockade

• IV undiluted, give over 1-2 min (only by qualified persons)

Additive compatibilities: Verapamil

Syringe compatibilities: Heparin

Y-site compatibilities: Aminophylline, cefazolin, cefuroxime, cimetidine, dobutamine, dopamine, epinephrine, esmolol, fentanyl, fluconazole, gentamicin, heparin, hydrocortisone, isoproterenol, lorazepam, midazolam, morphine, nitroglycerin, nitroprusside, ranitidine, trimethoprim-sulfamethoxazole, vancomycin

Perform/provide:

• Storage in refrigerator; do not store in plastic; use only fresh sol

• Reassurance if communication is difficult during recovery from neuromuscular blockade

• Frequent (q2h) instillation of artificial tears and covering eyes to prevent drying of cornea

Evaluate:

• Therapeutic response: paralysis of jaw, eyelid, head, neck, rest of body

Treatment of overdose: Edrophonium or neostigmine, atropine, monitor VS; may require mechanical ventilation

pantoprazole (R)

(pan-toe-pray´zole)

Protonix, Prontonix IV

Func. class.: Proton pump inhibitor

Chem. class.: Benzimidazole

Action: Suppresses gastric secretion by inhibiting hydrogen/potassium ATPase enzyme system in gastric parietal cell; characterized as gastric acid pump inhibitor, since it blocks final step of acid production

Uses: Gastroesophageal reflux disease (GERD), severe erosive esophagitis, maintenance

Dosage and routes:

• *Adult:* **PO** 40 mg qd × 8 wk, may repeat course; **IV**

Available forms: Tabs, delayed rel 20, 40 mg; pwd for inj, freeze-dried 40 mg/vial

Side effects/adverse reactions:

CNS: Headache, insomnia

GI: Diarrhea, abdominal pain, flatulence

INTEG: Rash

META: Hyperglycemia

Contraindications: Hypersensitivity

Precautions: Pregnancy (C), lactation, children

Pharmacokinetics: Peak 2.4 hr, duration >24 hr, half-life 1.5 hr, protein binding 97%, eliminated in urine as metabolites and in feces; in elderly elimination rate decreased

Interactions:

• May increase serum levels of pantoprazole: diazepam, phenytoin, flurazepam, triazolam, clarithromycin

• Possible increased bleeding: warfarin

• May delay absorption: sucralfate

◆ = Nursing alert   ✐ = Herb-drug interaction   ⊘ = Do not crush

NURSING CONSIDERATIONS
Assess:
• GI system: bowel sounds q8h, abdomen for pain, swelling, anorexia
• Hepatic enzymes: AST, ALT, alk phosphatase during treatment
Administer:
🚫 Do not crush del rel tabs, swallow whole
• May take with or without food
IV
• Reconstitute with 10 ml 0.9% NaCl, further dilute with 100 ml Ringer's, D₅ (0.4 mg/ml), give over 15 min (≤3 mg/min) using in-line filter provided
Evaluate:
• Therapeutic response: absence of epigastric pain, swelling, fullness
Teach patient/family:
• To report severe diarrhea; drug may have to be discontinued
• That diabetic patient should know hypoglycemia may occur
• To avoid hazardous activities; dizziness may occur
• To avoid alcohol, salicylates, ibuprofen; may cause GI irritation

---

RARELY USED

papaverine (℞)
(pa-pav′er-een)
Func. class.: Peripheral vasodilator

Uses: Arterial spasm resulting in cerebral and peripheral ischemia; myocardial ischemia associated with vascular spasm or dysrhythmias; angina pectoris; peripheral pulmonary embolism; visceral spasm as in ureteral, biliary, GI colic, peripheral vascular disease
Dosage and routes:
• *Adult:* **PO** 100-300 mg 3-5×/day; **SUS REL** 150-300 mg q8-12h; **IM/IV** 30-120 mg q3h prn

Contraindications: Hypersensitivity, complete AV heart block

RARELY USED

paraldehyde (℞)
(par-al′de-hyde)
Func. class.: Anticonvulsant

Uses: Refractory seizures, status epilepticus, sedation, insomnia, alcohol withdrawal, tetanus, eclampsia
Dosage and routes:
Seizures
• *Adult:* **IM** 5-10 ml; divide 10 ml into 2 inj; **IV** 0.2-0.4 ml/kg in **NS** inj
• *Child:* **IM** 0.15 ml/kg; **RECT** 0.3 ml/kg q4-6h or 1 ml/yr of age, not to exceed 5 ml; may repeat in 1 hr prn; **IV** 5 ml/90 ml **NS** inj; begin infusion at 5 ml/hr; titrate to patient response
Alcohol withdrawal
• *Adult:* **PO/RECT** 5-10 ml, not to exceed 60 ml; **IM** 5 ml q4-6h × 24 hr, then q6h on following days, not to exceed 30 ml
Sedation
• *Adult:* **PO/REC** 4-10 ml; **IM** 5 ml; **IV** 3-5 ml in emergency only; Child: **PO/REC/IM** 0.15 ml/kg
Tetanus
• *Adult:* **IV** 4-5 ml or 12 ml by gastric tube q4h diluted with water; **IM** 5-10 ml prn
Contraindications: Hypersensitivity, gastroenteritis with ulceration

P

---

paramethadione (℞)
(par-a-meth-a-dye'one)
Func. class.: Anticonvulsant

Uses: Refractory absence (petit mal) seizures
Dosage and routes:
• *Adult:* **PO** 300 mg tid; may increase by 300 mg/wk, not to exceed 600 mg qid
• *Child >6 yr:* **PO** 0.9 g/day in divided doses tid or qid
• *Child 2-6 yr:* **PO** 0.6 g/day in divided doses tid or qid
• *Child <2 yr:* **PO** 0.3 g/day in divided doses tid or qid
Contraindications: Hypersensitivity, blood dyscrasias, pregnancy (D), lactation

paricalcitol (℞)
(par-ih-cal'sih-tol)
Zemplar
Func. class.: Vit D analong
Chem. class.: Fat-soluble vitamin

Action: Reduces parathyroid hormone (PTH) levels; suppresses PTH levels in patients with chronic renal failure with absence of hypercalcemia/hyperphosphatemia. Serum PO_4, Ca, CaXP may increase
Uses: Hypoparathyroidism
Dosage and routes:
• *Adult:* **IV BOL** 0.04-0.1 μg/kg (2.8-7 μg) no more than qod during dialysis; may increase by 2-4 μg q2-4wk
Available forms: Inj μg/ml
Side effects/adverse reactions:
GI: Nausea, vomiting, anorexia, dry mouth
CNS: Lightheadedness

CV: Palpitations
OTHER: Pneumonia, edema, chills, fever, flu, *sepsis*
Contraindications: Hypersensitivity, hypercalcemia
Precautions: Cardiovascular disease, renal calculi, pregnancy (C), elderly, lactation, children
Interactions:
• Digitalis toxicity: digitalis
NURSING CONSIDERATIONS
Assess:
• Ca, PO_4, q2×/wk during initial therapy; after dose is established take calcium and phosphorus qmo
Administer:
IV
• By IV bolus only
Evaluate:
• Decreased hypoparathyroidism in chronic renal disease
Teach patient/family:
• To report weakness, lethargy, headache, anorexia, loss of weight
• To report nausea, vomiting, palpitations

paromomycin (℞)
(par-oh-moe-mye'sin)
Func. class.: Amebicide

Uses: Intestinal amebiasis, adjunct in hepatic coma
Dosage and routes:
Intestinal amebiasis
• *Adult and child:* **PO** 25-35 mg/kg/day in 3 divided doses × 5-10 day pc
Hepatic coma
• *Adult:* 4 g qd in divided doses × 5-6 day
Contraindications: Hypersensitivity, renal disease, GI obstruction

---

 = Nursing alert   = Herb-drug interaction   = Do not crush

paroxetine (℞)
(par-ox'e-teen)
Paxil

Func. class.: Antidepressant, SSRI

Chem. class.: Phenylpiperidine derivative

Action: Inhibits CNS neuron uptake of serotonin but not of norepinephrine or dopamine

Uses: Major depressive disorder, obsessive-compulsive disorder, panic disorder, generalized anxiety disorder

Investigational uses: Diabetic neuropathy, headaches, premature ejaculation, premenstrual disorders, bipolar depression with lithium, fibromyalgia, posttraumatic stress

Research note: Risperidone given with paroxetine resulted in an increase of risperidone levels[31]

Research note: One study has shown a decrease in thyroxine during treatment with paroxetine[32]

Dosage and routes:

Depression
• *Adult:* **PO** 20 mg qd in AM; after 4 wk if no clinical improvement is noted, dose may be increased by 10 mg/day qwk to desired response, not to exceed 50 mg/day
• *Geriatric:* **PO** 10 mg qd, increase by 10 mg to desired dose, max 40 mg/day

Renal dose
• *Adult:* **PO** 10 mg qd in AM, may increase by 10 mg/day qwk, max 40 mg qd

Obsessive-compulsive disorder
• *Adult:* **PO** 40 mg/day in AM, start with 20 mg/day, increase 10 mg/day increments, max 60 mg/day

Panic disorder
• *Adult:* **PO** 40 mg/day, start with 10 mg/day and increase in 10 mg/day increments, max 60 mg/day

Premenstrual disorders (off-label)
• *Adult:* **PO** 10-30 mg qd

Available forms: Tabs 10, 20, 30, 40 mg; oral susp 10 mg/5 ml

Side effects/adverse reactions:

CNS: Headache, nervousness, insomnia, drowsiness, anxiety, tremor, dizziness, fatigue, sedation, abnormal dreams, agitation, apathy, euphoria, hallucinations, delusions, psychosis

GI: Nausea, diarrhea, dry mouth, anorexia, dyspepsia, constipation, cramps, vomiting, taste changes, flatulence, decreased appetite

INTEG: Sweating, rash

RESP: Infection, pharyngitis, nasal congestion, sinus headache, sinusitis, cough, dyspnea

CV: Vasodilation, postural hypotension, palpitations

MS: Pain, arthritis, myalgia, myopathy, myosthenia

GU: Dysmenorrhea, decreased libido, urinary frequency, UTI, amenorrhea, cystitis, impotence, abnormal ejaculation

EENT: Visual changes

SYST: Asthenia, fever

Contraindications: Hypersensitivity, patients taking MAOIs

Precautions: Pregnancy (B), lactation, children, elderly, seizure history, patients with history of mania, renal and hepatic disease

Do not confuse:
paroxetine/paclitaxel
Paxil/paclitaxel
Paxil/Taxol

Pharmacokinetics:
PO: Peak 5.2 hr; metabolized in liver, unchanged drugs and metabolites excreted in feces and urine; half-life 21 hr; protein binding 95%

Interactions:
• Increased bleeding: warfarin

P

◆Do not use with MAOIs, potentially fatal reactions can occur
• Cimetidine increases paroxetine plasma levels
• Increased agitation: L-tryptophan
• Phenobarbital and phenytoin decrease paroxetine levels
• Increased side effects: highly protein-bound drugs
• Paroxetine may decrease digoxin levels
• Increased theophylline levels: theophylline

Lab test interferences:
Increase: Serum bilirubin, blood glucose, alk phosphatase
Decrease: VMA, 5-HIAA
False increase: Urinary catecholamines

NURSING CONSIDERATIONS
Assess:
• Mental status: mood, sensorium, affect, suicidal tendencies, increase in psychiatric symptoms, depression, panic
• B/P (lying/standing), pulse q4h; if systolic B/P drops 20 mm Hg, hold drug, notify prescriber; take vital signs q4h in patients with cardiovascular disease
• Blood studies: CBC, leukocytes, differential, cardiac enzymes if patient is receiving long-term therapy
• Hepatic studies: AST, ALT, bilirubin, creatinine
• Weight qwk; appetite may decrease with drug
• ECG for flattening of T wave, bundle branch, AV block, dysrhythmias in cardiac patients
• EPS primarily in elderly: rigidity, dystonia, akathisia
• Urinary retention, constipation
• Withdrawal symptoms: headache, nausea, vomiting, muscle pain, weakness; not usual unless drug discontinued abruptly
• Alcohol intake; if alcohol is consumed, hold dose until morning

Administer:
• Increased fluids, bulk in diet for constipation, urinary retention
• With food, milk for GI symptoms
• Crushed if patient is unable to swallow medication whole
• Dosage hs for oversedation during day; may take entire dose hs; elderly may not tolerate once/day dosing
• Gum, hard candy, frequent sips of water for dry mouth

Perform/provide:
• Storage at room temperature; do not freeze
• Assistance with ambulation during therapy, since drowsiness, dizziness occur
• Safety measures primarily in elderly
• Checking to see if PO medication swallowed

Evaluate:
• Therapeutic response: decreased depression

Teach patient/family:
• That therapeutic effect may take 1-4 wk
• To use caution in driving, other activities requiring alertness because of drowsiness, dizziness, blurred vision
• Not to discontinue medication quickly after long-term use; may cause nausea, headache, malaise
• To avoid alcohol ingestion, other CNS depressants

Treatment of overdose: Airway, for seizures give diazepam, symptomatic treatment

pegaspargase (℞)

(peg-as´per-gase)

Oncaspar, PEG-L-asparaginase

Func. class.: Antineoplastic

Chem. class.: Escherichia coli enzyme

Action: Indirectly inhibits protein synthesis in tumor cells; without amino acid, DNA, RNA synthesis is halted; asparagine, protein synthesis is halted; G₁ phase; cell-cycle specific; a nonvesicant; a modified version of L-asparaginase

Uses: Acute lymphocytic leukemia in combination with other antineoplastics

Dosage and routes:

In combination

• *Adult and child with BSA ≥0.6 m²:* **IV/IM** 2500 IU/m² q14d, run **IV** over 1-2 hr in 100 ml of NaCl or D₅ through a running **IV**; **IM** should be no more than 2 ml in one inj site

• *Child with BSA <0.6 m²:* **IV/IM** 82.5 IU/kg q14d

Sole induction

• *Adult:* **IV** 2500 IU/m² q14 days

Available forms: Inj 750 IU/ml in a phosphate buffered saline sol

Side effects/adverse reactions:

*SYST: **Anaphylaxis, hypersensitivity***

*HEMA: **Thrombocytopenia, leukopenia, myelosuppression, anemia, decreased clotting factors, pancytopenia***

*GI: Nausea, vomiting, anorexia, cramps, stomatitis, **hepatotoxicity, pancreatitis**, diarrhea*

*GU: Urinary retention, **renal failure**, glycosuria, polyuria, azotemia, uric acid neuropathy*

INTEG: Rash, urticaria, chills, fever

ENDO: Hyperglycemia

*RESP: **Fibrosis, pulmonary infiltrate, severe bronchospasm***

*CV: Chest pain, **hypertension***

*CNS: Neuritis, dizziness, headache, **coma**, depression, fatigue, confusion, hallucinations, **seizures***

Contraindications: Hypersensitivity, infant, lactation, pancreatitis

Precautions: Renal disease, hepatic disease, pregnancy (C), CNS disease

Pharmacokinetics: Half-life 5½ days, onset rapid, duration 2 wk, metabolized in reticuloendothelial system

Interactions:

• Decreased action of methotrexate

• Do not use with radiation

• Coagulation factor imbalances: heparin, warfarin, aspirin, NSAIDs

NURSING CONSIDERATIONS

Assess:

◆ For signs and symptoms of pancreatitis (nausea, vomiting, severe abdominal pain), anaphylaxis (bronchospasm, dyspnea), cyanosis

• CBC, differential, platelet count qwk; withhold drug if WBC count is <4000 or platelet count is <75,000; notify prescriber of results

• Pulmonary function tests, chest x-ray studies before and during therapy; chest x-ray film should be obtained q2wk during treatment, watch for severe bronchospasm, fibrosis, pulmonary infiltrate

• Renal function studies: BUN, serum uric acid, ammonia, urine CrCl, electrolytes before and during therapy

• I&O ratio; report fall in urine output of 30 ml/hr, may indicate renal failure

• Temp q4h (may indicate beginning infection)

• LFTs before and during therapy (bilirubin, AST, ALT, LDH) as needed or monthly, hepatotoxicity can occur; check for jaundiced skin,

P

sclera; dark urine, clay-colored stools, itchy skin, abdominal pain, fever, diarrhea

RBC, Hct, Hgb; may be decreased
Serum, urine glucose levels, glycosuria can occur

Bleeding: hematuria, stool guaiac, bruising or petechiae, mucosa or orifices q8h

Dyspnea, rales, nonproductive cough, chest pain, tachypnea, fatigue, increased pulse, pallor, lethargy, swelling around eyes or lips; anaphylaxis may occur

B/P, since hypertension can occur
Local irritation, pain, burning, discoloration at inj site

Symptoms of severe allergic reaction: rash, pruritus, urticaria, purpuric skin lesions, itching, flushing, dyspnea

Frequency of stools, characteristics; cramping, acidosis; signs of dehydration: rapid respirations, poor skin turgor, decreased urine output, dry skin, restlessness, weakness

Administer:
• Antispasmodic if GI symptoms occur
• Allopurinol or sodium bicarbonate to reduce uric acid levels, alkalinization of urine

IV infusion
• Using 21, 23, 25G needle; administer by slow IV infusion via Y-tube or 3-way stopcock of flowing D_5W or NS infusion over 2 hr after diluting
• Considered incompatible with other drugs in syringe or sol

Perform/provide:
• Deep-breathing exercises with patient tid-qid; place in semi-Fowler's position
• Increase fluid intake to 2-3 L/day to prevent urate deposits, calculi formation

• Diet low in purines: no organ meats (kidney, liver), dried beans, peas to maintain alkaline urine
• Rinsing of mouth tid-qid with water, club soda; brushing of teeth bid-tid with soft brush or cotton-tipped applicator for stomatitis; use unwaxed dental floss
• Warm compresses at injection site for inflammation
• Nutritious diet with iron, vitamin supplements
• HOB raised to facilitate breathing

Evaluate:
• Therapeutic response: decreased exacerbations in acute lymphocytic leukemia

Teach patient/family:
• To report nausea, vomiting, bruising, bleeding, stomatitis, severe diarrhea, jaundice, chest pain, abdominal pain, trouble breathing, rash
• To avoid vaccinations without advice of prescriber
• Not to use hard-bristled toothbrush, razors
• To avoid OTC medications, alcohol

Treatment of anaphylaxis: Administer epinephrine, diphenhydramine, IV corticosteroids

---

pemoline (℞)
(pem′oh-leen)
Cylert, Pem ADD, pemoline
Func. class.: Cerebral stimulant
Chem. class.: Oxazolidinone derivative

Controlled Substance Schedule IV
Action: Exact mechanism unknown; may act through dopaminergic mechanisms; produces CNS stimulation and a paradoxic effect in ADHD
Uses: Attention deficit hyperactiv-

 = Nursing alert   = Herb-drug interaction   = Do not crush

ity disorder when other treatment has failed

Investigational uses: Narcolepsy, fatigue, excessive daytime sleepiness

Dosage and routes:
• *Child >6 yr:* **PO** 37.5 mg in AM, increasing by 18.75 mg/wk, not to exceed 112.5 mg/day

Available forms: Tabs 18.75, 37.5, 75 mg; chewable tabs 37.5 mg

Side effects/adverse reactions:

MISC: Rashes, growth suppression in children

CNS: Hyperactivity, insomnia, restlessness, dizziness, depression, headache, stimulation, irritability, aggressiveness, hallucinations, *seizures, masking or worsening of Gilles de la Tourette's syndrome,* drowsiness, dyskinetic movements

GI: Nausea, anorexia, diarrhea, abdominal pain, increased liver enzymes, *hepatitis,* jaundice, weight loss, *life-threatening hepatic failure*

CV: Tachycardia

Contraindications: Hypersensitivity, hepatic insufficiency

Precautions: Renal disease, pregnancy (B), lactation, drug abuse, child <6 yr, psychosis, tics, seizure disorder

Pharmacokinetics:

PO: Peak 2-4 hr, duration 8 hr, metabolized (50%) by liver, excreted (40%) by kidneys, half-life 10-30 hr

Interactions:
• Increased CNS stimulation: other CNS stimulants
• Decreased seizure threshold: anticonvulsants

NURSING CONSIDERATIONS
Assess:
• For attention span, decreased hyperactivity in ADHD persons
◆ Hepatic function studies: ALT, AST, bilirubin; renal, creatinine, prior to treatment and periodically

thereafter; if life-threatening, hepatic failure has occurred; discontinue drug if hepatic symptoms occur
• Height, growth rate q3mo in child; growth rate may be decreased
• Mental status: mood, sensorium, affect, stimulation, insomnia, aggressiveness

PO
• In AM

Evaluate:
• Therapeutic response: decreased hyperactivity

Teach patient/family:
• To decrease caffeine consumption (coffee, tea, cola, chocolate); may increase irritability, stimulation
• To avoid OTC preparations unless approved by prescriber
• To withdraw over several wk
• To avoid alcohol ingestion
• To avoid hazardous activities until patient is stabilized
• That therapeutic effect may take 2-4 wk
• To notify prescriber if tremors, insomnia, palpitations, restlessness, jaundice, bleeding, dark urine occur
• Regarding the possibility of hepatotoxicity and need for blood work

P

PENICILLINS

penicillin G benzathine (℞)

(pen-i-sill'in)
Bicillin, Bicillin L-A, Megacillin*, Permapen

penicillin G potassium (℞)

Pfizerpen

penicillin G procaine (℞)

Ayercillin*, Crysticillin A.S., Pfizerpen-AS, Wycillin

penicillin G sodium (℞)

penicillin V potassium (℞)

Apo-Pen-VK*, Beepen-VK, Betapen-VK, Ledercillin-VK, Nadopen-V*, Novopen-VK*, Pen-Vee K*, PVFK*, Veetids

Func. class.: Broad-spectrum antiinfective
Chem. class.: Natural penicillin

Action: Interferes with cell wall replication of susceptible organisms; osmotically unstable cell wall swells, bursts from osmotic pressure, results in cell death

Uses: Respiratory infections, scarlet fever, erysipelas, otitis media, pneumonia, skin and soft tissue infections, gonorrhea; effective for gram-positive cocci *(Staphylococcus, Streptococcus pyogenes, S. viridans, S. faecalis, S. bovis, S. pneumoniae)*, gram-negative cocci *(Neisseria gonorrhoeae)*, gram-positive bacilli *(Actinomyces, Bacillus anthracis, Clostridium perfringens, C. tetani, Corynebacterium diphtheriae, Listeria monocytogenes)*, gram-negative bacilli *(Escherichia coli, Proteus mirabilis, Salmonella, Shigella, Enterobacter, Streptobacillus moniliformis)*, spirochetes *(Treponema pallidum)*

Dosage and routes:

Penicillin G benzathine
Early syphilis
• *Adult:* **IM** 2.4 million U in single dose

Congenital syphilis
• *Child <2 yr:* **IM** 50,000 U/kg in single dose

Prophylaxis of rheumatic fever, glomerulonephritis
• *Adult and child >27 kg:* **IM** 1.2 million U in single dose qmo or 600,000 U q2wk
• *Child <27 kg:* **IM** 600,000 U in single dose qmo

Upper respiratory infections (group A streptococcal)
• *Adult:* **IM** 1.2 million U in single dose
• *Child >27 kg:* **IM** 900,000 U in single dose
• *Child <27 kg:* **IM** 300,000-600,000 g in single dose

Available forms: Inj 300,000 U/ml; 600,000; 1,200,000; 2,400,000 U/dose

Penicillin G potassium
• Dosage reduction indicated in renal impairment (CrCl <50 ml/min)

Pneumococcal/streptococcal infections (mild to moderate)
• *Adult:* **IM/IV** 1.2-24 million U in divided doses q4h
• *Child <12 yr:* **IV** 100,000-400,000 U/kg/day in 4-6 divided doses

Available forms: Tabs 500,000 U*, oral susp 250,000, 500,000 U*; pwd for inj 1, 5, 10, 20 million U/vial

Penicillin G procaine
Renal dose
• CrCl 10-30 ml/min give q8-12h; CrCl <10 ml/min give q12-18h

Moderate to severe infections
• *Adult and child:* **IM** 600,000-1.2 million U in 1 or 2 doses/day for 10 days to 2 wk

 = Nursing alert   = Herb-drug interaction ⃠ = Do not crush

• *Newborn:* 50,000 U/kg **IM** once daily (avoid use in newborns)
Gonorrhea
• *Adult and child >12 yr:* **IM** 4.8 million U in two injections given 30 min after probenecid 1 g
Pneumococcal pneumonia
• *Adult and child >12 yr:* **IM** 600,000-1.2 million U/day × 7-10 days
Available forms: INJ 300,000, 500,000, 600,000, 1,200,000, 2,400,000 U/unit dose
Penicillin G sodium
• Dosage reduction indicated in renal impairment (CrCl <50 ml/min)
Moderate to severe infections
• *Adult:* **IM/IV** 2 million-24 million U/day in divided doses q4h
• *Child:* **IM/IV** 50,000-400,000 U/kg/day in divided doses q4-12h
Dental surgery prophylaxis for endocarditis
• *Adult:* **IM/IV** 2 million U ½-1 hr before procedure, then 1 million U 6 hr after procedure
Available forms: Inj 5 million U/vial
Penicillin V potassium
• Dosage reduction indicated in renal impairment (CrCl <50 ml/min)
Pneumococcal/staphylococcal infections
• *Adult:* **PO** 250-500 mg q6h
• *Child <12 yr:* **PO** 25-50 mg/kg/day in divided doses q6-8h
Streptococcal infections
• *Adult:* **PO** 125-250 mg q6-8h × 10 days
Prevention of recurrence of rheumatic fever/chorea
• *Adult:* **PO** 125 mg bid continuously
• *Child <5 yr:* **PO** 125 mg bid
• *Child >5 yr:* **PO** 250 mg bid
Vincent's gingivitis/pharyngitis
• *Adult:* **PO** 250 mg q6-8h
Available forms: Tabs 125, 250, 500 mg; pwd for oral sol 125, 250 mg/5 ml

Side effects/adverse reactions:
HEMA: Anemia; increased bleeding time; ***bone marrow depression, granulocytopenia***
GI: Nausea, vomiting, diarrhea, increased AST, ALT, abdominal pain, glossitis, colitis
GU: ***Oliguria, proteinuria, hematuria,*** vaginitis, moniliasis, ***glomerulonephritis***
CNS: Lethargy, hallucinations, anxiety, depression, twitching, ***coma, convulsions***
META: Hyperkalemia, hypokalemia, alkalosis, hypernatremia
MISC: ***Anaphylaxis,*** local pain, tenderness and fever with IM injection
Contraindications: Hypersensitivity to penicillins; neonates
Precautions: Hypersensitivity to cephalosporins, pregnancy (B), lactation, severe renal disease
Pharmacokinetics:
Penicillin G benzathine
IM: Very slow absorption, duration 21-28 days, half-life 30-60 min; excreted in urine, feces, breast milk; crosses placenta
Penicillin G potassium
IV: Peak immediate
IM: Peak ¼-½ hr
PO: Peak 1 hr, duration 6 hr
Excreted in urine unchanged, excreted in breast milk, crosses placenta, half-life 30-60 min
Penicillin G procaine
IM: Peak 1-4 hr, duration 15 hr, excreted in urine
Penicillin G sodium
IM: Peak 1-3 hr, duration 6 hr; excreted in urine
Penicillin V potassium
PO: Peak 30-60 min, duration 6-8 hr, half-life 30 min, excreted in urine, breast milk
Interactions:
• Decreased antimicrobial effect of penicillin: tetracyclines

P

Side effects: *italics* = common; ***bold italics*** = life-threatening

• Increased penicillin concentrations: aspirin, probenecid
• Decreased effect of oral contraceptives
• Increased effect of heparin

🍃 Delayed, reduced absorption of penicillin: khat, separate doses by 2 or more hr

Lab test interferences:

False positive: Urine glucose, urine protein

NURSING CONSIDERATIONS
Assess:
• For infection: temp, characteristics of sputum, wounds, urine, stools before, during, and after treatment
• I&O ratio; report hematuria, oliguria, since penicillin in high doses is nephrotoxic

◆ Any patient with compromised renal system, since drug is excreted slowly in poor renal system function; toxicity may occur rapidly
• Liver studies: AST, ALT
• Blood studies: WBC, RBC, Hct, Hgb, bleeding time
• Renal studies: urinalysis, protein, blood
• C&S before therapy; drug may be given as soon as culture is taken
• Bowel pattern before and during treatment
• Skin eruptions after administration of penicillin to 1 wk after discontinuing drug
• Respiratory status: rate, character, wheezing, tightness in chest
• Allergies before initiation of treatment, reaction of each medication; highlight allergies on chart; because of prolonged action, allergic reaction may be prolonged and severe; watch for anaphylaxis: rash, dyspnea, pruritus, laryngeal edema

Administer:

Penicillin G benzathine
• Drug after C&S completed
• After shaking well, deep IM inj in large muscle mass; avoid intravascular inj, aspirate

Penicillin G potassium
• Drug after C&S

Solution compatibility: Sterile H_2O for inj

Additive compatibilities: Ascorbic acid, calcium chloride, calcium gluconate, cephapirin, chloramphenicol, cimetidine, clindamycin, colistimethate, corticotropin, dimenhydrinate, diphenhydramine, ephedrine, erythromycin, furosemide, hydrocortisone, kanamycin, lidocaine, magnesium sulfate, methicillin, methylprednisolone, metronidazole, polymyxin B, prednisolone, potassium chloride, procaine, prochlorperazine, ranitidine, verapamil

Syringe compatibilities: Heparin

Y-site compatibilities: Acyclovir, amiodarone, cyclophosphamide, diltiazem, enalaprilat, esmolol, fluconazole, foscarnet, heparin, hydromorphone, labetalol, magnesium sulfate, meperidine, morphine, perphenazine, potassium chloride, tacrolimus, theophylline, verapamil, vit B/C

Penicillin G procaine
• Drug after C&S
• Deep IM inj avoid intravascular inj, aspirate

Penicillin G sodium
• IV after diluting with sterile H_2O; shake; follow manufacturer's instructions for dilution; may be added to 0.9% NaCl; give by continuous inf, usually over 12 hr
• Drug after C&S

Solution compatibility: Sterile H_2O for inj

Additive compatibilities: Calcium chloride, calcium gluconate, chloramphenicol, clindamycin, colistimethate, diphenhydramine, erythromycin, furosemide, gentamicin, hydrocortisone, kanamycin, methicillin,

---

◆ = Nursing alert   🍃 = Herb-drug interaction   🚫 = Do not crush

polymyxin B, prednisolone, procaine, ranitidine, verapamil, vit B/C
Syringe compatibilities: Aminoglycosides, chloramphenicol, cimetidine, colistimethate, gentamicin, heparin, kanamycin, lincomycin, polymyxin B, streptomycin
Penicillin V potassium
• Orally on empty stomach for best absorption
• Drug after C&S
Perform/provide:
• Adrenaline, suction, tracheostomy set, endotracheal intubation equipment
• Adequate fluid intake (2 L) during diarrhea episodes
• Scratch test to assess allergy after securing order from prescriber; usually done when penicillin is only drug of choice
• Storage in dry, tight container; oral susp refrigerated 2 wk, 1 wk at room temperature
Evaluate:
• Therapeutic response: absence of fever, draining wounds
• Allergies before initiation of treatment, reaction of each medication; highlight allergies on chart; hypersensitivity reaction may be delayed
Teach patient/family:
• To report sore throat, fever, fatigue; may indicate superinfection
• To wear or carry Medic Alert ID if allergic to penicillins
• To report diarrhea, prevent dehydration
• To shake susp well before each dose; store in refrigerator for up to 2 wk
• To use all medication prescribed
• To use additional contraception if using any of these drugs
Treatment of anaphylaxis: Withdraw drug; maintain airway; administer epinephrine, aminophylline, O₂, IV corticosteroids

pentamidine (℞)
(pen-tam'i-deen)
Nebupent, Pentam 300,
Pentacarinat*, Pneumopent*
Func. class.: Antiprotozoal
Chem. class.: Aromatic diamide derivative

Action: Interferes with DNA/RNA synthesis in protozoa
Uses: Treatment/prevention of *Pneumocystis carinii* infections
Dosage and routes:
• *Adult and child:* **IV/IM** 4 mg/kg/day × 2-3 wk; **NEB** 300 mg via specific nebulizer given q4wk for prevention
Available forms: Inj, aerosol 300 mg/vial; sol for aerosol 60 mg/vial*
Side effects/adverse reactions:
CV: Hypotension, ventricular tachycardia, ECG abnormalities, ***dysrhythmias***
HEMA: Anemia, ***leukopenia, thrombocytopenia***
INTEG: Sterile abscess, pain at injection site, pruritus, urticaria, *rash*
GU: ***Acute renal failure, increased serum creatinine, renal toxicity***
GI: Nausea, vomiting, anorexia; increased AST, ALT; ***acute pancreatitis,*** metallic taste
CNS: Disorientation, hallucinations, *dizziness,* confusion
RESP: Cough, shortness of breath, ***bronchospasm*** (with aerosol)
MISC: Fatigue, chills, night sweats, ***anaphylaxis, Stevens-Johnson syndrome***
META: Hyperkalemia, hypocalcemia, hypoglycemia
Precautions: Blood dyscrasias, hepatic disease, renal disease, diabetes mellitus, cardiac disease, hypocalcemia, pregnancy (C), hypertension, hypotension, lactation, children

P

Pharmacokinetics: Excreted unchanged in urine (66%)
Interactions:

• Nephrotoxicity: aminoglycosides, amphotericin B, colistin, cisplatin, foscarnet, methoxyflurane, polymyxin B, vancomycin

◆ Fatal dysrhythmias: erythromycin IV

• Increased myelosuppression: antineoplastics, radiation

NURSING CONSIDERATIONS
Assess:

• Blood studies, blood glucose, CBC, platelets, calcium, magnesium

• I&O ratio; report hematuria, oliguria

• ECG for cardiac dysrhythmias

• Patient should be lying down when receiving drug; severe hypotension may develop; monitor B/P during administration and until B/P stable

◆ Any patient with compromised renal system; drug is excreted slowly in poor renal system function; toxicity may occur rapidly

• Liver studies: AST, ALT

• Renal studies: urinalysis, BUN, creatinine; nephrotoxicity may occur

• Signs of infection, anemia

• Bowel pattern before, during treatment

• Sterile abscess, pain at injection site

• Respiratory status: rate, character, wheezing, dyspnea

• Dizziness, confusion, hallucination

• Allergies before treatment, reaction of each medication; place allergies on chart in bright red letters; notify all people giving drugs

Administer:

INH

• Through nebulizer; mix contents in 6 ml of sterile H_2O; do not use low pressure (<20 psi); flow rate

should be 5-7 L/min (40-50 psi) air or O_2 source over 30-45 min until chamber is empty

IM

• 300 mg diluted in 3 ml sterile H_2O; give deep IM by Z-track; painful by this route

IV

• Reconstitute 300 mg/3-5 ml of sterile water for inj, D_5W, withdraw dose and further dilute in 50-250 ml D_5W, give over 1-2 hr

Y-site compatibilities: Diltiazem, zidovudine

Perform/provide:

• Storage in refrigerator protected from light

Evaluate:

• Therapeutic response: decreased temp, increased ability to breathe

Teach patient/family:

• To report sore throat, fever, fatigue (may indicate superinfection)

• To maintain adequate fluid intake

---

pentazocine (℞)

(pen-taz'oh-seen)

Talwin, Talwin NX

Func. class.: Opiate analgesic, antagonist

Chem. class.: Synthetic benzomorphan

Controlled Substance Schedule IV

Action: Inhibits ascending pain pathways in CNS, increases pain threshold, alters pain perception

Uses: Moderate to severe pain

Dosage and routes:

• *Adult:* **PO** 50-100 mg q3-4h prn, not to exceed 600 mg/day; **IV/IM/SC** 30 mg q3-4h prn, not to exceed 360 mg/day

Labor

• *Adult:* **IM** 60 mg; **IV** 30 mg q2-3h when contractions are regular

---

◆ = Nursing alert   ∅ = Herb-drug interaction   ⊘ = Do not crush

Renal dose
• CrCl 10-50 ml/min give q24-36h; CrCl <10 ml/min give q48h
Available forms: Inj 30 mg/ml; tabs 50 mg
Side effects/adverse reactions:
CNS: Drowsiness, dizziness, confusion, headache, sedation, euphoria, hallucinations, dreaming
GI: Nausea, vomiting, anorexia, constipation, *cramps,* dry mouth
GU: Increased urinary output, dysuria, urinary retention
INTEG: Rash, urticaria, bruising, flushing, diaphoresis, pruritus, severe irritation at inj sites
EENT: Tinnitus, blurred vision, miosis, diplopia
CV: Palpitations, bradycardia, change in B/P, tachycardia, increased B/P (high doses)
RESP: Respiratory depression
Contraindications: Hypersensitivity, addiction (opiate)
Precautions: Addictive personality, pregnancy (C), lactation, increased intracranial pressure, MI (acute), severe heart disease, respiratory depression, hepatic disease, renal disease, seizure disorder, child <18 yr, head trauma
Pharmacokinetics:
SC/IM: Onset 15-30 min, peak 1-2 hr, duration 2-4 hr
IV: Onset 2-3 min, duration 4-6 hr
Metabolized by liver, excreted by kidneys, crosses placenta, half-life 2-3 hr, extensive first-pass metabolism with less than 20% entering circulation
Interactions:
◆ Unpredictable reactions: MAOIs
• Increased effects: CNS depressants; alcohol, sedative/hypnotics, antipsychotics, skeletal muscle relaxants
• Decreased effects: opiates
Lab test interferences:
Increase: Amylase

NURSING CONSIDERATIONS
Assess:
• For pain: intensity, duration, location prior to and 1 hr after dose
• I&O ratio; check for decreasing output; may indicate urinary retention
• For withdrawal symptoms in opiate-dependent patients
• Pulmonary embolism, abscesses, ulcerations, vascular occlusion, WBC
• CNS changes: dizziness, drowsiness, hallucinations, euphoria, LOC, pupil reaction
• Allergic reactions: rash, urticaria
• Respiratory dysfunction: respiratory depression, character, rate, rhythm; notify prescriber if respirations are <10/min
• Need for pain medication, physical dependence
Administer:
• With antiemetic if nausea, vomiting occur
• When pain is beginning to return; determine dosage interval by patient response
SC/IM
• Give IM deeply into large muscle mass, rotate sites; SC may cause necrosis with repeated inj
IV
• Undiluted or diluted 5 mg/ml of sterile H_2O for inj; give 5 mg or less over 1 min
Syringe compatibilities: Atropine, benzquinamide, butorphanol, chlorpromazine, cimetidine, dimenhydrinate, diphenhydramine, droperidol, fentanyl, hydromorphone, hydroxyzine, meperidine, metoclopramide, morphine, perphenazine, prochlorperazine, promazine, promethazine, ranitidine, scopolamine
Y-site compatibilities: Heparin, hydrocortisone, potassium chloride, vit B/C

P

Perform/provide:
• Storage in light-resistant area at room temperature
• Assistance with ambulation
• Safety measures: night-light, call bell within easy reach

Evaluate:
• Therapeutic response: decrease in pain

Teach patient/family:
• To report any symptoms of CNS changes, allergic reactions
• That physical dependency may result from extended use
• That withdrawal symptoms may occur: nausea, vomiting, cramps, fever, faintness, anorexia

Treatment of overdose: Naloxone (Narcan) 0.2-0.8 mg IV, O₂, IV fluids, vasopressors

---

pentobarbital (℞)
(pen-toe-bar′bi-tal)
Nembutal, Novopentobarb*, Nova-Rectal*, pentobarbital sodium
Func. class.: Sedative/hypnotic barbiturate; anticonvulsant
Chem. class.: Barbitone, short acting

Controlled Substance Schedule II (USA), Schedule G (Canada)
Action: Depresses activity in brain cells, primarily in reticular activating system in brain stem; selectively depresses neurons in posterior hypothalamus, limbic structures
Uses: Insomnia, sedation, preoperative medication, increased intracranial pressure, dental anesthetic
Dosage and routes:
Insomnia
• *Adult:* **PO** 100-200 mg hs; **IM** 150-200 mg hs; **IV** 100 mg initially, then up to 500 mg; **RECT** 120-200 mg hs

• *Child:* **IM** 2-6 mg/kg, not to exceed 100 mg; **PO** 2-6 mg/kg/day in divided doses; **PO** preoperatively 2-6 mg/kg, max 100 mg/dose; **IV** 100 mg (hypnotic/anticonvulsant)
Available forms: Caps 50, 100 mg; elix 20 mg/5 ml; rect supp 25, 30, 50, 60, 120, 200 mg; inj 50 mg/ml
Side effects/adverse reactions:
CNS: Lethargy, drowsiness, hangover, dizziness, paradoxical stimulation in elderly and children, light-headedness, dependence, *CNS depression,* mental depression, slurred speech
GI: Nausea, vomiting, diarrhea, constipation
INTEG: Rash, urticaria, pain, abscesses at inj site, angioedema, thrombophlebitis, *Stevens-Johnson syndrome*
CV: Hypotension, bradycardia
RESP: Respiratory depression, apnea, laryngospasm, bronchospasm
HEMA: Agranulocytosis, thrombocytopenia, megaloblastic anemia (long-term treatment)
Contraindications: Hypersensitivity to barbiturates, pregnancy (D), respiratory depression, addiction to barbiturates; severe liver, renal impairment; porphyria, uncontrolled pain
Precautions: Anemia, lactation, hepatic disease, renal disease, hypertension, elderly, acute/chronic pain
Do not confuse:
pentobarbital/phenobarbital
Pharmacokinetics:
PO: Onset 15-30 min, duration 4-6 hr
RECT: Onset slow, duration 4-6 hr
Metabolized by liver, excreted by kidneys (metabolites); half-life 15-48 hr
Interactions:
• Increased CNS depression: alcohol, MAOIs, sedatives, other CNS depressants, antihistamines, opiates

---

◆ = Nursing alert　　🖋 = Herb-drug interaction　　🚫 = Do not crush

- Decreased effect of oral anticoagulants, corticosteroids, griseofulvin, quinidine
- Increased half-life of doxycycline
/ Elevated pentobarbital levels: quinine

Lab test interferences:
False increase: Sulfobromophthalein

NURSING CONSIDERATIONS
Assess:
- VS q30min after parenteral route for 2 hr
- Blood studies: Hct, Hgb, RBCs, serum folate, vit D (long-term therapy); PT in patients receiving anticoagulants
- Hepatic studies: AST, ALT, bilirubin; if increased, drug is usually discontinued
- Mental status: mood, sensorium, affect, memory (long, short)
- Physical dependency: more frequent requests for medication, shakes, anxiety
◆ Barbiturate toxicity: hypotension; pupillary constriction; cold, clammy skin; cyanosis of lips; insomnia; nausea; vomiting; hallucinations; delirium; weakness; coma; mild symptoms may occur in 8-12 hr without drug
- Respiratory changes: respiratory depression, character, rate, rhythm; hold drug if respirations are <10/min or if pupils are dilated
- Blood dyscrasias: fever, sore throat, bruising, rash, jaundice, epistaxis

Administer:
- For <14 days, since not effective after that; tolerance develops
- After removal of cigarettes to prevent fires
- After trying conservative measures for insomnia

PO
- Use elixir alone or diluted in fluids

- ½-1 hr before hs for sleeplessness
- On empty stomach for best absorption
- Crushed or whole
- Alone; do not mix with other drugs or inject if there is precipitate

IM
- Inj deep in large muscle mass to prevent tissue sloughing and abscesses; do not inject more than 5 ml in one site

IV
- IV undiluted or dilute in sterile H₂O, LR, NaCl, give 50 mg or less/min; titrate to patient response; use only clear sol; avoid extravasation
- IV only with resuscitative equipment available; administer at <100 mg/min (only by qualified personnel)

Additive compatibilities: Amikacin, aminophylline, calcium chloride, cephapirin, chloramphenicol, dimenhydrinate, erythromycin lactobionate, lidocaine, thiopental, verapamil

Syringe compatibilities: Aminophylline, ephedrine, hydromorphone, neostigmine, scopolamine, sodium bicarbonate, thiopental

Y-site compatibilities: Acyclovir, insulin (regular), propofol

Perform/provide:
- Assistance with ambulation after receiving dose
- Safety measures: night-light, call bell within easy reach
- Checking to see if PO medication has been swallowed
- Storage of suppositories in refrigerator; do not use aqueous solutions that contain precipitate

Evaluate:
- Therapeutic response: ability to sleep at night, less early morning awakening if taking drug for insom-

nia, or decrease in number, severity of seizures if taking drug for seizure disorder

Teach patient/family:
• That hangover is common
• That drug is indicated only for short-term treatment of insomnia; probably ineffective after 2 wk
• That physical dependency may result from extended use (45-90 days depending on dose)
• To avoid driving, other activities requiring alertness
• To avoid alcohol ingestion, CNS depressants; serious CNS depression may result
• Not to discontinue medication quickly after long-term use; drug should be tapered over 1-2 wk
• To tell all prescribers that a barbiturate is being taken
• That withdrawal insomnia may occur after short-term use; not to start using drug again; insomnia will improve in 1-3 nights
• That effects may take 2 nights for benefits to be noticed
• Alternative measures to improve sleep (reading, exercise several hr before hs, warm bath, warm milk, TV, self-hypnosis, deep breathing)

Treatment of overdose: Lavage, activated charcoal, warming blanket, vital signs, hemodialysis, I&O ratio

---

pentostatin (℞)

(pen-toh-stat'in)
Nipent

Func. class.: Antineoplastic, enzyme inhibitor

Chem. class.: Streptomyces antibioticus derivative

Action: Inhibits the enzyme adenosine deaminase (ADA), which is able to block DNA synthesis and some RNA synthesis

Uses: α-Interferon-refractory hairy cell leukemia, chronic lymphocytic leukemia

Dosage and routes:
• *Adult:* **IV** 4 mg/m² every other wk; may be given **IV BOL,** or diluted in a larger volume and given over 20-30 min

Available forms: Inj 10 mg/vial

Side effects/adverse reactions:
CNS: Headache, anxiety, confusion, depression, dizziness, insomnia, nervousness, paresthesia
RESP: Cough, upper respiratory infection, bronchitis, dyspnea, epistaxis, pneumonia, pharyngitis, rhinitis, sinusitis
SYST: Fever, infection, fatigue, pain, allergic reaction, chills, ***death, sepsis,*** chest pain, flulike symptoms
*HEMA: **Leukopenia, anemia, thrombocytopenia,** ecchymosis, **lymphadenopathy,** petechiae*
GI: Nausea, vomiting, anorexia, diarrhea, constipation, flatulence, stomatitis, elevated LFTs
INTEG: Rash, eczema, dry skin, pruritus, sweating, herpes simplex/zoster
*GU: **Hematuria,** dysuria, increased BUN/creatinine*

Contraindications: Hypersensitivity to this drug or mannitol, pregnancy (D)

Precautions: Renal disease, lactation, children, bone marrow depression

Pharmacokinetics:
IV: Elimination half-life 5.7 hr, low protein binding, 90% excreted in urine unchanged or as metabolites

Interactions:
◆ Fatal pulmonary toxicity: fludarabine
• Increased adverse reactions: vidarabine

Lab test interferences:
Increase: Uric acid

◆ = Nursing alert   ⫽ = Herb-drug interaction   ⊘ = Do not crush

NURSING CONSIDERATIONS
Assess:
• CBC, differential, platelet count qwk; withhold drug if WBC is <2000/mm³ or platelet count is <75,000/mm³; notify prescriber
• Renal function studies; BUN, serum uric acid, urine CrCl, electrolytes before, during therapy
• I&O ratio; report fall in urine output to <30 ml/hr
• Monitor temp q4h; fever may indicate beginning infection
• Liver function tests before, during therapy: bilirubin, AST, ALT, alk phosphatase, prn or qmo; check for jaundiced skin and sclera, dark urine, clay-colored stools, itchy skin, abdominal pain, fever, diarrhea
• Bleeding: hematuria, guaiac stools, bruising, petechiae, mucosa or orifices q8h
• Effects of alopecia on body image; discuss feelings about body changes
• Inflammation of mucosa, breaks in skin
• Buccal cavity q8h for dryness, sores, ulceration, white patches, oral pain, bleeding, dysphagia
• Local irritation, pain, burning at inj site
• Symptoms of severe allergic reaction: rash, pruritus, urticaria, purpuric skin lesions, itching, flushing
• GI symptoms: frequency of stools, cramping
• Acidosis, signs of dehydration; rapid respiration, poor skin turgor, decreased urine output, dry skin, restlessness, weakness
Administer:
• Antiemetic 30-60 min before giving drug to prevent vomiting
• Antibiotics as ordered for prophylaxis of infection
IV
• After diluting, use with 5 ml sterile H₂O for injection and mix thoroughly (2 mg/ml); may be given by bolus or diluted in 25-50 ml 5% dextrose, or 0.9% NaCl (0.33 or 0.18 mg/ml)

Solution compatibilities: D₅W, 0.9% NaCl, LR

Y-site compatibilities: Fludarabine, melphalan, ondansetron, paclitaxel, sargramostim

Perform/provide:
• Hydrocortisone, sodium thiosulfate to infiltration area, and ice compress after stopping infusion
• Strict hand-washing technique, gloves, protective covering
• Liquid diet: carbonated beverages; gelatin may be added if patient is not nauseated or vomiting
• Rinsing of mouth tid-qid with water, club soda; brushing of teeth bid-qid with soft brush or cotton-tipped applicators for stomatitis; use unwaxed dental floss
• Storage in refrigerator; reconstituted or diluted sol may be stored at room temperature up to 8 hr
Evaluate:
• Therapeutic response: decrease in tumor size, spread of malignancy
Teach patient/family:
• To report any complaints, side effects to nurse or prescriber
• That hair may be lost during treatment and wig or hairpiece may make patient feel better; tell patient that new hair may be different in color, texture
• To avoid foods with citric acid, hot or rough texture
• To report any bleeding, white spots, ulcerations in mouth to prescriber; tell patient to examine mouth qd
• To avoid crowds and sources of infection when granulocyte count is low

pentoxifylline (R)

(pen-tox'ih-fill-in)
Trental
Func. class.: Hemorrheologic agent
Chem. class.: Dimethylxanthine derivative

Action: Decreases blood viscosity, stimulates prostacyclin formation, increases blood flow by increasing flexibility of RBCs; decreases RBC hyperaggregation; reduces platelet aggregation, decreases fibrinogen concentration

Uses: Intermittent claudication related to chronic occlusive vascular disease

Investigational uses: Cerebrovascular insufficiency, diabetic neuropathies, TIAs, leg ulcers, strokes, aphthous stomatitis

Dosage and routes:
• *Adult:* **PO** 400 mg tid with meals
Stomatitis (off-label)
• *Adult:* **PO** 400 mg tid × 1-6 mo
Available forms: Tabs, cont release 400 mg

Side effects/adverse reactions:
MISC: Epistaxis, flulike symptoms, laryngitis, nasal congestion, *leukopenia,* malaise, weight changes
EENT: Blurred vision, earache, increased salivation, sore throat, conjunctivitis
CNS: Headache, anxiety, *tremors,* confusion, *dizziness*
GI: Dyspepsia, nausea, vomiting, anorexia, bloating, belching, constipation, cholecystitis, dry mouth, thirst, bad taste
INTEG: Rash, pruritus, urticaria, brittle fingernails
CV: Angina, dysrhythmias, palpitation, hypotension, chest pain, dyspnea, edema

Contraindications: Hypersensitivity to this drug or xanthines, retinal/cerebral hemorrhage

Precautions: Pregnancy (C), angina pectoris, cardiac disease, lactation, children, impaired renal function, recent surgery, peptic ulceration

Pharmacokinetics:
PO: Peak 1 hr, half-life ½-1 hr, degradation in liver, excreted in urine

Interactions:
• Increased risk of bleeding: warfarin, salicylates, NSAIDs, thrombolytics, plicamycin, valproic acid
• Increased theophylline level: theophylline
• Increased hypotension: antihypertensives, nitrates

NURSING CONSIDERATIONS
Assess:
• B/P, respirations of patient also taking antihypertensives; intermittent claudication baseline and throughout

Administer:
• With meals to prevent GI upset
🚫 Do not break, crush, or chew ext rel tabs

Evaluate:
• Therapeutic response: decreased pain, cramping, increased ambulation

Teach patient/family:
• That therapeutic response may take 2-4 wk
• That decreased fats, increased cholesterol, increased exercise, decreased smoking are necessary to correct condition
• To observe feet for arterial insufficiency
• To use cotton socks, well-fitted shoes; not to go barefoot
• To watch for bleeding, bruises, petechiae, epistaxis
• To avoid smoking, to prevent blood vessel constriction

◆ = Nursing alert   🖋 = Herb-drug interaction   🚫 = Do not crush

perflutren lipid microsphere
See appendix a—selected new drugs

---

perindopril (℞)
(per-in'doe-pril)
Aceon

Func. class.: Antihypertensive
Chem. class.: Angiotensin-converting enzyme inhibitor

Action: Selectively suppresses renin-angiotensin-aldosterone system; inhibits ACE; prevents conversion of angiotensin I to angiotensin II, dilation of arterial, venous vessels

Uses: Hypertension
Dosage and routes:
Hypertension
• *Adult:* **PO** 4 mg/day, may increase or decrease to desired response range 4-8 mg/day; may give in 2 divided doses or as a single dose
Patients on diuretics
• Discontinue diuretic 2-3 days prior to perindopril then resume diuretic if needed
Renal impairment
• CrCl <30 ml/min 2 mg/day, max 8 mg/day
Available forms: Tabs scored 2, 4, 8 mg
Side effects/adverse reactions:
CV: Hypotension, chest pain, tachycardia, dysrhythmias, syncope
CNS: Insomnia, dizziness, paresthesias, headache, fatigue, anxiety
GI: Nausea, vomiting, colitis, cramps, diarrhea, constipation, flatulence, dry mouth, loss of taste
INTEG: Rash, purpura, alopecia, hyperhidrosis, *angioedema*
HEMA: Agranulocytosis, neutropenia

EENT: Tinnitus, visual changes, sore throat, double vision, dry burning eyes
GU: Proteinuria, renal failure, increased frequency of polyuria or oliguria
RESP: Dyspnea, dry cough, rales, angioedema
META: Hyperkalemia
Contraindications: Hypersensitivity, history of angioedema
Precautions: Renal disease, hyperkalemia, pregnancy (C), lactation, hepatic failure, dehydration, bilateral renal artery stenosis
Pharmacokinetics: Metabolized by liver, excreted in urine
Interactions:
• Hypersensitivity: allopurinol
• Severe hypotension: diuretics, other antihypertensives
• Increased K levels: salt substitutes, K-sparing diuretics, K supplements
• May increase effects of neuromuscular blocking agents, antihypertensives, lithium
• Effects may be increased by diuretics
Lab test interferences:
Interference: Glucose/insulin tolerance tests
NURSING CONSIDERATIONS
Assess:
• B/P, pulse q4h; note rate, rhythm, quality
• Electrolytes: K, Na, Cl during 1st 2 wk of therapy
• Baselines in renal, liver function tests before therapy begins and 1 wk into therapy
• Edema in feet, legs daily
• Skin turgor, dryness of mucous membranes for hydration status
• Symptoms of CHF: edema, dyspnea, wet rales
Administer:
• **PO** as a single dose or in 2 divided doses

Side effects: *italics* = common; ***bold italics*** = life-threatening

Evaluate:

• Therapeutic response: decreased B/P

Teach patient/family:

• Not to use OTC (cough, cold, or allergy) products unless directed by prescriber; to avoid salt substitutes

• To avoid sunlight or wear sunscreen for photosensitivity

• To comply with dosage schedule, even if feeling better

• To notify prescriber of mouth sores, sore throat, fever, swelling of hands or feet, irregular heartbeat, chest pains, signs of angioedema

• That excessive perspiration, dehydration, vomiting, diarrhea may lead to fall in blood pressure; consult prescriber if these occur

• That drug may cause dizziness, fainting; light-headedness may occur during 1st few days of therapy

• That drug may cause skin rash or impaired perspiration; angioedema may occur and to D/C if it occurs

• Not to discontinue drug abruptly

• That CV adverse reactions may reoccur

• To rise slowly to sitting or standing position to minimize orthostatic hypotension

Treatment of overdose: Lavage, IV atropine for bradycardia, IV theophylline for bronchospasm, digitalis, O_2, diuretic for cardiac failure

RARELY USED

permethrin (OTC, R)
(per-meth′rin)
Func. class.: Pediculicide

Uses: Lice, nits, ticks, flea nits
Dosage and routes:
Lice (head)
• *Adult and child:* Wash hair, towel dry; apply liberally to hair, leave on 10 min, rinse with water
Scabies
• *Adult and child:* **TOP** 5% cream applied and massaged into all skin surfaces; leave cream on 8-14 hr, then wash
Contraindications: Hypersensitivity

perphenazine (R)
(per-fen′a-zeen)
Apo-Perphenazine*, perphenazine, PMS Perphenazine*, Trilafon, Trilafon Concentrate
Func. class.: Antipsychotic, neuroleptic
Chem. class.: Phenothiazine piperidine

Action: Depresses cerebral cortex, hypothalamus, limbic system, which control activity, aggression; blocks neurotransmission produced by dopamine at synapse; exhibits strong α-adrenergic, anticholinergic blocking action; as antiemetic inhibits medullary chemoreceptor trigger zone; mechanism for antipsychotic effects is unclear
Uses: Psychotic disorders, schizophrenia, nausea, vomiting
Dosage and routes:
• *Geriatric:* **PO** 2-4 mg qd-bid, increase by 2-4 mg/wk to desired dose
Nausea/vomiting
• *Adult and child >12 yr:* **IM** 5-10

◆ = Nursing alert   🖊 = Herb-drug interaction   🚫 = Do not crush

• B/P standing and lying; also include pulse, respirations q4h during initial treatment; establish baseline before starting treatment; report drops of 30 mm Hg
• Dizziness, faintness, palpitations, tachycardia on rising
• EPS including akathisia (inability to sit still, no pattern to movements), tardive dyskinesia (bizarre movements of jaw, mouth, tongue, extremities), pseudoparkinsonism (rigidity, tremors, pill rolling, shuffling gait)
• Skin turgor daily
◆ For neuroleptic malignant syndrome: hyperthermia, altered mental status, increased CPK, muscle rigidity
• Constipation, urinary retention daily; increase bulk, water in diet

Administer:
• Antiparkinsonian agent on order from prescriber for EPS
• Concentrate mixed in water, orange, pineapple, apricot, prune, tomato, grapefruit juice; do not mix with caffeine beverages (coffee, cola), tannics (tea), or pectinates (apple juice), since incompatibility may result; use 60 ml diluent for each 5 ml of concentrate
• IM inj into large muscle mass
IV
• After diluting each 5 mg/9 ml of NaCl, shake, give 0.5 mg or less (1 ml = 0.5 mg) over 1 min; may be further diluted and infused

Additive compatibilities: Ascorbic acid, ethacrynate, netilmicin
Syringe compatibilities: Atropine, benztropine, butorphanol, chlorpromazine, cimetidine, dimenhydrinate, diphenhydramine, droperidol, fentanyl, hydroxyzine, meperidine, methotrimeprazine, metoclopramide, morphine, pentazocine, prochlorperazine, promethazine, ranitidine, scopolamine

Y-site compatibilities: Acyclovir, amikacin, ampicillin, azlocillin, cefamandole, cefazolin, cefotaxime, cefoxitin, cefuroxime, cephalothin, cephapirin, chloramphenicol, clindamycin, doxycycline, erythromycin, famotidine, gentamicin, kanamycin, metronidazole, mezlocillin, minocycline, moxalactam, nafcillin, oxacillin, penicillin G potassium, piperacillin, tacrolimus, ticarcillin, ticarcillin/clavulanate, tobramycin, trimethoprim-sulfamethoxazole, vancomycin

Perform/provide:
• Decreased sensory input by dimming lights, avoiding loud noises
• Supervised ambulation until stabilized on medication; do not involve in strenuous exercise program because fainting is possible; patient should not stand still for long periods
• Increased fluids to prevent constipation
• Sips of water, candy, gum for dry mouth
• Storage in tight, light-resistant container

Evaluate:
• Therapeutic response: decrease in emotional excitement, hallucinations, delusions, paranoia, reorganization of patterns of thought, speech

Teach patient/family:
• That orthostatic hypotension occurs frequently and to rise from sitting or lying position gradually; to avoid hazardous activities until stabilized on medication
• To remain lying down after IM inj for at least 30 min
• To avoid hot tubs, hot showers, tub baths, since hypotension may occur
• To avoid abrupt withdrawal of this drug, or EPS may result; drug should be withdrawn slowly

---

◆ = Nursing alert　　　🖋 = Herb-drug interaction　　　🚫 = Do not crush

• To avoid OTC preparations (cough, hay fever, cold) unless approved by prescriber, since serious drug interactions may occur; avoid use with alcohol or CNS depressants; increased drowsiness may occur
• To use a sunscreen
• About compliance with drug regimen
• About necessity for meticulous oral hygiene, since oral candidiasis may occur
• To report sore throat, malaise, fever, bleeding, mouth sores; if these occur, CBC should be drawn and drug discontinued
• In hot weather, that heat stroke may occur; to take extra precautions to stay cool

Treatment of overdose: Lavage if orally ingested; provide an airway; *do not induce vomiting*

RARELY USED

phenacemide (℞)
(fe-nass'e-mide)
Func. class.: Anticonvulsant

Uses: Refractory, generalized tonic-clonic (grand mal), complex-partial (psychomotor), absence (petit mal), atypical seizures
Dosage and routes:
• *Adult:* **PO** 500 mg tid, may increase by 500 mg/wk, not to exceed 5 g/day
• *Child 5-10 yr:* **PO** 250 mg tid, may increase by 250 mg/wk, not to exceed 1.5 g/day prn
Contraindications: Hypersensitivity, psychiatric condition, pregnancy (D), lactation

phenazopyridine (℞, OTC)
(fen-az-oh-peer'i-deen)
Azo-Standard, Baridium, Eridium, Geridium, Phenazo*, phenazopyridine, Phenazodine, Prodium, Pyridiate, Pyridium, Urodine, Urogesic, Viridium
Func. class.: Nonopioid analgesic (urinary system)
Chem. class.: Azodye

Action: Exerts analgesic, anesthetic action on the urinary tract mucosa
Uses: Urinary tract irritation, infection used with a urinary antiinfective
Dosage and routes:
• *Adult:* **PO** 200 mg tid × 2 days or less when used with antibacterial for UTI
• *Child 6-12 yr:* **PO** 4 mg/kg tid × 2 days
Renal dose
• Do not use in CrCl <50 ml/min
Available forms: Tabs 100, 200 mg
Side effects/adverse reactions:
HEMA: ***Thrombocytopenia, agranulocytosis, leukopenia, neutropenia, hemolytic anemia, methemoglobinemia***
CNS: Headache
GI: Nausea, vomiting, diarrhea, heartburn, anorexia, ***hepatic toxicity***
INTEG: Rash, skin pigmentation, pruritus
GU: ***Renal toxicity,*** *orange-red urine*
Contraindications: Hypersensitivity, renal insufficiency
Precautions: Pregnancy (B), lactation, children <12 yr
Pharmacokinetics:
Metabolized by liver, excreted by kidneys, crosses placenta, duration 6-8 hr
Lab test interferences:
Interference: Urinalysis

NURSING CONSIDERATIONS
Assess:
• Urinary status: burning, pain, itching, urgency, frequency, hematuria, before/after treatment completed
• Liver function studies: AST, ALT, bilirubin if patient is on long-term therapy
◆ Hepatotoxicity: dark urine, clay-colored stools, jaundiced skin and sclera, itching, abdominal pain, fever, diarrhea if patient is on long-term therapy
• Allergic reactions: rash, urticaria; drug may have to be discontinued
Administer:
PO
• To patient crushed or whole; chewable tablets may be chewed
• With food or milk to decrease gastric symptoms
Evaluate:
• Therapeutic response: decrease in urinary pain
Teach patient/family:
• Not to exceed recommended dosage and to take with meals
• To discontinue after pain is relieved but continue to take concurrent prescribed antiinfective until finished
• That urine may turn red-orange; may stain clothing or contact lenses
Treatment of overdose: Methylene blue 1-2 mg/kg IV or 100-200 mg vit C PO

RARELY USED

phendimetrazine (℞)
(fen-dye-me′tra-zeen)
Func. class.: Anorexiant

Uses: Exogenous obesity
Dosage and routes:
• *Adult:* **PO** 35 mg bid-tid 1 hr ac, not to exceed 70 mg tid; **SUS REL** 105 mg qd ac AM

Contraindications: Hypersensitivity, hyperthyroidism, hypertension, glaucoma, severe arteriosclerosis, severe cardiovascular disease, children <12 yr, agitated states, drug abuse, MAOI use within 14 days

---

phenelzine (℞)
(fen′el-zeen)
Nardil
Func. class.: Antidepressant, MAOI
Chem. class.: Hydrazine

Action: Increases concentrations of endogenous epinephrine, norepinephrine, serotonin, dopamine in storage sites in CNS by inhibition of MAO; increased concentration reduces depression
Uses: Depression, when uncontrolled by other means
Dosage and routes:
• *Adult:* **PO** 45 mg/day in divided doses; may increase to 60 mg/day; dose should be reduced to 15 mg/day, not to exceed 90 mg/day
• *Geriatric:* **PO** 7.5 mg qd, increase by 7.5-15 mg q3-4 days
Available forms: Tabs 15 mg
Side effects/adverse reactions:
*HEMA: **Anemia***
CNS: Dizziness, drowsiness, confusion, headache, anxiety, tremors, stimulation, weakness, hyperreflexia, mania, insomnia, fatigue, weight gain
GI: Constipation, dry mouth, nausea, vomiting, *anorexia,* diarrhea, weight gain
GU: Change in libido, urinary frequency
INTEG: Rash, flushing, increased perspiration
*CV: Orthostatic hypotension, hypertension, dysrhythmias, **hypertensive crisis***

◆ = Nursing alert   🖋 = Herb-drug interaction   🚫 = Do not crush

EENT: Blurred vision
ENDO: SIADH-like syndrome

Contraindications: Hypersensitivity to MAOIs, hypertension, CHF, severe hepatic disease, pheochromocytoma, severe renal disease, severe cardiac disease

Precautions: Suicidal patients, convulsive disorders, severe depression, schizophrenia, hyperactivity, diabetes mellitus, pregnancy (C)

Pharmacokinetics: Metabolized by liver, excreted by kidneys

Interactions:

• Increased hypotension: thiazide diuretics

• Confusion, shivering, hyperreflexia: L-tryptophan

• Toxicity: sumatriptan, sulfonamides

• Decreased serotonin, norepinephrine: rauwolfia alkaloids

• Increased pressor effects: guanethidine, clonidine, indirect-acting or mixed sympathomimetics (ephedrine)

• Increased effects of direct-acting sympathomimetics (epinephrine): alcohol, barbiturates, benzodiazepines, CNS depressants, levodopa

◆ Hyperpyretic crisis, convulsions, hypertensive episode: tricyclics, SSRIs, meperidine, methylphenidate

• Increased hypoglycemic effect: antidiabetics

• Drug/food: avoid tyramine foods, caffeine

🖉 Increased sympathomimetic action: ephedra

🖉 Hypertension: brewer's yeast

🖉 Tension headaches, irritability, visual hallucinations: ginseng

NURSING CONSIDERATIONS
Assess:

• B/P (lying, standing), pulse; if systolic B/P drops 20 mm Hg, hold drug, notify prescriber

• Blood studies: CBC, leukocytes, cardiac enzymes (long-term therapy)

• Hepatic studies: ALT, AST, bilirubin; hepatotoxicity may occur

◆ Toxicity: increased headache, palpitation; discontinue drug immediately; prodromal signs of hypertensive crisis

• Mental status changes: mood, sensorium, affect, memory (long, short); increase in psychiatric symptoms

• Urinary retention, constipation, edema; take weight qwk

• Withdrawal symptoms: headache, nausea, vomiting, muscle pain, weakness

Administer:
PO

• Increased fluids, bulk in diet for constipation

• With food, milk for GI symptoms

• Crushed if patient cannot swallow medication whole

• Dosage hs for oversedation during day

• Gum, hard candy, or frequent sips of water for dry mouth

• Phentolamine for severe hypertension

Perform/provide:

• Storage in tight container in cool environment

• Ambulation assistance at start of therapy, since drowsiness/dizziness occurs, especially elderly

• Safety measures including side rails

• Checking to see if PO medication swallowed

Evalute:

• Therapeutic response: decreased depression

Teach patient/family:

• That therapeutic effects may take 1-4 wk

• To avoid driving, other activities requiring alertness

• To avoid alcohol ingestion, CNS

depressants, OTC medications: cold, weight loss, hay fever, cough syrup
• Not to discontinue medication quickly after long-term use
• To avoid high-tyramine foods: cheese (aged), sour cream, beer, wine, pickled products, liver, raisins, bananas, figs, avocados, meat tenderizers, chocolate, yogurt; increased caffeine
• To report headache, palpitation, neck stiffness, dizziness, constriction in chest, throat

Treatment of overdose: Lavage, activated charcoal, monitor electrolytes, vital signs, diazepam IV, NaHCO₃

---

phenobarbital (℞)

(fee-noe-bar'bi-tal)
Ancalixir*, Barbita, Luminal, phenobarbital sodium, Solfoton
Func. class.: Anticonvulsant
Chem. class.: Barbiturate

Controlled Substance Schedule IV
Action: Decreases impulse transmission; increases seizure threshold at cerebral cortex level
Uses: All forms of epilepsy, status epilepticus, febrile seizures in children, sedation, insomnia
Investigational uses: Hyperbilirubinemia, chronic cholestasis
Dosage and routes:
Seizures
• *Adult:* **PO** 60-200 mg/day in divided doses tid or total dose hs
• *Child:* **PO** 4-6 mg/kg/day in divided doses q12h; may be given as single dose
Status epilepticus
• *Adult:* **IV INF** 10 mg/kg; run no faster than 50 mg/min; may give up to 20 mg/kg
• *Child:* **IV INF** 5-10 mg/kg; may repeat q10-15min up to 20 mg/kg; run no faster than 50 mg/min
Insomnia
• *Adult:* **PO/IM** 100-320 mg
• *Child:* **PO/IM** 3-5 mg/kg
Sedation
• *Adult:* **PO** 30-120 mg/day in 2-3 divided doses
• *Child:* **PO** 3-5 mg/kg/day in 3 divided doses
Preoperative sedation
• *Adult:* **IM** 100-200 mg 1-1½ hr before surgery
• *Child:* **IM** 16-100 mg or **PO/IM/IV** 1-3 mg/kg 1-1½ hr before surgery
Available forms: Caps 15 mg; elix 20 mg/5 ml; tabs 8, 15, 30, 60, 100 mg; inj 30, 60, 65, 130 mg/ml
Side effects/adverse reactions:
CNS: Paradoxic excitement (elderly), drowsiness, lethargy, hangover headache, flushing, hallucinations, *coma*
GI: Nausea, vomiting, diarrhea, constipation
INTEG: Rash, urticaria, ***Stevens-Johnson syndrome, angioedema,*** local pain, swelling, necrosis, ***thrombophlebitis***
Contraindications: Hypersensitivity to barbiturates, porphyria, hepatic disease, respiratory disease, nephritis, hyperthyroidism, diabetes mellitus, elderly, lactation, pregnancy (D)
Precautions: Anemia
Do not confuse:
phenobarbital/pentobarbital
Pharmacokinetics:
IV: Onset 5 min, peak 30 min, duration 4-6 hr
IM/SC: Onset 10-30 min, duration 4-6 hr
PO: Onset 20-60 min, peak 8-12 hr, duration 6-10 hr
Metabolized by liver; crosses placenta; excreted in urine, breast milk; half-life 53-118 hr

---

⬥ = Nursing alert   ◢ = Herb-drug interaction   ⊘ = Do not crush

Interactions:

• Increased effects: CNS depression, alcohol, chloramphenicol, valproic acid, disulfiram, nondepolarizing skeletal muscle relaxants, sulfonamides

• Decreased effects: theophylline, oral anticoagulants, corticosteroids, metronidazole, doxycycline, quinidine

• Increased orthostatic hypotension: furosemide

🖉 Increased phenobarbital levels: quinine

NURSING CONSIDERATIONS
Assess:

• Mental status: mood, sensorium, affect, memory (long, short)

• For respiratory depression

• Blood dyscrasias: fever, sore throat, bruising, rash, jaundice

• Convulsion activity: type, duration, precipitating factors

• Blood studies, liver function tests during long-term treatment

• Therapeutic blood level periodically: 15-40 µg/ml

• Respiratory status: rate, rhythm, depth

Administer:

• IM inj deep in large muscle mass to prevent tissue sloughing; use <5 ml in each site

IV

• Slow IV after dilution with at least 10 ml sterile H_2O for inj regardless of dose; give 65 mg or less/min; titrate to patient response

Additive compatibilities: Amikacin, aminophylline, calcium chloride, calcium gluconate, cephapirin, colistimethate, dimenhydrinate, meropenem, polymyxin B, sodium bicarbonate, thiopental, verapamil

Solution compatibilities: D_5W, $D_{10}W$, 0.45% NaCl, 0.9% NaCl, Ringer's, dextrose/saline combinations, dextrose/Ringer's, dextrose/LR combinations, sodium lactate

Syringe compatibilities: Heparin

Y-site compatibilities: Enalaprilat, meropenem, propofol, sufentanil

Perform/provide:

• Supervision of ambulation for dizziness, drowsiness

Evaluate:

• Therapeutic response: decreased seizures, increased sedation

Teach patient/family:

• To use exactly as ordered

• To avoid other CNS depressants, including alcohol

• To avoid hazardous activities until stabilized on drug; drowsiness may occur

• Never to withdraw drug abruptly; withdrawal symptoms may occur

• That therapeutic effects (PO) may not be seen for 2-3 wk

Treatment of overdose: Lavage, activated charcoal, warming blanket, vital signs, hemodialysis, I&O ratio

---

RARELY USED

phenoxybenzamine (℞)

(fen-ox-ee-ben′za-meen)
Func. class.: Antihypertensive

P

Uses: Pheochromocytoma
Dosage and routes:

• *Adult:* PO 10 mg qd, increase by 10 mg qod, usual range: 20-40 mg bid-tid

• *Child:* PO 0.2 mg/kg or 6 mg/m^2/day, max 10 mg; may increase q4d; maintenance dose 0.4-1.2 mg/kg/day or 12-36 mg/m^2/day divided doses tid or qid

Contraindications: Hypersensitivity, CHF, angina, cerebral vascular insufficiency, coronary arteriosclerosis

---

RARELY USED

phentermine (R)
(fen'ter-meen)
Func. class.: Cerebral stimulant

Uses: Exogenous obesity
Dosage and routes:
• *Adult:* PO 8 mg tid 30 min before meals or 15-37.5 mg qd before breakfast

Contraindications: Hypersensitivity, hyperthyroidism, hypertension, glaucoma, severe arteriosclerosis, angina pectoris, cardiovascular disease, pregnancy (C), child <12 yr

---

phentolamine (R)
(fen-tole'a-meen)
Regitine, Rogitine*
Func. class.: Antihypertensive
Chem. class.: α-Adrenergic blocker

Action: α-Adrenergic blocker, binds to α-adrenergic receptors, dilating peripheral blood vessels, lowering peripheral resistances, lowering blood pressure
Uses: Hypertension, pheochromocytoma, prevention, treatment of dermal necrosis following extravasation of norepinephrine or dopamine, impotence
Dosage and routes:
Treatment of hypertensive episodes in pheochromocytoma
• *Adult:* IV/IM, 5 mg, repeat if necessary
• *Child:* IV/IM, 1 mg, repeat if necessary
Prevention, treatment of necrosis
• *Adult:* 5-10 mg/10 ml NS injected into area of norepinephrine extravasation within 12 hr
• *Child:* 0.1-0.2 mg/kg, max 10 mg

Available forms: Inj 5 mg/ml
Side effects/adverse reactions:
GI: Dry mouth, nausea, vomiting, diarrhea, abdominal pain
*CV: Hypotension, tachycardia, angina, dysrhythmias, **MI***
CNS: Dizziness, flushing, weakness, ***cerebrovascular spasm***
EENT: Nasal congestion
Contraindications: Hypersensitivity, MI, coronary insufficiency, angina
Precautions: Pregnancy (C), lactation
Pharmacokinetics:
IV: Peak 2 min, duration 10-15 min
IM: Peak 15-20 min, duration 3-4 hr
Metabolized in liver, excreted in urine
Interactions:
• Increased effects of epinephrine, antihypertensives
NURSING CONSIDERATIONS
Assess:
• Electrolytes: K, Na, Cl, CO_2; weight qd, I&O
• B/P lying, standing before starting treatment, q4h after
• Nausea, vomiting, diarrhea, edema in feet, legs daily; skin turgor, dryness of mucous membranes for hydration status, postural hypotension, cardiac system: pulse, ECG
Administer:
• Gum, frequent rinsing of mouth, or hard candy for dry mouth
• With vasopressor available
• After discontinuing all medication for 24 hr
IV
• After diluting 5 mg/1 ml sterile H_2O for inj; give 5 mg or less/min; patient to remain recumbent during administration
Cont Inf
• Dilute 5-10 mg/500 ml D_5W, titrate to patient response

• 10 mg/L may be added to norepinephrine in IV sol for prevention of dermal necrosis

Additive compatibilities: Dobutamine, verapamil

Syringe compatibilities: Papaverine

Y-site compatibilities: Amiodarone

Evaluate:

• Therapeutic response: decreased B/P

Teach patient/family:

• That bed rest is required during treatment, 1 hr after

Treatment of overdose: Administer norepinephrine; discontinue drug

---

phenylephrine (℞)

(fen-ill-ef′rin)

Neo-Synephrine

Func. class.: Adrenergic, direct-acting

Chem. class.: Substituted phenylethylamine

Action: Powerful and selective (α_1) receptor agonist causing contraction of blood vessels

Uses: Hypotension, paroxysmal supraventricular tachycardia, shock, maintain B/P for spinal anesthesia

Dosage and routes:

Hypotension

• *Adult:* **SC/IM** 2-5 mg, may repeat q10-15 min if needed, do not exceed initial dose; **IV** 0.1-0.5 mg, may repeat q10-15 min if needed, do not exceed initial dose

• *Child:* **IM/SC** 0.1 mg/kg/dose q1-2h prn

PVCs

• *Adult:* **IV BOL** 0.5 mg given rapidly, not to exceed prior dose by >0.1 mg, total dose >1 mg

Shock

• *Adult:* **IV INF** 10 mg/500 ml D_5W given 100-180 µg/min (if 20 gtt/ml inf device), then maintenance of 40-60 µg/min (if 20 gtt/ml inf device)

• *Child:* **IV BOL** 5-20 µg/kg/dose q10-15 min; **IV INF** 0.1-0.5 µg/kg/min

Available forms: Inj 1% (10 mg/ml)

Side effects/adverse reactions:

CNS: Headache, anxiety, tremor, insomnia, dizziness

*CV: Palpitations, tachycardia, hypertension, ectopic beats, angina, reflex bradycardia, **dysrhythmias***

GI: Nausea, vomiting

*INTEG: Necrosis, tissue sloughing with extravasation, **gangrene***

*SYST: **Anaphylaxis***

Contraindications: Hypersensitivity, ventricular fibrillation, tachydysrhythmias, pheochromocytoma, narrow-angle glaucoma

Precautions: Pregnancy (C), lactation, arterial embolism, peripheral vascular disease, elderly, hyperthyroidism, bradycardia, myocardial disease, severe arteriosclerosis

Pharmacokinetics:

IV: Duration 20-30 min

IM/SC: Duration 45-60 min

Interactions:

• Do not use within 2 wk of MAOIs, or hypertensive crisis may result

• Dysrhythmias: general anesthetics, bretylium

• Decreased action of phenylephrine: α-blockers

• Increase in B/P: oxytocics

• Increased pressor effect: tricyclics, MAOIs, guanethidine

NURSING CONSIDERATIONS

Assess:

• I&O ratio; notify prescriber if output <30 ml/hr

• ECG during administration continuously; if B/P increases, drug is decreased

• B/P and pulse q5min after parenteral route

• CVP or PWP during inf if possible

P

• For paresthesias and coldness of extremities; peripheral blood flow may decrease

Administer:

IV

• Plasma expanders for hypovolemia

• IV after diluting 1 mg/9 ml sterile H_2O for inj; give dose over ½-1 min; may be diluted 10 mg/500 ml of D_5W or NS; titrate to response (normal B/P); check for extravasation, check site for infiltration, use infusion pump

Additive compatibilities: Chloramphenicol, dobutamine, lidocaine, potassium chloride, sodium bicarbonate

Y-site compatibilities: Amiodarone, amrinone, cisatracurium, famotidine, haloperidol, remifentanil, zidovudine

Perform/provide:

• Storage of reconstituted sol if refrigerated for no longer than 24 hr

• Discard discolored sol

Evaluate:

• Therapeutic response: increased B/P with stabilization

Teach patient/family:

• The reason for administration

• To report pain at infusion site or other adverse reactions immediately

Treatment of overdose: Administer an α-blocker

---

phenytoin (R℞)

(fen'i-toh-in)

Dilantin, Dilantin Infatab, Dilantin Kapseals, Dilantin-125, diphenylhydantoin, Phenytex

Func. class.: Anticonvulsant; antidysrhythmic (IB)

Chem. class.: Hydantoin

Action: Inhibits spread of seizure activity in motor cortex by altering ion transport; increases AV conduction

Uses: Generalized tonic-clonic seizures; status epilepticus; nonepileptic seizures associated with Reye's syndrome or after head trauma; migraines, trigeminal neuralgia, Bell's palsy, ventricular dysrhythmics uncontrolled by antidysrhythmics

Research note: Increased dose of quetiapine may be necessary when used with phenytoin[33]

Dosage and routes:

Renal dose

• Do not use loading dose CrCl <10 ml/min or hepatic failure

Seizures

• *Adult:* PO 1 g or 20 mg/kg (ext rel) in 3-4 divided doses given q2h, or 400 mg, then 300 mg q2h × 2 doses, maintenance 300-400 mg/day, max 600 mg/day; IV 15-20 mg/kg, max 25-50 mg/min, then 100 mg q6-8h

• *Child:* PO 5 mg/kg/day in 2-3 divided doses, maintenance 4-8 mg/kg/day in 2-3 divided doses, max 300 mg/day; IV 15-20 mg/kg at 1-3 mg/kg/min

Status epilepticus

• *Adult:* IV 10-15 mg/kg, max 25-50 mg/min, may give 100 mg q6-8h thereafter

• *Child:* IV 15-20 mg/kg, max in divided doses 1-3 mg/kg/min

Neuritic pain

• *Adult:* PO 200-600 mg/day in divided doses

Ventricular dysrhythmias

• *Adult:* PO loading dose 1 g divided over 24 hr, then 500 mg/day × 2 days; IV 250 mg over 5 min until dysrhythmias subside or until 1 g is given, or 100 mg q15min until dysrhythmias subside or until 1 g given

• *Child:* PO 3-8 mg/kg or 250 mg/m^2/day as single dose or 2 divided doses; IV 3-8 mg/kg over several

◆ = Nursing alert   ✐ = Herb-drug interaction   ⊘ = Do not crush

min, or 250 mg/m^2/day as single dose or 2 divided doses

Available forms: Susp 30, 125 mg/5 ml; tabs, chewable 50 mg; inj 50 mg/ml; caps ext rel 30, 100 mg; caps prompt rel 30, 100 mg

Side effects/adverse reactions:

CNS: Drowsiness, dizziness, insomnia, paresthesias, depression, suicidal tendencies, aggression, headache, confusion, slurred speech

CV: Hypotension, ***ventricular fibrillation***

EENT: Nystagmus, diplopia, blurred vision

GI: Nausea, vomiting, constipation, anorexia, weight loss, *hepatitis,* jaundice, gingival hyperplasia

*GU: **Nephritis,*** urine discoloration

*HEMA: **Agranulocytosis, leukopenia, aplastic anemia, thrombocytopenia, megaloblastic anemia***

INTEG: Rash, ***lupus erythematosus, Stevens-Johnson syndrome,*** hirsutism

SYST: Hypocalcemia

Contraindications: Hypersensitivity, psychiatric condition, pregnancy (D), bradycardia, SA and AV block, Stokes-Adams syndrome, hepatic failure

Precautions: Allergies, hepatic disease, renal disease, elderly, petit mal seizures

Pharmacokinetics:

PO-ER: Onset 2-24 hr, peak 4-12 hr, duration 12-36 hr

IV: Onset 1-2 hr, duration 12-24 hr

PO: Onset 2-24 hr, peak 1½-2½ hr, duration 6-12 hr

Metabolized by liver, excreted by kidneys; highly protein-bound, half-life 22 hr

Interactions:

• Decreased effects of phenytoin: alcohol (chronic use), antihistamines, antacids, antineoplastics, CNS depressants, rifampin, folic acid

• Increased effect of phenytoin: low plasma albumin levels

/ Increased potassium loss, increased antidysrhythmic action: aloe, buckthorn, cascara sagrada, senna

Lab test interferences:

Decrease: Dexamethasone, metyrapone test serum, PBI, urinary steroids

Increase: Glucose, alk phosphatase, BSP

NURSING CONSIDERATIONS
Assess:

➡ For phenytoin hypersensitivity syndrome 3-12 wk after start of treatment: rash, temp, lymphadenopathy; may cause hepatotoxicity, renal failure, rhabdomyolysis

➡ For beginning rash that may lead to Stevens-Johnson syndrome or toxic epidermal necrolysis; phenytoin should not be used again

• Drug level: toxic level 30-50 µg/ml, ther level: 7.5-20 µg/ml, wait ≥1 wk to draw levels

• For seizures: duration, type, intensity precipitating factors

• Blood studies: CBC, platelets q2wk until stabilized, then qmo × 12, then q3mo; discontinue drug if neutrophils <1600/mm^3; renal function: albumin conc

• Mental status: mood, sensorium, affect, memory (long, short)

• Respiratory depression; rate, depth, character

• Blood dyscrasias: fever, sore throat, bruising, rash, jaundice

Administer:

• Do not interchange chewable product with caps, not equivalent

• Shake susp well before each dose G tube/NG tube: dilute susp prior to administration, flush tube with 20 ml H$_2$O after dose

IV

• After diluting with diluent provided (2.2 ml/100 mg, 5.2 ml/250 mg, 1 ml/50 mg); shake; place vial

P

in warm water to dissolve powder; give through Y-tube or 3-way stopcock; inject slowly <50 mg/min; clear IV tubing first with NS sol; use in-line filter; discard 4 hr after preparation; inject into large veins to prevent purple glove syndrome

Additive compatibilities: Bleomycin, sodium bicarbonate, verapamil

Y-site compatibilities: Esmolol, famotidine, fluconazole, foscarnet, tacrolimus

Evaluate:

• Therapeutic response; decrease in severity of seizures, ventricular dysrhythmias

Teach patient/family:

• To take PO doses divided with or after meals to decrease adverse effects

• That if diabetic, urine glucose should be monitored

• That urine may turn pink

• Not to discontinue drug abruptly; seizures may occur

• Proper brushing of teeth using a soft toothbrush, flossing to prevent gingival hyperplasia; need to see dentist frequently

• To avoid hazardous activities until stabilized on drug

• To carry Medic Alert ID stating drug use

• That heavy use of alcohol may diminish effect of drug; to avoid OTC medications; not to use antacids or antidiarrheals within 2 hr of this product

• Not to change brands or forms once stabilized on therapy; brands may vary

---

RARELY USED

physostigmine (℞)

(fi-zoe-stig'meen)

Antilirium

Func. class.: Antidote, reversible anticholinesterase

Uses: To reverse CNS effects of diazepam; anticholinergic, tricyclics, Alzheimer's disease, hereditary ataxia

Dosage and routes:

Overdose of anticholinergics

• *Adult:* **IM/IV** 2 mg; give no more than 1 mg/min; may repeat

• *Child:* **IM/IV** inj 0.02 mg/kg, not more than 0.5 mg/min; may repeat at 5-10 min intervals until max dose of 2 mg

Postanesthesia

• *Adult:* **IM/IV** 0.5-1 mg; give no more than 1 mg/min **(IV)**; can repeat at 10 to 30 min intervals

Contraindications: Hypotension, obstruction of intestine or renal system, asthma, gangrene, CV disease, choline esters, depolarizing neuromuscular blocking agents, diabetes

---

phytonadione (vit K₁) (℞)

(fye-toe-na-dye'one)

AquaMEPHYTON, Konakion, Mephyton

Func. class.: Vit K₁, fat-soluble vitamin

Action: Needed for adequate blood clotting (factors II, VII, IX, X)

Uses: Vit K malabsorption, hypoprothrombinemia, prevention of hypoprothrombinemia caused by oral anticoagulants, prevention of hemorrhagic disease of the newborn

---

◆ = Nursing alert   ∥ = Herb-drug interaction   ⊘ = Do not crush

Dosage and routes:
Hypoprothrombinemia caused by vit K malabsorption
• *Adult:* **PO/IM** 2.5-25 mg, may repeat or increase to 50 mg
• *Child:* **PO/IM** 5-10 mg
• *Infant:* **PO/IM** 2 mg
Prevention of hemorrhagic disease of the newborn
• *Neonate:* **IM** 0.5-1 mg within 1 hr after birth, repeat in 2-3 wk if required
Hypoprothrombinemia caused by oral anticoagulants
• *Adult and child:* **PO/SC/IM** 2.5-10 mg, may repeat 12-48 hr after **PO** dose or 6-8 hr after **SC/IM** dose, based on PT
Available forms: Tabs 5 mg; inj 2 mg, 10 ml aqueous colloidal; inj aqueous dispersion 10 mg/ml, (IM)
Side effects/adverse reactions:
CNS: Headache, ***brain damage*** (large doses)
GI: Nausea, decreased LFTs
HEMA: ***Hemolytic anemia, hemoglobinuria, hyperbilirubinemia***
INTEG: Rash, urticaria
Contraindications: Hypersensitivity, severe hepatic disease, last few wk of pregnancy
Precautions: Pregnancy (C), neonates
Pharmacokinetics:
PO/INJ: Metabolized, crosses placenta
Interactions:
• Decreased action of phytonadione: cholestyramine, mineral oil
• Decreased action of oral anticoagulants
NURSING CONSIDERATIONS
Assess:
• For bleeding: emesis, stools, urine
• PT during treatment (2-sec deviation from control time, bleeding time, and clotting time); monitor for bleeding, pulse, and B/P

• Nutritional status: liver (beef), spinach, tomatoes, coffee, asparagus, broccoli, cabbage, lettuce, greens
Administer:
IV
• After diluting with D₅NS 10 ml or more; give 1 mg/min or more
◆ IV only when other routes not possible (deaths have occurred)
Additive compatibilities: Amikacin, calcium gluceptate, cephapirin, chloramphenicol, cimetidine, netilmicin, sodium bicarbonate
Syringe compatibilities: Doxapram
Y-site compatibilities: Ampicillin, epinephrine, famotidine, heparin, hydrocortisone, potassium chloride, tolazoline, vit B/C
Perform/provide:
• Storage in tight, light-resistant container
Evaluate:
• Therapeutic response: decreased bleeding tendencies, decreased PT, decreased clotting time
Teach patient/family:
• Not to take other supplements unless directed by prescriber
• The necessary foods for diet
• To avoid IM injections, use soft toothbrush, don't floss, use electric razor until coagulation defect corrected
• To report symptoms of bleeding
• Not to use OTC medications unless approved by prescriber
• The importance of frequent lab tests to monitor coagulation factors

RARELY USED

pinacidil (℞)
(pye-na′si-dill)
Func. class.: Antihypertensive

Uses: Severe hypertension not responsive to other therapy
Dosage and routes:
• *Adult:* **PO** 12.5-25 mg bid
Contraindications: Acute MI, dissecting aortic aneurysm, hypersensitivity, pheochromocytoma

pindolol (℞)
(pin′doe-lole)
Novo-Pindol*, Syn-Pindolol*,
Visken
Func. class.: Antihypertensive
Chem. class.: Nonselective β-blocker

Action: Competitively blocks stimulation of β-adrenergic receptor within vascular smooth muscle; decreases rate of SA node discharge, increases recovery time, slows conduction of AV node, decreases heart rate, which decreases O_2 consumption in myocardium; also decreases renin-aldosterone-angiotensin system, at high doses inhibits $β_2$ receptors in bronchial system
Uses: Mild to moderate hypertension
Investigational uses: angina pectoris
Dosage and routes:
• *Adult:* **PO** 5 mg bid, usual dose 15 mg/day (5 mg tid), may increase by 10 mg/day q3-4wk to a max of 60 mg/day
• *Geriatric:* **PO** 5 mg qd, increase by 5 mg q3-4wk
Available forms: Tabs 5, 10 mg

Side effects/adverse reactions:
CV: Hypotension, bradycardia, ***CHF,*** edema, chest pain, palpitation, claudication, tachycardia, *AV block*
CNS: Insomnia, *dizziness,* hallucinations, anxiety, fatigue
GI: Nausea, vomiting, ***ischemic colitis,*** diarrhea, *abdominal pain,* ***mesenteric arterial thrombosis***
INTEG: Rash, alopecia, pruritus, fever
HEMA: ***Agranulocytosis, thrombocytopenia, purpura***
EENT: Visual changes, sore throat, *double vision;* dry, burning eyes
GU: Impotence, urinary frequency
RESP: ***Bronchospasm,*** *dyspnea,* cough, rales
MISC: Joint pain, muscle pain
Contraindications: Hypersensitivity to β-blockers, cardiogenic shock; 2nd, 3rd degree heart block; sinus bradycardia, CHF, cardiac failure, bronchial asthma
Precautions: Major surgery, pregnancy (B), lactation, diabetes mellitus, renal disease, thyroid disease, COPD, well-compensated heart failure, CAD, nonallergic bronchospasm
Do not confuse:
pindolol/Parlodel
pindolol/Plendil
Pharmacokinetics:
PO: Peak 2-4 wk; half-life 3-4 hr, excreted 30%-45% unchanged; 60%-65% metabolized by liver; excreted in breast milk; protein binding 40%
Interactions:
• Increased hypotension, bradycardia: reserpine, hydralazine, methyldopa, prazosin, anticholinergics
• Decreased antihypertensive effects: NSAIDs, sympathomimetics, thyroid
• Increased hypoglycemic effect: insulin, oral hypoglycemics

⬧ = Nursing alert   🖋 = Herb-drug interaction   🚫 = Do not crush

• Decreased bronchodilation: theophyllines, β₂-agonists

Lab test interferences:

Increase: LFTs, renal function tests

NURSING CONSIDERATIONS

Assess:

• I&O, weight qd

• B/P during initial treatment, periodically thereafter; pulse q4h, note rate, rhythm, quality; apical, radial pulse before administration; notify prescriber of any significant changes

• Baselines in renal, liver function tests before therapy begins

• Skin turgor, dryness of mucous membranes for hydration status; edema in feet, legs qd

Administer:

• PO ac, hs; tablet may be crushed or swallowed whole

• Reduced dosage in renal dysfunction

Perform/provide:

• Storage in dry area at room temperature; do not freeze

Evaluate:

• Therapeutic response: decreased B/P after 1-2 wk

Teach patient/family:

• To take with or immediately after meals

• Not to discontinue drug abruptly; taper over 2 wk; may cause precipitate angina

• Not to use OTC products containing α-adrenergic stimulants (nasal decongestants, OTC cold preparations) unless directed by prescriber

• To report bradycardia, dizziness, confusion, depression, fever, sore throat, shortness of breath to prescriber

• To take pulse at home; to notify prescriber if pulse <60 bpm

• To avoid alcohol, smoking, Na

• To comply with weight control, dietary adjustments, modified exercise program

• To carry Medic Alert ID to identify drug, allergies

• To avoid hazardous activities if dizziness is present

• To report symptoms of CHF: difficult breathing, especially on exertion or when lying down, night cough, swelling of extremities

• To take medication at bedtime to prevent orthostatic hypotension

• To wear support hose to minimize effects of orthostatic hypotension

Treatment of overdose: Lavage, IV atropine for bradycardia, IV theophylline for bronchospasm, digitalis, O₂, diuretic for cardiac failure, hemodialysis, hypotension; give vasopressor (norepinephrine)

---

pioglitazone (℞)

(pie-oh-glye'ta-zone)

Actos

Func. class.: Antidiabetic, oral

Chem. class.: Thiazolidinedione

Action: Improves insulin resistance by hepatic glucose metabolism, insulin receptor kinase activity, insulin receptor phosphorylation

Uses: Stable adult-onset diabetes mellitus (type II) NIDDM

Dosage and routes:

Monotherapy

• *Adult:* **PO** 15-30 qd, may increase to 45 mg/day

Combination therapy

• *Adult:* **PO** 15-30 mg qd with a sulfonylurea, metformin, or insulin. Decrease sulfonylurea dose if hypoglycemia occurs. Decrease insulin dose by 10%-25% if hypoglycemia occurs or if plasma glucose is <100 mg/dl, max 45 mg/day

Hepatic dose

• Do not use in active liver disease or if ALT >2.5 times ULN

Available forms: Tabs 15, 30, 45 mg
Side effects/adverse reactions:
MISC: Myalgia, sinusitis, URI, pharyngitis
CNS: Headache
ENDO: Aggravated diabetes mellitus
Contraindications: Hypersensitivity to thiazolidinedione, lactation, children, diabetic ketoacidosis
Precautions: Pregnancy (C), elderly, thyroid disease, hepatic, renal disease, edema, CHF
Pharmacokinetics: Maximal reduction in FBS after 12 wk; half-life 3-7 hr, terminal 16-24 hr
Interactions:
• Decreased effect of: oral contraceptives, use an alternative contraceptive method
• Decreased effort of pioglitazone: ketoconazole
NURSING CONSIDERATIONS
Assess:
• For hypoglycemic reactions (sweating, weakness, dizziness, anxiety, tremors, hunger), hyperglycemic reactions soon after meals
• CBC (baseline, q3mo) during treatment; check LFTs periodically AST, LDH, renal studies: BUN, creatinine, urinary glucose
• FBS, glycosylated Hgb, fasting plasma insulin, plasma lipids/lipoproteins, B/P, body weight during treatment
Administer:
• Once a day; give with meals to decrease GI upset and provide best absorption
• Tabs crushed and mixed with food or fluids for patients with difficulty swallowing
Perform/provide:
• Conversion from other oral hypoglycemic agents; change may be made without gradual dosage change; monitor serum or urine glucose and ketones tid during conversion
• Storage in tight container in cool environment
Teach patient/family:
• To use capillary blood glucose test or Chemstrip tid; that periodic LFTs are mandatory
• The symptoms of hypo/hyperglycemia, what to do about each
• That the drug must be continued on daily basis; explain consequence of discontinuing drug abruptly
• To avoid OTC medications or herbal preparations unless approved by prescriber
• That diabetes is lifelong illness; that this drug is not a cure; only controls symptoms
• That all food included in diet plan must be eaten to prevent hypoglycemia
• To carry Medic Alert ID and glucagon emergency kit for emergencies
• To notify prescriber if oral contraceptives are used
• Not to use if breast-feeding
Evaluate:
• Therapeutic response: Decrease in polyuria, polydipsia, polyphagia; clear sensorium; absence of dizziness; stable gait, blood glucose at normal level

---

pipecuronium (R)
(pip-e-kyoor-oh'nee-um)
Arduran
Func. class.: Neuromuscular blocker (nondepolarizing)
Chem. class.: Synthetic curariform
Action: Inhibits transmission of nerve impulses by binding with cho-

---

 = Nursing alert   = Herb-drug interaction   🚫 = Do not crush

linergic receptor sites, antagonizing action of acetylcholine

Uses: Facilitation of endotracheal intubation; skeletal muscle relaxation during mechanical ventilation, surgery, or general anesthesia

Dosage and routes:
• *Adult:* IV dosage is individualized; in patients with normal renal function who are not obese, initial dose is 70-85 µg/kg; maintenance dose ranges from 10-15 µg/kg
• *Child 1-14 yr:* IV 57 µg/kg
• *Child 3 mo-1 yr:* IV 40 µg/kg

Available forms: Inj 10 mg vials

Side effects/adverse reactions:
CV: Bradycardia, tachycardia, increased or decreased B/P, ventricular extrasystole, ***myocardial ischemia, cardiovascular accident, thrombosis, atrial fibrillation***
RESP: ***Prolonged apnea, bronchospasm, cyanosis, respiratory depression***
GU: ***Anuria***
EENT: Increased secretions
CNS: Hypesthesia, CNS depression
MS: Weakness to prolonged skeletal muscle relaxation
INTEG: Rash, urticaria
META: Hypoglycemia, hyperkalemia, increased creatinine

Contraindications: Hypersensitivity to bromide ion

Precautions: Pregnancy (C), renal disease, cardiac disease, lactation, children <3 mo, fluid and electrolyte imbalances, neuromuscular diseases, respiratory disease, obesity

Pharmacokinetics:
IV: Onset 30-45 sec, peak 3-5 min: metabolized (small amounts), excreted in urine (unchanged), crosses placenta

Interactions:
• Increased neuromuscular blockade: aminoglycosides, quinidine, local anesthetics, polymyxin antibiotics, enflurane, isoflurane, tetracyclines, halothane, magnesium, colistin

NURSING CONSIDERATIONS
Assess:
• For electrolyte imbalances (K, Mg); may lead to increased action of this drug
• Vital signs (B/P, pulse, respirations, airway) until fully recovered; rate, depth, pattern of respirations; strength of hand grip
• I&O ratio; check for urinary retention, frequency, hesitancy
• Recovery: decreased paralysis of face, diaphragm, leg, arm, rest of body
• Allergic reactions: rash, fever, respiratory distress, pruritus; drug should be discontinued

Administer:
• Using nerve stimulator by anesthesiologist to determine neuromuscular blockade
• Atropine to counteract muscarinic effects
• After succinylcholine effects subside
• Anticholinesterase to reverse neuromuscular blockade
IV
• By slow IV over 1-2 min (only by qualified persons, usually an anesthesiologist)
• Only fresh sol

Perform/provide:
• Storage in refrigerator; do not store in plastic container or syringe
• Reassurance if communication is difficult during recovery from neuromuscular blockade
• Use of reconstituted sol within 24 hr or discard
• Frequent (q2h) instillation of artificial tears and covering eyes to prevent drying of cornea

P

Evaluate:
• Therapeutic response: paralysis of jaw, eyelid, head, neck, rest of body
Treatment of overdose: Neostigmine, atropine; monitor VS; may require mechanical ventilation

---

piperacillin (R)

(pip′er-ah-sill′in)
Pipracil
Func. class.: Broad-spectrum antiinfective
Chem. class.: Extended-spectrum penicillin

Action: Interferes with cell wall replication of susceptible organisms; osmotically unstable cell wall swells and bursts from osmotic pressure
Uses: Respiratory, skin, urinary tract, bone infections; gonorrhea; pneumonia; effective for gram-positive cocci *(Staphylococcus aureus, Streptococcus pyogenes, Streptococcus viridans, Streptococcus faecalis, Streptococcus bovis, Streptococcus pneumoniae),* gram-negative cocci *(Neisseria gonorrhoeae, Neisseria meningitidis),* gram-positive bacilli *(Acinetobacter, Clostridium perfringens, Clostridium tetani),* gram-negative bacilli *(Bacteroides, Citrobacter, Enterobacter, Escherichia coli, Eubacterium, Fusobacterium nucleatum, Klebsiella, Morganella morganii, Peptococcus, Peptostreptococcus, Proteus mirabilis, Proteus vulgaris, Providencia rettgeri, Pseudomonas aeruginosa, Serratia)*
Dosage and routes:
Renal dose
• CrCl 20-40 ml/min give q8h; CrCl <20 ml/min give q12h; CrCl 10-50 ml/min give q6-8h; CrCl <10 ml/min give q8h

Urinary tract infections
• *Adult:* IV 8-16 g/day (125-200 mg/kg/day) in divided doses q6-8h
Serious systemic infections
• *Adult and child >12 yr:* **IM/IV** 2-4 g q4-6h (2 g/site **IM**)
• *Child <12 yr:* **IM/IV** 200-300 mg/kg/day in divided doses q4-6h
• *Neonates <36 wk:* **IV** 75 mg/kg q12h in the 1st wk of life, then q8h in 2nd wk
• *Full-term infants:* **IV** 75 mg/kg q8h in 1st wk of life; q6h thereafter
Prophylaxis of surgical infections
• *Adult:* **IV** 2 g ½-1 hr before procedure; may be repeated during surgery or after surgery
Available forms: Pwd for inj 2, 3, 4, 40 g
Side effects/adverse reactions:
HEMA: Anemia, increased bleeding time, *bone marrow depression,* thrombocytopenia
GI: Nausea, vomiting, diarrhea; increased AST, ALT; abdominal pain, glossitis, *pseudomembranous colitis*
GU: *Oliguria, proteinuria, hematuria,* vaginitis, moniliasis, *glomerulonephritis*
CNS: Lethargy, hallucinations, anxiety, depression, twitching, *coma, seizures*
META: Hypokalemia, hypernatremia
SYST: *Serum sickness, anaphylaxis*
Contraindications: Hypersensitivity to penicillins
Precautions: Pregnancy (B), lactation, hypersensitivity to cephalosporins; CHF, renal disease, seizures
Pharmacokinetics:
IM: Peak 30-50 min
IV: Peak 20-30 min
Half-life 0.7-1.33 hr; excreted in urine, bile, breast milk; crosses placenta
Interactions:
• Decreased antimicrobial effect of

⬥ = Nursing alert   〃 = Herb-drug interaction   🚫 = Do not crush piperacillin: tetracyclines (with high concentrations of piperacillin), aminoglycosides

• Increased piperacillin concentrations: aspirin, probenecid

🖉 Delayed/reduced absorption: khat, separate by ≥2 hr:

Lab test interferences:

False positive: Urine glucose, urine protein, Coombs' test

NURSING CONSIDERATIONS
Assess:

• For infection: temp, WBC, sputum, stools, urine, wounds

• I&O ratio; report hematuria, oliguria, since penicillin in high doses is nephrotoxic

◆ Any patient with compromised renal system, since drug is excreted slowly in poor renal system function; toxicity may occur rapidly

• Liver studies: AST, ALT

• Blood studies: WBC, RBC, Hgb, Hct, bleeding time prior to and periodically during treatment

• Renal studies: urinalysis, protein, blood, BUN, creatinine prior to and periodically during treatment

• C&S before drug therapy; drug may be taken as soon as culture is taken

• Bowel pattern before and during treatment

• Skin eruptions after administration of penicillin to 1 wk after discontinuing drug

• Respiratory status: rate, character, wheezing, tightness in chest

• Allergies before initiation of treatment, reaction of each medication

Administer:

• Drug after C&S completed

IM

• 2 g/4 ml, 3 g/6 ml, 4 g/8 ml of sterile water, 0.9% NaCl max 2 g/site

IV

• After diluting 1 g or less/5 ml or more sterile H_2O or 0.9% NaCl; shake; give dose over 3-5 min; may

further dilute to 50-100 ml with D_5W, 0.9% NS, and give over ½ hr; discontinue primary IV

Additive compatibilities: Ciprofloxacin, clindamycin, flucloxacillin, fluconazole, hydrocortisone, ofloxacin, potassium chloride, verapamil

Syringe compatibilities: Heparin

Y-site compatibilities: Acyclovir, allopurinol, amifostine, aztreonam, ciprofloxacin, cyclophosphamide, diltiazem, doxorubicin liposome, enalaprilat, esmolol, famotidine, fludarabine, foscarnet, gallium, granisetron, heparin, hydromorphone, IL-2, labetalol, lorazepam, magnesium sulfate, melphalan, meperidine, midazolam, morphine, perphenazine, propofol, ranitidine, remifentanil, tacrolimus, teniposide, theophylline, thiotepa, verapamil, zidovudine

Perform/provide:

• Adrenaline, suction, tracheostomy set, endotracheal intubation equipment on unit

• Adequate intake of fluids (2 L) during diarrhea episodes

• Scratch test to assess allergy after securing order from prescriber; usually done when penicillin is only drug of choice

• Storage of reconstituted sol 24 hr at room temperature or 7 days refrigerated

Evaluate:

• Therapeutic response: absence of fever, purulent drainage, redness, inflammation

Teach patient/family:

• That culture may be taken after completed course of medication

• To report sore throat, fever, fatigue; may indicate superinfection

• To wear or carry Medic Alert ID if allergic to penicillins

• To notify nurse of diarrhea

Treatment of anaphylaxis: Withdraw drug, maintain airway, administer epinephrine, aminophylline, O_2, IV corticosteroids

---

piperacillin/ tazobactam (℞)

(pip'er-ah-sill'in & ta-zoe-bak'tam)

Zosyn

Func. class.: Antiinfective, broad-spectrum

Chem. class.: Extended-spectrum penicillin, β-lactamase inhibitor

Action: Interferes with cell wall replication of susceptible organisms; osmotically unstable cell wall swells and bursts from osmotic pressure

Uses: Moderate to severe infections: piperacillin-resistant, β-lactamase-producing strains causing infections in respiratory, skin, urinary tract, bone, gonorrhea, pneumonia; effective for resistant *Staphylococcus aureus,* resistant *Escherichia coli, Bacteroides fragilis, Bacteroides ovatus, Bacteroides thetaiotaomicron, Bacteroides vulgatus, Haemophilus influenzae*

Dosage and routes:

Renal dose

• CrCl 20-40 ml/min give 2.25 g q6h; CrCl <20 ml/min give 2.25 g q8h

Nosocomial pneumonia

• *Adult:* 3.375g q6-8h with an aminoglycoside × 1-2 wk; continue aminoglycoside only if *Pseudomonas aeruginosa* is isolated

Other infections

• *Adult:* **IV INF** 6-12 g/day given 2.25 g q8h to 3.375 g q6h over 30 min × 7-10 days

Available forms: Pwd for inj 2 g piperacillin/0.25 g tazobactam, 3 g piperacillin/0.375 g tazobactam, 4 g piperacillin/0.5 g tazobactam, 36 g piperacillin/4.5 g tazobactam

Side effects/adverse reactions:

CNS: Lethargy, hallucinations, anxiety, depression, twitching, *coma, seizures,* insomnia, headache, fever, dizziness

GI: Nausea, vomiting, diarrhea; increased AST, ALT; abdominal pain, glossitis, *pseudomembranous colitis,* constipation

GU: Oliguria, proteinuria, hematuria, vaginitis, moniliasis, glomerulonephritis

HEMA: Anemia, increased bleeding time, *bone marrow depression*

META: Hypokalemia, hypernatremia

CV: Hypertension

INTEG: Rash, pruritus

SYST: Serum sickness, anaphylaxis

Contraindications: Hypersensitivity to penicillins, neonates

Precautions: Pregnancy (B), lactation, hypersensitivity to cephalosporins, CHF, renal insufficiency in children, seizures

Pharmacokinetics:

IV: Peak completion of IV, duration 6 hr

Half-life 0.7-1.2 hr; excreted in urine, bile, breast milk; crosses placenta; 33% bound to plasma proteins

Interactions:

• Increased effect of neuromuscular blockers, heparin

• Decreased antimicrobial effect of piperacillin: tetracyclines, aminoglycosides IV

• Increased piperacillin concentrations: aspirin, probenecid

🖊 Delayed/reduced absorption: khat, separate by ≥2 hr

Lab test interferences:

False positive: Urine glucose, urine protein, Coombs' test

Decrease: Hct, Hgb, electrolytes

Increase: Platelet count, eosino-

---

philia, neutropenia, leukopenia, serum creatinine, PTT, AST, ALT, alk phosphatase, bilirubin, BUN, electrolytes

NURSING CONSIDERATIONS
Assess:
• For infection: temp, stools, urine, sputum, wounds
• I&O ratio; report hematuria, oliguria, since penicillin in high doses is nephrotoxic

⬧ Any patient with compromised renal system, since drug is excreted slowly in poor renal system function; toxicity may occur rapidly
• Liver studies: AST, ALT prior to and periodically thereafter
• Blood studies: WBC, RBC, Hct, Hgb, bleeding time prior to and periodically thereafter
• Renal studies: urinalysis, protein, blood, BUN, creatinine prior to and periodically thereafter
• C&S before drug therapy; drug may be given as soon as culture is taken
• Bowel pattern before and during treatment
• Skin eruptions after administration of penicillin to 1 wk after discontinuing drug
• Respiratory status: rate, character, wheezing, tightness in chest
• Allergies before initiation of treatment, reaction of each medication

Administer:
• Drug after C&S is complete

IV
• After diluting 5 ml 0.9% NaCl for injection or sterile H_2O for injection, dextran 6% in NS, dextrose 5%, KCl 40 mEq, bacteriostatic saline/parabens, bacteriostatic saline/benzyl alcohol, bacteriostatic H_2O/benzyl alcohol per 1 g piperacillin; shake well; further dilute in at least 50 ml compatible IV sol and run as int inf over at least 30 min

Y-site compatibilities: Aminoph-

ylline, aztreonam, bleomycin, bumetanide, buprenorphine, butorphanol, calcium gluconate, carboplatin, carmustine, cefepime, cimetidine, clindamycin, cyclophosphamide, cytarabine, dexamethasone, diphenhydramine, dopamine, enalaprilat, etoposide, floxuridine, fluconazole, fludarabine, fluorouracil, furosemide, gallium, granisetron, heparin, hydrocortisone, hydromorphone, ifosfamide, leucovorin, lorazepam, magnesium sulfate, mannitol, meperidine, mesna, methotrexate, methylprednisolone, metoclopramide, metronidazole, morphine, ondansetron, plicamycin, potassium chloride, ranitidine, remifentanil, sargramostim, sodium bicarbonate, thiotepa, trimethoprim-sulfamethoxazole, vinblastine, vincristine, zidovudine

Perform/provide:
• Adrenaline, suction, tracheostomy set, endotracheal intubation equipment on unit
• Adequate intake of fluids (2 L) during diarrhea episodes
• Scratch test to assess allergy on order from prescriber; usually when penicillin is only drug of choice
• Discard after 24 hr if stored at room temperature or after 48 hr if refrigerated; use single-dose vials immediately after reconstitution; stable in ambulatory IV pump for 12 hr

Evaluate:
• Therapeutic response: absence of fever, purulent drainage, redness, inflammation; culture shows decreased organisms

Teach patient/family:
• That culture may be taken after completed course of medication
• To report sore throat, fever, fatigue (may indicate superinfection)
• To wear or carry Medic Alert ID if allergic to penicillins
• To notify nurse of diarrhea

Treatment of overdose: Withdraw drug, maintain airway, administer epinephrine, aminophylline, O₂, IV corticosteroids for anaphylaxis

---

pirbuterol (℞)

(peer-byoo'ter-ole)
Maxair
Func. class.: Bronchodilator
Chem. class.: β-Adrenergic agonist

Action: Causes bronchodilation with little effect on heart rate by action on β-receptors, causing increased cAMP and relaxation of smooth muscle

Uses: Reversible bronchospasm (prevention, treatment) including asthma; may be given with theophylline or steroids

Dosage and routes:
• *Adult and child >12 yr:* **INH** 1-2 puffs (0.4 mg) q4-6h; max 12 **INH/** day

Available forms: Aerosol delivery 0.2 mg pirbuterol/actuation

Side effects/adverse reactions:
CNS: Tremors, anxiety, insomnia, headache, dizziness, stimulation, restlessness, hallucinations, drowsiness, irritability
EENT: Dry nose and mouth, irritation of nose, throat
CV: Palpitations, tachycardia, hypertension, angina, hypotension, dysrhythmias
GI: Gastritis, nausea, vomiting, anorexia
MS: Muscle cramps
RESP: **Paradoxical bronchospasm,** dyspnea, coughing

Contraindications: Hypersensitivity to sympathomimetics, tachycardia

Precautions: Lactation, pregnancy (C), cardiac disorders, hyperthyroidism, diabetes mellitus, prostatic hypertrophy

Pharmacokinetics:
INH: Onset 3 min, peak ½-1 hr, duration 5 hr

Interactions:
• Increased action of other aerosol bronchodilators
• Increased action of pirbuterol: tricyclic antidepressants, antihistamines, levothyroxine
• Decreased action of pirbuterol: β-blockers
◆ Hypertensive crisis: MAOIs
⚫ Increased action of both: ephedra

NURSING CONSIDERATIONS
Assess:
• Respiratory function: vital capacity, forced expiratory volume, ABGs, B/P, lung sounds, pulse, characteristics of sputum
◆ Paradoxical bronchospasm, that can occur rapidly, hold drug, notify prescriber

Administer:
• After shaking; exhale, place mouthpiece in mouth, inhale slowly, hold breath, remove, exhale slowly
• Gum, sips of water for dry mouth

Perform/provide:
• Storage in light-resistant container; do not expose to temperatures over 86° F (30° C)

Evaluate:
• Therapeutic response: absence of dyspnea, wheezing over 1 hr

Teach patient/family:
• Not to use OTC medications; extra stimulation may occur
• Use of inhaler; review package insert with patient
• To avoid getting aerosol in eyes
• To wash inhaler in warm water and dry qd, rinse mouth after use; if used with inhalers containing glucocorticosteroids, wait 5 min before using steroid inhaler
• About all aspects of drug; avoid

◆ = Nursing alert   ⚫ = Herb-drug interaction   ⊘ = Do not crush smoking, smoke-filled rooms, persons with respiratory infections

• To keep fluid intake >2 L/day to liquefy thick secretions

Treatment of overdose: Administer a β-adrenergic blocker

---

piroxicam (R)

(peer-ox'i-kam)
Apo-Piroxicam*, Feldene, Novopirocam*, Nu-Pirox, PMS-Piroxicam

Func. class.: Nonsteroidal antiinflammatory

Chem. class.: Oxicam derivative

Action: Inhibits prostaglandin synthesis by decreasing an enzyme needed for biosynthesis; has analgesic, antiinflammatory, antipyretic properties

Uses: Mild to moderate pain, osteoarthritis, rheumatoid arthritis

Dosage and routes:

• *Adult:* **PO** 20 mg qd or 10 mg bid

Available forms: Caps 10, 20 mg

Side effects/adverse reactions:

GI: Nausea, anorexia, vomiting, diarrhea, jaundice, *cholestatic hepatitis,* constipation, flatulence, cramps, dry mouth, peptic ulcer, *bleeding, ulceration, perforation*

CNS: Dizziness, *drowsiness,* fatigue, tremors, confusion, insomnia, anxiety, depression, *headache*

CV: Tachycardia, peripheral edema, palpitations, dysrhythmias

INTEG: Purpura, rash, pruritus, sweating, photosensitivity

GU: Nephrotoxicity: dysuria, hematuria, oliguria, azotemia

HEMA: Blood dyscrasias

EENT: Tinnitus, hearing loss, blurred vision

Contraindications: Hypersensitivity, asthma, severe renal disease, severe hepatic disease, ulcer disease, cardiac disease

Precautions: Pregnancy (B), lactation, children, bleeding disorders, GI disorders, cardiac disorders, hypersensitivity to other antiinflammatory agents, CHF

Pharmacokinetics:

PO: Peak 2 hr; duration 48-72 hr, half-life 30-80 hr; metabolized in liver; excreted in urine (metabolites), breast milk; 99% protein binding

Interactions:

• Increased toxicity: cyclosporine, methotrexate, lithium, alcohol, oral anticoagulants, aspirin, corticosteroids

• Decreased effects of: antihypertensives, diuretics

• Hypoglycemia: oral antidiabetics

NURSING CONSIDERATIONS

Assess:

• For pain: location, duration, type, ROM before and 1-2 hr after administration

• Renal, liver, blood studies: BUN, creatinine, AST, ALT, Hgb, before treatment, periodically thereafter

• Audiometric, ophthalmic exam before, during, after treatment

• For eye, ear problems: blurred vision, tinnitus (may indicate toxicity)

◆ Those with aspirin sensitivity, asthma, nasal polyps may develop allergic reactions

Administer:

• With food to decrease GI symptoms; take on empty stomach to facilitate absorption; take drug same time qd

Perform/provide:

• Storage at room temperature

Evaluate:

• Therapeutic response: decreased pain, stiffness, swelling in joints; ability to move more easily

---

Side effects: *italics* = common; *bold italics* = life-threatening

Teach patient/family:

🚫 Not to break, crush, or chew caps

• To report blurred vision or ringing, roaring in ears (may indicate toxicity)

• To avoid driving, other hazardous activities if dizzy or drowsy

• That patient should drink at least 6-8 glasses of water/day

• To report change in urine pattern, weight increase, edema, pain increase in joints, fever, blood in urine (indicates nephrotoxicity)

• That therapeutic effects may take up to 1 mo

• To avoid ASA, other OTC meds, alcohol; advise patient to use sunscreen

---

plasma protein fraction (℞)

Plasmanate, Plasma Plex, Plasmatein, Protenate

Func. class.: Blood derivative

Chem. class.: Human plasma in NaCl

Action: Exerts similar oncotic pressure as human plasma, expands blood volume

Uses: Hypovolemic shock, hypoproteinemia, ARDS, preoperative cardiopulmonary bypass, acute liver failure, nephrotic syndrome

Dosage and routes:

Hypovolemia

• *Adult:* **IV INF** 250-500 ml (12.5-25 g protein), not to exceed 10 ml/min

• *Child:* **IV INF** 22-33 ml/kg at 5-10 ml/min

Hypoproteinemia

• *Adult:* **IV INF** 1000-1500 ml qd, not to exceed 8 ml/min

Available forms: Inj 5%

Side effects/adverse reactions:

GI: Nausea, vomiting, increased salivation

INTEG: Rash, urticaria, cyanosis

CNS: Fever, chills, headache, paresthesias, flushing

RESP: Altered respirations, dyspnea, **pulmonary edema**

CV: **Fluid overload,** hypotension, erratic pulse

Contraindications: Hypersensitivity, CHF, severe anemia, renal insufficiency

Precautions: Decreased salt intake, decreased cardiac reserve, lack of albumin deficiency, hepatic disease, renal disease, pregnancy (C)

Pharmacokinetics: Metabolized as a protein/energy source

Lab test interferences:

False increase: Alk phosphatase

NURSING CONSIDERATIONS

Assess:

• Blood studies: Hct, Hgb, electrolytes, serum protein; if serum protein declines, dyspnea, hypoxemia can result

• B/P (decreased), pulse (erratic), respiration during infusion

• I&O ratio; urinary output may decrease

• CVP, pulmonary wedge pressure (increases if overload occurs), jugular vein distention

• Allergy: fever, rash, itching, chills, flushing, urticaria, nausea, vomiting, or hypotension requires discontinuation of infusion; use new lot if therapy reinstituted, premedicate with diphenhydramine

◆ Increased CVP reading: distended neck veins indicate circulatory overload; SOB, anxiety, insomnia, expiratory rales, frothy blood-tinged cough, cyanosis indicate pulmonary overload

Administer:

IV

• No dilution required; use infusion

◆ = Nursing alert   🖋 = Herb-drug interaction   🚫 = Do not crush

pump, use large-gauge needle (≥20G), discard unused portion, infuse slowly

• Within 4 hr of opening

Additive compatibilities: Carbohydrate and electrolyte sol, whole blood, packed red blood cells, chloramphenicol, tetracycline

Perform/provide:

• Adequate hydration before administration

• Storage—check type of albumin, date; may have to refrigerate

Evaluate:

• Therapeutic response: increased B/P, decreased edema, increased serum albumin

---

plicamycin (℞)

(ply-ka-my′sin)

Mithramycin, Mithracin

Func. class.: Antineoplastic, antibiotic; hypocalcemic

Chem. class.: Crystalline aglycone

Action: Inhibits DNA, RNA, protein synthesis; derived from *Streptomyces plicatus;* replication is decreased by binding to DNA; demonstrates calcium-lowering effect not related to its tumoricidal activity; also acts on osteoclasts and blocks action of parathyroid hormone; a vesicant

Uses: Testicular cancer, hypercalcemia, hypercalciuria, symptomatic treatment of advanced neoplasms

Dosage and routes:

Testicular tumors

• *Adult:* IV 25-30 µg/kg/day × 8-10 days, not to exceed 30 µg/kg/day

Hypercalcemia/hypercalciuria

• *Adult:* IV 25 µg/kg/day × 3-4 days, repeat at intervals of 1 wk

Available forms: Inj 2500 µg/vial pwd

Side effects/adverse reactions:

META: Decreased serum Ca, P, K

HEMA: ***Hemorrhage, thrombocytopenia,*** decreased PT, WBC count

GI: Nausea, vomiting, anorexia, diarrhea, stomatitis, increased liver enzymes

GU: Increased BUN, creatinine; ***proteinuria***

INTEG: Rash, cellulitis, ***extravasation,*** facial flushing

CNS: Drowsiness, weakness, lethargy, headache, flushing, fever, depression

Contraindications: Hypersensitivity, thrombocytopenia, bone marrow depression, bleeding disorders, pregnancy (X), lactation, child <15 yr

Precautions: Renal disease, hepatic disease, electrolyte imbalances

Pharmacokinetics: Crosses blood-brain barrier, excreted in urine; little known about pharmacokinetics

Interactions:

• Increased toxicity: other antineoplastics or radiation

NURSING CONSIDERATIONS

Assess:

• CBC, differential, platelet count qwk; withhold drug if WBC is <4000/mm^3 or platelet count is <50,000/mm^3; notify prescriber

• Renal function studies: BUN, serum uric acid, urine CrCl, electrolytes before, during therapy

• I&O ratio; report urine output <30 ml/hr

• Monitor temp q4h; fever may indicate beginning infection

• LFTs before, during therapy: bilirubin, AST, ALT, alk phosphatase prn or qmo; jaundiced skin, sclera; dark urine, clay-colored stools, itchy skin, abdominal pain, fever, diarrhea

• Alkalosis if severe vomiting is present

P

◆ Toxicity: facial flushing, epistaxis, increased PT, thrombocytopenia; drug should be discontinued

◆ Bleeding: hematuria, guaiac stools, bruising or petechiae, mucosa or orifices q8h; may progress to severe bleeding

• Inflammation of mucosa, breaks in skin

• Buccal cavity q8h for dryness, sores, ulceration, white patches, oral pain, bleeding, dysphagia

• Local irritation, pain, burning at inj site

• Frequency of stools, characteristics, cramping

• Acidosis, signs of dehydration: rapid respirations, poor skin turgor, decreased urine output, dry skin, restlessness, weakness

Administer:

• Antiemetic 30-60 min before giving drug and 4-10 hr after treatment to prevent vomiting

• Transfusion for anemia

• Antispasmodic for diarrhea, phenothiazine for nausea and vomiting

IV

• Dilute 2.5 mg/4.9 ml of sterile H_2O; (500 µg/ml) dilute single dose in 1000 ml of D_5W run over 4-6 hr

• EDTA for extravasation, apply ice compress

• Slow IV infusion using 20G, 21G needle

Y-site compatibilities: Allopurinol, amifostine, aztreonam, filgrastim, granisetron, melphalan, piperacillin/tazobactam, teniposide, thiotepa, vinorelbine

Perform/provide:

• Liquid diet: carbonated beverages; gelatin may be added if patient is not nauseated or vomiting

• Rinsing of mouth tid-qid with water; brushing of teeth qid with baking soda bid-tid with soft brush or cotton-tipped applicator for stomatitis; unwaxed dental floss

• Usage immediately after mixing

Evaluate:

• Therapeutic response: decreased tumor size, spread of malignancy

Teach patient/family:

• To report any complaints or side effects to nurse or prescriber

• To avoid foods with citric acid, hot or rough texture

• To report to prescriber any bleeding, white spots, ulcerations in the mouth; tell patient to examine mouth qd

• To avoid driving, activities requiring alertness; drowsiness may occur

• To report leg cramps, tingling of fingertips, weakness; may indicate hypocalcemia

• To avoid crowds, persons with infections when granulocyte count is low

---

poractant alfa (℞)
Curosurf

Func. class.: Lung surfactant extract

Action: Replenishes surfactant and restores surface activity to the lungs in premature infants

Uses: Treatment (rescue) of respiratory distress syndrome in premature infants

Investigational uses: Prophylaxis of RDS, adult RDS due to viral pneumonia, HIV-infected infants with *Pneumocystis carinii* pneumonia, treatment of adult RDS in near drowning

Dosage and routes:

• **INTRATRACHEAL INSTILL**

Available forms: Susp 120 mg (1.5 ml); 240 mg (3 ml), phospholipids

Side effects/adverse reactions: (Concurrent illnesses that have occurred during treatment are in bold)

*RESP: **Pulmonary air leaks, pul-***

◆ = Nursing alert   🌿 = Herb-drug interaction   ⃠ = Do not crush

monary interstitial emphysema, apnea, pulmonary hemorrhage
SYST: **Patent ductus arteriosus, intracranial hemorrhage, severe intracranial hemorrhage, necrotizing enterocolitis, posttreatment sepsis, posttreatment infection,** bradycardia, oxygen desaturation, pallor, vasoconstriction, hypotension, hypertension

Precautions: Bradycardia, rales, infections

Pharmacokinetics: Becomes lung associated within hours of administration

NURSING CONSIDERATIONS
Assess:

• Respiratory rate, rhythm, character, chest expansion, color, transcutaneous saturation, ABGs

• Endotracheal tube placement before dosing; for apnea after endotracheal administration

• Reflux of drug into the endotracheal tube during administration; stop drug if this occurs, and if needed, increase peak inspiratory pressure on the ventilator by 4-5 cm H_2O until tube is cleared

• Infant for repeat dosing using radiographic confirmation of RDS; repeat doses should be given as above; ventilator settings for repeat doses FIo_2 were decreased by 0.2 or amount to prevent cyanosis; ventilator rate of 30/min; inspiratory time <1 sec; if infant's pretreatment rate was >30, it was left unchanged during dosing; resume usual ventilator management after dosing

Administer:

• After suctioning

• By endotracheal administration only by persons trained in neonatal intubation and ventilation

• After using a No. 5 Fr end-hole catheter inserted into the endotracheal tube with the tip at distal end of endotracheal tube just beyond the end of the endotracheal tube; shorten the catheter before insertion; insert the drug into the main bronchi by positioning infant with either right or left side dependent

Divide doses and administer with infant in different positions

Determine dosing by weight of infant; slowly withdraw contents into plastic syringe through 20G needle; do not filter or shake; attach premeasured No. 5 Fr catheter to syringe; fill with drug and discard excess through catheter so only dose to be given remains in syringe

For prevention dosing, stabilize, weigh, and intubate infant; give drug within 15 min of birth if possible; position infant and inject first dose through catheter over 2-3 sec; remove catheter and manually ventilate with O_2 to prevent cyanosis (60 bpm) and sufficient positive pressure to promote adequate air exchange and chest wall excursion

For rescue dosing, give dosing as soon as infant is placed on ventilator after birth; immediately before administering dose, change ventilator settings to 60/min, inspiratory time 0.5 sec, FIo_2 1; position infant and inject first dose through catheter over 2-3 sec; remove catheter; return to mechanical ventilator

Ventilate infant for >30 sec or until stable after prevention or rescue strategy; reposition for next dose; same procedure for subsequent dosing; do not suction for at least 1 hr after dosing unless airway obstruction is evident; resume ventilator therapy after dosing

Perform/provide:

• Reduction in peak ventilator inspiratory pressures immediately if chest expansion improves substantially after dose

• Reduction in FIo_2 in small, repeated steps when infant becomes

pink and transcutaneous oxygen saturation is in excess of 95%; oxygen saturation should remain between 90% and 95%
• Suctioning of all infants before administration to prevent mucus plugging; if endotracheal tube obstruction is suspected, remove obstruction and replace tube immediately
• Storage in refrigeration; protect from light; warm to room temperature for >20 min or warm in hand >8 min before giving; do not use artificial warming methods; enter a vial only once; unopened, unused vials that have been warmed to room temperature may be rerefrigerated within 8 hr of warming; do not warm and return to refrigerator more than once

Evaluate:
• Therapeutic response: significant improvement in respiratory status

---

porfimer (℞)

(pour′fih-mur)
Photofrin
Func. class.: Antineoplastic-miscellaneous

Action: Used in photodynamic treatment of tumors (PDT); antitumor and cytotoxic actions are light and O_2 dependent; used with 630 nm laser light

Uses: Esophageal cancer (completely obstructing), endobronchial non–small cell lung cancer

Dosage and routes:
• Refer to Optiguide for complete instructions
• *Adult:* IV 2 mg/kg, then illumination with laser light 40-50 hr after inj; a second laser light application may be given 96-120 hr after inj; may repeat q30 days × 3

Endobronchial cancer
• *Adult:* 200 joules/cm of tumor length

Available forms: Cake/pwd for inj 75 mg

Side effects/adverse reactions:

CV: Hypotension, hypertension, atrial fibrillation, **cardiac failure,** *tachycardia*

GI: Abdominal pain, constipation, diarrhea, dyspepsia, dysphagia, eructation, esophageal edema/ bleeding, hematemesis, melena, nausea, vomiting, anorexia

CNS: Anxiety, confusion, insomnia

RESP: **Pleural effusion,** *pneumonia, dyspnea, respiratory insufficiency,* **tracheoesophageal fistula**

MISC: Dehydration, weight decrease, anemia, photosensitivity reaction, UTI, moniliasis

Contraindications: Porphyria, porphyrin allergy (porfimer); tracheoesophageal, bronchoesophageal fistula; major blood vessels with eroding tumors (PDT)

Precautions: Elderly, pregnancy (C), lactation, children

Pharmacokinetics: Half-life 250 hr, 90% protein bound

Interactions:
• Increased photosensitivity: tetracyclines, sulfonamides, phenothiazines, sulfonylureas, thiazides, griseofulvin

NURSING CONSIDERATIONS
Assess:
• Ocular sensitivity: sensitivity to sun, bright lights, car headlights, patients should wear dark sunglasses with an average light transmittance of <4%
• Chest pain: may be so severe as to necessitate opiate analgesics
• For extravasation at inj site: take care to protect from light

Administer:
• As a single slow IV inj over 3-5 min at 2 mg/kg; reconstitute each

---

⬧ = Nursing alert   ⫽ = Herb-drug interaction   🚫 = Do not crush

vial with 31.8 ml D$_5$ or 0.9% NaCl (2.5 mg/ml), shake well; do not mix with other drugs or sol; protect from light and use immediately
• Laser light is initiated 630 nm wave length laser light
Perform/provide:
• Wiping of spills with damp cloth, avoid skin/eye contact, use rubber gloves, eye protection, dispose of material in polyethylene bag according to policy
Teach patient/family:
• To report chest pain, eye sensitivity
• To wear sunglasses with average white light transmittance of <4%; avoid exposure to sunlight or bright light for 30 days

potassium acetate
potassium bicarbonate (OTC, ℞)
K+ Care ET, K-Electrolyte, K-Ide, Klor-Con EF, K-Lyte, K-Vescent
potassium bicarbonate and potassium chloride (OTC, ℞)
Klorvess, Klorvess Effervescent Granules, K-Lyte/Cl, Neo-K*
potassium bicarbonate and potassium citrate (OTC, ℞)
Effer-K, K-Lyte DS
potassium chloride (OTC, ℞)
Apo-K*, Cena-K, Gen-K, K+ Care, K+ 10, Kalium Durules*, Kaochlor, Kaochlor S-F, Kaon-Cl, Kay Ciel, KCl, K-Dur, K-Lease, K-Long*, K-Lor, Klor-Con, Klorvess, Klotrix, K-Lyte/C1 powder, K-med, K-Norm, K-Sol, K-tab, Micro-K, Micro-LS, Potasalan, Roychlor, Rum-K, Slow-K, Ten-K
potassium chloride/ potassium bicarbonate/ potassium citrate (OTC, ℞)
Kaochlor Eff
potassium gluconate (OTC, ℞)
Kaon, Kaylixir, K-G Elixir, Potassium-Rougier*
potassium gluconate/ potassium chloride (OTC, ℞)
Kolyum
potassium gluconate/ potassium citrate (OTC, ℞)
Twin-K
Func. class.: Electrolyte
Chem. class.: Potassium

P

Action: Needed for adequate transmission of nerve impulses and cardiac contraction, renal function, intracellular ion maintenance

Uses: Prevention and treatment of hypokalemia

Dosage and routes:

Potassium bicarbonate

• *Adult:* **PO** dissolve 25-50 mEq in water qd-qid

Potassium acetate—hypokalemia

• *Adult and child:* **PO** 40-100 mEq/day in divided doses 2-4 days

Hypokalemia (prevention)

• *Adult and child:* **PO** 20 mEq/day in 2-4 divided doses

Potassium chloride

• *Adult:* **PO** 40-100 mEq in divided doses tid-qid; **IV** 20 mEq/hr when diluted as 40 mEq/1000 ml, not to exceed 150 mEq/day

• *Child:* **PO** 2-4 mEq/kg/day

Potassium gluconate

• *Adult:* **PO** 40-100 mEq in divided doses tid-qid

Potassium phosphate

• *Adult:* **IV** 1 mEq/hr in sol of 60 mEq/L, not to exceed 150 mEq/day; **PO** 40-100 mEq/day in divided doses

• *Child:* **IV** max rate of inf 1 mEq/kg/hr

Available forms: Tabs for sol 6.5, 25 mEq; caps, ext rel 8, 10 mEq; powder for sol 3.3, 5, 6.7, 10, 13.3 mEq/5 ml; tabs 2, 4, 5, 13.4 mEq; tabs, ext 6.7, 8, 10 mEq; elix 6.7 mEq/5 ml; oral sol 2.375 mEq/5 ml; inj for prep of IV 1.5, 2, 2.4, 3, 3.2, 4.4, 4.7 mEq/ml

Side effects/adverse reactions:

CNS: Confusion

CV: Bradycardia, *cardiac depression, dysrhythmias, arrest, peaking T waves, lowered R and depressed RST, prolonged P-R interval, widened QRS complex*

GI: Nausea, vomiting, cramps, pain, *diarrhea,* ulceration of small bowel

GU: Oliguria

INTEG: Cold extremities, rash

Contraindications: Renal disease (severe), severe hemolytic disease, Addison's disease, hyperkalemia, acute dehydration, extensive tissue breakdown

Precautions: Cardiac disease, K-sparing diuretic therapy, systemic acidosis, pregnancy (C)

Pharmacokinetics:

PO: Excreted by kidneys and in feces; onset of action ≈30 min

IV: Immediate onset of action

Interactions:

• Hyperkalemia: potassium phosphate IV and products containing Ca or Mg; K-sparing, diuretic, or other K products

NURSING CONSIDERATIONS

Assess:

• ECG for peaking T waves, lowered R, depressed RST, prolonged P-R interval, widening QRS complex, hyperkalemia; drug should be reduced or discontinued

• K level during treatment (3.5-5 mg/dl is normal level)

• I&O ratio; watch for decreased urinary output; notify prescriber immediately

• Cardiac status: rate, rhythm, CVP, PWP, PAWP, if being monitored directly

Administer:

PO

• With meal or pc; dissolve effervescent tabs, pwd in 8 oz cold water or juice; do not give IM, SC

IV

• Through large-bore needle to decrease vein inflammation; check for extravasation

• In large vein, avoiding scalp vein in child (IV)

• IV after diluting in large volume of IV sol and give as an inf, slowly by IV inf to prevent toxicity; never give IV bolus or IM

Potassium acetate

Additive compatibilities: Metoclopramide

Y-site compatibilities: Ciprofloxacin

Potassium chloride

Additive compatibilities: Aminophylline, amiodarone, atracurium, bretylium, calcium gluconate, cefepime, cephalothin, cephapirin, chloramphenicol, cimetidine, ciprofloxacin, cisatracurium, clindamycin, cloxacillin, corticotropin, cytarabine, dimenhydrinate, dopamine, doxorubicin liposome, enalaprilat, erythromycin, floxacillin, fluconazole, fosphenytoin, furosemide, heparin, hydrocortisone, isoproterenol, lidocaine, metaraminol, methicillin, methyldopa, metoclopramide, mitoxantrone, nafcillin, netilmicin, norepinephrine, oxacillin, penicillin G potassium, phenylephrine, piperacillin, ranitidine, sodium bicarbonate, thiopental, vancomycin, verapamil, vit B/C

Y-site compatibilities: Acyclovir, aldesleukin, allopurinol, amifostine, aminophylline, amiodarone, ampicillin, amrinone, atropine, aztreonam, betamethasone, calcium gluconate, cefmetazole, cephalothin, cephapirin, chlordiazepoxide, chlorpromazine, ciprofloxacin, cladribine, cyanocobalamin, dexamethasone, digoxin, diltiazem, diphenhydramine, dobutamine, dopamine, droperidol, edrophonium, enalaprilat, epinephrine, esmolol, estrogens, ethacrynate, famotidine, fentanyl, filgrastim, fludarabine, fluorouracil, furosemide, gallium, granisetron, heparin, hydralazine, idarubicin, indomethacin, insulin (regular), isoproterenol, kanamycin, labetalol, lidocaine, lorazepam, magnesium sulfate, melphalan, meperidine, methicillin, methoxamine, methylergonovine, midazolam, minocy-cline, morphine, neostigmine, norepinephrine, ondansetron, oxacillin, oxytocin, paclitaxel, penicillin G potassium, pentazocine, phytonadione, piperacillin/tazobactam, prednisolone, procainamide, prochlorperazine, propofol, propranolol, pyridostigmine, remifentanil, sargramostim, scopolamine, sodium bicarbonate, succinylcholine, tacrolimus, teniposide, theophylline, thiotepa, trimethaphan, trimethobenzamide, vinorelbine, warfarin, zidovudine

Perform/provide:

• Storage at room temperature

Evaluate:

• Therapeutic response: absence of fatigue, muscle weakness; decreased thirst and urinary output; cardiac changes

Teach patient/family:

• To add K-rich foods to diet: bananas, orange juice, avocados; whole grains, broccoli, carrots, prunes, cocoa after this medication is discontinued

• To avoid OTC products: antacids, salt substitutes, analgesics, vitamin preparations, unless specifically directed by prescriber

• To report hyperkalemia symptoms (lethargy, confusion, diarrhea, nausea, vomiting, fainting, decreased output) or continued hypokalemia symptoms (fatigue, weakness, polyuria, polydipsia, cardiac changes)

• To take capsules with full glass of liquid

• To dissolve powder or tablet completely in at least 120 ml water or juice

🚫 Not to chew time-rel or ext-rel preparations

• Importance of regular follow-up visits

potassium iodide (℞)
Pima, potassium iodide solution, SSKI, Thyro-Block
Func. class.: Thyroid hormone antagonist
Chem. class.: Iodine product

Action: Inhibits secretion of thyroid hormone, fosters colloid accumulation in thyroid follicles, decreases vascularity of gland

Uses: Preparation for thyroidectomy, thyrotoxic crisis, neonatal thyrotoxicosis, radiation protectant, thyroid storm

Dosage and routes:
Thyrotoxic crisis
• *Adult and child:* **PO** 1 ml in water tid after meals (strong iodine sol)
Preparation for thyroidectomy
• *Adult and child:* **PO** 0.1-0.3 ml tid (strong iodine sol) or 5 gtt in water tid pc × 2-3 wk before surgery (potassium iodide sol)
Available forms: Sol 5%, 10%, 21 mg/gtt; tabs 130, 300 mg; inj 10%, 20%; oral syr 325 mg/5 ml; tabs 130 mg*

Side effects/adverse reactions:
ENDO: Hypothyroidism, hyperthyroid adenoma
INTEG: Rash, urticaria, *angineurotic edema,* acne, mucosal hemorrhage, fever
CNS: Headache, confusion, paresthesias
GI: Nausea, diarrhea, vomiting, small-bowel lesions, upper gastric pain
MS: Myalgia, arthralgia, weakness
EENT: Metallic taste, stomatitis, salivation, periorbital edema, sore teeth and gums, cold symptoms
Contraindications: Hypersensitivity to iodine, pulmonary edema, pulmonary TB, pregnancy (D)
Precautions: Lactation, children

Pharmacokinetics:
PO: Onset 24-48 hr, peak 10-15 days after continuous therapy, uptake by thyroid gland or excreted in urine; crosses placenta
Interactions:
• Hypothyroidism: lithium, other antithyroid agents
Lab test interferences:
Interference: Urinary 17-OHCS
NURSING CONSIDERATIONS
Assess:
• Pulse, B/P, temp
• I&O ratio; check for edema: puffy hands, feet, periorbit; indicate hypothyroidism
• Weight qd; same clothing, scale, time of day
• T_3, T_4, which is increased; serum TSH, which is decreased; free thyroxine index, which is increased if dosage is too low; discontinue drug 3-4 wk before RAIU
◆ Overdose: peripheral edema, heat intolerance, diaphoresis, palpitations, dysrhythmias, severe tachycardia, fever, delirium, CNS irritability
• Hypersensitivity: rash; enlarged cervical lymph nodes may indicate drug should be discontinued
• Hypoprothrombinemia: bleeding, petechiae, ecchymosis
• Clinical response: after 3 wk should include increased weight, pulse; decreased T_4
Administer:
• Strong iodine solution after diluting with water or juice to improve taste
• Through straw to prevent tooth discoloration
• With meals to decrease GI upset
• At same time each day to maintain drug level
• Lowest dose that relieves symptoms, discontinue before RAIU

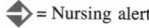 ◆ = Nursing alert　　∥ = Herb-drug interaction　　⊘ = Do not crush

Perform/provide:
• Fluids to 3-4 L/day, unless contraindicated
Evaluate:
• Therapeutic response: weight gain, decreased pulse, T_4, size of thyroid gland
Teach patient/family:
• To abstain from breastfeeding after delivery
• To keep graph of weight, pulse, mood
• To avoid OTC products that contain iodine
• That seafood, other iodine products may be restricted
• Not to discontinue this medication abruptly; thyroid crisis may occur; stress response
• That response may take several mo if thyroid is large
• To discontinue drug, notify prescriber of fever, rash, metallic taste, swelling of throat; burning of mouth, throat; sore gums, teeth; severe GI distress, enlargement of thyroid, cold symptoms

---

RARELY USED

pralidoxime (℞)
(pra-li-dox'eem)
Protopam Chloride
Func. class.: Cholinesterase reactivator

Uses: Cholinergic crisis in myasthenia gravis, organophosphate poisoning antidote (early), relief of paralysis of respiratory muscles; used as an adjunct to systemic atropine administration
Dosage and routes:
Anticholinesterase overdose
• *Adult:* IV 1-2 g, then 250 mg q5min until desired response

Organophosphate poisoning
• *Adult:* IV INF 1-2 g/100 ml 0.9% NaCl over 15-30 min; may repeat in 1 hr; PO 1-3 g q5h
• *Child:* IV INF 20-40 mg/kg/dose diluted in 100 ml 0.9% NaCl over 15-30 min
Contraindications: Hypersensitivity, carbamate insecticide poisoning

---

pramipexole (℞)
(pra-mi-pex'ol)
Mirapex
Func. class.: Antiparkinson agent
Chem. class.: Dopamine-receptor agonist, non-ergot

Action: Selective agonist for D_2 receptors (presynaptic/postsynaptic sites); binding at D_3 receptor contributes to antiparkinson effects
Uses: Parkinsonism
Investigational uses: Restless leg syndrome
Dosage and routes:
Initial treatment
• *Adult:* PO from a starting dose of 0.375 mg/day given in 3 divided doses; increase gradually by 0.125 mg/dose at 5-7 day intervals until total daily dose of 4.5 mg is reached
Maintenance treatment
• *Adult:* PO 1.5-4.5 mg qd in 3 divided doses
Renal dose
• *Adult:* PO CrCl 35-59 ml/min-0.125 mg bid, may increase q5-7 days to 1.5 mg bid; CrCl 15-34 ml/min 0.125 mg qd, increase q5-7 days to 1.5 mg qd
Restless leg syndrome (off-label)
• *Adult:* PO 0.125-0.375 mg 1-2 hr prior to hs, increase gradually
Available forms: Tabs 0.125, 0.25, 1, 1.5 mg

P

Side effects/adverse reactions:
*HEMA: **Hemolytic anemia, leukopenia, agranulocytosis***
CNS: Agitation, insomnia, psychosis, hallucination, depression, dizziness, headache, confusion
GI: Nausea, anorexia, constipation, dysphagia, dry mouth
CV: Orthostatic hypotension, edema, syncope, tachycardia
GU: Impotence, urinary frequency
EENT: Blurred vision
Contraindications: Hypersensitivity
Precautions: Renal disease, cardiac disease, MI with dysrhythmias, affective disorders, psychosis, pregnancy (C), preexisting dyskinesias
Pharmacokinetics: Minimally metabolized, peak 2 hr, half-life 8 hr, 12-14 hr in elderly
Interactions:
• Increased pramipexole levels: levodopa, cimetidine, ranitidine, diltiazem, triamterene, verapamil, quinidine
• Decreased pramipexole levels: dopamine antagonists, phenothiazines, metoclopramide, butyrophenones
⁄ Decreased effect of pramipexole: chaste tree fruit
NURSING CONSIDERATIONS
Assess:
• Renal function studies
• Involuntary movements in parkinsonism: akinesia, tremors, staggering gait, muscle rigidity, drooling
• B/P, respiration during initial treatment; hypo/hypertension should be reported
• Mental status: affect, mood, behavioral changes, depression; complete suicide assessment
Administer:
• Drug until NPO before surgery
• Adjust dosage to patient response
• With meals

Perform/provide:
• Assistance with ambulation during beginning therapy
• Testing for diabetes mellitus, acromegaly if on long-term therapy
Evaluate:
• Therapeutic response: decrease in akathisia, increased mood
Teach patient/family:
• That therapeutic effects may take several wk to a few mo
• To change positions slowly to prevent orthostatic hypotension
• To use drug exactly as prescribed: if drug is discontinued abruptly, parkinsonian crisis may occur, avoid alcohol, OTC sleeping products

---

pravastatin (℞)
(pra′va-sta-tin)
Pravachol
Func. class.: Antilipidemic
Chem. class.: HMG-CoA reductase enzyme

Action: Inhibits HMG-CoA reductase enzyme, which reduces cholesterol synthesis
Uses: As an adjunct in primary hypercholesterolemia (types IIa, IIb), apolipoprotein B (apo B), to reduce the risk of recurrent MI, atherosclerosis
Dosage and routes:
• *Adult:* **PO** 10-20 mg qd at hs (range 10-40 mg qd)
• *Elderly/renal hepatic disease:* **PO** 10 mg/day
Available forms: Tabs 10, 20, 40 mg
Side effects/adverse reactions:
INTEG: Rash, pruritus
GI: Nausea, constipation, diarrhea, dyspepsia, flatus, abdominal pain, heartburn, *liver dysfunction,* pancreatitis, *hepatitis*
EENT: Lens opacities, common cold, rhinitis, cough

◆ = Nursing alert   *⁄* = Herb-drug interaction   ⊘ = Do not crush

MS: Muscle cramps, myalgia, ***myositis, rhabdomyolysis***

CNS: Headache, dizziness, psychic disturbances

Contraindications: Hypersensitivity, pregnancy (X), lactation, active liver disease

Precautions: Past liver disease, alcoholism, severe acute infections, trauma, hypotension, uncontrolled seizure disorders, severe metabolic disorders, electrolyte imbalances

Do not confuse:

Pravacho/Prevacid

Pharmacokinetics: Peak 1-1½ hr; metabolized by the liver, highly protein bound; excreted in urine, feces, breast milk; crosses placenta

Interactions:

• Increased risk for myopathy: erythromycin, niacin, cyclosporine, gemfibrozil, clofibrate, clarithromycin, itraconazole, protease inhibitors

• Increased effects of warfarin

• Decreased bioavailability of pravastatin: bile acid sequestrants

Lab test interferences:

Increase: CPK, LFTs

NURSING CONSIDERATIONS

Assess:

• Whether patient is pregnant

• Fasting lipid profile: LDL, HDL, TG, cholesterol q8wk, then q3-6mo when stable; obtain diet history

• Liver function studies: baseline, q6wk during the first 3 mo, q8wk for remainder of yr, then q6mo; AST, ALT, LFTs may increase

• Ophthalmic status qyr

• Renal studies in patients with compromised renal system: BUN, I&O ratio, creatinine

• For muscle tenderness, pain, obtain CPK, rhabdomyolysis may occur

Administer:

• Without regard to meals, hs

Perform/provide:

• Storage in cool environment in tight container protected from light

Evaluate:

• Therapeutic response: decrease in cholesterol to desired level after 8 wk

Teach patient/family:

• That blood work will be necessary during treatment

• To report blurred vision, severe GI symptoms, dizziness, headache, muscle pain, weakness, fever

• That regimen will continue: low-cholesterol diet, exercise program

• To report suspected pregnancy, not to use during pregnancy

---

prazosin (℞)

(pray'zoe-sin)

Minipress, prazosin

Func. class.: Antihypertensive

Chem. class.: α_1-Adrenergic blocker

Action: Blocks α-mediated vasoconstriction of adrenergic receptors, inducing peripheral vasodilation

Uses: Hypertension, refractory CHF, Raynaud's vasospasm

Investigational uses: Benign prostatic hypertrophy to decrease urine outflow obstruction

Dosage and routes:

• *Adult:* **PO** 1 mg bid or tid, increasing to 20 mg qd in divided doses if required; usual range 6-15 mg/day, not to exceed 1 mg initially; max 20-40 mg/day

• *Child:* **PO** 0.5-7 mg tid

Available forms: Caps 1, 2, 5 mg

Side effects/adverse reactions:

CV: Palpitations, orthostatic hypotension, tachycardia, edema, rebound hypertension

CNS: Dizziness, headache, drowsiness, anxiety, depression, vertigo, weakness, fatigue

---

808 prednisolone

GI: Nausea, vomiting, diarrhea, constipation, abdominal pain

GU: Urinary frequency, incontinence, impotence, priapism, H_2O, sodium retention

EENT: Blurred vision, epistaxis, tinnitus, dry mouth, red sclera

Contraindications: Hypersensitivity

Precautions: Pregnancy (C), children

Pharmacokinetics:

PO: Onset 2 hr, peak 1-3 hr, duration 6-12 hr; half-life 2-3 hr, metabolized in liver, excreted via bile, feces (>90%), in urine (<10%)

Interactions:
• Increased hypotensive effects: β-blockers, nitroglycerin
• Decreased effect: indomethacin

Lab test interferences:

Increase: Urinary norepinephrine, VMA

NURSING CONSIDERATIONS
Assess:
• B/P (sitting, standing) during initial treatment, periodically thereafter; pulse, jugular venous distention q4h
• BUN, uric acid if on long-term therapy
• Weight qd, I&O; edema in feet, legs qd
• Skin turgor, dryness of mucous membranes for hydration status
• Rales, dyspnea, orthopnea q30min

Perform/provide:
• Storage in tight container in cool environment

Evaluate:
• Therapeutic response: decreased B/P

Teach patient/family:
• That fainting occasionally occurs after 1st dose; do not drive or operate machinery for 4 hr after 1st dose, or take 1st dose at bedtime
• To change positions slowly, to prevent orthostatic hypotension
• To avoid OTC medications unless approved by prescriber

Treatment of overdose: Administer volume expanders or vasopressors, discontinue drug, place in supine position

---

prednisolone (℞)
(pred-niss'oh-lone)
Articulose-50, Delta-Cortef, Hydeltrasol, Hydeltra-T.B.A., Key-Pred 25, Key-Pred 50, Key-Pred-SP, Pediapred, Predaject-50, Predalone 50, Predalone-T.B.A., Predcor-25, Predcor-50, prednisolone, Prednisolone Acetate, Prednisol TBA, Prelone
Func. class.: Corticosteroid
Chem. class.: Glucocorticoid, immediate acting

Action: Decreases inflammation by suppression of migration of polymorphonuclear leukocytes, fibroblasts; reversal to increase capillary permeability and lysosomal stabilization

Uses: Severe inflammation, immunosuppression, neoplasms

Dosage and routes:
• *Adult:* **PO** 2.5-15 mg bid-qid; **IM** 2-30 mg (acetate, phosphate) q12h; **IV** 2-30 mg (phosphate) q12h; 2-30 mg in joint or soft tissue (phosphate), 4-40 mg in joint of lesion (tebutate)

Asthma/antiinflammatory
• *Child:* **PO** 1-2 mg/kg/day; **IV** 2-4 mg/kg/day

Available forms: Tabs 5 mg; syr 5 mg/5 ml, 15 mg/15 ml; acetate:

◆ = Nursing alert   ∥ = Herb-drug interaction   ⊘ = Do not crush

inj 25, 50 mg/ml; tebutate: inj 20
mg/ml; phosphate: inj 20 mg/ml,
oral liquid 5 mg/ml, tabs 1, 2.5,
5, 10, 20, 50 mg, oral sol 5 mg/ml,
5 mg/5 ml, syr 5 mg/5 ml
Side effects/adverse reactions:
INTEG: Acne, poor wound healing,
ecchymosis, petechiae
CNS: Depression, flushing, sweating, headache, mood changes
*CV: Hypertension, **circulatory collapse, thrombophlebitis, embolism,***
tachycardia
*HEMA: **Thrombocytopenia***
MS: Fractures, osteoporosis, weakness
*GI: Diarrhea, nausea, abdominal
distention, **GI hemorrhage,*** increased appetite, ***pancreatitis***
EENT: Fungal infections, increased
intraocular pressure, blurred vision
Contraindications: Psychosis, hypersensitivity, idiopathic thrombocytopenia, acute glomerulonephritis, amebiasis, fungal infections, nonasthmatic bronchial disease, child
<2 yr
Precautions: Pregnancy (C), diabetes mellitus, glaucoma, osteoporosis, seizure disorders, ulcerative
colitis, CHF, myasthenia gravis
Do not confuse:
prednisolone/prednisone
Pharmacokinetics:
PO: Peak 1-2 hr, duration 2 days
IM: Peak 3-45 hr
Interactions:
• Decreased action of prednisolone:
cholestyramine, colestipol, barbiturates, rifampin, ephedrine, phenytoin, theophylline
• Decreased effects of anticoagulants, anticonvulsants, antidiabetics, ambenonium, neostigmine, isoniazid, toxoids, vaccines, anticholinesterases, salicylates, somatrem
• Increased side effects: alcohol, sa-

licylates, indomethacin, amphoter-
icin B, digitalis, cyclosporine, di-
uretics
• Increased action of prednisolone:
salicylates, estrogens, indometha-
cin, oral contraceptives, ketocona-
zole, macrolide antibiotics
🍃 K deficiency: aloe, buckthorn,
cascara sagrada, senna
Lab test interferences:
Increase: Cholesterol, Na, blood glu-
cose, uric acid, Ca, urine glucose
Decrease: Ca, K, T_4, T_3, thyroid^{131}I
uptake test, urine 17-OHCS, 17-
KS, PBI
False negative: Skin allergy tests
NURSING CONSIDERATIONS
Assess:
• K, blood sugar, urine glucose while
on long-term therapy; hypokalemia
and hyperglycemia
• Weight qd; notify prescriber if
weekly gain >5 lb
• B/P q4h, pulse; notify prescriber
if chest pain occurs
• I&O ratio; be alert for decreasing
urinary output, increasing edema
• Plasma cortisol levels (long-term
therapy) (normal level: 138-635
nmol/L SI units when drawn at 8 AM)
• Infection: increased temp, WBC,
even after withdrawal of medication; drug masks infection
• K depletion: paresthesias, fatigue,
nausea, vomiting, depression, polyuria, dysrhythmias, weakness
• Edema, hypertension, cardiac
symptoms
• Mental status: affect, mood, behavioral changes, aggression
Administer:
• After shaking suspension (parenteral)
• Titrated dose; use lowest effective
dose
• IM inj deep in large muscle mass;
rotate sites; avoid deltoid; use 21G
needle

Side effects: *italics* = common; ***bold italics*** = life-threatening

• In 1 dose in AM to prevent adrenal suppression; avoid SC administration; may damage tissue
• With food or milk to decrease GI symptoms

IV
• Undiluted or added to NaCl or D_5 and given by IV inf; give 10 mg or less/1 min; decrease rate if burning occurs

Additive compatibilities: Ascorbic acid, cephalothin, cytarabine, erythromycin, fluorouracil, heparin, methicillin, penicillin G potassium, penicillin G sodium, vit B/C
Y-site compatibilities: Ciprofloxacin, heparin/hydrocortisone, potassium chloride, vit B/C

Perform/provide:
• Assistance with ambulation to patient with bone tissue disease to prevent fractures

Evaluate:
• Therapeutic response: ease of respirations, decreased inflammation

Teach patient/family:
• That ID as steroid user should be carried
• To notify prescriber if therapeutic response decreases; dosage adjustment may be needed
• Not to discontinue abruptly; adrenal crisis can result
• To avoid OTC products: salicylates, alcohol in cough products, cold preparations unless directed by prescriber
• About cushingoid symptoms
• The symptoms of adrenal insufficiency: nausea, anorexia, fatigue, dizziness, dyspnea, weakness, joint pain

---

prednisone (R)
(pred′ni-sone)
Apo-Prednisone*, Deltasone*, Liquid Pred, Meticorten, Orasone, Panasol-S, Prednicen-M, Prednisone, Sterapred, Winpred
Func. class.: Corticosteroid
Chem. class.: Intermediate-acting glucocorticoid

Action: Decreases inflammation by suppression of migration of polymorphonuclear leukocytes, fibroblasts, reversal to increase capillary permeability, and lysosomal stabilization

Uses: Severe inflammation, immunosuppression, neoplasms, multiple sclerosis, collagen disorders, dermatologic disorders

Dosage and routes:
• *Adult:* **PO** 1.5-2.5 mg bid-qid, then qd or qod; maintenance up to 250 mg/day
• *Child:* **PO** 0.05-2 mg/kg/day divided 1-4 ×/day

Nephrosis
• *Child 18 mo-4 yr:* 7.5-10 mg qid initially
• *Child 4-10 yr:* 15 mg qid initially
• *Child >10 yr:* 20 mg qid initially

Multiple sclerosis
• *Adult:* **PO** 200 mg/day × 1 wk, then 80 mg qod × 1 mo

Available forms: Tabs 1, 2.5, 5, 10, 20, 50 mg; oral sol 5 mg/5 ml; syr 5 mg/5 ml

Side effects/adverse reactions:
CNS: Depression, flushing, sweating, headache, mood changes
CV: Hypertension, *circulatory collapse, thrombophlebitis, embolism,* tachycardia
EENT: Fungal infections, increased intraocular pressure, blurred vision
GI: Diarrhea, nausea, abdominal dis-

---

tention, *GI hemorrhage,* increased appetite, pancreatitis

*HEMA: **Thrombocytopenia***

INTEG: Acne, poor wound healing, ecchymosis, petechiae

MS: Fractures, osteoporosis, weakness

Contraindications: Psychosis, hypersensitivity, idiopathic thrombocytopenia, acute glomerulonephritis, amebiasis, fungal infections, nonasthmatic bronchial disease, child <2 yr, AIDS, TB

Precautions: Pregnancy (C), diabetes mellitus, glaucoma, osteoporosis, seizure disorders, ulcerative colitis, CHF, myasthenia gravis, renal disease, esophagitis, peptic ulcer

Do not confuse:
prednisone/methylprednisolone
prednisone/prednisolone
prednisone/Prilosec

Pharmacokinetics:

PO: Well absorbed PO, peak 1-2 hr, duration 1-1½ days, half-life 3½-4 hr

Crosses placenta, enters breast milk, metabolized by liver after conversion

Interactions:

• Decreased action of prednisone: cholestyramine, colestipol, barbiturates, rifampin, ephedrine, phenytoin, theophylline

• Decreased effects of anticoagulants, anticonvulsants, antidiabetics, ambenonium, neostigmine, isoniazid, toxoids, vaccines, anticholinesterases, salicylates, somatrem

• Increased side effects: alcohol, salicylates, indomethacin, amphotericin B, digitalis, cyclosporine, diuretics

• Increased action of prednisone: salicylates, estrogens, indomethacin, oral contraceptives, ketoconazole, macrolide antiinfectives

🌿 Potassium deficiency: aloe, buckthorn, rhubarb, senna

Lab test interferences:

Increase: Cholesterol, Na, blood glucose, uric acid, Ca, urine glucose

Decrease: Ca, K, T_4, T_3, thyroid ^{131}I uptake test, urine 17-OHCS, 17-KS, PBI

False negative: Skin allergy tests

NURSING CONSIDERATIONS

Assess:

• Adrenal insufficiency: nausea, vomiting, anorexia, confusion, hypotension

• K, blood sugar, urine glucose while on long-term therapy; hypokalemia and hyperglycemia

• Weight qd; notify prescriber of weekly gain >5 lb

• B/P q4h, pulse; notify prescriber of chest pain; monitor for rales, crackles, dyspnea if edema is present

• I&O ratio; be alert for decreasing urinary output, increasing edema

• Plasma cortisol (long-term therapy) (normal: 138-635 nmol/L SI units drawn at 8 AM)

• Infection: increased temp, WBC, even after withdrawal of medication; drug masks infection

• K depletion: paresthesias, fatigue, nausea, vomiting, depression, polyuria, dysrhythmias, weakness

• Edema, hypertension, cardiac symptoms

• Mental status: affect, mood, behavioral changes, aggression

Administer:

• Titrated dose; use lowest effective dose

• With food or milk to decrease GI symptoms

Perform/provide:

• Assistance with ambulation to patient with bone tissue disease to prevent fractures

Evaluate:

• Therapeutic response: ease of respirations, decreased inflammation

P

---

* = Canada only   Side effects: *italics* = common; ***bold italics*** = life-threatening

Teach patient/family:

• That ID as steroid user should be carried; information on drug being taken and condition
• To notify prescriber if therapeutic response decreases; dosage adjustment may be needed
• To avoid vaccinations
• Not to discontinue abruptly, or adrenal crisis can result
• To avoid OTC products: salicylates, alcohol in cough products, cold preparations unless directed by prescriber
• About cushingoid symptoms: moon face, weight gain
• That drug causes immunosuppression; to report any symptoms of infection (fever, sore throat, cough)
• The symptoms of adrenal insufficiency: nausea, anorexia, fatigue, dizziness, dyspnea, weakness, joint pain

---

primaquine (℞)
(prim'a-kween)

Func. class.: Antimalarial
Chem. class.: Synthetic 8-amino-quinolone

Action: Unknown; thought to destroy exoerythrocytic forms by gametocidal action

Uses: Malaria caused by *Plasmodium vivax,* in combination with clindamycin for *Pneumocystis carinii* pneumonia

Dosage and routes:
• *Adult:* PO 15 mg (base) qd × 2 wk; 26.3-mg tab is 15-mg base
• *Child:* PO 0.5 mg/kg (0.3 mg/base/day) qd × 2 wk

Available forms: Tabs 26.3 mg, pwd

Side effects/adverse reactions:
INTEG: Pruritus, skin eruptions, pallor, weakness

CNS: Headache, dizziness
EENT: Blurred vision, difficulty focusing
GI: Nausea, vomiting, anorexia, cramps
CV: Hypertension
HEMA: Agranulocytosis, granulocytopenia, leukopenia, hemolytic anemia, leukocytosis, mild anemia, *methemoglobinemia*

Contraindications: Hypersensitivity, anemia, lupus erythematosus, methemoglobinemia, porphyria, rheumatoid arthritis, methemoglobin reductase deficiency, G6PD deficiency, iodine hypersensitivity

Precautions: Pregnancy (C), bone marrow suppression

Pharmacokinetics:
PO: Metabolized by liver (metabolites), half-life 3.7-9.6 hr

Interactions:
• Toxicity: quinacrine

NURSING CONSIDERATIONS
Assess:
• Ophthalmic test if long-term treatment or drug dosage >150 mg/day
• Liver studies qwk: AST, ALT, bilirubin, if on long-term therapy
• Blood studies: CBC; blood dyscrasias occur
• Allergic reactions: pruritus, rash, urticaria
• Blood dyscrasias: malaise, fever, bruising, bleeding (rare)
• For renal status: dark urine, hematuria, decreased output
◆ For hemolytic reaction: chills, fever, chest pain, cyanosis; drug should be discontinued immediately

Administer:
PO
• Before or after meals at same time each day to maintain drug level

Evaluate:
• Therapeutic response: decreased symptoms of malaria

◆ = Nursing alert   ∥ = Herb-drug interaction   ⊘ = Do not crush

Teach patient/family:
• To report visual problems, fever, fatigue, dark urine, bruising, bleeding; may indicate blood dyscrasias
• To complete full course of therapy

---

primidone (℞)

(pri'mi-done)
Apo-Primidone*, Mysoline, PMS-Primidone*, primidone, Sertan*
Func. class.: Anticonvulsant
Chem. class.: Barbiturate derivative

Action: Raises seizure threshold by conversion of drug to phenobarbital, decreases neuron firing
Uses: Generalized tonic-clonic (grand mal), complex-partial psychomotor seizures
Dosage and routes:
• *Adult and child >8 yr:* **PO** 100-125 mg hs on days 1, 2, 3; then 100-125 mg bid on days 4, 5, 6; then 100-125 mg tid on days 7, 8, 9, then maintenance 250 mg tid-qid, max 2 g/day in divided doses
• *Child <8 yr:* **PO** 50 mg hs on days 1, 2, 3; then 50 mg bid on days 4, 5, 6; then 100 mg bid on days 7, 8, 9, maintenance 125-250 mg tid
Available forms: Tabs 50, 250 mg; susp 250 mg/5 ml; chew tabs 125 mg*
Side effects/adverse reactions:
HEMA: **Thrombocytopenia, leukopenia, neutropenia, eosinophilia, megaloblastic anemia,** decreased serum folate level, lymphadenopathy
CNS: Stimulation, drowsiness, dizziness, confusion, sedation, headache, flushing, hallucinations, **coma,** psychosis, ataxia, vertigo
GI: Nausea, vomiting, anorexia, **hepatitis**
INTEG: Rash, edema, alopecia, lupuslike syndrome

EENT: Diplopia, nystagmus, edema of eyelids
GU: Impotence
Contraindications: Hypersensitivity, porphyria, pregnancy (D)
Precautions: COPD, hepatic disease, renal disease, hyperactive children
Pharmacokinetics:
PO: Peak 4 hr; excreted by kidneys, in breast milk; half-life 3-24 hr
Interactions:
• Primidone levels are decreased by acetazolamide, succinimides, carbamazepine
• Primidone levels are increased by: isoniazid, nicotinamide, hydantoins
• Increased blood levels: alcohol, heparin, CNS depressants, isoniazid, phenytoin, phenobarbital
• May decrease effect of: oral contraceptives, acebutolol, metoprolol, propranolol, tricyclics, phenothiazines

NURSING CONSIDERATIONS
Assess:
• For seizures: location, duration, type; folic acid deficiency; fatigue, weakness, neuropathy, depression
• Drug level: therapeutic level 5-12 µg/ml; CBC should be done q6mo
• Mental status: mood, sensorium, affect, memory (long, short)
• Respiratory depression, wheezing
• Blood dyscrasias: fever, sore throat, bruising, rash, jaundice
Administer:
PO
• After shaking liquid susp well
• With food for GI upset
• Tablets crushed and mixed with food or fluid for swallowing difficulties
Evaluate:
• Therapeutic response: decreased seizures

P

---

* = Canada only   Side effects: *italics* = common; ***bold italics*** = life-threatening

Teach patient/family:

• Not to withdraw drug quickly; withdrawal symptoms may occur

• To avoid hazardous activities until stabilized on drug; drowsiness, dizziness may occur

• To carry Medic Alert ID with condition and medication

• To recognize the signs of blood dyscrasias; when to notify prescriber

• To avoid alcohol, CNS depressants

---

probenecid (R℞)
(proe-ben′e-sid)
Benemid, Benuryl*, probenecid, Probalan
Func. class.: Uricosuric
Chem. class.: Sulfonamide derivative

Action: Inhibits tubular reabsorption of urates, with increased excretion of uric acids

Uses: Hyperuricemia in gout, gouty arthritis, adjunct to cephalosporin or penicillin treatment

Dosage and routes:

Renal dose

• Avoid use if CrCl <30 ml/min

Gonorrhea

• *Adult:* **PO** 1 g with 3.5 g ampicillin or 1 g ½ hr before 4.8 million U of aqueous penicillin G procaine injected into 2 sites **IM**

Gout/gouty arthritis

• *Adult:* **PO** 250 mg bid for 1 wk, then 500 mg bid, not to exceed 2 g/day; maintenance: 500 mg/day × 6 mo

Adjunct in penicillin/cephalosporin treatment

• *Adult and child >50 kg:* **PO** 500 mg qid

• *Child <50 kg:* **PO** 25 mg/kg, then 40 mg/kg in divided doses qid

Available forms: Tabs 0.5 g

Side effects/adverse reactions:

CNS: Drowsiness, headache

CV: Bradycardia

GU: Glycosuria, thirst, frequency, *nephrotic syndrome*

*GI: Gastric irritation, nausea, vomiting, anorexia, **hepatic necrosis***

INTEG: Rash, dermatitis, pruritus, fever

META: Acidosis, hypokalemia, hyperchloremia, hyperglycemia

*RESP: **Apnea,** irregular respirations*

Contraindications: Hypersensitivity, severe hepatic disease, severe renal disease, CrCl <50 mg/min, history of uric acid calculus

Precautions: Pregnancy (B), child <2 yr

Pharmacokinetics:

PO: Peak 2-4 hr, duration 8 hr, half-life 5-8 hr; metabolized by liver; excreted in urine

Interactions:

• Increased effect of acyclovir, barbiturates, allopurinol, benzodiazepines, dyphylline, zidovudine

• Increased toxicity: sulfa drugs, dapsone, clofibrate, indomethacin, rifampin, naproxen, methotrexate

• Decreased action of probenecid: salicylates

Lab test interferences:

False positive: Urine glucose with copper sulfate test (Clinitest)

Increase: BSP/urinary PSP, theophylline levels

NURSING CONSIDERATIONS

Assess:

• Uric acid levels (3-7 mg/dl); mobility, joint pain, swelling

• Respiratory rate, rhythm, depth; notify prescriber of abnormalities

• Electrolytes, CO_2 before, during treatment

• Urine pH, output, glucose during beginning treatment

◆ For CNS symptoms: confusion, twitching, hyperreflexia, stimula-

---

◆ = Nursing alert   ✒ = Herb-drug interaction   ⊘ = Do not crush

tion, headache; may indicate overdose

Administer:
• After meals or with milk if GI symptoms occur
• Increase fluid intake to 2-3 L/day to prevent urinary calculi

Evaluate:
• Therapeutic response: absence of pain, stiffness in joints

Teach patient/family:
• To avoid OTC preparations (aspirin) unless directed by prescriber; increase water intake, avoid alcohol, caffeine

---

procainamide (℞)

(proe-kane-ah′mide)
procainamide, Procanbid, Promine, Pronestyl, Pronestyl-SR

Func. class.: Antidysrhythmic (Class IA)

Chem. class.: Procaine HCl amide analog

Action: Depresses excitability of cardiac muscle to electrical stimulation and slows conduction in atrium, bundle of His, and ventricle

Uses: Ventricular dysrhythmias

Dosage and routes:
Renal dose
• CrCl 10-50 ml/min give q6-12h; CrCl <10 ml/min give q8-24h
• *Adult:* **IV BOL** 100 mg q5min, given 25-50 mg/min, not to exceed 500 mg; or 17 mg/kg total then **IV INF** 2-6 mg/min

Available forms: Caps 250, 375, 500 mg; tabs 250, 375, 500 mg; tabs sus rel 250, 500, 750, 1000 mg; inj 100, 500 mg/ml

Side effects/adverse reactions:
CNS: Headache, dizziness, confusion, psychosis, restlessness, irritability, weakness, *seizures*

GI: Nausea, vomiting, anorexia, diarrhea, hepatomegaly
CV: Hypotension, **heart block, cardiovascular collapse, arrest**
HEMA: SLE syndrome, **agranulocytosis, thrombocytopenia, neutropenia, hemolytic anemia**
INTEG: Rash, urticaria, edema, swelling (rare), pruritus

Contraindications: Hypersensitivity, myasthenia gravis, severe heart block

Precautions: Pregnancy (C), lactation, children, renal disease, liver disease, CHF, respiratory depression

Pharmacokinetics:
PO: Peak 1-2 hr, duration 3 hr (8 hr extended)
IM: Peak 10-60 min, duration 3 hr; half-life 3 hr
Metabolized in liver to active metabolites, excreted unchanged by kidneys (60%)

Interactions:
• Increased effects of neuromuscular blockers, anticholinergics, antihypertensives, antihistamines, antidepressants, atropine, haloperidol, phenothiazines
• Increased procainamide effects: cimetidine, quinidine, trimethoprim
• Decreased effects of procainamide: barbiturates
• Increased toxicity: other antidysrhythmics
⚘ Increased anticholinergic effect: henbane

NURSING CONSIDERATIONS
Assess:
◆ECG continuously if using IV to determine increased PR or QRS segments; discontinue immediately; watch for increased ventricular ectopic beats, maximum need to rebolus
• Blood levels, 3-10 μg/ml or NAPA levels
• CBC q2wk × 3 mo

• B/P continuously for fluctuations
• I&O ratio; electrolytes (K, Na, Cl)
◆ Malignant hyperthermia: tachypnea, tachycardia, changes in B/P, fever
• Cardiac rate, rhythm, character
• Respiratory status: rate, rhythm, character, lung fields; bilateral rales may occur in CHF patient; watch for respiratory depression
• CNS effects: dizziness, confusion, psychosis, paresthesias, convulsions; drug should be discontinued
• Increased respiration, increased pulse; drug should be discontinued

Administer:

IM

• IM injection in deltoid; aspirate to avoid intravascular administration

IV

• After diluting 100 mg/ml of D_5W or sterile H_2O for inj; give 20 mg or less/1 min; may dilute 1 g/250-500 ml D_5W, run at 2-6 mg/min
• Check IV site q8h for infiltration or extravasation

Additive compatibilities: Amiodarone, atracurium, dobutamine, flumazenil, lidocaine, netilmicin, verapamil

Solution compatibilities: D_5W, D_5/0.9% NaCl, 0.45% NaCl, 0.9% NaCl, water for inj

Y-site compatibilities: Amiodarone, cisatracurium, famotidine, heparin, hydrocortisone, potassium chloride, ranitidine, remifentanil, vit B/C

Evaluate:

• Therapeutic response: decreased dysrhythmias

Teach patient/family:

• That wax matrix may appear in stools
• Not to discontinue without healthcare provider's advice

---

procaine (℞)
(proe'kane)
Novocain, Unicaine
Func. class.: Local anesthetic
Chem. class.: Ester

Action: Competes with calcium for sites in nerve membrane that control sodium transport across cell membrane; decreases rise of depolarization phase of action potential

Uses: Spinal anesthesia, epidural, peripheral nerve block, perineum, lower extremities, infiltration

Dosage and routes:
Vary by route of anesthesia

Available forms: Inj 1%, 2%, 10%

Side effects/adverse reactions:

CNS: Anxiety, restlessness, *convulsions, loss of consciousness,* drowsiness, disorientation, tremors, shivering

CV: Myocardial depression, cardiac arrest, dysrhythmias, bradycardia, hypotension, hypertension, fetal bradycardia

GI: Nausea, vomiting

EENT: Blurred vision, tinnitus, pupil constriction

INTEG: Rash, urticaria, allergic reactions, edema, burning, skin discoloration at inj site, tissue necrosis

RESP: Status asthmaticus, respiratory arrest, anaphylaxis

Contraindications: Hypersensitivity, child <12 yr, severe liver disease

Precautions: Elderly, severe drug allergies, pregnancy (C)

Pharmacokinetics: Onset 2-5 min, duration 1 hr; metabolized by liver, excreted in urine (metabolites)

Interactions:

• Dysrhythmias: epinephrine, halothane, enflurane
• Hypertension: MAOIs, tricyclics, phenothiazines

◆ = Nursing alert   ✐ = Herb-drug interaction   ⊘ = Do not crush

• Decreased action of procaine: chloroprocaine

NURSING CONSIDERATIONS

Assess:

• B/P, pulse, respiration during treatment

• Fetal heart tones if drug is used during labor

• Allergic reactions: rash, urticaria, itching

• Cardiac status: ECG for dysrhythmias, pulse, B/P during anesthesia

Administer:

• Only drugs that are not cloudy, do not contain precipitate

• Only with crash cart, resuscitative equipment nearby

• Only drugs without preservatives for epidural or caudal anesthesia

Additive compatibilities: Ascorbic acid, cephalothin, hydrocortisone, methicillin, penicillin G potassium, penicillin G sodium, vit B/C

Syringe compatibilities: Ampicillin, cloxacillin, glycopyrrolate, hydroxyzine, methicillin

Perform/provide:

• Use of new sol; discard unused portions

Evaluate:

• Therapeutic response: anesthesia necessary for procedure

Treatment of overdose: Airway, O_2, vasopressor, IV fluids, anticonvulsants for seizures

---

procarbazine (℞)

(proe-kar′ba-zeen)

Matulane, Natulan*

Func. class.: Antineoplastic, alkylating agent

Chem. class.: Hydrazine derivative

Action: Inhibits DNA, RNA, protein synthesis; has multiple sites of action; a nonvesicant

Uses: Lymphoma, Hodgkin's disease, cancers resistant to other therapy

Investigational uses: Brain, lung malignancies, other lymphomas, multiple myeloma, malignant melanoma, polycythemia vera

• *Adult:* **PO** 2-4 mg/kg/day for first wk; maintain dosage of 4-6 mg/kg/day until platelets and WBC fall; after recovery, 1-2 mg/kg/day

• *Child:* **PO** 50 mg/m²/day for 7 days, then 100 mg/m² until desired response, leukopenia, or thrombocytopenia occurs; 50 mg/day is maintenance after bone marrow recovery

Available forms: Caps 50 mg

Side effects/adverse reactions:

HEMA: ***Thrombocytopenia, anemia, leukopenia, myelosuppression, bleeding tendencies,*** purpura, petechiae, epistaxis

GI: Nausea, vomiting, anorexia, diarrhea, constipation, dry mouth, stomatitis

EENT: Retinal hemorrhage, nystagmus, photophobia, diplopia

INTEG: Rash, pruritus, dermatitis, alopecia, herpes, hyperpigmentation

CNS: Headache, dizziness, insomnia, hallucinations, confusion, ***coma,*** pain, chills, fever, sweating, paresthesias, ***seizures***

RESP: Cough, pneumonitis

MS: Arthralgias, myalgias

GU: Azoospermia, cessation of menses

Contraindications: Hypersensitivity, pregnancy (D), thrombocytopenia, bone marrow depression

Precautions: Renal disease, hepatic disease, radiation therapy

Pharmacokinetics: Half-life 1 hr; concentrates in liver, kidney, skin; metabolized in liver, excreted in urine

P

---

* = Canada only   Side effects: *italics* = common; ***bold italics*** = life-threatening

Interactions:
• Increased CNS depression: barbiturates, antihistamines, opioids, hypotensive agents, phenothiazines
• Disulfiram-like reaction: ethyl alcohol, MAOIs, tricyclics, tyramine foods, sympathomimetic drugs
• Hypertension: guanethidine, levodopa, methyldopa, reserpine
• Increased hypoglycemia: insulin, oral hypoglycemics
• Life-threatening hypertension: sympathomimetics

NURSING CONSIDERATIONS
Assess:
• CBC, differential, platelet count qwk; withhold drug if WBC is <4000/mm^3 or platelet count is <100,000/mm^3; notify prescriber
• Renal function studies: BUN, serum uric acid, urine CrCl, electrolytes before, during therapy
• I&O ratio, report fall in urine output to <30 ml/hr
• Monitor temp q4h; fever may indicate beginning infection
• LFTs before, during therapy: bilirubin, AST, ALT, alk phosphatase prn or qmo
• CNS changes: confusion, paresthesias, neuropathies, drug should be discontinued
◆ For tyramine foods in diet, hypertensive crisis can occur
◆ Toxicity: facial flushing, epistaxis, increased PT, thrombocytopenia; drug should be discontinued
• Bleeding: hematuria, guaiac stools, bruising or petechiae, mucosa or orifices q8h
• Effects of alopecia on body image; discuss feelings about body changes
• Jaundiced skin, sclera; dark urine, clay-colored stools, itchy skin, abdominal pain, fever, diarrhea
• Buccal cavity q8h for dryness, sores or ulceration, white patches, oral pain, bleeding, dysphagia

• Alkalosis if vomiting is severe
• GI symptoms: frequency of stools, cramping
• Acidosis, signs of dehydration: rapid respirations, poor skin turgor, decreased urine output, dry skin, restlessness, weakness
Administer:
• In divided doses and at hs to minimize nausea and vomiting
• Nonphenothiazine antiemetic 30-60 min before giving drug and 4-10 hr after treatment to prevent vomiting
• Transfusion for anemia
• Antispasmodic for GI symptoms
Perform/provide:
• Liquid diet: carbonated beverages; gelatin may be added if patient is not nauseated or vomiting
• Storage in tight, light-resistant container in cool environment
Evaluate:
• Therapeutic response: decreased tumor size, spread of malignancy
Teach patient/family:
• To report any complaints, side effects to nurse or prescriber; cough, shortness of breath, fever, chills, sore throat, bleeding, bruising, vomiting blood; black, tarry stools
• That hair may be lost during treatment and wig or hairpiece may make patient feel better; tell patient that new hair may be different in color, texture
• To avoid foods with citric acid, hot or rough texture
• To report any bleeding, white spots, ulcerations in mouth to prescriber; tell patient to examine mouth qd
• To avoid driving, activities requiring alertness; dizziness may occur
• That contraceptive measures are recommended during therapy
• To avoid ingestion of alcohol, tyramine-containing foods; cold, hay fever, weight-reducing products may cause serious drug interactions

◆ = Nursing alert 📷 = Herb-drug interaction 🚫 = Do not crush

• To avoid crowds, persons with infections if granulocytes are low

prochlorperazine (℞)

(proe-klor-pair'a-zeen)
Chlorpazine, Compa-Z, Compazine, Contranzine, Provacin*, Stemetil*, Ultrazine
Func. class.: Antiemetic, antipsychotic
Chem. class.: Phenothiazine, piperazine derivative

Action: Acts centrally by blocking chemoreceptor trigger zone, which in turn acts on vomiting center
Uses: Nausea, vomiting, psychotic disorders
Dosage and routes:
Postoperative nausea/vomiting
• *Adult:* IM 5-10 mg 1-2 hr before anesthesia; may repeat in 30 min; IV 5-10 mg 15-30 min before anesthesia; IV INF 20 mg/L D$_5$W or NS 15-30 min before anesthesia, not to exceed 40 mg/day
Severe nausea/vomiting
• *Adult:* PO 5-10 mg tid-qid; SUS REL 15 mg qd in AM or 10 mg q12h; RECT 25 mg/bid; IM 5-10 mg; may repeat q4h, not to exceed 40 mg/day
• *Child 18-39 kg:* PO 2.5 mg tid or 5 mg bid, not to exceed 15 mg/day; IM 0.132 mg/kg
• *Child 14-17 kg:* PO/RECT 2.5 mg bid-tid, not to exceed 10 mg/day; IM 0.132 mg/kg
• *Child 9-13 kg:* PO/RECT 2.5 mg qd-bid, not to exceed 7.5 mg/day; IM 0.132 mg/kg
Antipsychotic
• *Adult and child ≥12 yr:* PO 5-10 mg tid-qid; may increase q2-3day, max 150 mg/day; IM 10-20 mg q2-4hr up to 4 doses, then 10-20 mg

q4-6h, max 200 mg/day; RECT 10 mg tid-qid, may increase by 5-10 mg q2-3 days as needed
• *Child 2-12 yr:* PO 2.5 mg bid-tid; IM 132 µg/kg, max 10 mg/dose
Antianxiety
• *Adult and child ≥12 yr:* 5 mg tid-qid, max 20 mg/day or >12 wk; IM 5-10 mg q3-4hr, max 40 mg/day; IV 2.5-10 mg; max 40 mg/day
• *Child 2-12 yr:* IM 132 µg/kg
Available forms: Syr 5 mg/ml; inj 5 mg/ml; tabs 5, 10, 25 mg; caps, sus rel 10, 15 mg; supp 2.5, 5, 25 mg
Side effects/adverse reactions:
CNS: **Neuroleptic malignant syndrome,** *extrapyramidal reactions, tardive dyskinesia, euphoria, depression, EPS,* restlessness, tremor, dizziness
GI: Nausea, vomiting, anorexia, dry mouth, diarrhea, constipation, weight loss, metallic taste, cramps
CV: **Circulatory failure, tachycardia**
RESP: **Respiratory depression**
Contraindications: Hypersensitivity to phenothiazines, coma, seizure, encephalopathy, bone marrow depression
Precautions: Children <2 yr, pregnancy (C), elderly, lactation
Do not confuse:
Compazine/Coumadin
prochlorperazine/chlorpromazine
Pharmacokinetics:
PO: Onset 30-40 min, duration 3-4 hr
SUS REL: Onset 30-40 min, duration 10-12 hr
RECT: Onset 60 min, duration 3-4 hr
IM: Onset 10-20 min, duration 12 hr
Metabolized by liver; excreted in urine, breast milk; crosses placenta
Interactions:
• Decreased effect of prochlorperazine: barbiturates, antacids
• Increased anticholinergic action: anticholinergics, antiparkinson drugs, antidepressants

/ Increased anticholinergic effect: henbane

Lab test interferences:

Increase: LFTs, cardiac enzymes, cholesterol, blood glucose, prolactin, bilirubin, PBI, ^{131}I, alk phosphatase, leukocytes, granulocytes, platelets

Decrease: Hormones (blood and urine)

False-positive: Pregnancy tests, PKU, urine bilirubin

False-negative: Urinary steroids, 17-OHCS, pregnancy tests

NURSING CONSIDERATIONS

Assess:
• EPS: abnormal movement, tardive dyskinesia, akathisia
• VS, B/P; check patients with cardiac disease more often
• Respiratory status before, during, after administration of emetic; check rate, rhythm, character; respiratory depression can occur rapidly with elderly or debilitated patients

Administer:

IM
• IM injection in large muscle mass; aspirate to avoid IV administration
• Keep patient recumbent for ½ hr

IV
• IV after diluting 5 mg/9 ml of NaCl for inj (0.5 mg/ml); give 5 mg or less/min; may dilute 10-20 mg/L NaCl and give as infusion; can cause contact dermatitis

Additive compatibilities: Amikacin, ascorbic acid, dexamethasone, dimenhydrinate, erythromycin, ethacrynate, lidocaine, nafcillin, sodium bicarbonate, vit B/C

Syringe compatibilities: Atropine, butorphanol, chlorpromazine, cimetidine, diamorphine, diphenhydramine, droperidol, fentanyl, glycopyrrolate, hydroxyzine, meperidine, metoclopramide, nalbuphine, pentazocine, perphenazine, promazine, promethazine, ranitidine, scopolamine, sufentanil

Y-site compatibilities: Amsacrine, calcium gluconate, cisatracurium, cisplatin, cladribine, cyclophosphamide, cytarabine, doxorubicin, doxorubicin liposome, fluconazole, granisetron, heparin, hydrocortisone, melphalan, methotrexate, ondansetron, paclitaxel, potassium chloride, propofol, remifentanil, sargramostim, sufentanil, teniposide, thiotepa, vinorelbine, vit B/C

Evaluate:
• Therapeutic response: absence of nausea, vomiting; reduced anxiety, agitation, excitability

Teach patient/family:
• To avoid hazardous activities, activities requiring alertness; dizziness may occur
• To avoid alcohol
• Not to double or skip doses
• That urine may be pink to reddish brown
• To report dark urine, clay-colored stools, bleeding, bruising, rash, blurred vision

---

progesterone (℞)

(proe-jess'ter-one)

Crinone, progesterone, Progesterone in Oil, Prometrium

Func. class.: Progestogen

Chem. class.: Progesterone derivative

Action: Inhibits secretion of pituitary gonadotropins, which prevents follicular maturation, ovulation; stimulates growth of mammary tissue; antineoplastic action against endometrial cancer

Uses: Contraception, amenorrhea, premenstrual syndrome, abnormal

---

◆ = Nursing alert   */* = Herb-drug interaction   Ⓢ = Do not crush

uterine bleeding, endometrial hyperplasia prevention
Investigational uses: Corpus luteum dysfunction
Dosage and routes:
Infertility
• *Adult:* **VAG** 90 mg qd
Amenorrhea/uterine bleeding
• *Adult:* **IM** 5-10 mg qd × 6-8 doses
Endometrial hyperplasia prevention
• *Adult:* **PO** 200 mg/day
Available forms: Inj 50 mg/ml; pwd micronized, vag gel 8%; caps 100, 200 mg
Side effects/adverse reactions:
CNS: Dizziness, headache, migraines, depression, fatigue
CV: Hypotension, ***thrombophlebitis,*** edema, ***thromboembolism, stroke, pulmonary embolism, MI***
GI: Nausea, vomiting, anorexia, cramps, increased weight, ***cholestatic jaundice***
EENT: Diplopia
GU: Amenorrhea, cervical erosion, breakthrough bleeding, dysmenorrhea, vaginal candidiasis, breast changes, *gynecomastia, testicular atrophy, impotence,* endometriosis, ***spontaneous abortion***
INTEG: Rash, urticaria, acne, hirsutism, alopecia, oily skin, seborrhea, purpura, melasma
META: Hyperglycemia
SYST: ***Angioedema, anaphylaxis***
Contraindications: Breast cancer, hypersensitivity, thromboembolic disorders, reproductive cancer, genital bleeding (abnormal, undiagnosed), cerebral hemorrhage, pregnancy (D)
Precautions: Lactation, hypertension, asthma, blood dyscrasias, gallbladder disease, CHF, diabetes mellitus, bone disease, depression, migraine headache, convulsive dis-

orders, hepatic disease, renal disease, family history of breast or reproductive tract cancer
Pharmacokinetics:
IM, Rect, Vag: Duration 24 hr
Excreted in urine, feces; metabolized in liver
Lab test interferences:
Increase: Alk phosphatase, nitrogen (urine), pregnanediol, amino acids, factors VII, VIII, IX, X
Decrease: GTT, HDL
NURSING CONSIDERATIONS
Assess:
• Weight qd; notify prescriber of weekly weight gain >5 lb
• B/P at beginning of treatment and periodically
• I&O ratio; be alert for decreasing urinary output, increasing edema
• Liver function studies: ALT, AST, bilirubin periodically during long-term therapy
• Edema, hypertension, cardiac symptoms, jaundice
• Mental status: affect, mood, behavioral changes, depression
• Hypercalcemia
Administer:
• Titrated dose; use lowest effective dose
• Oil solution deep in large muscle mass IM; rotate sites
• After warming to dissolve crystals
• In one dose in AM
• With food or milk to decrease GI symptoms
Perform/provide:
• Storage in dark area
Evaluate:
• Therapeutic response: decreased abnormal uterine bleeding, absence of amenorrhea
Teach patient/family:
◆ To report breast lumps, vaginal bleeding, edema, jaundice, dark urine, clay-colored stools, dyspnea,

headache, blurred vision, abdominal pain, numbness or stiffness in legs, chest pain
- To report suspected pregnancy
- To monitor blood sugar if diabetic

---

promethazine (℞)

(proe-meth′a-zeen)
Anergan 50, Phenergan, Phenergan Fortis, Phenergan Plain, promethazine HCl

Func. class.: Antihistamine, H₁-receptor antagonist

Chem. class.: Phenothiazine derivative

Action: Acts on blood vessels, GI, respiratory system by competing with histamine for H_1-receptor site; decreases allergic response by blocking histamine

Uses: Motion sickness, rhinitis, allergy symptoms, sedation, nausea, preoperative and postoperative sedation

Dosage and routes:

Nausea
- *Adult:* **PO/IM/IV** 10-25 mg; may repeat 12.5-25 mg q4-6h
- *Child >2 yr:* **PO/IM** 0.25-0.5 mg/kg q4-6h

Motion sickness
- *Adult:* **PO** 25 mg bid, give ½-1 hr before departure
- *Child >2 yr:* **PO/IM/RECT** 12.5-25 mg bid, give ½-1 hr before departure

Allergy/rhinitis
- *Adult:* **PO** 12.5 mg qid, or 25 mg hs
- *Child >2 yr:* **PO** 6.25-12.5 mg tid or 25 mg hs

Sedation
- *Adult:* **PO/IM** 25-50 mg hs
- *Child >2 yr:* **PO/IM/RECT** 12.5-25 mg hs

Sedation (preoperative/postoperative)
- *Adult:* **PO/IM/IV** 25-50 mg
- *Child >2 yr:* **PO/IM/IV** 12.5-25 mg

Available forms: Tabs 12.5, 25, 50 mg; supp 12.5, 25, 50 mg; inj 25, 50 mg/ml, syr 6.25 mg/5 ml, 10 mg/5 ml*, 25 mg/5 ml

Side effects/adverse reactions:

CNS: Dizziness, drowsiness, poor coordination, fatigue, anxiety, euphoria, confusion, paresthesia, neuritis, EPS, *neuroleptic malignant syndrome*

CV: Hypotension, palpitations, tachycardia

RESP: Increased thick secretions, wheezing, chest tightness, *apnea in neonates, infants, young children*

HEMA: Thrombocytopenia, agranulocytosis, hemolytic anemia

GI: Constipation, dry mouth, nausea, vomiting, anorexia, diarrhea

INTEG: Rash, urticaria, photosensitivity

GU: Urinary retention, dysuria, frequency

EENT: Blurred vision, dilated pupils, tinnitus, nasal stuffiness; dry nose, throat, mouth; photosensitivity

Contraindications: Hypersensitivity to H_1-receptor antagonist, acute asthma attack, lower respiratory tract disease

Precautions: Increased intraocular pressure, renal disease, cardiac disease, hypertension, bronchial asthma, seizure disorder, stenosed peptic ulcers, hyperthyroidism, prostatic hypertrophy, bladder neck obstruction, pregnancy (C)

Do not confuse:

Phenergan/Theragran

Pharmacokinetics:

PO: Onset 20 min, duration 4-6 hr; metabolized in liver; excreted by

---

◆ = Nursing alert   ⫘ = Herb-drug interaction   ⊘ = Do not crush kidneys, GI tract (inactive metabolites)

Interactions:

• Increased CNS depression: barbiturates, narcotics, hypnotics, tricyclics, alcohol

• Decreased effect of oral anticoagulants, heparin

• Increased effect of promethazine: MAOIs

⚕ Increased anticholinergic effect: henbane

Lab test interferences:

False-negative: Skin allergy test

False-positive: Urine pregnancy test

NURSING CONSIDERATIONS

Assess:

• I&O ratio; be alert for urinary retention, frequency, dysuria; drug should be discontinued

• CBC during long-term therapy; blood dyscrasias

• Respiratory status: rate, rhythm, increase in bronchial secretions, wheezing, chest tightness

• Cardiac status: palpitations, increased pulse, hypotension

Administer:

• With meals for GI symptoms; absorption may slightly decrease

• When used for motion sickness, 30 min before travel

IM

• IM inj deep in large muscle; rotate site

IV

• After diluting each 25-50 mg/9 ml of NaCl for inj; give 25 mg or less/2 min

Additive compatibilities: Amikacin, ascorbic acid, chloroquine, hydromorphone, netilmicin, vit B/C

Syringe compatibilities: Atropine, butorphanol, chlorpromazine, cimetidine, diphenhydramine, droperidol, fentanyl, glycopyrrolate, hydromorphone, hydroxyzine, meperidine, metoclopramide, midazolam, pentazocine, perphenazine, prochlorperazine, promazine, ranitidine, scopolamine

Y-site compatibilities: Amifostine, amsacrine, aztreonam, ciprofloxacin, cisatracurium, cisplatin, cladribine, cyclophosphamide, cytarabine, doxorubicin, filgrastim, fluconazole, fludarabine, granisetron, melphalan, ondansetron, remifentanil, sargramostim, teniposide, thiotepa, vinorelbine

Perform/provide:

• Hard candy, gum, frequent rinsing of mouth for dryness

• Storage in tight, light-resistant container

Evaluate:

• Therapeutic response: absence of running, congested nose, rashes, absence of motion sickness, nausea; sedation

Teach patient/family:

• That drug may cause photosensitivity; to avoid prolonged sunlight

• To notify prescriber of confusion, sedation, hypotension

• To avoid driving, other hazardous activity if drowsy

• To avoid concurrent use of alcohol, other CNS depressants

Treatment of overdose: Administer ipecac syrup or lavage, diazepam, vasopressors, barbiturates (short-acting)

P

---

propafenone (℞)

(pro-paff'e-nown)

Rythmol

Func. class.: Antidysrhythmic, (Class Ic)

Action: Slows conduction velocity; reduces membrane responsiveness; inhibits automaticity; increases ratio of effective refractory period to action potential duration; β-blocking activity

---

Uses: Life-threatening dysrhythmias, sustained ventricular tachycardia

Dosage and routes:
• *Adult:* **PO** 300-900 mg/day in divided doses, 150 mg q8h; allow a 3-4 day interval before increasing dose

Available forms: Tabs 150, 225, 300 mg

Side effects/adverse reactions:
INTEG: Rash

*CV: **Dysrhythmias, bradycardia,*** pro-dysrhythmia, palpitations, AV block, intraventricular conduction delay, AV dissociation, ***CHF, sudden death, atrial flutter***

*HEMA: **Leukopenia, agranulocytosis, granulocytopenia, thrombocytopenia,*** anemia

CNS: Headache, dizziness, abnormal dreams, syncope, confusion, ***seizures***

*GI: **Nausea, vomiting,*** constipation, dyspepsia, cholestasis, ***hepatitis,*** abnormal liver function studies, dry mouth

RESP: Dyspnea

EENT: Blurred vision, altered taste, tinnitus

Contraindications: 2nd-, 3rd-degree AV block, right bundle branch block, cardiogenic shock, hypersensitivity, bradycardia, uncontrolled CHF, sick-sinus syndrome, marked hypotension, bronchospastic disorders

Precautions: CHF, hypokalemia, hyperkalemia, recent MI, nonallergic bronchospasm, pregnancy (C), lactation, children, hepatic or renal disease

Pharmacokinetics: Peak 3-5 hr, half-life 2-10 hr; metabolized in liver; excreted in urine (metabolite)

Interactions:
• Increased effect of propafenone: cimetidine, quinidine
• Increased anticoagulation: warfarin
• Increased digoxin level: digoxin
• Increased β-blocker effect: propranolol, metoprolol
• Increased cyclosporine levels: cyclosporine
• Decreased propafenone effect: rifampin

▰ Decreased potassium, increased antidysrhythmic action: aloe, buckthorn, cascara sagrada, senna pod/leaf

Lab test interferences:
Increase: CPK

NURSING CONSIDERATIONS
Assess:
• GI status: bowel pattern, number of stools
• Cardiac status: rate, rhythm, quality
• Chest x-ray film, pulmonary function test during treatment
• I&O ratio; check for decreasing output
• B/P for fluctuations
• Lung fields; bilateral rales may occur in CHF patient
• Increased respiration, increased pulse; drug should be discontinued
◆ Toxicity: fine tremors, dizziness
• Cardiac function: respiratory rate, rhythm, character continuously

Evaluate:
• Therapeutic response: absence of dysrhythmias

Teach patient/family:
• To avoid hazardous activities until response is known
• To report fever, chills, sore throat, bleeding, shortness of breath
• To carry emergency ID identifying medication and prescriber

Treatment of overdose: O_2, artificial ventilation, ECG; administer dopamine for circulatory depression, diazepam or thiopental for convulsions

◆ = Nursing alert　　*▰* = Herb-drug interaction　　⊘ = Do not crush

propantheline (℞)

(pro-pan'the-leen)
Pro-Banthine, Propanthel*,
propantheline bromide
Func. class.: GI anticholinergic
Chem. class.: Synthetic quaternary ammonium compound

Action: Inhibits muscarinic actions of acetylcholine at postganglionic parasympathetic neuroeffector sites

Uses: Treatment of peptic ulcer disease, irritable bowel syndrome, duodenography, urinary incontinence

Investigational uses: Antispasmodic uses

Dosage and routes:
• *Adult:* **PO** 15 mg tid ac, 30 mg hs
• *Elderly:* **PO** 7.5 mg tid ac
• *Child:* 1.5 mg/kg/day divided in 3-4 doses (antisecretory); 2-3 mg/kg/day divided q4-6hr and hs (antispasmodic)

Available forms: Tabs 7.5, 15 mg

Side effects/adverse reactions:
CNS: Confusion, stimulation in elderly, headache, insomnia, dizziness, drowsiness, anxiety, weakness, hallucinations
*GI: Dry mouth, constipation, **paralytic ileus,** heartburn, nausea, vomiting, dysphagia, absence of taste
GU: Urinary hesitancy, retention, impotence
CV: Palpitations, tachycardia, orthostatic hypotension (elderly)
EENT: Blurred vision, photophobia, mydriasis, cycloplegia, increased ocular tension
INTEG: Urticaria, rash, pruritus, anhidrosis, fever, allergic reactions

Contraindications: Hypersensitivity to anticholinergics, narrow-angle glaucoma, GI obstruction, myasthenia gravis, paralytic ileus, GI atony, toxic megacolon

Precautions: Hyperthyroidism, coronary artery disease, dysrhythmias, CHF, ulcerative colitis, hypertension, hiatal hernia, hepatic disease, renal disease, pregnancy (C), urinary retention, prostatic hypertrophy, elderly

Pharmacokinetics:
PO: Onset 30-45 min, duration 6 hr; metabolized by liver, GI system; excreted in urine, bile

Interactions:
• Increased anticholinergic effect: amantadine, tricyclics, MAOIs, H_1-antihistamines
• Decreased effect of phenothiazines, levodopa, ketoconazole

NURSING CONSIDERATIONS
Assess:
• VS, cardiac status: checking for dysrhythmias, increased rate, palpitations
• I&O ratio; check for urinary retention or hesitancy
• GI complaints: pain, bleeding (frank or occult), nausea, vomiting, anorexia

Administer:
• ½-1 hr ac for better absorption
• Decreased dose to elderly patients; metabolism may be slowed
• Gum, hard candy, frequent rinsing for dry mouth

Perform/provide:
• Storage in tight container protected from light
• Increased fluids, bulk, exercise to decrease constipation

Evaluate:
• Therapeutic response: absence of epigastric pain, bleeding, nausea, vomiting

Teach patient/family:
• To avoid driving, other hazardous activities until stabilized on medication; may cause blurred vision; to use caution when standing due to orthostatic hypotension
• To avoid alcohol, other CNS de-

P

Side effects: *italics* = common; ***bold italics*** = life-threatening

pressants; will enhance sedating properties of this drug
• To drink plenty of fluids
• To report dysphagia

propofol (℞)

(pro'poh-fole)

Diprivan, Disoprofol

Func. class.: General anesthetic

Action: Produces dose-dependent CNS depression; action is unknown

Uses: Induction or maintenance of anesthesia as part of balanced anesthetic technique; sedation in mechanically ventilated patients

Dosage and routes:

Induction

• *Adult:* **IV** 2-2.5 mg/kg, approximately 40 mg q10sec until induction onset

• *Child ≥3 yr:* **IV** 2.5-3.5 mg/kg over 20-30 sec

• *Elderly:* **IV** 1-1.5 mg/kg, approximately 20 mg q10sec until induction onset

Maintenance

• *Adult:* **IV** 0.1-0.2 mg/kg/min (6-12 mg/kg/hr)

• *Child ≥3 yr:* **IV** 0.125-0.3 mg/kg/min (7.5-18 mg/kg/hr)

• *Elderly:* **IV** 0.05-0.1 mg/kg/min (3-6 mg/kg/hr)

ICU sedation

• *Adult:* **IV** 5 µg/kg/min over 5 min; may give 5-10 µg/kg/min over 5-10 min until desired response

Available forms: Inj 10 mg/ml in 20 ml ampule, 50 ml and 100 ml vials; inj emulsion 10 mg/ml

Side effects/adverse reactions:

CNS: Movement, headache, jerking, fever, dizziness, shivering, tremor, confusion, somnolence, paresthesia, agitation, abnormal dreams, euphoria, fatigue

GI: Nausea, vomiting, abdominal

cramping, dry mouth, swallowing, hypersalivation

MS: Myalgia

GU: Urine retention, green urine

EENT: Blurred vision, tinnitus, eye pain, strange taste

CV: Bradycardia, hypotension, hypertension, PVC, PAC, tachycardia, abnormal ECG, ST segment depression, *asystole*

*RESP: **Apnea,** cough, hiccups,* dyspnea, hypoventilation, sneezing, wheezing, tachypnea, hypoxia

INTEG: Flushing, phlebitis, hives, burning/stinging at injection site

Contraindications: Hypersensitivity, hyperlipidemia

Precautions: Elderly, respiratory depression, severe respiratory disorders, cardiac dysrhythmias, pregnancy (B), labor and delivery, lactation, children

Pharmacokinetics: Onset 40 sec, rapid distribution, half-life 1-8 min, terminal elimination half-life 5-10 hr; 70% excreted in urine; metabolized in liver by conjugation to inactive metabolites

Interactions:

• Increased CNS depression: alcohol, narcotics, sedative/hypnotics, antipsychotics, skeletal muscle relaxants, inhalational anesthetics

• Do not administer with other drugs

NURSING CONSIDERATIONS

Assess:

• Injection site: phlebitis, burning, stinging

• ECG for changes: PVC, PAC, ST segment changes

• CNS changes: movement, jerking, tremors, dizziness, LOC, pupil reaction

• Allergic reactions: hives

 Respiratory dysfunction: respiratory depression, character, rate, rhythm; notify prescriber if respirations are <10/min

Administer:
IV
• After diluting with D₅W mixed in lipid base; use only glass containers when mixing, not stable in plastic
• Alone; do not mix with other agents before using
• Only with resuscitative equipment available
• Only by qualified persons trained in anesthesia
Syringe compatibilities: Thiopental
Y-site compatibilities: Acyclovir, alfentanil, amikacin, aminophylline, ampicillin, amrinone, aztreonam, bumetanide, buprenorphine, butorphanol, calcium gluconate, carboplatin, cefazolin, cefonicid, cefoperazone, cefotaxime, cefotetan, cefoxitin, ceftazidime, ceftizoxime, ceftriaxone, cefuroxime, chlorpromazine, cimetidine, ciprofloxacin, cisplatin, clindamycin, cyclophosphamide, cyclosporine, cytarabine, dexamethasone, digoxin, diphenhydramine, dobutamine, dopamine, doxorubicin, doxycycline, droperidol, enalaprilat, ephedrine, epinephrine, esmolol, famotidine, fentanyl, fluconazole, fluorouracil, furosemide, ganciclovir, glycopyrrolate, granisetron, haloperidol, heparin, hydrocortisone, hydromorphone, hydroxyzine, ifosfamide, imipenem/cilastatin, insulin, isoproterenol, ketamine, labetalol, levorphanol, lidocaine, lorazepam, magnesium sulfate, mannitol, meperidine, metoclopramide, mezlocillin, miconazole, morphine, nafcillin, nalbuphine, naloxone, nitroglycerin, norepinephrine, ofloxacin, paclitaxel, pentobarbital, phenobarbital, piperacillin, potassium chloride, prochlorperazine, propranolol, ranitidine, scopolamine, sodium bicarbonate, sodium nitroprusside, succinylcholine, sufentanil, ticarcillin, ticarcillin/clavulanate, vancomycin, vecuronium, verapamil
Perform/provide:
• Storage in light-resistant area at room temperature
• Safety measures: night-light, call bell within easy reach
Evaluate:
• Therapeutic response: induction of anesthesia
Treatment of overdose: Discontinue drug; administer vasopressor agents or anticholinergics, artificial ventilation

---

propoxyphene (℞)
(proe-pox'i-feen)
Darvon, Darvon-N, Dolene, Novapropoxyn*
Func. class.: Opiate analgesic
Chem. class.: Synthetic opiate
Controlled Substance Schedule IV
Action: Depresses pain impulse transmission at the spinal cord level by interacting with opioid receptors
Uses: Mild to moderate pain
Dosage and routes:
• *Adult:* **PO** 65 mg q4h prn (HCl)
• *Adult:* **PO** 100 mg q4h prn (napsylate)
Available forms: Propoxyphene HCl Caps 32, 65 mg; propoxyphene napsylate tabs 100 mg; oral susp 50 mg/5 ml
Side effects/adverse reactions:
CNS: Drowsiness, dizziness, confusion, headache, sedation, euphoria, **convulsions, hyperthermia** (elderly)
GI: Nausea, vomiting, anorexia, constipation, cramps
GU: Urinary retention, dysuria
INTEG: Rash, urticaria, bruising, flushing, diaphoresis, pruritus
EENT: Tinnitus, blurred vision, miosis, diplopia

P

---

* = Canada only   Side effects: *italics* = common; ***bold italics*** = life-threatening

CV: Palpitations, bradycardia, change in B/P, *dysrhythmias*
RESP: Respiratory depression
Contraindications: Hypersensitivity to ASA products (some preparations), addiction (opioid)
Precautions: Addictive personality, pregnancy (C), lactation, increased intracranial pressure, MI (acute), severe heart disease, respiratory depression, hepatic disease, renal disease, child <18 yr, elderly
Pharmacokinetics:
PO: Onset ½-1 hr, peak 2-2½ hr, duration 4-6 hr
Metabolized by liver, excreted by kidneys (as metabolites), crosses placenta, excreted in breast milk, half-life 6-12 hr (metabolites)
Interactions:
• Increased effects with other CNS depressants: alcohol, narcotics, sedative/hypnotics, antipsychotics, skeletal muscle relaxants
Lab test interferences:
Increase: Amylase
NURSING CONSIDERATIONS
Assess:
• For pain: duration, location, type
• I&O ratio; check for decreasing output; may indicate retention
• CNS changes: dizziness, drowsiness, hallucinations, euphoria, loss of consciousness, pupil reaction
• Allergic reactions: rash, urticaria
• Respiratory dysfunction: respiratory depression, character, rate, rhythm; notify prescriber if respirations are <10/min
• Need for pain medication; physical dependence
Administer:
• With antiemetic for nausea, vomiting
• When pain is beginning to return; determine dosage interval by response

Perform/provide:
• Storage in light-resistant area at room temperature
• Assistance with ambulation
• Safety measures: night-light, call bell within easy reach
Evaluate:
• Therapeutic response: decrease in pain
Teach patient/family:
• To report any symptoms of CNS changes, allergic reactions
• That physical dependency may result when used for extended periods; not to exceed dose
• That withdrawal symptoms may occur: nausea, vomiting, cramps, fever, faintness, anorexia
Treatment of overdose: Naloxone (Narcan) 0.2-0.8 mg IV, O₂, IV fluids, vasopressors

propranolol (Rx)
(proe-pran'oh-lole)
Apo-Propranolol*, Detensol*, Inderal, Inderal LA, propranolol HCl, Propranolol Intensol, Novo-Pranol*
Func. class.: Antihypertensive, antianginal
Chem. class.: β-Adrenergic blocker

Action: Nonselective β-blocker with negative inotropic, chronotropic, dromotropic properties
Uses: Chronic stable angina pectoris, hypertension, supraventricular dysrhythmias, migraine, prophylaxis, MI, pheochromocytoma, essential tremor, cyanotic spells related to hypertrophic subaortic stenosis, tetralogy of Fallot, dysrhythmias associated with thyrotoxicosis, alcohol withdrawal
Investigational uses: Mitral valve prolapse, anxiety, hyperthyroidism

= Nursing alert   = Herb-drug interaction   = Do not crush

adjunct therapy; Parkinson's tremor, prevention of variceal bleeding caused by pork, hypertension, akathisia

Dosage and routes:

Dysrhythmias

• *Adult:* PO 10-30 mg tid-qid; **IV BOL** 0.5-3 mg give 1 mg/min; may repeat in 2 min, may repeat q4h thereafter

• *Child:* PO 0.5-1 mg/kg/day divided q6-8h; **IV** 0.01-0.1 mg/kg

Hypertension

• *Adult:* PO 40 mg bid or 80 mg qd (ext rel) initially; usual dose 120-240 mg/day bid-tid or 120-160 mg qd (ext rel)

• *Child:* PO 0.5-1 mg/kg/day divided q6-12h

Angina

• *Adult:* PO 80-320 mg in divided doses bid-qid or 80 mg qd (ext rel); usual dose 160 mg qd (ext rel)

MI prophylaxis

• *Adult:* PO 180-240 mg/day tid-qid starting 5 day to 2 wk after MI

Pheochromocytoma

• *Adult:* PO 60 mg/day × 3 days preoperatively in divided doses or 30 mg/day in divided doses (inoperable tumor)

Migraine

• *Adult:* PO 80 mg/day (ext rel) or in divided doses; may increase to 160-240 mg/day in divided doses

• *Child:* PO 0.6-1.5 mg/kg/day divided q8h PO

Essential tremor

• *Adult:* PO 40 mg bid; usual dose 120 mg/day

Tetralogy of Fallot

• *Child:* PO 1-2 mg/kg/dose q6h

Available forms: Caps, sus rel 60, 80, 120, 160 mg; tabs 10, 20, 40, 60, 80, 90 mg; inj 1 mg/ml; oral sol 4 mg/ml, 8 mg/ml; conc oral sol 80 mg/ml

Side effects/adverse reactions:

RESP: Dyspnea, respiratory dysfunction, *bronchospasm,* cough

CV: Bradycardia, hypotension, **CHF,** palpitations, AV block, peripheral vascular insufficiency, vasodilation

HEMA: **Agranulocytosis, thrombocytopenia**

GI: Nausea, vomiting, diarrhea, colitis, constipation, cramps, dry mouth, hepatomegaly, gastric pain, acute pancreatitis

GU: Impotence, decreased libido, UTIs

MS: Joint pain, arthralgia, muscle cramps, pain

MISC: Facial swelling, weight change, Raynaud's phenomenon

INTEG: Rash, pruritus, fever

CNS: Depression, hallucinations, dizziness, fatigue, lethargy, paresthesias, bizarre dreams, disorientation

EENT: Sore throat, *laryngospasm,* blurred vision, dry eyes

META: Hyperglycemia, hypoglycemia

Contraindications: Hypersensitivity to this drug; cardiac failure; cardiogenic shock, 2nd-, 3rd-degree heart block; bronchospastic disease; sinus bradycardia; CHF

Precautions: Diabetes mellitus, pregnancy (C), renal disease, lactation, hyperthyroidism, COPD, hepatic disease, children, myasthenia gravis, peripheral vascular disease, hypotension, CHF

Do not confuse:

Inderal/Toradol

Inderal/LA/IMDUR

Pharmacokinetics:

PO: Onset 30 min, peak 1-1½ hr, duration 6-12 hr

PO-ER: Peak 6 hr, duration 24 hr

IV: Onset 2 min, peak 15 min, duration 3-6 hr; immediate rel half-life 3-5 hr; ext rel half-life 8-11 hr; metabolized by liver; crosses placenta, blood-brain barrier; excreted in breast milk, protein binding 90%

Interactions:

- AV block: digitalis, calcium channel blockers
- Increased negative inotropic effects: verapamil, disopyramide
- Increased effects of reserpine, digitalis, neuromuscular blocking agents
- Decreased β-blocking effects: norepinephrine, isoproterenol, barbiturates, rifampin, dopamine, dobutamine, smoking
- Increased β-blocking effect: cimetidine
- Increased hypotension: quinidine, haloperidol, hydralazine

Lab test interferences:

Increase: Serum K, serum uric acid, ALT, AST, alk phosphatase, LDH
Decrease: Blood glucose

NURSING CONSIDERATIONS

Assess:

- B/P, pulse, respirations during beginning therapy; notify prescriber if pulse <50 BPM
- Weight qd; report gain of 5 lb
- I&O ratio, CrCl if kidney damage is diagnosed
- ECG if using as antidysrhythmic
- Hepatic enzymes: AST, ALT, bilirubin
- Angina pain: duration, time started, activity being performed, character
- Tolerance (long-term use)
- Headache, light-headedness, decreased B/P; may indicate a need for decreased dosage

Administer:

- With 8 oz water on empty stomach
- Do not give with aluminum-containing antacid; may decrease GI absorption

IV

- IV undiluted or diluted 10 ml D₅W for inj; give 1 mg or less/min; may be diluted in 50 ml NaCl and run 1 mg over 10-15 min

Additive compatibilities: Dobutamine, verapamil

Solution compatibilities: 0.9% NaCl, 0.45 NaCl, Ringer's, D₅W, D₅/0.9% NaCl, D₅/0.45% NaCl

Syringe compatibilities: Amrinone, benzquinamide, milrinone

Y-site compatibilities: Alteplase, amrinone, heparin, hydrocortisone, meperidine, milrinone, morphine, potassium chloride, propofol, tacrolimus, vit B/C

Perform/provide:

- Protection from light (injection)

Evaluate:

- Therapeutic response: decreased B/P, dysrhythmias

Teach patient/family:

- Not to discontinue abruptly, to take drug at same time each day; to decrease dosage over 2 wk to prevent cardiac damage
- To avoid OTC drugs unless approved by prescriber
- To avoid hazardous activities if dizzy
- The importance of compliance with complete medical regimen
- To make position changes slowly to prevent fainting

---

propylthiouracil (℞)
(proe-pill-thye-oh-yoor′a-sill)
propylthiouracil, Propyl-Thyracil*, PTU
Func. class.: Thyroid hormone antagonist (antithyroid)
Chem. class.: Thioamide

Action: Blocks synthesis peripherally of T₃, T₄ (triiodothyronine, thyroxine), inhibits organification of iodine

Uses: Preparation for thyroidectomy, thyrotoxic crisis, hyperthyroidism, thyroid storm

◆ = Nursing alert   ✦ = Herb-drug interaction   ⊘ = Do not crush

Dosage and routes:

Thyrotoxic crisis

• *Adult and child:* PO same as hyperthyroidism with iodine and propranolol

Preparation for thyroidectomy

• *Adult:* 600-1200 mg/day

• *Child:* 10 mg/kg/day in divided doses

Hyperthyroidism

• *Adult:* **PO** 100 mg tid increasing to 300 mg q8h if condition is severe; continue to euthyroid state, then 100 mg qd-tid

• *Child >10 yr:* **PO** 100 mg tid; continue to euthyroid state, then 25 mg tid to 100 mg bid

• *Child 6-10 yr:* **PO** 50-150 mg in divided doses q8h

• *Neonate:* **PO** 10 mg/kg/day in divided doses

Available forms: Tabs 50, 100 mg

Side effects/adverse reactions:

INTEG: Rash, urticaria, pruritus, alopecia, hyperpigmentation, lupuslike syndrome

*GU: **Nephritis***

CNS: Drowsiness, headache, vertigo, fever, paresthesias, neuritis

*HEMA: **Agranulocytosis, leukopenia, thrombocytopenia, hypothrombinemia, lymphadenopathy,*** bleeding, vasculitis, periarteritis

*GI: Nausea, diarrhea, vomiting, **jaundice, hepatitis,*** loss of taste

MS: Myalgia, arthralgia, nocturnal muscle cramps, osteoporosis

Contraindications: Hypersensitivity, pregnancy (D), lactation

Precautions: Infection, bone marrow depression, hepatic disease

Pharmacokinetics:

PO: Onset up to 3 wk, peak 6-10 wk, duration 1 wk to 1 mo, half-life 1-2 hr; excreted in urine, bile, breast milk; crosses placenta; concentration in thyroid gland

Interactions:

• Increased anticoagulant effect: heparin, oral anticoagulants

• Bone marrow depression: radiation, antineoplastics

• Additive effects: potassium/sodium iodide, lithium

• Agranulocytosis: phenothiazines

Lab test interferences:

Increase: PT, AST, ALT, alk phosphatase

NURSING CONSIDERATIONS

Assess:

• Pulse, B/P, temp

• I&O ratio; check for edema: puffy hands, feet, periorbits; indicates hypothyroidism

• Weight qd; same clothing, scale, time of day

• T_3, T_4, which are increased; serum TSH, which is decreased; free thyroxine index, which is increased if dosage is too low; discontinue drug 3-4 wk before RAIU

◆ Blood work: CBC for blood dyscrasias: leukopenia, thrombocytopenia, agranulocytosis; LFTs

◆ Overdose: peripheral edema, heat intolerance, diaphoresis, palpitations, dysrhythmias, severe tachycardia, increased temp, delirium, CNS irritability

◆ Hypersensitivity: rash, enlarged cervical lymph nodes; drug may have to be discontinued

• Hypoprothrombinemia: bleeding, petechiae, ecchymosis

• Clinical response: after 3 wk should include increased weight, pulse; decreased T_4

• Bone marrow depression: sore throat, fever, fatigue

Administer:

• With meals to decrease GI upset

• At same time each day to maintain drug level

• Lowest dose that relieves symptoms

P

Side effects: *italics* = common; ***bold italics*** = life-threatening

Perform/provide:
• Storage in light-resistant container
• Fluids to 3-4 L/day, unless contraindicated

Evaluate:
• Therapeutic response: weight gain, decreased pulse, decreased T₄, decreased B/P

Teach patient/family:
• To abstain from breastfeeding after delivery
• To take pulse qd
• To report redness, swelling, sore throat, mouth lesions, which indicate blood dyscrasias
• To keep graph of weight, pulse, mood
• To avoid OTC products that contain iodine
• That seafood, other iodine products may be restricted
• Not to discontinue this medication abruptly; thyroid crisis may occur; stress response
• That response may take several months if thyroid is large
• The symptoms/signs of overdose: periorbital edema, cold intolerance, mental depression
• The symptoms of inadequate dose: tachycardia, diarrhea, fever, irritability
• To take medication as prescribed; not to skip or double dose; missed doses should be taken when remembered up to 1 hr before next dose
• To carry Medic Alert ID listing condition, medication

---

protamine (R)
(proe'ta-meen)

Func. class.: Heparin antagonist

Chem. class.: Low-molecular-weight protein

Action: Binds heparin, making it ineffective

Uses: Heparin overdose

Dosage and routes:
• *Adult and child:* **IV** 1 mg of protamine/90-115 U heparin given; administer slowly 1-3 min; not to exceed 50 mg/10 min

Available forms: Inj 10 mg/ml

Side effects/adverse reactions:
CV: Hypotension, bradycardia, *circulatory collapse*
GI: Nausea, vomiting, anorexia
INTEG: Rash, dermatitis, urticaria
CNS: Lassitude
HEMA: Bleeding, *anaphylaxis*
RESP: Dyspnea, *pulmonary edema, severe respiratory distress*

Contraindications: Hypersensitivity

Precautions: Pregnancy (C), lactation, children, allergy to salmon

Pharmacokinetics:
IV: Onset 5 min, duration 2 hr

NURSING CONSIDERATIONS
Assess:
• Blood studies (Hct, platelets, occult blood in stools) q3mo
• Coagulation tests (APTT, ACT) 15 min after dose, then in several hours
• VS, B/P, pulse after 30 min; plus 3 hr after dose
• Skin rash, urticaria, dermatitis
◆ Allergy to fish; use with caution

Administer:
IV
• After diluting 50 mg/5 ml sterile bacteriostatic H₂O for inj; shake; give 20 mg or less over 1-3 min; may further dilute with equal volume of NaCl or D₅W and run over 2-3 hr; titrate to APTT, ACT; use infusion pump

Additive compatibilities: Cimetidine, ranitidine, verapamil

Perform/provide:
• Storage at 36°-46° F (2°-8° C)

Evaluate:
• Therapeutic response: reversal of heparin overdose

◆ = Nursing alert   🌿 = Herb-drug interaction   ⊘ = Do not crush

pseudoephedrine
(OTC, ℞)

(soo-doh-eh-fed'rin)

Afrin, Allermed, Canafed, Cenafed, Children's Congestion Relief, Children's Silfedrine, Congestion Relief, Decofed Syrup, DeFed-60, Dorcol Children's Decongestant, Drixoral Non-Drowsy Formula, Dynafed, Efidac/24, Eltor*, Genaphed, Halofed, Mini Thin Pseudo, PediaCare Infant's Decongestant, Pseudo, pseudoephedrine HCl, Pseudogest, Seudotabs, Sinustop Pro, Sudafed, Sudafed 12 Hour, Sudex, Triaminic AM Decongestant Formula

Func. class.: Adrenergic

Chem. class.: Substituted phenylethylamine

Action: Primary activity through α-effects on respiratory mucosal membranes reducing congestion hyperemia, edema; minimal bronchodilation secondary to β-effects

Uses: Nasal decongestant, adjunct in otitis media; with antihistamines

Dosage and routes:
• *Adult:* PO 60 mg q6h; ext rel 60-120 mg q12h or q24h
• *Geriatric:* PO 30-60 mg q6h prn
• *Child 6-12 yr:* PO 30 mg q6h, not to exceed 120 mg/day
• *Child 2-6 yr:* PO 15 mg q6h, not to exceed 60 mg/day

Available forms: Caps, ext rel 120, 240 mg; oral sol 15 mg, 30 mg/5 ml; drops 7.5 mg/0.8 ml; tabs 30, 60 mg; caps 60 mg; tabs, ext rel 120, 240 mg

Side effects/adverse reactions:
CNS: Tremors, anxiety, insomnia, headache, dizziness, hallucinations, *seizures* (elderly)

EENT: Dry nose, irritation of nose and throat

CV: Palpitations, tachycardia, hypertension, chest pain, ***dysrhythmias, CV collapse***

GI: Anorexia, nausea, vomiting, dry mouth

GU: Dysuria

Contraindications: Hypersensitivity to sympathomimetics, narrow-angle glaucoma

Precautions: Pregnancy (C), cardiac disorders, hyperthyroidism, diabetes mellitus, prostatic hypertrophy, lactation, hypertension

Pharmacokinetics:
PO: Onset 15-30 min, duration 4-6 hr, 8-12 hr (ext rel); metabolized in liver, excreted in feces and breast milk

Interactions:
◆ Do not use with MAOIs or tricyclics; hypertensive crisis may occur
• Decreased effect of this drug: methyldopa, urinary acidifiers, rauwolfia alkaloids
• Increased effect of this drug: urinary alkalizers

NURSING CONSIDERATIONS
Assess:
• For nasal congestion; auscultate lung sounds; check for tenacious bronchial secretions
• B/P, pulse throughout treatment
• For CNS side effects in the elderly: excitation, seizures, hallucinations

Perform/provide:
• Storage at room temperature

Evaluate:
• Therapeutic response: decreased nasal congestion

Teach patient/family:
• The reason for drug administration
• Not to use continuously, or more than recommended dose; rebound congestion may occur

• To check with prescriber before using other drugs, as drug interactions may occur
• To avoid taking near hs; stimulation can occur
• Not to use if stimulation, restlessness, or tremors occur
• That use in children may cause excessive agitation

---

psyllium (OTC, ℞)
(sill´ee-um)

Alramucil, Fiberall, Fiberall Natural Flavor and Orange Flavor, Genifiber, Hydrocil Instant, Karacil*, Konsyl, Konsyl Orange, Maalox Daily Fiber Therapy, Metamucil, Metamucil Lemon Lime, Metamucil Orange Flavor, Metamucil Sugar Free, Metamucil Sugar Free Orange Flavor, Modane Bulk, Mylanta Natural Fiber Supplement, Natural Fiber Laxative, Natural Fiber Laxative Sugar Free, Natural Vegetable Reguloid, Perdiem, Prodiem Plain*, Reguloid Natural, Reguloid Orange, Reguloid Sugar Free Orange, Reguloid Sugar Free Regular, Restore, Restore Sugar Free, Serutan, Syllact, V-Lax

Func. class.: Bulk laxative
Chem. class.: Psyllium colloid

Action: Bulk-forming laxative
Uses: Chronic constipation, ulcerative colitis, irritable bowel syndrome
Dosage and routes:
• *Adult:* **PO** 1-2 tsp in 8 oz H_2O bid or tid, then 8 oz H_2O or 1 premeasured packet in 8 oz H_2O bid or tid, then 8 oz H_2O
• *Child >6 yr:* **PO** 1 tsp in 4 oz H_2O hs

Available forms: Chew pieces 1.7, 3.4 g/piece; effervescent pwd 3.4, 3.7 g/packet; pwd 3.3, 3.4, 3.5, 4.94 g/tsp; granules 2.5, 4.03 g/tsp; wafers 3.4 g/wafer
Side effects/adverse reactions:
GI: Nausea, vomiting, anorexia, diarrhea, cramps
Contraindications: Hypersensitivity, intestinal obstruction, abdominal pain, nausea/vomiting, fecal impaction
Precautions: Pregnancy (C)
Pharmacokinetics: Excreted in feces, not absorbed in GI tract
NURSING CONSIDERATIONS
Assess:
• Blood, urine electrolytes if used often
• I&O ratio to identify fluid loss
• Cause of constipation; fluids, bulk, exercise missing
• Cramping, rectal bleeding, nausea, vomiting; drug should be discontinued
Administer:
PO
• Alone for better absorption
• In morning or evening (oral dose)
• Immediately after mixing with H_2O
• With 8 oz H_2O or juice followed by another 8 oz of fluid
Evaluate:
• Therapeutic response: decrease in constipation or decreased diarrhea in colitis
Teach patient/family:
• To maintain adequate fluid consumption
• That normal bowel movements do not always occur daily
• Not to use in presence of abdominal pain, nausea, vomiting
• To notify prescriber if constipation unrelieved or if symptoms of electrolyte imbalance occur: mus-

◆ = Nursing alert　　🌿 = Herb-drug interaction　　🚫 = Do not crush

cle cramps, pain, weakness, dizziness, excessive thirst

pyrantel (OTC)

(pie-ran'tel)
Antiminth, Combantrin*, Pin-Rid, Pin-X, Reese's Pinworm
Func. class.: Anthelmintic
Chem. class.: Pyrimidine derivative

Action: Causes paralysis in worm by neuroblockade via stimulation of ganglionic receptors; worms expelled by normal peristalsis
Uses: Pinworms, roundworms, hookworms
Dosage and routes:
• *Adult and child >2 yr:* **PO** 11 mg/kg as single dose, not to exceed 1 g; repeat in 2 wk for pinworms
Available forms: Oral susp 50 mg/ml; liquid 50 mg/ml; caps, soft gel 180 mg
Side effects/adverse reactions:
INTEG: Rash
CNS: Dizziness, headache, drowsiness, insomnia, fever, weakness
GI: Nausea, vomiting, anorexia, diarrhea, distention, abdominal cramps
Contraindications: Hypersensitivity
Precautions: Seizure disorders, hepatic disease, dehydration, anemia, child <2 yr, pregnancy (C), malnutrition
Pharmacokinetics:
PO: Peak 1-3 hr; metabolized in liver; excreted in feces, urine (unchanged/metabolites)
Interactions:
• Antagonizes effect of pyrantel: piperazine
NURSING CONSIDERATIONS
Assess:
• Stools during entire treatment; specimens must be sent to lab while still warm

• For diarrhea during expulsion of worms
• For allergic reaction: rash
Administer:
PO
• After meals to avoid GI symptoms
• After shaking suspension
Perform/provide:
• Storage in tight, light-resistant container in cool environment
Evaluate:
• Therapeutic response: expulsion of worms, 3 negative stool cultures after completion of treatment
Teach patient/family:
• Proper hygiene after BM, including hand-washing technique; tell patient not to put fingers in mouth
• That infected person should sleep alone; not to shake bed linen; to change bed linen qd, wash in hot water; that all family members should be treated for pinworms; treat dogs/cats; keep children away from animal's feces
• To clean toilet qd with disinfectant (green soap solution)
• The need for compliance with dosage schedule, duration of treatment
• To drink fruit juice to help expel worms
• To wear shoes, wash all fruits, vegetables well before eating

pyrazinamide (R)

(peer-a-zin'a-mide)
PMS Pyrazinamide*, pyrazinamide, Tebrazid*
Func. class.: Antitubercular agent
Chem. class.: Pyrazinoic acid amine, nicoturimide analog

Action: Bactericidal interference with lipid, nucleic acid biosynthesis
Uses: Tuberculosis, as an adjunct when other drugs are not feasible

Dosage and routes:
• *Adult and child:* **PO** 15-30 mg/kg/day not to exceed 2 g/day
Available forms: Tabs 500 mg
Side effects/adverse reactions:
INTEG: Photosensitivity, urticaria
CNS: Headache
*GI: **Hepatotoxicity,** abnormal liver function tests, peptic ulcer
GU: Urinary difficulty, increased uric acid, nausea, vomiting, anorexia, cramps, diarrhea
*HEMA: **Hemolytic anemia***
Contraindications: Hypersensitivity, severe hepatic damage, acute gout
Precautions: Pregnancy (C), child <13 yr, renal failure, diabetes, porphyria, chronic gout
Pharmacokinetics:
PO: Peak 2 hr, half-life 9-10 hr; metabolized in liver, excreted in urine (metabolites/unchanged drug)
Lab test interferences:
Increase: PBI
Decrease: 17-KS
NURSING CONSIDERATIONS
Assess:
• Signs of anemia: Hct, Hgb, fatigue
• Temp; if >101° F (38° C), drug should be reduced
◆ Liver studies qwk: ALT, AST, bilirubin
• Renal status before, qmo: BUN, creatinine, output, sp gr, urinalysis, uric acid
• Hepatic status: decreased appetite, jaundice, dark urine, fatigue
Administer:
PO
• With meals for GI symptoms
• After C&S is completed; qmo to detect resistance
Evaluate:
• Therapeutic response: decreased symptoms of TB, culture negative

Teach patient/family:
• That compliance with dosage schedule, length is necessary
• To avoid alcohol
• To report fever, loss of appetite, malaise, nausea, vomiting, darkened urine, pale stools

---

pyridostigmine (℞)
(peer-id-oh-stig'meen)
Mestinon, Mestinon SR, Mestinon Timespan, Regonol
Func. class.: Cholinergic; anticholinesterase
Chem. class.: Tertiary amine carbamate

Action: Inhibits destruction of acetylcholine, which increases concentration at sites where acetylcholine is released; this facilitates transmission of impulses across myoneural junction
Uses: Nondepolarizing muscle relaxant antagonist, myasthenia gravis
Dosage and routes:
Myasthenia gravis
• *Adult:* **PO** 60-180 mg bid-qid, not to exceed 1.5 g/day; **IM/IV** 2 mg or ¹⁄₃₀ of **PO** dose; **SUS REL** 180-540 mg qd or bid at intervals of at least 6 hr
• *Child:* 7 mg/kg/day in 5-6 divided doses
Nondepolarizing neuromuscular blocker antagonist
• *Adult:* 0.6-1.2 mg **IV** atropine, then 10-30 mg
• *Child:* **IV** 0.1-0.25 mg/kg/dose
Available forms: Tabs 60 mg; tabs, ext rel 180 mg; syr 60 mg/5 ml; inj 5 mg/ml
Side effects/adverse reactions:
INTEG: Rash, urticaria, flushing
CNS: Dizziness, headache, sweating, weakness, ***convulsions,*** inco-

---

◆ = Nursing alert   🖋 = Herb-drug interaction   🚫 = Do not crush

ordination, *paralysis,* drowsiness, LOC

GI: Nausea, diarrhea, vomiting, cramps, increased salivary and gastric secretions, peristalsis

CV: Tachycardia, dysrhythmias, bradycardia, AV block, hypotension, ECG changes, *cardiac arrest,* syncope

GU: Urinary frequency, incontinence, urgency

RESP: Respiratory depression, bronchospasm, constriction, laryngospasm, respiratory arrest

EENT: Miosis, blurred vision, lacrimation, visual changes

Contraindications: Bradycardia; hypotension; obstruction of intestine, renal system; bromide sensitivity

Precautions: Seizure disorders, bronchial asthma, coronary occlusion, hyperthyroidism, dysrhythmias, peptic ulcer, megacolon, poor GI motility, pregnancy (C)

Pharmacokinetics:

PO: Onset 20-30 min, duration 3-6 hr

IM/IV/SC: Onset 2-15 min, duration 2½-4 hr; metabolized in liver, excreted in urine

Interactions:

• Decreased action: gallamine, metocurine, pancuronium, tubocurarine, atropine

• Increased action: decamethonium, succinylcholine

• Decreased action of pyridostigmine: aminoglycosides, anesthetics, procainamide, quinidine, mecamylamine, polymyxin, magnesium, corticosteroids, antidysrhythmics

NURSING CONSIDERATIONS
Assess:

• VS, respiration q8h

• I&O ratio; check for urinary retention or incontinence

• Bradycardia, hypotension, bronchospasm, headache, dizziness, convulsions, respiratory depression; drug should be discontinued if toxicity occurs

Administer:

• Only with atropine sulfate available for cholinergic crisis

• Only after all other cholinergics have been discontinued

• Increased doses for tolerance, as ordered

• Larger doses after exercise or fatigue, as ordered

• On empty stomach for better absorption

IV

• Undiluted, give through Y-tube or 3-way stopcock, give 0.5 mg or less/min

Syringe compatibilities: Glycopyrrolate

Y-site compatibilities: Heparin, hydrocortisone, potassium chloride, vit B/C

Perform/provide:

• Storage at room temperature

Evaluate:

• Therapeutic response: increased muscle strength, hand grasp, improved gait, absence of labored breathing (if severe)

Teach patient/family:

🚫 Not to break, crush, or chew sus rel tabs

• That drug is not a cure, only relieves symptoms

• To wear Medic Alert ID specifying myasthenia gravis, drugs taken

Treatment of overdose: Discontinue drug, atropine 1-4 mg IV

P

pyridoxine (vit B$_6$)
(R̶, OTC)
(peer-i-dox′een)
Beesix, Doxine, Nestrex, pyridoxine HCl, Pyri, Rodex, Vitabee 6, vitamin B$_6$
Func. class.: Vit B$_6$, water soluble

Action: Needed for fat, protein, carbohydrate metabolism; enhances glycogen release from liver and muscle tissue; needed as coenzyme for metabolic transformations of a variety of amino acids

Uses: Vit B$_6$ deficiency of inborn errors of metabolism, seizures, isoniazid therapy, oral contraceptives, alcoholic polyneuritis

Investigational uses: Palmar-Plantar erythrodysesthesia syndrome

Dosage and routes:

Vit B$_6$ deficiency
• *Adult:* **PO/IM/IV** 10-20 mg qd × 3wk
• *Child:* **PO/IM/IV** 100 mg until desired response

Deficiency caused by isoniazid
• *Adult:* **PO** 6-100 mg qd
• *Child:* **PO** 5-25 mg/day

Prevention of deficiency caused by isoniazid
• *Adult:* **PO** 6-50 mg qd
• *Child:* **PO** 0.5-1.5 mg qd
• *Infant:* **PO** 0.1-0.5 mg qd

Palmar-Plantar erythrodysesthesia syndrome (off-label)
• *Adult:* **PO** 50-150 mg qd

Available forms: Tabs 10, 25, 50, 100 mg; tabs, time rel 100 mg; inj 100 mg/ml

Side effects/adverse reactions:
CNS: Paresthesia, flushing, warmth, lethargy (rare with normal renal function)
INTEG: Pain at inj site

Contraindications: Hypersensitivity

Precautions: Pregnancy (A), lactation, children, Parkinson's disease

Pharmacokinetics:
PO/Inj: Half-life 2-3 wk, metabolized in liver, excreted in urine

Interactions:
• Decreased effects of levodopa
• Decreased effects of pyridoxine: oral contraceptives, isoniazid, cycloserine, hydralazine, penicillamine

NURSING CONSIDERATIONS

Assess:
• Pyridoxine levels throughout treatment
• Nutritional status: yeast, liver, legumes, bananas, green vegetables, whole grains

Administer:

IM
• Rotate sites; burning or stinging at site may occur
• Z-track to minimize pain

IV
• Undiluted or added to most IV sol; give 50 mg or less/1 min if undiluted

Syringe compatibilities: Doxapram

Perform/provide:
• Storage in tight, light-resistant container

Evaluate:
• Therapeutic response: absence of nausea, vomiting, anorexia, skin lesions, glossitis, stomatitis, edema, convulsions, restlessness, paresthesia

Teach patient/family:
• To avoid vitamin supplements unless directed by prescriber
• To keep out of children's reach
• To increase meat, bananas, potatoes, lima beans, whole grain cereals in diet
• To discuss birth control status with prescriber

◆ = Nursing alert   ∥ = Herb-drug interaction   ⊘ = Do not crush

pyrimethamine (℞)
(peer-i-meth′a-meen)
Daraprim, Fansidar (with sulfadoxine)
Func. class.: Antimalarial
Chem. class.: Folic acid antagonist

Action: Inhibits folic acid metabolism in parasite, prevents transmission by stopping growth of fertilized gametes

Uses: Malaria prophylaxis, *Plasmodium vivax*

Investigational uses: *Pneumocystis carinii* pneumonia as an adjunct

Dosage and routes:
Prophylaxis of malaria
• *Adult and child >10 yr:* **PO** 25 mg qwk
• *Child 4-10 yr:* **PO** 12.5 mg qwk
• *Child <4 yr:* **PO** 6.25 mg qwk
Toxoplasmosis
• *Adult:* **PO** 100 mg, then 25 mg qd × 4-5 wk, with 1 g sulfadoxine q6h
• *Child:* **PO** 1 mg/kg/day in 2 divided doses or 2 mg/kg/day × 3 days, then 1 mg/kg/day or divided twice qd × 4 wk, max 25 mg/day
Toxoplasmosis in AIDS patients
• *Adult:* **PO** 100-200 mg/day × 1-2 days, then 50-100 mg/day × 3-6 wk, then 25-50 mg/day for life (given with clindamycin or sulfadiazine)
Available forms: Tabs 25 mg; combo tabs 500 mg sulfadoxine/25 mg pyrimethamine

Side effects/adverse reactions:
*RESP: **Respiratory failure***
INTEG: Skin eruptions, photosensitivity
CNS: Stimulation, irritability, *seizures,* tremors, ataxia, fatigue
GI: Nausea, vomiting, cramps, anorexia, diarrhea, atrophic glossitis, gastritis
*CV: **Dysrhythmias***

*HEMA: **Thrombocytopenia, leukopenia, pancytopenia, megaloblastic anemia,*** decreased folic acid, ***agranulocytosis***

Contraindications: Hypersensitivity, chloroquine-resistant malaria, megaloblastic anemia caused by folate deficiency

Precautions: Blood dyscrasias, seizure disorder, pregnancy (C), lactation, G6PD disease, renal, hepatic disease

Pharmacokinetics:
PO: Peak 2 hr, half-life 111 hr; metabolized in liver, highly protein bound, excreted in urine (metabolites)

Interactions:
• Synergistic action: folic acid
• Increased bone marrow suppression: bone marrow depressants, radiation therapy

NURSING CONSIDERATIONS
Assess:
• Folic acid level; megaloblastic anemia occurs
◆ Blood studies, CBC, platelets, since blood dyscrasias occur; twice weekly if dosage is increased
◆ For toxicity: vomiting, anorexia, seizure, blood dyscrasia, glossitis; drug should be discontinued immediately

Administer:
• Leucovorin IM 3-9 mg/day × 3 days if folic acid deficiency occurs
• Before or after meals at same time each day to maintain drug level, to decrease GI symptoms

Perform/provide:
• Storage in tight, light-resistant container

Evaluate:
• Therapeutic response: decreased symptoms of malaria

Teach patient/family:
• To report visual problems, fever, fatigue, bruising, bleeding; may indicate blood dyscrasias

P

Treatment of overdose: Gastric lavage, short-acting barbiturate, leucovorin, respiratory support if needed

---

quetiapine (℞)
(kwe-tie′a-peen)
Seroquel
Func. class.: Antipsychotic

Action: Functions as an antagonist at multiple neurotransmitter receptors in the brain including $5HT_{1A}$, $5HT_2$, dopamine D_1, D_2, H_1, and adrenergic α_1, α_2 receptors
Uses: Psychotic disorders
Research note: Increased dose of quetiapine may be necessary when used with phenytoin[34]
Dosage and routes:
• *Adult:* **PO** 25 mg bid, with incremental increases of 25 mg bid-tid on days 2 and 3 to a dose of 300-400 mg qd given bid-tid
Available forms: Tabs 25, 100, 200 mg
Side effects/adverse reactions:
CNS: EPS, pseudoparkinsonism, akathisia, dystonia, tardive dyskinesia; drowsiness, insomnia, agitation, anxiety, *headache, **seizures, neuroleptic malignant syndrome,** dizziness*
CV: Orthostatic hypotension, ***tachycardia***
GI: Nausea, anorexia, constipation, abdominal pain, dry mouth
RESP: Rhinitis
INTEG: Rash
MISC: Asthenia, back pain, fever, ear pain
Contraindications: Hypersensitivity
Precautions: Children, pregnancy (C), hepatic disease, elderly, breast cancer, lactation, long-term use, seizures, dementia

Pharmacokinetics:
PO: Extensively metabolized by liver half-life ≥6 hr; peak 1½ hr
Interactions:
• Decreased clearance of quetiapine: cimetidine
• Increased clearance of quetiapine: phenytoin, thioridazine, barbiturates, glucocorticoids, carbamazepine, rifampin
• Decreased clearance of lorazepam: lorazepam
• Decreased clearance of levodopa: levodopa
• Decreased effects of dopamine agonists: dopamine agonists
• May be increased by ketoconazole, fluconazole, itraconazole
NURSING CONSIDERATIONS
Assess:
• Mental status before initial administration
• Swallowing of PO medication: check for hoarding or giving of medication to other patients
• I&O ratio; palpate bladder if urinary output is low
• Bilirubin, CBC, liver function studies qmo
• Urinalysis before, during prolonged therapy
• Affect, orientation, LOC, reflexes, gait, coordination, sleep pattern disturbances
• B/P standing and lying; also pulse, respirations; take these q4h during initial treatment; establish baseline before starting treatment; report drops of 30 mm Hg; watch for ECG changes
• Dizziness, faintness, palpitations, tachycardia on rising
• EPS, including akathisia (inability to sit still, no pattern to movements), tardive dyskinesia (bizarre movements of the jaw, mouth, tongue, extremities), pseudoparkinsonism (rigidity, tremors, pill rolling, shuffling gait)

◆ = Nursing alert   🖋 = Herb-drug interaction   ⊘ = Do not crush

◆ For neuroleptic malignant syndrome: hyperthermia, increased CPK, altered mental status, muscle rigidity

• Skin turgor qd

• Constipation, urinary retention qd; if these occur, increase bulk and water in the diet

Administer:

• Reduced dose in elderly

• Antiparkinsonian agent on order from prescriber, to be used for EPS

Perform/provide:

• Decreased stimulus by dimming lights, avoiding loud noises

• Supervised ambulation until patient is stabilized on medication; do not involve in strenuous exercise program because fainting is possible; patient should not stand still for a long time

• Increased fluids to prevent constipation

• Sips of water, candy, gum for dry mouth

• Storage in tight, light-resistant container

Evaluate:

• Therapeutic response: decrease in emotional excitement, hallucinations, delusions, paranoia; reorganization of patterns of thought, speech

---

quinapril (℞)

(kwin'a-pril)
Accupril

Func. class.: Antihypertensive
Chem. class.: Angiotensin-converting enzyme (ACE) inhibitor

Action: Selectively suppresses renin-angiotensin-aldosterone system; inhibits ACE, prevents conversion of angiotensin I to angiotensin II; results in dilation of arterial, venous vessels

Uses: Hypertension, alone or in combination with thiazide diuretics; systolic CHF

Dosage and routes:
Renal dose
• CrCl 30-60 ml/min 5 mg/day initially; CrCl <30 ml/min 2.5 mg/day initially

Hypertension (alone)
• *Adult:* **PO** 10-20 mg qd initially, then 20-80 mg/day divided bid or qd
• *Geriatric:* **PO** 10 mg qd, titrate to desired response

Congestive heart failure
• *Adult:* **PO** 2.5 mg initially, then 5-40 mg/day maintenance qd or in 2 divided doses

Available forms: Tabs 5, 10, 20, 40 mg

Side effects/adverse reactions:

CV: Hypotension, postural hypotension, syncope, palpitations, angina pectoris, *MI, tachycardia,* vasodilation

GU: Increased BUN, creatinine, decreased libido, impotence, urinary tract infection

HEMA: **Thrombocytopenia, agranulocytosis**

INTEG: **Angioedema,** rash, sweating, photosensitivity, pruritus

RESP: Cough, bronchitis

META: Hyperkalemia

GI: Nausea, constipation, vomiting, gastritis, *GI hemorrhage,* dry mouth

CNS: Headache, dizziness, fatigue, somnolence, depression, malaise, nervousness, vertigo

MISC: Back pain, amblyopia, pharyngitis

MS: Arthralgia, arthritis, myalgia

Contraindications: Hypersensitivity to ACE inhibitors, pregnancy (D) 2nd, 3rd trimester, children

Precautions: Impaired renal, liver function, dialysis patients, hypovolemia, blood dyscrasias, COPD, asthma, elderly, lactation

Pharmacokinetics:

PO: Peak ½-1 hr, serum protein binding 97%, half-life 2 hr, metabolized by liver (metabolites), metabolites excreted in urine

Interactions:

• Increased hypotension: diuretics, other antihypertensives, ganglionic blockers, adrenergic blockers, phenothiazines, nitrates, acute alcohol ingestion

• Use caution with vasodilators, hydralazine, prazosin, potassium-sparing diuretics, sympathomimetics, K supplements

• Decreased absorption of tetracycline

• Reduced hypotensive effect of quinapril: indomethacin

• Increased toxicity: lithium, digoxin

Lab test interferences:

False-positive: Urine acetone, ANA titer

NURSING CONSIDERATIONS

Assess:

• Blood studies: neutrophils, decreased platelets; WBC with diff baseline and periodically q3mo; if neutrophils <1000/mm³, discontinue treatment

• B/P, orthostatic hypotension, syncope

• Renal studies: protein, BUN, creatinine; watch for increased levels; may indicate nephrotic syndrome

• Baselines in renal, liver function tests before therapy begins and periodically; increased LFTs; uric acid and glucose may be increased

• K levels; hyperkalemia is rare

• Edema in feet, legs qd, weight daily in CHF

• Allergic reactions: rash, fever, pruritus, urticaria; drug should be discontinued if antihistamines fail to help

• Renal symptoms: oliguria, urinary frequency, dysuria

Administer:

• IV infusion of 0.9% NaCl (as ordered) to expand fluid volume if severe hypotension occurs

Perform/provide:

• Supine or Trendelenburg position for severe hypotension

Evaluate:

• Therapeutic response: decrease in B/P

Teach patient/family:

• To take 1 hr before meals; not to take antacids within 1-2 hr of quinapril

• Not to discontinue drug abruptly

• Not to use OTC products (cough, cold, allergy); not to use salt substitutes containing K unless directed by prescriber

• To comply with dosage schedule, even if feeling better

• To rise slowly to sitting or standing position to minimize orthostatic hypotension

• To notify prescriber of mouth sores, sore throat, fever, swelling of hands or feet, irregular heartbeat, chest pain, persistent dry cough

• To report excessive perspiration, dehydration, vomiting, diarrhea; may lead to fall in B/P

• That drug may cause dizziness, fainting, light-headedness; may occur during first few days of therapy

• That drug may cause skin rash or impaired taste perception

• How to take B/P, and normal readings for age group

Treatment of overdose: 0.9% NaCl IV inf

◆ = Nursing alert   / = Herb-drug interaction   ⃠ = Do not crush

quinidine (℞)

(kwin′i-deen)
Apo-Quinidine*, Cardioquin;
Cin-Quin*, Novoquinidin*,
Quinaglute, Quinalan, Quinidex Extentabs, quinidine gluconate; quinidine sulfate

Func. class.: Antidysrhythmic (Class Ia)

Chem. class.: Quinine dextroisomer

Action: Prolongs duration of action potential and effective refractory period, thus decreasing myocardial excitability; anticholinergic properties

Uses: PVCs, atrial fibrillation, PAT, ventricular tachycardia, atrial flutter
Investigational uses: Malaria/IV quinidine gluconate
Dosage and routes:
Quinidine sulfate
Atrial fibrillation/flutter
• *Adult:* PO 200 mg q2-3h × 5-8 doses; may increase qd until sinus rhythm is restored; max 4 g/day given only after digitalization
Paroxysmal supraventricular tachycardia
• *Adult:* PO 400-600 mg q2-3h, then 200-300 mg q6-8h or 300-600 mg q8-12h (sus rel)
Premature atrial/ventricular contraction
• *Adult:* PO 200-300 mg q6-8h or 300-600 mg (sus rel) q8-12h; max 4 g/day
• *Child:* PO 30 mg/kg/day or 900 mg/m^2/day in 5 divided doses
Quinidine gluconate
• *Adult:* PO 324-660 mg q6-12h (sus rel); IM 600 mg, then 400 mg q2h; IV give 16 mg/min
Quinidine polygalacturonate
• *Adult:* PO 275-825 mg q3-4h × 4 doses, then increase by 137.5-275

mg; repeat up to 4× until dysrhythmias decreased
• *Child:* PO 8.25 mg/kg (247.5 mg/m^2) 5×/day
Available forms: Gluconate tabs sus rel 324, 330 mg; inj gluconate 80 mg/ml; sulfate tabs 200, 300 mg; tabs sus rel 300 mg; polygalacturonate tabs 275 mg
Side effects/adverse reactions:
CNS: Headache, dizziness, involuntary movement, confusion, psychosis, restlessness, irritability, syncope, excitement
EENT: Cinchonism: tinnitus, blurred vision, hearing loss, mydriasis, disturbed color vision
GI: Nausea, vomiting, anorexia, abdominal pain, *diarrhea, hepatotoxicity*
CV: Hypotension, bradycardia, PVCs, **heart block, cardiovascular collapse, arrest,** torsades de pointes
HEMA: **Thrombocytopenia,** hemolytic anemia, agranulocytosis, hypoprothrombinemia
RESP: Dyspnea, **respiratory depression**
INTEG: Rash, urticaria, angioedema, swelling, photosensitivity
Contraindications: Hypersensitivity, blood dyscrasias, severe heart block, myasthenia gravis
Precautions: Pregnancy (C), lactation, children, renal disease, K imbalance, liver disease, CHF, respiratory depression
Pharmacokinetics:
PO: Peak 0.5-6 hr, duration 6-8 hr; half-life 6-7 hr, metabolized in liver, excreted unchanged by kidneys
Interactions:
• Increased effects of neuromuscular blockers, digoxin, warfarin
• Increased effects of quinidine: cimetidine, propranolol, thiazides, sodium bicarbonate, carbonic anhydrase inhibitors, antacids, hydroxide suspensions, amiodarone

• May decrease effects of quinidine: barbiturates, phenytoin, rifampin, nifedipine

• Additive vagolytic effect: anticholinergic blockers

• Additive cardiac depression: other antidysrhythmics, phenothiazines, reserpine

␥ K deficiency, increased antidysrhythmic action: aloe, buckthorn, cascara sagrada, senna

• Food/drug: delayed absorption, decreased metabolism: grapefruit juice

Lab test interferences:
Increase: CPK

NURSING CONSIDERATIONS
Assess:

♦ ECG continuously to determine increased PR or QRS segments, QT interval; discontinue or reduce dose

• Blood levels (therapeutic level 2-6 µg/ml)

• B/P continuously for fluctuations

• For cinchonism: tinnitus, headache, nausea, dizziness, fever, vertigo, tremor; may lead to hearing loss

• Cardiac status: rate, rhythm, character, continuously

• Respiratory status: rate, rhythm, lung fields for rales; increased respiration, increased pulse; drug should be discontinued

• CNS effects: dizziness, confusion, psychosis, paresthesias, convulsions; drug should be discontinued

Administer:

• AV node blocker (digoxin, verapamil) before starting quinidine to avoid increased ventricular rate

IM

• IM inj in deltoid; aspirate to avoid intravascular administration

IV

• After diluting 800 mg/40 ml or more D_5; give 16 mg or less over 1 min as inf; use infusion pump

Additive compatibilities: Brety-

lium, cimetidine, milrinone, ranitidine, verapamil

Y-site compatibilities: Diazepam, milrinone

Evaluate:

• Therapeutic response: decreased dysrhythmias

Treatment of overdose: O_2, artificial ventilation, ECG, administer dopamine for circulatory depression, diazepam or thiopental for convulsions

---

quinine (OTC, ℞)
(kwye'nine)
Novoquine*, quinine sulfate
Func. class.: Antimalarial
Chem. class.: Cinchona tree alkaloid

Action: Inhibits parasite replications, transcription of DNA to RNA by forming complexes with DNA of parasite

Uses: *Plasmodium falciparum,* malaria, nocturnal leg cramps

Dosage and routes:

• *Adult:* **PO** 650 mg q8h × 10 days, given with pyrimethamine 25 mg q12h × 3 days, with sulfadiazine 500 mg qid × 5 days

• *Child:* **PO** 25 mg/kg/day divided q8h for 3-7 days in conjunction with another agent

Leg cramps

• *Adult:* **PO** 250-300 mg hs

Available forms: Caps 200, 260, 325 mg; tabs 260 mg

Side effects/adverse reactions:
RESP: Dyspnea
INTEG: Pruritus, pigmentary changes, skin eruptions, lichen planuslike eruptions, flushing, facial edema, sweating
HEMA: ***Thrombocytopenia, purpura, hypothrombinemia, hemolysis***

♦ = Nursing alert   ␥ = Herb-drug interaction   ⊘ = Do not crush

CNS: Headache, stimulation, fatigue, irritability, ***convulsions,*** bad dreams, dizziness, fever, confusion, anxiety

EENT: *Blurred vision, corneal changes, retinal changes, difficulty focusing,* tinnitus, vertigo, deafness, photophobia, diplopia, night blindness

GU: Renal tubular damage, ***anuria***

GI: *Nausea, vomiting, anorexia,* diarrhea, epigastric pain

CV: Angina, dysrhythmias, tachycardia, hypotension, ***acute circulatory failure***

ENDO: Hypoglycemia

Contraindications: Hypersensitivity, G6PD deficiency, retinal field changes, pregnancy (X)

Precautions: Blood dyscrasias, severe GI disease, neurologic disease, severe hepatic disease, psoriasis, cardiac dysrhythmias, tinnitus

Pharmacokinetics:

PO: Peak 1-3 hr, metabolized in liver, excreted in urine, half-life 8-14 hr

Interactions:

• Toxicity: $NaHCO_3$, acetazolamide

• Decreased absorption: magnesium or aluminum salts

• Increased levels of digoxin, digitoxin, neuromuscular blockers, other anticoagulants

Lab test interferences:

Increase: 17-KS

Interference: 17-OHCS

NURSING CONSIDERATIONS

Assess:

• B/P, pulse, watch for hypotension, tachycardia

• Liver studies qwk: ALT, AST, bilirubin

• Blood studies, CBC, since blood dyscrasias occur

• For cinchonism: nausea, blurred vision, tinnitus, headache, difficulty focusing

Administer:

• Before or after meals at same time each day to maintain level

Perform/provide:

• Storage in tight, light-resistant container

Evaluate:

• Therapeutic response: decreased symptoms of malaria

Teach patient/family:

• To avoid OTC preparations: cold preparations, tonic water

---

rabeprazole (℞)

(rah-bep′rah-zole)

Aciphex

Func. class.: Antiulcer, proton pump inhibitor

Chem. class.: Benzimidazole

Action: Suppresses gastric secretion by inhibiting hydrogen/potassium ATPase enzyme system in gastric parietal cell; characterized as gastric acid pump inhibitor, since it blocks final step of acid production

Uses: Gastroesophageal reflux disease (GERD), severe erosive esophagitis, poorly responsive systemic GERD, pathologic hypersecretory conditions (Zollinger-Ellison syndrome, systemic mastocytosis, multiple endocrine adenomas); treatment of active duodenal ulcers with or without antiinfectives for *Helicobacter pylori*

Dosage and routes:

Healing of duodenal ulcers

• *Adult:* **PO** 20 mg qd × ≤4 wk to be taken after breakfast

Healing of erosive esophagitis or ulcerative GERD

• *Adult:* **PO** 20 mg qd × 4-8 wk

Pathologic hypersecretory conditions

• *Adult:* **PO** 60 mg/day; may increase to 120 mg in 2 divided doses

Available forms: Tabs, del rel 20 mg

R

Side effects/adverse reactions:
CNS: Headache, dizziness, asthenia
GI: Diarrhea, abdominal pain, vomiting, nausea, constipation, flatulence, acid regurgitation, abdominal swelling, anorexia, irritable colon, esophageal candidiasis, dry mouth
RESP: Upper respiratory infections, cough, epistaxis
INTEG: Rash, dry skin, urticaria, pruritus, alopecia
META: Hypoglycemia, increased hepatic enzymes, weight gain
EENT: Tinnitus, taste perversion
CV: Chest pain, angina, tachycardia, bradycardia, palpitations, peripheral edema
GU: UTI, urinary frequency, increased creatinine, *proteinuria, hematuria,* testicular pain, glycosuria
HEMA: Pancytopenia, thrombocytopenia, neutropenia, leukocytosis, anemia
MISC: Back pain, fever, fatigue, malaise

Contraindications: Hypersensitivity

Precautions: Pregnancy (C), lactation, children

Pharmacokinetics: Eliminated in urine as metabolites and in feces

Interactions:
• Increased serum levels of rabeprazole: benzodiazepines, phenytoin, clarithromycin
• Decreased levels of rabeprazole: sucralfate

NURSING CONSIDERATIONS
Assess:
• GI system: bowel sounds q8h, abdomen for pain, swelling, anorexia
• Hepatic enzymes: AST, ALT, alk phosphatase during treatment

Administer:
🚫 After breakfast qd; do not crush, break, chew delayed rel tab

Evaluate:
• Therapeutic response: absence of epigastric pain, swelling, fullness

Teach patient/family:
• To report severe diarrhea; drug may have to be discontinued
• That diabetic patient should know hypoglycemia may occur
• To avoid hazardous activities; dizziness may occur
• To avoid alcohol, salicylates, ibuprofen; may cause GI irritation

---

radioactive iodine (sodium iodide) ^{131}I (R)

Func. class.: Antithyroid
Chem. class.: Radiopharmaceutical

Action: Converted to protein-bound iodine by thyroid gland for use when needed

Uses: *High dose:* Thyroid cancer, hyperthyroidism
Low dose: Visualization to determine thyroid cancer, diagnostic aid in thyroid function studies

Dosage and routes:
Thyroid cancer
• *Adult:* **PO** 50-150 mCi, may repeat depending on clinical status
Hyperthyroidism
• *Adult:* **PO** 4-10 mCi, depending on serum thyroxine level

Available forms: Caps 1-50, 0.8-100 mCi; oral sol 7.05 mCi/ml, 3.5-150 mCi/vial

Side effects/adverse reactions:
ENDO: Hypothyroidism, *hyperthyroid adenoma,* transient thyroiditis
INTEG: Alopecia
HEMA: Eosinophilia, lymphedema, leukemia, bone marrow depression, leukopenia, anemia
GI: Nausea, diarrhea, vomiting
EENT: Sore throat, cough

◆ = Nursing alert   🌿 = Herb-drug interaction   🚫 = Do not crush

Contraindications: Recent MI, lactation, large nodular goiter, pregnancy (X), age <30 yr, vomiting/diarrhea, acute hyperthyroidism, use of thyroid drugs, lactation

Pharmacokinetics:

PO: Onset 3-6 days; excreted in urine, sweat, feces, breast milk; crosses placenta; excreted in 56 days

Interactions:

• Hypothyroidism: lithium

• Decreased uptake if recent intake of stable iodine, thyroid, antithyroid drugs

NURSING CONSIDERATIONS

Assess:

• Weight qd in same clothing, scale, time of day

• Blood work, including CBC for blood dyscrasias (leukopenia, thrombocytopenia, agranulocytosis)

• Overdose: peripheral edema, heat intolerance, diaphoresis, palpitations, dysrhythmias, severe tachycardia, increased temp, delirium, CNS irritability

• Hypersensitivity: rash, enlarged cervical lymph nodes; drug may have to be discontinued

• Hypoprothrombinemia: bleeding, petechiae, ecchymosis

• Clinical response: after 3 wk should include increased weight, pulse; decreased T_4

• Bone marrow depression: sore throat, fever, fatigue

Administer:

• Only after discontinuing all other antithyroid agents × 5-7 days

• After NPO overnight, food delays action

• During or within 10 days after menstruation

Perform/provide:

• Limited contact with patient ½ hr/day for each person

• Adequate rest after treatment

• Fluids to 3-4 L/day for 48 hr to remove agent from body

Evaluate:

• Therapeutic response: weight gain, decreased pulse, decreased T_4, B/P

Teach patient/family:

• To empty bladder often during treatment; avoid irradiation of gonads

• To report redness, swelling, sore throat, mouth lesions; indicate blood dyscrasias

• To avoid extended contact with children, spouse for 1 wk

• That bathroom may be used by entire family

• Not to take antithyroid agents but propranolol, which decreases hyperthyroid symptoms, until total effect of taking ^{131}I has occurred (about 6 wk)

• To avoid coughing, expectorating for 24 hr (saliva and vomitus are highly radioactive for 6-8 hr)

---

raloxifene (Rx)

(ral-ox'ih-feen)

Evista

Func. class.: Bone resorption inhibitor, selective estrogen receptor modulator (SERM)

Chem. class.: Benzthiophene

Action: Reduces resorption of bone and decreases bone turnover; mediated through estrogen receptor binding

Uses: Prevention of osteoporosis in postmenopausal women

Dosage and routes:

• *Adult:* PO 60 mg qd

Available forms: Tabs 60 mg

Side effects/adverse reactions:

CNS: Insomnia, migraines, depression

CV: Hot flashes

GI: Nausea, vomiting, diarrhea, anorexia, cramps

GU: Vaginitis, UTI, leukorrhea, endometrial disorder, breast pain

---

INTEG: Rash, sweating

META: Weight gain, peripheral edema

MS: Arthralgia, myalgia, leg cramps, arthritis

RESP: Sinusitis, pharyngitis, increased cough, pneumonia, laryngitis

Contraindications: Hypersensitivity, pregnancy (X), lactation

Precautions: Lactation, venous thromboembolic events, hepatic disease

Pharmacokinetics: Elimination half-life 28-32 hr; excreted in feces; excreted in breast milk; highly bound to plasma proteins

Interactions:

• Decreased action of: anticoagulants

• Decreased action of raloxifene: ampicillin, cholestyramine

• Administer cautiously with other highly protein-bound drugs

Lab test interferences:

Increase: Apolipoprotein A$_1$, B, liporotein, fibrinogen, LDL cholesterol, total cholesterol, corticosteroid-binding globulin, thyroxine-binding globulin (TBG)

Decrease: Calcium, total protein, albumin, platelets

NURSING CONSIDERATIONS
Assess:

• Blood glucose of diabetic patient

• Weight daily, notify prescriber of weekly weight gain >5 lb

• B/P q4h, watch for increase caused by H$_2$O and Na retention

• I&O ratio; decreasing urinary output, increasing edema

• Liver function studies, including AST, ALT, bilirubin, alk phosphatase

• Bone density test baseline and throughout treatment

Administer:
PO

• Without regard to meals

Evaluate:

• Therapeutic response: prevention of osteoporosis

Teach patient/family:

• To weigh weekly, report gain >5 lb

• To discontinue 72 hr before prolonged bedrest; advise to avoid one position for long periods

• To take calcium supplements, vit D if intake is inadequate

• To increase exercise using weights

• To stop smoking and to decrease alcohol consumption

• That this drug does not help control hot flashes

• To report fever, acute migraine, insomnia, emotional distress; urinary tract infection, or vaginal burning/itching; swelling, warmth, or pain in calves

---

ramipril (R)

(ra-mi'pril)

Altace

Func. class.: Antihypertensive

Chem. class.: Angiotensin-converting enzyme inhibitor (ACE)

Action: Selectively suppresses renin-angiotensin-aldosterone system; inhibits ACE, prevents conversion of angiotensin I to angiotensin II; results in dilation of arterial, venous vessels

Uses: Hypertension, alone or in combination with thiazide diuretics; CHF (post MI), reduction in risk of MI, stroke, death from CV disorders

Dosage and routes:

• *Adult:* **PO** 2.5 mg qd initially, then 2.5-20 mg/day divided bid or qd; *renal impairment:* 1.25 mg qd with CrCl <40 ml/min/1.73 m^2, increase as needed to max or 5 mg/day

---

◆ = Nursing alert   ✱ = Herb-drug interaction   ⊘ = Do not crush

CHF

• *Adult:* **PO** 1.25-2.5 mg bid; may increase to 5 mg bid

Available forms: Caps 1.25, 2.5, 5, 10 mg

Side effects/adverse reactions:

CV: Hypotension, chest pain, palpitations, angina, syncope, dysrhythmia

GU: Proteinuria, increased BUN, creatinine, impotence

HEMA: Decreased Hct, Hgb, *eosinophilia, leukopenia*

INTEG: Angioedema, rash, sweating, photosensitivity, pruritus

RESP: Cough, dyspnea

META: Hyperkalemia

GI: Nausea, constipation, vomiting, dyspepsia, dysphagia, anorexia, diarrhea, abdominal pain

CNS: Headache, dizziness, anxiety, insomnia, paresthesia, fatigue, depression, malaise, vertigo, *seizures,* hearing loss

MS: Arthralgia, arthritis, myalgia

Contraindications: Hypersensitivity to ACE inhibitors, pregnancy (D), lactation, children

Precautions: Impaired renal, liver function; dialysis patients, hypovolemia, blood dyscrasias, CHF, COPD, asthma, elderly, renal artery stenosis

Do not confuse:

Altace/alteplase

Altace/Artane

ramipril/enalapril

Pharmacokinetics:

PO: Peak ½-1 hr, serum protein binding 97%, half-life 1-2 hr, metabolized by liver (metabolites excreted in urine, feces)

Interactions:

• Increased hypotension: diuretics, other antihypertensives, ganglionic blockers, adrenergic blockers, nitrates, acute alcohol ingestion

• Increased toxicity: vasodilators, hydralazine, prazosin, K-sparing diuretics, sympathomimetics, K supplements

• Decreased absorption: antacids

• Decreased antihypertensive effect: indomethacin

• Increased serum levels of digoxin, lithium

• Increased hypersensitivity: allopurinol

Lab test interferences:

False-positive: Urine acetone, ANA titer

NURSING CONSIDERATIONS
Assess:

• Blood studies: neutrophils, decreased platelets; WBC with diff baseline and periodically q3mo, if neutrophils <1000/mm^3, discontinue treatment

• B/P, orthostatic hypotension, syncope

• Renal studies: protein, BUN, creatinine; increased levels may indicate nephrotic syndrome

• Baselines in renal, liver function tests before therapy begins and periodically; increased LFTs; uric acid and glucose may be increased

• Potassium levels, although hyperkalemia rarely occurs

• Dipstick of urine for protein qd in first morning specimen; if protein is increased, a 24-hr urinary protein should be collected

• Edema in feet, legs qd, weight daily in CHF

• Allergic reactions: rash, fever, pruritus, urticaria; drug should be discontinued if antihistamines fail to help

• Renal symptoms: polyuria, oliguria, urinary frequency, dysuria

Administer:

• Caps can be opened and added to food

Perform/provide:

• Storage in tight container at 86° F (30° C) or less

• Supine position for severe hypotension

Evaluate:
• Therapeutic response: decrease in B/P

Teach patient/family:
• Not to discontinue drug abruptly
• Not to use OTC products (cough, cold, allergy) unless directed by prescriber; not to use salt substitutes containing potassium without consulting prescriber
• To comply with dosage schedule, even if feeling better
• To rise slowly to sitting or standing position to minimize orthostatic hypotension
• To notify prescriber of mouth sores, sore throat, fever, swelling of hands or feet, irregular heartbeat, chest pain
• To report excessive perspiration, dehydration, vomiting, diarrhea; may lead to fall in B/P
• That drug may cause dizziness, fainting, light-headedness; may occur during first few days of therapy
• That drug may cause skin rash or impaired perspiration
• How to take B/P, and normal readings for age group

Treatment of overdose: 0.9% NaCl IV inf, hemodialysis

---

ranitidine (℞, OTC)
(ra-nit′i-deen)
Apo-Ranitidine*, Zantac, Zantac C*, Zantac EFFERdose, Zantac GELdose
ranitidine bismuth citrate
Tritec
Func. class.: H$_2$-histamine receptor antagonist

Action: Inhibits histamine at H$_2$-receptor site in parietal cells, which inhibits gastric acid secretion

Uses: Duodenal ulcer, Zollinger-Ellison syndrome, gastric ulcers, hypersecretory conditions, gastroesophageal reflux disease, stress ulcers, erosive esophagitis (maintenance), active duodenal ulcers with *Helicobacter pylori* in combination with clarithromycin

Investigational uses: Prevention of aspiration pneumonitis, stress ulcers, upper GI bleeding

Dosage and routes:
Renal dose
• CrCl <50 ml/min give **PO** q24h give **IM/IV** q8-24h
Duodenal ulcer
• *Adult:* **PO** 150 mg bid, maintenance 150 mg hs
Zollinger-Ellison syndrome
• *Adult:* **PO** 150 mg bid, may increase if needed
Gastric ulcer
• *Adult:* **PO** 150 mg bid × 6 wk, then 150 mg hs
GERD
• *Adult:* **PO** 150 mg bid
Erosive esophagitis
• *Adult:* **PO** 150 mg qid
• *Adult:* **PO** 150 mg bid, 300 mg hs; **IM** 50 mg q6-8h; **IV BOL** 50 mg diluted to 20 ml over 5 min q6-8h; **IV INT INF** 50 mg/100 ml D$_5$ over 15-20 min q6-8h
• *Child:* **PO** 4-5 mg/kg/day divided q8-12h, max 6 mg/kg/day or 300 mg; **IV** 2-4 mg/kg/day divided q6-8h
ranitidine bismuth citrate
• *Adult:* **PO** 400 mg bid × 4 wk with clarithromycin 500 mg tid × 1st 2 wk

Available forms: Tabs 75, 150, 300 mg; sol for inj 25 mg/ml; tabs, effervescent 75, 150 mg; inj 0.5, 25 mg/ml; caps 150, 300 mg; syr 15 mg/ml; granules, effervescent 150 mg/packet; ranitidine bismuth citrate: tabs 400 mg

◆ = Nursing alert   〆 = Herb-drug interaction   ⊘ = Do not crush

Side effects/adverse reactions:

CNS: Headache, sleeplessness, dizziness, confusion, agitation, depression, hallucination (elderly)

GI: Constipation, abdominal pain, diarrhea, nausea, vomiting, ***hepatotoxicity***

GU: Impotence, gynecomastia

CV: Tachycardia, bradycardia, PVCs

EENT: Blurred vision, increased ocular pressure

INTEG: Urticaria, rash, fever

Contraindications: Hypersensitivity

Precautions: Pregnancy (B), lactation, child <12 yr, hepatic disease, renal disease

Do not confuse:

Zantac/Xanax

Zantac/Zofran

ranitidine/amantadine

Pharmacokinetics:

PO: Peak 2-3 hr, duration 8-12 hr; metabolized by liver; excreted in urine, breast milk; half-life 2-3 hr

Interactions:

• Increased absorption, toxicity: anticoagulants, sulfonylureas, procainamide

• Decreased absorption of ranitidine: antacids, diazepam, anticholinergics, metoclopramide

Lab test interferences:

Increase: AST, ALT, alk phosphatase, creatinine, LDH, bilirubin

False positive: Urine protein

NURSING CONSIDERATIONS

Assess:

• Gastric pH (>5 should be maintained)

• I&O ratio, BUN, creatinine

• Mental status: confusion, dizziness, depression, anxiety, weakness, tremors, psychosis, diarrhea, abdominal discomfort, jaundice; report immediately

• GI complaints: nausea, vomiting, diarrhea, cramps

Administer:

• With meals for prolonged effect

• Antacids 1 hr before or 1 hr after ranitidine

IV

• IV after diluting 50 mg/20 ml 0.9% NaCl, D_5W, $D_{10}W$, LR, $NaCO_3$ 5% and give 50 mg or less/5 min or more; may dilute 50 mg/50-100 ml of 0.9% NaCl, D_5W, $D_{10}W$, LR, $NaCO_3$ 5% and give over 15-20 min

Additive compatibilities: Acetazolamide, amikacin, aminophylline, chloramphenicol, chlorothiazide, ciprofloxacin, colistimethate, dexamethasone, digoxin, dobutamine, dopamine, doxycycline, epinephrine, erythromycin, floxacillin, fluconazole/ondansetron, flumazenil, furosemide, gentamicin, heparin, insulin (regular), isoproterenol, lidocaine, lincomycin, meropenem, methylprednisolone, moxalactam, penicillin G potassium, penicillin G sodium, polymyxin B, potassium chloride, protamine, quinidine, sodium nitroprusside, ticarcillin, tobramycin, vancomycin

Syringe compatibilities: Atropine, cyclizine, dexamethasone, dimenhydrinate, diphenhydramine, dobutamine, dopamine, fentanyl, glycopyrrolate, hydromorphone, isoproterenol, meperidine, metoclopramide, morphine, nalbuphine, oxymorphone, pentazocine, perphenazine, prochlorperazine, promethazine, scopolamine

Y-site compatibilities: Acyclovir, aldesleukin, allopurinol, amifostine, aminophylline, amsacrine, atracurium, aztreonam, bretylium, cefepime, cefmetazole, ceftazidime, ciprofloxacin, cisatracurium, cisplatin, cladribine, cyclophosphamide, cytarabine, diltiazem, dobutamine, dopamine, doxorubicin, doxorubicin liposome, enalaprilat, epinephrine, esmolol, fentanyl,

R

filgrastim, fluconazole, fludarabine, foscarnet, furosemide, gallium, granisetron, heparin, hydromorphone, idarubicin, labetalol, lorazepam, melphalan, meperidine, methotrexate, midazolam, milrinone, morphine, nicardipine, nitroglycerin, norepinephrine, ondansetron, paclitaxel, pancuronium, piperacillin, piperacillin/tazobactam, procainamide, propofol, remifentanil, sargramostim, tacrolimus, teniposide, theophylline, thiopental, thiotepa, vecuronium, vinorelbine, warfarin, zidovudine

Perform/provide:
• Storage at room temperature
Evaluate:
• Therapeutic response: decreased abdominal pain
Teach patient/family:
• That gynecomastia, impotence may occur but are reversible
• To avoid driving, other hazardous activities until stabilized on this medication
• To avoid black pepper, caffeine, alcohol, harsh spices, extremes in temperature of food
• That drug must be continued for prescribed time to be effective

---

remifentanil (R)
(rem-ih-fin'ta-nill)
Ultiva
Func. class.: Opiate agonist analgesic
Chem. class.: μ-Opioid agonist
Controlled Substance Schedule II
Action: Inhibits ascending pain pathways in limbic system, thalamus, midbrain, hypothalamus
Uses: In combination with other drugs in general anesthesia, as a primary anesthetic in general surgery

Dosage and routes:
• *Adult:* Induction **IV** 0.5-1 μg/kg/min with a hypnotic or volatile agent; maintenance with isoflurane (0.4-1.5 MAC) or propofol (100-200 μg/kg/min); cont inf 0.25 μg/kg/min
Available forms: Pwd for inj-lyophilized 1 mg/ml after reconstitution
Side effects/adverse reactions:
CNS: Drowsiness, *dizziness,* confusion, *headache,* sedation, euphoria, delirium, agitation, anxiety
GI: Nausea, vomiting, anorexia, constipation, cramps, dry mouth
GU: Urinary retention, dysuria
INTEG: Rash, urticaria, bruising, flushing, diaphoresis, pruritus
EENT: Tinnitus, blurred vision, miosis, diplopia
CV: Palpitations, *bradycardia,* change in B/P, facial flushing, syncope, *asystole*
*RESP: **Respiratory depression, apnea***
MS: Rigidity
Contraindications: Child <12 yr, hypersensitivity
Precautions: Pregnancy (C), lactation, increased intracranial pressure, acute MI, severe heart disease, renal disease, hepatic disease, asthma, respiratory conditions, convulsive disorders, elderly
Pharmacokinetics: Unknown
Interactions:
• Respiratory depression, hypotension, profound sedation: alcohol, sedatives, hypnotics, or other CNS depressants; antihistamines, phenothiazines
⚘ Increased CNS depression: kava
NURSING CONSIDERATIONS
Assess:
• I&O ratio, check for decreasing output; may indicate urinary retention, especially in elderly

---

◆ = Nursing alert   ⚘ = Herb-drug interaction   ⊘ = Do not crush

• CNS changes; dizziness, drowsiness, hallucinations, euphoria, LOC, pupil reaction
• Allergic reactions: rash, urticaria
• Respiratory dysfunction: respiratory depression, character, rate, rhythm; notify prescriber if respirations are <12/min; CV status; bradycardia, syncope
• Use pain scoring to determine pain perception

Administer:
• Direct IV over 1½-3 min; use tuberculin syringe

Y-site compatibilities: Acyclovir, alfentanil, amikacin, aminophylline, ampicillin, ampicillin/sulbactam, amrinone, aztreonam, bretylium, bumetanide, buprenorphine, butorphanol, calcium gluconate, cefazolin, cefotaxime, cefotetan, cefoxitin, ceftazidime, ceftizoxime, ceftriaxone, cefuroxime, cimetidine, ciprofloxacin, cisatracurium, clindamycin, dexamethasone, digoxin, diphenhydramine, dobutamine, dopamine, doxycycline, droperidol, enalaprilat, epinephrine, esmolol, famotidine, fentanyl, fluconazole, furosemide, ganciclovir, gentamicin, haloperidol, heparin, hydrocortisone sodium succinate, hydromorphone, hydroxyzine, imipenem/cilastatin, isoproterenol, ketorolac, lidocaine, lorazepam, magnesium sulfate, mannitol, meperidine, methyl prednisolone, sodium succinate, metoclopramide, metronidazole, mezlocillin, midazolam, minocycline, morphine, nalbuphine, netilmicin, nitroglycerin, norepinephrine, ofloxacin, ondansetron

Perform/provide:
• Storage in light-resistant area at room temperature

Evaluate:
• Therapeutic response: maintenance of anesthesia

repaglinide (℞)
(re-pag'lih'nide)
Prandin
Func. class.: Antidiabetic
Chem. class.: Meglitinide

Action: Causes functioning β-cells in pancreas to release insulin, leading to drop in blood glucose levels; closes ATP-dependent potassium channels in the β-cell membrane; this leads to opening of calcium channels; increased calcium influx induces insulin secretion

Uses: Stable adult-onset diabetes mellitus (type II) NIDDM

Research note: Repaglinide given with rifampin resulted in the decrease of repaglinide levels[35]

Dosage and routes:
• *Adult:* **PO** 1-2 mg with each meal, max 16 mg/day, adjust at weekly intervals

Available forms: Tabs 0.5, 1, 2 mg

Side effects/adverse reactions:
CNS: Headache, weakness, paresthesia
*ENDO: **Hypoglycemia***
GI: Nausea, vomiting, diarrhea, constipation, dyspepsia
INTEG: Rash, allergic reactions
MS: Back pains, arthralgia
RESP: URI, sinusitis, rhinitis, bronchitis

Contraindications: Hypersensitivity to meglitinides, diabetic ketoacidosis, type I diabetes

Precautions: Pregnancy (C), elderly, cardiac disease, severe renal disease, severe hepatic disease, thy-

R

roid disease, severe hypoglycemic reactions, lactation, children

Pharmacokinetics:

PO: Competely absorbed by GI route; onset 2-4 hr, peak 2-8 hr, duration 24 hr; half-life 1 hr; metabolized in liver; excreted in urine, feces (metabolites); crosses placenta; 98% plasma protein bound

Interactions:

• Increased repaglinide metabolism: rifampin, barbiturates, carbamazepine

• Decreased repaglinide metabolism: antifungals (ketoconazole, miconazole), erythromycin

• Increased effect of repaglinide: NSAIDs, salicylates, sulfonamides, chloramphenicol, MAOIs, coumarins, β-blockers, probenecid

• Decreased action of repaglinide: calcium channel blockers, corticosteroids, oral contraceptives, thizide diuretics, thyroid preparations, estrogens, phenothiazines, phenytoin, rifampin, isoniazid, phenobarbital, sympathomimetics

🌿 May decrease hypoglycemic effect: broom, buchu, dandelion, juniper

🌿 May increase or decrease hypoglycemic effect: chromium, fenugreek, ginseng

🌿 May improve glucose tolerance: karela

NURSING CONSIDERATIONS

Assess:

• Hypo/hyperglycemic reaction that can occur soon after meals

Administer:

• 15 min before meals; 2, 3, or 4×/day preprandially

• Skip dose if meal is skipped; add dose if meal is added

Perform/provide:

• Storage in tight container in cool environment

Evaluate:

• Therapeutic response: decrease in polyuria, polydipsia, polyphagia, clear sensorium, absence of dizziness, stable gait

Teach family/patient:

• To avoid alcohol; explain disulfiram-like reaction

• To use a capillary blood glucose test while on this drug

• The symptoms of hypo/hyperglycemia; what to do about each

• That drug must be continued on daily basis; explain consequences of discontinuing drug abruptly

• To avoid OTC medications unless ordered by prescriber

• That diabetes is a lifelong illness; drug will not cure disease

• That all food included in diet plan must be eaten to prevent hypoglycemia; to have glucagon emergency kit available

• To carry a MedicAlert ID for emergency purposes

Treatment of overdose: Glucose 25 g IV via dextrose 50% solution, 50 ml or 1 mg glucagon

---

reserpine (℞)

(re-ser'peen)

Novoreserpine*, Reserfia*, reserpine

Func. class.: Antihypertensive, antiadrenergic agent, peripheral action

Chem. class.: Rauwolfia derivative

Action: Inhibits norepinephrine release, depleting norepinephrine stores in adrenergic nerve endings; therapeutic effect due to peripheral effect

Uses: Hypertension

Dosage and routes:

• *Adult:* **PO** 0.25-0.5 mg qd × 1-2

 = Nursing alert   = Herb-drug interaction   🚫 = Do not crush

wk, then 0.1-0.25 mg qd maintenance

• *Geriatric:* **PO** 0.05 mg qd, increase by 0.05 weekly to desired dose

Available forms: Tabs 0.1, 0.25 mg

Side effects/adverse reactions:

CV: Bradycardia, chest pain, dysrhythmias, prolonged bleeding time, ***thrombocytopenia,*** purpura

CNS: Drowsiness, fatigue, lethargy, dizziness, depression, anxiety, headache, increased dreaming, nightmares, **convulsions,** parkinsonism, EPS (high doses)

GI: Nausea, vomiting, cramps, peptic ulcer, dry mouth, increased appetite, anorexia

INTEG: Rash, purpura, alopecia, flushing, warm feeling, pruritus, ecchymosis

EENT: Lacrimation, miosis, blurred vision, ptosis, dry mouth, epistaxis

GU: Impotence, dysuria, nocturia, Na and H_2O retention, edema, breast engorgement, galactorrhea, gynecomastia

RESP: ***Bronchospasm,*** dyspnea, cough, rales

Contraindications: Hypersensitivity, depression, suicidal patients, active peptic ulcer disease, ulcerative colitis, pregnancy (D), Parkinson's disease

Precautions: Lactation, seizure disorders, renal disease

Do not confuse:

reserpine/Risperdal

Pharmacokinetics:

PO: Peak 4 hr, duration 2-6 wk; half-life 50-100 hr; metabolized by liver; excreted in urine, feces, breast milk; crosses placenta; blood-brain barrier

Interactions:

• Increased hypotension: diuretics, hypotension, β-blockers, methotrimeprazine

• Dysrhythmias: cardiac glycosides

• Increased cardiac depression: quinidine, procainamide

• Excitation, hypertension: MAOIs, avoid use

• Increased CNS depression: barbiturates, alcohol, opioids

• Increased pressor effects: epinephrine, isoproterenol, norepinephrine

• Decreased pressor effects: ephedrine, amphetamine

Lab test interferences:

Increase: VMA excretion, 5-HIAA excretion

Interferences: 17-OHCS, 17-KS

NURSING CONSIDERATIONS

Assess:

• Renal function studies in renal impairment (BUN, creatinine)

• Bleeding time; check for ecchymosis, thrombocytopenia, purpura

• I&O in renal disease patient

• Cardiac status: B/P, pulse; watch for hypotension, bradycardia

• Edema in feet, legs qd; take weight qd

• Skin turgor, dryness of mucous membranes for hydration status

• Symptoms of CHF: edema, dyspnea, wet rales

Evaluate:

• Therapeutic response: decreased hypertension

Teach patient/family:

• To avoid driving, hazardous activities if drowsiness occurs

• Not to discontinue drug abruptly

• Not to use OTC products (cough, cold preparations) unless directed by prescriber

• To report bradycardia, dizziness, confusion, depression, fever, sore throat

• That impotence, gynecomastia may occur but are reversible

• To rise slowly to sitting or standing position to minimize orthostatic hypotension

• That therapeutic effect may take 2-4 wk

R

Treatment of overdose: Lavage, IV atropine for bradycardia, supportive therapy

---

Rh$_o$(D) immune globulin standard dose IM$_o$ (℞)

Gamulin Rh, Hydro Rho-D, Rho-Gam

Rh$_o$(D) globulin microdose IM$_a$ (℞)

HypRho-D Mini-Dose, MiCRhoGAM, Mini-Gamulin

Rh$_o$(D) globulin IV (℞)

WinRho SD, WinRho SDF

Func. class.: Immune globulins

Action: Suppresses immune response of nonsensitized Rh$_o$ (D or D^u)-negative patients who are exposed to Rh$_o$ (D or D^u)-positive blood

Uses: Prevention of isoimmunization in Rh-negative women given Rh-positive blood after abortions, miscarriages, amniocentesis

Dosage and routes:

Prior delivery
• *Adult:* **IM** 1 vial (standard dose) at 26-28 wk, 1 vial (standard dose) 72 hr after delivery

Pregnancy termination <13 wk
• *Adult:* **IM** 1 vial (microdose) within 72 hr

Following delivery
• *Adult:* **IM** 1 vial (standard dose) if fetal-packed RBCs <15 ml, or 2 vials if fetal-packed RBCs >15 ml; given within 72 hr of delivery or miscarriage

Transfusion error
• *Adult:* **IM** (standard dose) give within 72 hr

After 34 wk gestation
• *Adult:* **IM/IV** 120 µg given within 72 hr (IV dose)

Available forms: Inj single-dose vial (50 µg/vial-microdose; 300 µg/vial-standard); inj 120, 300 µg Rh$_o$ (D) immune globulin IV, human

Side effects/adverse reactions:
INTEG: Irritation at inj site, fever
CNS: Lethargy
MS: Myalgia

Contraindications: Previous immunization with this drug, Rh$_o$ (O)-positive/D^u-positive patient

Do not confuse:
Gamulin Rh/MICRh$_o$GAM

NURSING CONSIDERATIONS
Assess:
• Allergies, reactions to immunizations; previous immunization with this drug
• For intravascular hemolysis: back pain, chills, hemoglobinuria (ITP)

Administer:
IM
• Reconstitute Rh$_o$(D) immune globulin IV using 1.25 ml of 0.9% NaCl, swirl
• After sending newborn's cord blood to lab after delivery for crossmatch, type; infant must be Rh-positive, with Rh-negative mother
• IM inj in deltoid; aspirate within 3 hr if possible
• Only equal lot numbers of drug, cross-match
• Only MICRhoGAM for abortions or miscarriages <12 wk unless fetus or father is Rh negative; unless patient is Rh$_o$ (D)-positive, D^u-positive, Rh antibodies are present
• Do not use Rh$_o$(D) immune globulin or Rh$_o$(D) immune globulin micro dose by IV

IV, direct
• Reconstitute Rh$_o$(D) immune globulin IV using 2.5 ml of 0.9% NaCl, swirl, give over 3-5 min

---

◆ = Nursing alert   🖉 = Herb-drug interaction   ⊘ = Do not crush

Perform/provide:
• Storage in refrigerator
Evaluate:
• Rh_o (D) sensitivity in transfusion error, prevention of erythroblastosis fetalis
Teach patient/family:
• How drug works; that drug must be given after subsequent deliveries if subsequent babies are Rh positive

---

riboflavin (vit B₂)
(OTC)
(rye'boh-flay-vin)
Func. class.: Vit B_2, water soluble

Action: Needed for respiratory reactions by catalyzing proteins and for normal vision
Uses: Vit B_2 deficiency or polyneuritis; cheilosis adjunct with thiamine
Dosage and routes:
• *Adult and child >12 yr:* **PO** 5-25 mg qd
• *Child <12 yr:* **PO** 2-10 mg qd, then 0.6 mg/1000 calories ingested
RDA
• *Adult:* males 1.4-1.8 mg, females 1.2-1.3 mg
Available forms: Tabs 5, 10, 25, 50, 100, 250 mg
Side effects/adverse reactions:
GU: Yellow discoloration of urine (large doses)
Contraindications: Child <12 yr
Precautions: Pregnancy (A)
Pharmacokinetics:
PO: Half-life 65-85 min, 60% protein bound, unused amounts excreted in urine (unchanged)
Interactions:
• Decreased action of tetracyclines
Lab test interferences:
• May cause false elevations of urinary catecholamines

NURSING CONSIDERATIONS
Assess:
• Nutritional status: liver, eggs, dairy products, yeast, whole grain, green vegetables
Administer:
• With food for better absorption
Perform/provide:
• Storage in airtight, light-resistant container
Evaluate:
• Therapeutic response: absence of headache, GI problems, cheilosis, skin lesions, depression, burning, itchy eyes, anemia
Teach patient/family:
• That urine may turn bright yellow
• About addition of needed foods that are rich in riboflavin
• To avoid alcohol

---

rifabutin (℞)
(riff'a-byoo-ten)
Mycobutin
Func. class.: Antimycobacterial agent
Chem. class.: Rifamycin S derivative

Action: Inhibits DNA-dependent RNA polymerase in susceptible strains of *Escherichia coli* and *Bacillus subtilis;* mechanism of action against *Mycobacterium avium* unknown
Uses: Prevention of *Mycobacterium avium* complex (MAC) in patients with advanced HIV infection
Dosage and routes:
• *Adult:* 300 mg qd (may take as 150 mg bid)
Available forms: Caps 150 mg
Side effects/adverse reactions:
INTEG: Rash
MS: Asthenia, arthralgia, myalgia
MISC: Flulike symptoms, shortness of breath, chest pressure

GI: Nausea, vomiting, anorexia, diarrhea, heartburn, ***hepatitis***
GU: Hematuria, *discolored urine*
CNS: Headache, fatigue, anxiety, confusion, insomnia
HEMA: ***Hemolytic anemia, eosinophilia, thrombocytopenia, leukopenia***
Contraindications: Hypersensitivity, active TB, WBC <1000 or platelet count <50,000
Precautions: Pregnancy (B), lactation, hepatic disease, blood dyscrasias, children
Do not confuse:
rifabutin/rifampin
Pharmacokinetics:
PO: Peak 2-3 hr, duration >24 hr, half-life 3 hr; metabolized in liver (active/inactive metabolites), excreted in urine primarily as metabolites
Interactions:
• Decreased action of: barbiturates, clofibrate, corticosteroids, dapsone, anticoagulants, sulfonylureas, estrogens, digitoxin and digoxin, oral contraceptives, theophylline, β-blockers, verapamil, cyclosporine, zidovudine, ketoconazole
• Increased levels of rifabutin: ritonavir
• Drug/food: high-fat diet decreases absorption
Lab test interferences:
Interference: Folate level, vit B_{12}, BSP, gallbladder studies
NURSING CONSIDERATIONS
Assess:
• CBC for neutropenia, thrombocytopenia, eosinophilia
• For acute TB: chest x-ray, sputum culture, blood culture, biopsy of lymph nodes, PPD; drug should not be given for active TB
• Signs of anemia: Hct, Hgb, fatigue
• Liver studies qwk: ALT, AST, bilirubin

• Renal status before, qmo: BUN, creatinine, output, specific gravity, urinalysis
• Hepatic studies: decreased appetite, jaundice, dark urine, fatigue
Administer:
• With food if GI upset occurs; better to take on empty stomach 1 hr ac or 2 hr pc, high-fat foods slow absorption
• Antiemetic if vomiting occurs
• After C&S is completed; qmo to detect resistance
Evaluate:
• Therapeutic response: not used for active TB because of risk of development of resistance to rifampin; culture negative
Teach patient/family:
• That patients using oral contraceptives should consider using nonhormonal methods of birth control, since rifabutin may decrease their efficacy
• That compliance with dosage schedule, duration is necessary
• That scheduled appointments must be kept; relapse may occur
• That urine, feces, saliva, sputum, sweat, tears may be colored redorange; soft contact lenses may be permanently stained
• To report flulike symptoms: excessive fatigue, anorexia, vomiting, sore throat; unusual bleeding, yellowish discoloration of skin, eyes
• To report myositis: muscle or bone pain

◆ = Nursing alert   ⫽ = Herb-drug interaction   ⊘ = Do not crush

rifampin (R)

(rif'am-pin)
Rifadin, Rimactane, Rofact*
Func. class.: Antitubercular
Chem. class.: Rifamycin B derivative

Action: Inhibits DNA-dependent polymerase, decreases tubercle bacilli replication

Uses: Pulmonary tuberculosis, meningococcal carriers (prevention)

Research note: Repaglinide given with rifampin resulted in the decrease of repaglinide levels[36]

Dosage and routes:

Tuberculosis

• *Adult:* **PO/IV** max 600 mg/day as single dose 1 hr ac or 2 hr pc or 10 mg/kg/day 2-3 ×/wk

• *Child >5 yr:* **PO/IV** 10-20 mg/kg/day as single dose 1 hr ac or 2 hr pc, not to exceed 600 mg/day, with other antituberculars

• 6-mo regimen: 2 mo treatment of isoniazid, rifampin, pyrazinamide and possibly streptomycin or ethambutol; then rifampin and isoniazid × 4 mo

• 9-mo regimen: rifampin and isoniazid supplemented with pyrazinamide, or streptomycin or ethambutol

Meningococcal carriers

• *Adult:* **PO/IV** 600 mg bid × 2 days

• *Child >5 yr:* **PO/IV** 10-20 mg/kg not to exceed 600 mg/dose

• *Infant 3 mo-1 yr:* 5 mg/kg **PO** bid for 2 days

Available forms: Caps 150, 300 mg; powder for inj 600 mg/vial

Side effects/adverse reactions:

INTEG: Rash, pruritus, urticaria
EENT: Visual disturbances
MS: Atoxia, weakness
MISC: Flulike symptoms, menstrual disturbances, edema, shortness of breath

GI: Nausea, vomiting, anorexia, diarrhea, **pseudomembranous colitis,** *heartburn,* sore mouth and tongue, **pancreatitis,** increased LFTs

GU: **Hematuria, acute renal failure, hemoglobinuria**

CNS: Headache, fatigue, anxiety, drowsiness, confusion

HEMA: **Hemolytic anemia, eosinophilia, thrombocytopenia, leukopenia**

Contraindications: Hypersensitivity

Precautions: Pregnancy (C), lactation, hepatic disease, blood dyscrasias

Do not confuse:

rifampin/rifabutin

Pharmacokinetics:

PO: Peak 2-3 hr, duration >24 hr, half-life 3 hr; metabolized in liver (active/inactive metabolites), excreted in urine as free drug (30% crosses placenta) and breast milk

Interactions:

• Decreased action of: barbiturates, clofibrate, corticosteroids, dapsone, anticoagulants, antidiabetics, hormones, digoxin, alcohol, oral contraceptives, verapamil, diltiazem, nifedipine, cyclosporine, haloperidol, theophylline, chloramphenicol, acetaminophen, benzodiazepines, phenytoin, sulfonamides, β-blockers, doxycycline, fluoroquinolones, zidovudine, imidazole antifungals

• Lithium toxicity: lithium

• Hepatotoxicity: isoniazid

• Incompatible with sodium lactate

Lab test interferences:

Interference: Folate level, vit B_{12}, gallbladder studies

NURSING CONSIDERATIONS

Assess:

• For infection: sputum culture, lung sounds

R

• Signs of anemia: Hct, Hgb, fatigue
• Liver studies qwk: ALT, AST, bilirubin
• Renal status before, qmo: BUN, creatinine, output, specific gravity, urinalysis
• Hepatic status: decreased appetite, jaundice, dark urine, fatigue
Administer:
• After C&S is completed; qmo to detect resistance
PO
• On empty stomach, 1 hr ac or 2 hr pc
• Antiemetic if vomiting occurs
IV
• After diluting each 600 mg/10 ml of sterile water for inj (60 mg/ml), agitate, withdraw dose and dilute in 100 ml or 500 ml of D_5W or 0.9% NaCl given as an inf over 3 hr, or if diluted in 100 ml, give over ½ hr
Evaluate:
• Therapeutic response: decreased symptoms of TB, culture negative
Teach patient/family:
• That compliance with dosage schedule, duration is necessary
• That scheduled appointments must be kept; relapse may occur
• To avoid alcohol
• That urine, feces, saliva, sputum, sweat, tears may be colored red-orange; soft contact lenses may be permanently stained
• To report flulike symptoms: excessive fatigue, anorexia, vomiting, sore throat; unusual bleeding, yellowish discoloration of skin, eyes

rifapentine (℞)

(riff'ah-pen-teen)
Priftin
Func. class.: Antitubercular
Chem. class.: Rifamycin derivative

Action: Inhibits DNA-dependent polymerase, decreases tubercle bacilli replication
Uses: Pulmonary tuberculosis, must be used with at least one other antitubercular
Dosage and routes:

Intensive phase
• *Adult:* **PO** 600 mg (four 150 mg tabs 2×/wk), with an interval of 72 hr between doses × 2 mo; must be given with at least one other antitubercular

Continuation phase
• *Adult:* **PO** continue with 1×/wk × 4 mo in combination with isoniazid or other appropriate antitubercular
Available forms: Tabs 150 mg
Side effects/adverse reactions:

INTEG: Rash, pruritus, urticaria, acne
EENT: Visual disturbances
MS: Gout, arthrosis
MISC: Edema, aggressive reaction, increased B/P
GI: Nausea, vomiting, anorexia, diarrhea, bilirubinemia, hepatitis, increased ALT, AST, *heartburn, pancreatitis*
GU: Hematuria, pyuria, *proteinuria,* urinary casts, urine discoloration
CNS: Headache, fatigue, anxiety, dizziness
HEMA: Thrombocytopenia, leukopenia, neutropenia, lymphopenia, anemia, *leukocytosis,* purpura, hematoma
Contraindications: Hypersensitivity to rifamycins, porphyria

⬥ = Nursing alert   ⫸ = Herb-drug interaction   🚫 = Do not crush

Precautions: Pregnancy (C), lactation, hepatic disease, blood dyscrasias, children <12 yr, HIV, elderly

Pharmacokinetics:
PO: Peak 5-6 hr, half-life 13 hr; metabolized in liver (active/inactive metabolites), excreted in urine and feces, excreted in breast milk, protein binding 97%, steady state 10 days

Interactions:
• Use with extreme caution with protease inhibitors
• Decreased action of: amitriptyline, anticoagulants, antidiabetics, barbiturates, β-blockers, chloramphenicol, clarithromycin, clofibrate, corticosteroids, cyclosporine, dapsone, delavirdine, diazepam, digoxin, diltiazem, disopyramide, doxyclycline, fentanyl, fluconazole, fluoroquinolones, haloperidol, indinavir, itraconazole, ketoconazole, methadone, mexiletine, nelfinavir, nifedipine, nortriptyline, oral contraceptives, phenothiazines, phenytoin, progestins, quinidine, quinine, ritonavir, saquinavir, sildenafil, tacrolimus, theophylline, thyroid preparations, tocainide, verapamil, warfarin, zidovudine
• Drug/food: increased absorption with food

Lab test interferences:
Interference: Folate level, vit B_{12}

NURSING CONSIDERATIONS
Assess:
• Baselines in CBC, AST, ALT, bilirubin, platelets
• For infection: sputum culture, lung sounds
• Signs of anemia: Hct, Hgb, fatigue
• Liver studies qmo: ALT, AST, bilirubin
• Renal status qmo: BUN, creatinine, output, specific gravity, urinalysis
• Hepatic status: decreased appetite, jaundice, dark urine, fatigue

Administer:
PO
• May give with food for GI upset
• Antiemetic if vomiting occurs
• After C&S is completed; qmo to detect resistance

Evaluate:
• Therapeutic response: decreased symptoms of TB, culture negative

Teach patient/family:
• That compliance with dosage schedule, duration is necessary
• That scheduled appointments must be kept; relapse may occur
• That urine, feces, saliva, sputum, sweat, tears may be colored red-orange; soft contact lenses, dentures may be permanently stained
• To use alternative method of contraception, oral contraceptive action may be decreased
• To report flulike symptoms: excessive fatigue, anorexia, vomiting, sore throat; unusual bleeding, yellowish discoloration of skin, eyes

---

riluzole (℞)
(rill'you-zole)
Rilutek
Func. class.: ALS agent
Chem. class.: Benzathiazole

Action: Unknown; may act by inhibiting glutamate, interfering with binding of amino acid receptors, and inactivating of voltage-dependent sodium channels

Uses: Amyotropic lateral sclerosis (ALS)

Dosage and routes:
• *Adult:* PO 50 mg q12h, take 1 hr ac or 2 hr pc
Available forms: Tabs 50 mg

Side effects/adverse reactions:
GI: Nausea, vomiting, dyspepsia, anorexia, diarrhea, flatulence, stomatitis, dry mouth

*HEMA: **Neutropenia***

CNS: Hypertonia, depression, dizziness, insomnia, somnolence, vertigo

INTEG: Pruritus, eczema, alopecia, ***exfoliative dermatitis***

RESP: Decreased lung function, rhinitis, increased cough

CV: Hypertension, tachycardia, phlebitis, palpitation, postural hypertension

GU: UTI, dysuria

Contraindications: Hypersensitivity

Precautions: Neutropenia, renal disease, hepatic disease, elderly, pregnancy (C), lactation, children

Pharmacokinetics: Well absorbed, extensively metabolized by the liver, excretion in urine/feces

Interactions:
• Decreased elimination of riluzole: caffeine, theophylline, amitriptyline, quinolones
• Increased elimination of riluzole: cigarette smoking, rifampin, omeprazole, charcoal-broiled food

NURSING CONSIDERATIONS
Assess:
• LFTs: AST, ALT, bilirubin, GGT, baseline and qmo × 3 mo, then q3mo; monitor liver chemistries
• For neutropenia <500/mm

Administer:
• 1 hr ac or 2 hr pc; a high-fat meal decreases absorption

Teach patient/family:
• To report febrile illness, which may indicate neutropenia
• The reason for drug and expected results

---

rimantadine (R̞)
(ri-man'tah-deen)
Flumadine
Func. class.: Synthetic antiviral
Chem. class.: Tricyclic amine

Action: Prevents uncoating of nucleic acid in viral cell, preventing penetration of virus to host; causes release of dopamine from neurons

Uses: Prophylaxis or treatment of influenza type A

Dosage and routes:
Renal/hepatic dose
• Reduce dose as needed
Influenza type A
Prophylaxis
• *Adult and child >10 yr:* **PO** 100 mg bid; in renal, hepatic disease, lower dose to 100 mg/day
• *Child <10 yr:* **PO** 5 mg/kg/day, not to exceed 150 mg
Treatment
• *Adult:* **PO** 100 mg bid; in renal or hepatic disease, lower dose to 100 mg/day; start treatment at onset of symptoms, continue for at least 1 wk
• *Geriatric:* **PO** 100 mg/day
Available forms: Tabs 100 mg; syr 50 mg/5 ml

Side effects/adverse reactions:
CNS: Headache, dizziness, fatigue, depression, hallucinations, tremors, ***seizures,*** insomnia, *poor concentration,* asthenia, gait abnormalities, *anxiety, confusion*

CV: Pallor, palpitations, *hypotension, edema*

EENT: Tinnitus, taste abnormality, eye pain

GI: Nausea, vomiting, constipation, dry mouth, anorexia, abdominal pain, diarrhea, dyspepsia

INTEG: Rash

Contraindications: Hypersensitivity to drugs of adamantance class (this drug, amantadine)

◆ = Nursing alert   🌿 = Herb-drug interaction   🚫 = Do not crush

Precautions: Epilepsy, hepatic disease, renal disease, pregnancy (C), lactation, children <1 yr

Do not confuse:
rimantadine/amantadine

Pharmacokinetics:
PO: Peak 6 hr, elimination half-life 25½ hr, plasma protein binding (40%)

Interactions:
• Decreased peak concentration of rimantadine: acetaminophen, aspirin
• Increased rimantadine concentration: cimetidine

NURSING CONSIDERATIONS
Assess:
• Assess for seizures; if seizures occur, drug should be discontinued
• I&O ratio; report urinary frequency, hesitancy in renal disease
• Bowel pattern before, during treatment
• CNS effect in elderly or patients with severe hepatic/renal disease
• Skin eruptions, photosensitivity after administration of drug
• Respiratory status: rate, character, wheezing, tightness in chest
• Allergies before initiation of treatment, reaction of each medication; list allergies on chart in bright red letters
• Signs of infection

Administer:
• Within 48 hr of exposure to influenza; continue for 10 days after contact
• At least 4 hr before hs to prevent insomnia
• After meals for better absorption, to decrease GI symptoms
• In divided doses to prevent CNS disturbances: headache, dizziness, fatigue, drowsiness

Perform/provide:
• Storage in tight, dry container

Evaluate:
• Therapeutic response: absence of fever, malaise, cough, dyspnea in infection

Teach patient/family:
• About aspects of drug therapy: need to report dyspnea, dizziness, poor concentration, behavioral changes
• To avoid hazardous activities if dizziness occurs

Treatment of overdose: Withdraw drug, maintain airway, administer epinephrine, aminophylline, O$_2$, IV corticosteroids, physostigmine

---

risedronate (℞)
(rih-sed′roh-nate)
Actonel
Func. class.: Bone resorption inhibitor
Chem. class.: Biphosphonate

Action: Absorbs calcium phosphate crystal in bone and may directly block dissolution of hydroxyapatite crystals of bone; inhibits bone resorption, apparently without inhibiting bone formation, mineralization

Uses: Paget's disease, osteoporosis in postmenopausal women, glucocorticoid-induced osteoporosis

Dosage and routes:
Paget's disease
• *Adult:* **PO** 30 mg qd × 2 mo; patients with Paget's disease should receive calcium and vit D if dietary intake is lacking; if relapse occurs, retreatment is advised

Treatment/prevention of postmenopausal osteoporosis/glucocorticoid-induced osteoporosis
• *Adult:* **PO** 5 mg qd

Available forms: Tabs 5, 30 mg

Side effects/adverse reactions:
CNS: Dizziness, heacache

R

Side effects: *italics* = common; ***bold italics*** = life-threatening

GI: Abdominal pain, anorexia, diarrhea, nausea
MS: Bone pain, arthralgia
CV: Chest pain

Contraindications: Hypersensitivity to biphosphonates

Precautions: Children, lactation, pregnancy (C), renal disease

Pharmacokinetics: Rapidly cleared from circulation, taken up mainly by bones, eliminated primarily through kidneys

Interactions:
• Decreased absorption of risedronate: calcium supplements, antacids
• Drug/food: decreased bioavailability: take ½ hr before food or drinks

NURSING CONSIDERATIONS

Assess:
• Symptoms of Paget's disease: headache, bone pain, increased head circumference
• Electrolytes: renal function studies; Ca, P, Mg, K
• For hypercalcemia: paresthesia, twitching, laryngospasm, Chvostek's, Trousseau's signs

Administer:
• PO for 2 months to be effective in Paget's disease
• With a full glass of water, patient should be in upright position for ½ hr
• Supplemental Ca and vit D in Paget's disease
• Give qd ≥30 min ac

Perform/provide:
• Storage in cool environment, out of direct sunlight

Evaluate:
• Therapeutic response: increased bone mass, absence of fractures

Teach patient/family:
• To sit upright for ½ hr after dose to prevent irritation
• To comply with diet

• To notify prescriber if pregnancy is suspected

---

risperidone (Ŗ)
(ris-pehr'ih-dohn)
Risperdal
Func. class.: Antipsychotic
Chem. class.: Benzisoxazole derivative

Action: Unknown; may be mediated through both dopamine type 2 (D^2) and serotonin type 2 (5-HT_2) antagonism

Uses: Psychotic disorders

Research note: Risperidone given with paroxetine resulted in an increase of risperidone levels[37]

Dosage and routes:
• *Adult:* **PO** 1 mg bid, with incremental increases of 1 mg bid on days 2 and 3 to a dose of 3 mg bid by day 3; then do not increase dose for at least 1 wk
• *Geriatric:* **PO** 0.5 mg qd-bid, increase by 1 mg qwk
Hepatic dose
• *Adult:* **PO** 0.5 mg bid, increase by 0.5 mg bid, increase to 1.5 mg bid

Available forms: Tabs 1, 2, 3, 4 mg; oral sol 1 mg/ml

Side effects/adverse reactions:
*CNS: EPS, pseudoparkinsonism, akathisia, dystonia, tardive dyskinesia; drowsiness, insomnia, agitation, anxiety, headache, **seizures, neuroleptic malignant syndrome***
*CV: Orthostatic hypotension, **tachycardia***
EENT: Blurred vision
GI: Nausea, vomiting, anorexia, constipation, jaundice, weight gain
RESP: Rhinitis

Contraindications: Hypersensitivity, lactation, seizure disorders

Precautions: Children, renal dis-

◆ = Nursing alert   ✐ = Herb-drug interaction   ⊘ = Do not crush

ease, pregnancy (C), hepatic disease, elderly, breast cancer

Do not confuse:

Risperdal/reserpine

Pharmacokinetics:

PO: Extensively metabolized by liver to a major active metabolite, plasma protein binding 90%

Interactions:

• Increased sedation: other CNS depressants, alcohol

• Increased EPS: other antipsychotics, lithium

• Increased excretion of risperidone: carbamazepine

🍴 Increased CNS depression: kava

Lab test interferences: Not known

NURSING CONSIDERATIONS

Assess:

• Mental status before initial administration

• Swallowing of PO medication; check for hoarding or giving of medication to other patients

• I&O ratio; palpate bladder if urinary output is low

• Bilirubin, CBC, liver function studies qmo

• Urinalysis before, during prolonged therapy

• Affect, orientation, LOC, reflexes, gait, coordination, sleep pattern disturbances

• B/P standing and lying; also pulse, respirations; take these q4h during initial treatment; establish baseline before starting treatment; report drops of 30 mm Hg; watch for ECG changes

• Dizziness, faintness, palpitations, tachycardia on rising

• EPS, including akathisia (inability to sit still, no pattern to movements), tardive dyskinesia (bizarre movements of the jaw, mouth, tongue, extremities), pseudoparkinsonism (rigidity, tremors, pill rolling, shuffling gait)

◆ For neuroleptic malignant syndrome: hyperthermia, increased CPK, altered mental status, muscle rigidity

• Skin turgor qd

• Constipation, urinary retention qd; if these occur, increase bulk and water in diet

Administer:

• Reduced dose in elderly

• Antiparkinsonian agent on order from prescriber, to be used for EPS

Perform/provide:

• Decreased stimulus by dimming lights, avoiding loud noises

• Supervised ambulation until patient is stabilized on medication; do not involve in strenuous exercise program because fainting is possible; patient should not stand still for a long time

• Increased fluids to prevent constipation

• Sips of water, candy, gum for dry mouth

• Storage in tight, light-resistant container

Evaluate:

• Therapeutic response: decrease in emotional excitement, hallucinations, delusions, paranoia; reorganization of patterns of thought, speech

Teach patient/family:

• That orthostatic hypotension may occur and to rise from sitting or lying position gradually

• To avoid hot tubs, hot showers, tub baths; hypotension may occur

• To avoid abrupt withdrawal of this drug; EPS may result; drug should be withdrawn slowly

• To avoid OTC preparations (cough, hay fever, cold) unless approved by prescriber, since serious drug interactions may occur; avoid use with alcohol, CNS depressants; increased drowsiness may occur

• To avoid hazardous activities if drowsy or dizzy

R

Side effects: *italics* = common; ***bold italics*** = life-threatening

• Compliance with drug regimen
• To report impaired vision, tremors, muscle twitching
• In hot weather, that heat stroke may occur; take extra precautions to stay cool
• To use contraception, inform prescriber if pregnancy is planned or suspected

Treatment of overdose: Lavage if orally ingested; provide airway; *do not induce vomiting*

---

ritodrine (Ḃ)
(rih'toh-dreen)
ritodrine, Yutopar
Func. class.: Tocolytic, uterine relaxant
Chem. class.: β_2-Adrenergic agonist

Action: Reduces frequency, intensity of uterine contractions by stimulation of the β_2-receptors in uterine smooth muscle

Uses: Management of preterm labor

Dosage and routes:
• *Adult:* **IV INF** 150 mg/500 ml (0.3 mg/ml) given 0.1 mg/min, increased gradually by 0.05 mg/min q10min until desired response

Available forms: Inj 10 mg/ml, 15 mg/ml

Side effects/adverse reactions:
MISC: Erythema, rash, dyspnea, hyperventilation, glycosuria, *lactic acidosis*
META: Hyperglycemia, hypokalemia
CNS: Headache, restlessness, anxiety, nervousness, sweating, chills, drowsiness, tremor
GI: Nausea, vomiting, anorexia, malaise, bloating, constipation, diarrhea
CV: Altered maternal, fetal heart rate, B/P, dysrhythmias, palpitations, chest pain, maternal pulmonary edema

Contraindications: Hypersensitivity, eclampsia, hypertension, dysrhythmias, thyrotoxicosis, before 20th wk of pregnancy, antepartum hemorrhage, intrauterine fetal death, maternal cardiac disease, pulmonary hypertension, uncontrolled diabetes, pheochromocytoma, bronchial asthma

Precautions: Migraine, sulfite sensitivity, pregnancy-induced hypertension, diabetes, pregnancy (B)

Pharmacokinetics:
IV: Immediate, distribution half-life 6 min, 2nd phase 1½-2½ hr, elimination phase >10 hr; metabolized in liver; 90% excreted in urine; crosses placenta

Interactions:
• Pulmonary edema: corticosteroids
• Increased CV effects of ritodrine: magnesium sulfate, diazoxide, meperidine, potent general anesthetics
• Increased effects of sympathomimetic amines
• Systemic hypertension: atropine
• Decreased action of ritodrine: β-blockers

Lab test interferences:
Increase: Blood glucose, free fatty acids, insulin, GTT
Decrease: K

NURSING CONSIDERATIONS
Assess:
• Maternal, fetal heart tones during infusion; maternal ECG to determine CV disease
• Intensity, length of uterine contractions
• Fluid intake to prevent fluid overload; discontinue if this occurs
• Blood glucose in diabetics

Administer:
• Only clear sol
• After dilution: 150 mg/500 ml D_5W or NS, give at 0.3 mg/ml
• Using infusion pump

• Considered incompatible with any drug in sol or syringe

Perform/provide:

• Positioning of patient in left lateral recumbent position to decrease hypotension, increase renal blood flow

Evaluate:

• Therapeutic response: decreased intensity, length of contraction, absence of preterm labor, decreased B/P

Teach patient/family:

• To remain in bed during infusion

---

ritonavir (℞)

(ri-toe′na-veer)

Norvir

Func. class.: Antiretroviral

Chem. class.: Protease inhibitor

Action: Inhibits human immunodeficiency virus (HIV) protease and prevents maturation of the infectious virus

Uses: HIV in combination with zidovudine, ddc, or alone

Dosage and routes:

• *Adult:* PO 600 mg bid. If nausea occurs begin dose at ½ and gradually increase

• *Child:* PO 250 mg/m^2 bid, titrate upward to 400 mg/m^2 bid

Available forms: Caps 100 mg; oral sol 80 mg/ml

Side effects/adverse reactions:

GI: Diarrhea, buccal mucosa ulceration, abdominal pain, *nausea,* taste perversion, dry mouth, dizziness, insomnia, headache, vomiting

CNS: Paresthesia, *headache,* vomiting, *seizures*

INTEG: Rash

MS: Pain

MISC.: Asthenia, *angioedema, anaphylaxis, Stevens-Johnson syndrome*

Contraindications: Hypersensitivity

Precautions: Liver disease, pregnancy (B), lactation, children

Pharmacokinetics: Well absorbed; 98% protein binding, hepatic metabolism

Interactions:

• Increased ritonavir levels: fluconazole

• Decreased ritonavir levels: rifamycins, nevirapine, barbiturates, phenytoin

• Increased level of both drugs: clarithromycin, ddI

• Toxicity: amiodarone, benzodiazepines, bepridil, bupropion, clozapine, desipramine, flecainide, meperidine, piroxicam, propafenone, propoxyphene, quinidine, saquinavir, terfenadine, zolpidem

• Decreased ethinyl estradiol, sulfamethoxazole, theophylline, zidovudine levels when used with ritonavir

Lab test interferences:

Increase: ALT, GGT, PT, triglycerides

Decrease: Hct, RBC

NURSING CONSIDERATIONS

Assess:

• Signs of infection, anemia

• Liver studies: ALT, AST

• Viral load and CD4 baseline and throughout therapy

• C&S before drug therapy; drug may be taken as soon as culture is taken; repeat C&S after treatment; determine the presence of other sexually transmitted diseases

• Bowel pattern before, during treatment; if severe abdominal pain with bleeding occurs, drug should be discontinued; monitor hydration

• Skin eruptions; rash

• Allergies before treatment, reaction to each medication; place allergies on chart

R

Side effects: *italics* = common; ***bold italics*** = life-threatening

Administer:
• With food; mix oral powder with high-calorie drink such as Ensure
• Store caps in refrigerator
Teach patient/family:
• To take as prescribed; if dose is missed, take as soon as remembered up to 1 hr before next dose; do not double dose
• That drug must be taken in equal intervals around the clock to maintain blood levels for duration of therapy
• To take with food; mix liquid formulation with chocolate milk or liquid nutritional supplement

---

rituximab

(rih-tuks'ih-mab)

Rituxan

Func. class.: Misc. antineoplastic

Chem. class.: Murine/human monoclonal antibody

Action: Directed against the CD20 antigen that is found on malignant B lymphocytes; CD20 regulates a portion of cell-cycle initiation/differentiation
Uses: Non-Hodgkin's lymphoma (CD20 positive, B-cell), bulky disease (tumors >10 cm)
Dosage and routes:
• *Adult:* IV INF 375 mg/m² qwk × 4 doses; give at 50 mg/hr for 1st inf; if hypersensitivity does not occur, increase rate by 50 mg/hr q½h, max 400 mg/hr; slow/interrupt inf if hypersensitivity occurs; other inf can be given at 100 mg/hr and increased by 100 mg/hr, max 400 mg/hr
Available forms: Inj 10 mg/ml
Side effects/adverse reactions:
CV: Cardiac dysrhythmias
GU: Renal failure
SYST: Stevens-Johnson syndrome
GI: Nausea, vomiting, anorexia

INTEG: Irritation at site, rash, *fatal mucocutaneous infections (rare)*
HEMA: Leukopenia, neutropenia, thrombocytopenia
OTHER: Fever, chills, asthenia, headache, angioedema, hypotension, myalgia, *bronchospasm*
Contraindications: Hypersensitivity, murine proteins
Precautions: Lactation, children, elderly, pregnancy (C), cardiac conditions
Pharmacokinetics: Half-life 42-79 min
NURSING CONSIDERATIONS
Assess:
◆ For signs of fatal infusion reaction: hypoxia, pulmonary infiltrates, acute respiratory distress syndrome, MI, ventricular fibrillation, cardiogenic shock; most fatal infusion reactions occur with first infusion; potentially fatal
◆ For signs of severe mucocutaneous reactions: Stevens-Johnson syndrome, lichenoid dermatitis, toxic epidermal lysis; occur 1-13 wk after drug was given
◆ Tumor lysis syndrome: acute renal failure requiring hemodialysis, hyperkalemia, hypocalcemia, hyperuricemia, hyperphosphatemia
• CBC, differential, platelet count weekly; withhold drug if WBC is <3500/mm³, or platelet count <100,000/mm³; notify prescriber of these results; drug should be discontinued
• Food preferences: list likes, dislikes
• GI symptoms: frequency of stools
• Signs of dehydration: rapid respirations, poor skin turgor, decreased urine output, dry skin, restlessness, weakness
Administer:
IV inf
• After diluting to a final conc. of 1-4 mg/ml; use 0.9% NaCl, D₅W,

◆ = Nursing alert   ✦ = Herb-drug interaction   ⊘ = Do not crush

gently invert bag to mix; do not mix with other drugs

Perform/provide:
• Increased fluid intake to 2-3 L/day to prevent dehydration, unless contraindicated
• Changing of IV site q48h
• Nutritious diet with iron, vitamin supplement, low fiber, few dairy products
• Storage of vials at 36°-40° F, protect vials from direct sunlight, inf sol is stable at 36°-46° F × 24 hr and room temperature for another 12 hr

Evaluate:
• Therapeutic response: decrease in tumor size, decrease in spread of cancer

Teach patient/family:
• To report adverse reactions

---

rivastigmine (℞)
(riv-as-tig′mine)
Exelon
Func. class.: Cholinesterase inhibitor

Action: May enhance cholinergic functioning by increasing acetylcholine

Uses: Alzheimer's dementia

Dosage and routes:
• *Adult:* PO 1.5 mg bid, after 2 wk or more, may increase to 3 mg bid after 2 wk or more; may increase to 4.5 mg bid and thereafter 6 mg bid

Available forms: Caps 1.5, 3, 4.5, 6 mg; solution 2 mg/ml

Side effects/adverse reactions:
CNS: Tremors, confusion, insomnia, psychosis, hallucination, depression, dizziness, headache, anxiety, somnolence, fatigue, syncope
GI: Nausea, vomiting, anorexia, abdominal distress, flatulence, diarrhea, constipation
MISC: Urinary tract infection, asthenia, increased sweating, hypertension, influenza-like symptoms, weight change

Contraindications: Hypersensitivity to this drug, other carbamates; narrow-angle glaucoma, undiagnosed skin lesions

Precautions: Renal disease, hepatic disease, respiratory disease, seizure disorder, peptic ulcer, cardiac disease, urinary obstruction, asthma, pregnancy (B), asthma, lactation, children, peptic ulcer

Pharmacokinetics:
Rapidly and completely absorbed, metabolized to decarbamylated metabolite, half-life is 1.5 hr, excreted via kidneys (metabolites), clearance is lowered in the elderly, hepatic disease, and increased in nicotine use

Interactions:
• Synergistic effect: cholinomimetics, other cholinesterase inhibitors

NURSING CONSIDERATIONS
Assess:
• Liver function enzymes: AST, ALT, alk phosphatase, LDH, bilirubin, CBC
• For severe GI effects: nausea, vomiting, anorexia, weight loss
• B/P, respiration during initial treatment; hypo/hypertension should be reported
• Mental status: affect, mood, behavioral changes, depression; complete suicide assessment

Administer:
• With meals; take with morning and evening meal even though absorption may be decreased

Perform/provide:
• Assistance with ambulation during beginning therapy

Evaluate:
• Therapeutic response

R

Teach patient/family:

• The procedure for giving oral solution; use instruction sheet provided

• To notify prescriber of severe GI effects

---

rizatriptan (R)

(rye-zah-trip'tan)
Maxalt, Maxalt-MLT
Func. class.: Migraine agent
Chem. class.: 5-HT₁ receptor agonist

Action: Binds selectively to the vascular 5-HT_1 receptor subtype, exerts antimigraine effect; causes vasoconstriction in cranial arteries

Uses: Acute treatment of migraine

Dosage and routes:

• *Adult:* **PO** 5-10 mg single dose, redosing separate by 2 hr or more; max 30 mg/24 hr

Available forms: Maxalt: tabs 5, 10 mg; Maxalt-MLT: tabs, orally disintegrating 5, 10 mg

Side effects/adverse reactions:

CNS: Dizziness, headache, fatigue, warm/cold sensations, flushing, hot flashes

RESP: Chest tightness, pressure, dyspnea

GI: Nausea, dry mouth, diarrhea

CV: MI, ventricular fibrillation, ventricular tachycardia, coronary artery vasospasm

Contraindications: Angina pectoris, history of MI, documented silent ischemia, Prinzmetal's angina, ischemic heart disease, concurrent ergotamine-containing preparations, uncontrolled hypertension, hypersensitivity, basilar or hemiplegic migraine

Precautions: Postmenopausal women, men >40 yr, risk factors for CAD, hypercholesterolemia, obesity, diabetes, impaired hepatic or renal function, pregnancy (C), lactation, children, elderly

Pharmacokinetics: Onset of pain relief 10 min-2 hr, 14% plasma protein binding, metabolized in the liver (metabolite), excreted in urine, feces, half-life 2-3 hr

Interactions:

• Extended vasospastic effects: ergot, ergot derivatives, other 5-HT receptor agonists

• Increased action of rizatriptan: cimetidine, oral contraceptives, MAOIs, nonselective MAOI (type A and B), isocarboxazid, pargyline, phenelzine, propranolol, tranylcypromine

• Weakness, hyperreflexia, incoordination: SSRIs

NURSING CONSIDERATIONS

Assess:

• Tingling, hot sensation, burning, feeling of pressure, numbness, flushing, inj site reaction

• For stress level, activity, recreation, coping mechanisms

• Neurologic status: LOC, blurring vision, nausea, vomiting, tingling in extremities preceding headache

• Ingestion of tyramine foods (pickled products, beer, wine, aged cheese), food additives, preservatives, colorings, artificial sweeteners, chocolate, caffeine, which may precipitate these types of headaches

Perform/provide:

• Quiet, calm environment with decreased stimulation for noise, bright light, excessive talking

Evaluate:

• Therapeutic response: decrease in frequency, severity of headache

Teach patient/family:

• Use of orally disintegrating tab: instruct patient not to open blister until use, to peel blister open with

---

◆ = Nursing alert   ✿ = Herb-drug interaction   Ⓢ = Do not crush dry hands, to place tab on tongue, where it will dissolve, and to swallow with saliva (contains phenylalanine)

• To report any side effects to prescriber

• To use alternative contraception while taking drug if oral contraceptives are being used

rocuronium (R)

(ro-kyur-oh'nium)

Zemuron

Func. class.: Neuromuscular blocker (nondepolarizing)

Chem. class.: Biquaternary ammonium ester

Action: Inhibits transmission of nerve impulses by binding with cholinergic receptor sites, antagonizing action of acetylcholine

Uses: Facilitation of endotracheal intubation, skeletal muscle relaxation during mechanical ventilation, surgery, or general anesthesia

Dosage and routes:

Intubation

• *Adult and child:* IV 0.6 mg/kg

Available forms: Inj 10 mg/ml

Side effects/adverse reactions:

CV: Bradycardia, tachycardia, change in B/P

*RESP: **Prolonged apnea, bronchospasm, cyanosis, respiratory depression***

GI: Nausea, vomiting

INTEG: Rash, flushing, pruritus, urticaria

Contraindications: Hypersensitivity

Precautions: Pregnancy (C), cardiac disease, lactation, child <2 yr, electrolyte imbalances, dehydration, neuromuscular disease, respiratory disease

Pharmacokinetics: Half-life 71-203 min, duration ½ hr

Interactions:

• Blocked action of rocuronium: phenylephrine

• Increased effect of rocuronium: anesthetics

NURSING CONSIDERATIONS

Assess:

• For electrolyte imbalances (K, Mg), before drug is used; electrolyte imbalances may lead to increased action of this drug

• Vital signs (B/P, pulse, respirations, airway) until fully recovered; rate, depth, pattern of respirations, strength of hand grip; patient should be intubated before use

• Recovery: decreased paralysis of face, diaphragm, leg, arm, rest of body; residual weakness and respiratory problems may occur during recovery

• Allergic reactions: rash, fever, respiratory distress, pruritus; drug should be discontinued

Administer:

• Using peripheral nerve stimulator by anesthesiologist to determine neuromuscular blockade; deep tendon reflexes should be monitored during extended use

• Undiluted direct IV over 2 min (only by qualified person, usually anesthesiologist); do not administer IM

• Maintenance q20-45min after 1st dose; titrate to response

Perform/provide:

• Storage in light-resistant area

• Reassurance if communication is difficult during recovery from neuromuscular blockade

Evaluate:

• Therapeutic response: paralysis of jaw, eyelid, head, neck, rest of body as evaluated by peripheral nerve stimulator

R

Teach patient/family:
• About all procedures or treatments; patient will remain conscious if anesthesia is not given also

Treatment of overdose: Edrophonium or neostigmine, atropine, monitor VS; may require mechanical ventilation

rofecoxib (R)

(roh-fih-kox'ib)
Vioxx
Func. class.: Nonsteroidal antiinflammatory
Chem. class.: COX-2 inhibitor

Action: May inhibit prostaglandin synthesis by decreasing enzyme needed for biosynthesis; analgesic, antiinflammatory, antipyretic properties

Uses: Acute, chronic osteoarthritis pain, primary dysmenorrhea

Dosage and routes:
Osteoarthritis
• *Adult:* **PO** 12.5 mg/day as a single dose may increase to 25 mg if needed
Primary dysmenorrhea
• *Adult:* **PO** 50 mg qd, use for <5 days
Available forms: Tabs 12.5, 25 mg; susp 12.5, 25 mg/5 ml

Side effects/adverse reactions:
CNS: Fatigue, anxiety, depression, nervousness, paresthesia
*CV: **Tachycardia,** angina, **MI,** palpitations, **dysrhythmias,** hypertension, fluid retention*
EENT: Tinnitus, hearing loss, blurred vision, glaucoma, cataract, conjunctivitis, eye pain
*GI: Nausea, anorexia, vomiting, constipation, dry mouth, diverticulitis, gastritis, gastroenteritis, hemorrhoids, hiatal hernia, stomatitis, **GI bleeding***
*GU: **Nephrotoxicity: dysuria,** he-*

maturia, oliguria, azotemia, cystitis, UTI
*HEMA: **Blood dyscrasias,** epistaxis, bruising, anemia*
INTEG: Purpura, rash, pruritus, sweating, erythema, petechiae, photosensitivity, alopecia
RESP: Pharyngitis, shortness of breath, pneumonia, coughing

Contraindications: Hypersensitivity to aspirin, iodides, other NSAIDs, asthma

Precautions: Pregnancy (C), lactation, children, bleeding disorders, GI disorders, cardiac disorders, hypersensitivity to other antiinflammatory agents

Pharmacokinetics: Well absorbed, crosses placenta, bound to plasma proteins

Interactions:
• Decreased effect, increased adverse reactions: aspirin, ACE inhibitors
• Increased bleeding: aspirin, other NSAIDs, anticoagulants
• Decreased effect of: diuretics
• Increased toxicity: lithium, antineoplastics
• Increased adverse reaction: glucocorticosteroids

NURSING CONSIDERATIONS

Assess:
• For patients with asthma, aspirin allergy, or nasal polyps; they may be hypersensitive
• For pain of rheumatoid arthritis, osteoarthritis; check ROM, inflammation of joints, characteristics of pain
• Blood counts during therapy; watch for decreasing platelets; if low, therapy may need to be discontinued, restarted after hematologic recovery; and for blood dyscrasias (thrombocytopenia): bruising, fatigue, bleeding, poor healing

◆ = Nursing alert   🖊 = Herb-drug interaction   ⊘ = Do not crush

Administer:

PO

• With food or milk to decrease gastric symptoms

🚫 Do not crush, dissolve, or chew

Evaluate:

• Therapeutic response: decreased pain in arthritic conditions; decreased inflammation in arthritic conditions

Teach patient/family:

• That drug must be continued for prescribed time to be effective; to avoid other NSAIDs, aspirin, alcohol

• To report bleeding, bruising, fatigue, malaise, since blood dyscrasia do occur

• To take with a full glass of water to enhance absorption

---

ropinirole (℞)

(roh-pin′ih-role)

Requip

Func. class.: Antiparkinson agent

Chem. class.: Dopamine-receptor agonist, non-ergot

Action: Selective agonist for D_2 receptors (presynaptic/postsynaptic sites); binding at D_3 receptor contributes to antiparkinson effects

Uses: Parkinsonism

Dosage and routes:

• *Adult:* **PO** 0.25 mg tid, titrate weekly to a max of 24 mg/day

Available forms: Tabs 0.25, 0.5, 1, 2, 4, 5 mg

Side effects/adverse reactions:

*HEMA: **Hemolytic anemia, leukopenia, agranulocytosis***

CNS: Agitation, insomnia, psychosis, hallucination, dystonia, depression, dizziness, somnolence

GI: Nausea, vomiting, anorexia, dry mouth, constipation, dyspepsia, flatulence

INTEG: Rash, sweating

CV: Orthostatic hypotension, tachycardia, hypertension, hypotension, syncope, palpitations

EENT: Blurred vision

GU: Impotence, urinary frequency

RESP: Pharyngitis, rhinitis, sinusitis, bronchitis, dyspnea

Contraindications: Hypersensitivity

Precautions: Renal disease, cardiac disease, dysrhythmias, affective disorder, psychosis, pregnancy (C), hepatic disease

Pharmacokinetics:

PO: Half-life 6 hr

Interactions:

• Increased ropinirole effect: cimetidine, ciprofloxacin, diltiazem, enoxacin, erythromycin, fluvoxamine, mexiletine, norfloxacin, tacrine, digoxin, theophylline, L-dopa

🌿 Decreased ropinirole action: chaste tree fruit

NURSING CONSIDERATIONS

Assess:

• Involuntary movements in parkinsonism: akinesia, tremors, staggering gait, muscle rigidity, drooling

• B/P, respiration during initial treatment; hypo/hypertension should be reported

• Mental status: affect, mood, behavioral changes, depression; complete suicide assessment

Administer:

• Drug until NPO before surgery

• Adjust dosage to patient response

• With meals

Perform/provide:

• Assistance with ambulation during beginning therapy

• Testing for diabetes mellitus, acromegaly if on long-term therapy

Evaluate:

• Therapeutic response: decrease in akathisia, increased mood

R

Side effects: *italics* = common; ***bold italics*** = life-threatening

Teach patient/family:
• That therapeutic effects may take several wk to a few mo
• To change positions slowly to prevent orthostatic hypotension
• To use drug exactly as prescribed; if drug is discontinued abruptly, parkinsonian crisis may occur

ropivacaine (℞)

(roe-pi′va-kane)
Naropin
Func. class.: Local anesthetic
Chem. class.: Amide

Action: Competes with calcium for sites in nerve membrane that control sodium transport across cell membrane; decreases rise of depolarization phase of action potential
Uses: Peripheral nerve block, caudal anesthesia, central neural block, vaginal block
Dosage and routes:
• Varies with route of anesthesia
Available forms: Inj 2, 5, 7.5 mg/ml
Side effects/adverse reactions:
CNS: Anxiety, restlessness, ***convulsions, loss of consciousness,*** drowsiness, disorientation, tremors, shivering
*CV: **Myocardial depression, cardiac arrest, dysrhythmias,*** bradycardia, hypotension, hypertension, ***fetal bradycardia***
GI: Nausea, vomiting
EENT: Blurred vision, tinnitus, pupil constriction
INTEG: Rash, urticaria, allergic reactions, edema, burning, skin discoloration at inj site, tissue necrosis
*RESP: **Status asthmaticus, respiratory arrest, anaphylaxis***
Contraindications: Hypersensitivity, child <12 yr, elderly, severe liver disease

Precautions: Severe drug allergies, pregnancy (B)
Pharmacokinetics: Onset 2-8 min, duration 3-6 hr; metabolized by liver, excreted in urine (metabolites)
Interactions:
• Dysrhythmias: epinephrine, halothane, enflurane
• Hypertension: MAOIs, tricyclics, phenothiazines
• Decreased action of ropivacaine: chloroprocaine
NURSING CONSIDERATIONS
Assess:
• B/P, pulse, respiration during treatment
• Fetal heart tones during labor
• Allergic reactions: rash, urticaria, itching
• Cardiac status: ECG for dysrhythmias, pulse, B/P during anesthesia
Administer:
• Only with crash cart, resuscitative equipment nearby
• Only drugs without preservatives for epidural or caudal anesthesia
Perform/provide:
• Use of new sol; discard unused portions
Evaluate:
• Therapeutic response: anesthesia necessary for procedure
Treatment of overdose: Airway, O_2, vasopressor, IV fluids, anticonvulsants for seizures

rosiglitazone (℞)

(ros-ih-glit′ah-zone)
Avandia
Func. class.: Antidiabetic, oral
Chem. class.: Thiazolidinedione

Action: Improves insulin resistance by hepatic glucose metabolism, insulin receptor kinase activity, insulin receptor phosphorylation

---

◆ = Nursing alert　　🖉 = Herb-drug interaction　　🚫 = Do not crush

Uses: Stable adult-onset diabetes mellitus (type II) NIDDM, alone or in combination with sulfonylureas, metformin, or insulin

Dosage and routes:

Monotherapy

• *Adult:* **PO** 4 mg qd or in 2 divided doses, may increase to 8 mg qd or in 2 divided doses after 12 wk

Combination therapy

• *Adult:* **PO** This drug should be added to metformin, sulfonylurea at the adult dose

Available forms: Tabs 2, 4, 8 mg

Side effects/adverse reactions:

MISC: Accidental injury, URI, sinusitis, anemia, back pain, diarrhea, edema

CNS: Fatigue, headache

ENDO: Hyper/hypoglycemia

Contraindications: Hypersensitivity to thiazolidinediones, children, lactation, diabetic ketoacidosis

Precautions: Pregnancy (C), elderly, thyroid disease, hepatic, renal disease

Pharmacokinetics: Maximal reductions in FBS after 6-12 wk, protein binding 99.8%, excreted in urine, feces, elimination half-life 3-4 hr, may be excreted in breast milk

Interactions:

• May decrease effect of: oral contraceptives, alternative method advised

NURSING CONSIDERATIONS

Assess:

• For hypoglycemic reactions (sweating, weakness, dizziness, anxiety, tremors, hunger), hyperglycemic reactions soon after meals

• CBC (baseline, q3mo) during treatment; check liver function tests periodically AST, ALT (if ALT >2.5 × ULN, do not use), LDH, renal studies: BUN, creatinine, urinary glucose

• FBS, HbA$_{1C}$, fasting plasma insulin, plasma lipids/lipoproteins, B/P, body weight during treatment

Administer:

• Once or in 2 divided doses

• Tabs crushed and mixed with food or fluids for patients with difficulty swallowing

Perform/provide:

• Conversion from other oral hypoglycemic agents if needed; change may be made without gradual dosage change; monitor serum or urine glucose and ketones tid during conversion

• Storage in tight container in cool environment

Teach patient/family:

• To use capillary blood glucose test or Chemstrip tid; that periodic LFTs mandatory

• The symptoms of hypo/hyperglycemia, what to do about each

• That the drug must be continued on daily basis: explain consequence of discontinuing drug abruptly

• To avoid OTC medications or herbal preparations unless approved by prescriber

• That diabetes is lifelong illness; that this drug is not a cure; only controls symptoms

• That all food included in diet plan must be eaten to prevent hypoglycemia

• To carry Medic Alert ID and glucagon emergency kit for emergencies

• To notify prescriber if oral contraceptives are used

• Not to use if breast-feeding, may be secreted in breast milk

Evaluate:

• Therapeutic response: Decrease in polyuria, polydipsia, polyphagia; clear sensorium; absence of dizziness; stable gait, blood glucose at normal level

R

---

* = Canada only   Side effects: *italics* = common; ***bold italics*** = life-threatening

salmeterol (R̵)

(sal-met′er-ole)

Serevent

Func. class.: β₂-Adrenergic agonist

Action: Causes bronchodilation by action on β₂ (pulmonary) receptors by increasing levels of cAMP, which relaxes smooth muscle; with very little effect on heart rate, maintains improvement in FEV from 3 to 12 hr; prevents nocturnal asthma symptoms

Uses: Prevention of exercise-induced asthma, bronchospasm, COPD

Dosage and routes:

• *Adult:* **INH** 2 puffs bid (AM and PM)

Available forms: Aerosol 25 µg/actuation; inhalation pwd 50 µg

Side effects/adverse reactions:

CNS: Tremors, anxiety, insomnia, headache, dizziness, stimulation, restlessness, hallucinations, flushing, irritability

CV: Palpitations, tachycardia, hypertension, angina, hypotension, dysrhythmias

EENT: Dry nose, irritation of nose and throat

GI: Heartburn, nausea, vomiting

MS: Muscle cramps

*RESP: **Bronchospasm***

Contraindications: Hypersensitivity to sympathomimetics, tachydysrhythmias, severe cardiac disease

Precautions: Lactation, pregnancy (C), cardiac disorders, hyperthyroidism, diabetes mellitus, hypertension, prostatic hypertrophy, narrow-angle glaucoma, seizures

Pharmacokinetics:

INH: Onset 5-15 min, peak 4 hr, duration 12 hr, metabolized in liver, excreted in urine, breast milk; crosses placenta; blood-brain barrier

Interactions:

• Increased action of aerosol bronchodilators

• Increased action of salmeterol: tricyclics, MAOIs

• May inhibit action of salmeterol: other β-blockers

NURSING CONSIDERATIONS

Assess:

• Respiratory function: vital capacity, forced expiratory volume, ABGs, lung sounds, heart rate and rhythm

Administer:

• After shaking; exhale, place mouthpiece in mouth, inhale slowly, hold breath, remove, exhale slowly

• Gum, sips of water for dry mouth

• Using spacing device for pediatric/geriatric patients

Perform/provide:

• Storage in light-resistant container; do not expose to temperatures over 86° F (30° C)

Evaluate:

• Therapeutic response: absence of dyspnea, wheezing

Teach patient/family:

• Not to use OTC medications; extra stimulation may occur

• Use of inhaler; review package insert with patient

• To avoid getting aerosol in eyes

• To wash inhaler in warm water qd and dry

• To avoid smoking, smoke-filled rooms, persons with respiratory infections

Treatment of overdose: β₂-adrenergic blocker

◆ = Nursing alert   🌿 = Herb-drug interaction   ⊘ = Do not crush

salsalate (℞)

(sal'sah-late)
Amigesic, Argesic-SA,
Arthra-G, Disalcid, Marthritic,
Mono-Gesic, Salflex, salsalate,
Salsitab

Func. class.: Nonnarcotic analgesic, nonsteroidal antiinflammatory

Chem. class.: Salicylate

Action: Blocks formation of peripheral prostaglandins, which cause pain and inflammation; antipyretic action results from inhibition of hypothalamic heat-regulating center; does not inhibit platelet aggregation

Uses: Mild to moderate pain or fever, including arthritis, juvenile rheumatoid arthritis

Dosage and routes:

• *Adult:* **PO** 3 g/day in divided doses

Available forms: Caps 500 mg; tabs 500, 750 mg

Side effects/adverse reactions:

*HEMA: **Thrombocytopenia, agranulocytosis, leukopenia, neutropenia, hemolytic anemia,** increased pro-time*

*CNS: Stimulation, drowsiness, dizziness, confusion, **convulsions,** headache, flushing, hallucinations, **coma***

*GI: Nausea, vomiting, GI bleeding, diarrhea, heartburn, anorexia, **hepatotoxicity***

INTEG: Rash, urticaria, bruising

EENT: Tinnitus, hearing loss

*CV: Rapid pulse, **pulmonary edema***

RESP: Wheezing, hyperpnea

ENDO: Hypoglycemia, hyponatremia, hypokalemia, alteration in acid-base balance

Contraindications: Hypersensitivity to salicylates, NSAIDs, GI bleeding, bleeding disorders, children <3 yr, vit K deficiency

Precautions: Anemia, hepatic disease, renal disease, Hodgkin's disease, pregnancy (C), lactation, elderly

Pharmacokinetics: Metabolized by liver; excreted by kidneys; half-life 1 hr; highly protein bound; crosses blood-brain barrier and placenta slowly

Interactions:

• Decreased effects of salsalate: antacids, steroids, urinary alkalizers

• Increased blood loss: alcohol, heparin, ibuprofen, warfarin

• Increased effects of anticoagulants, insulin, methotrexate, probenecid, penicillins, phenytoin

• Decreased effects of spironolactone, sulfinpyrazone, sulfonamides, loop diuretics

• Toxic effects: PABA

• Decreased blood sugar levels: salicylates

• Drug/food: foods that cause acidic urine, may increase salsalate levels

Lab test interferences:

Increase: Coagulation studies, liver function studies, serum uric acid, amylase, CO_2, urinary protein

Decrease: Serum K, PBI, cholesterol, blood glucose

Interference: Urine catecholamines, pregnancy test

NURSING CONSIDERATIONS

Assess:

• Pain: frequency, intensity, characteristics; relief of pain after medication

• For asthma, aspirin hypersensitivity, nasal polyps; may develop hypersensitivity to this product

• Liver function studies: AST, ALT, bilirubin (long-term therapy)

• Renal function studies: BUN, urine creatinine (long-term therapy)

• Blood studies: CBC, Hct, Hgb, PT (long-term therapy)

S

• I&O ratio; decreasing output may indicate renal failure (long-term therapy)
• Hepatotoxicity: dark urine, clay-colored stools; jaundiced skin, sclera; itching, abdominal pain, fever, diarrhea (long-term therapy)
• Allergic reactions: rash, urticaria; drug may have to be discontinued
• Ototoxicity: tinnitus, ringing, roaring in ears; audiometric testing is needed before, after long-term therapy
• Visual changes: blurring, halos, corneal and retinal damage
• Edema in feet, ankles, legs
• Drug history; many interactions
Administer:
• To patient crushed or whole; chewable tablets may be chewed
• With food or milk to decrease gastric symptoms; give 30 min before or 2 hr after meals
Evaluate:
• Therapeutic response: decreased pain, fever
Teach patient/family:
• To report any symptoms of hepatotoxicity, renal toxicity, visual changes, ototoxicity, allergic reactions (long-term therapy)
• Not to exceed recommended dosage; acute poisoning may result
• To read label on other OTC drugs; many contain aspirin
• That therapeutic response takes 2 wk (arthritis)
• To avoid alcohol ingestion; GI bleeding may occur
• To watch for signs of bleeding: dark stools
Treatment of overdose: Lavage, activated charcoal, monitor electrolytes, VS

---

saquinavir (℞)

(sa-quen'ah-veer)
Invirase, Fortovase
Func. class.: Antiretroviral
Chem. class.: Protease inhibitor

Action: Inhibits human immunodeficiency virus (HIV) protease, which prevents maturation of the infectious virus
Uses: HIV in combination with AZT, zalcitabine, ddc
Dosage and routes:
• *Adult:* **PO** 600 mg (hard cap-Invirase) or 1200 mg (soft cap-Fortovase) tid within 2 hr after a full meal; given with either zalcitabine 0.75 mg tid or zidovudine 200 mg tid
Available forms: Caps 200 mg (soft); 200 mg (hard)
Side effects/adverse reactions:
GI: Diarrhea, buccal mucosa ulceration, *abdominal pain, nausea*
CNS: Paresthesia, headache
INTEG: Rash
MS: Pain
MISC.: Asthenia, hyperglycemia
Contraindications: Hypersensitivity
Precautions: Liver disease, pregnancy (B), lactation, children
Pharmacokinetics: Absorption increased with food, protein binding 98%, extensive first-pass metabolism
Interactions:
• Toxicity: ergots, midazolam, triazolam, dapsone, quinidine, calcium channel blockers, clindamycin
• Increased saquinavir levels: ketoconazole, indinavir, delaviridine, nelfinavir, ritonavir, clarithromycin
• Decreased saquinavir levels: rifamycins, carbamazepine, phenobarbital, phenytoin, nevirapine, dexamethasone

---

◆ = Nursing alert   ∥ = Herb-drug interaction   ⊘ = Do not crush

• Avoid use with HmG-CoA reductase inhibitors

◆ Increased vasoconstriction: ergots, do not use concurrently

◆ Increased CNS depression: midazolam, triazolam, do not use concurrently

• Drug/food: increased bioavailability after high-fat meal

🖉 St. John's wort may decrease saquinavir levels, avoid concurrent use

Lab test interferences:

CPK, glucose (low)

NURSING CONSIDERATIONS

Assess:

• Signs of infection, anemia

• Liver function studies: ALT, AST

• C&S before drug therapy; drug may be taken as soon as culture is taken; repeat C&S after treatment; determine the presence of other sexually transmitted diseases

• Bowel pattern before, during treatment; if severe abdominal pain with bleeding occurs, drug should be discontinued; monitor hydration

• Skin eruptions, rash, urticaria, itching

• Allergies before treatment, reaction of each medication; place allergies on chart

Teach patient/family:

• To take as prescribed within 2 hr of a full meal; if dose is missed, take as soon as remembered up to 1 hr before next dose; do not double dose

• That drug must be taken in equal intervals around the clock to maintain blood levels for duration of therapy

• That Invirase and Fortovase are not interchangeable

---

sargramostim (℞)

(sar-gram'oh-stim)

Leukine, rhu GM-CSF recombinant human

Func. class.: Biologic modifier: cytokine

Action: Stimulates proliferation and differentiation of hematopoietic progenitor cells (granulocytes, macrophages)

Uses: Acceleration of myeloid recovery in patients with non-Hodgkin's lymphoma, acute lymphoblastic leukemia, autologous bone marrow transplantation in Hodgkin's disease; bone marrow transplantation failure or engraftment delay, mobilization and transplant of peripheral blood progenitor cells (PBPCs)

Dosage and routes:

Myeloid reconstitution after autologous bone marrow transplantation

• *Adult:* IV 250 μg/m²/day × 3 wk; give over 2 hr, 2-4 hr after autologous bone marrow infusion, not less than 24 hr after last dose of antineoplastics and 12 hr after last dose of radiotherapy, bone marrow transplantation failure, or engraftment delay

Acceleration of myeloid recovery

• *Adult:* IV 250 μg/m²/day × 14 days; give over 2 hr; may repeat in 7 days, may repeat 500 μg/m²/day × 14 days after another 7 days if no improvement

Mobilization of PBPCs

• *Adult:* IV/SC 250 μg/m²/day during collection of PBPCs

After PBPC transplantation

• *Adult:* IV/SC 250 μg/m²/day until ANC >1500 cells/mm³ × 3 days

Available forms: Pwd for inj lyophilized 250, 500 μg

S

Side effects/adverse reactions:

CNS: Fever, malaise, CNS disorder, weakness, chills

GI: Nausea, vomiting, diarrhea, anorexia, ***GI hemorrhage,*** stomatitis, ***liver damage***

HEMA: ***Blood dyscrasias, hemorrhage***

INTEG: Alopecia, rash, peripheral edema

GU: Urinary tract disorder, abnormal kidney function

RESP: Dyspnea

CV: ***Supraventricular tachycardia,*** peripheral edema, ***pericardial effusion***

Contraindications: Hypersensitivity to GM-CSF, yeast products; excessive leukemic myeloid blast in bone marrow, peripheral blood

Precautions: Pregnancy (C), lactation, child; renal, hepatic, lung disease; cardiac disease; pleural, pericardial effusions

Do not confuse:

Leukine/leucovorin

Leukine/Leukeran

Pharmacokinetics: Half-life 2 hr, detected within 5 min after administration, peak 2 hr

Interactions:

• Do not use this drug concomitantly with antineoplastics

• Increased myeloproliferation: lithium, corticosteroids

NURSING CONSIDERATIONS

Assess:

• Blood studies: CBC, differential count before treatment and twice weekly; leukocytosis may occur (WBC >50,000 cells/mm^3, ANC >20,000 cells/mm^3), platelets; if ANC >20,000/mm^3 or 10,000/mm^3 after nadir has occurred, or platelets >500,000/mm^3 reduce dose by $\frac{1}{2}$ or discontinue; if blast cells occur, discontinue

• Renal and hepatic studies before treatment: BUN, creatinine, urinalysis; AST, ALT, alk phosphatase; twice weekly monitoring is needed in renal, hepatic disease

• For hypersensitivity, rashes, local inj site reactions; usually transient

• For increased fluid retention in cardiac disease

• For myalgia, arthralgia in legs, feet, use analgesics

Administer:

SC

• Use reconstituted sol

IV

• After reconstituting with 1 ml sterile water for inj without preservative; do not reenter vial; discard unused portion; direct reconstitution sol at side of vial; rotate contents; do not shake

• Dilute in 0.9% NaCl inj to prepare IV inf; if final concentration is <10 µg/ml, add human albumin to make a final concentration of 0.1% to NaCl before adding sargramostim to prevent adsorption; for a final concentration of 0.1% albumin, add 1 mg human albumin/1 ml 0.9% NaCl inj run over 2 hr (bone marrow transplant or failure of graft); over 4 hr (chemotherapy for AML); over 24 hr as cont inf (PBPCs); give within 6 hr after reconstitution

Y-site compatibilities: Amikacin, aminophylline, aztreonam, bleomycin, butorphanol, calcium gluconate, carboplatin, carmustine, cefazolin, cefepime, cefotaxime, cefotetan, ceftizoxime, ceftriaxone, cefuroxime, cimetidine, cisplatin, clindamycin, cyclophosphamide, cyclosporine, cytarabine, dacarbazine, dactinomycin, dexamethasone, diphenhydramine, dopamine, doxorubicin, doxycycline, droperidol, etoposide, famotidine, fentanyl, floxuridine, fluconazole, fluorouracil, furosemide, gentamicin, granisetron, heparin, idarubicin, ifosfamide, immune globulin, mag-

---

◆ = Nursing alert   ∥ = Herb-drug interaction   ⊘ = Do not crush

nesium sulfate, mannitol, mechlorethamine, meperidine, mesna, methotrexate, metoclopramide, metronidazole, mezlocillin, miconazole, minocycline, mitoxantrone, netilmicin, pentostatin, piperacillin/tazobactam, potassium chloride, prochlorperazine, promethazine, ranitidine, teniposide, ticarcillin, ticarcillin/clavulanate, trimethoprim-sulfamethoxazole, vinblastine, vincristine, zidovudine

Perform/provide:

• Storage in refrigerator; do not freeze

Evaluate:

• Therapeutic response: WBC and differential recovery

---

scopolamine (R)

(skoe-pol′a-meen)

Func. class.: Cholinergic blocker
Chem. class.: Belladonna alkaloid

Action: Inhibits acetylcholine at receptor sites in autonomic nervous system, which controls secretions, free acids in stomach; blocks central muscarinic receptors, which decreases involuntary movements

Uses: Reduction of secretions before surgery, calm delirium, motion sickness, parkinsonian symptoms

Dosage and routes:

Parkinsonian symptoms

• *Adult:* **IM/SC/IV** 0.3-0.6 mg tid-qid using dilution provided

Preoperatively

• *Adult:* **SC** 0.4-0.6 mg

Nausea and vomiting

• *Child:* **SC** 0.006 mg/kg or 0.2 mg/m^2

Available forms: Inj 0.3, 0.4, 0.86, 1 mg/ml

Side effects/adverse reactions:

CNS: Confusion, anxiety, restlessness, irritability, delusions, hallucinations, headache, sedation, depression, incoherence, dizziness, excitement, delirium, flushing, weakness

INTEG: Urticaria

MISC: Suppression of lactation, nasal congestion, decreased sweating

EENT: Blurred vision, photophobia, dilated pupils, difficulty swallowing, mydriasis, cycloplegia

CV: Palpitations, tachycardia, postural hypotension, paradoxic bradycardia

GI: Dryness of mouth, constipation, nausea, vomiting, abdominal distress, ***paralytic ileus***

GU: Urinary hesitancy, retention

Contraindications: Hypersensitivity, narrow-angle glaucoma, myasthenia gravis, GI/GU obstruction, hypersensitivity to belladonna, barbiturates

Precautions: Pregnancy (C), elderly, lactation, prostatic hypertrophy, CHF, hypertension, dysrhythmia, children, gastric ulcer

Pharmacokinetics:

SC/IM: Peak 30-45 min, duration 7 hr

IV: Peak 10-15 min, duration 4 hr Excreted in urine, bile, feces (unchanged)

Interactions:

• Increased anticholinergic effect: alcohol, opioids, antihistamines, phenothiazines, tricyclics

NURSING CONSIDERATIONS

Assess:

• I&O ratio; retention commonly causes decreased urinary output

• Parkinsonism, EPS: shuffling gait, muscle rigidity, involuntary movements

• Urinary hesitancy, retention; palpate bladder if retention occurs

• Constipation; increase fluids, bulk, exercise if this occurs

S

Side effects: *italics* = common; ***bold italics*** = life-threatening

• For tolerance over long-term therapy; dose may have to be increased or changed
• Mental status: affect, mood, CNS depression, worsening of mental symptoms during early therapy
Administer:
• Parenteral dose with patient recumbent to prevent postural hypotension
• Parenteral dose slowly; keep in bed for at least 1 hr after dose
• With or after meals for GI upset; may give with fluids other than H_2O
• At hs to avoid daytime drowsiness in patient with parkinsonism
• With analgesic to avoid behavioral changes when given as a preop
Additive compatibilities: Floxacillin, furosemide, meperidine, succinylcholine
Syringe compatibilities: Atropine, benzquinamide, butorphanol, chlorpromazine, cimetidine, diamorphine, dimenhydrinate, diphenhydramine, droperidol, fentanyl, glycopyrrolate, hydromorphone, hydroxyzine, meperidine, metoclopramide, midazolam, morphine, nalbuphine, pentazocine, pentobarbital, perphenazine, prochlorperazine, promazine, promethazine, ranitidine, sufentanil, thiopental
Y-site compatibilities: Heparin, hydrocortisone, potassium chloride, propofol, sufentanil, vit B/C
Perform/provide:
• Storage at room temperature in light-resistant container
• Hard candy, frequent drinks, sugarless gum to relieve dry mouth
Evaluate:
• Therapeutic response: decreased secretions
Teach patient/family:
• Not to discontinue this drug abruptly; to taper off over 1 wk
• To avoid driving, other hazardous activities; drowsiness may occur

• To avoid OTC medication: cough, cold preparations with alcohol, antihistamines unless directed by prescriber

scopolamine (Rx) (transdermal)
(skoe-pol'-a-meen)
Transderm-Scop, Transderm-V
Func. class.: Antiemetic, anticholinergic
Chem. class.: Belladonna alkaloid

Action: Competitive antagonism of acetylcholine at receptor site in eye, smooth muscle, cardiac muscle, glandular cells; inhibition of vestibular input to the CNS, resulting in inhibition of vomiting reflex
Uses: Prevention of motion sickness
Investigational uses: Drooling
Dosage and routes:
• *Adult:* **PATCH** 1 placed behind ear 4-5 hr before travel, reapply q3d, alternate ears
Not recommended for children
Drooling (off-label)
• *Adult:* **TD** 1.5 mg patch q3d
Available forms: Patch, 0.5, 1 mg delivered in 72 hr
Side effects/adverse reactions:
INTEG: Rash, erythema
GU: Difficult urination
CNS: Dizziness, drowsiness, confusion, disorientation, memory disturbances, hallucinations
EENT: Blurred vision, altered depth perception, *dilated pupils,* photophobia, *dry mouth;* dry, itchy, red eyes; acute narrow-angle glaucoma
Contraindications: Hypersensitivity, glaucoma
Precautions: Children, elderly, pregnancy (C); pyloric, urinary, bladder

◆ = Nursing alert   〆 = Herb-drug interaction   Ⓢ = Do not crush neck, intestinal obstruction; liver, kidney disease

Pharmacokinetics:

Patch: Onset 4-5 hr, duration 72 hr

Interactions:

• Increased anticholinergic effects: antihistamines, antidepressants

NURSING CONSIDERATIONS

Teach patient/family:

• To avoid hazardous activities, activities requiring alertness; dizziness may occur

• To wash, dry hands before and after applying to surface behind ear

• To change patch q72h

• To apply at least 4 hr before traveling

• If blurred vision, severe dizziness, drowsiness occurs, to discontinue use, use another type of antiemetic or rotate the patch to other ear

• To read label of all OTC medications; if any scopolamine is found in product, avoid use

• To keep out of children's reach

---

secobarbital (℞)

(see-koe-bar´bi-tal)

Secogen Sodium*, Seconal Sodium Pulvules, Seral*

Func. class.: Sedative/hypnotic-barbiturate

Chem. class.: Barbitone (short acting)

Controlled Substance Schedule II (USA), Schedule G (Canada)

Action: Depresses activity in brain cells primarily in reticular activating system in brain stem; selectively depresses neurons in posterior hypothalamus, limbic structures; decreases seizure activity by inhibition of epileptic activity in CNS

Uses: Insomnia, sedation, preoperative medication, status epilepticus, acute tetanus convulsions

Dosage and routes:

Insomnia

• *Adult:* **PO/IM** 100-200 mg hs

• *Child:* **IM** 3-5 mg/kg, not to exceed 100 mg, not to inject >5 ml in one site

Sedation/preoperatively

• *Adult:* **PO** 200-300 mg 1-2 hr preoperatively

• *Child:* **PO** 50-100 mg 1-2 hr preoperatively

Status epilepticus

• *Adult and child:* **IM/IV** 250-350 mg

Acute psychotic agitation

• *Adult and child:* **IM/IV** 5.5 mg/kg q3-4h

Available forms: Caps 100 mg; inj 50 mg/ml

Side effects/adverse reactions:

CNS: Lethargy, drowsiness, hangover, dizziness, paradoxical stimulation in elderly and children, lightheadedness, dependency, CNS depression, mental depression, slurred speech

GI: Nausea, vomiting, diarrhea, constipation

INTEG: Rash, urticaria, pain, abscesses at inj site, angioedema, thrombophlebitis, *Stevens-Johnson syndrome*

CV: Hypotension, bradycardia

RESP: Depression, *apnea, laryngospasm, bronchospasm*

HEMA: Agranulocytosis, thrombocytopenia, megaloblastic anemia (long-term treatment)

Contraindications: Hypersensitivity to barbiturates, pregnancy (D), respiratory depression, addiction to barbiturates, severe liver impairment, porphyria, uncontrolled severe pain

Precautions: Anemia, lactation, hepatic disease, renal disease, hypertension, elderly, acute/chronic pain

Pharmacokinetics:

IM: Onset 10-15 min, duration 4-

6 hr, metabolized by liver, excreted by kidneys (metabolites); half-life 15-40 hr

Interactions:
• Do not mix with other drugs in sol or syringe
• Increased CNS depression: alcohol, MAOIs, sedatives, opioids
• Decreased effect of oral anticoagulants, corticosteroids, griseofulvin, quinidine
• Decreased half-life of doxycycline

🌿 Increased CNS depression: kava
Lab test interferences:
False increase: Sulfobromophthalein

NURSING CONSIDERATIONS
Assess:
• VS q30min after parenteral route for 2 hr
• Blood studies: Hct, Hgb, RBCs, serum folate, vit D (if on long-term therapy); PT in patients receiving anticoagulants
• Hepatic studies: AST, ALT, bilirubin; if increased, drug is usually discontinued
• Unresolved pain; drug may cause severe stimulation if pain is present
• Mental status: mood, sensorium, affect, memory (long, short)
• Physical dependency: frequent requests for medication, shakes, anxiety

◆ Barbiturate toxicity: hypotension; pulmonary constriction; cold, clammy skin; cyanosis of lips; insomnia; nausea; vomiting; hallucinations; delirium; weakness; mild symptoms may occur in 8-12 hr without drug
• Respiratory dysfunction: depression, character, rate, rhythm; hold drug if respirations <10/min or if pupils dilated
• Blood dyscrasias: fever, sore throat, bruising, rash, jaundice, epistaxis

• Perianal irritation if rectal forms used
Administer:
• After removal of cigarettes to prevent fires
• IM inj deep in large muscle mass to prevent tissue sloughing and abscesses
• After conservative measures for insomnia have been tried
• ½-1 hr before hs for sleeplessness
• On empty stomach for best absorption
• For <14 days, since drug is not effective after that; tolerance develops
• Crushed or whole
• Alone; do not mix with other drugs or inject if there is precipitate
• After cleansing enema is given rectally preoperatively in children
IV
• After diluting with sterile H_2O for inj; rotate; give 50 mg or less over 1 min; titrate to response
• Within 30 min of mixing with sterile water for inj; reconstitute after rotating ampule; do not shake; do not use cloudy sol; may be given directly or indirectly
• IV only with resuscitative equipment available; administer at <100 mg/min (only by qualified personnel)
Additive compatibilities: Amikacin, aminophylline
Perform/provide:
• Assistance with ambulation after receiving dose
• Safety measures: night-light, call bell within easy reach
• Checking to see if PO medication has been swallowed
• Storage of suppositories in refrigerator; do not use aqueous sol containing precipitate
Evaluate:
• Therapeutic response: ability to sleep at night, decreased early morn-

◆ = Nursing alert   🌿 = Herb-drug interaction   🚫 = Do not crush

ing awakening if taking drug for insomnia, or decrease in number, severity of seizures if taking drug for seizure disorder

Teach patient/family:
• That morning hangover is common
• That drug is indicated only for short-term treatment of insomnia, probably ineffective after 2 wk
• That physical dependency may result when used for extended periods (45-90 days depending on dose)
• To avoid driving, other activities requiring alertness
• To avoid alcohol ingestion, CNS depressants; serious CNS depression may result
• Not to discontinue medication quickly after long-term use; drug should be tapered over 1-2 wk
• To tell all prescribers that barbiturate is being taken
• That withdrawal insomnia may occur after short-term use; not to start using drug again; insomnia will improve in 1-3 nights; may experience increased dreaming
• That effects may take 2 nights for benefits to be noticed
• Alternative measures to improve sleep (reading, exercise several hr before hs, warm bath, warm milk, TV, self-hypnosis, deep breathing)

Treatment of overdose: Lavage, activated charcoal, warming blanket, vital signs, hemodialysis, I&O ratio

selegiline (℞)

(se-le'ji-leen)
Carbex, Eldepryl, Novo-Selegiline*, SD-Deprenyl
Func. class.: Antiparkinson agent
Chem. class.: Levorotatory acetylenic derivative of phenethylamine

Action: Increased dopaminergic activity by inhibition of MAO type B activity; not fully understood
Uses: Adjunct management of Parkinson's disease in patients being treated with levodopa/carbidopa who had poor response to therapy
Investigational uses: Alzheimer's disease

Dosage and routes:
• *Adult:* **PO** 10 mg/day given with levodopa/carbidopa in divided doses 5 mg at breakfast and lunch; after 2-3 days begin to reduce dose of levodopa/carbidopa 10%-30%
Available forms: Tabs 5 mg, caps 5 mg

Side effects/adverse reactions:
CNS: Increased tremors, chorea, restlessness, blepharospasm, increased bradykinesia, grimacing, tardive dyskinesia, dystonic symptoms, involuntary movements, increased apraxia, hallucinations, *dizziness,* mood changes, nightmares, delusions, lethargy, apathy, overstimulation, sleep disturbances, headache, migraine, numbness, muscle cramps, confusion, anxiety, tiredness, vertigo, personality change, back/leg pain
CV: Orthostatic hypotension, hypertension, dysrhythmia, palpitations, angina pectoris, hypotension, ***tachycardia,*** edema, ***sinus bradycardia,*** syncope
GI: Nausea, vomiting, constipation,

weight loss, anorexia, diarrhea, heartburn, rectal bleeding, poor appetite, dysphagia, xerostomia

GU: Slow urination, nocturia, prostatic hypertrophy, urinary hesitation, retention, frequency, sexual dysfunction

INTEG: Increased sweating, alopecia, hematoma, rash, photosensitivity, facial hair

RESP: Asthma, shortness of breath

EENT: Diplopia, dry mouth, blurred vision, tinnitus

Contraindications: Hypersensitivity

Precautions: Pregnancy (C), lactation, children

Do not confuse:

Eldepryl/enalapril

Pharmacokinetics: Rapidly absorbed, peak ½-2 hr; rapidly metabolized (active metabolites: *N*-desmethyldeprenyl, amphetamine, methamphetamine), metabolites excreted in urine, half-life 9 min

Interactions:

◆ **Fatal interaction:** Opioids (especially meperidine); do not administer together

• Increased side effects of: levodopa/carbidopa

• **Serotonin syndrome** (confusion, seizures, fever, hypertension, agitation): fluoxetine, paroxitine, sertraline, fluvoxamine (discontinue 5 wk prior to selegiline); do not use together

• Do not use with tricyclics

🌿 May decrease selegiline action: chaste tree fruit

Lab test interferences:

False positive: Urine ketones, urine glucose

False negative: Urine glucose (glucose oxidase)

False increase: Uric acid, urine protein

Decrease: VMA

NURSING CONSIDERATIONS

Assess:

• Decreased parkinsonian symptoms: rigidity, unsteady gait, weakness, tremors

• B/P, respiration throughout treatment

• Mental status: affect, mood behavioral changes, depression; perform suicide assessment

Administer:

• Drug until NPO before surgery

• Adjusting dosage to response

• With meals; limit protein taken with drug

• At doses <10 mg/day, because of risks associated with nonselective inhibition of MAO

Perform/provide:

• Assistance with ambulation during beginning therapy

Evaluate:

• Therapeutic response: decrease in akathisia, improved mood

Teach patient/family:

• To change positions slowly to prevent orthostatic hypotension

• To report side effects: twitching, eye spasms; indicate overdose

• To use drug exactly as prescribed; if discontinued abruptly, parkinsonian crisis may occur

• To avoid foods high in tyramine: cheese, pickled products, wine, beer, large amounts of caffeine

• Not to exceed recommended dose of 10 mg; might precipitate hypertensive crisis; report severe headache, other unusual symptoms

Treatment of overdose: IV fluids for hypertension, IV dilute pressure agent for B/P titration

---

senna, sennosides
(OTC)

(sen'na)

Black Draught, Dr. Caldwell Dosalax, Ex-Lax Gentle, Fletcher's Castoria, Gentlax, Senexon, Senna-Gen, Senokot, Senokotxtra, Senolax

Func. class.: Laxative-stimulant
Chem. class.: Anthraquinone

Action: Stimulates peristalsis by action on Auerbach's plexus; softens feces by increasing water, electrolytes in large intestine

Uses: Acute constipation; bowel preparation for surgery or examination

Dosage and routes:

• *Adult:* **PO** 1-8 tabs (Senokot)/day or ½ to 4 tsp of granules (1 tsp-4 ml) added to water or juice; **RECT SUPP** 1-2 hs; **SYR** 1-4 tsp hs, 7.5-15 ml; (Black Draught) ¾ oz dissolved in 2.5 oz liquid given between 2-4 PM the day before procedure (X-Prep)

• *Child >27 kg:* **PO** ½ adult dose; do not use Black Draught for children

• *Child 1 mo-1 yr:* **SYR** 1.25-2.5 ml (Senokot) hs

Available forms: Supp 625 mg, 30 mg sennosides; pwd 662 mg/g, 6, 15 mg sennosides/3g; tabs 8.6 mg sennosides, 180 mg; oral sol 3 mg sennosides/ml

Side effects/adverse reactions:

GI: Nausea, vomiting, anorexia, cramps, diarrhea, flatulence

META: Hypocalcemia, enteropathy, alkalosis, hypokalemia, ***tetany***

GU: Pink, red or brown, black urine

Contraindications: Hypersensitivity, GI bleeding, obstruction, CHF, lactation, abdominal pain, nausea/vomiting, appendicitis, acute surgical abdomen

Precautions: Pregnancy (C)

Pharmacokinetics:

PO: Onset 6-24 hr; metabolized by liver, excreted in feces

Interactions:

• Do not use with disulfiram (Antabuse)

NURSING CONSIDERATIONS

Assess:

• Stool: color, consistency, amount
• Blood, urine electrolytes if drug is used often
• I&O ratio to identify fluid loss
• Cause of constipation; fluids, bulk, exercise missing
• Cramping, rectal bleeding, nausea, vomiting; drug should be discontinued

Administer:

• In morning or evening (oral dose) with full glass of water
• Dissolve granules in water or juice before administration
• On empty stomach for more rapid results
• Shake oral sol before giving

Evaluate:

• Therapeutic response: decrease in constipation

Teach patient/family:

• That urine, feces may turn yellow-brown to red
• Not to use laxatives for long-term therapy; bowel tone will be lost
• That normal bowel movements do not always occur daily
• Not to use in presence of abdominal pain, nausea, vomiting
• To notify prescriber if constipation unrelieved or of symptoms of electrolyte imbalance: muscle cramps, pain, weakness, dizziness, excessive thirst

S

---

sertraline (Rx)

(ser'tra-leen)

Zoloft

Func. class.: Antidepressant

Chem. class.: SSRI

Action: Inhibits serotonin reuptake in CNS; increases action of serotonin; does not affect dopamine, norepinephrine

Uses: Major depression, obsessive-compulsive disorder (OCD), post-traumatic stress disorder (PTSD), panic disorder

Investigational uses: Extended-interval dosing, premenstrual disorders

Dosage and routes:

• *Adult:* **PO** 50 mg qd; may increase to max of 200 mg/day; do not change dose at intervals of <1 wk; administer qd in AM or PM; or 100 mg 3 ×/wk (off-label)

• *Geriatric:* **PO** 25 mg qd, increase by 25 mg q3 days to desired dose

• *Child 6-12 yr:* **PO** 25 mg qd

• *Child 13-17 yr:* **PO** 50 mg qd

Premenstrual disorders (off-label)

• *Adult:* **PO** 50-150 mg qhs

Available forms: Tabs 25, 50, 100 mg; liq 20 mg/ml

Side effects/adverse reactions:

CNS: Insomnia, agitation, somnolence, dizziness, headache, tremor, fatigue, paresthesia, twitching, confusion, ataxia, gait abnormality (elderly)

GU: Male sexual dysfunction, micturition disorder

GI: Diarrhea, nausea, constipation, anorexia, dry mouth, dyspepsia, *vomiting, flatulence*

CV: Palpitations, chest pain

EENT: Vision abnormalities

INTEG: Increased sweating, rash, hot flashes

ENDO: SIADH (elderly)

Contraindications: Hypersensitivity to this drug or SSRIs

Precautions: Pregnancy (B), lactation, elderly, hepatic, renal disease, epilepsy

Do not confuse:

Zoloft/Zocor

Pharmacokinetics:

PO: Peak 4.5-8.4 hr; steady state 1 wk; plasma protein binding 99%, elimination half-life 1-4 days, extensively metabolized, metabolite excreted in urine, bile

Interactions:

• Increased effects of: antidepressants (tricyclics), diazepam, tolbutamide, warfarin, benzodiazepines

◆ **Fatal reactions:** MAOIs

• Increased sertraline levels: cimetidine, warfarin, other highly protein-bound drugs

• Altered lithium levels: lithium

 Potentiation of SSRI: St. John's wort; do not use together

Lab test interferences:

Increase: AST, ALT

NURSING CONSIDERATIONS

Assess:

• Mental status: mood, sensorium, affect, suicidal tendencies, increase in psychiatric symptoms, depression, panic

• B/P (lying/standing), pulse q4h; if systolic B/P drops 20 mm Hg, hold drug, notify prescriber; take vital signs q4h in patients with cardiovascular disease

• Weight qwk; appetite may decrease with drug

• Urinary retention, constipation, especially in elderly

• Alcohol consumption; hold dose until morning

Administer:

• Increased fluids, bulk in diet for constipation, urinary retention

• With food, milk for GI symptoms

◆ = Nursing alert   = Herb-drug interaction   🚫 = Do not crush

• Crushed if patient is unable to swallow medication whole
• Gum, hard candy, frequent sips of water for dry mouth
Perform/provide:
• Storage at room temperature; do not freeze
• Assistance with ambulation during therapy, since drowsiness, dizziness occur
• Safety measures, including side rails, primarily for elderly
• Checking to see that PO medication is swallowed
Evaluate:
• Therapeutic response: significant improvement in depression, OCS
Teach patient/family:
• That therapeutic effect may take 1 wk
• To use caution in driving, other activities requiring alertness; drowsiness, dizziness, blurred vision may occur
• Not to discontinue medication quickly after long-term use; may cause nausea, headache, malaise
• To avoid alcohol, other CNS depressants
• To notify prescriber if pregnant or plan to become pregnant or breastfeed

RARELY USED

sevelamer (℞)
(seh-vel'ah-mer)
Renagel
Func. class.: Polymeric phosphate binder

Uses: End-stage renal disease (ESRD)
Dosage and routes:
Reduction of serum phosphorus in adults not taking phosphate binders

• *Adult:* **PO** initially 800-1600 mg tid with meals based on serum phosphorus level (see below); adjust dose gradually at 2-wk intervals until serum phosphorus 6 mg/dl
• *Adult, serum phosphorus 9 mg/dl:* 1600 mg tid with meals
• *Adult, serum phosphorus 7.5 and <9 mg/dl:* 1200-1600 mg tid with meals
• *Adult, serum phosphorus >6 and <7.5 mg/dl:* 800 mg tid with meals
Contraindications: Hypophosphatemia, bowel obstruction, hypersensitivity

RARELY USED

sibutramine (℞)
(si-byoo'tra-meen)
Meridia
Func. class.: Appetite suppressant

Controlled Substance Schedule IV
Uses: Obesity in conjunction with other treatments
Dosage and routes:
• *Adult:* **PO** 10 mg qd; may be increased to 15 mg qd after 4 wk, or lowered to 5 mg qd depending on response
Contraindications: Hypersensitivity, hypothyroidism, anorexia nervosa, severe hepatic/renal disease, uncontrolled hypertension, history of CAD, CHF, dysrhythmias, lactation, CVA

sildenafil (R)

(sil-den'a-fill)
Viagra
Func. class: Erectile agent
Chem. class: Selective inhibitor
of cGMP-PDE5

Action: Enhances the effect of nitric oxide (NO) by inhibiting phosphodiesterase type 5 (PDE5), which is necessary for degrading cGMP in the corpus cavernosum

Uses: Treatment of erectile dysfunction

Dosage and routes:
• *Adult:* **PO** 50 mg 1 hr before sexual activity, may be taken ½-4 hr before sexual activity; may be increased to 100 mg or decreased to 25 mg; max once/day

Available forms: Tabs 25, 50, 100 mg

Side effects/adverse reactions:
CV: MI, sudden death, CV collapse
CNS: Headache, flushing, dizziness
MISC.: Dyspepsia, nasal congestion, UTI, abnormal vision, diarrhea, rash

Contraindication: Hypersensitivity

Precautions: Anatomical penile deformities, sickle cell anemia, leukemia, multiple myeloma, pregnancy (B)

Pharmacokinetics: Rapidly absorbed; bioavailability 40%; metabolized by liver (active metabolites); terminal half-life 4 hr, peak ½-1½ hr; reduced absorption with high-fat meal; excreted feces, urine

Interactions:
• Increased sildenafil levels: cimetidine, erythromycin, ketoconazole, itraconazole
• Decreased sildenafil levels: rifampin
• Decreased B/P: amlodipine

◆ Do not use with nitrates; fatal fall in B/P

NURSING CONSIDERATIONS
Assess:
• Use of organic nitrates that should not be used with this drug
Administer:
PO
• Approximately 1 hr before sexual activity, do not use more than once a day
Teach patient/family:
• That drug does not protect against sexually transmitted diseases, including HIV
• That drug absorption is reduced with a high-fat meal
• That drug should not be used with nitrates in any form
• That tabs may be split

silver nitrate (R)

Func. class.: Keratolytic

Action: Antiinfective, astringent, caustic

Uses: Cauterization of lesions, warts, burns (low concentrations)

Dosage and routes:
• *Adult and child:* **TOP** apply to area to be treated

Available forms: Sticks, sol 10%, 25%, 50%

Side effects/adverse reactions:
INTEG: Skin discoloration

Contraindications: Hypersensitivity

Interactions:
• Not to be used with alkalies, phosphates, thimerosal, benzalkonium chloride, halogenated acids

NURSING CONSIDERATIONS
Administer:
• After moistening stick with water
• To burns using a wet dressing (low concentrations 0.125%)
Perform/provide:
• Storage in cool area

 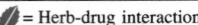

Evaluate:
• Therapeutic response: absence of lesions, healing of burned areas
Teach patient/family:
• To avoid contact with clothing, unaffected areas; discoloration may occur

---

silver protein, mild (R, OTC)
Argyrol S.S. 10%, Argyrol S.S. 20%
Func. class.: Disinfectant
Chem. class.: Silver colloidal compound

Action: Destroys gram-positive, gram-negative organisms
Uses: Eye, nose, throat, swelling, infection
Dosage and routes:
• *Adult and child:* **TOP** sol use as needed
Available forms: Top sol 5%, 10%, 25%; eyedrops 20%
Side effects/adverse reactions:
INTEG: Irritation, discolored tissue
Contraindications: Hypersensitivity
Precautions: Pregnancy (C)
NURSING CONSIDERATIONS
Administer:
• To area to be treated only; do not apply to healthy skin
Perform/provide:
• Storage in tight container
Evaluate:
• Area of body involved: irritation, rash, breaks, dryness, scales

---

simethicone (OTC, R)
(si-meth'i-kone)
Extra Strength Gas-X, Extra Strength Maalox Anti-Gas, Extra Stength Maalox GRFGas Relief Formula*, Flatulex, Gas-Relief, Gas-X, Genasyme, Maalox Anti-Gas, Maalox GRF Gas Relief Formula*, Maximum Strength Gas Relief, Maximum Strength Mylanta Gas Relief, Maximus Strength Phazyme, Mylanta Gas, Mylicon, Ovol*, Phazyme, Phazyme 95, Phazyme 125
Func. class.: Antiflatulent

Action: Disperses, prevents gas pockets in GI system; does not decrease gas production
Uses: Flatulence
Dosage and routes:
• *Adult and child >12 yr:* **PO** 40-100 mg pc, hs
Available forms: Chew tabs 40, 80, 125 mg; tabs 60, 80, 95 mg; drops 40 mg/0.6 ml, 40 mg/ml, 95 mg/1.425 ml; caps 95, 125 mg; caps, soft gel 125 mg
Side effects/adverse reactions:
GI: Belching, rectal flatus
Contraindications: Hypersensitivity
Precautions: Pregnancy (C)
Do not confuse:
Mylicone/Mylanta Gas
NURSING CONSIDERATIONS
Assess:
• Reason for excess gas production, decreased bowel sounds, recent surgery, other GI conditions
Administer:
• After meals, hs; shake susp well before giving; chew tabs should be chewed

S

Evaluate:
• Therapeutic response: absence of flatulence
Teach patient/family:
• That tablets must be chewed
• To shake suspension well before pouring

---

simvastatin (Rx)

(sim-va-sta'tin)
Zocor
Func. class.: Antilipidemic
Chem. class.: HMG-CoA reductase inhibitor

Action: Inhibits HMG-CoA reductase enzyme, which reduces cholesterol synthesis
Uses: As an adjunct in primary hypercholesterolemia (types IIa, IIb), isolated hypertriglyceridemia (Frederickson type IV) and type III hyperlipoproteinemia, coronary artery disease
Dosage and routes:
• *Adult:* **PO** 5-10 mg qd in PM initially; usual range 5-40 mg/day qd in PM, not to exceed 40 mg/day; dosage adjustments may be made in 4-wk intervals or more
• *Elderly/renal disease:* **PO** 5 mg/day
Available forms: Tabs 5, 10, 20, 40, 80 mg
Side effects/adverse reactions:
INTEG: Rash, pruritus, alopecia
GI: Nausea, constipation, diarrhea, dyspepsia, flatus, abdominal pain, heartburn, *liver dysfunction,* pancreatitis
EENT: Lens opacities
MS: Muscle cramps, myalgia, *myositis, rhabdomyolysis*
CNS: Headache, tremor, vertigo, peripheral neuropathy
Contraindications: Hypersensitivity, pregnancy (X), lactation, active liver disease
Precautions: Past liver disease, alcoholism, severe acute infections, trauma, hypotension, uncontrolled seizure disorders, severe metabolic disorders, electrolyte imbalances
Do not confuse:
Zocor/Cozaar
Zocor/Zoloft
Pharmacokinetics: Peak 1-2½ hr, metabolized in liver (active metabolites), highly protein bound, excreted primarily in bile, feces
Interactions:
• Increased effects of warfarin
• Increased myalgia, myositis: cyclosporine, gemfibrozil, niacin, erythromycin
• Increased serum level of digoxin
Lab test interferences:
Increase: CPK, LFTs
NURSING CONSIDERATIONS
Assess:
• 12-hr fasting lipid profile: LDL, ADL, TG, cholesterol at 6-8 wk, and q6mo
• Liver function studies q1-2mo during the first 1½ yr of treatment; AST, ALT, LFTs may increase
• Renal studies in patients with compromised renal system: BUN, I&O ratio, creatinine
• Eyes with slit lamp before, 1 mo after treatment begins, annually; lens opacities may occur
Administer:
• Total daily dose in evening
Perform/provide:
• Storage in cool environment in tight container protected from light
Evaluate:
• Therapeutic response: decrease in cholesterol to desired level after 8 wk
Teach patient/family:
• That blood work and eye exam will be necessary during treatment

---

 = Nursing alert    = Herb-drug interaction $\bigcirc$ = Do not crush

• To report blurred vision, severe GI symptoms, dizziness, headache
• That previously prescribed regimen will continue: low-cholesterol diet, exercise program

---

sirolimus (℞)

(seer-oh-lie′mus)

Rapamune

Func. class.: Immunosuppressant

Chem. class.: Macrolide

Action: Produces immunosuppression by inhibiting T-lymphocyte activation and proliferation

Uses: Organ transplants to prevent rejection, recommended use is with cyclosporine and corticosteroids

Investigational uses: Psoriasis

Dosage and routes:
• *Adult:* **PO** 2 mg qd with a 6 mg loading dose, may use 5 mg qd with a 15 mg loading dose
• *Child >13 yr weighing <40 kg (88 lb):* to 1 mg/m²/day, 3 mg/m² loading dose

Hepatic dose
• Reduce by 33% in maintenance dose

Available forms: Oral sol 1 mg/ml

Side effects/adverse reactions:

HEMA: **Anemia, leukopenia, thrombocytopenia, purpura**

GI: Nausea, vomiting, diarrhea, constipation

CV: Hypertension, *atrial fibrillation, CHF, hypotension, palpitation, tachycardia*

CNS: *Tremors, headache,* insomnia, *paresthesia,* chills, fever

GU: UTIs, **albuminuria, hematuria, proteinuria, renal failure**

META: Hyperglycemia, increased creatinine, edema, hypercholesterolemia, hyperlipemia, hypophospha-

temia, weight gain, hyperkalemia, hyperuricemia, hypokalemia, hypomagnesemia

RESP: **Pleural effusion, atelectasis, dyspnea**

INTEG: Rash, acne

EENT: Blurred vision, photophobia

SYST: **Lymphoma**

Contraindications: Hypersensitivity to this drug or to components of the drug

Precautions: Severe renal, hepatic disease; pregnancy (C), diabetes mellitus, hyperkalemia, hyperuricemia, lymphomas, lactation, children <13 yr, hypertension

Pharmacokinetics: Rapidly absorbed, peak 1 hr single dose, 2 hr multiple dosing, protein binding 92%

Interactions:
• Increased blood levels: antifungals, calcium channel blockers, cimetidine, danazol, erythromycin, cyclosporine, metoclopramide, bromocriptine, HIV-protease inhibitors
• Decreased blood levels: carbamazepine, phenobarbital, phenytoin, rifamycin, rifapentine
• Decreased effect of: vaccines
• Drug/food: alters bioavailability; use consistently with or without food; do not use with grapefruit juice

NURSING CONSIDERATIONS

Assess:
• Blood levels in those that may have altered metabolism, trough level ≥15 ng/ml are associated with increased adverse reactions
• Lipid profile: cholesterol, triglycerides, a lipid-lowering agent may be needed
• For infection and development of lymphoma
• Blood studies: Hgb, WBC, platelets during treatment qmo; if leukocytes <3000/mm³ or platelets <100,000/mm³, drug should be dis-

continued or reduced; decreased hemoglobulin level may indicate bone marrow suppression

• Liver function studies: alk phosphatase, AST, ALT, amylase, bilirubin, and for hepatotoxicity: dark urine, jaundice, itching, light-colored stools; drug should be discontinued

Administer:

• Prophylaxis for *Pneumocystis carinii* pneumonia for 1 yr after transplantation; prophylaxis for cytomegalovirus (CMV) is recommended for 90 days after transplantation in those at increased risk for CMV

• All medications PO if possible, avoiding IM injections; bleeding may occur

• For 3 days before transplant surgery; patients should be placed in protective isolation

• Use amber oral dose syringe and withdraw amount needed oral sol from the bottle, empty correct dose into plastic/glass container holding 60 ml of water/orange juice, stir vigorously and have patient drink at once, refill container with additional 120 ml water/orange juice, stir vigorously and drink at once, if using a pouch squeeze entire contents into container and follow above directions

• Store protected from light, refrigerate, stable for 24 mo

Evaluate:

• Therapeutic response: absence of graft rejection; immunosuppression in autoimmune disorders

Teach patient/family:

• To report fever, rash, severe diarrhea, chills, sore throat, fatigue; serious infections may occur; claycolored stools, cramping (hepatotoxicity)

• To avoid crowds, persons with known infections to reduce risk of infection

• To use contraception before, during and 12 wk after drug has been discontinued

---

sodium bicarbonate (℞, OTC)
Arm & Hammer Pure Baking Soda, Bellans, Citrocarbonate, Soda Mint, Neut
Func. class.: Alkalinizer
Chem. class.: $NaHCO_3$

Action: Orally neutralizes gastric acid, which forms water, NaCl, CO_2; increases plasma bicarbonate, which buffers H^+-ion concentration; reverses acidosis IV

Uses: Acidosis (metabolic), cardiac arrest, alkalinization (systemic/urinary) antacid

Dosage and routes:

Acidosis, metabolic

• *Adult and child:* **IV INF** 2-5 mEq/kg over 4-8 hr depending on CO_2, pH

Cardiac arrest

• *Adult and child:* **IV BOL** 1 mEq/kg of 7.5% or 8.4% sol, then 0.5 mEq/kg q10 min, then doses based on ABGs

• *Infant:* **IV INF** not to exceed 8 mEq/kg/day based on ABGs (4.2% sol)

Alkalinization of urine

• *Adult:* **PO** 325 mg-2 g qid or 48 mEq (4g), then 12-24 mEq q4h

• *Child:* **PO** 12-120 mg/kg/day (1-10 mEq/kg)

Antacid

• *Adult:* **PO** 300 mg-2 g chewed, taken with H_2O qd-qid

Available forms: Tabs 300, 325, 600, 650 mg; inj 4.2%, 5%, 7.5%, 8.4%

Side effects/adverse reactions:

CNS: Irritability, headache, confusion, stimulation, tremors, *twitching, hyperreflexia, tetany,* weakness, **convulsions** of alkalosis

---

◆ = Nursing alert   🖊 = Herb-drug interaction   ⊘ = Do not crush

CV: Irregular pulse, ***cardiac arrest,*** water retention, edema, weight gain

GI: Flatulence, ***belching, distention, paralytic ileus,*** acid rebound

META: Alkalosis

GU: Calculi

RESP: Shallow, slow respirations; cyanosis, ***apnea***

Contraindications: Hypertension, peptic ulcer, renal disease, hypocalcemia

Precautions: CHF, cirrhosis, toxemia, renal disease, pregnancy (C)

Pharmacokinetics:

PO: Onset 2 min, duration 10 min

IV: Onset 15 min, duration 1-2 hr, excreted in urine

Interactions:

• Increased effects: amphetamines, mecamylamine, quinine, quinidine, pseudoephedrine, flecainide, anorexiants

• Decreased effects: lithium, chlorpropamide, barbiturates, salicylates, benzodiazepines

• Increased Na and decreased K: corticosteroids

⊘ Decreased action of sodium bicarbonate: oak bark

Lab test interferences:

Increase: Urinary urobilinogen

False positive: Urinary protein, blood lactate

NURSING CONSIDERATIONS

Assess:

• Respiratory and pulse rate, rhythm, depth, lung sounds; notify prescriber of abnormalities

• Fluid balance (I&O, weight qd, edema); notify prescriber of fluid overload

• Electrolytes, blood pH, PO_2, HCO_3^-, during treatment; ABGs frequently during emergencies

• Urine pH, urinary output, during beginning treatment

• Extravasation with IV administration (tissue sloughing, ulceration, and necrosis)

• Weight qd with initial therapy

• Alkalosis: irritability, confusion, twitching, hyperreflexia stimulation, slow respirations, cyanosis, irregular pulse

• Milk-alkali syndrome: confusion, headache, nausea, vomiting, anorexia, urinary stones, hypercalcemia

• For GI perforation secondary to CO_2 in GI tract; may lead to perforation if ulcer is severe enough

Administer:

IV

• In prepared sol or diluted in an equal amount of compatible sol given 2-5 mEq/kg over 4-8 hr, not to exceed 50 mEq/hr; slower rate in children

Additive compatibilities: Amikacin, aminophylline, amobarbital, amphotericin B, atropine, bretylium, calcium chloride, calcium gluceptate, cefoxitin, ceftazidime, cephalothin, cephapirin, chloramphenicol, chlorothiazide, cimetidine, clindamycin, cytarabine, droperidol/fentanyl, ergonovine, erythromycin, esmolol, floxacillin, furosemide, heparin, hyaluronidase, hydrocortisone, kanamycin, lidocaine, mannitol, metaraminol, methotrexate, methyldopa, multivitamins, nafcillin, nalmefene, netilmicin, nizatidine, ofloxacin, oxacillin, oxytocin, phenobarbital, phenylephrine, phenytoin, phytonadione, potassium chloride, prochlorperazine, thiopental, verapamil

Syringe compatibilities: Milrinone, pentobarbital

Y-site compatibilities: Acyclovir, amifostine, asparaginase, aztreonam, cefepime, cefmetazole, ceftriaxone, cladribine, cyclophosphamide, cytarabine, daunorubicin, dexamethasone, dexchlorpheniramine, doxorubicin, etoposide, famotidine, filgrastim, fludarabine, gallium, granisetron, heparin, ifosfamide, indomethacin sodium trihydrate, insulin, melphalan, mesna, methylprednisolone, morphine, paclitaxel, piperacillin/tazobactam, potassium chloride, propofol, remifentanil, tacrolimus, teniposide, thiotepa, tolazoline, vancomycin, vit B/C

Evaluate:

• Therapeutic response: ABGs, electrolytes, blood pH, HCO$_3^-$ WNL

Teach patient/family:

• To chew antacid tablets and drink 8 oz water

• Not to take antacid with milk, or milk-alkali syndrome may result

• Not to use antacid for more than 2 wk

• To notify prescriber if indigestion is accompanied by chest pain, dyspnea, diarrhea, dark, tarry stools

• About sodium-restricted diet; to avoid use of baking soda for indigestion

---

sodium biphosphate/ sodium phosphate
(OTC)

Fleet Enema, Phospho-Soda
Func. class.: Laxative, saline

Action: Increases water absorption in the small intestine by osmotic action, laxative effect occurs by increased peristalsis and water retention

Uses: Constipation, bowel or rectal preparation for surgery, exam

Dosage and routes:

• *Adult:* **PO** 20-30 ml (Phospho-Soda)

• *Child:* **PO** 5-15 ml (Phospho-Soda)

• *Adult and child >12 yr:* **RECT** 1 enema (118 ml)

• *Child 2-12 yr:* **RECT** ½ enema (59 ml)

Available forms: Enema 7 g phosphate/19 g biphosphate/118 ml; oral sol 18 g phosphate/48 g biphosphate/100 ml

Side effects/adverse reactions:

GI: Nausea, cramps, diarrhea

META: Electrolyte, fluid imbalances

Contraindications: Hypersensitivity, rectal fissures, abdominal pain, nausea/vomiting, appendicitis, acute surgical abdomen, ulcerated hemorrhoids, Na-restricted diets (Phospho-Soda)

Precautions: Pregnancy (C)

Pharmacokinetics: Excreted in feces

NURSING CONSIDERATIONS

Assess:

• Stools: color, amount, consistency

• Bowel pattern, bowel sounds, flatulence, distention, fever, dietary patterns, exercise

• Blood, urine electrolytes if drug is used often by patient

• Cramping, rectal bleeding, nausea, vomiting; if these symptoms occur, drug should be discontinued

Administer:

• Alone for better absorption; do not take within 1 hr of other drugs

Evaluate:

• Therapeutic response: decrease in constipation

Teach patient/family:

• Not to use laxatives for long-term therapy; bowel tone will be lost

• That normal bowel movements do not always occur daily

• Not to use in presence of abdominal pain, nausea, vomiting

• To notify prescriber if constipation unrelieved or if symptoms of electrolyte imbalance occur: muscle cramps, pain, weakness, dizziness, excessive thirst

• To maintain fluid consumption

◆ = Nursing alert   ✿ = Herb-drug interaction   ⊘ = Do not crush

sodium polystyrene sulfonate (℞)

(po-lee-stye'reen)
Kayexalate, K-Exit*, Kionex, PMS Sodium Polystyrene Sulfonate*, SPS

Func. class.: Potassium-removing resin

Chem. class.: Cation exchange resin

Action: Removes potassium by exchanging sodium for potassium in body primarily in large intestine

Uses: Hyperkalemia in conjunction with other measures

Dosage and routes:
• *Adult:* **PO** 15 g qd-qid; **RECT** enema 30-50 g/100 ml of sorbitol warmed to body temp q6h
• *Child:* **PO/RECT** 1 mEq of K exchanged/g of resin, approximate dose 1g/kg q6h

Available forms: Susp 15 g polystyrene sulfonate, 21.5 ml sorbitol, 15 g (65 mEq) Na/60 ml; pwd 15 g/4 level tsp

Side effects/adverse reactions:
GI: Constipation, anorexia, nausea, vomiting, diarrhea (sorbitol), fecal impaction, gastric irritation
META: Hypocalcemia, hypokalemia, hypomagnesemia, Na retention

Precautions: Pregnancy (C), renal failure, CHF, severe edema, severe hypertension

Interactions:
• Decreased effect of sodium polystyrene: antacids, laxatives

NURSING CONSIDERATIONS
Assess:
• Hyperkalemia: confusion, dyspnea, weakness, dysrhythmias
• ECG for spiked T waves, depressed ST segments, prolonged QT and widening QRS complex
• Bowel function qd, note consistency of stools, times/day
• Hypotension: confusion, irritability, muscular pain, weakness
• Serum K, Ca, Mg, Na, acid-base balance
• I&O ratio, weight qd

Administer:
• Oral dose as susp mixed with H_2O or syr (20-100 ml)
• Mild laxative as ordered to prevent constipation, fecal impaction
• Sorbitol as ordered to prevent constipation
• Retention enema after mixing with warm water; introduce by gravity, continue stirring, flush with 100 ml of fluid, clamp, and leave in place

Perform/provide:
• Retention of enema for at least ½-1 hr
• Irrigation of colon after enema with 1-2 qt nonsodium sol, drain
• Storage of freshly prepared sol 24 hr at room temperature

Evaluate:
• Therapeutic response: K level 3.5-5 mg/dl

Teach patient/family:
• Reason for medication and expected results

somatropin (℞)

(soe-ma-troe'pin)
Genotropin, Humatrope, Norditropin, Nutropin, Nutropin Depot, Nutropin AQ, Saizen, Serostim

Func. class.: Pituitary hormone

Chem. class.: Growth hormone

Action: Stimulates growth; somatropin similar to natural growth hormone; both preparations developed by recombinant DNA

Uses: Pituitary growth hormone deficiency (hypopituitary dwarfism),

S

children with human growth hormone deficiency, AIDS wasting syndrome, cachexia, adults with somatropin deficiency syndrome (SDS)

Dosage and routes:

Genotropin

SC 0.16-0.24 mg/kg/wk divided into 6 or 7 inj, give in abdomen, thigh, buttocks

Humatrope

SC/IM 0.18 mg/kg divided into equal doses either on 3 alternate days or 6×/wk, max wk dose is 0.3 mg/kg

Nutropin/Nutropin AQ (growth hormone deficiency)

SC 0.3 mg/kg/wk

Serostim

SC at hs >55 kg, 6 mg; 45-55 kg, 5 mg; 35-45 kg, 4 mg

Norditropin

SC 0.024-0.034 mg/kg 6-7 ×/wk

Nutropin depot

Available forms: Pwd for inj (lyophilized) 1.5 mg (4 IU/ml), 4 mg (12 IU/vial), 5 mg (13 IU/vial), 5 mg (15 IU/vial), 5 mg (15 IU/vial) rDNA origin, 5.8 mg (15 IU/ml), 6 mg (18 IU/ml), 8 mg (24 IU/vial), 10 mg (26 IU/vial); inj 10 mg (30 IU/vial), 5 mg/1.5 ml, 10 mg/1.5 ml, 15 mg/1.5 ml

Side effects/adverse reactions:

GU: Hypercalciuria

INTEG: Rash, urticaria, pain; inflammation at inj site

CNS: Headache, growth of intracranial tumor

ENDO: Hyperglycemia, ketosis, hypothyroidism

SYST: Antibodies to growth hormone

MS: Tissue swelling, joint and muscle pain

Contraindications: Hypersensitivity to benzyl alcohol, closed epiphyses, intracranial lesions

Precautions: Diabetes mellitus, hypothyroidism, pregnancy (C)

Pharmacokinetics: Half-life 15-60 min, duration 7 days; metabolized in liver

Interactions:

• Decreased growth: glucocorticosteroids

• Epiphyseal closure: androgens, thyroid hormones

NURSING CONSIDERATIONS

Assess:

• Growth hormone antibodies if patient fails to respond to therapy

• Thyroid function tests: T_3, T_4, T_7, TSH to identify hypothyroidism

• Allergic reaction: rash, itching, fever, nausea, wheezing

• Hypercalciuria: urinary stones; groin, flank pain; nausea, vomiting, urinary frequency, hematuria, chills

• Growth rate of child at intervals during treatment

Administer:

IM

• Rotate inj site

• Norditropin: after reconstituting 4 or 8 mg/2 ml diluent

• Humatrope: 5 mg/1.5-5 ml diluent, do not shake

• Nutropin/Nutropin AQ: reconstitute 5 mg/1-5 ml or 10 mg/1-10 ml bacteriostatic water for inj (benzyl alcohol preserved)

Perform/provide:

• Storage in refrigerator for <1 mo, if reconstituted <1 wk; do not use discolored or cloudy sol

Evaluate:

• Therapeutic response: growth in children

Teach patient/family:

• That treatment may continue for years; regular assessments are required

---

◆ = Nursing alert   ▨ = Herb-drug interaction   ⊘ = Do not crush

sotalol (℞)

(sot'ah-lahl)
Betapace, Betapace AF,
Sotacar*

Func. class.: Antidysrhythmic
group II, III
Chem. class.: Nonselective
β-blocker

Action: Blockade of $β_1$- and $β_2$-receptors leads to antidysrhythmic effect, prolongs action potential in myocardial fibers without affecting conduction, prolongs QT interval, no effect on QRS duration

Uses: Life-threatening ventricular dysrhythmias; Betapace AF: to maintain sinus rhythm in symptomatic atrial fibrillation/flutter

Dosage and routes:

• *Adult:* **PO** initial 80 mg bid, may increase to 240-320 mg/day

Renal dose

• *CrCl 30-60 ml/min:* Give q24h; *CrCl 10-29 ml/min:* give q36-48h; *CrCl <10 ml/min:* individualize dose

Betapace AF

• *Adult:* **PO** initial 80 mg, titrate upward to 120 mg during initial hospitalization

Renal dose (Betapace AF)

• *CrCl >60 ml/min:* Give q12h; *CrCl 40-60 ml/min:* give q24h; *CrCl <40 ml/min:* do not use

Available forms: Tabs 80, 120, 160, 240 mg; Betapace AF 80, 120, 160 mg

Side effects/adverse reactions:

*CV: **Prodysrhythmia,*** orthostatic hypotension, bradycardia, ***CHF,*** chest pain, ventricular dysrhythmias, AV block, peripheral vascular insufficiency, palpitations, prodysrhythmia, torsades de pointes; ***life-threatening ventricular arrhythmias (Betapace AF)***

CNS: Dizziness, mental changes, drowsiness, fatigue, headache, catatonia, depression, anxiety, nightmares, paresthesia, lethargy, insomnia, decreased concentration

GI: Nausea, vomiting, diarrhea, dry mouth, flatulence, constipation, anorexia

INTEG: Rash, alopecia, urticaria, pruritus, fever

*HEMA: **Agranulocytosis, thrombocytopenic purpura** (rare), **thrombocytopenia, leukopenia***

EENT: Tinnitus, visual changes, sore throat, double vision; dry, burning eyes

GU: Impotence, dysuria, ejaculatory failure, urinary retention

*RESP: **Bronchospasm,*** dyspnea, wheezing, nasal stuffiness, pharyngitis

MS: Joint pain, arthralgia, muscle cramps, pain

MISC.: Facial swelling, decreased exercise tolerance, weight change, Raynaud's disease

Contraindications: Hypersensitivity to β-blockers, cardiogenic shock, heart block (2nd or 3rd degree), sinus bradycardia, CHF, bronchial asthma, congenital or acquired long QT syndrome

Precautions: Major surgery, pregnancy (B), lactation, diabetes mellitus, renal disease, thyroid disease, COPD, well-compensated heart failure, CAD, nonallergic bronchospasm, electrolyte disturbances, bradycardia, cardiac dysrhythmias, peripheral vascular disease

Pharmacokinetics:

PO: Onset 1-2 hr, peak 2-4 hr, duration 8-12 hr, half-life 12 hr; metabolized by liver (metabolites inactive), excreted unchanged in urine, crosses placenta, excreted in breast milk, protein binding 0%

S

Interactions:

• Increased hypotension: diuretics, other antihypertensives, nitroglycerin, prazosin

• Decreased β-blocker effects: sympathomimetics, nonsteroidal antiinflammatory agents, salicylates

• Increased hypoglycemia effect: insulin

• Increased effects of lidocaine

• Decreased bronchodilating effects of theophylline

• Decreased hypoglycemic effects of sulfonylureas

🍃 Potassium deficiency, increased antidysrhythmic effect: aloe, buckthorn, cascara sagrada, senna

Lab test interferences:

• *False increase:* Urinary catecholamines

• *Interference:* Glucose, insulin tolerance tests

NURSING CONSIDERATIONS
Assess:

• I&O, weight qd

• B/P, pulse q4h; note rate, rhythm, quality

• Apical/radial pulse before administration: notify prescriber of any significant changes; monitor ECG continuously (Betapace AF); use QT interval to determine patient eligibility; baseline QT must be ≤450 msec; if the QT prolongs to 500 msec, reduce or stop drug

• Baselines in renal, LFTs before therapy begins

• Edema in feet, legs qd

• Skin turgor, dryness of mucous membranes for hydration status

Administer:

• PO: ac, hs; tablet may be crushed or swallowed whole

• Reduced dosage in renal dysfunction

Perform/provide:

• Storage in dry area at room temperature; do not freeze

Evaluate:

• Therapeutic response: absence of life-threatening dysrhythmias

Teach patient/family:

• Not to discontinue drug abruptly; taper over 2 wk or may precipitate angina

• Not to use OTC products containing α-adrenergic stimulants (nasal decongestants, OTC cold preparations) unless directed by prescriber

• To report bradycardia, dizziness, confusion, depression, fever

• To take pulse at home; advise when to notify prescriber

• To avoid alcohol, smoking, sodium intake

• To carry Medic Alert ID to identify drug being taken, allergies

• To avoid hazardous activities if dizziness is present

• To report symptoms of CHF including: difficulty in breathing, especially on exertion or when lying down; night cough, swelling of extremities

• To take medication to minimize orthostatic hypotension

• To wear support hose to minimize effects of orthostatic hypotension

Treatment of overdose: Lavage, IV atropine for bradycardia, IV theophylline for bronchospasm, digitalis, O_2, diuretic for cardiac failure; hemodialysis is useful for removal; administer vasopressor (norepinephrine) for hypotension, isoproterenol for heart block

---

⬥ = Nursing alert   🍃 = Herb-drug interaction   🚫 = Do not crush

sparfloxacin

(spar-floks'a-sin)
Zagam
Func. class.: Antiinfective
Chem. class.: Fluoroquinolone

Action: Interferes with conversion of intermediate DNA fragments into high-molecular-weight DNA in bacteria; DNA-gyrase inhibitor

Uses: Community-acquired pneumonia; chronic bronchitis caused by *Klebsiella pneumoniae, Haemophilus influenzae, Haemophilus parainfluenzae, Moraxella catarrhalis*

Dosage and routes:
• *Adult:* **PO** 400 mg loading dose, then 200 mg q24h × 10 days

Renal dose
• CrCl <50 ml/min day 400 mg on 1st day then 200 mg qod day 2-10

Available forms: Tabs 200 mg

Side effects/adverse reactions:
HEMA: **Leukopenia,** eosinophilia, anemia

CNS: Headache, dizziness, insomnia

GI: Nausea, flatulence, *vomiting,* diarrhea, *abdominal pain,* **pseudomembranous colitis**

CV: QT interval prolongation, vasodilation

INTEG: Rash, pruritus, photosensitivity

SYST: **Anaphylaxis, Stevens-Johnson syndrome**

Contraindications: Hypersensitivity to quinolones, photosensitivity

Precautions: Pregnancy (C), lactation, children, renal disease, seizure disorders

Pharmacokinetics: Slow, erratic absorption, widely distributed; metabolized by liver, excreted in urine, feces; half-life 20 hr

Interactions:
• Decreased absorption of sparfloxacin: antacids with aluminum, magnesium, iron products, zinc, sucralfate, give 4 hr apart
• Torsades de pointes: amiodarone, bepridil, disopyramide, erythromycin, pentamidine, phenothiazines, tricyclics, class Ia antidysrhythmics, class III antidysrhythmics
• May increase theophylline level, lead to toxicity
• May increase warfarin level
• Nephrotoxicity may occur with cyclosporine

Lab test interferences:
Increase: AST, ALT

NURSING CONSIDERATIONS
Assess:
• For previous sensitivity reaction
• For signs and symptoms of infection: characteristics of sputum, WBC >10,000/mm^3, fever; obtain baseline information before and during treatment
• C&S before beginning drug therapy to identify if correct treatment has been initiated
◆ For allergic reactions, anaphylaxis: rash, urticaria, pruritus, chills, fever, joint pain; may occur a few days after therapy begins; epinephrine and resuscitation equipment should be available for anaphylactic reaction
• Blood studies: AST, ALT, alk phosphatase if patient is on long-term therapy
• Bowel pattern qd; if severe diarrhea occurs, drug should be discontinued
• For overgrowth of infection: perineal itching, fever, malaise, redness, pain, swelling, drainage, rash, diarrhea, change in cough, sputum

Administer:
• As directed only
• 4 hr before or 2 hr after antacids, zinc, calcium

S

Evaluate:
• Therapeutic response: absence of signs/symptoms of infection (WBC <10,000/mm^3, temp WNL)

Teach patient/family:
• To avoid hazardous activities until response is known
• To contact prescriber if vaginal itching, loose, foul-smelling stools, furry tongue occur (may indicate superinfection); report itching, rash, pruritus, urticaria
• To take all medication prescribed for the length of time ordered; drug must be taken as directed to maintain blood levels; do not give medication to others
• To notify prescriber of diarrhea with blood or pus
• To increase fluid intake to 2 L/day to prevent crystalluria
• To take 4 hr before or 2 hr after antacids, dairy products, zinc products
• To avoid direct sunlight or use sunscreen to prevent phototoxicity
• Not to use theophylline with this product unless approved by prescriber
• To use frequent rinsing of mouth, sugarless candy, or gum for dry mouth

---

spectinomycin (℞)
(spek-ti-noe-mye′sin)
Trobicin
Func. class.: Antiinfective
Chem. class.: Aminocyclitol

Action: Inhibits bacterial synthesis by binding to 30S subunit on ribosomes

Uses: Gonococcal urethritis, proctitis in men and cervicitis and proctitis, disseminated gonococcal infection

Dosage and routes:
• *Adult:* **IM** 2-4 g as single dose
• *Child <45 kg:* **IM** 40 mg/kg single dose

Gonococcal infections in pregnancy
• *Adult:* **IM** 2 g to treat those allergic to cephalosporins

Available forms: Pwd for inj 400 mg/ml when reconstituted

Side effects/adverse reactions:
CNS: Dizziness, chills, fever, insomnia, headache, anxiety
HEMA: Anemia
GI: Nausea, vomiting, increased BUN
GU: Decreased urine output
INTEG: Pain at injection site, urticaria, rash, pruritus, fever
*SYST: **Anaphylaxis***

Contraindications: Hypersensitivity, syphilis

Precautions: Pregnancy (B), infants, children, lactation

Pharmacokinetics:
IM: Peak 1-2 hr, duration >8 hr, half-life 1-3 hr, excreted in urine (active form)

NURSING CONSIDERATIONS
Assess:
• Gonorrhea culture after treatment
• I&O ratio; report decreased output
• Liver studies: AST, ALT, serum alk phosphatase following multiple doses
• Blood studies: Hct, Hgb, BUN if multiple doses given
• Serologic test for gonorrhea 3 mo after treatment
• Allergies before treatment, reaction of each medication

Administer:
IM
• After shaking vial
• IM inj deep into large muscle mass (gluteus muscle only)
• With 20G needle; no more than 5 ml per site

◆ = Nursing alert   ⫻ = Herb-drug interaction   ⊘ = Do not crush

Perform/provide:
• Storage at room temperature; discard reconstituted sol after 24 hr
• Treatment of partner; report infection

Evaluate:
• Therapeutic response: negative gonorrhea culture after treatment

---

spironolactone (R)

(speer'on-oh-lak'tone)
Aldactone, Novo-Spiroton*
Func. class.: Potassium-sparing diuretic
Chem. class.: Aldosterone antagonist

Action: Competes with aldosterone at receptor sites in distal tubule, resulting in excretion of sodium chloride, water, retention of potassium, phosphate

Uses: Edema of CHF, hypertension, diuretic-induced hypokalemia, primary hyperaldosteronism (diagnosis, short-term treatment, long-term treatment), edema of nephrotic syndrome, cirrhosis of the liver with ascites

Investigational uses: CHF

Edema/hypertension
• *Adult:* **PO** 25-400 mg/qd in single or divided doses

CHF
• *Adult:* **PO** 12.5-25 mg/day

Edema
• *Child:* **PO** 3.3 mg/kg/day in single or divided doses

Hypertension
• *Child:* **PO** 1-2 mg/kg bid

Hypokalemia
• *Adult:* **PO** 25-100 mg/day; if **PO**, K supplements must not be used

Primary hyperaldosteronism diagnosis
• *Adult:* **PO** 400 mg/day × 4 days

or 4 wk depending on test, then 100-400 mg/day maintenance
Available forms: Tabs 25, 50, 100 mg

Side effects/adverse reactions:
CNS: Headache, confusion, drowsiness, lethargy, ataxia
GI: Diarrhea, cramps, **bleeding,** gastritis, *vomiting,* anorexia, nausea
INTEG: Rash, pruritus, urticaria
ENDO: Impotence, gynecomastia, irregular menses, amenorrhea, postmenopausal bleeding, hirsutism, deepening voice
HEMA: Agranulocytosis
ELECT: Hyperchloremic metabolic acidosis, **hyperkalemia,** hyponatremia

Contraindications: Hypersensitivity, anuria, severe renal disease, hyperkalemia, pregnancy (D)
Precautions: Dehydration, hepatic disease, lactation, renal impairment
Pharmacokinetics:
PO: Onset 24-48 hr, peak 48-72 hr; metabolized in liver, excreted in urine, crosses placenta
Interactions:
• Decreased effect of anticoagulants
• Increased action of antihypertensives, digitalis, lithium
• Increased hyperkalemia: K-sparing diuretics, K products, ACE inhibitors, salt substitutes
• Decreased effect of spironolactone: ASA
✐ Hypokalemic alkalosis: licorice
Lab test interferences:
Interference: 17-OHCS, 17-KS, radioimmunoassay, digoxin assay
NURSING CONSIDERATIONS
Assess:
• Electrolytes: Na, Cl, K, BUN, serum creatinine, ABGs, CBC
• Weight, I&O qd to determine fluid loss; effect of drug may be decreased if used qd; ECG periodically (long-term therapy)

• Signs of metabolic acidosis: drowsiness, restlessness
• Rashes, temp qd
• Confusion, especially in elderly; take safety precautions if needed
• Hydration: skin turgor, thirst, dry mucous membranes

Administer:
• In AM to avoid interference with sleep
• With food; if nausea occurs, absorption may be decreased slightly

Evaluate:
• Therapeutic response: improvement in edema of feet, legs, sacral area qd if medication is being used in CHF

Teach patient/family:
• To avoid foods with high K$^+$ content: oranges, bananas, salt substitutes, dried apricots, dates
• That drowsiness, ataxia, mental confusion may occur; observe caution in driving
• To notify prescriber of cramps, diarrhea, lethargy, thirst, headache, skin rash, menstrual abnormalities, deepening voice, breast enlargement

Treatment of overdose: Lavage if taken orally; monitor electrolytes, administer IV fluids, monitor hydration, renal, CV status

---

stavudine (R)

(sta'vyoo-deen)
Zerit
Func. class.: Antiretroviral
Chem. class.: Thymidine nucleoside

Action: Prevents replication of HIV by the inhibition of the enzyme reverse transcriptase, causes DNA chain termination

Uses: Treatment of advanced HIV infection not responsive to other antivirals

Dosage and routes:
• *Adult >60 kg:* **PO** 40 mg q12h
• *Adult <60 kg:* **PO** 30 mg q12h
• *Child <30 kg:* **PO** 2 mg/kg/day divided q12h

Renal dose
• *Adult: >60 kg:* **PO** CrCl 26-50 ml/min 20 mg q12h; CrCl 10-25 ml/min 20 mg q24h
• *Adult: <60 kg:* **PO** CrCl 26-50 ml/min 15 mg q12h; CrCl 10-25 ml/min 15 mg q24h

Available forms: Caps 15, 20, 30, 40 mg; pwd for oral sol 1 mg/ml

Side effects/adverse reactions:
HEMA: **Bone marrow suppression**
CNS: Peripheral neuropathy, insomnia, anxiety, neuropathy, depression, dizziness, confusion, headache, chills/fever, malaise
GI: **Hepatotoxicity,** diarrhea, nausea, vomiting, anorexia, dyspepsia, constipation, stomatitis
MS: Myalgia, arthralgia
CV: Chest pain, vasodilation, hypertension
MISC: **Lactic acidosis**
RESP: Dyspnea, pneumonia, asthma
INTEG: Rash, sweating, pruritus, benign neoplasms
EENT: Conjunctivitis, abnormal vision

Contraindications: Hypersensitivity to this drug or zidovudine, didanosine, zalcitabine; severe peripheral neuropathy

Precautions: Advanced HIV infection, pregnancy (C), lactation, bone marrow suppression; renal, liver disease, peripheral neuropathy

Interactions:
• Increased myelosuppression: other myelosuppressants
• Increased peripheral neuropathy: lithium, dapsone, chloramphenicol didanosine, ethambutol, hydralazine, phenytoin, vincristine, zalcitabine

---

♦ = Nursing alert   ∥ = Herb-drug interaction   ⃠ = Do not crush

Pharmacokinetics: Excreted in urine, breast milk; peak 1 hr; half-life: elimination: 1-1.6 hr, intracellular: 3-3.5 hr

NURSING CONSIDERATIONS
Assess:

◆ For lactic acidosis and severe hepatomegaly with steatosis, death may result

• Blood studies: WBC, differential, RBC, Hct, Hgb, platelets

• Renal studies: urinalysis, protein, blood

• C&S before drug therapy; drug may be given as soon as culture is taken

• Bowel pattern before, during treatment

• Weakness, tremors, confusion, dizziness; drug may have to be decreased or discontinued

• Viral load and CD4 counts baseline and throughout treatment

• For peripheral neuropathy: tingling, pain, in extremities; discontinue drug

◆ For pancreatitis: severe upper abdominal pain, nausea, vomiting throughout treatment, discontinue drug

Administer:

• With or without meals; absorption does not appear to be lowered when taken with food

Teach patient/family:

• The signs of peripheral neuropathy: burning, weakness, pain, prickling feeling in the extremities

• That drug should not be given with antineoplastics

• That drug is not a cure for AIDS, but will control symptoms

• To call prescriber if sore throat, swollen lymph nodes, malaise, fever occur; other drugs may be needed to prevent other infections

• That even with this drug, patient may pass AIDS virus to others

• That follow-up visits are necessary; serious toxicity may occur; blood counts must be done q2wk

• To take q12h around clock

• That serious drug interactions may occur if other medications are ingested; see prescriber before taking chloramphenicol, dapsone, cisplatin, didanosine, ethambutol, lithium, antifungals, antineoplastics

• That drug may cause fainting or dizziness

Evaluate:

• Therapeutic response: decreased symptoms of HIV

---

streptokinase (℞)

(strep-toe-kye′nase)
Kabikinase, Streptase
Func. class.: Thrombolytic enzyme
Chem. class.: β-Hemolytic streptococcus filtrate (purified)

Action: Activates conversion of plasminogen to plasmin (fibrinolysin): plasmin breaks down clots (fibrin), fibrinogen, factors V, VII; occlusion of venous access lines

Uses: Deep-vein thrombosis, pulmonary embolism, arterial thrombosis, arterial embolism, arteriovenous cannula occlusion, lysis of coronary artery thrombi after MI, acute evolving transmural MI

Dosage and routes:

Lysis of coronary artery thrombi

• *Adult:* IC 20,000 IU, then 2000 IU/min over 1 hr as **IV INF**

Arteriovenous cannula occlusion

• *Adult:* **IV INF** 250,000 IU/2 ml sol into occluded limb of cannula run over ½ hr; clamp for 2 hr; aspirate contents; flush with NaCl sol and reconnect

Thrombosis/embolism/DVT/ pulmonary embolism

• *Adult:* **IV INF** 250,000 IU over ½

---

hr, then 100,000 IU/hr for 72 hr for deep-vein thrombosis; 100,000 IU/hr over 24-72 hr for pulmonary embolism; 100,000 IU/hr × 24-72 hr for arterial thrombosis or embolism

Acute evolving transmural MI

• *Adult:* **IV INF** 1,500,000 IU diluted to a volume of 45 ml; give within 1 hr; intracoronary **INF** 20,000 IU by **BOL**, then 2,000 IU/min × 1 hr, total dose 140,000 IU

Available forms: Pwd for inj, lyophilized, 250,000, 600,000, 750,000, 1,500,000 IU/vial

Side effects/adverse reactions:

CV: Dysrhythmias, hypotension, noncardiogenic pulmonary edema, ***pulmonary embolism***

CNS: Headache, fever

EENT: Periorbital edema

GI: Nausea

HEMA: Decreased Hct, ***bleeding***

INTEG: Rash, urticaria, phlebitis at IV inf site, itching, flushing

MS: Low back pain

RESP: Altered respirations, SOB, ***bronchospasm***

*SYST: **GI, GU, intracranial, retroperitoneal bleeding, surface bleeding, anaphylaxis***

Contraindications: Hypersensitivity, active bleeding, intraspinal surgery, CNS neoplasms, ulcerative colitis, enteritis, severe hypertension, severe renal disease, hepatic disease, hypocoagulation, COPD, subacute bacterial endocarditis, rheumatic valvular disease, cerebral embolism/thrombosis/hemorrhage, intraarterial diagnostic procedure or surgery (10 days), recent major surgery

Precautions: Arterial emboli from left side of heart, pregnancy (C)

Pharmacokinetics:

IV: Onset immediate, duration <12 hr; half-life <20 min; excreted in bile, urine

Interactions:

• Bleeding potential: aspirin, indomethacin, phenylbutazone, anticoagulants, other NSAIDs, abciximab, eptifibatide, tirofiban, clopidogrel, ticlopidine, some cephalosporins, plicamycin, valproic acid

Lab test interferences:

Increase: PT, aPTT, TT

Decrease: Plasminogen, fibrinogen

NURSING CONSIDERATIONS

Assess:

• Allergy: fever, rash, itching, chills; mild reaction may be treated with antihistamines

◆ For bleeding during 1st hr of treatment; hematuria, hematemesis, bleeding from mucous membranes, epistaxis, ecchymosis; may require tranfusion (rare), continue to assess for bleeding for 24 hr

• Blood studies (Hct, platelets, PTT, PT, TT, aPTT) before starting therapy; PT or aPTT must be less than 2× control before starting therapy; PTT or PT q3-4h during treatment

◆ For hypersensitive reactions: fever, rash, dyspnea, facial swelling; drug should be discontinued; for streptokinase reactions previously; notify prescriber immediately, stop drug, keep resuscitative equipment nearby

• VS, B/P, pulse, respirations, neurologic signs, temp at least q4h; temp >104° F (40° C) indicates internal bleeding; cardiac rhythm following intracoronary administration; systolic pressure increase >25 mm Hg should be reported to prescriber; assess neurologic status, neurologic change may indicate intracranial bleeding

◆ For neurologic changes that may indicate intracranial bleeding

◆ Retroperitoneal bleeding: back pain, leg weakness, diminished pulses

• For Guillain-Barré syndrome that

◆ = Nursing alert   ✎ = Herb-drug interaction   ⊘ = Do not crush may occur after treatment with this drug

• ECG continuously, cardiac enzymes, radionuclide myocardial scanning/coronary angiography

• For respiratory depression

Administer:

IV

• As soon as thrombi identified; not useful for thrombi over 1 wk old

• Cryoprecipitate or fresh frozen plasma if bleeding occurs

• Loading dose at beginning of therapy; may require increased loading doses

• Heparin after fibrinogen level >100 mg/dl; heparin infusion to increase PTT to 1.5-2 × baseline for 3-7 days; IV heparin with loading dose is recommended after discontinuing streptokinase to prevent redevelopment of thrombi

• After reconstituting with 5 ml NS or D₅W; do not shake; further dilute to total volume of 45 ml; may be diluted to 500 ml in 45 ml increments; may dilute vial in 15 ml NS, further dilute 750,000 IU/50 ml NS or D₅W; further dilute 1,500,000 IU dose/100 ml or more

• About 10% patients have high streptococcal antibody titers requiring increased loading doses

• IV therapy using 0.8-μm filter

Y-site compatibilities: Dobutamine, dopamine, heparin, lidocaine, nitroglycerin

Perform/provide:

• Storage of reconstituted sol in refrigerator; discard after 24 hr

• Bed rest during entire course of treatment

• Avoidance of venous or arterial puncture, inj, rectal temp; any invasive treatment

• Treatment of fever with acetaminophen or aspirin

• Pressure for 30 sec to minor bleeding sites; inform prescriber if this does not attain hemostasis; apply pressure dressing

Evaluate:

• Therapeutic response: resolution of thrombosis, embolism

Teach patient/family:

• Reason for medication and expected results

---

streptomycin (℞)
(strep-toe-mye′sin)

Func. class.: Antiinfective/antitubercular

Chem. class.: Aminoglycoside

Action: Interferes with protein synthesis in bacterial cell by binding to ribosomal subunit, causing inaccurate peptide sequence to form in protein chain, causing bacterial death

Uses: Sensitive strains of *Mycobacterium tuberculosis,* nontuberculous infections caused by sensitive strains of *Yersinia pestis, Brucella, Haemophilus influenzae, Klebsiella pneumoniae, Escherichia coli, Escherichia aerogenes, Streptococcus viridans, Francisella tularensis, Proteus*

Dosage and routes:

Tuberculosis

• *Adult:* **IM** 15 mg/kg (max 1 g) qd × 2-3 mo, then 1 g 2-3 ×/week with other antitubercular drugs

• *Child:* **IM** 20-40 mg/kg/day in divided doses with other antitubercular drugs; max 15 mg/kg/day

Streptococcal endocarditis

• *Adult:* **IM** 1 g q12h × 1 wk with penicillin, then 500 mg bid × 1 wk

Enterococcal endocarditis

• *Adult:* **IM** 1 g q12h × 2 wk, then

S

500 mg q12h × 4 wk with penicillin, max 15 mg/kg/day

Available forms: Inj 500 mg, 1 g/ml

Side effects/adverse reactions:

*GU: **Oliguria, hematuria, renal damage, azotemia, renal failure, nephrotoxicity***

CNS: Confusion, depression, numbness, tremors, ***convulsions,*** muscle twitching, ***neurotoxicity,*** dizziness

*EENT: **Ototoxicity,*** deafness, visual disturbances, tinnitus

*HEMA: **Agranulocytosis, thrombocytopenia, leukopenia, eosinophilia, anemia***

GI: Nausea, vomiting, anorexia, increased ALT, AST, bilirubin; hepatomegaly, ***hepatic necrosis,*** splenomegaly

CV: Hypotension, myocarditis, palpitations

INTEG: Rash, burning, urticaria, dermatitis, alopecia

Contraindications: Severe renal disease, hypersensitivity, pregnancy (D)

Precautions: Neonates, mild renal disease, myasthenia gravis, lactation, hearing deficit, elderly, Parkinson's disease

Pharmacokinetics:

IM: Onset rapid, peak 1-2 hr; plasma half-life 2-2½ hr; not metabolized, excreted unchanged in urine, crosses placental barrier, poor penetration into CSF, small amounts enter breast milk

Interactions:

• Increased ototoxicity, neurotoxicity, nephrotoxicity: other aminoglycosides, amphotericin B, polymyxin, vancomycin, ethacrynic acid, furosemide, mannitol, methoxyflurane, cisplatin, cephalosporins, bacitracin

• Increased effects: nondepolarizing muscle relaxants, succinylcholine, warfarin

NURSING CONSIDERATIONS
Assess:

• Weight before treatment; calculation of dosage is usually based on ideal body weight, but may be calculated on actual body weight

• I&O ratio, urinalysis qd for proteinuria, cells, casts; report sudden change in urine output

• Serum peak 20-30 min after IM injection, trough level drawn 8 hr; acceptable levels—peak 5-25 µg/ml, trough should not be >5 µg/ml

• Urine pH if drug is used for UTI; urine should be kept alkaline

• Renal impairment by collecting urine for CrCl testing, BUN, serum creatinine; lower dosage should be given in renal impairment (CrCl <80 ml/min), monitor electrolytes: K, Na, Cl, Mg

• Deafness by audiometric testing, ringing, roaring in ears, vertigo; assess hearing before, during, after treatment

• Dehydration: high specific gravity, decrease in skin turgor, dry mucous membranes, dark urine

• Overgrowth of infection: fever, malaise, redness, pain, swelling, perineal itching, diarrhea, stomatitis, change in cough, sputum

• C&S before starting treatment to identify infecting organism

• Vestibular dysfunction: nausea, vomiting, dizziness, headache; drug should be discontinued if severe

• Inj sites for redness, swelling, abscesses; use warm compresses at site

Administer:

• IM inj in large muscle mass; rotate inj sites

• Drug in evenly spaced doses to maintain blood level

Additive compatibilities: Bleomycin

Syringe compatibilities: Penicillin G sodium

Y-site compatibilities: Esmolol

⬥ = Nursing alert   🖋 = Herb-drug interaction   🚫 = Do not crush

Perform/provide:
• Adequate fluids of 2-3 L/day unless contraindicated to prevent irritation of tubules
• Supervised ambulation, other safety measures with vestibular dysfunction
Evaluate:
• Therapeutic effect: absence of fever, draining wounds, negative C&S after treatment
Teach patient/family:
• To report headache, dizziness, symptoms of overgrowth of infection, renal impairment
• To report loss of hearing, ringing, roaring in ears, fullness in head
Treatment of overdose: Hemodialysis; monitor serum levels of drug

---

RARELY USED

streptozocin (℞)
(strep-toe-zoe'sin)
Zanosar
Func. class.: Antineoplastic alkylating agent

Uses: Metastatic islet cell carcinoma of pancreas
Dosage and routes:
• *Adult:* **IV** 500 mg/m² × 5 days q6wk until desired response; or 1 g/m² qwk × 2 wk, not to exceed 1.5 g/m² in 1 dose
Investigational uses: Prevention of spread of Hodgkin's disease, metastatic carcinoid tumor, pancreatic adenocarcinoma, colon malignancies
Contraindications: Hypersensitivity

succimer (℞)
(sux'i-mer)
Chemet
Func. class.: Heavy metal antagonist
Chem. class.: Chelating agent

Action: Binds with ions of lead to form a water-soluble complex excreted by kidneys
Uses: Lead poisoning in children with lead levels above 45 µg/dl; may be beneficial in mercury, arsenic poisoning
Dosage and routes:
• *Child:* **PO** 10 mg/kg or 350 mg/m² q8h × 5 days, then 10 mg/kg or 350 mg/m² q12h × 2 wk; another course may be required depending on lead levels; allow 2 wk between courses
Available forms: Caps 100 mg
Side effects/adverse reactions:
SYST: Back, stomach, head, rib, flank pain; abdominal cramps, chills, fever, flulike symptoms, head cold, headache
HEMA: **Increased platelets, intermittent eosinophilia**
GU: **Proteinuria,** decreased urination, voiding difficulties
INTEG: Rash, urticaria, pruritus
META: Increased AST, ALT, alk phosphatase, cholesterol
GI: Nausea, vomiting, diarrhea, metallic taste, anorexia
CNS: Drowsiness, dizziness, paresthesia, sensorimotor neuropathy
EENT: Otitis media, watery eyes, film in eyes, plugged ears
RESP: Sore throat, rhinorrhea, nasal congestion, cough
Contraindications: Hypersensitivity
Precautions: Pregnancy (C), lactation, children <1 yr

S

Pharmacokinetics:
PO: Peak 1-2 hr, 49% excreted (39% in feces, 9% urine, 1% as CO_2 from lungs)

Interactions:
• Not recommended concurrently with other chelating agents

NURSING CONSIDERATIONS
Assess:
• Hepatic, renal studies: ALT, AST, alk phosphatase, BUN, creatinine, serum lead level
• I&O
• For lead sources in home, school
• Allergic reactions: rash, pruritus, urticaria; drug should be discontinued if antihistamines fail to help

Administer:
PO
• To children who cannot swallow capsule by separating the capsule and sprinkling content on food or in a spoon followed by a drink

Perform/provide:
• Adequate fluids; check hydration status qd

Evaluate:
• Therapeutic response: decrease in serum lead level

Teach patient/family:
• That therapeutic effect may take 1-3 mo
• To report urticaria, rash
• To increase fluid intake

---

succinylcholine (℞)
(suk-sin-ill-koe'leen)
Anectine, Anectine Flo-Pack, Quelicin, succinylcholine chloride, Sucostrin, Suxamethonium
Func. class.: Neuromuscular blocker (depolarizing–ultra short)

Action: Inhibits transmission of nerve impulses by binding with cholinergic receptor sites, antagonizing action of acetylcholine; causes release of histamine

Uses: Facilitation of endotracheal intubation, skeletal muscle relaxation during orthopedic manipulations

Dosage and routes:
• *Adult:* **IV** 0.6 mg/kg, then 2.5 mg/min as needed; **IM** 2.5 mg/kg, not to exceed 150 mg
• *Child:* **IV/IM** 1-2 mg/kg, not to exceed 150 mg **IM**
Available forms: Inj 20, 50, 100 mg/ml; pwd for inj 100, 500 mg/vial, 1 g/vial

Side effects/adverse reactions:
CV: Bradycardia, tachycardia; increased, decreased B/P; *sinus arrest, dysrhythmias*
RESP: Prolonged apnea, bronchospasm, cyanosis, respiratory depression
EENT: Increased secretions, increased intraocular pressure
MS: Weakness, muscle pain, fasciculations, prolonged relaxation
HEMA: Myoglobulinemia
INTEG: Rash, flushing, pruritus, urticaria

Contraindications: Hypersensitivity, malignant hyperthermia, decreased plasma pseudocholinesterase, penetrating eye injuries, acute narrow-angle glaucoma

Precautions: Pregnancy (C), cardiac disease, severe burns, fractures—fasciculations may increase damage—lactation, children <2 yr, electrolyte imbalances, dehydration, neuromuscular disease, respiratory disease, collagen diseases, glaucoma, eye surgery, elderly or debilitated patients

Pharmacokinetics:
IV: Onset 1 min, peak 2-3 min, duration 6-10 min
IM: Onset 2-3 min

◆ = Nursing alert   🌿 = Herb-drug interaction   🚫 = Do not crush

Hydrolyzed in urine (active/inactive metabolites)
Interactions:
• Increased neuromuscular blockade: aminoglycosides, clindamycin, lincomycin, quinidine, local anesthetics, polymyxin antibiotics, lithium, opioids, thiazides, enflurane, isoflurane, Mg salts, oxytocin
• Dysrhythmias: theophylline
⊘ Blocks succinylcholine: melatonin

NURSING CONSIDERATIONS
Assess:
• For electrolyte imbalances (K, Mg); may lead to increased action of this drug
• Vital signs (B/P, pulse, respirations, airway) until fully recovered; rate, depth, pattern of respirations, strength of hand grip
• I&O ratio; check for urinary retention, frequency, hesitancy
• Recovery: decreased paralysis of face, diaphragm, leg, arm, rest of body
• Allergic reactions: rash, fever, respiratory distress, pruritus; drug should be discontinued
Administer:
• Deep IM inj, preferably high in deltoid muscle
IV
• Using nerve stimulator by anesthesiologist to determine neuromuscular blockade
• Anticholinesterase to reverse neuromuscular blockade
• IV inf; dilute 1-2 mg/ml in D₅, isotonic saline sol, give 0.5-10 mg/min, titrate to response; may be given directly over 1 min
Additive compatibilities: Amikacin, cephapirin, isoproterenol, meperidine, methyldopate, morphine, norepinephrine, scopolamine
Syringe compatibilities: Heparin

Y-site compatibilities: Etomidate, heparin, potassium chloride, propofol, vit B/C
Perform/provide:
• Storage in refrigerator, powder at room temperature; close tightly
• Reassurance if communication is difficult during recovery from neuromuscular blockade; postoperative stiffness is normal, soon subsides
Evaluate:
• Therapeutic response: paralysis of jaw, eyelid, head, neck, rest of body
Treatment of overdose: Edrophonium or neostigmine, atropine, monitor VS; may require mechanical ventilation

sucralfate (℞)
(soo-kral'fate)
Carafate, Sulcrate*
Func. class.: Protectant, antiulcer
Chem. class.: Aluminum hydroxide, sulfated sucrose

Action: Forms a complex that adheres to ulcer site, adsorbs pepsin
Uses: Duodenal ulcer, oral mucositis, stomatitis after radiation of head and neck
Investigational uses: Gastric ulcers, gastroesophageal reflux
Dosage and routes:
Ulcers
• *Adult:* **PO** 1 g qid 1 hr ac, hs
• *Child:* **PO** 40-80 mg/kg/day
Prevention of ulcers
• *Adult:* **PO** 1 g bid, 1 hr ac
GERD
• *Adult:* **PO** 1 g qid 1 hr ac and hs
• *Child:* **PO** 500 mg-1 g qid, 1 hr ac and hs
Available forms: Tabs 1 g; oral susp 500 mg/5 ml

Side effects/adverse reactions:
CNS: Drowsiness, dizziness
GI: Dry mouth, constipation, nausea, gastric pain, vomiting
INTEG: Urticaria, rash, pruritus
Contraindications: Hypersensitivity
Precautions: Pregnancy (B), lactation, children, renal failure
Do not confuse:
Carafate/Cafergot
Pharmacokinetics:
PO: Duration up to 6 hr
Interactions:
• Decreased action of tetracyclines, phenytoin, fat-soluble vitamins, cimetidine, digoxin, ketoconazole, ranitidine, theophylline
• Decreased absorption of fluoroquinolones
• Decreased absorption of sucralfate: antacids

NURSING CONSIDERATIONS
Assess:
• Gastric pH (>5 should be maintained); blood in stools
Administer:
PO
• On an empty stomach, 1 hr before meals and hs
🚫 Do not crush, chew tabs
Perform/provide:
• Storage at room temperature
Evaluate:
• Therapeutic response: absence of pain, GI complaints
Teach patient/family:
• To take on empty stomach
• To take full course of therapy, not to use over 8 wk, to avoid smoking
• To avoid antacids within ½ hr of drug

sufentanil (℞)
(soo-fen'ta-nil)
Sufenta
Func. class.: Opiate analgesic

Controlled Substance Schedule II
Action: Inhibits ascending pain pathways in CNS, increases pain threshold, alters pain perception
Uses: Primary anesthetic, adjunct to general anesthetic
Dosage and routes:
Primary anesthetic
• *Adult:* **IV** 8-30 µg/kg given with 100% O₂, a muscle relaxant
Adjunct
• *Adult:* **IV** 1-8 µg/kg given with nitrous oxide/O₂
Available forms: Inj 50 µg/ml
Side effects/adverse reactions:
CNS: Drowsiness, dizziness, confusion, headache, sedation, euphoria
GI: Nausea, vomiting, anorexia, constipation, cramps
GU: Increased urinary output, dysuria, urinary retention
INTEG: Rash, urticaria, bruising, flushing, diaphoresis, pruritus
EENT: Tinnitus, blurred vision, miosis, diplopia
CV: Palpitations, bradycardia, change in B/P
RESP: **Respiratory depression**
Contraindications: Hypersensitivity, addiction (opiate)
Precautions: Addictive personality, pregnancy (C), lactation, increased intracranial pressure, MI (acute), severe heart disease, respiratory depression, hepatic disease, renal disease, child <18 yr
Pharmacokinetics: Onset 1½-3 hr, half-life 2½ hr
Interactions:
• Increased effects with other CNS depressants: alcohol, opioids,

---

◆ = Nursing alert /// = Herb-drug interaction 🚫 = Do not crush sedative/hypnotics, antipsychotics, skeletal muscle relaxants, antihistamines

🖋 Increased CNS depression: kava

Lab test interferences:

Increase: Amylase

NURSING CONSIDERATIONS

Assess:

• I&O ratio; decreasing output may indicate urinary retention

• CNS changes: dizziness, drowsiness, hallucinations, euphoria, LOC, pupil reaction

• Allergic reactions: rash, urticaria

• Respiratory dysfunction: respiratory depression, character, rate, rhythm; notify prescriber if respirations are <10/min

• Need for pain medication, physical dependence

Administer:

• With antiemetic if nausea, vomiting occur

IV

• Undiluted over 1-2 min or give as inf

Y-site compatibilities: Amphotericin B cholesteryl, cisatracurium, remifentanil

Perform/provide:

• Storage in light-resistant area at room temperature

• Safety measures: side rails, nightlight, call bell within easy reach

Evaluate:

• Therapeutic response: maintenance of anesthesia

Teach patient/family:

• To report any symptoms of CNS changes, allergic reactions

Treatment of overdose: Naloxone (Narcan) 0.2-0.8 mg IV, O₂, IV fluids, vasopressors

sulfadiazine (℞)

(sul-fa-dye′a-zeen)
Coptin, sulfadiazine
Func. class.: Antiinfective
Chem. class.: Sulfonamide, intermediate acting

Action: Interferes with bacterial biosynthesis of proteins by competitive antagonism of PABA

Uses: UTIs, rheumatic fever prophylaxis, with pyrimethamine for *Toxoplasma gondii* encephalitis, chancroid, inclusion conjunctivitis, malaria, meningitis, *Haemophilus influenzae,* meningococeal meningitis, nocardiosis, acute otitis media, trachoma

Dosage and routes:

Meningococcal carriers (asymptomatic)

• *Adult:* **PO** 1 g q12h × 2 days

• *Child 1-12 yr:* **PO** 500 mg q12h × 2 days

• *Child 2-12 mo:* **PO** 500 mg qd × 2 days

Rheumatic fever prophylaxis

• *Child >30 kg:* **PO** 1 g qd

• *Child <30 kg:* **PO** 500 mg qd

Available forms: Tabs 500 mg

Side effects/adverse reactions:

*SYST: **Anaphylaxis***

GI: Nausea, vomiting, abdominal pain, stomatitis, ***hepatitis,*** glossitis, pancreatitis, diarrhea, ***enterocolitis,*** anorexia

CNS: Headache, insomnia, hallucinations, depression, vertigo, fatigue, anxiety, ***convulsions,*** drug fever, chills, drowsiness

*HEMA: **Leukopenia, thrombocytopenia, agranulocytosis, hemolytic anemia, aplastic anemia***

INTEG: Rash, dermatitis, urticaria, ***Stevens-Johnson syndrome,*** erythema, photosensitivity, alopecia

*GU: **Renal failure, toxic nephrosis,***

S

increased BUN, creatinine, crystalluria, hematuria, proteinuria

*CV: **Allergic myocarditis***

Contraindications: Hypersensitivity to sulfonamides, sulfonylureas, thiazide and loop diuretics, salicylates, sunscreens with PABA, lactation, infants <2 mo (except congenital toxoplasmosis), pregnancy at term, porphyria

Precautions: Pregnancy (B), impaired hepatic function, severe allergy, bronchial asthma, renal dysfunction

Pharmacokinetics:

PO: Rapidly absorbed, onset ½ hr; peak 3-6 hr, 30%-50% bound to plasma proteins, half-life 8-10 hr; excreted in urine, breast milk; crosses placenta, metabolized in liver

Interactions:

• Increased hypoglycemic response: sulfonylurea agents

• Increased anticoagulant effects: warfarin

• Decreased renal excretion of: methotrexate

• Decreased hepatic clearance of: phenytoin

• Increased effects of: barbiturates, tolbutamide, uricosurics

• Increased drug-free concentrations: indomethacin, probenecid, salicylates

• Increased thrombocytopenia: thiazide diuretics

• Increased nephrotoxicity; cyclosporine

Lab test interferences:

False positive: Urinary glucose test (Benedict's method)

NURSING CONSIDERATIONS

Assess:

• I&O ratio; note color, character, pH of urine if drug administered for UTIs; output should be 800 ml less than intake; if urine is highly acidic, alkalization may be needed

• Kidney function studies: BUN, creatinine, urinalysis (long-term therapy)

• Blood dyscrasias: skin rash, fever, sore throat, bruising, bleeding, fatigue, joint pain, monitor CBC before and periodically

• Allergic reaction: rash, dermatitis, urticaria, pruritus, dyspnea, bronchospasm

Administer:

• On an empty stomach

• With full glass of H_2O to maintain adequate hydration; increase fluids to 2 L/day to decrease crystallization in kidneys

• Medication after C&S; repeat C&S after full course of medication

Perform/provide:

• Storage in tight, light-resistant container at room temperature

Evaluate:

• Therapeutic response: absence of pain, fever, C&S negative

Teach patient/family:

• To take each oral dose with full glass of water to prevent crystalluria

• To complete full course of treatment to prevent superinfection

• To avoid sunlight or use sunscreen to prevent burns

• To avoid OTC medication (aspirin, vit C) unless directed by prescriber

• To notify prescriber of skin rash, sore throat, fever, mouth sores, unusual bruising, bleeding

---

◆ = Nursing alert   ∥ = Herb-drug interaction   Ⓢ = Do not crush

---

sulfamethoxazole (Ŗ)

(sul-fa-meth-ox′a-zole)
Apo-Sulfamethoxazole*,
Gantanol, Urobak
Func. class.: Antiinfective
Chem. class.: Sulfonamide, intermediate acting

Action: Interferes with bacterial biosynthesis of proteins by competitive antagonism of PABA

Uses: UTIs, chancroid, inclusion conjunctivitis, malaria, meningococcal meningitis, nocardiosis, acute otitis media, toxoplasmosis, trachoma

Dosage and routes:
• *Adult:* **PO** 2 g, then 1 g bid or tid for 7-10 days
• *Child >2 mo:* **PO** 50-60 mg/kg × 1 dose then 25-30 mg/kg bid, not to exceed 75 mg/kg/day
Renal dose
• CrCl <50 ml/min give 50% of dose
Available forms: Tabs 500 mg, oral susp 500 mg/5 ml

Side effects/adverse reactions:
SYST: Anaphylaxis
GI: Nausea, vomiting, abdominal pain, stomatitis, ***hepatitis,*** glossitis, pancreatitis, diarrhea, ***enterocolitis,*** anorexia
*CNS: Headache, insomnia, hallucinations, depression, vertigo, fatigue, anxiety, **convulsions, drug fever,** chills, drowsiness*
*HEMA: **Leukopenia, thrombocytopenia, agranulocytosis, hemolytic anemia, aplastic anemia***
INTEG: Rash, dermatitis, urticaria, ***Stevens-Johnson syndrome,*** erythema, photosensitivity, alopecia
*GU: **Renal failure, toxic nephrosis,*** increased BUN, creatinine, crystalluria, hematuria, proteinuria
*CV: **Allergic myocarditis***

Contraindications: Hypersensitivity to sulfonamides, sulfonylureas, thiazide and loop diuretics, salicylates, sunscreens with PABA, infants <2 mo (except congenital toxoplasmosis), pregnancy at term, porphyria, lactation, G6PD deficiency

Precautions: Pregnancy (C), lactation, impaired hepatic/renal function, severe allergy, bronchial asthma

Pharmacokinetics:
PO: Poorly absorbed, peak 3-4 hr, 50%-70% bound to plasma proteins, half-life 7-12 hr; excreted in urine (unchanged 90%), breast milk; crosses placenta

Interactions:
• Increased effects of: barbiturates, uricosurics
• Increased drug-free concentrations: indomethacin, probenecid, salicylates
• Increased thrombocytopenia: thiazide diuretics
• Increased nephrotoxicity: cyclosporine
• Increased hypoglycemic response: sulfonylurea agents
• Increased anticoagulant effects: warfarin
• Decreased renal excretion of methotrexate
• Decreased hepatic clearance of phenytoin

Lab test interferences:
False positive: Urinary glucose test (Benedict's method)

NURSING CONSIDERATIONS
Assess:
• I&O ratio; note color, character, pH of urine if drug administered for UTIs; output should be 800 ml less than intake; if urine is highly acidic, alkalization may be needed
• Kidney function studies: BUN, creatinine, urinalysis (long-term therapy)
• Blood dyscrasias: skin rash, fever,

S

---

sore throat, bruising, bleeding, fatigue, joint pain, monitor CBC before and periodically

• Allergic reaction: rash, dermatitis, urticaria, pruritus, dyspnea, bronchospasm

Administer:

PO

• On empty stomach

• With full glass of H_2O to maintain adequate hydration; increase fluids to 2 L/day to decrease crystallization in kidneys

• Medication after C&S; repeat C&S after full course of medication

Perform/provide:

• Storage in tight, light-resistant container at room temperature

Evaluate:

• Therapeutic response: absence of pain, fever, C&S negative

Teach patient/family:

• To take each oral dose with full glass of H_2O to prevent crystalluria

• To complete full course of treatment to prevent superinfection

• To avoid sunlight or use sunscreen to prevent burns

• To avoid OTC medication (aspirin, vit C) unless directed by prescriber

◆ To notify prescriber of skin rash, sore throat, fever, mouth sores, unusual bruising, bleeding

---

sulfasalazine (Ɍ)

(sul-fa-sal′a-zeen)
Azulfidine, Azulfidine EN-tabs, PMS-Sulfasalazine*, S.A.S.*, Salazopyrin*, sulfasalazine
Func. class.: Antiinflammatory
Chem. class.: Sulfonamide

Action: Prodrug to deliver sulfapyridine and 5-aminosalicylic acid to colon; antiinflammatory in connective tissue also

Uses: Ulcerative colitis; rheumatoid arthritis in patients who inadequately respond to or are intolerant of analgesics/NSAIDs; juvenile, rheumatoid arthritis (Azulfidine EN-tabs)

Investigational uses: Ankylosing spondylitis, Crohn's disease, psoriasis

Dosage and routes:

Bowel disease

• *Adult:* PO 3-4 g/day in divided doses; maintenance 2 g/day in divided doses q6h

• *Child >2 yr:* PO 40-60 mg/kg/day in 4-6 divided doses, then 30 mg/kg/day in 4 doses, max 2 g/day

Rheumatoid arthritis

• *Adult:* PO 2g/day in evenly divided doses, initiate treatment with a lower dose of enteric-coated tab

• *Child ≥2 yr:* PO 30 mg/kg/24 hr, divided into 4 doses

Renal dose

• CrCl 10-30 ml/min give bid; CrCl <10 ml/min give qd

Available forms: Tabs 500 mg; oral susp 250 mg/5 ml; tabs, del rel 500 mg

Side effects/adverse reactions:

SYST: Anaphylaxis

GI: Nausea, vomiting, abdominal pain, stomatitis, ***hepatitis,*** glossitis, pancreatitis, diarrhea

CNS: Headache, confusion, insomnia, hallucinations, depression, vertigo, fatigue, anxiety, ***convulsions,*** drug fever, chills

*HEMA: **Leukopenia, neutropenia, thrombocytopenia, agranulocytosis, hemolytic anemia***

INTEG: Rash, dermatitis, urticaria, ***Stevens-Johnson syndrome,*** erythema, photosensitivity

*GU: **Renal failure, toxic nephrosis,*** increased BUN, creatinine, crystalluria

*CV: **Allergic myocarditis***

Contraindications: Hypersensitivity to sulfonamides or salicylates,

---

◆ = Nursing alert   🌿 = Herb-drug interaction   🚫 = Do not crush

pregnancy at term, child <2 yr, intestinal, urinary obstruction

Precautions: Pregnancy (C), lactation, impaired hepatic function, severe allergy, bronchial asthma, impaired renal function

Do not confuse:
sulfasalazine/sulfisoxazole

Pharmacokinetics:
PO: Partially absorbed, peak 1½-6 hr, duration 6-12 hr, half-life 6 hr, excreted in urine as sulfasalazine (15%), sulfapyridine (60%), 5-aminosalicylic acid and metabolites (20%-33%), in breast milk; crosses placenta

Interactions:
• Decreased absorption of digoxin
• Increased hypoglycemic response: oral hypoglycemics
• Increased anticoagulant effects: oral anticoagulants
• Decreased renal excretion of methotrexate
• Decreased hepatic clearance of phenytoin
• Drug/food: decreased iron/folic acid absorption

Lab test interferences:
False positive: Urinary glucose test

NURSING CONSIDERATIONS
Assess:
• Kidney function studies: BUN, creatinine, urinalysis (long-term therapy)
• Blood dyscrasias: skin rash, fever, sore throat, bruising, bleeding, fatigue, joint pain; monitor CBC before and q3mo
• Allergic reaction: rash, dermatitis, urticaria, pruritus, dyspnea, bronchospasm

Administer:
• With full glass of H_2O to maintain adequate hydration; increase fluids to 2 L/day to decrease crystallization in kidneys

• Total daily dose in evenly spaced doses and after meals to help minimize GI intolerance

Perform/provide:
• Storage in tight, light-resistant container at room temperature

Evaluate:
• Therapeutic response: absence of fever, mucus in stools, pain in joints

Teach patient/family:
• To take each oral dose with full glass of H_2O to prevent crystalluria
• That contact lens, urine/skin may be yellow-orange
• To avoid sunlight or use sunscreen to prevent burns
• To notify prescriber of skin rash, sore throat, fever, mouth sores, unusual bruising, bleeding

---

sulfinpyrazone (℞)
(sul-fin-peer'a-zone)
Anturan*, Anturane, sulfinpyrazone
Func. class.: Uricosuric
Chem. class.: Pyrazolone

Action: Inhibits tubular reabsorption of urates, with increased excretion of uric acid; inhibits prostaglandin synthesis, which decreases platelet aggregation

Uses: Inhibition of platelet aggregation, gout

Dosage and routes:
Inhibition of platelet aggregation
• *Adult:* **PO** 200 mg qid
Gout/gouty arthritis
• *Adult:* **PO** 100-200 mg bid × 1 wk, then 200-400 mg bid, not to exceed 800 mg/day

Available forms: Tabs 100 mg; caps 200 mg

Side effects/adverse reactions:
CNS: Dizziness, ***convulsions, coma***
EENT: Tinnitus
GU: Renal calculi, hypoglycemia

*GI: Gastric irritation, nausea, vomiting, anorexia, **hepatic necrosis, GI bleeding***
INTEG: Rash, dermatitis, pruritus, fever, photosensitivity
*HEMA: **Agranulocytosis*** (rare)
*RESP: **Apnea,*** irregular respirations
Contraindications: Hypersensitivity to pyrazolone derivatives, blood dyscrasias, CrCl <50 ml/min, active peptic ulcer, GI inflammation
Precautions: Pregnancy (C)
Pharmacokinetics:
PO: Peak 1-2 hr, duration 4-6 hr, half-life 4 hr; metabolized by liver, excreted in urine
Interactions:
• Increased toxicity: acetaminophen
• Increased effects of: warfarin, tolbutamide
• Decreased effects of: verapamil, theophylline
• Decreased effects of sulfinpyrazone: salicylates, niacin
Lab test interferences:
Increase: PSP, aminohippuric acid
False positive: Clinitest
NURSING CONSIDERATIONS
Assess:
• Uric acid levels (3-7 mg/dl); joint mobility, pain, swelling
• Respiratory rate, rhythm, depth; notify prescriber of abnormalities
• Renal function
• Bleeding tendencies, RBC, Hct
• I&O
• Electrolytes, CO_2 before, during treatment
• Urine pH, output, glucose during beginning treatment
Administer:
• With glass of milk
• With food for GI symptoms
• Increased fluids to prevent calculi; alkalinization of urine may be required
Evaluate:
• Therapeutic response: absence of pain, stiffness in joints

Teach patient/family:
• To avoid aspirin, alcohol, high-purine diet

---

sulfisoxazole (℞)

(sul-fi-sox′a-zole)
Gantrisin, Novo-Soxazole*, sulfisoxazole, Gantrisin Pediatric
Func. class.: Antiinfective
Chem. class.: Sulfonamide, short acting

Action: Interferes with bacterial biosynthesis of proteins by competitive antagonism of PABA
Uses: Urinary tract, systemic infections; chancroid; trachoma; toxoplasmosis; acute otitis media, malaria, *Haemophilus influenzae* meningitis, meningococcal meningitis, nocardiosis, eye infections
Dosage and routes:
UTIs, other systemic infections
• *Adult:* **PO** 2-4 g loading dose, then 1-2 g qid × 7-10 days
• *Child >2 mo:* **PO** 75 mg/kg or 2 g/m² loading dose, then 120-150 mg/kg/day or 4 g/m²/day in divided doses q6h, not to exceed 6 g/day
Chlamydia trachomatis
• *Adult:* **PO** 500 mg-1 g qid × 3 wk
Renal dose
• CrCl 10-50 ml/min give q8-12h; CrCl <10 ml/min give q12-24h
Available forms: Tabs 500 mg; liquid 500 mg/5 ml
Side effects/adverse reactions:
*SYST: **Anaphylaxis***
GI: Nausea, vomiting, abdominal pain, stomatitis, ***hepatitis,*** glossitis, pancreatitis, diarrhea, ***enterocolitis,*** anorexia
CNS: Headache, insomnia, hallucinations, depression, vertigo, fatigue, anxiety, ***convulsions,*** drug fever, chills, drowsiness

---

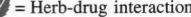

HEMA: ***Leukopenia, thrombocytopenia, agranulocytosis, hemolytic anemia, aplastic anemia***
INTEG: Rash, dermatitis, urticaria, ***Stevens-Johnson syndrome,*** erythema, photosensitivity, alopecia
GU: ***Renal failure, toxic nephrosis,*** increased BUN, creatinine, crystalluria, hematuria, proteinuria
CV: ***Allergic myocarditis***

Contraindications: Hypersensitivity to sulfonamides and sulfonylureas, thiazide and loop diuretics, salicylates; sunscreen with PABA, lactation, infants < 2 mo (except congenital toxoplasmosis), pregnancy at term, porphyria

Precautions: Pregnancy (B), lactation, impaired hepatic/renal function, severe allergy, bronchial asthma

Do not confuse:
sulfisoxazole/sulfasalazine

Pharmacokinetics:
PO: Rapidly absorbed, peak 2-4 hr, 85% protein bound; half-life 4-7 hr, excreted in urine, crosses placenta

Interactions:
• Increased effects of: barbiturates, tolbutamide, uricosurics
• Increased drug-free concentrations: indomethacin, probenecid, salicylates
• Increased thrombocytopenia: thiazides
• Increased nephrotoxicity: cyclosporine
• Increased hypoglycemic response: sulfonylurea agents
• Increased anticoagulant effect: warfarin
• Decreased renal excretion of methotrexate
• Decreased hepatic clearance of phenytoin

Lab test interferences:
False positive: Urinary glucose test

NURSING CONSIDERATIONS
Assess:
• I&O ratio; note color, charac-

ter, pH of urine if drug administered for UTIs; output should be 800 ml less than intake; if urine is highly acidic, alkalization may be needed
• Renal function studies: BUN, creatinine, urinalysis (long-term therapy)
• Blood dyscrasias: skin rash, fever, sore throat, bruising, bleeding, fatigue, joint pain, monitor CBC before and periodically
• Allergic reaction: rash, dermatitis, urticaria, pruritus, dyspnea, bronchospasm

Administer:
• On an empty stomach
• With full glass of H_2O to maintain adequate hydration; increase fluids to 2 L/day to decrease crystallization in kidneys
• Medication after C&S; repeat C&S after full course of medication

Perform/provide:
• Storage in tight, light-resistant container at room temperature

Evaluate:
• Therapeutic response: absence of pain, fever, C&S negative

Teach patient/family:
• To take each oral dose with full glass of H_2O to prevent crystalluria
• To complete full course of treatment to prevent superinfection
• To avoid sunlight or use sunscreen to prevent burns; avoid hazardous activities if dizziness occurs
• To avoid OTC medication (aspirin, vit C) unless directed by prescriber
• To notify prescriber of skin rash, sore throat, fever, mouth sores, unusual bruising, bleeding

Side effects: *italics* = common; ***bold italics*** = life-threatening

sulindac (R)

(sul-in'dak)

Apo-Sulin*, Clinoril , NovoSundac*, sulindac

Func. class.: Nonsteroidal antiinflammatory

Chem. class.: Indeneacetic acid derivative

Action: Inhibits prostaglandin synthesis by decreasing an enzyme needed for biosynthesis; analgesic, antiinflammatory, antipyretic

Uses: Mild to moderate pain, osteoarthritis; rheumatoid, gouty arthritis; ankylosing spondylitis

Dosage and routes:

Arthritis

• *Adult:* **PO** 150 mg bid, may increase to 200 mg bid

Bursitis/acute arthritis

• *Adult:* **PO** 200 mg bid × 1-2 wk, then reduce dose

Available forms: Tabs 150, 200 mg

Side effects/adverse reactions:

GI: Nausea, anorexia, vomiting, diarrhea, jaundice, **cholestatic hepatitis,** constipation, flatulence, cramps, dry mouth, peptic ulcer, **bleeding, ulceration, perforation**

CNS: Dizziness, drowsiness, fatigue, tremors, confusion, insomnia, anxiety, depression, headache

CV: Tachycardia, peripheral edema, palpitations, dysrhythmias

INTEG: Purpura, *rash, pruritus,* sweating, photosensitivity

GU: Nephrotoxicity: dysuria, hematuria, oliguria, azotemia

HEMA: Blood dyscrasias with prolonged use

EENT: Tinnitus, hearing loss, blurred vision

Contraindications: Hypersensitivity, asthma, severe renal disease, severe hepatic disease, active ulcers

Precautions: Pregnancy (C), lactation, children, bleeding disorders, GI disorders, cardiac disorders, hypersensitivity to other antiinflammatory agents, renal disease

Do not confuse:

Clinoril/Clozaril

Clinoril/Oruvail

Pharmacokinetics:

PO: Peak 2 hr, half-life 3-3½ hr; metabolized in liver; excreted in urine (metabolites), breast milk; 93% protein binding

Interactions:

• Increased risk of bleeding: anticoagulants

• Increased nephrotoxicity: cyclosporine

• Decreased sulindac effect: diflunisal, do not use together

• Increased toxicity: methotrexate, sulfonamides, sulfonylureas, probenecid

• GI side effects: aspirin

NURSING CONSIDERATIONS

Assess:

• Pain: frequency, intensity, characteristics, relief after med

• Asthma, aspirin hypersensitivity, nasal polyps; increased hypersensitivity

• Renal, liver, blood studies: BUN, creatinine, AST, ALT, Hgb, before treatment, periodically thereafter

• Have B/P checked qmo; drug causes Na retention

• Audiometric, ophthalmic exam before, during, after treatment

• For eye, ear problems: blurred vision, tinnitus may indicate toxicity

Administer:

• With food to decrease GI symptoms; take on empty stomach to facilitate absorption; tablet may be crushed

Perform/provide:

• Storage at room temperature

 = Nursing alert　　 = Herb-drug interaction　　⊘ = Do not crush

Evaluate:

- Therapeutic response: decreased pain, stiffness, swelling in joints, ability to move more easily

Teach patient/family:

- To report blurred vision or ringing, roaring in ears (may indicate toxicity)
- To avoid driving, other hazardous activities if dizzy or drowsy
- To report change in urine pattern, weight increase, edema, pain increase in joints, fever, blood in urine (indicates nephrotoxicity)
- That therapeutic effects may take up to 1 mo
- To avoid alcohol and aspirin
- To take with full glass of water
- To use sunscreen

---

sumatriptan (R)

(soo-ma-trip′tan)
Imitrex
Func. class.: Antimigraine agent
Chem. class.: 5-HT$_1$ receptor agonist

Action: Binds selectively to the vascular 5-HT$_1$ receptor subtype, exerts antimigraine effect; causes vasoconstriction in cranial arteries

Uses: Acute treatment of migraine with or without aura and cluster headache

Dosage and routes:

- *Adult:* **SC** 6 mg or less; may repeat in 1 hr; not to exceed 12 mg/24 hr; **PO** 25 mg with fluids, max 100 mg; **NASAL** one dose of 5, 10, or 20 mg in one nostril, may repeat in 2 hr, max 40 mg/24 hr

Hepatic dose

- *Adult:* **PO** 25 mg, if no response after 2 hr, give up to 50 mg

Available forms: Inj 12 mg/ml; tabs 25, 50, 100 mg, nasal spray 5 mg/ 100 mcl-U dose spray device, 20 mg/100 mcl-U

Side effects/adverse reactions:

NEURO: Tingling, hot sensation, burning, feeling of pressure, tightness, numbness, dizziness, sedation, headache, anxiety, fatigue, cold sensation
CV: Flushing, **MI**
RESP: Chest tightness, pressure
EENT: Throat, mouth, nasal discomfort; vision changes
GI: Abdominal discomfort
MS: Weakness, neck stiffness, myalgia
INTEG: Inj site reaction, sweating

Contraindications: Angina pectoris, history of MI, documented silent ischemia, Prinzmetal's angina, ischemic heart disease, IV use, concurrent ergotamine-containing preparations, uncontrolled hypertension, hypersensitivity, basilar or hemiplegic migraine

Precautions: Postmenopausal women, men >40 yr, risk factors for CAD, hypercholesterolemia, obesity, diabetes, impaired hepatic or renal function, pregnancy (C), lactation, children, elderly

Pharmacokinetics: Onset of pain relief 10 min-2 hr, peak 10-20 min, 10%-20% plasma protein binding, metabolized in the liver (metabolite), excreted in urine, feces

Interactions:

- Extended vasospastic effects: ergot, ergot derivatives
- Increased sumatriptan effect: MAOIs, SSRIs

NURSING CONSIDERATIONS

Assess:

- B/P; signs/symptoms of coronary vasospasms
- Tingling, hot sensation, burning, feeling of pressure, numbness, flushing, inj site reaction
- For stress level, activity, recreation, coping mechanisms

• Neurologic status: LOC, blurring vision, nausea, vomiting, tingling in extremities preceding headache
• Ingestion of tyramine foods (pickled products, beer, wine, aged cheese), food additives, preservatives, colorings, artificial sweeteners, chocolate, caffeine, which may precipitate these types of headaches

Administer:
• SC only just below the skin; avoid IM or IV administration, use only for actual migraine attack

🚫 PO, swallow whole; take with fluids as soon as symptoms appear; may take a second dose >4 hr; max 200 mg/24 hr

Perform/provide:
• Quiet, calm environment with decreased stimulation for noise, bright light, excessive talking

Evaluate:
• Therapeutic response: decrease in frequency, severity of migraine

Teach patient/family:
• To report chest pain, tightness; sudden, severe abdominal pain to prescriber immediately
• To use contraception while taking drug
• To use nasal spray: one spray in one nostril, may repeat if headache returns, do not repeat if pain continues after 1st dose
• To have dark, quiet environment

---

tacrine (℞)
(tack'rin)
Cognex
Func. class.: Reversible cholinesterase inhibitor

Action: Elevates acetylcholine concentrations (cerebral cortex) by slowing degradation of acetylcholine released in cholinergic neurons; does not alter underlying dementia

Uses: Treatment of mild to moderate dementia in Alzheimer's disease
Dosage and routes:
• *Adult:* **PO** 10 mg qid × 6 wk, then 20 mg qid × 6 wk, increase at 6-wk intervals if patient tolerating drug well and if transaminase is WNL
Available forms: Caps 10, 20, 30, 40 mg
Side effects/adverse reactions:
CNS: Dizziness, confusion, insomnia, tremor, *ataxia, somnolence, anxiety, agitation, depression, hallucinations, hostility, abnormal thinking,* chills, fever
CV: Hypotension or hypertension
GI: Nausea, vomiting, anorexia, abdominal pain, constipation, dyspepsia, flatulence, ***hepatotoxicity, GI bleeding***
GU: Urinary frequency, UTI, incontinence
INTEG: Rash, flushing
RESP: Rhinitis, URI, cough, pharyngitis
Contraindications: Hypersensitivity to this drug or acridine derivatives, patients treated with this drug who developed jaundice with a total bilirubin of >3 mg/dl
Precautions: Sick sinus syndrome, history of ulcers, GI bleeding, hepatic disease, bladder obstruction, asthma, pregnancy (C), lactation, children, seizure disorders
Do not confuse:
Cognex/Corgard
Pharmacokinetics: Rapidly absorbed PO, 55% bound to plasma proteins, extensively metabolized to metabolites, elimination half-life 2-4 hr
Interactions:
• Decreased activity of anticholinergics
• Increased levels of tacrine: cimetidine
• Increased elimination half-life of theophylline

◆ = Nursing alert   🌿 = Herb-drug interaction   🚫 = Do not crush

• Synergistic effect: succinylcholine, cholinesterase inhibitors, cholinergic agonists

NURSING CONSIDERATIONS
Assess:
• B/P: hypotension, hypertension
• Mental status: affect, mood, behavioral changes, depression; complete suicide assessment; hallucinations, confusion
• GI status: nausea, vomiting, anorexia, constipation, abdominal pain; add bulk, increase fluids for constipation
• GU status: urinary frequency, incontinence
• Serum ALT qo wk × 4-16 wk, then q3mo
Administer:
• Between meals; may be given with meals for GI symptoms
• Dosage adjusted to response no more than q6wk
Perform/provide:
• Assistance with ambulation during beginning therapy; dizziness, ataxia may occur
Evaluate:
• Therapeutic response: decrease in confusion, improved mood
Teach patient/family:
• To report side effects: twitching, eye spasms; indicate overdose
• To use drug exactly as prescribed: at regular intervals, preferably between meals; may be taken with meals for GI upset; drug is not a cure
• To notify prescriber of nausea, vomiting, diarrhea (dose increase or beginning treatment), or rash; very dark or very light stools, jaundice (delayed onset)
• Not to increase or abruptly decrease dose; serious consequences may result
Treatment of overdose: Withdraw drug, administer tertiary anticholinergics, provide supportive care

tacrolimus (℞)
(tak-roe-li′mus)
Prograf
Func. class.: Immunosuppressant
Chem. class.: Macrolide

Action: Produces immunosuppression by inhibiting T-lymphocytes
Uses: Organ transplants to prevent rejection
Dosage and routes:
• *Adult and child:* **IV** 0.03-0.05 mg/kg/day × 3 days then **PO** 0.15 mg/kg bid; adjust dose in renal impairment
Available forms: Inj 5 mg/ml; caps 1, 5 mg
Side effects/adverse reactions:
*HEMA: **Anemia, leukocytosis, thrombocytopenia, purpura***
GI: Nausea, vomiting, diarrhea, constipation, *GI bleeding*
CV: Hypertension
CNS: Tremors, headache, insomnia, paresthesia, chills, fever
GU: UTIs, ***albuminuria, hematuria, proteinuria, renal failure***
META: Hirsutism, hyperglycemia, hyperkalemia, hyperuricemia, hypokalemia, hypomagnesemia
*RESP: **Pleural effusion, atelectasis,*** dyspnea
INTEG: Rash, flushing, itching, alopecia
EENT: Blurred vision, photophobia
*SYST: **Anaphylaxis***
Contraindications: Hypersensitivity to this drug or to some kinds of castor oil
Precautions: Severe renal, hepatic disease; pregnancy (C), diabetes mellitus, hyperkalemia, hyperuricemia, lymphomas, lactation, children <12, hypertension
Pharmacokinetics: Extensively metabolized, half-life 10 hr, 75% protein binding

T

Interactions:
• Increased toxicity: aminoglycosides, cisplatin, cyclosporine
• Increased blood levels: antifungals, calcium channel blockers, cimetidine, danazol, erythromycin
• Decreased blood levels: carbamazepine, phenobarbital, phenytoin, rifamycin
• Decreased effect of: vaccines

NURSING CONSIDERATIONS
Assess:
• Blood studies: Hgb, WBC, platelets during treatment qmo; if leukocytes <3000/mm³ or platelets <100,000/mm³, drug should be discontinued or reduced; decreased hemoglobulin level may indicate bone marrow suppression
• Liver function studies: alk phosphatase, AST, ALT, amylase, bilirubin, and for hepatotoxicity: dark urine, jaundice, itching, light-colored stools; drug should be discontinued

Administer:
• All medications PO if possible, avoiding IM injections; bleeding may occur
• With meals to reduce GI upset; nausea is common
• For several days before transplant surgery; patients should be placed in protective isolation

IV
• After diluting in 0.9% NaCl or D₅W to 0.004 to 0.02 mg/ml as a continuous infusion

Additive compatibilities: Cimetidine

Y-site compatibilities: Acyclovir, aminophylline, amphotericin B, ampicillin, ampicillin/sulbactam, benztropine, calcium gluconate, cefazolin, cefotetan, ceftazidime, ceftriaxone, cefuroxime, chloramphenicol, cimetidine, ciprofloxacin, clindamycin, dexamethasone, digoxin, diphenhydramine, dobutamine, dopamine, doxycycline, erythromycin, esmolol, fluconazole, furosemide, ganciclovir, gentamicin, haloperidol, heparin, hydrocortisone, imipenem/cilastatin, insulin (regular), isoproterenol, leucovorin, lorazepam, methylprednisolone, metoclopramide, metronidazole, mezlocillin, multivitamins, nitroglycerin, oxacillin, penicillin G potassium, perphenazine, phenytoin, piperacillin, potassium chloride, propranolol, ranitidine, sodium bicarbonate, sodium nitroprusside, trimethoprimsulfamethoxazole, vancomycin

Evaluate:
• Therapeutic response: absence of graft rejection; immunosuppression in autoimmune disorders

Teach patient/family:
• To report fever, rash, severe diarrhea, chills, sore throat, fatigue; serious infections may occur; clay-colored stools, cramping (hepatotoxicity)
• To avoid crowds, persons with known infections to reduce risk of infection

---

tamoxifen (℞)
(ta-mox'i-fen)
Alpha-Tamoxifen*, Med Tamoxifen*, Nolvadex, Nolvadex-D*, Novo-Tamoxifen*, Tamofen*, Tamone*, Tamoplex*
Func. class.: Antineoplastic
Chem. class.: Antiestrogen hormone

Action: Inhibits cell division by binding to cytoplasmic estrogen receptors; resembles normal cell complex but inhibits DNA synthesis and estrogen response of target tissue
Uses: Advanced breast carcinoma not responsive to other therapy in estrogen-receptor-positive patients

---

 = Nursing alert   = Herb-drug interaction   = Do not crush

(usually postmenopausal), prevention of breast cancer, following breast surgery/radiation in ductal carcinoma in situ

Investigational uses: Mastalgia, to reduce pain/size of gynecomastia

Dosage and routes:

Breast cancer
• *Adult:* **PO** 20-40 mg qd; doses >20 mg/day, divide AM/PM

High risk for breast cancer
• *Adult:* **PO** 20 mg qd × 5 yr

DCIS
• *Adult:* **PO** 20 mg qd × 5 yr

Available forms: Tabs 10, 20 mg

Side effects/adverse reactions:

*HEMA: **Thrombocytopenia, leukopenia,** DVT, PE*

GI: Nausea, vomiting, altered taste (anorexia)

GU: Vaginal bleeding, pruritus vulvae

INTEG: Rash, alopecia

CV: Chest pain

CNS: Hot flashes, headache, lightheadedness, depression

META: Hypercalcemia

EENT: Ocular lesions, retinopathy, corneal opacity, blurred vision (high doses)

Contraindications: Hypersensitivity, pregnancy (D)

Precautions: Leukopenia, thrombocytopenia, lactation, cataracts

Pharmacokinetics:

PO: Peak 4-7 hr, half-life 7 days (1 wk terminal), excreted primarily in feces

Interactions:
• Increased chance of bleeding: anticoagulants
• Increased tamoxifen levels: bromocriptine
• Increased thromboembolic events: cytotoxics

Lab test interferences:
Increase: Serum Ca

NURSING CONSIDERATIONS
Assess:
• CBC, differential, platelet count qwk; withhold drug if WBC is <3500 or platelet count is <100,000; notify prescriber
• Bleeding q8h: hematuria, guaiac, bruising, petechiae, mucosa or orifices
• Food preferences; list likes, dislikes
• Effects of alopecia on body image; discuss feelings about body changes
◆ Symptoms indicating severe allergic reactions: rash, pruritus, urticaria, purpuric skin lesions, itching, flushing

Administer:
• Antacid before oral agent; give drug after evening meal, before bedtime
• Antiemetic 30-60 min before giving drug to prevent vomiting

Perform/provide:
• Liquid diet, if needed, including cola, Jell-O; dry toast or crackers may be added if patient is not nauseated or vomiting
• Increase fluid intake to 2-3 L/day to prevent dehydration
• Nutritious diet with iron, vitamin supplements as ordered
• Storage in light-resistant container at room temperature

Evaluate:
• Therapeutic response: decreased tumor size, spread of malignancy

Teach patient/family:
• To report any complaints, side effects to prescriber
• To increase fluids to 2 L/day unless contraindicated
• To wear sun screen, protective clothing, sunglasses
• That vaginal bleeding, pruritus, hot flashes are reversible after discontinuing treatment

• To report immediately decreased visual acuity, which may be irreversible; stress need for routine eye exams; care providers should be told about tamoxifen therapy

• To report vaginal bleeding immediately

• That tumor flare—increase in size of tumor, increased bone pain—may occur and will subside rapidly; may take analgesics for pain

• That premenopausal women must use mechanical birth control because ovulation may be induced

• That hair may be lost during treatment; a wig or hairpiece may make patient feel better; new hair may be different in color, texture

---

tamsulosin (℞)

(tam-sue-lo'sen)
Flomax
Func. class.: Selective α_1-adrenergic blocker
Chem. class.: Sulfamoylphenethylamine derivative

Action: Binds preferentially to α_{1A}-adrenoceptor subtype located mainly in the prostate

Uses: Symptoms of benign prostatic hyperplasia

Dosage and routes:

• *Adult:* PO 0.4 mg qd, increasing up to 0.8 mg qd if required

Available forms: Caps 0.4 mg

Side effects/adverse reactions:

CV: Chest pain

CNS: Dizziness, headache, asthenia

GI: Nausea, diarrhea

GU: Decreased libido, abnormal ejaculation

EENT: Amblyopia

MS: Back pain

RESP: Rhinitis, pharyngitis, cough

Contraindications: Hypersensitivity

Precautions: Pregnancy (C), children, lactation, hepatic disease, coronary artery disease, severe renal disease

Pharmacokinetics:

PO: Onset 2 hr, peak 2-6 hr, duration 6-12 hr; half-life 9-15 hr; metabolized in liver; excreted via urine; extensively protein bound (98%)

Interactions:

• Not to be taken with: prazosin, terazosin, doxazosin

NURSING CONSIDERATIONS
Assess:

• Prostatic hyperplasia: change in urinary patterns, baseline and throughout treatment

• CBC with diff and liver function studies; B/P and heart rate

• BUN, uric acid, urodynamic studies (urinary flow rates, residual volume)

• I&O ratios, weight qd, edema, report weight gain or edema

Administer:

PO

🚫 Whole; do not chew or crush tablets; may be given with food

Perform/provide:

• Storage in tight container in cool environment

Evaluate:

• Therapeutic response: decreased symptoms of benign prostatic hyperplasia

Teach patient/family:

• Not to drive or operate machinery for 4 hr after first dose or after dosage increase

---

⬥ = Nursing alert   🌿 = Herb-drug interaction   🚫 = Do not crush

telmisartan (Ŗ)

(tel-mih-sar'tan)
Micardis
Func. class.: Antihypertensive
Chem. class.: Angiotensin II receptor (Type AT_1)

Action: blocks the vasoconstrictor and aldosterone-secreting effects of angiotensin II; selectively blocks the binding of angiotensin II to the AT_1 receptor found in tissues

Uses: Hypertension, alone or in combination

Investigational uses: Heart failure

Research note: Telmisartan administered with digoxin resulted in an increased digoxin level[38]

Dosage and routes:
• *Adult:* **PO** 40 mg qd; range 20-80 mg

Available forms: Tabs 40, 80 mg

Side effects/adverse reactions:
CNS: Dizziness, insomnia, *anxiety*
GI: Diarrhea, dyspepsia, *anorexia, vomiting*
MS: Myalgia, pain
RESP: Cough, *upper respiratory infection*

Contraindications: Hypersensitivity, pregnancy (D) 2nd and 3rd trimesters

Precautions: Hypersensitivity to ACE inhibitors: pregnancy (C) 1st trimester, lactation, children, elderly

Pharmacokinetics: Extensively metabolized, terminal half-life 24 hr, highly bound to plasma proteins, excreted in urine and feces

Interactions:
• Increased digoxin peak concentrations, and in trough concentrations: digoxin
• Decreased antihypertensive action: NSAIDs, barbiturates
• Increased antihypertensive action: diuretics, other antihypertensives

NURSING CONSIDERATIONS
Assess:
• B/P, pulse q4h; note rate, rhythm, quality
• Electrolytes: K, Na, Cl
• Baselines in renal, liver function tests before therapy begins
• Edema in feet, legs qd
• Skin turgor, dryness of mucous membranes for hydration status
Administer:
• Without regard to meals
• Increased dose to black patients, B/P response may be reduced
Evaluate:
• Therapeutic response: decreased B/P
Teach patient/family:
• To comply with dosage schedule, even if feeling better
• To notify prescriber of mouth sores, fever, swelling of hands or feet, irregular heartbeat, chest pain
• That excessive perspiration, dehydration, vomiting, diarrhea may lead to fall in blood pressure; consult prescriber if these occur
• That drug may cause dizziness, fainting; light-headedness may occur
• To use contraception while taking this drug
• To notify prescriber of all prescriptions, OTC, and supplements taken

temazepam (Ŗ)

T

(te-maz'e-pam)
Razepam, Restoril, temazepam
Func. class.: Sedative-hypnotic
Chem. class.: Benzodiazepine

Controlled Substance Schedule IV (USA), Schedule F (Canada)

Action: Produces CNS depression at limbic, thalamic, hypothalamic levels of the CNS; may be mediated by neurotransmitter γ-aminobutyric

---

acid (GABA); results are sedation, hypnosis, skeletal muscle relaxation, anticonvulsant activity, anxiolytic action

Uses: Insomnia

Dosage and routes:
• *Adult:* **PO** 15-30 mg hs
• *Geriatric:* **PO** 7.5 mg hs

Available forms: Caps 7.5, 15, 30 mg

Side effects/adverse reactions:
HEMA: **Leukopenia, granulocytopenia** (rare)

CNS: Lethargy, drowsiness, daytime sedation, dizziness, confusion, lightheadedness, headache, anxiety, irritability

GI: Nausea, vomiting, diarrhea, heartburn, abdominal pain, constipation, anorexia

CV: Chest pain, pulse changes

Contraindications: Hypersensitivity to benzodiazepines, pregnancy (X), lactation, intermittent porphyria

Precautions: Anemia, hepatic disease, renal disease, suicidal individuals, drug abuse, elderly, psychosis, children <15 yr, acute narrow-angle glaucoma, seizure disorders

Pharmacokinetics:
PO: Onset 30-45 min, duration 6-8 hr, half-life 10-20 hr; metabolized by liver, excreted by kidneys, crosses placenta, excreted in breast milk

Interactions:
• Increased effects of cimetidine, disulfiram, oral contraceptives
• Increased action of both drugs: alcohol, CNS depressants
• Decreased effect of antacids, theophylline, rifampin
⚕ Increased CNS depression: kava

Lab test interferences:
Increase: ALT, AST, serum bilirubin
Decrease: RAI uptake
False increase: Urinary 17-OHCS

NURSING CONSIDERATIONS
Assess:
• Blood studies: Hct, Hgb, RBCs (long-term therapy)
• Hepatic studies: AST, ALT, bilirubin (long-term therapy)
• Mental status: mood, sensorium, affect, memory (long, short)
• Blood dyscrasias: fever, sore throat, bruising, rash, jaundice, epistaxis (rare)
• Type of sleep problem: falling asleep, staying asleep

Administer:
• After removal of cigarettes to prevent fires
• After trying conservative measures for insomnia
• ½-1 hr before hs for sleeplessness
• On empty stomach for fast onset, but may be taken with food if GI symptoms occur

Perform/provide:
• Assistance with ambulation after receiving dose
• Safety measures: night-light, call bell within easy reach
• Checking to see if PO medication has been swallowed
• Storage in tight container in cool environment

Evaluate:
• Therapeutic response: ability to sleep at night, decreased early morning awakening if taking drug for insomnia

Teach patient/family:
• To avoid driving, other activities requiring alertness until stabilized
• To avoid alcohol ingestion, CNS depressants; serious CNS depression may result
• That effects may take 2 nights for benefits to be noticed
• Alternative measures to improve sleep: reading, exercise several hours before hs, warm bath, warm milk, TV, self-hypnosis, deep breathing

---

◆ = Nursing alert   ⚕ = Herb-drug interaction   ⊘ = Do not crush

• That hangover, memory impairment are common in elderly but less common than with barbiturates

• To use contraception while taking this product

Treatment of overdose: Lavage, activated charcoal; monitor electrolytes, VS

---

temozolomide (℞)

(tem-oh-zole'oh-mide)

Temodar

Func. class.: Antineoplastic-alkylating agent

Chem. class.: Imidazotetrazine derivative

Action: A prodrug that undergoes conversion to MTIC. MTIC action prevents DNA transcription

Uses: Anaplastic astrocytoma with relapse

Dosage and routes:

• *Adult:* PO Adjust dose based on nadir neutrophil and platelet counts 150 mg/m^2/day × 5 days during a 28-day cycle

Available forms: Caps 5, 20, 100, 250 mg

Side effects/adverse reactions:

HEMA: ***Thrombocytopenia, leukopenia,*** anemia

GI: *Nausea, anorexia, vomiting*

CNS: ***Seizures,*** *hemiparesis, dizziness, poor coordination, amnesia, insomnia, paresthesia, somnolence, paresis, ataxia, anxiety, dysphagia, depression, confusion*

INTEG: *Rash, pruritus*

GU: Urinary incontinence, UTI, frequency

RESP: URI, pharyngitis, sinusitis, coughing

MISC: Headache, fatigue, asthenia, fever, edema, back pain, weight increase, diplopia

Contraindications: Hypersensitivity to this drug or carbazine, pregnancy (D), lactation

Precautions: Radiation therapy, renal, hepatic disease

Pharmacokinetics: Absorption complete, rapid; crosses blood-brain barrier, excreted urine/feces, half-life 1.8 hr, peak 1 hr

Interactions:

• Increased myelosuppression: radiation, other antineoplastics

• Decreased antibody reaction: live virus vaccines

NURSING CONSIDERATIONS

Assess:

• CBC on day 22 (21 days after 1st dose), CBC weekly until recovery if ANC is <1.5 × 10^9/L and platelets <100 × 10^9/L, do not administer to patients that do not tolerate 100 mg/m^2, myelosuppression usually occurs late in the treatment cycle

• For seizures throughout treatment

• Monitor temp q4h (may indicate beginning of infection)

• LFTs before, during therapy (bilirubin, AST, ALT, LDH), as needed or monthly

• Bleeding: hematuria, guaiac, bruising or petechiae, mucosa or orifices q8h

Administer:

• Antiemetic 30-60 min before giving drug to prevent vomiting

🚫 Caps one at a time with 8 oz of water at same time of day; do not open, break, chew

• Fluids IV or PO before chemotherapy to hydrate patient

• Caps should not be opened; if accidentally damaged, do not allow contact with skin, or inhale

• Give on empty stomach to prevent nausea/vomiting

Perform/provide:

• Storage in light-resistant container, dry area

Evaluate:

• Therapeutic response: decreased tumor size, spread of malignancy

Teach patient/family:

• To report signs of infection: fever, sore throat, flulike symptoms

• To report signs of anemia: fatigue, headache, faintness, shortness of breath, irritability

• To report bleeding; avoid use of razors, commercial mouthwash

• To avoid use of aspirin products or ibuprofen

---

tenecteplase (Ⓡ)

(ten-ek′ta-place)

TNKase

Func. class.: Thrombolytic enzyme

Chem. class.: β-Hemolytic streptococcus filtrate (purified)

Action: Activates conversion of plasminogen to plasmin (fibrinolysin): plasmin breaks down clots (fibrin), fibrinogen, factors V, VII; occlusion of venous access lines

Uses: Acute myocardial infarction

Dosage and routes:

• *Adult <60 kg:* **IV BOL** 30 mg, give over 6 sec

• *Adult ≥60-<70 kg:* **IV BOL** 35 mg, give over 7 sec

• *Adult ≥70-<80 kg:* **IV BOL** 40 mg, give over 8 sec

• *Adult ≥80-<90 kg:* **IV BOL** 45 mg, give over 9 sec

• *Adult ≥90 kg:* **IV BOL** 50 mg, give over 10 sec

Available forms: Pwd for inj, lyophilized 50 mg

Side effects/adverse reactions:

CV: Dysrhythmias, hypotension, pulmonary edema, *pulmonary embolism, cardiogenic shock, cardiac arrest, heart failure, myocardial reinfarction, myocardial rupture,*

tamponade, pericarditis, pericardial effusion, thrombosis

HEMA: Decreased Hct, *bleeding*

INTEG: Rash, urticaria, phlebitis at IV inf site, itching, flushing

SYST: **GI, GU, intracranial, retroperitoneal bleeding, surface bleeding, anaphylaxis**

Contraindications: Hypersensitivity, active bleeding, intraspinal surgery, CNS neoplasms, ulcerative colitis, enteritis, severe hypertension, severe renal disease, hepatic disease, hypocoagulation, COPD, subacute bacterial endocarditis, rheumatic valvular disease, cerebral embolism/thrombosis/hemorrhage, intraarterial diagnostic procedure or surgery (10 days), recent major surgery

Precautions: Arterial emboli from left side of heart, pregnancy (C), lactation, children

Pharmacokinetics:

IV: Onset immediate, half-life 20-24 min; metabolized by the liver

Interactions:

• Bleeding potential: aspirin, indomethacin, phenylbutazone, anticoagulants, antithrombolytics

Lab test interferences:

Increase: PT, aPTT, TT

Decrease: Plasminogen, fibrinogen

NURSING CONSIDERATIONS

Assess:

• Allergy: fever, rash, itching, chills; mild reaction may be treated with antihistamines

◆For bleeding during 1st hr of treatment; hematuria, hematemesis, bleeding from mucous membranes, epistaxis, ecchymosis; may require tranfusion (rare), continue to assess for bleeding for 24 hr

• Blood studies (Hct, platelets, PTT, PT, TT, aPTT) before starting therapy; PT or aPTT must be less than 2× control before starting therapy; PTT or PT q3-4h during treatment

---

◆ = Nursing alert   𝕸 = Herb-drug interaction   ⊘ = Do not crush

• For hypersensitive reactions: fever, rash, dyspnea; drug should be discontinued; for streptokinase reactions previously
• VS, B/P, pulse, respirations, neurologic signs, temp at least q4h; temp >104° F (40° C) indicates internal bleeding; cardiac rhythm following intracoronary administration; systolic pressure increase >25 mm Hg should be reported to prescriber
◆ For neurologic changes that may indicate intracranial bleeding
◆ Retroperitoneal bleeding: back pain, leg weakness, diminished pulses
• For respiratory depression

Administer:
IV
• As soon as thrombi identified; not useful for thrombi over 1 wk old
• Cryoprecipitate or fresh frozen plasma if bleeding occurs
• Loading dose at beginning of therapy; may require increased loading doses
• Heparin after fibrinogen level >100 mg/dl; heparin infusion to increase PTT to 1.5-2 × baseline for 3-7 days; IV heparin with loading dose is recommended after discontinuing streptokinase to prevent redevelopment of thrombi
• Aseptically withdraw 10 ml of sterile H_2O for inj from diluent vial, use red cannula syringe-filling device, inject all contents of syringe into drug vial, direct into powder, swirl, withdraw correct dose, discard any unused solution; stand the shield with dose vertically on flat surface and passively recap the red cannula, remove entire shield assembly by twisting counter-clockwise, give by IV BOL
• About 10% patients have high streptococcal antibody titers requiring increased loading doses

• IV therapy: use upper extremity vessel that is accessible to manual compression
Y-site compatibilities: Dobutamine, dopamine, heparin, lidocaine, nitroglycerin
Perform/provide:
• Bed rest during entire course of treatment
• Avoidance of venous or arterial puncture, inj, rectal temp; any invasive treatment
• Treatment of fever with acetaminophen or aspirin
• Pressure for 30 sec to minor bleeding sites; inform prescriber if this does not attain hemostasis; apply pressure dressing
Evaluate:
• Therapeutic response: resolution of myocardial infarction

RARELY USED

teniposide (℞)
(ten-i-poe'side)
Vumon, VM 26
Func. class.: Antineoplastic

Uses: Childhood acute lymphoblastic leukemia (ALL), refractory childhood acute lymphocytic leukemia
Dosage and routes:
• *Child:* IV INF combo teniposide 165 mg/m² and cytarabine 300 mg/m² 2×/wk × 8-9 doses or combo teniposide 250 mg/m² and vincristine 1.5 mg/m² qwk × 4-8 wk and prednisone 40 mg/m² **PO** × 28 days
Contraindications: Hypersensitivity, bone marrow depression, severe hepatic disease, severe renal disease, bacterial infection, pregnancy (D)

tenofovir
See appendix a—selected new drugs

terazosin (℞)
(ter-ay′zoe-sin)
Hytrin
Func. class.: Antihypertensive
Chem. class.: Peripherally acting adrenergic blocker

Action: Decreases total vascular resistance, which is responsible for a decrease in B/P; this occurs by blockade of α_1-adrenoreceptors
Uses: Hypertension, as a single agent or in combination with diuretics or β-blockers, BPH
Dosage and routes:
• *Adult:* **PO** 1 mg hs, may increase dose slowly to desired response; not to exceed 20 mg/day
Available forms: Caps 1, 2, 5, 10 mg
Side effects/adverse reactions:
CV: Palpitations, orthostatic hypotension, tachycardia, edema, rebound hypertension
CNS: Dizziness, headache, drowsiness, anxiety, depression, vertigo, weakness, fatigue
GI: Nausea, vomiting, diarrhea, constipation, abdominal pain
GU: Urinary frequency, incontinence, impotence, priapism
EENT: Blurred vision, epistaxis, tinnitus, dry mouth, red sclera, nasal congestion, sinusitis
RESP: Dyspnea
Contraindications: Hypersensitivity
Precautions: Pregnancy (C), children, lactation
Pharmacokinetics: Peak 1 hr, half-life 9-12 hr, highly bound to plasma proteins; metabolized in liver, excreted in urine, feces

Interactions:
• Increased hypotensive effects: β-blockers, nitroglycerin, verapamil, nifedipine
NURSING CONSIDERATIONS
Assess:
• Urinary symptoms associated with BPH
• Orthostatic B/P, pulse, jugular venous distention q4h
• BUN, uric acid if on long-term therapy
• Weight qd, I&O
• Skin turgor, dryness of mucous membranes for hydration status
• Rales, dyspnea, orthopnea q30min
Perform/provide:
• Cool storage in tight container
Evaluate:
• Therapeutic response: decreased B/P, edema in feet, legs, decreased symptoms of BPH
Teach patient/family:
• That fainting occasionally occurs after first dose; not to drive or operate machinery for 4 hr after first dose or after an increase in dose; or take first dose hs
• To rise slowly from sitting/lying position

terbinafine (℞)
(ter-bin′a-feen)
Lamisil
Func. class.: Topical antifungal
Chem. class.: Synthetic allylamine derivative

Action: Interferes with cell membrane permeability in fungi such as *Trichophyton rubrum, Trichophyton mentagrophytes, Trichophyton tonsurans, Epidermophyton floccosum, Microsporum canis, Microsporum audouinii, Microsporum gypseum, Candida,* broad-spectrum antifungal

 = Nursing alert ⬥ = Herb-drug interaction 🚫 = Do not crush

Uses: (TOP) Tinea cruris, tinea corporis, tinea pedis; (oral) onychomycosis of the toenail or fingernail due to dermatophytes

Investigational uses: Cutaneous candidiasis, tinea versicolor

Dosage and routes:

Topical

• Massage into affected area, surrounding area qd or bid, continue for 7-14 days, not to exceed 4 wk

Oral

• *Fingernail:* 250 mg/day × 6 wk
• *Toenail:* 250 mg/day × 12 wk

Available forms: Cream 1%, tabs 250 mg

Side effects/adverse reactions:

Topical

INTEG: Burning, stinging, dryness, itching, local irritation

Oral

HEME: Neutropenia

GI: Diarrhea, dyspepsia, abdominal pain, nausea

INTEG: Rash, pruritus, urticaria, **Stevens-Johnson syndrome**

MISC: Headache, liver enzyme changes, taste, visual disturbance

Contraindications: Hypersensitivity, chronic/active liver disease

Precautions: Pregnancy (B), lactation, children, renal disease

Interactions:

• Increased levels of: dextromethorphan
• Decreased terbinafine clearance: cimetidine
• Increased terbinafine clearance: rifampin
• Increased clearance of: cyclosporine

NURSING CONSIDERATIONS

Assess:

• LFTs (ALT, AST) prior to beginning treatment; do not use in presence of liver disease
• CBC in treatment >6 wk
• For continuing infection: increased size, number of lesions

Administer:

• To affected area, surrounding area; do not cover with occlusive dressings

Perform/provide:

• Storage below 30° C (86° F)

Evaluate:

• Therapeutic response: decrease in size, number of lesions

Teach patient/family:

Topical

• To wear cotton clothing
• To use clean towel, dry well
• To avoid contact with mucous membranes
• Not to cover areas unless directed by prescriber
• To report excessive itching, burning
• How to apply; massage cream into affected area and surrounding skin in AM, PM; effects observed within 1 wk, continue 1-2 wk after symptoms decrease

Oral

• To notify prescriber of nausea, vomiting, fatigue, jaundice, dark urine, clay-colored stool, RUQ pain, that may indicate liver dysfunction

---

terbutaline (℞)

(ter-byoo′te-leen)

Brethaire, Brethine, Bricanyl

Func. class.: Selective β₂-agonist; bronchodilator

Chem. class.: Catecholamine

Action: Relaxes bronchial smooth muscle by direct action on β₂-adrenergic receptors through accumulation of cAMP at β-adrenergic receptor sites; bronchodilation, diuresis, CNS, cardiac stimulation occur; relaxes uterine smooth muscle

Uses: Bronchospasm, hyperkalemia

Investigational uses: Premature labor

Dosage and routes:

Bronchodilation

• *Adult and child >15 yr:* 2.5-5 mg q6h during the day, max 15 mg/24 hr

• *Child 12-15 yr:* **PO** 2.5 mg tid q6h

Bronchospasm

• *Adult and child >12 yr:* **INH** 2 puffs q1min, then q4-6h; **PO** 2.5-5 mg q8h; **SC** 0.25 mg q8h

Available forms: Tabs 2.5, 5 mg; aerosol 0.2 mg/actuation; inj 1 mg/ml

Side effects/adverse reactions:

CNS: Tremors, anxiety, insomnia, headache, dizziness, stimulation

CV: Palpitations, tachycardia, hypertension, dysrhythmias, *cardiac arrest*

GI: Nausea, vomiting

Contraindications: Hypersensitivity to sympathomimetics, narrow-angle glaucoma, tachydysrhythmias

Precautions: Pregnancy (B), cardiac disorders, hyperthyroidism, diabetes mellitus, prostatic hypertension, lactation, elderly, hypertension, glaucoma

Pharmacokinetics:

PO: Onset ½ hr, peak 1-2 hr, duration 4-8 hr

SC: Onset 6-15 min, peak ½-1 hr, duration 1½-4 hr

INH: Onset 5-30 min, peak 1-2 hr, duration 3-6 hr

Interactions:

• Increased effects of both drugs: other sympathomimetics

• Decreased action: β-blockers

• Hypertensive crisis: MAOIs

• Incompatible with bleomycin

NURSING CONSIDERATIONS

Assess:

• Respiratory function: vital capacity, forced expiratory volume, ABGs, B/P, pulse, respiratory pattern, lung sounds, sputum before and after treatment

• Tolerance over long-term therapy; dose may have to be changed; monitor for rebound bronchospasm

• Paradoxical bronchospasm: dyspnea, wheezing, keep emergency equipment nearby

• Labor: maternal heart rate, B/P, contraction, fetal heart rate

Administer:

• With food; may be crushed

• 2 hr before hs to avoid sleeplessness

IV

• IV after diluting each 5 mg/1 L D₅W for inf

• IV, run 5 μg/min; may increase 5 μg q10min, titrate to response; after ½-1 hr taper dose by 5 μg; switch to PO as soon as possible

Additive compatibilities: Aminophylline

Syringe compatibilities: Doxapram

Y-site compatibilities: Insulin (regular)

Perform/provide:

• Storage at room temperature; do not use discolored sol

Evaluate:

• Therapeutic response: absence of dyspnea, wheezing

Teach patient/family:

• Not to use OTC medications; extra stimulation may occur

• The use of inhaler; review package insert with patient

• To avoid getting aerosol in eyes; burning, stinging will occur

• To wash inhaler in warm water and dry qd, rinse mouth after use

• All aspects of drug; avoid smoking, smoke-filled rooms, persons with respiratory infections

• To increase fluids >2 L/day; allow 15 min between inhalation of this drug and inhaler containing steroid

• To take on time; if missed, do not

◆ = Nursing alert   ⫸ = Herb-drug interaction   ⃠ = Do not crush make up after 1 hr; wait until next dose

Treatment of overdose: Administer an α-blocker, then norepinephrine for severe hypotension

---

testolactone (℞)
(tess-toe-lak'tone)
Teslac
Func. class.: Antineoplastic
Chem. class.: Androgen hormone

Controlled Substance Schedule III
Action: Acts on adrenal cortex to suppress activity; reduces estrone synthesis

Uses: Advanced breast carcinoma in postmenopausal women; prostatic cancer

Dosage and routes:
• *Adult:* **PO** 250 mg qid
Available forms: Tabs 50 mg
Side effects/adverse reactions:
GI: Nausea, vomiting, anorexia, glossitis
GU: Urinary retention, ***renal failure***
INTEG: Rash, nail changes, facial hair growth
CV: Orthostatic hypertension, edema
CNS: Paresthesias, dizziness
EENT: Deepening voice
META: Hypercalcemia
Contraindications: Hypersensitivity, premenopausal women, carcinoma of male breast
Precautions: Renal disease, hypercalcemia, cardiac disease, pregnancy (C)
Pharmacokinetics: None known
Interactions:
• Enhanced effects of oral anticoagulants
Lab test interferences:
Increase: Urinary 17-OHCS
Decrease: Estradiol

NURSING CONSIDERATIONS
Assess:
• CA$^+$ levels
• B/P q4h; tell patient to rise slowly from sitting or lying down
• Food preferences; list likes, dislikes
• Edema in feet; joint, stomach pain; shaking
◆ Symptoms indicating severe allergic reaction: rash, pruritus, urticaria, purpuric skin lesions, itching, flushing
• Anorexia, nausea, vomiting, constipation, weakness, loss of muscle tone (indicating hypercalcemia)
Administer:
PO
• For 1 mo or longer for desired response
Evaluate:
• Therapeutic response: decreased tumor size, spread of malignancy
Teach patient/family:
• To recognize and report signs of hepatotoxicity, hypercalcemia, virilization (in females), bleeding if on anticoagulants

T

**testosterone
cypionate (R)**
Depo-Testosterone
**testosterone
enanthate (R)**
Delatestryl
testosterone gel (R)
AndroGel 1%
**testosterone, long-
acting (R)**
**testosterone
pellets (R)**
Testopel
**testosterone
transdermal (R)**
Testoderm, Testoderm TTS,
Testoderm with Adhesive,
Androderm
Func. class.: Androgenic anabolic steroid
Chem. class.: Halogenated testosterone derivative

Controlled Substance Schedule III
Action: Increases weight by building body tissue, increases potassium, phosphorus, chloride, nitrogen levels, bone development
Uses: Female breast cancer, eunuch-
oidism, male climacteric, oligo-
spermia, impotence, osteoporosis,
weight loss in AIDS patients, vul-
var dystrophies, low testosterone
levels

Dosage and routes:
Replacement
• *Adult:* **IM** 25-50 mg 2-3 ×/wk
(base or propionate) or 50-400 mg
q2-4wk (enanthate or cypionate)
• *Adult:* **Trans Testoderm** 4-6 mg
applied q24h; **Androderm, Andro-
Gel** 5 mg applied q24h; once qd
(gel)
Breast cancer
• *Adult:* **IM** 50-100 mg 3 ×/wk (pro-

pionate) or 200-400 mg q2-4wk (cypionate or enanthate)
Delayed male puberty
• *Child >12 yr:* **IM** up to 100 mg/mo
for up to 6 mo
Available forms: Enanthate: inj 200
mg/ml; *cypionate:* inj 100, 200 mg/
ml; pellets 75 mg; transdermal 2.5,
4, 5, 6 mg/24 hr; gel 1%
Side effects/adverse reactions:
INTEG: Rash, acneiform lesions, oily
hair and skin, flushing, sweating,
acne vulgaris, alopecia, hirsutism
CNS: Dizziness, headache, fatigue,
tremors, paresthesias, flushing,
sweating, anxiety, lability, insomnia, carpal tunnel syndrome
MS: Cramps, spasms
CV: Increased B/P
GU: Hematuria, amenorrhea, vaginitis, decreased libido, decreased
breast size, clitoral hypertrophy, testicular atrophy
GI: Nausea, vomiting, constipation,
weight gain, *cholestatic jaundice*
EENT: Conjunctival edema, nasal
congestion
ENDO: Abnormal GTT
Contraindications: Severe renal,
severe cardiac, severe hepatic dis-
ease, hypersensitivity, pregnancy
(X), lactation, genital bleeding (rare)
Precautions: Diabetes mellitus, CV
disease, MI
Pharmacokinetics:
PO: Metabolized in liver, excreted
in urine, breast milk; crosses pla-
centa
Interactions:
• Increased effects of oral antidia-
betics, oxyphenbutazone
• Increased PT: anticoagulants
• Edema: ACTH, adrenal steroids
• Decreased effects of insulin
Lab test interferences:
Increase: Serum cholesterol, blood
glucose, urine glucose
Decrease: Serum Ca, serum K, T₄,

◆ = Nursing alert   ∥ = Herb-drug interaction   ⊘ = Do not crush

T_3, thyroid ^{131}I uptake test, urine 17-OHCS, 17-KS, PBI

NURSING CONSIDERATIONS
Assess:

• Weight qd; notify prescriber if weekly weight gain is >5 lb

• B/P q4h

• I&O ratio; be alert for decreasing urinary output, increasing edema

• Growth rate in children; growth rate may be uneven (linear/bone growth) with extended use

• Electrolytes: K, Na, Cl, Ca; cholesterol

• Liver function studies: ALT, AST, bilirubin

• Edema, hypertension, cardiac symptoms, jaundice

• Mental status: affect, mood, behavioral changes, aggression

• Signs of masculinization in female: increased libido, deepening of voice, decreased breast tissue, enlarged clitoris, menstrual irregularities; male: gynecomastia, impotence, testicular atrophy

• Hypercalcemia: lethargy, polyuria, polydipsia, nausea, vomiting, constipation; drug may have to be decreased

• Hypoglycemia in diabetics; oral antidiabetic action is increased

Administer:

• Titrated dose; use lowest effective dose

• IM inj deep into upper outer quadrant of gluteal muscle

• Transdermal patches: Testoderm to skin of scrotum; Androderm to skin of back, upper arms, thighs, abdomen; area must be dry-shaved; may be reapplied after bathing, swimming

• Gel: apply qd to clean, dry area on shoulders, upper arms or abdomen

Perform/provide:

• Diet with increased calories, protein; decrease Na if edema occurs

Evaluate:

• Therapeutic response: 4-6 wk in osteoporosis

Teach patient/family:

• That drug must be combined with complete health plan: diet, rest, exercise

• To notify prescriber if therapeutic response decreases; if edema occurs

• Not to discontinue abruptly

• About changes in sex characteristics

• That women should report menstrual irregularities, voice changes, acne, facial hair growth

• That 1-3-mo course is necessary for response in breast cancer

• The proper application of patches

---

tetracaine (℞)
(tet′ra-kane)
Pontocaine
Func. class.: Local anesthetic
Chem. class.: Ester

Action: Competes with calcium for sites in nerve membrane that control sodium transport across cell membrane; decreases rise of depolarization phase of action potential

Uses: Spinal anesthesia, epidural and peripheral nerve block, perineum, lower extremities

Dosage and routes:
Varies with route of anesthesia
Available forms: Inj 0.2%, 0.3%, 1%; powder

Side effects/adverse reactions:
CNS: Anxiety, restlessness, ***convulsions, LOC,*** drowsiness, disorientation, tremors, shivering
CV: ***Myocardial depression, cardiac arrest, dysrhythmias,*** bradycardia, hypotension, hypertension, fetal bradycardia
GI: Nausea, vomiting

EENT: Blurred vision, tinnitus, pupil constriction
INTEG: Rash, urticaria, allergic reactions, edema, burning, skin discoloration at inj site, tissue necrosis
RESP: **Status asthmaticus, respiratory arrest, anaphylaxis**
Contraindications: Hypersensitivity, severe liver disease, heart block
Precautions: Elderly, severe drug allergies, pregnancy (C), lactation, children
Pharmacokinetics: Onset 15 min, duration 3 hr; metabolized by liver, excreted in urine (metabolites)
Interactions:
• Dysrhythmias: epinephrine, halothane, enflurane
• Hypertension: MAOIs, tricyclics, phenothiazines
• Decreased action of tetracaine: chloroprocaine
• Decreased action of sulfonamides
NURSING CONSIDERATIONS
Assess:
• B/P, pulse, respiration during treatment
• Fetal heart tones during labor
• Allergic reactions: rash, urticaria, itching
• Cardiac status: ECG for dysrhythmias, pulse, B/P, during anesthesia
Administer:
• Only if not cloudy, does not contain precipitate
• Only with crash cart, resuscitative equipment nearby
• Only without preservatives for epidural or caudal anesthesia
Perform/provide:
• Use of new sol, discard unused portions, store in refrigerator
Evaluate:
• Therapeutic response: anesthesia necessary for procedure
Treatment of overdose: Airway, O₂, vasopressor, IV fluids, anticonvulsants for seizures

---

tetracycline (℞)
(tet-ra-sye′kleen)
Achromycin V, Alatel, Apo-Tetra*, Novotetra*, Nu-Tetra*, Panmycin, Robitet, Sumycin, Teline, Tetracap, tetracycline HCl, Tetracyn, Tetralan, Tetram
Func. class.: Broad-spectrum antiinfective
Chem. class.: Tetracycline

Action: Inhibits protein synthesis and phosphorylation in microorganisms; bacteriostatic
Uses: Syphilis, *Chlamydia trachomatis,* gonorrhea, lymphogranuloma venereum; uncommon gram-positive, gram-negative organisms; rickettsial infections
Dosage and routes:
• *Adult:* **PO** 250-500 mg q6h
• *Child >8 yr:* **PO** 25-50 mg/kg/day in divided doses q6h
Gonorrhea
• *Adult:* **PO** 1.5 g, then 500 mg qid for a total of 9 g over 7 days
Chlamydia trachomatis
• *Adult:* **PO** 500 mg qid × 7 days
Syphilis
• *Adult:* **PO** 2-3 g in divided doses × 10-15 days; if syphilis duration >1 yr, must treat 30 days
Brucellosis
• *Adult:* **PO** 500 mg qid × 3 wk with 1 g streptomycin **IM** 2 ×/day × 1 wk, and 1 ×/day the second wk
Urethral syndrome in women
• *Adult:* **PO** 500 mg qid × 7 days
Acne
• *Adult:* 1 g/day in divided doses; maintenance 125-500 mg/day
Available forms: Oral susp 125 mg/5 ml; caps 100, 250, 500 mg; tabs 250, 500 mg

---

◆ = Nursing alert   ∥ = Herb-drug interaction   ⊗ = Do not crush

Side effects/adverse reactions:

CNS: Fever, headache, paresthesia

HEMA: ***Eosinophilia, neutropenia, thrombocytopenia, leukocytosis, hemolytic anemia***

EENT: Dysphagia, glossitis, decreased calcification, discoloration of deciduous teeth, oral candidiasis, oral ulcers

GI: Nausea, abdominal pain, *vomiting, diarrhea,* anorexia, enterocolitis, ***hepatotoxicity,*** flatulence, abdominal cramps, epigastric burning, stomatitis

CV: Pericarditis

GU: Increased BUN

*INTEG: Rash, urticaria, photosensitivity, increased pigmentation, **exfoliative dermatitis,*** pruritus, ***angioedema***

Contraindications: Hypersensitivity to tetracyclines, children <8 yr, pregnancy (D), lactation

Precautions: Renal disease, hepatic disease

Pharmacokinetics:

PO: Peak 2-3 hr, duration 6 hr, half-life 6-10 hr; excreted in urine, breast milk; crosses placenta; 20%-60% protein bound

Interactions:

• Decreased effect of tetracycline: antacids, $NaHCO_3$, dairy products, alkali products, iron, kaolin/pectin, cimetidine

• Increased effect: warfarin, digoxin

• Decreased effect of penicillins, oral contraceptives

• Nephrotoxicity: methoxyflurane

Lab test interferences:

False negative: Urine glucose with Clinistix or Tes-Tape

False increase: Urinary catecholamines

NURSING CONSIDERATIONS

Assess:

• Signs of anemia: Hct, Hgb, fatigue

• I&O ratio

• Blood studies: PT, CBC, AST, ALT, BUN, creatinine

• Allergic reactions: rash, itching, pruritus, angioedema

• Nausea, vomiting, diarrhea; administer antiemetic, antacids as ordered

• Overgrowth of infection: fever, malaise, redness, pain, swelling, drainage, perineal itching, diarrhea, changes in cough or sputum

Administer:

• After C&S obtained

• 2 hr before or after iron products; 3 hr after antacid or kaolin/pectin products

• Oral form should be given on an empty stomach

Perform/provide:

• Storage in tight, light-resistant container at room temperature

Evaluate:

• Therapeutic response: decreased temp, absence of lesions, negative C&S

Teach patient/family:

• To avoid sun exposure; sunscreen does not seem to decrease photosensitivity

• That diabetic should avoid use of Clinistix, Diastix, or Tes-Tape for urine glucose testing

• That all prescribed medication must be taken to prevent superinfection

• To avoid milk products, antacids, or separate by 2 hr; take with a full glass of water

theophylline (℞)

(thee-off'i-lin)

Accurbron, Aquaphyllin, Asmalix, Bronkodyl, Elixomin, Elixophyllin, Lanophyllin, Quibron-T Dividose, Quibron-T/SR Dividose, Respbid, Slo-bid Gyrocaps, Slo-Phyllin, Sustaire, Theo-24, Theobid Duracaps, Theochron, Theoclear-80, Theoclear L.A., Theo-Dur, Theolair-SR, Theo-Sav, Theospan-SR, Theostat 80, Theovent, Theo-X, T-Phyl, Uni-Dur, Uniphyl

Func. class.: Spasmolytic
Chem. class.: Xanthine, ethylenediamide

Action: Relaxes smooth muscle of respiratory system by blocking phosphodiesterase, which increases cAMP

Uses: Bronchial asthma, bronchospasm of COPD, chronic bronchitis

Dosage and routes:

Bronchospasm, bronchial asthma
• *Adult:* **PO** 100-200 mg q6h; dosage must be individualized; **RECT** 250-500 mg q8-12h
• *Child:* **PO** 50-100 mg q6h, not to exceed 12 mg/kg/24 hr

COPD, chronic bronchitis
• *Adult:* **PO** 330-660 mg q6-8h pc (sodium glycinate)
• *Child 1-9 yr:* **PO** 5 mg/kg loading dose, then 4 mg/kg q6h
• *Child 9-16 yr:* **PO** 5 mg/kg loading dose, then 3 mg/kg q6h

Apnea of prematurity
• *Neonate:* 2-10 mg/kg/day divided q8-12h (usual loading dose is 4 mg/kg **PO**)

Available forms: Caps 50, 100, 200, 250 mg; tabs 100, 125, 200, 225, 250, 300 mg; tabs, time rel 100, 200, 250, 300, 400, 500 mg; caps, time rel 50, 65, 100, 125, 130, 200, 250, 260, 300, 400, 500 mg; elix 80, 11.25 mg/15 ml; sol 80 mg/15 ml; liquid 80, 150, 160 mg/15 ml; susp 300 mg/15 ml

Side effects/adverse reactions:

CNS: Anxiety, restlessness, insomnia, dizziness, **convulsions,** headache, light-headedness, muscle twitching, tremors
CV: Palpitations, sinus tachycardia, hypotension, other dysrhythmias, fluid retention with tachycardia
ENDO: Hyperglycemia
GI: Nausea, vomiting, anorexia, diarrhea, bitter taste, dyspepsia, gastric distress
RESP: Increased rate
INTEG: Flushing, urticaria

Contraindications: Hypersensitivity to xanthines, tachydysrhythmias
Precautions: Elderly, CHF, cor pulmonale, hepatic disease, active peptic ulcer disease, diabetes mellitus, hyperthyroidism, hypertension, children, pregnancy (C)

Pharmacokinetics:
PO: Peak 2 hr
SOL: Peak 1 hr
Metabolized in liver, excreted in urine and breast milk, crosses placenta

Interactions:
• Decreased theophylline level: phenytoin, phenobarbital, carbamazepine, rifampin, smoking
• Increased action of theophylline: cimetidine, propranolol, erythromycin, troleandomycin, ciprofloxacin, oral contraceptives
• May increase effects of anticoagulants
• Cardiotoxicity: β-blockers
• Decreased effect of lithium
⚞ Toxicity: ephedra (ma huang)

NURSING CONSIDERATIONS
Assess:
◆ Theophylline blood levels (therapeutic level is 5-15 µg/ml); toxic-

ity may occur with small increase above 20 µg/ml

• Monitor I&O; diuresis occurs; elderly or child may be dehydrated

• Signs of toxicity: irritability, insomnia, restlessness, tremors, nausea, vomiting

• Respiratory rate, rhythm, depth; auscultate lung fields bilaterally; notify prescriber of abnormalities

• Allergic reactions: rash, urticaria; drug should be discontinued

Administer:

• PO after meals for GI symptoms; absorption may be affected

IV

Additive compatibilities: Cefepime, chlorpromazine, fluconazole, furosemide, hydrocortisone, lidocaine, methylprednisolone, verapamil

Y-site compatibilities: Acyclovir, ampicillin, ampicillin/sulbactam, aztreonam, cefazolin, cefotetan, ceftazidime, ceftriaxone, cimetidine, cisatracurium, clindamycin, dexamethasone, diltiazem, dobutamine, dopamine, doxycycline, erythromycin, famotidine, fluconazole, gentamicin, haloperidol, heparin, hydrocortisone, lidocaine, methyldopate, methylprednisolone, metronidazole, midazolam, nafcillin, nitroglycerin, penicillin G potassium, piperacillin, potassium chloride, ranitidine, remifentanil, sodium nitroprusside, ticarcillin, ticarcillin/clavulanate, tobramycin, vancomycin

Evaluate:

• Therapeutic response: ability to breathe more easily

Teach patient/family:

• To check OTC medications, current prescription medications for ephedrine, which will increase stimulation; to avoid alcohol, caffeine

• To avoid hazardous activities; dizziness may occur

• That if GI upset occurs, to take

drug with 8 oz H_2O; avoid food; absorption may be decreased

🚫 Not to break, crush, chew, or dissolve slow-release products

• That contents of bead-filled capsule may be sprinkled over food for children's use

• To notify prescriber of toxicity: nausea, vomiting, anxiety, insomnia, convulsions

• To notify prescriber of change in smoking habit; dosage may have to be changed

---

thiabendazole (℞)

(thye-a-ben'da-zole)

Mintezol

Func. class.: Anthelmintic

Chem. class.: Benzimidazole derivative

Action: Inhibits anaerobic metabolism, disrupts microtubules

Uses: Pinworm, roundworm, threadworm, whipworm, trichinosis, hookworm, cutaneous larva migrans (creeping eruption)

Dosage and routes:

• *Adult and child:* PO 25 mg/kg in 2 doses qd × 2-5 days, not to exceed 3 g/day

Available forms: Tabs, chew 500 mg; oral susp 500 mg/5 ml

Side effects/adverse reactions:

*SYST: **Anaphylaxis***

*GU: **Hematuria, nephrotoxicity,** enuresis, abnormal smell of urine*

INTEG: Rash, pruritus, erythema, ***Stevens-Johnson syndrome***

CNS: Dizziness, headache, drowsiness, fever, flushing, ***convulsions,*** behavioral changes

EENT: Tinnitus, blurred vision, xanthopsia

GI: Nausea, vomiting, anorexia, diarrhea, jaundice, ***liver damage,*** epigastric distress

CV: Hypotension, bradycardia

T

---

* = Canada only   Side effects: *italics* = common; ***bold italics*** = life-threatening

Contraindications: Hypersensitivity

Precautions: Severe malnutrition, hepatic disease, renal disease, anemia, severe dehydration, child <14 kg, pregnancy (C), lactation

Pharmacokinetics:

PO: Peak 1-2 hr, metabolized completely by liver, excreted in feces and urine

Interactions

• Increased theophylline toxicity: theophylline, dose reduction may be necessary

NURSING CONSIDERATIONS
Assess:

• Stools periodically during entire treatment

Administer:

• Susp after shaking

• PO after meals to avoid GI symptoms

Perform/provide:

• Storage in tight container

Evaluate:

• Therapeutic response: stools negative for helminths

Teach patient/family:

• Proper hygiene after BM, including hand-washing technique; tell patient not to put fingers in mouth

• That infected person should sleep alone; not to shake bed linen; to change bed linen qd

• To clean toilet qd with disinfectant (green soap solution)

• The need for compliance with dosage schedule, duration of treatment

• To drink fruit juice to remove mucus that intestinal tapeworms burrow in; aids in expulsion of worms

• To avoid hazardous activities if drowsiness occurs

Treatment of overdose: Induce emesis or gastric lavage

---

thiamine (vit B$_1$)
(PO-OTC, IM-℞)

Betaxin*, Betalin S, Biamine, Revitonus, Thiamilate, thiamine HCl

Func. class.: Vit B$_1$
Chem. class.: Water soluble

Action: Needed for pyruvate metabolism, carbohydrate metabolism

Uses: Vit B$_1$ deficiency or polyneuritis, cheilosis adjunct with thiamine beriberi, Wernicke-Korsakoff syndrome, pellagra, metabolic disorders

Dosage and routes:
Beriberi

• *Adult:* **IM** 10-20 mg tid × 2 wk, then 5-10 mg qd × 1 mo

Beriberi with cardiac failure

• *Adult and child:* **IV** 10-30 mg tid

Available forms: Tabs 50, 100, 250, 500 mg; inj 100 mg/ml; enteric coated tabs 20 mg

Side effects/adverse reactions:

CNS: Weakness, restlessness

GI: Hemorrhage, *nausea, diarrhea*

CV: Collapse, pulmonary edema, hypotension

INTEG: Angioneurotic edema, cyanosis, sweating, warmth

SYST: Anaphylaxis

EENT: Tightness of throat

Contraindications: Hypersensitivity

Precautions: Pregnancy (A)

Do not confuse:

thiamine/Tenormin

Pharmacokinetics:

PO/INJ: Unused amounts excreted in urine (unchanged)

NURSING CONSIDERATIONS
Assess:

• Thiamine levels throughout treatment

• Nutritional status: yeast, beef, liver, whole or enriched grains, legumes

---

 = Nursing alert   = Herb-drug interaction   = Do not crush

Administer:

- By IM injection; rotate sites if pain and inflammation occur; do not mix with alkaline sols; Z-track to minimize pain

IV

- Undiluted over 5 min or diluted with IV sol and given as an inf at 100 mg or less/5 min or more

Syringe compatibilities: Doxapram

Y-site compatibilities: Famotidine

Perform/provide:

- Storage in tight, light-resistant container
- Application of cold to help decrease pain

Evaluate:

- Therapeutic response: absence of nausea, vomiting, anorexia, insomnia, tachycardia, paresthesias, depression, muscle weakness

Teach patient/family:

- The necessary foods to be included in diet: yeast, beef, liver, legumes, whole grain

---

thiethylperazine (℞)

(thye-eth-il-per′a-zeen)

Norzine, Torecan

Func. class.: Antiemetic

Chem. class.: Phenothiazine, piperazine derivative

Action: Acts centrally by blocking chemoreceptor trigger zone, which in turn acts on vomiting center

Uses: Nausea, vomiting

Dosage and routes:

- *Adult:* **PO/IM** 10 mg/qd-tid

Available forms: Tabs 10 mg; inj 5 mg/ml

Side effects/adverse reactions:

GU: Urinary retention, dark urine

CNS: Euphoria, depression, restlessness, tremor, EPS, ***convulsions,*** drowsiness, confusion

GI: Nausea, vomiting, anorexia, dry mouth, diarrhea, constipation, weight loss, metallic taste, cramps

*CV: **Circulatory failure, tachycardia,*** postural hypotension, ECG changes

*RESP: **Respiratory depression***

Contraindications: Hypersensitivity to phenothiazines, coma, seizure, encephalopathy, bone marrow depression, pregnancy (X)

Precautions: Children <2 yr, elderly, lactation

Do not confuse:

Torecan/Toradol

Pharmacokinetics:

PO: Onset 45-60 min

RECT: Onset 45-60 min, metabolized by liver, crosses placenta, excreted in urine, breast milk

Interactions:

- Decreased effect of thiethylperazine: barbiturates, antacids
- Increased anticholinergic action: anticholinergics, antiparkinson drugs, antidepressants

NURSING CONSIDERATIONS

Assess:

- VS, B/P; check patients with cardiac disease more often
- Respiratory status before, during, after administration of emetic; check rate, rhythm, character; respiratory depression can occur rapidly with elderly or debilitated patients

Administer:

- IM inj in large muscle mass; aspirate to avoid IV administration; patient should remain recumbent 1 hr after inj

Syringe compatibilities: Butorphanol, hydromorphone, midazolam, ranitidine

Y-site compatibilities: Aldesleukin

Evaluate:

- Therapeutic response: absence of nausea, vomiting

Teach patient/family:

- To avoid hazardous activities, ac-

T

tivities requiring alertness; dizziness may occur

RARELY USED

thioguanine (6-TG) (℞)

(thye-oh-gwah′neen)
thioguanine, Lanvis*
Func. class.: Antineoplastic-antimetabolite

Uses: Acute leukemias, chronic granulocytic leukemia, lymphomas, multiple myeloma, solid tumors

Dosage and routes:
• *Adult and child:* **PO** 2 mg/kg/day, then increase slowly to 3 mg/kg/day after 4 wk

Contraindications: Prior drug resistance, leukopenia (<2500/mm^3), thrombocytopenia (<100,000/mm^3), anemia, pregnancy (D)

---

thiopental (℞)

(thye-oh-pen′tal)
Pentothal, thiopental sodium
Func. class.: General anesthetic
Chem. class.: Barbiturate
Controlled Substance Schedule III

Action: Acts in reticular-activating system to produce anesthesia, raises seizure threshold

Uses: Short, general anesthesia; narcoanalysis, induction anesthesia before other anesthetics

Investigational uses: Increased intracranial pressure

Dosage and routes:
Induction
• *Adult:* **IV** 210-280 mg or 3-5 mg/kg

General anesthetic
• *Child:* **IV** 3-8 mg/kg then 1 mg/kg as needed
• *Adult:* **IV** 50-75 mg given at 20-40 sec intervals

Narcoanalysis
• *Adult:* **IV** 100 mg/min, not to exceed 50 ml/min

Sedation or narcosis
• *Adult:* **RECT** 12-20 mg/lb

Available forms: Pwd for inj 2%, 2.5%

Side effects/adverse reactions:
*RESP: **Respiratory depression, bronchospasm***
CNS: Retrograde amnesia, prolonged somnolence
CV: Tachycardia, hypotension, ***myocardial depression, dysrhythmias***
EENT: Sneezing, coughing
INTEG: Chills, *shivering*, necrosis, pain at inj site
MS: Muscle irritability

Contraindications: Hypersensitivity, status asthmaticus, hepatic/intermittent porphyrias

Precautions: Severe cardiovascular disease, renal disease, hypotension, liver disease, myxedema, myasthenia gravis, asthma, increased intracranial pressure, pregnancy (C)

Pharmacokinetics:
IV: Onset 30-40 sec; half-life 11½ hr; crosses placenta

Interactions:
• Increased action: CNS depressants
🥢 Increased CNS depression: kava

NURSING CONSIDERATIONS
Assess:
• VS q3-5min during IV administration, after dose, q4h postoperatively
• Extravasation; if it occurs, use nitroprusside or chloroprocaine to decrease pain, increase circulation
• Dysrhythmias or myocardial depression

Administer:
• Only with crash cart, resuscitative equipment nearby
IV
• After diluting 500 mg/20 ml sterile H$_2$O for inj; give each 25 mg or less/min, titrate to response

---

◆ = Nursing alert   🥢 = Herb-drug interaction   🚫 = Do not crush

Additive compatibilities: Chloramphenicol, hydrocortisone sodium succinate, oxytocin, pentobarbital, phenobarbital, potassium chloride, sodium bicarbonate

Solution compatibilities: D_5/0.45% NaCl, D_5W, multiple electrolyte sol, 0.45% NaCl, 0.9% NaCl, 1/6 M sodium lactate

Syringe compatibilities: Aminophylline, hyaluronidase, hydrocortisone sodium succinate, neostigmine, pentobarbital, propofol, scopolamine, tubocurarine

Y-site compatibilities: Doxacurium, fentanyl, heparin, milrinone, mivacurium, nitroglycerin, ranitidine, remifentanil

Evaluate:

• Therapeutic response: maintenance of anesthesia

---

thioridazine (Rx)

(thye-or-rid′a-zeen)
Apo-Thioridazine*, Mellaril, Mellaril Concentrate, Mellaril-5, Novo-Ridazine*, PMS-Thioridazine*, thioridazine HCl

Func. class.: Antipsychotic, neuroleptic

Chem. class.: Phenothiazine piperidine

Action: Depresses cerebral cortex, hypothalamus, limbic system, which control activity, aggression; blocks neurotransmission produced by dopamine at synapse; exhibits strong α-adrenergic, anticholinergic blocking action; mechanism for antipsychotic effects is unclear

Uses: Psychotic disorders, schizophrenia, behavioral problems in children, anxiety, major depressive disorders, organic brain syndrome

Dosage and routes:
Psychosis
• *Adult:* **PO** 25-100 mg tid, max dose 800 mg/day; dose is gradually increased to desired response, then reduced to minimum maintenance
Depression/behavioral problems/organic brain syndrome
• *Adult:* **PO** 25 mg tid, range from 10 mg bid-qid to 50 mg tid-qid; decreased dose in elderly
• *Geriatric:* **PO** 10-25 mg qd-bid, increase 4-7 days by 10-25 mg to desired dose
• *Child 2-12 yr:* **PO** 0.5-3 mg/kg/day in divided doses
Available forms: Tabs 10, 15, 25, 50, 100, 150, 200 mg; conc 30, 100 mg/ml; susp 25, 100 mg/5 ml; syr 10 mg/15 ml

Side effects/adverse reactions:
RESP: **Laryngospasm,** dyspnea, *respiratory depression*
CNS: EPS (rare): *pseudoparkinsonism, akathisia, dystonia, tardive dyskinesia,* **seizures,** headache, confusion, **neuroleptic malignant syndrome**
HEMA: Anemia, **leukopenia, leukocytosis, agranulocytosis**
INTEG: *Rash,* photosensitivity, dermatitis
EENT: Blurred vision, glaucoma, dry eyes
GI: *Dry mouth, nausea, vomiting, anorexia, constipation,* diarrhea, jaundice, weight gain
GU: Urinary retention, urinary frequency, enuresis, impotence, amenorrhea, gynecomastia
CV: Orthostatic hypotension, **cardiac arrest,** ECG changes, **tachycardia**

Contraindications: Hypersensitivity, blood dyscrasias, coma, children <2 yr, brain damage, bone marrow depression

Precautions: Pregnancy (C), lactation, seizure disorders, hypertension, hepatic disease, cardiac disease

Do not confuse:

Mellaril/Elavil

Pharmacokinetics:

PO: Onset erratic, peak 2-4 hr; metabolized by liver, excreted in urine, breast milk; crosses placenta, half-life 26-36 hr

Interactions:

• Oversedation: other CNS depressants, alcohol, barbiturate anesthetics

• Decreased thioridazine effect: lithium, barbiturates

• Decreased antihypertensive effect: centrally acting antihypertensives

• Decreased absorption: aluminum hydroxide, magnesium hydroxide antacids

• Increased anticholinergic effects: anticholinergics

 Increased CNS depression: kava

Lab test interferences:

Increase: LFTs, cardiac enzymes, cholesterol, blood glucose, prolactin, bilirubin, PBI, cholinesterase, ^{131}I

Decrease: Hormones (blood, urine)

False positive: Pregnancy test, PKU

False negative: Urinary steroid, pregnancy test

NURSING CONSIDERATIONS

Assess:

• Mental status before first dose

• Swallowing of PO medication; check for hoarding or giving of medication to other patients

• I&O ratio; palpate bladder if low urinary output occurs

• Bilirubin, CBC, liver function studies qmo

• Urinalysis is recommended before and during prolonged therapy

• Affect, orientation, LOC, reflexes, gait, coordination, sleep pattern disturbances

• B/P standing and lying; also include pulse and respirations q4h during initial treatment; establish baseline before starting treatment; report drops of 30 mm Hg

• Dizziness, faintness, palpitations, tachycardia on rising

• EPS including akathisia (inability to sit still, no pattern to movements), tardive dyskinesia (bizarre movements of jaw, mouth, tongue, extremities), pseudoparkinsonism (rigidity, tremors, pill rolling, shuffling gait)

◆ For neuroleptic malignant syndrome: altered mental status, muscle rigidity, increased CPK, hyperthermia

• Skin turgor qd

• Constipation, urinary retention qd; increase bulk, water in diet

Administer:

• Antiparkinsonian agent on order from prescriber for EPS

• Concentrate mixed in citrus juices or distilled or acidified tap water

• Decreased dose in elderly

Perform/provide:

• Decreased sensory input by dimming lights, avoiding loud noises

• Supervised ambulation until stabilized on medication if needed; do not involve in strenuous exercise program because fainting is possible; patient should not stand still for long periods

• Increased fluids to prevent constipation

• Sips of water, candy, gum for dry mouth

• Storage in tight, light-resistant container; avoid contact with skin

Evaluate:

• Therapeutic response: decrease in emotional excitement, hallucinations, delusions, paranoia, reorganization of patterns of thought, speech

Teach patient/family:

• That orthostatic hypotension occurs frequently, to rise from sitting

---

◆ = Nursing alert   = Herb-drug interaction   ⊘ = Do not crush

or lying position gradually; to avoid hazardous activities until stabilized on medication
• To remain lying down after IM injection for at least 30 min
• To avoid hot tubs, hot showers, tub baths; hypotension may occur
• To avoid abrupt withdrawal of thioridazine, or EPS may result; drug should be withdrawn slowly
• To avoid OTC preparations (cough, hay fever, cold) unless approved by prescriber; serious drug interactions may occur; avoid use with alcohol, CNS depressants; increased drowsiness may occur
• To use a sunscreen
• About compliance with drug regimen
• About the necessity for meticulous oral hygiene, since oral candidiasis may occur
• To report sore throat, malaise, fever, bleeding, mouth sores; if these occur, CBC should be drawn and drug discontinued
• That in hot weather, heat stroke may occur; take extra precautions to stay cool

Treatment of overdose: Lavage if orally ingested, provide an airway; do not induce vomiting, CV monitoring, continuous EKG

RARELY USED

thiotepa (℞)
(thye-oh-tep'a)
Thioplex
Func. class.: Antineoplastic

Uses: Hodgkin's disease, lymphomas; breast, ovarian, lung, bladder cancer; neoplastic effusions
Dosage and routes:
• *Adult:* **IV** 0.3-0.4 mg/kg at 1-4 wk intervals

Neoplastic effusions
• *Adult:* **INTRACAVITY** 0.6-0.8 mg/kg
Bladder cancer
• *Adult:* **INSTILL** 60 mg/30-60 ml water for inj instilled in bladder for 2 hr once weekly × 4 wk
Contraindications: Hypersensitivity, pregnancy (D)

RARELY USED

thiothixene (℞)
(thye-oh-thix'een)
Navane, thiothixene
Func. class.: Antipsychotic, neuroleptic

Uses: Psychotic disorders, schizophrenia, acute agitation
Dosage and routes:
• *Adult:* **PO** 2-5 mg bid-qid depending on severity of condition; dose gradually increased to 15-30 mg if needed; **IM** 4 mg bid-qid; max dose 30 mg qd; administer **PO** dose as soon as possible
• *Geriatric:* **PO** 1-2 mg qd-bid, increase by 1-2 mg q4-7 days to desired dose
Contraindications: Hypersensitivity, blood dyscrasias, child <12 yr, bone marrow depression, circulatory collapse, CNS depression, coma, alcoholism, CV disease, hepatic disease, Reye's syndrome, narrow-angle glaucoma
Do not confuse:
Navane/Norvasc

thyroid USP (desiccated) (R)

(thye'roid)

Armour Thyroid, Cholaxin*, S-P-T, Thyrar, Thyroid Strong, Thyroid USP

Func. class.: Thyroid hormone

Chem. class.: Active thyroid hormone in natural state and ratio

Action: Increases metabolic rates, increases cardiac output, O_2 consumption, body temp, blood volume, growth, development at cellular level

Uses: Hypothyroidism, cretinism (juvenile hypothyroidism), myxedema

Dosage and routes:

Hypothyroidism

• *Adult:* **PO** 65 mg qd, increased by 65 mg q30d until desired response; maintenance dose 65-195 mg qd

• *Elderly:* **PO** 7.5-15 mg qd, double dose q6-8wk until desired response

Cretinism/juvenile hypothyroidism

• *Child over 1 yr:* **PO** up to 180 mg qd titrated to response

• *Child 4-12 mo:* **PO** 30-60 mg qd

• *Child 1-4 mo:* **PO** 15-30 mg qd; may increase q2wk; titrated to response; maintenance dose 30-45 mg qd

Myxedema

• *Adult:* **PO** 16 mg qd, double dose q2wk, maintenance 65-195 mg/day

Available forms: Tabs 16, 32, 65, 98, 130, 195, 260, 325 mg; tabs enteric coated 32, 65, 130 mg; sugar-coated tabs 32, 65, 130, 195 mg; caps 65, 130, 195, 325 mg

Side effects/adverse reactions:

CNS: Insomnia, tremors, headache, *thyroid storm*

CV: Tachycardia, palpitations, angina, dysrhythmias, hypertension, *cardiac arrest*

GI: Nausea, diarrhea, increased or decreased appetite, cramps

MISC: Menstrual irregularities, weight loss, sweating, heat intolerance, fever

Contraindications: Adrenal insufficiency, MI, thyrotoxicosis

Precautions: Elderly, angina pectoris, hypertension, ischemia, cardiac disease, pregnancy (A), lactation

Do not confuse:

Thyrar/Thyrolar

Pharmacokinetics:

PO: Peak 12-48 hr, half-life 6-7 days

Interactions:

• Decreased absorption of thyroid: cholestyramine

• Increased effects of anticoagulants, sympathomimetics, tricyclics, catecholamines

• Decreased effects of digitalis drugs, insulin, hypoglycemics

• Decreased effects of thyroid: estrogens

 Do not use with: bugleweed

Lab test interferences:

Increase: CPK, LDH, AST, PBI, blood glucose

Decrease: Thyroid function tests

NURSING CONSIDERATIONS

Assess:

• B/P, pulse before each dose

• I&O ratio

• Weight qd in same clothing, using same scale, at same time of day

• Height, growth rate of child

• T_3, T_4, which are decreased; radioimmunoassay of TSH, which is increased; radio uptake, which is decreased if dosage is too low

• PT may require decreased anticoagulant; check for bleeding, bruising

• Increased nervousness, excitabil-

 = Nursing alert   = Herb-drug interaction   🚫 = Do not crush

ity, irritability; may indicate too high dose of medication, usually after 1-3 wk of treatment

• Cardiac status: angina, palpitation, chest pain, change in VS

Administer:

• In AM if possible as a single dose to decrease sleeplessness

• At same time each day to maintain drug level

• Only for hormone imbalances; not to be used for obesity, male infertility, menstrual disorders, lethargy

• Lowest dose that relieves symptoms

Perform/provide:

• Removal of medication 4 wk before RAIU test

Evaluate:

• Therapeutic response: absence of depression; increased weight loss, diuresis, pulse, appetite; absence of constipation, peripheral edema, cold intolerance; pale, cool, dry skin; brittle nails, alopecia, coarse hair, menorrhagia, night blindness, paresthesias, syncope, stupor, coma, rosy cheeks

Teach patient/family:

• That hair loss will occur in child, is temporary

• To report excitability, irritability, anxiety; indicates overdose

• Not to switch brands unless directed by prescriber

• That hypothyroid child will show almost immediate behavior/personality change

• That treatment drug is not to be taken to reduce weight

• To avoid OTC preparations with iodine; read labels

• To avoid iodine food, iodized salt, soybeans, tofu, turnips, some seafood, some bread

tiagabine (℞)

(tie-ah-ga'been)
Gabitril
Func. class.: Anticonvulsant

Action: Mechanism unknown; may increase seizure threshold; structurally similar to GABA; tiagabine binding sites in neocortex, hippocampus

Uses: Adjunct treatment of partial seizures

Dosage and routes:

• *Adult:* **PO** 4 mg qd, may increase by 4-8 mg qwk until desired response, max 32 mg/day

• *Child 12-18 yr:* **PO** 4 mg qd, may increase by 4 mg at beginning of wk 2; may increase by 4-8 mg qwk until desired response; max 32 mg/day

Available forms: Tabs 2, 4, 12, 16, 20 mg

Side effects/adverse reactions:

CNS: Dizziness, anxiety, somnolence, ataxia, amnesia, unsteady gait, depression

CV: Vasodilation

GI: Nausea, vomiting, diarrhea

INTEG: Pruritus, rash

RESP: Pharyngitis, coughing

Contraindications: Hypersensitivity to this drug

Precautions: Hepatic disease, renal disease, pregnancy (C), lactation, children <12 yr, elderly

Pharmacokinetics: Absorption >95%, half-life 7-9 hrs

Interactions:

Unknown

NURSING CONSIDERATIONS

Assess:

• Renal studies: urinalysis, BUN, urine creatinine q3mo

• Hepatic studies: ALT, AST, bilirubin

• Description of seizures: location, duration, presence of aura

T

• Mental status: mood, sensorium, affect, behavioral changes; if mental status changes, notify prescriber
• Eye problems, need for ophthalmic examinations before, during, after treatment (slit lamp, funduscopy, tonometry)
• Allergic reaction: purpura, red raised rash; if these occur, drug should be discontinued

Perform/provide:
• Storage at room temperature away from heat and light
• Hard candy, frequent rinsing of mouth, gum for dry mouth
• Assistance with ambulation during early part of treatment; dizziness occurs
• Seizure precautions: padded side rails; move objects that may harm patient
• Increased fluids, bulk in diet for constipation

Evaluate:
• Therapeutic response: decreased seizure activity; document on patient's chart

Teach patient/family:
• To carry Medic Alert ID stating patient's name, drugs taken, condition, prescriber's name and phone number
• To avoid driving, other activities that require alertness
• Not to discontinue medication quickly after long-term use

Treatment of overdose: Lavage, VS

ticarcillin (Ŗ)
(tye-kar-sill'in)
Ticar
Func. class.: Broad-spectrum antiinfective
Chem. class.: Extended-spectrum penicillin

Action: Interferes with cell wall replication of susceptible organisms; osmotically unstable cell wall swells, bursts from osmotic pressure.

Uses: Respiratory, soft tissue, urinary tract infections, bacterial septicemia; effective for gram-positive cocci *(Staphylococcus aureus, Streptococcus faecalis, Streptococcus pneumoniae),* gram-negative cocci *(Neisseria gonorrhoeae),* gram-positive bacilli *(Clostridium perfringens, Clostridium tetani),* gram-negative bacilli *(Bacteroides, Fusobacterium nucleatum, Escherichia coli, Proteus mirabilis, Salmonella, Morganella morganii, Proteus rettgeri, Enterobacter, Pseudomonas aeruginosa, Serratia, Peptococcus, Peptostreptococcus, Eubacterium)*

Dosage and routes:
• Dosage reduction needed for renal impairment CrCl <30 ml/min
• *Adult:* **IV/IM** 4-24 g/day in divided doses q4-6h; infuse over ½-2 hr
• *Child:* **IV/IM** 50-300 mg/kg/day in divided doses q4-8h
• *Neonate:* **IV INF** 75-100 mg/kg/8-12 hr

Available forms: Inj 1, 3, 6, 20, 30 g
Side effects/adverse reactions:
HEMA: Anemia, increased bleeding time, ***bone marrow depression, granulocytopenia***
GI: Nausea, vomiting, diarrhea; increased AST, ALT; abdominal pain, glossitis, colitis

---

 = Nursing alert   = Herb-drug interaction   = Do not crush

GU: Oliguria, proteinuria, hematuria, *vaginitis, moniliasis, **glomerulonephritis***

CNS: Lethargy, hallucinations, anxiety, depression, twitching, ***coma, convulsions***

INTEG: Rash

META: Hypokalemia

Contraindications: Hypersensitivity to penicillins

Precautions: Hypersensitivity to cephalosporins, pregnancy (B), lactation, renal disease

Pharmacokinetics:

IM: Peak 1 hr, duration 4-6 hr

IV: Peak 30-45 min, duration 4 hr, half-life 70 min; small amount metabolized in liver; excreted in urine, breast milk

Interactions:

• Decreased antimicrobial effect of ticarcillin: tetracyclines, aminoglycosides IV

• Increased effect of: neuromuscular blockers, heparin

• Increased ticarcillin concentrations: aspirin, probenecid

• Decreased effect: oral contraceptives

🌿 Delayed/reduced absorption: khat, separate by ≥2 hr

Lab test interferences:

False positive: Urine glucose, urine protein

NURSING CONSIDERATIONS

Assess:

• I&O ratio; report hematuria, oliguria, since penicillin in high doses is nephrotoxic

◆ Any patient with compromised renal system, since drug is excreted slowly in poor renal system function; toxicity may occur rapidly

• Liver studies: AST, ALT

• Blood studies: WBC, RBC, Hgb, Hct, bleeding time

• Renal studies: urinalysis, protein, blood, BUN, creatinine

• C&S before drug therapy; drug may be given as soon as culture is taken

• Bowel pattern before, during treatment

• Skin eruptions after administration of penicillin to 1 wk after discontinuing drug

• Respiratory status: rate, character, wheezing, tightness in chest

• Allergies before initiation of treatment, reaction of each medication; highlight allergies on chart

Administer:

• Drug after C&S has been completed

IV

• After diluting 1 g or less/4 ml sterile H_2O for inj; dilute further with 10-20 ml or more D_5W, NS, or sterile H_2O for inj sol; give 1 g or less/5 min or more or by intermittent inf over ½-2 hr or by continuous inf at prescribed rate

Additive compatibilities: Ranitidine, verapamil

Y-site compatibilities: Acyclovir, allopurinol, amifostine, aztreonam, cisatracurium, cyclophosphamide, diltiazem, doxorubicin, famotidine, filgrastim, fludarabine, granisetron, heparin, hydromorphone, IL-2, insulin (regular), magnesium sulfate, melphalan, meperidine, morphine, ondansetron, perphenazine, propofol, remifentanil, sargramostim, teniposide, theophylline, thiotepa, verapamil, vinorelbine

Perform/provide:

• Adrenalin, suction, tracheostomy set, endotracheal intubation equipment

• Adequate fluid intake (2 L) during diarrhea episodes

• Scratch test to assess allergy on order from prescriber; done when penicillin is only drug of choice

• Storage at room temperature, reconstituted sol 72 hr at room temperature

T

Evaluate:
• Therapeutic response: absence of fever, purulent drainage, redness, inflammation
Teach patient/family:
• That culture may be taken after completed course of medication
• To report sore throat, fever, fatigue (may indicate superinfection)
• To wear or carry Medic Alert ID if allergic to penicillins
• To notify nurse of diarrhea
Treatment of overdose: Withdraw drug, maintain airway, administer epinephrine, aminophylline, O_2, IV corticosteroids for anaphylaxis

---

ticarcillin/ clavulanate (R)

Timentin
Func. class.: Broad-spectrum antiinfective
Chem. class.: Extended-spectrum penicillin

Action: Interferes with cell wall replication of susceptible organisms; osmotically unstable cell wall swells, bursts from osmotic pressure
Uses: Respiratory, soft tissue, and urinary tract infections, bacterial septicemia; effective for gram-positive cocci *(Staphylococcus aureus, Streptococcus faecalis, Streptococcus pneumoniae),* gram-negative cocci *(Neisseria gonorrhoeae),* gram-positive bacilli *(Clostridium perfringens, C. tetani),* gram-negative bacilli *(Bacteroides, Fusobacterium nucleatum, Escherichia coli, Proteus mirabilis, Salmonella, Morganella morganii, Proteus rettgeri, Enterobacter, Pseudomonas aeruginosa, Serratia, Peptococcus, Peptostreptococcus, Eubacterium)*
Dosage and routes:
• Dosage reduction indicated in renal impairment (CrCl <30 ml/min)

• *Adult:* **IV INF** 1 vial containing ticarcillin 3 g, clavulanate 0.1 g q4-6h, infuse over 30 min
• *Child <60 kg:* **IV INF** 200-300 mg ticarcillin/kg/day in divided doses q4-6h
Available forms: Inj 3 g ticarcillin, 0.1 g clavulanate; IV inf 3 g ticarcillin, 0.1 g clavulanate; discs 75 µg ticarcillin, 10 µg clavulanate; powder for inj 3 g ticarcillin, 0.1 g clavulanate; 30 g ticarcillin, 1 g clavulanate
Side effects/adverse reactions:
HEMA: Anemia, increased bleeding time, ***bone marrow depression, granulocytopenia***
GI: Nausea, vomiting, diarrhea; increased AST, ALT; abdominal pain, glossitis, colitis
GU: Oliguria, proteinuria, hematuria, *vaginitis, moniliasis,* ***glomerulonephritis***
CNS: Lethargy, hallucinations, anxiety, depression, twitching, ***coma, convulsions***
META: Hyperkalemia, hypokalemia, alkalosis, hypernatremia
Contraindications: Hypersensitivity to penicillins; neonates
Precautions: Hypersensitivity to cephalosporins, pregnancy (B), renal disease
Pharmacokinetics:
IV: Peak 30-45 min, duration 4 hr, half-life 64-68 min; excreted in urine
Interactions:
• Decreased antimicrobial effect of ticarcillin: tetracyclines, aminoglycosides IV
• Decreased effect: oral contraceptives
• Increased effect of: neuromuscular blockers, heparin
• Increased ticarcillin concentrations: aspirin, probenecid
⚫ Delayed/reduced absorption: khat, separate by ≥2 hr

⬥ = Nursing alert   ⫽ = Herb-drug interaction   ⊘ = Do not crush

Lab test interferences:

False positive: Urine glucose, urine protein, Coombs' test

NURSING CONSIDERATIONS

Assess:

• I&O ratio; report hematuria, oliguria, since penicillin in high doses is nephrotoxic

◆ Any patient with compromised renal system, since drug is excreted slowly in poor renal system function; toxicity may occur rapidly

• Liver studies: AST, ALT

• Blood studies: WBC, RBC, Hct, Hgb, bleeding time

• Renal studies: urinalysis, protein, blood, BUN, creatinine

• C&S before drug therapy; drug may be given as soon as culture is taken

• Bowel pattern before, during treatment

• Skin eruptions after administration of penicillin to 1 wk after discontinuing drug

• Respiratory status: rate, character, wheezing, and tightness in chest

• Allergies before initiation of treatment, reaction of each medication; highlight allergies on chart

Administer:

• Drug after C&S

IV

• After diluting 3.1 g or less/13 ml of sterile H_2O or NaCl (200 mg/ml), shake; may further dilute in 50-100 ml or more NS, D_5W, or LR sol and run over ½ hr

Y-site compatibilities: Allopurinol, amifostine, aztreonam, cefepime, cyclophosphamide, diltiazem, doxorubicin liposome, famotidine, filgrastim, fluconazole, fludarabine, foscarnet, gallium, granisetron, heparin, insulin (regular) melphalan, meperidine, morphine, ondansetron, perphenazine, propofol, remifentanil, sargramostim, teniposide, theophylline, thiotepa, vinorelbine

Perform/provide:

• Adrenaline, suction, tracheostomy set, endotracheal intubation equipment

• Adequate fluid intake (2 L) during diarrhea episodes

• Scratch test to assess allergy on order from prescriber; usually done when penicillin is only drug of choice

• Storage of reconstituted sol 12-24 hr at room temperature, or 3-7 days refrigerated

Evaluate:

• Therapeutic response: absence of fever, purulent drainage, redness, inflammation

Teach patient/family:

• To report persistent diarrhea

• That culture may be taken after completed course of medication

• To report sore throat, fever, fatigue (may indicate superinfection)

• To wear or carry Medic Alert ID if allergic to penicillins

Treatment of overdose: Withdraw drug, maintain airway, administer epinephrine, O_2, IV corticosteroids for anaphylaxis

---

ticlopidine (R)

(tye-cloe'pi-deen)

Ticlid

Func. class.: Platelet aggregation inhibitor

Action: Inhibits first and second phases of ADP-induced effects in platelet aggregation

Uses: Reducing the risk of stroke in high-risk patients

Investigational uses: Intermittent claudication, chronic arterial occlusion, subarachnoid hemorrhage, uremic patients with AV shunts/fistulas, open heart surgery, coronary artery bypass grafts, primary glomerulonephritis, sickle cell disease

T

Dosage and routes:
• *Adult:* **PO** 250 mg bid with food
Available forms: Tabs 250 mg
Side effects/adverse reactions:
INTEG: Rash, pruritus
GI: Nausea, vomiting, *diarrhea,* GI discomfort, ***cholestatic jaundice, hepatitis,*** increased cholesterol, LDL, VLDL, TG
*HEMA: **Bleeding (epistaxis, hematuria, conjunctival hemorrhage, GI bleeding), agranulocytosis, neutropenia, thrombocytopenia, thrombotic thombocytopenic purpura***
CNS: Dizziness
Contraindications: Hypersensitivity, active liver disease, blood dyscrasias, active bleeding
Precautions: Past liver disease, renal disease, elderly, pregnancy (B), lactation, children, increased bleeding risk
Pharmacokinetics: Peak 1-3 hr, metabolized by liver, excreted in urine, feces; half-life increases with repeated dosing
Interactions:
• Increased bleeding tendencies: anticoagulants, aspirin
• Decreased plasma levels of ticlopidine: antacids
• Decreased plasma levels of digoxin
• Increased effects of ticlopidine: cimetidine
• Increased effects of theophylline
NURSING CONSIDERATIONS
Assess:
• Liver function studies: AST, ALT, bilirubin, creatinine (long-term therapy)
◆ Blood studies: CBC; CBC q2 wk × 3 mo, Hct, Hgb, PT (long-term therapy)
◆ Bleed time baseline and throughout, levels may be 2-5 × normal limit

Administer:
• With food to decrease gastric symptoms
Evaluate:
• Therapeutic response: absence of stroke
Teach patient/family:
• That blood work will be necessary during treatment
• To report any unusual bleeding to prescriber
• To take with food or just after eating to minimize GI discomfort
• To report side effects such as diarrhea, skin rashes, subcutaneous bleeding, signs of cholestasis (jaundiced skin and sclera, dark urine, light-colored stools)

---

tiludronate (℞)

(till-oo′droe-nate)

Skelid

Func. class.: Bone resorption inhibitor

Chem. class.: Bisphosphonate

Action: Decreases bone resorption and new bone development
Uses: Paget's disease
Dosage and routes:
• *Adult:* **PO** 400 mg qd, with 8 oz water × 3 mo
Available forms: Tabs 400 mg
Side effects/adverse reactions:
GI: Nausea, diarrhea, dry mouth, gastritis, vomiting, flatulence, gastric ulcers
RESP: Rhinitis, rales, sinusitis, URI
CNS: Headache, somnolence, dizziness, anxiety, vertigo, nervousness, involuntary movements
ENDO: Hyperparathyroidism
INTEG: Rash, epidermal necrosis, pruritus, sweating
*GU: **Nephrotoxicity,*** UTI
MS: Bone pain, decreased mineral-

◆ = Nursing alert   🌿 = Herb-drug interaction   🚫 = Do not crush

ization of nonaffected bones, pathological fractures

Contraindications: Hypersensitivity to bisphosphonates, pathologic fractures, children, colitis, severe renal disease with creatinine >5 mg/dl

Precautions: Pregnancy (C), renal disease, lactation, restricted vit D/Ca, GI disease

Pharmacokinetics:

Half-life 150 hr; duration 6 mo

Interactions:

• Decreased absorption of tiludronate: antacids, mineral supplements with magnesium, calcium, aluminum, aspirin

• Increased effect of tiludronate: indomethacin

NURSING CONSIDERATIONS

Assess:

• GI symptoms, polyuria, flushing, head swelling, tingling, headache—may indicate hypercalcemia; nervousness, irritability, twitching, seizures, spasm, paresthesia indicates hypocalcemia at start of treatment

• Nutritional status; evaluate diet for sources of vit D (milk, some seafood), calcium (dairy products, dark green vegetables), phosphates

• BUN, creatinine, uric acid, chloride, electrolytes, urine pH, urinary Ca, Mg, phosphate, urinalysis (Ca should be kept at 9-10 mg/dl), albumin, alk phosphatase baseline and q3-6 mo; check urine sediment for casts throughout treatment

• For increased drug level—toxic reactions occur rapidly; have calcium chloride or gluconate on hand if Ca level drops too low; check for tetany

Administer:

• On empty stomach to improve absorption (2 hr ac), with 6-8 oz water

Evaluate:

• Therapeutic response: Ca levels 9-10 mg/dl; decreasing symptoms of Paget's disease

Teach patient/family:

• To notify prescriber of hypercalcemic relapse: renal calculi, nausea, vomiting, thirst, lethargy, deep bone or flank pain

• To follow a low-calcium diet as prescribed (Paget's disease, hypercalcemia)

• To notify prescriber of diarrhea, nausea; dose may be divided to lessen these symptoms

---

timolol (Rx)

(tye'moe-lole)
Apo-Timol*, Blocadren, Novo-Timol*, timolol maleate
Func. class.: Antihypertensive
Chem. class.: Nonselective β-blocker

Action: Competitively blocks stimulation of β-adrenergic receptor within vascular smooth muscle (decreases rate of SA node discharge, increases recovery time), slows conduction of AV node, decreases heart rate, which decreases O_2 consumption in myocardium; also decreases renin-aldosterone-angiotensin system, at high doses inhibits $β_2$-receptors in bronchial system

Uses: Mild to moderate hypertension, sinus tachycardia, persistent atrial extrasystoles, tachydysrhythmias, prophylaxis of angina pectoris, reduction of mortality after MI, migraine prevention

Investigational uses: Mitral valve prolapse, hypertrophic cardiomyopathy, thyrotoxicosis, tremors, anxiety, pheochromocytoma, tachydysrhythmias, angina pectoris

Dosage and routes:

Hypertension

• *Adult:* **PO** 10 mg bid, or 20 mg qd, may increase by 10 mg q2-3d, not to exceed 60 mg/day

---

T

Myocardial infarction
- *Adult:* **PO** 10 mg bid beginning 1-4 wks after MI

Migraine headache prevention
- *Adult:* **PO** 10 mg bid or 20 mg qd; may increase to 30 mg/day, 20 mg in AM, 10 mg in PM

Available forms: Tabs 5, 10, 20 mg

Side effects/adverse reactions:
CV: Hypotension, bradycardia, ***CHF,*** edema, chest pain, claudication
CNS: Insomnia, dizziness, hallucinations, anxiety
GI: Nausea, vomiting, ***ischemic colitis,*** diarrhea, *abdominal pain,* ***mesenteric arterial thrombosis***
INTEG: Rash, alopecia, pruritus, fever
HEMA: ***Agranulocytosis, thrombocytopenia, purpura***
EENT: Visual changes, sore throat, *double vision,* dry burning eyes
GU: Impotence, urinary frequency
RESP: ***Bronchospasm,*** *dyspnea,* cough, rales
META: Hypoglycemia
MUSC: Joint pain, muscle pain

Contraindications: Hypersensitivity to β-blockers, cardiogenic shock, heart block (2nd or 3rd degree), sinus bradycardia, CHF, cardiac failure

Precautions: Major surgery, pregnancy (C), lactation, diabetes mellitus, renal disease, thyroid disease, COPD, well-compensated heart failure, CAD, nonallergic bronchospasm

Do not confuse:
Timoptic/Viroptic

Pharmacokinetics:
PO: Peak 2-4 hr; half-life 4 hr; excreted 30%-45% unchanged; 60%-65% metabolized by liver; excreted in urine, breast milk, protein binding <10%

Interactions:
- Increased hypotension, bradycardia: reserpine, hydralazine, methyldopa, prazosin, anticholinergics, alcohol, reserpine, nitrates
- Decreased antihypertensive effects: indomethacin, thyroid
- Increased hypoglycemic effects: insulin, sulfonylureas
- Decreased bronchodilation: theophyllines

Lab test interferences:
Increase: LFTs, renal function tests, K, uric acid
Decrease: Hct, Hgb, HDL

NURSING CONSIDERATIONS
Assess:
- Headaches: location, severity, duration, frequency baseline and throughout treatment
- I&O, weight qd
- B/P during initial treatment, periodically thereafter, pulse q4h; note rate, rhythm, quality
- Apical/radial pulse before administration; notify prescriber of any significant changes
- Baselines in renal, LFTs before therapy begins
- Edema in feet, legs qd
- Skin turgor, dryness of mucous membranes for hydration status

Administer:
- PO ac, hs, tablet may be crushed or swallowed whole
- Reduced dosage in renal dysfunction

Perform/provide:
- Dry storage at room temperature; do not freeze

Evaluate:
- Therapeutic response: decreased B/P after 1-2 wk

Teach patient/family:
- To take with or immediately after meals
- Not to discontinue drug abruptly; taper over 2 wk; may cause precipitate angina
- Not to use OTC products containing α-adrenergic stimulants (nasal

$\Diamondsuit$ = Nursing alert $\text{\textit{\textbf{/}}}$ = Herb-drug interaction $\bigcirc$ = Do not crush

decongestants, cold preparations) unless directed by prescriber

• To report bradycardia, dizziness, confusion, depression, fever, sore throat, shortness of breath to prescriber

• To take pulse at home; advise when to notify prescriber

• To avoid alcohol, smoking, sodium intake

• To comply with weight control, dietary adjustments, modified exercise program

• To carry Medic Alert ID to identify drug, allergies

• To avoid hazardous activities if dizziness is present

• To report symptoms of CHF: difficult breathing, especially on exertion or when lying down; night cough; swelling of extremities

• To take medication hs to minimize effect of orthostatic hypotension

• To wear support hose to minimize effects of orthostatic hypotension

Treatment of overdose: Lavage, IV atropine for bradycardia, IV theophylline for bronchospasm, digitalis, O_2, diuretic for cardiac failure, hemodialysis; administer vasopressor (norepinephrine)

tinzaparin (℞)
(tin-zay-par'in)
Innohep
Func. class.: Anticoagulant
Chem. class.: Unfractionated porcine heparin

Action: Prevents conversion of fibrinogen to fibrin and prothrombin to thrombin by enhancing inhibitory effects of antithrombin III; produces higher ratio of antifactor Xa to antifactor IIa

Uses: Treatment of deep-vein thrombosis, pulmonary emboli when given with warfarin

Dosage and routes:
• *Adult:* SC 175 anti-Xa IU/kg qd ≥6 days and until adequate anticoagulation with warfarin (INR ≥2 for 2 consecutive days)

Available forms: Inj 40,000 IU/2 ml

Side effects/adverse reactions:
CNS: Fever, confusion
GI: Nausea
GU: Edema, peripheral edema
HEMA: **Hypochromic anemia, thrombocytopenia,** bleeding
INTEG: Ecchymosis

Contraindications: Hypersensitivity to this drug, heparin, or pork; hemophilia, leukemia with bleeding, peptic ulcer disease, thrombocytopenic purpura, heparin-induced thrombocytopenia

Precautions: Alcoholism, elderly, pregnancy (C), hepatic disease (severe), renal disease (severe), blood dyscrasias, severe hypertension, subacute bacterial endocarditis, acute nephritis, lactation, children

Pharmacokinetics:
SC: Maximum antithrombin activity (3-5 hr), elimination half-life 4.5 hr

Interactions:
• Increased action of tinzaparin oral anticoagulants, salicylates
• Do not mix with other drugs or infusion fluids

⚠ Increased risk of bleeding: bromelain, cinchona bark

NURSING CONSIDERATIONS
Assess:
• Blood studies (Hct, platelets, occult blood in stools), anti-Xa; thrombocytopenia may occur
• Bleeding gums, petechiae, ecchymosis, black tarry stools, hematuria

T

Administer:
• Only after screening patient for bleeding disorders
• SC only; do not give IM
• To recumbent patient; give SC; rotate inj sites (left/right anterolateral, left-right posterolateral abdominal wall)
• Insert whole length of needle into skin fold held with thumb and forefinger
◆ Only this drug when ordered; not interchangeable with heparin
• At same time each day to maintain steady blood levels
• Do not massage area or aspirate when giving SC injection
• Avoiding all IM injections that may cause bleeding

Perform/provide:
• Storage at 77° F (25° C); do not freeze

Evaluate:
• Therapeutic response: resolution of deep vein thrombosis

Teach patient/family:
• To use soft-bristle toothbrush to avoid bleeding gums, to use electric razor
• To report any signs of bleeding: gums, under skin, urine, stools

Treatment of overdose: Protamine SO_4 1% sol; dose should equal dose of enoxaparin

---

tirofiban (℞)

(tie-roh-fee'ban)
Aggrastat
Func. class.: Antiplatelet
Chem. class.: Nonpeptide antagonist

Action: Antagonist of platelet glycoprotein (GP) IIb/IIIa receptor that leads to binding of fibrinogen and von Willebrand's factor, which inhibits platelet aggregation

Uses: Acute coronary syndrome

Dosage and routes:
• *Adult:* **IV** 0.4 µg/kg/min × 30 min, then 0.1 µg/kg/min

Renal dose
• *Adult:* **IV** CrCl <30 ml/min 0.2 µg/kg/min × 30 min, then 0.05 µg/kg/min, during angiography and for up to 24 hr after angioplasty

Available forms: Inj for sol 250 µg/ml, inj 50 µg/ml

Side effects/adverse reactions:
CV: Bradycardia
CNS: Dizziness
INTEG: Rash
*HEMA: **Bleeding, thrombocytopenia***
OTHER: Dissection, coronary artery edema, pain in legs/pelvis, sweating

Contraindications: Hypersensitivity, active internal bleeding, stroke, major surgery, severe trauma, intracranial neoplasm, aneurysm, hemorrhage

Precautions: Pregnancy (B), lactation, elderly, renal disease, bleeding tendencies

Pharmocokinetics: Half-life 2 hr, excretion via urine/feces; plasma clearance 20%-25% lower in elderly; renal insufficiency decreases plasma clearance

Interactions:
• Increased bleeding: aspirin, heparin, NSAIDs, abciximab, eptifibatide, clopidogrel, ticlopidine, dipyridamole, cefamandole, cefotetan, cefoperazone, plicamycin, valproic acid

NURSING CONSIDERATIONS
Assess:
• B/P pulse during treatment until stable; take B/P lying, standing; orthostatic hypotension is common
◆ Platelet counts, Hct, Hgb, prior to treatment, within 6 hr of loading dose and at least qd thereafter; watch for bleeding from puncture sites, catheters or in stools, urine

---

◆ = Nursing alert   ⧪ = Herb-drug interaction   ⊘ = Do not crush

Administer:

• IV: Give ½ dose in renal disease

• Dilute inj: withdraw and discard 100 ml from a 500 ml bag of sterile 0.9% NaCl or D₅W and replace this vol with 50 ml of tirofiban inj from one vial

• Tirofiban inj for sol is premixed in containers of 500 ml 0.9% NaCl (50 mg/ml)

• Minimize other arterial/venous punctures; IM inj, catheter use, intubation, to reduce bleeding risks

Evaluate:

• Therapeutic response: decreased platelet count

Teach patient/family:

• That it is necessary to quit smoking to prevent excessive vasoconstriction

• To avoid hazardous activities; dizziness may occur

---

tizanidine

(ti-za′nih-deen)

Zanaflex

Func. class.: Skeletal muscle relaxant, α₂-adrenergic agonist

Chem. class.: Imidazoline

Action: Increases presynaptic inhibition of motor neurons and reduces spasticity by α₂-adrenergic agonism

Uses: Acute/intermittent management of increased muscle tone associated with spasticity

Dosage and routes:

• *Adult:* **PO** 4-8 mg, increase gradually by 2-4 mg increments, may repeat dose q6-8h, not to exceed 36 mg/24 hr

Available forms: Tabs 4 mg

Side effects/adverse reactions:

GI: Dry mouth, vomiting, increased ALT, abnormal liver function studies, constipation

CNS: Somnolence, dizziness, speech disorder, dyskinesia, nervousness, hallucination, psychosis

OTHER: UTI, infection, blurred vision, urinary frequency, flulike symptoms, pharyngitis, rhinitis

Contraindications: Hypersensitivity

Precautions: Hypotension, liver disease, pregnancy (C), lactation, elderly, children, renal disease

Pharmacokinetics: Completely absorbed, widely distributed; half-life 2.5 hr, peak 1½ hr; protein binding 30%; metabolized by liver, excreted in urine, feces

Interactions:

• Increased CNS depression: alcohol

• Decreased clearance of tizanidine: oral contraceptives

NURSING CONSIDERATIONS

Assess:

• For muscle spasticity baseline and throughout treatment

• For hypotension, gradual dosage increase should lessen hypotensive effects; have patient rise slowly from supine to upright; watch those patients receiving antihypertensives for increased effects

• For increased sedation, dizziness, hallucinations, psychosis; drug may need to be discontinued

• Vision by ophthalmic exam, corneal opacities may occur

• Liver function studies: 1, 3, 6 mo during treatment and periodically thereafter

Teach patient/family:

• To rise slowly from lying or sitting to upright position

• To ask for assistance if dizziness, sedation occur; to avoid drinking alcohol, to avoid operating machinery or driving until effects are known

---

tobramycin (℞)

(toe-bra-mye'sin)
Nebcin, TOBI, tobramycin
sulfate, Tobrax
Func. class.: Antiinfective
Chem. class.: Aminoglycoside

Action: Interferes with protein synthesis in bacterial cell by binding to ribosomal subunit, causing inaccurate peptide sequence to form in protein chain, causing bacterial death

Uses: Severe systemic infections of CNS, respiratory, GI, urinary tract, bone, skin, soft tissues caused by *Pseudomonas aeruginosa, Escherichia coli, Enterobacter, Providencia, Citrobacter, Staphylococcus, Proteus, Klebsiella, Serratia;* cystic fibrosis (nebulizer) for *Pseudomonas aeruginosa*

Dosage and routes:

• *Adult:* **IM/IV** 3 mg/kg/day in divided doses q8h; may give up to 5 mg/kg/day in divided doses q6-8h; once qd dosing is an option

• *Child:* **IM/IV** 6-7.5 mg/kg/day in 3-4 equal divided doses

• *Child ≥6 yr:* **NEB** 300 mg bid in repeating cycles of 28 days on/28 days off of drug; give **INH** over 10-15 min using a handheld PARI LC PLUS reusable nebulizer with a DeVilbiss Pulmo-Aid compressor

• *Neonate <1 wk:* **IM** up to 4 mg/kg/day in divided doses q12h; **IV** up to 4 mg/kg/day in divided doses q12h diluted in 50-100 mg NS or D_5W; give over 30-60 min

Available forms: Inj 10, 40 mg/ml; pwd for inj 1.2 g; inj 20 mg/2 ml; neb sol 300 mg/5 ml

Side effects/adverse reactions:

GU: Oliguria, hematuria, renal damage, azotemia, renal failure, nephrotoxicity

CNS: Confusion, depression, numbness, tremors, *convulsions,* muscle twitching, *neurotoxicity,* dizziness, vertigo

EENT: Ototoxicity, deafness, visual disturbances, tinnitus

HEMA: Agranulocytosis, thrombocytopenia, leukopenia, eosinophilia, anemia

GI: Nausea, vomiting, anorexia; increased ALT, AST, bilirubin, hepatomegaly, *hepatic necrosis,* splenomegaly

CV: Hypotension, hypertension, palpitation

INTEG: Rash, burning, urticaria, dermatitis, alopecia

Contraindications: Severe renal disease, hypersensitivity to aminoglycosides, pregnancy (D)

Precautions: Neonates, mild renal disease, myasthenia gravis, lactation, hearing deficits, Parkinson's disease, elderly

Do not confuse:

Tobrex/Tobra Dex

Pharmacokinetics:

IM: Onset rapid, peak 1 hr

IV: Onset immediate, peak 1 hr Plasma half-life 2-3 hr prolonged in neonates; not metabolized, excreted unchanged in urine, crosses placental barrier, poor penetration into CSF

Interactions:

• Increased ototoxicity, neurotoxicity, nephrotoxicity: other aminoglycosides, amphotericin B, polymyxin, vancomycin, ethacrynic acid, furosemide, mannitol, methoxyflurane, cisplatin, cephalosporins, bacitracin, acyclovir, penicillins

NURSING CONSIDERATIONS

Assess:

• Weight before treatment; dosage is usually based on ideal body weight, but may be calculated on actual body weight

• I&O ratio, urinalysis qd for proteinuria, cells, casts; report sudden change in urine output

---

◆ = Nursing alert   🖊 = Herb-drug interaction   🚫 = Do not crush

- VS during infusion; watch for hypotension, change in pulse
- IV site for thrombophlebitis, including pain, redness, swelling q30min; change site if needed; apply warm compresses to discontinued site
- Serum peak, drawn at 30-60 min after IV infusion or 60 min after IM injection, trough drawn just before next dose, peak 4-12 µg/ml, trough 1-2 µg/ml
- Urine pH if drug is used for UTI; urine should be kept alkaline
- Renal impairment by securing urine for CrCl testing, BUN, serum creatinine; lower dosage should be given in renal impairment (CrCl <80 ml/min); monitor electrolytes: potassium, sodium, chloride, magnesium monthy, if patient is on long-term therapy
- Deafness by audiometric testing; ringing, roaring in ears; vertigo; assess hearing before, during, after treatment
- Dehydration: high specific gravity, decrease in skin turgor, dry mucous membranes, dark urine
- Overgrowth of infection: fever, malaise, redness, pain, swelling, perineal itching, diarrhea, stomatitis, change in cough, sputum
- C&S before starting treatment to identify infecting organism
- Vestibular dysfunction: nausea, vomiting, dizziness, headache; drug should be discontinued if severe
- Inj sites for redness, swelling, abscesses; use warm compresses at site

Administer:
- IM inj in large muscle mass; rotate inj sites
- Drug in evenly spaced doses to maintain blood level; separate aminoglycosides and penicillins by ≥1 hr

- Bicarbonate to alkalinize urine if ordered in treating UTI, as drug is most active in an alkaline environment

IV
- Diluted in 50-100 ml 0.9% NaCl or D₅W (adult), infuse over 20-60 min

Additive compatibilities: Aztreonam, bleomycin, calcium gluconate, cefoxitin, ciprofloxacin, clindamycin, furosemide, metronidazole, ofloxacin, ranitidine, verapamil
Syringe compatibilities: Doxapram
Y-site compatibilities: Acyclovir, amifostine, amiodarone, amsacrine, aztreonam, ciprofloxacin, cisatracurium, cyclophosphamide, diltiazem, doxorubicin liposome, enalaprilat, esmolol, filgrastim, fluconazole, fludarabine, foscarnet, furosemide, granisetron, hydromorphone, IL-2, insulin (regular), labetalol, magnesium sulfate, melphalan, meperidine, midazolam, morphine, perphenazine, remifentanil, tacrolimus, teniposide, theophylline, thiotepa, tolazoline, vinorelbine, zidovudine

Nebulizer
- Give as close to q12hr apart as possible; do not use <6 hr apart
- Do not mix with dornase alfa in the nebulizer

Perform/provide:
- Adequate fluids of 2-3 L/day unless contraindicated to prevent irritation of tubules
- Flush of IV line with NS or D₅W after infusion
- Supervised ambulation, other safety measures with vestibular dysfunction

Evaluate:
- Therapeutic response: absence of fever, draining wounds, negative C&S after treatment

Teach patient/family:
- To report headache, dizziness,

symptoms of overgrowth of infection, renal impairment

• To report loss of hearing; ringing, roaring in ears; feeling of fullness in head

Nebulizer

• Have patient inhale sitting or standing, breathe normally through the mouthpiece; may use noseclips

• To use multiple therapies first, then tobramycin

Treatment of overdose: Hemodialysis; monitor serum levels of drug

---

tocainide (℞)

(toe-kay′nide)
Tonocard
Func. class.: Antidysrhythmic (Class Ib)
Chem. class.: Lidocaine analog

Action: Suppresses automaticity of tissue conduction and spontaneous depolarization of ventricles during diastole; does not affect heart rate

Uses: Life-threatening ventricular dysrhythmias (multifocal/unifocal PVCs), ventricular tachycardia

Dosage and routes:

• *Adult:* **PO** 400 mg q8h, may increase to 1.2-1.8 g/day in divided doses q8-12h

Available forms: Tabs 400, 600 mg

Side effects/adverse reactions:

CNS: Headache, dizziness, involuntary movement, confusion, psychosis, restlessness, irritability, paresthesias, tremors, *seizures*

EENT: Tinnitus, blurred vision, hearing loss

GI: Nausea, vomiting, anorexia, diarrhea, hepatitis

CV: Hypotension, bradycardia, angina, PVCs, **heart block, cardiovascular collapse, arrest, CHF,** chest pain, tachycardia, prodysrhythmia

RESP: Dyspnea, *respiratory depression, pulmonary fibrosis*

INTEG: Rash, urticaria, edema, swelling

*HEMA: **Blood dyscrasias: leukopenia, agranulocytosis, hypoplastic anemia, thrombocytopenia***

Contraindications: Hypersensitivity to amides, severe heart block

Precautions: Pregnancy (C), lactation, children, renal disease, liver disease, CHF, respiratory depression, myasthenia gravis, blood dyscrasias

Pharmacokinetics:

PO: Peak 0.5-3 hr; half-life 10-17 hr; metabolized by liver, excreted in urine

Interactions:

• Increased effects: propranolol, quinidine, all other antidysrhythmics

• Decreased tocainide effects: cimetidine, rifampin

🍃 Potassium deficiency, antidysrhythmic action: aloe, buckthorn, cascara sagrada, senna

Lab test interferences:

Increase: CPK

False positive: ANA titer

NURSING CONSIDERATIONS

Assess:

◆Chest x-ray film, pulmonary function tests, liver enzymes during treatment, monitor for lung sounds, sputum, SOB after 3-18 wk

• CBC, with diff and platelet count during beginning treatment and q3mo

• I&O ratio; check for decreasing output

• Blood levels (therapeutic level 4-10 μg/ml)

• B/P continuously for fluctuations

• Lung fields; bilateral rales may occur in CHF patient

• Increased respiration, increased pulse; drug should be discontinued

• Toxicity: fine tremors, dizziness

◆ = Nursing alert   🍃 = Herb-drug interaction   🚫 = Do not crush

• Blood dyscrasias: fatigue, sore throat, fever, bruising
• Cardiac status, respiration: rate, rhythm, character

Evaluate:
• Therapeutic response: decreased dysrhythmia

Treatment of overdose: O₂, artificial ventilation, ECG; administer dopamine for circulatory depression, diazepam or thiopental for convulsions

---

RARELY USED

tolazamide (R)
(tole-az′a-mide)
Tolamide, tolazimide,
Tolinase
Func. class.: Antidiabetic

Uses: Type II (NIDDM) diabetes mellitus
Dosage and routes:
• *Adult:* **PO** 100 mg/day for FBS <200 mg/dl or 250 mg/day for FBS >200 mg/dl; dose should be titrated to response (1 g or less/day)
Contraindications: Hypersensitivity to sulfonylureas, juvenile or type I diabetes

---

RARELY USED

tolbutamide (R)
(tole-byoo′ta-mide)
Mobenol*, Novobutamide*,
Orinase, tolbutamide,
Tolbutone*
Func. class.: Antidiabetic

Uses: Type II (NIDDM) diabetes mellitus
Dosage and routes:
• *Adult:* **PO** 1-2 g/day in divided doses, titrated to patient response;

IV 1 g (Fajans test) over 2-3 min
Contraindications: Hypersensitivity to sulfonylureas, juvenile or type I diabetes

---

tolcapone (R)
(toll′cah′pone)
Tasmar
Func. class.: Antiparkinson agent
Chem. class.: Catecholamine inhibitor (comt)

Action: Selective, reversible inhibitor of catecholamine; used as adjunct to levodopa/carbidopa therapy
Uses: Parkinsonism
Dosage and routes:
• *Adult:* **PO** 100-200 mg tid, with levodopa/carbidopa therapy; max 600 mg/day, discontinue if no benefit in 3 wk
Renal dose
• *Adult:* **PO** Use 100 mg tid or less
Available forms: Tabs 100, 200 mg
Side effects/adverse reactions:
CNS: Dystonia, dyskinesia, dreaming, *fatigue, headache, confusion,* psychosis, hallucination, dizziness
CV: Orthostatic hypotension, chest pain, hypotension
EENT: Cataract, eye inflammation
GI: Nausea, vomiting, anorexia, abdominal distress, diarrhea, constipation, ***fatal liver failure,*** increased LFTs
GU: UTI, urine discoloration, uterine tumor, micturition disorder, hematuria
*HEMA: **Hemolytic anemia, leukopenia, agranulocytosis***
INTEG: Sweating, alopecia
Contraindications: Hypersensitivity, hepatic disease
Precautions: Renal disease, cardiac disease, hepatic disease, hy-

---

pertension, pregnancy (C), asthma, lactation

Pharmacokinetics: Rapidly absorbed, peak 2 hr, protein binding 99%, extensively metabolized, half-life 2-3 hr, excreted in urine (60%), feces (40%)

Interactions:
• Inhibition of normal catecholamine metabolism: MAOIs, MAO-B inhibitor may be used
• May influence pharmacokinetics of: α-methyldopa, dobutamine, apomorphine, isoproterenol

NURSING CONSIDERATIONS
Assess:
• Liver function enzymes: AST, ALT, alk phosphatase, LDH, bilirubin, CBC, monitor ALT, AST q2wk × 1 yr, then q4wk × 6 mo, and q8wk thereafter; if LFTs are elevated, this drug should not be used
• Involuntary movements in parkinsonism: akinesia, tremors, staggering gait, muscle rigidity, drooling
• B/P, respiration during initial treatment; hypo/hypertension should be reported
• Mental status: affect, mood, behavioral changes

Administer:
• PO tid with levodopa/carbidopa therapy, only to be used if levodopa/carbidopa does not provide satisfactory result

Perform/provide:
• Assistance with ambulation during beginning therapy

Evaluate:
• Therapeutic response: decrease in akathisia, increased mood

Teach patient/family:
• To change positions slowly to prevent orthostatic hypotension
• That urine, sweat may change color
• That food taken within 1 hr ac or 2 hr pc decreases action of drug by 20%

• To report signs of liver injury: clay-colored stools, jaundice, fatigue, appetite loss, lethargy
• To report nausea, vomiting, anorexia

---

tolmetin (R)
(tole'met-in)
Tolectin, Tolectin DS, Tolectin 200, Tolectin 600, tolmetin sodium
Func. class.: Nonsteroidal antiinflammatory
Chem. class.: Pyrrole acetic acid derivative

Action: Inhibits prostaglandin synthesis by decreasing an enzyme needed for biosynthesis; analgesic, antiinflammatory, antipyretic

Uses: Mild to moderate pain, osteoarthritis, rheumatoid arthritis

Dosage and routes:
• *Adult:* **PO** 400 mg tid-qid, not to exceed 2 g/day
• *Child >2 yr:* **PO** 15-30 mg/kg/day in 3 or 4 divided doses

Available forms: Caps 400 mg; tabs 200, 600 mg

Side effects/adverse reactions:
GI: Nausea, anorexia, vomiting, diarrhea, jaundice, ***cholestatic hepatitis,*** constipation, flatulence, cramps, dry mouth, peptic ulcer, ulceration, bleeding, perforation
CNS: Dizziness, drowsiness, fatigue, tremors, confusion, insomnia, anxiety, depression, headache
CV: Tachycardia, peripheral edema, palpitations, dysrhythmias, hypertension
INTEG: Purpura, rash, pruritus, sweating
GU: **Nephrotoxicity: dysuria, hematuria, oliguria, azotemia, pseudoproteinuria**
HEMA: **Blood dyscrasias**

♦ = Nursing alert   🌿 = Herb-drug interaction   ⊘ = Do not crush

EENT: Tinnitus, hearing loss, blurred vision

Contraindications: Hypersensitivity, asthma, severe renal disease, severe hepatic disease, ulcer disease

Precautions: Pregnancy (B), lactation, children, bleeding disorders, GI disorders, cardiac disorders, hypersensitivity to other antiinflammatory agents, peptic ulcer disease

Pharmacokinetics:

PO: Peak 2 hr, half-life 3-3½ hr; metabolized in liver, excreted in urine (metabolites), excreted in breast milk, 99% protein binding

Interactions:

• Increased action of warfarin, phenytoin, sulfonamides

NURSING CONSIDERATIONS

Assess:

• Renal, liver, blood studies: BUN, creatinine, AST, ALT, Hgb before treatment, periodically thereafter

• For asthma, nasal polyp, or aspirin allergy, may have hypersensitivity to this product

• I&O ratio

• Audiometric, ophthalmic exam before, during, after treatment

• For eye, ear problems: blurred vision, tinnitus (may indicate toxicity)

Administer:

• With food to decrease GI symptoms; take on empty stomach to facilitate absorption; tab may be crushed

Perform/provide:

• Storage at room temperature

Evaluate:

• Therapeutic response: decreased pain, stiffness, swelling in joints, ability to move more easily

Teach patient/family:

• To report blurred vision, ringing, roaring in ears (may indicate toxicity)

• To avoid driving, other hazardous activities if dizzy or drowsy

• To report change in urine pattern, weight increase, edema, pain increase in joints, fever, blood in urine (indicates nephrotoxicity)

• That therapeutic effects may take up to 1 mo

• To drink 8 glasses water daily

• About drug interactions, to avoid ASA, alcohol

---

tolterodine (Rx)

(toll-tehr'oh-deen)

Detrol, Detrol LA

Func. class.: Overactive bladder product

Chem. class.: Muscarinic receptor antagonist

Action: Relaxes smooth muscles in urinary tract by inhibiting acetylcholine at postganglionic sites

Uses: Overactive bladder (urinary frequency, urgency)

Dosage and routes:

• *Adult:* **PO** 2 mg bid, hepatic disease 1 mg bid; 4 mg qd, may decrease to 2 mg if needed

Available forms: Tabs 1, 2 mg; cap, ext rel 2, 4 mg

Side effects/adverse reactions:

CNS: Anxiety, paresthesia, fatigue, *dizziness,* headache

CV: Chest pain, hypertension

EENT: Vision abnormalities, xerophthalmia

GI: Nausea, vomiting, anorexia, abdominal pain, constipation, dry mouth, dyspepsia

GU: Dysuria, urinary retention, frequency, UTI

INTEG: Rash, pruritus

RESP: Bronchitis, cough, pharyngitis, URI

Contraindications: hypersensitivity, uncontrolled narrow-angle glaucoma, urinary retention, gastric retention

T

Precautions: Pregnancy (C), lactation, children, renal/hepatic disease, controlled narrow-angle glaucoma

Pharmacokinetics: Rapidly absorbed, highly protein bound, extensively metabolized, excreted in urine/feces

Interactions:

• Increased action of tolterodine: macrolide antiinfectives, antifungals

• Drug/food: food increases the bioavailability of tolterodine

NURSING CONSIDERATIONS

Assess:

• Urinary patterns: distention, nocturia, frequency, urgency, incontinence

• Allergic reactions: rash; if this occurs, drug should be discontinued

Evaluate:

• Urinary status: dysuria, frequency, nocturia, incontinence

Teach patient/family:

• To avoid hazardous activities; dizziness may occur

---

topiramate (R)

(toh-pire′ah-mate)
Topamax
Func. class.: Anticonvulsant, miscellaneous
Chem. class.: Carbamate derivative

Action: Mechanism of action unknown; may prevent seizure spread as opposed to an elevation of seizure threshold

Uses: Partial seizures, with or without generalization in adults; tonic-clonic seizures; seizures in Lennox-Gastaut syndrome

Investigational uses: Bipolar disorder, cluster headache, infantile spasms

Dosage and routes:
Renal dose
• CrCl <70 ml/min give ½ dose
Adjunctive therapy
• *Adult:* **PO** add 400 mg in 2 divided doses
Bipolar disorder (off-label)
• *Adult:* **PO** 50-200 mg/day, max 400 mg/day
Available forms: Tabs 25, 100, 200 mg; sprinkle cap 15, 25 mg

Side effects/adverse reactions:
RESP: URI, pharyngitis, sinusitis
EENT: Diplopia, vision abnormality
INTEG: Rash
MISC: Weight loss, leukopenia
CNS: Dizziness, fatigue, cognitive disorder, insomnia, anxiety, depression, paresthesia
ENDO: Weight loss
GI: Diarrhea, anorexia, nausea, dyspepsia, abdominal pain, constipation, dry mouth
GU: Breast pain, dysmenorrhea, menstrual disorder

Contraindications: Hypersensitivity

Precautions: Hepatic, renal, cardiac disease, elderly, lactation, children, pregnancy (C)

Pharmacokinetics: Well absorbed, terminal half-life 21 hr; excreted in urine (55%-97% unchanged), crosses placenta, excreted in breast milk, protein binding (9%-17%); steady state 4 days

Interactions:
• Decreased levels of: oral contraceptives, digoxin
• Increased levels of: alcohol, CNS depressants, carbonic anhydrase inhibitors
• Decreased levels of topiramate: food, phenytoin, carbamazepine, valproic acid

NURSING CONSIDERATIONS

Assess:
• Renal studies: urinalysis, BUN, urine creatinine q3mo

◆ = Nursing alert   🖋 = Herb-drug interaction   ⊘ = Do not crush

• Hepatic studies: ALT, AST, bilirubin if on long-term treatment
• CBC during long-term therapy
• Description of seizures: location, type, duration, aura
• Mental status: mood, sensorium, affect, behavioral changes; if mental status changes, notify prescriber
• Body weight, evidence of cognitive disorder

Administer:
🚫 Whole; do not break, crush, or chew tabs, very bitter
• May take with food
• Sprinkle cap can be given whole or opened and sprinkled on soft food; do not chew

Perform/provide:
• Storage at room temperature away from heat and light
• Assistance with ambulation during early part of treatment; dizziness occurs
• Seizure precautions: padded side rails, move objects that may harm patient

Evaluate:
• Therapeutic response: decreased seizure activity

Teach patient/family:
• To carry ID stating patient's name, drugs taken, condition, prescriber's name, phone number
• To avoid driving, other activities that require alertness
• Not to discontinue medication quickly after long-term use

Treatment of overdose: Lavage, VS

topotecan
(toh-poh-tee′kan)
Hycamtin
Func. class.: Antineoplastic hormone
Chem. class.: Semi-synthetic derivative of camptothecin (topoisomerase inhibitor)

Action: Antitumor drug with topoisomerase I–inhibitory activity topoisomerase I relieves torsional strain in DNA by causing single-strand breaks; causes double-strand DNA damage

Uses: Metastatic carcinoma of the ovary after failure of traditional chemotherapy

Dosage and routes:
• *Adult:* **IV INF** 1.5 mg/m^2 over 30 min qd × 5 days starting on day 1 of a 21-day course × 4 courses; may be reduced to 0.25 mg/m^2 for subsequent courses if severe neutropenia occurs

Renal dose
• *Adult:* **IV** CrCl 20-39 ml/min 0.75 mg/m^2/day × 5 days starting on day 1 of a 21 day course

Available forms: Lyophilized pwd for inj 4 mg

Side effects/adverse reactions:
*HEMA: **Neutropenia, leukopenia, thrombocytopenia, anemia, sepsis***
GI: Abdominal pain, constipation, diarrhea, obstruction, nausea, stomatitis, vomiting; increased ALT, AST; anorexia
CNS: Arthralgia, asthenia, headache, myalgia, pain
RESP: Dyspnea
INTEG: Total alopecia

Contraindications: Hypersensitivity, lactation, severe bone marrow depression, pregnancy (D)
Precautions: Children

T

Interactions:
• Increased duration of neutropenia when used with: G-CSF
• Increased myelosuppression when used with: cisplatin

Pharmacokinetics: Rapidly and completely absorbed; excreted in urine and feces as metabolites; half-life 6 hr, geriatric half-life 8 hr; 94% bound to plasma proteins

NURSING CONSIDERATIONS
Assess:
• Liver function studies: AST, ALT, alk phosphatase, which may be elevated
• For CNS symptoms: drowsiness, confusion, depression, anxiety
• CBC, differential, platelet count weekly; withhold drug if WBC is <3500/mm³ or platelet count is <100,000/mm³; notify prescriber of these results; drug should be discontinued
• Buccal cavity q8h for dryness, sores or ulceration, white patches, oral pain, bleeding, dysphagia
• GI symptoms: frequency of stools, cramping
• Signs of dehydration: rapid respiration, poor skin turgor, decreased urine output, dry skin, restlessness, weakness

Perform/provide:
• Increased fluid intake to 2-3 L/day to prevent dehydration, unless contraindicated
• Changing of IV site q48h
• Rinsing of mouth tid-qid with water, club soda; brushing of teeth bid-tid with soft brush or cotton-tipped applicator for stomatitis; use unwaxed dental floss
• Nutritious diet with iron, vit K supplements, low fiber, few dairy products

Evaluate:
• Therapeutic response: decreased tumor size, spread of malignancy

Teach patient/family:
• To avoid foods with citric acid or hot or rough texture if stomatitis is present; to drink adequate fluids
• To report stomatitis; any bleeding, white spots, ulcerations in mouth; tell patient to examine mouth qd; report symptoms
• To report signs of anemia: fatigue, headache, faintness, shortness of breath, irritability
• To use contraception during therapy

---

toremifene (℞)
(tor-em'ih-feen)
Fareston
Func. class.: Antineoplastic
Chem. class.: Antiestrogen hormone

Action: Inhibits cell division by binding to cytoplasmic estrogen receptors; resembles normal cell complex but inhibits DNA synthesis and estrogen response of target tissue

Uses: Advanced breast carcinoma not responsive to other therapy in estrogen-receptor-positive patients (usually postmenopausal)

Dosage and routes:
• *Adult:* **PO** 60 mg qd
Available forms: Tabs 60 mg

Side effects/adverse reactions:
*HEMA: **Thrombocytopenia, leukopenia***
*CV: **CHF, MI, pulmonary embolism***
GI: Nausea, vomiting, altered taste (anorexia)
GU: Vaginal bleeding, pruritus vulvae
INTEG: Rash, alopecia
CV: Chest pain
CNS: Hot flashes, headache, lightheadedness, depression
META: Hypercalcemia
EENT: Ocular lesions, retinopathy,

◆ = Nursing alert   🖋 = Herb-drug interaction   🚫 = Do not crush

corneal opacity, blurred vision (high doses)

Contraindications: Hypersensitivity, pregnancy (D)

Precautions: Leukopenia, thrombocytopenia, lactation, cataracts

Pharmacokinetics:

PO: Peak 3 hr, excreted primarily in feces

Interactions:

• May increase the effect of: warfarin

Lab test interferences:

Increase: Serum Ca

NURSING CONSIDERATIONS

Assess:

• CBC, differential, platelet count qwk; withhold drug if WBC is <3500/mm³ or platelet count is <100,000/mm³; notify prescriber

• Bleeding: hematuria, guaiac, bruising, petechiae, mucosa or orifices q8h

• Effects of alopecia on body image; discuss feelings about body changes

◆ Symptoms indicating severe allergic reactions: rash, pruritus, urticaria, purpuric skin lesions, itching, flushing

Administer:

• Antacid before oral agent; give drug after evening meal, before bedtime

• Antiemetic 30-60 min before giving drug to prevent vomiting

Perform/provide:

• Liquid diet, if needed, including cola, Jell-O; dry toast or crackers may be added if patient is not nauseated or vomiting

• Increase fluid intake to 2-3 L/day to prevent dehydration

• Nutritious diet with iron, vitamin supplements as ordered

• Storage in light-resistant container at room temperature

Evaluate:

• Therapeutic response: decreased tumor size, spread of malignancy

Teach patient/family:

• To report any complaints, side effects to prescriber

• That vaginal bleeding, pruritus, hot flashes are reversible after discontinuing treatment

• To report immediately decreased visual acuity, which may be irreversible; stress need for routine eye exams; care providers should be told about tamoxifen therapy

• To report vaginal bleeding immediately

• That tumor flare—increase in size of tumor, increased bone pain—may occur and will subside rapidly; may take analgesics for pain

• That premenopausal women must use mechanical birth control because ovulation may be induced

• That hair may be lost during treatment; a wig or hairpiece may make patient feel better; new hair may be different in color, texture

---

torsemide (℞)

(tor′suh-mide)

Demadex

Func. class.: Loop diuretic

Chem. class.: Sulfonamide derivative

Action: Acts on loop of Henle, proximal, distal tubule by inhibiting absorption of chloride, sodium, water

Uses: Treatment of hypertension and edema in CHF, hepatic disease, renal disease

Dosage and routes:

CHF

• *Adult:* PO/IV 10-20 mg/day, may increase as needed up to 200 mg/day

Chronic renal failure

• *Adult:* PO/IV 20 mg/day, may increase up to 200 mg/day

T

Side effects: *italics* = common; **bold italics** = life-threatening

Hepatic cirrhosis
• *Adult:* **PO/IV** 5-10 mg/day may increase as needed up to 40 mg/day
Hypertension
• *Adult:* **PO** 5 mg/day may increase to 10 mg/day
Available forms: Tabs 5, 10, 20, 100 mg; inj 10 mg/ml
Side effects/adverse reactions:
CNS: Headache, dizziness, asthenia, insomnia, nervousness
CV: Orthostatic hypotension, chest pain, ECG changes, *circulatory collapse,* ventricular tachycardia
EENT: Loss of hearing, ear pain, tinnitus, blurred vision
ENDO: Hyperglycemia, hyperuricemia
ELECT: Hypokalemia, hypochloremic alkalosis, hypomagnesemia, hypocalcemia, hyponatremia, metabolic alkalosis
GI: Nausea, diarrhea, dyspepsia, GI hemorrhage, rectal bleeding, cramps
*GU: Polyuria, **renal failure,*** glycosuria
INTEG: Rash, photosensitivity
MS: Cramps, stiffness
RESP: Rhinitis, cough increase
Contraindications: Hypersensitivity to sulfonamides, anuria, hypovolemia, infants, lactation, electrolyte depletion
Precautions: Diabetes mellitus, dehydration, severe renal disease, pregnancy (C)
Pharmacokinetics:
PO: Rapidly absorbed; duration 6 hr; excreted in urine, feces, breast milk; crosses placenta; half-life 2-4 hr, plasma protein binding 97%-99%
Interactions:
• Increased toxicity: lithium, nondepolarizing skeletal muscle relaxants, digitalis
• Increased action of antihypertensives, oral anticoagulants, nitrates
• Increased ototoxicity: aminoglycosides, cisplatin, vancomycin
• Decreased antihypertensive effect of torsemide: indomethacin, metolazone
• Incompatible with acidic sol, vit C, corticosteroids, diphenhydramine, dobutamine, esmolol, epinephrine, gentamicin, meperidine, milrinone, netilmicin, norepinephrine, reserpine, spironolactone, tetracyclines in sol
• Incompatible with any drug in syringe
Lab test interferences:
Interference: GTT
NURSING CONSIDERATIONS
Assess:
• Hearing when giving high doses
• Weight, I&O daily to determine fluid loss; effect of drug may be decreased if used qd
• Rate, depth, rhythm of respiration, effect of exertion
• B/P lying, standing; postural hypotension may occur
• Electrolytes: K, Na, Cl; include BUN, blood sugar, CBC, serum creatinine, blood pH, ABGs, uric acid, Ca, Mg
• Glucose in urine of diabetic
• Signs and symptoms of metabolic alkalosis: drowsiness, restlessness
• Signs and symptoms of hypokalemia: postural hypotension, malaise, fatigue, tachycardia, leg cramps, weakness
• Rashes, temp elevation qd
• Confusion, especially in elderly; take safety precautions if needed
Administer:
• In AM to avoid interference with sleep if using drug as a diuretic
• K replacement if K <3 mg/dl
• With food if nausea occurs; absorption may be decreased slightly
Evaluate:
• Therapeutic response: improvement in edema of feet, legs, sacral

➡ = Nursing alert   ⫻ = Herb-drug interaction   🚫 = Do not crush area qd if medication is being used in CHF

Teach patient/family:

• To rise slowly from lying, sitting position

• To recognize adverse reactions: muscle cramps, weakness, nausea, dizziness

• To take with food or milk for GI symptoms

• To take early in day to prevent nocturia

Treatment of overdose: Lavage if taken orally; monitor electrolytes, administer dextrose in saline; monitor hydration, CV, renal status

---

trace elements (℞)

Concentrated Multiple Trace Elements, ConTE-PAK-4, M.T.E.-4, M.T.E.-4 Concentrated, M.T.E.-5, M.T.E.-5 Concentrated, M.T.E.-6, M.T.E.-6 Concentrated, M.T.E.-7, MulTE-PAK-4, MulTE-PAK-5, Multiple Trace Element, Multiple Trace Element Neonatal, Multiple Trace Element Pediatric, Neotrace 4, PedTE-PAK-4, Pedtrace-4, P.T.E.-4, P.T.E.-5

Func. class.: Mineral supplements

Action: Needed for adequate absorption and synthesis of amino acids

Uses: Prevention of trace element deficiency

Dosage and routes:

Usual dosage may be given in TPN sol

Chromium

• *Adult:* IV 10-15 μg qd

• *Child:* IV 0.14-0.20 μg/kg/day

Copper

• *Adult:* IV 0.5-1.5 mg/day

• *Child:* IV 0.05-0.2 mg/kg/day

Iodine

• *Adult:* IV 1 μg/kg/day

Manganese

• *Adult:* IV 1-3 mg/day

Selenium

• *Adult:* 40-120 μg/day

• *Child:* 3 μg/kg/day

Zinc

• *Adult:* IV 2-4 mg/day

• *Child:* IV 0.05 mg/kg/day

Available forms: Many forms available—see particular elements

Side effects/adverse reactions: Depends on element

Precautions: Liver, biliary disease, pregnancy (C), lactation, vomiting, diarrhea

NURSING CONSIDERATIONS

Assess:

• Trace element levels; notify prescriber if low; copper 0.07-0.15 mg/ml, zinc 0.05-0.15 mg/100 ml, manganese 4-20 μg/100 ml, selenium 0.1-0.19 μg/ml

• Trace element deficiency of patient receiving TPN for extended period

Administer:

• By IV infusion, often mixed with TPN solution

Evaluate:

• Therapeutic response: absence of element deficiency

---

tramadol (℞)

(tram'a-dole)

Ultram

Func. class.: Central analgesic

Action: Not completely understood, binds to opioid receptors, inhibits reuptake of norepinephrine, serotonin; does not cause histamine release or affect heart rate

Uses: Management of moderate to severe pain

T

Dosage and routes:
Renal dose
• CrCl <30 ml/min give q12h, max 200 mg/day
• *Adult:* **PO** 50-100 mg prn q4-6h; not to exceed 400 mg/day
• *Elderly (>75 years):* **PO** <300 mg/day in divided doses
Hepatic impairment
• **PO** 50 mg q12h
Available forms: Tabs 50 mg
Side effects/adverse reactions:
CNS: Dizziness, CNS stimulation, somnolence, headache, anxiety, confusion, euphoria, *seizures,* hallucinations
GI: Nausea, constipation, vomiting, dry mouth, diarrhea, abdominal pain, anorexia, flatulence, *GI bleeding*
CV: Vasodilation, orthostatic hypotension, tachycardia, hypertension, abnormal ECG
INTEG: Pruritus, rash, urticaria, vesicles
GU: Urinary retention/frequency, menopausal symptoms, dysuria, menstrual disorder
Interactions:
• Decreased levels of tramadol: carbamazepine
• Inhibition of norepinephrine and serotonin reuptake: MAO inhibitors, use together with caution
• Increased CNS depression: alcohol, sedatives, hypnotics, opiates
🖋 Increased CNS depression: kava
Lab test interferences:
Increase: Creatinine, liver enzymes
Decrease: Hgb
Contraindications: Hypersensitivity, acute intoxication with any CNS depressant
Precautions: Seizure disorder, pregnancy (C), lactation, children, elderly, renal or hepatic disease, respiratory depression, head trauma, increased intracranial pressure, acute abdominal condition, drug abuse
Do not confuse:
tramadol/Toradol
Pharmacokinetics: Rapidly and almost completely absorbed, steady state 2 days, may cross blood-brain barrier, extensively metabolized, 30% excreted in the urine as unchanged drug

NURSING CONSIDERATIONS
Assess:
• Pain: location, type, character, give before pain becomes extreme
• I&O ratio: check for decreasing output; may indicate urinary retention
• Need for drug
• Bowel pattern; for constipation increase fluids, bulk in diet
• CNS changes: dizziness, drowsiness, hallucinations, euphoria, LOC, pupil reaction
• Allergic reactions: rash, urticaria
Administer:
PO
• With antiemetic for nausea, vomiting
• When pain is beginning to return; determine dosage interval by patient response
Perform/provide:
• Storage in cool environment, protected from sunlight
• Assistance with ambulation
• Safety measures: side rails, nightlight, call bell within easy reach
Evaluate:
• Therapeutic response: decrease in pain
Teach patient/family:
• To report any symptoms of CNS changes, allergic reactions
• That drowsiness, dizziness, and confusion may occur, to call for assistance
• To make position changes slowly, orthostatic hypotension may occur

---

◆ = Nursing alert   🖋 = Herb-drug interaction   🚫 = Do not crush

• To avoid OTC medications and alcohol unless approved by prescriber

trandolapril (℞)
(tran-doe'la-prill)
Mavik
Func. class.: Antihypertensive
Chem. class.: Angiotension-converting enzyme inhibitor

Action: Selectively suppresses renin-angiotensin-aldosterone system; inhibits ACE; prevents conversion of angiotensin I to angiotensin II, dilates arterial and venous vessels, lowers B/P

Uses: Hypertension, heart failure, post-MI/left ventricular dysfunction post MI

Dosage and routes:
Hypertension
• *Adult:* PO 1 mg/day, 2 mg/day in African-Americans, make dosage adjustment ≥wk; up to 8 mg/day
Heart failure post MI/left ventricular dysfunction post MI
• *Adult:* PO 1 mg/day, titrate upward to 4 mg/day if tolerated
Renal dose
• CrCl <30 ml/min give 0.5 mg/day, may increase gradually
Available forms: Tabs 1, 2, 4 mg
Side effects/adverse reactions:
*CV: Hypotension, **MI,** palpitations, angina, TIAs, **stroke,** bradycardia, dysrhythmias
CNS: Dizziness, paresthesias, headache, fatigue, drowsiness, depression, sleep disturbances
GI: Nausea, vomiting, cramps, diarrhea, constipation, ileus, pancreatitis, hepatitis, *dyspepsia*
INTEG: Rash, purpura
*HEMA: **Agranulocytosis, neutropenia, leukopenia, anemia***
*GU: **Proteinuria, renal failure***
RESP: Dyspnea, *cough*
MISC: Hyperkalemia, hyponatremia, impotence, *myalgia*

Contraindications: Hypersensitivity, history of angioedema, pregnancy (D) (2nd, 3rd trimester)
Precautions: Renal disease, hyperkalemia, hepatic disease, bilateral renal stenosis, post kidney transplant, aorta/mitral valve stenosis, cirrhosis, severe renal disease, untreated CHF, autoimmune disease, severe hypertension
Pharmacokinetics:
PO: Peak 4-10 hr; half-life 0.6-1.1 hr, 16-24 hr; metabolized by liver, excreted in urine
Interactions:
• Hypersensitivity: allopurinol
• Severe hypotension: diuretics, other antihypertensives
• Decreased effects of trandolapril: aspirin, antacids
• Increased K levels: salt substitutes, K-sparing diuretics, K supplements
• May increase effects of ergots, neuromuscular blocking agents, antihypertensives, hypoglycemics, barbiturates, reserpine, levodopa
• Effects may be increased by phenothiazines, diuretics, phenytoin, quinidine, nifedipine
NURSING CONSIDERATIONS
Assess:
• B/P, pulse q4h; note rate, rhythm, quality
• Electrolytes: K, Na, Cl
• Baselines in renal, LFTs before therapy begins
• Edema in feet, legs daily
• Skin turgor, dryness of mucous membranes for hydration status
• Symptoms of CHF: edema, dyspnea, wet rales
Evaluate:
• Therapeutic response: decreased B/P

Teach patient/family:

• Not to use OTC (cough, cold, or allergy) products unless directed by prescriber

• To avoid sunlight or wear sunscreen for photosensitivity

• To comply with dosage schedule, even if feeling better

• To notify prescriber of mouth sores, sore throat, fever, swelling of hands or feet, irregular heartbeat, chest pain, signs of angioedema

• That excessive perspiration, dehydration, vomiting, diarrhea may lead to fall in blood pressure; consult prescriber if these occur

• That drug may cause dizziness, fainting; light-headedness may occur during 1st few days of therapy

• That drug may cause skin rash or impaired perspiration

• Not to discontinue drug abruptly

• Not to use OTC products unless directed by prescriber

• To rise slowly to sitting or standing position to minimize orthostatic hypotension

---

tranylcypromine (R)

(tran-ill-sip′roe-meen)
Parnate

Func. class.: Antidepressant-MAOI

Chem. class.: Nonhydrazine

Action: Increases concentrations of endogenous epinephrine, norepinephrine, serotonin, dopamine in storage sites in CNS by inhibition of MAO; increased concentration reduces depression

Uses: Depression, when uncontrolled by other means

Investigational uses: Bulimia, cocaine addiction, migraines, seasonal affective disorder, panic disorder

Dosage and routes:

• *Adult:* PO 10 mg bid; may increase to 30 mg/day after 2 wk; up to 60 mg/day

Available forms: Tabs 10 mg

Side effects/adverse reactions:

HEMA: Anemia

CNS: Dizziness, drowsiness, confusion, headache, anxiety, tremors, stimulation, weakness, hyperreflexia, mania, insomnia, fatigue

GI: Constipation, dry mouth, nausea, vomiting, *anorexia,* diarrhea, weight gain

GU: Change in libido, urinary frequency

INTEG: Rash, flushing, increased perspiration

CV: Orthostatic hypotension, hypertension, dysrhythmias, **hypertensive crisis**

EENT: Blurred vision

*ENDO: **SIADH-like syndrome***

Contraindications: Hypersensitivity to MAOIs, elderly, hypertension, CHF, severe hepatic disease, pheochromocytoma, severe renal disease, severe cardiac disease

Precautions: Suicidal patients, convulsive disorders, severe depression, schizophrenia, hyperactivity, diabetes mellitus, pregnancy (C), lactation

Pharmacokinetics: Metabolized by liver, excreted by kidneys, crosses placenta, excreted in breast milk

Interactions:

• Increased pressor effects: guanethidine, clonidine, indirect-acting sympathomimetics (ephedrine), buspirone

• Increased effects of: direct-acting sympathomimetics (epinephrine), alcohol, barbiturates, benzodiazepines, CNS depressants, levodopa, β-blockers, antidiabetics, sulfonamide, rauwolfia alkaloids, methyldopa, L-tryptophan, thiazide diuretics, sumatriptan

---

◆ = Nursing alert   🖋 = Herb-drug interaction   🚫 = Do not crush

◆ *Serotonin-syndrome:* fluoxetine, fluvoxamine, sertraline, paroxetine

◆ *Hypertensive crisis:* tricyclics, meperidine, dibenzazepine agents, methylphenidate, dextromethorphan

⬧ Increased sympathomimetic action: ephedra

⬧ Increased B/P: brewer's yeast

NURSING CONSIDERATIONS
Assess:
• B/P (lying, standing), pulse; if systolic B/P drops 20 mm Hg, stop drug, notify prescriber
• Blood studies: CBC, leukocytes, cardiac enzymes (long-term therapy)
• Hepatic studies: ALT, AST, bilirubin; hepatotoxicity may occur
◆ Toxicity: increased headache, palpitation; discontinue drug immediately; prodromal signs of hypertensive crisis
• Mental status changes: mood, sensorium, affect, memory (long, short), increase in psychiatric symptoms
• Urinary retention, constipation, edema: take weight weekly
• Withdrawal symptoms: headache, nausea, vomiting, muscle pain, weakness

Administer:
• Increased fluids, bulk in diet if constipation occurs
• With food or milk for GI symptoms
• Crushed if patient is unable to swallow medication whole
• Dosage hs if oversedation occurs during day
• Gum, hard candy, frequent sips of water for dry mouth
• Phentolamine for severe hypertension

Perform/provide:
• Cool storage in tight container
• Assistance with ambulation during beginning therapy for drowsiness/dizziness

• Safety measures including side rails
• Checking to see if PO medication swallowed

Evaluate:
• Therapeutic response: decreased depression

Teach patient/family:
• That therapeutic effects may take 48 hr-3 wks
• To avoid driving, other activities requiring alertness
• To avoid alcohol ingestion, CNS depressants, OTC medications: cold, weight loss, hay fever, cough syrup
• Not to discontinue medication quickly after long-term use
◆ To avoid high-tyramine foods: cheese (aged), sour cream, yogurt, beer, wine, pickled products, liver, raisins, bananas, figs, avocados, meat tenderizers, chocolate, increased caffeine, ginseng
• To report headache, palpitation, neck stiffness

Treatment of overdose: Lavage, activated charcoal; monitor electrolytes, vital signs; diazepam IV, $NaHCO_3$

trastuzumab (R)
(tras-tuz'uh-mab)
Herciptin
Func. class.: Miscellaneous antineoplastic
Chem. class.: Humanized monoclonal antibody

Action: DNA-derived monoclonal antibody selectively binds to extracellular portion of human epidermal growth factor receptor 2; it inhibits proliferation of cancer cells

Uses: Breast cancer; metastatic with overexpression of HER2

Dosage and routes:
• *Adult:* **IV** 4 mg/kg given over 90

T

min, then maintenance 2 mg/kg given over 30 min; do not give as IV push or BOL

Available forms: Lyophilized pwd 440 mg

Side effects/adverse reactions:

CNS: Dizziness, numbness, paresthesias, depression, insomnia, neuropathy, peripheral neuritis

*CV: **Tachycardia, CHF***

INTEG: Rash, acne, herpes simplex

GI: Nausea, vomiting, anorexia, diarrhea

MISC: Flulike symptoms; fever, headache, chills

HEMA: Anemia, ***leukopenia***

MS: Arthralgia, bone pain

META: Edema, peripheral edema

RESP: Cough, dyspnea, pharyngitis, rhinitis, sinusitis

*SYST: **Anaphylaxis, angioedema***

Contraindications: Hypersensitivity to this drug, Chinese hamster ovary cell protein

Precautions: Pregnancy (B), lactation, children, elderly, cardiac disease, anemia, leukopenia

Pharmacokinetics: Half-life 1.7-12 days

Interactions:

• Increased chance of cardiomyopathy: anthracyclines, cyclophosphamide, avoid use

NURSING CONSIDERATIONS

Assess:

 CHF and other cardiac symptoms: dyspnea, coughing; gallop; obtain a full cardiac workup including ECG, echo, MUGA

• For symptoms of infection; may be masked by drug

• CNS reaction: LOC, mental status, dizziness, confusion

For hypersensitive reactions, anaphylaxis

For infusion reactions that may be fatal: fever, chills, nausea, vomiting, pain, headache, dizziness, hypotension, discontinue drug

Administer:

• Acetaminophen as ordered to alleviate fever and headache

IV

• After reconstituting vial with 20 ml bacteriostatic water for inj, 1.1% benzyl alcohol preserved (supplied) to yield 21 mg/ml, mark date on vial 28 days from reconstitution date, if patient is allergic to benzyl alcohol, reconstitute with sterile water for inj—use immediately

• Do not mix or dilute with other drugs or dextrose sol

Perform/provide:

• Increased fluid intake to 2-3 L/day

Evaluate:

• Therapeutic response: decrease in size of tumors

Teach patient/family:

• To take acetaminophen for fever

• To avoid hazardous tasks, since confusion, dizziness may occur

• To report signs of infection: sore throat, fever, diarrhea, vomiting

• Emotional lability is common; notify presriber if severe or incapacitating

---

trazodone (℞)

(tray′zoe-done)

Desyrel, Desyrel Dividose, Trazon, trazodone HCl, Trialodine

Func. class.: Antidepressant, miscellaneous

Chem. class.: Triazolopyridine

Action: Selectively inhibits serotonin uptake by brain, potentiates behavioral changes

Uses: Depression

Investigational uses: Chronic pain

Dosage and routes:

• *Adult:* **PO** 150 mg/day in divided doses; may increase by 50 mg/day q3-4d, not to exceed 600 mg/day

---

 = Nursing alert   = Herb-drug interaction   ⊘ = Do not crush

• *Child 6-18 yr:* **PO** 1.5-2 mg/kg/day in divided dose, may increase q3-4d, up to 6 mg/kg/day

• *Geriatric:* **PO** 25-50 mg hs, increase by 25-50 mg q3-7d to desired dose

Available forms: Tabs 50, 100, 150, 300 mg

Side effects/adverse reactions:

HEMA: **Agranulocytosis, thrombocytopenia, eosinophilia, leukopenia**

CNS: Dizziness, drowsiness, confusion, headache, anxiety, tremors, stimulation, weakness, insomnia, nightmares, EPS (elderly), increase in psychiatric symptoms

GI: Diarrhea, dry mouth, nausea, vomiting, **paralytic ileus,** increased appetite, cramps, epigastric distress, jaundice, **hepatitis,** stomatitis

*GU: Urinary retention, **acute renal failure,** priapism*

INTEG: Rash, urticaria, sweating, pruritus, photosensitivity

CV: Orthostatic hypotension, ECG changes, tachycardia, **hypertension,** palpitations

EENT: Blurred vision, tinnitus, mydriasis

Contraindications: Hypersensitivity to tricyclics, recovery phase of MI, convulsive disorders, prostatic hypertrophy

Precautions: Suicidal patients, severe depression, increased intraocular pressure, narrow-angle glaucoma, urinary retention, cardiac disease, hepatic disease, hyperthyroidism, electroshock therapy, elective surgery, pregnancy (C)

Pharmacokinetics: Metabolized by liver, excreted by kidneys, feces; half-life 4.4-7.5 hr

Interactions:

• Decreased effects of guanethidine, clonidine, indirect-acting sympathomimetics (ephedrine)

• Increased effects of direct-acting sympathomimetics (epinephrine), alcohol, barbiturates, benzodiazepines, CNS depressants

⬥ Hyperpyretic crisis, convulsions, hypertensive episode: MAOI (pargyline [Eutonyl])

🗲 Increased CNS depression: kava

Lab test interferences:

Increase: Serum bilirubin, blood glucose, alk phosphatase

False increase: Urinary catecholamines

Decrease: VMA, 5-HIAA

NURSING CONSIDERATIONS

Assess:

• Pain: location, duration, intensity before and 1-2 hr after medication

• B/P (lying, standing), pulse q4h; if systolic B/P drops 20 mm Hg, hold drug, notify prescriber; take vital signs q4h in patients with cardiovascular disease

• Blood studies: CBC, leukocytes, differential, cardiac enzymes if patient is receiving long-term therapy

• Hepatic studies: AST, ALT, bilirubin

• Weight qwk; appetite may increase with drug

• ECG for flattening of T wave, bundle branch block, AV block, dysrhythmias in cardiac patients

• EPS, primarily in elderly: rigidity, dystonia, akathisia

• Mental status changes: mood, sensorium, affect, suicidal tendencies, increase in psychiatric symptoms, depression, panic

• Urinary retention, constipation; constipation most likely in children

• Withdrawal symptoms: headache, nausea, vomiting, muscle pain, weakness; not usual unless drug discontinued abruptly

• Alcohol consumption; hold dose until morning

Administer:
• Increased fluids, bulk in diet if constipation occurs, especially in elderly
• With food, milk for GI symptoms
• Dosage hs for oversedation during day; may take entire dose hs; elderly may not tolerate qd dosing
• Gum, hard candy, frequent sips of water for dry mouth

Perform/provide:
• Storage in tight, light-resistant container at room temperature
• Assistance with ambulation during beginning therapy for drowsiness/dizziness
• Safety measures, including side rails, primarily for elderly
• Checking to see if PO medication swallowed

Evaluate:
• Therapeutic response: decreased depression

Teach patient/family:
• That therapeutic effects may take 2-3 wk
• To use caution in driving, other activities requiring alertness because of drowsiness, dizziness, blurred vision
• To avoid alcohol ingestion, other CNS depressants
• Not to discontinue medication quickly after long-term use; may cause nausea, headache, malaise
• To wear sunscreen or large hat, since photosensitivity occurs
• Signs of suicidal ideation

Treatment of overdose: ECG monitoring; induce emesis; lavage, activated charcoal; administer anticonvulsant

---

tretinoin (vit A acid, retinoic acid) (Ŗ)

(tret'i-noyn)
Retin-A, Stievaa*, Tretinoin LF, IV, Vesanoid
Func. class.: Vit A acid, acne product; antineoplastic (misc.)
Chem. class.: Tretinoin derivative

Action: Decreases cohesiveness of follicular epithelium, decreases microcomedone formation (TOP); induces maturation of acute promyelocytic leukemia, exact action is unknown (PO)

Uses: Acne vulgaris (grades 1-3) (top); (PO) acute promyelocytic leukemia

Investigational uses: Skin cancer

Dosage and routes:
• *Adult and child:* **TOP** cleanse area, apply hs; cover lightly

Promyelocytic leukemia
• *Adult:* **PO** 45 mg/m^2/day given as 2 evenly divided doses until remission, discontinue treatment 30 days after remission or 90 days of treatment, whichever is first

Available forms: Cream 0.01%, 0.05%; gel 0.01%, 0.025%; liquid 0.05%; caps 10 mg

Side effects/adverse reactions:
INTEG: (top) Rash, stinging, warmth, redness, erythema, blistering, crusting, peeling, contact dermatitis, hypopigmentation, hyperpigmentation

Oral
CNS: Headache, fever, sweating
*GI: Nausea, vomiting, **hemorrhage**, abdominal pain, diarrhea, constipation, dyspepsia, distention, hepatitis*

Contraindications: Hypersensitivity to retinoids or sensitivity to parabens, pregnancy (D) (PO)

◆ = Nursing alert   ⬮ = Herb-drug interaction   ⊘ = Do not crush

Precautions: Lactation, eczema, sunburn, pregnancy (C) (top)
Pharmacokinetics:
TOP: Poor systemic absorption
Interactions:
• Increase peeling: medication containing agents such as sulfur, benzoyl peroxide, resorcinol, salicylic acid (top)
• Use with caution: medicated, abrasive soaps, cleansers that have drying effect, products with high concentrations of alcohol astringents (top)
• Increased plasma concentrations of tretinoin: ketoconazole (oral)
NURSING CONSIDERATIONS
Assess:
Topical
• Area of body involved, what helps or aggravates condition; cysts, dryness, itching; lesions may worsen at beginning of treatment
Oral
• Liver function, coagulation, hematologic parameters, also cholesterol, triglyceride
Administer:
Topical
• Once daily before hs; cover area lightly using gauze; use gloves to apply
Perform/provide:
Topical
• Storage at room temperature
• Hand washing after application
Evaluate:
• Therapeutic response: decrease in size and number of lesions
Teach patient/family:
Topical
• To avoid application on normal skin, getting cream in eyes, nose, other mucous membranes
• To avoid sunlight, sunlamps, or use protective clothing, sunscreen
• That treatment may cause warmth, stinging, dryness, peeling will occur

• That cosmetics may be used over drug; not to use shaving lotions
• That rash may occur during first 1-3 wk of therapy
• That drug does not cure condition; only relieves symptoms
• That therapeutic results may be seen in 2-3 wk but may not be optimal until after 6 wk

---

triamcinolone (℞)

(trye-am-sin'oh-lone)
Amcort, Aristocort, Aristocort Forte, Aristocort Intralesional, Aristospan Intra-Articular, Aristospan Intralesional, Articulose L.A., Atolone, Azmacort, Cenocort A-40, Cenocort Forte, Kenacort, Kenaject-40, Kenalog, Kenalog-10, Kenalog-40, Tac-3, Tac-40, Triam-A, triamcinolone, triamcinolone acetonide, Triam Forte, Triamolone 40, Triamonide 40, Tri-Kort, Trilog, Trilone, Trisoject

Func. class.: Corticosteroid
Chem. class.: Glucocorticoid, intermediate-acting

Action: Decreases inflammation by suppression of migration of polymorphonuclear leukocytes, fibroblasts, reversal to increase capillary permeability and lysosomal stabilization
Uses: Severe inflammation, immunosuppression, neoplasms, asthma (steroid dependent), collagen, respiratory, dermatologic disorders
Dosage and routes:
• *Adult:* **PO** 4-12 mg/day in divided doses qd-qid; **IM** 40 mg qwk (acetonide, or diacetate), 5-48 mg into neoplasms (diacetate, acetonide), 2-40 mg into joint or soft tissue (diacetate, acetonide), 0.5 mg/in^2 of

---

affected intralesional skin (hexacetonide), 2-20 mg into joint or soft tissue (hexacetonide)

• *Child:* **PO** 117 µg/kg/day as a single or divided dose

Asthma

• *Adult:* **INH** 2 tid-qid, not to exceed 16 **INH**/day

• *Child 6-12 yr:* **INH** 1-2 tid-qid, not to exceed 12 **INH**/day

Available forms: Tabs 1, 2, 4, 8 mg; syr 2 mg/5 ml, 4.85 mg/5 ml; inj 25, 40 mg/ml diacetate; inj 3, 10, 40 mg/ml acetonide; inj 20, 5 mg/ml hexacetonide; aerosol actuation/100 µg (acetonide)

Side effects/adverse reactions:

INTEG: Acne, poor wound healing, ecchymosis, petechiae

CNS: Depression, flushing, sweating, headache, mood changes

*CV: Hypertension, **circulatory collapse, thrombophlebitis, embolism,*** tachycardia, edema

*HEMA: **Thrombocytopenia***

MS: Fractures, osteoporosis, weakness

*GI: Diarrhea, nausea, abdominal distention, **GI hemorrhage,*** increased appetite, **pancreatitis**

EENT: Fungal infections, increased intraocular pressure, blurred vision

Contraindications: Psychosis, hypersensitivity, idiopathic thrombocytopenia, acute glomerulonephritis, amebiasis, fungal infections, nonasthmatic bronchial disease, child <2 yr, AIDS, TB, adrenal insufficiency

Precautions: Pregnancy (C), diabetes mellitus, glaucoma, osteoporosis, seizure disorders, ulcerative colitis, CHF, myasthenia gravis, renal disease, esophagitis, peptic ulcer

Pharmacokinetics:

PO/IM: Peak 1-2 hr, half-life 2-5 hr

Interactions:

• Decreased action of triamcinolone: cholestyramine, colestipol, barbiturates, rifampin, ephedrine, phenytoin, theophylline

• Decreased effects of anticoagulants, anticonvulsants, antidiabetics, ambenonium, neostigmine, isoniazid, toxoids, vaccines, anticholinesterases, salicylates, somatrem

• Increased side effects: alcohol, salicylates, indomethacin, amphotericin B, digitalis, cyclosporine, diuretics

• Increased action of triamcinolone: salicylates, estrogens, indomethacin, oral contraceptives, ketoconazole, macrolide antiinfectives

🌿 Increased potassium loss: aloe, buckthorn, rhubarb, senna

Lab test interferences:

Increase: Cholesterol, Na, blood glucose, uric acid, Ca, urine glucose

Decrease: Ca, K, T_4, T_3, thyroid ^{131}I uptake test, urine 17-OHCS, 17-KS, PBI

False negative: Skin allergy tests

NURSING CONSIDERATIONS

Assess:

• K, blood sugar, urine glucose while on long-term therapy; hypokalemia and hyperglycemia

• Weight qd; notify prescriber if weekly gain >5 lb

• B/P q4h, pulse; notify prescriber if chest pain occurs

• I&O ratio; be alert for decreasing urinary output, increasing edema

• Plasma cortisol levels during long-term therapy (normal level: 138-635 nmol/L SI units when drawn at 8 AM)

• Infection: increased temp, WBC, even after withdrawal of medication; drug masks infection

• K depletion: paresthesias, fatigue, nausea, vomiting, depression, polyuria, dysrhythmias, weakness

---

◆ = Nursing alert   🌿 = Herb-drug interaction   🚫 = Do not crush

• Edema, hypertension, cardiac symptoms
• Mental status: affect, mood, behavioral changes, aggression
Administer:
• After shaking susp (parenteral)
• Titrated dose; use lowest effective dose
• IM injection deep in large muscle mass; rotate sites; avoid deltoid; use 21G needle
• In one dose in AM to prevent adrenal suppression; avoid SC administration; may damage tissue
• With food or milk to decrease GI symptoms
Perform/provide:
• Assistance with ambulation for patient with bone tissue disease to prevent fractures
• Use of spacer device for elderly patients with inhaler
Evaluate:
• Therapeutic response: ease of respirations, decreased inflammation
Teach patient/family:
• That ID as steroid user should be carried
• To notify prescriber if therapeutic response decreases; dosage adjustment may be needed
• Not to discontinue abruptly; adrenal crisis can result
• To avoid OTC products: salicylates, alcohol in cough products, cold preparations unless directed by prescriber
• About cushingoid symptoms
• The symptoms of adrenal insufficiency: nausea, anorexia, fatigue, dizziness, dyspnea, weakness, joint pain

triamcinolone (topical-oral) (OTC)
(trye-am-sin′oh-lone)
Kenalog in Orabase, Oralone Dental
Func. class.: Topical anesthetic
Chem. class.: Synthetic fluorinated adrenal corticosteroid

Action: Inhibits nerve impulses from sensory nerves
Uses: Oral pain
Dosage and routes:
• *Adult and child:* **TOP** press ¼ inch into affected area until film appears, repeat bid-tid
Available forms: Paste 0.1%
Side effects/adverse reactions:
INTEG: Rash, irritation, sensitization
Contraindications: Hypersensitivity, infants <1 yr, application to large areas, presence of fungal, viral, or bacterial infections of mouth or throat
Precautions: Child <6 yr, sepsis, pregnancy (C), denuded skin
NURSING CONSIDERATIONS
Assess:
• Allergy: rash, irritation, reddening, swelling
• Infection: if affected area is infected, do not apply
Administer:
• After cleansing oral cavity
Evaluate:
• Therapeutic response: absence of pain in affected area
Teach patient/family:
• To report rash, irritation, redness, swelling
• How to apply paste

triamterene (℞)

(trye-am′ter-een)

Dyrenium

Func. class.: Potassium-sparing diuretic

Chem. class.: Pteridine derivative

Action: Acts on distal tubule to inhibit reabsorption of sodium, chloride; increase potassium retention

Uses: Edema, may be used with other diuretics; hypertension

Dosage and routes:

• *Adult:* **PO** 100 mg bid pc, not to exceed 300 mg/day

• *Geriatric:* **PO** 50 mg qd, max 100 mg/day

Available forms: Caps 50, 100 mg

Side effects/adverse reactions:

GI: Nausea, diarrhea, vomiting, dry mouth, jaundice, ***liver disease***

ELECT: Hyperkalemia, hyponatremia, hypochloremia

CNS: Weakness, headache, dizziness, fatigue

INTEG: Photosensitivity, rash

*HEMA: **Thrombocytopenia, megaloblastic anemia,*** low folic acid levels

*GU: **Azotemia, interstitial nephritis,*** increased BUN, creatinine, renal stones, bluish discoloration of urine

Contraindications: Hypersensitivity, anuria, severe renal disease, severe hepatic disease, hyperkalemia, lactation

Precautions: Dehydration, hepatic disease, CHF, renal disease, pregnancy (B), cirrhosis

Pharmacokinetics:

PO: Onset 2 hr, peak 6-8 hr, duration 12-16 hr; half-life 3 hr; metabolized in liver, excreted in bile and urine

Interactions:

• Nephrotoxicity: indomethacin

• Enhanced action of antihypertensives, amantadine

• Increased hyperkalemia: other K-sparing diuretics, K products, ACE inhibitors, salt substitutes

• Decreased renal clearance of triamterene: cimetidine

Lab test interferences:

Interference: Quinidine serum levels, LDH

NURSING CONSIDERATIONS

Assess:

• Weight, I&O qd to determine fluid loss; effect of drug may be decreased if used qd

• Electrolytes: K, Na, Cl; include BUN, blood sugar, CBC, serum creatinine, blood pH, ABGs, LFTs

• Improvement in CVP q8h

• Signs of metabolic acidosis: drowsiness, restlessness

• Rashes, temp qd

• Confusion, especially in elderly; take safety precautions if needed

• Hydration: skin turgor, thirst, dry mucous membranes

Administer:

• In AM to avoid interference with sleep

• With food if nausea occurs; absorption may be decreased slightly

Evaluate:

• Therapeutic response: improvement in edema of feet, legs, sacral area qd if medication is being used in CHF

Teach patient/family:

• To take medication after meals for GI upset

• To avoid prolonged exposure to sunlight; photosensitivity may occur; may turn urine blue

• To avoid foods high in K: oranges, bananas, salt substitutes, dried apricots, dates

• To notify prescriber of weakness, headache, nausea, vomiting, dry

---

 = Nursing alert   = Herb-drug interaction   ⊘ = Do not crush

mouth, fever, sore throat, mouth sores, unusual bleeding or bruising
Treatment of overdose: Lavage if taken orally; monitor electrolytes; administer IV fluids, dialysis; monitor hydration, CV, renal status

---

triazolam (℞)
(trye-ay'zoe-lam)
Apo-Triazo*, Gen-Triazolam*, Halcion, Novo-Triolam*, Nu-Triazol*
Func. class.: Sedative-hypnotic, antianxiety
Chem. class.: Benzodiazepine

Controlled Substance Schedule IV (USA), Schedule F (Canada)
Action: Produces CNS depression at limbic, thalamic, hypothalamic levels of CNS; may be mediated by neurotransmitter γ-aminobutyric acid (GABA); results are sedation, hypnosis, skeletal muscle relaxation, anticonvulsant activity, anxiolytic action
Uses: Insomnia, sedative, hypnotic
Dosage and routes:
• *Adult:* **PO** 0.125-0.5 mg hs
• *Elderly:* **PO** 0.625-0.125 mg hs
Available forms: Tabs 0.125, 0.25 mg
Side effects/adverse reactions:
HEMA: **Leukopenia, granulocytopenia** (rare)
CNS: *Headache, lethargy, drowsiness, daytime sedation,* dizziness, confusion, light-headedness, anxiety, irritability, amnesia, poor coordination
GI: Nausea, vomiting, diarrhea, heartburn, abdominal pain, constipation
CV: Chest pain, pulse changes
Contraindications: Hypersensitivity to benzodiazepines, pregnancy

(X), lactation, intermittent porphyria
Precautions: Anemia, hepatic disease, renal disease, suicidal individuals, drug abuse, elderly, psychosis, child <15 yr, acute narrow-angle glaucoma, seizure disorders
Pharmacokinetics:
PO: Onset 30-45 min, duration 6-8 hr; metabolized by liver, excreted by kidneys (inactive metabolites), crosses placenta, excreted in breast milk; half-life 2-3 hr
Interactions:
• Increased effects of cimetidine, disulfiram, erythromycin, macrolides, probenecid, isoniazid, oral contraceptives; do not use concurrently
• Increased action of both drugs: alcohol, CNS depressants
• Decreased effect of antacids, theophylline, rifampin, smoking
🌿 Increased CNS depression: kava
Lab test interferences:
Increase: ALT, AST, serum bilirubin
Decrease: RAI uptake
False increase: Urinary 17-OHCS
NURSING CONSIDERATIONS
Assess:
• Blood studies: Hct, Hgb, RBC if blood dyscrasias suspected (rare)
• Hepatic studies: AST, ALT, bilirubin if liver damage has occurred
• Mental status: mood, sensorium, affect, memory (long, short)
• Blood dyscrasias: fever, sore throat, bruising, rash, jaundice, epistaxis (rare)
• Type of sleep problem: falling asleep, staying asleep
Administer:
• After removal of cigarettes to prevent fires
• After trying conservative measures for insomnia
• ½ hr before hs for sleeplessness

• On empty stomach for fast onset, but may be taken with food if GI symptoms occur

Perform/provide:

• Assistance with ambulation after receiving dose
• Safety measures: side rails, night-light, call bell within easy reach
• Checking to see if PO medication has been swallowed
• Cool storage in tight container

Evaluate:

• Therapeutic response: ability to sleep at night, decreased amount of early morning awakening if taking drug for insomnia

Teach patient/family:

• That dependence is possible after long-term use
• To avoid driving, other activities requiring alertness until drug is stabilized
• To avoid alcohol ingestion, CNS depressants; serious CNS depression may result
• That effects may take 2 nights for benefits to be noticed; for short-term use only
• Alternative measures to improve sleep: reading, exercise several hours before hs, warm bath, warm milk, TV, self-hypnosis, deep breathing
• That hangover is common in elderly but less common than with barbiturates; rebound insomnia may occur for 1-2 nights after discontinuing drug

Treatment of overdose: Lavage, activated charcoal; monitor electrolytes, VS

RARELY USED

trientine (R̲)
(tri′en-teen)
Syprine
Func. class.: Heavy-metal antagonist

Uses: Wilson's disease, chelating agent if other agents are not tolerated

Dosage and routes:

• *Adult:* **PO** 750-1250 mg in divided doses bid-qid, max 2000 mg/day
• *Child:* **PO** 500-1500 mg in divided doses bid-qid

Contraindications: Hypersensitivity, cystinuria, rheumatoid arthritis, biliary cirrhosis

---

trifluoperazine (R̲)
(trye-floo-oh-per′a-zeen)
Apo-Trifluoperazine*, Novofluorazine*, Solazine*, Stelazine, Suprazine, Terfluzine, trifluoperazine HCl, Triflurin
Func. class.: Antipsychotic, neuroleptic
Chem. class.: Phenothiazine, piperazine

Action: Depresses cerebral cortex, hypothalamus, limbic system, which control activity, aggression; blocks neurotransmission produced by dopamine at synapse; exhibits strong α-adrenergic, anticholinergic blocking action; mechanism for antipsychotic effects is unclear

Uses: Psychotic disorders, nonpsychotic anxiety, schizophrenia

Dosage and routes:

Psychotic disorders

• *Adult:* **PO** 2-5 mg bid, usual range

15-20 mg/day, may require 40 mg/day or more; **IM** 1-2 mg q4-6h

• *Geriatric:* **PO** 0.5-1 mg qd-bid, increase q4-7d by 0.5-1 mg/day to desired dose

• *Child >6 yr:* **PO** 1 mg qd or bid; **IM** not recommended for children, but 1 mg may be given qd or bid

Nonpsychotic anxiety

• *Adult:* **PO** 1-2 mg bid, not to exceed 5 mg/day; do not give longer than 12 wk

Available forms: Tabs 1, 2, 5, 10 mg; conc 10 mg/ml; inj 2 mg/ml

Side effects/adverse reactions:

RESP: ***Laryngospasm,*** dyspnea, ***respiratory depression***

CNS: *EPS: pseudoparkinsonism, akathisia, dystonia, tardive dyskinesia,* ***seizures,*** *headache,* ***neuroleptic malignant syndrome***

HEMA: Anemia, ***leukopenia, leukocytosis, agranulocytosis***

INTEG: *Rash,* photosensitivity, dermatitis

EENT: Blurred vision, glaucoma, dry eyes

GI: Dry mouth, nausea, vomiting, anorexia, constipation, diarrhea, jaundice, weight gain

GU: Urinary retention, urinary frequency, enuresis, impotence, amenorrhea, gynecomastia

CV: *Orthostatic hypotension,* hypertension, ***cardiac arrest,*** ECG changes, ***tachycardia***

Contraindications: Hypersensitivity, cardiovascular disease, coma, blood dyscrasias, severe hepatic disease, child <6 yr, glaucoma

Precautions: Breast cancer, seizure disorders, pregnancy (C), lactation, diabetes mellitus, respiratory conditions, prostatic hypertrophy, elderly

Do not confuse:

trifluoperazine/trihexyphenidyl

Pharmacokinetics:

PO: Onset rapid, peak 2-3 hr, duration 12 hr

IM: Onset immediate, peak 1 hr, duration 12 hr

Metabolized by liver, excreted in urine, breast milk; crosses placenta

Interactions:

• Oversedation: other CNS depressants, alcohol, barbiturate anesthetics

• Decreased absorption: aluminum hydroxide, magnesium hydroxide antacids

• Decreased effects of lithium, levodopa

• Increased effects of both drugs: β-adrenergic blockers, alcohol

• Increased anticholinergic effects: anticholinergics

🍂 Increased CNS depression: kava

Lab test interferences:

Increase: LFTs, cardiac enzymes, cholesterol, blood glucose, prolactin, bilirubin, PBI, cholinesterase, ^{131}I

Decrease: Hormones (blood, urine)

False positive: Pregnancy tests, PKU

False negative: Urinary steroids, 17-OHCS, pregnancy tests

NURSING CONSIDERATIONS

Assess:

◆ For neuroleptic malignant syndrome: seizures, hyper/hypotension, dyspnea, diaphoresis, fatigue, muscle stiffness; notify prescriber immediately

• Mental status before initial administration

• Swallowing of PO medication; check for hoarding or giving of medication to other patients

• I&O ratio; palpate bladder if low urinary output occurs

• Bilirubin, CBC, liver function studies qmo

• Urinalysis is recommended before and during prolonged therapy

T

• Affect, orientation, LOC, reflexes, gait, coordination, sleep pattern disturbances
• For hypo/hyperglycemia; appetite patterns
• B/P standing and lying; also include pulse, respirations q4h during initial treatment; establish baseline before starting treatment; report drops of 30 mm Hg
• Dizziness, faintness, palpitations, tachycardia on rising
• EPS including akathisia (inability to sit still, no pattern to movements), tardive dyskinesia (bizarre movements of jaw, mouth, tongue, extremities), pseudoparkinsonism (rigidity, tremors, pill rolling, shuffling gait)
• Skin turgor qd
• Constipation, urinary retention qd; if these occur increase bulk, water in diet

Administer:
• Reduced dose in elderly
• Antiparkinsonian agent on order from prescriber for EPS
PO
• Conc in 60 ml of tomato or fruit juice, milk, orange, carbonated beverage, coffee, tea, water, or semisolid foods (soup, pudding)
Perform/provide:
• Decreased stimulus by dimming lights, avoiding loud noises
• Supervised ambulation until stabilized on medication if needed; do not involve in strenuous exercise program because fainting is possible; patient should not stand still for long periods
• Increased fluids and bulk in diet to prevent constipation
• Sips of water, candy, gum for dry mouth
• Storage in tight, light-resistant container, oral sol in amber bottles; slight yellowing of inj or conc is common, does not affect potency

Evaluate:
• Therapeutic response: decrease in emotional excitement, hallucinations, delusions, paranoia, reorganization of patterns of thought, speech
Teach patient/family:
• That orthostatic hypotension occurs frequently, and to rise from sitting or lying position gradually; avoid hazardous activities until stabilized on medication
• To remain lying down after IM injection for at least 30 min
• To avoid hot tubs, hot showers, tub baths; hypotension may occur
• To avoid abrupt withdrawal of this drug, or EPS may result; drug should be withdrawn slowly
• To avoid OTC preparations (cough, hay fever, cold) unless approved by prescriber, since serious drug interactions may occur; avoid use with alcohol, CNS depressants; increased drowsiness may occur
• To use a sunscreen
• About compliance with drug regimen
• About the necessity for meticulous oral hygiene; oral candidiasis may occur
• To report sore throat, malaise, fever, bleeding, mouth sores; CBC should be drawn and drug discontinued
◆ That in hot weather, heat stroke may occur; take extra precautions to stay cool
Treatment of overdose: Lavage if orally ingested; provide an airway; do not induce vomiting

---

◆ = Nursing alert   / = Herb-drug interaction   ⊘ = Do not crush

trihexyphenidyl (℞)

(trye-hex-ee-fen'i-dill)
Apo-Trihex*, Artane, Artane
Sequels, Novohexidyl*, PMS-
Trihexyphenidyl*, Trihexane,
Trihexy-2, Trihexy-5,
trihexyphenidyl HCl
Func. class.: Cholinergic blocker
Chem. class.: Synthetic tertiary
amine

Action: Blocks central muscarinic receptors, which decreases involuntary movements, sweating, salivation

Uses: Parkinson symptoms, drug-induced EPS

Dosage and routes:
Parkinson symptoms
• *Adult:* **PO** 1 mg, increased by 2 mg q3-5d to a total of 6-10 mg/day; give ext rel q12h
Drug-induced EPS
• *Adult:* **PO** 1 mg/day; usual dose 5-15 mg/day; give ext rel q12h
Available forms: Tabs 2, 5 mg; caps ext rel 5 mg; elix 2 mg/5 ml

Side effects/adverse reactions:
CNS: Confusion, anxiety, restlessness, irritability, delusions, hallucinations, headache, sedation, depression, incoherence, dizziness, flushing, weakness
EENT: Blurred vision, photophobia, dilated pupils, difficulty swallowing, dry eyes, increased intraocular tension, angle-closure glaucoma
CV: Palpitations, tachycardia, postural hypotension
INTEG: Urticaria, rash
MISC: Suppression of lactation, nasal congestion, decreased sweating, increased temp, hyperthermia, heat stroke, numbness of fingers
MS: Weakness, cramping
GI: Dryness of mouth, constipation,

nausea, vomiting, abdominal distress, *paralytic ileus*
GU: Urinary hesitancy, retention, dysuria

Contraindications: Hypersensitivity, narrow-angle glaucoma, myasthenia gravis, GI/GU obstruction, myocardial ischemia, unstable CV disease, prostatic hypertrophy

Precautions: Pregnancy (C), elderly, lactation, tachycardia, abdominal obstruction, infection, children, gastric ulcer

Do not confuse:
tryhexyphenidyl/trifluoperazine
Artane/Altace

Pharmacokinetics:
PO: Onset 1 hr, peak 2-3 hr, duration 6-12 hr, excreted in urine, half-life 5-10 hr

Interactions:
• Increased anticholinergic effects: antihistamines, phenothiazines, amantadine
• Decreased action of haloperidol
• Increased CNS depression: analgesics, alcohol, sedatives/hypnotics, antihistamines, opioids
• Increased levels of: digoxin

NURSING CONSIDERATIONS
Assess:
• For Parkinson's and EPS baseline and throughout treatment
• I&O ratio; retention commonly causes decreased urinary output
• B/P, pulse frequently while dose is being determined
• Urinary hesitancy, retention; palpate bladder if retention occurs
• Constipation; increase fluids, bulk, exercise
• For tolerance over long-term therapy; dosage may have to be increased or medication changed
• Mental status: affect, mood, CNS depression, worsening of mental symptoms during early therapy

T

Administer:

• With or after meals for GI upset; may give with fluids other than water

• At hs to avoid daytime drowsiness in patient with parkinsonism

Perform/provide:

• Storage at room temperature in light-resistant container

• Hard candy, frequent drinks, sugarless gum to relieve dry mouth

Evaluate:

• Therapeutic response: parkinsonism: shuffling gait, muscle rigidity, involuntary movements

Teach patient/family:

• Not to discontinue this drug abruptly; to taper off over 1 wk

• To avoid driving, other hazardous activities; drowsiness may occur

• To avoid OTC medications: cough, cold preparations with alcohol, antihistamines unless directed by prescriber

• To avoid sudden position changes

• To avoid hot climates; overheating may occur

---

trimethobenzamide (R)

(trye-meth-oh-ben'za-mide)
Arrestin, Benzacot, Brogan, Stemetic, T-Gen, Tebamide, Ticon, Tigan, Tiject-20, Triban, Trimazide, Trimethobenzamide, trimethobenzamide HCl

Func. class.: Antiemetic, anticholinergic

Chem. class.: Ethanolamine derivative

Action: Acts centrally by blocking chemoreceptor trigger zone, which in turn acts on vomiting center

Uses: Nausea, vomiting, prevention of postoperative vomiting

Dosage and routes:

Postoperative vomiting

• *Adult:* IM/RECT 200 mg before or during surgery; may repeat 3 hr after

Discontinuing anesthesia

• *Child 13-40 kg:* PO/RECT 100-200 mg tid-qid

• *Child <13 kg:* PO/RECT 100 mg tid-qid

Nausea/vomiting

• *Adult:* PO 250 mg tid-qid; IM/RECT 200 mg tid-qid

Available forms: Caps 100, 250 mg; supp 100, 200 mg; inj 100 mg/ml

Side effects/adverse reactions:

CNS: Drowsiness, restlessness, headache, dizziness, insomnia, confusion, nervousness, tingling, *vertigo,* EPS

GI: Nausea, anorexia, diarrhea, vomiting, constipation

CV: Hypertension, hypotension, palpitation

INTEG: Rash, urticaria, fever, chills, flushing

EENT: Dry mouth, blurred vision, diplopia, nasal congestion, photosensitivity

Contraindications: Hypersensitivity to narcotics, shock, children (parenterally)

Precautions: Children, cardiac dysrhythmias, elderly, asthma, pregnancy (C), prostatic hypertrophy, bladder-neck obstruction, narrow-angle glaucoma, stenosing peptic ulcer, pyloroduodenal obstruction

Pharmacokinetics:

PO: Onset 20-40 min, duration 3-4 hr

IM: Onset 15 min, duration 2-3 hr
Metabolized by liver, excreted by kidneys

Interactions:

• Increased effect: CNS depressants

• May mask ototoxic symptoms associated with antibiotics

⬧ = Nursing alert   🌿 = Herb-drug interaction   🚫 = Do not crush

NURSING CONSIDERATIONS
Assess:
• For nausea, vomiting before, after treatment
• VS, B/P; check patients with cardiac disease more often
• Signs of toxicity of other drugs or masking of symptoms of disease: brain tumor, intestinal obstruction
• Observe for drowsiness, dizziness

Administer:
• IM inj in large muscle mass; aspirate to avoid IV administration
• Tablets may be swallowed whole, chewed, allowed to dissolve

Syringe compatibilities: Glycopyrrolate, hydromorphone, midazolam, nalbuphine

Y-site compatibilities: Heparin, hydrocortisone, potassium chloride, vit B/C

Evaluate:
• Therapeutic response: decreased nausea, vomiting

Teach patient/family:
• To avoid hazardous activities, activities requiring alertness; dizziness may occur; to request assistance with ambulation
• To avoid alcohol, other depressants
• To keep out of children's reach

---

trimethoprim (℞)
(trye-meth'oh-prim)
Proloprim, trimethoprim, Trimpex
Func. class.: Urinary antiinfective
Chem. class.: Folate antagonist

Action: Prevents bacterial synthesis by blocking enzyme reduction of dihydrofolic acid

Uses: *Escherichia coli, Proteus mirabilis, Klebsiella, Enterobacter* UTIs

Dosage and routes:
• *Adult:* **PO** 100 mg q12h × 10 days
• *Child:* 4 mg/kg/day divided q12h
Renal dose
• CrCl 15-30 ml/min 50 mg q12h; CrCl <15 ml/min avoid use
Available forms: Tabs 100, 200 mg

Side effects/adverse reactions:
INTEG: **Exfoliative dermatitis,** pruritus, rash
HEMA: **Thrombocytopenia, leukopenia, neutropenia, megaloblastic anemia** (rare)
GI: *Nausea, vomiting,* abdominal pain, abnormal taste, increased AST, ALT, bilirubin, creatinine
CNS: Fever

Contraindications: Hypersensitivity, CrCl <15 ml/min, megaloblastic anemia

Precautions: Folate deficiency, pregnancy (C), lactation, fragile X chromosome, child <12 yr old, renal disease, hepatic disease

Pharmacokinetics:
PO: Peak 1-4 hr, half-life 8-11 hr; metabolized in liver, excreted in urine (unchanged 60%), breast milk; crosses placenta

Interactions:
• Increased action of phenytoin

NURSING CONSIDERATIONS
Assess:
• For symptoms of UTI: fever, frequency, burning or pain when urinating; baseline and throughout
• Nocturia; may indicate drug resistance
• Signs of infection, anemia
• AST, ALT, BUN, bilirubin, creatinine, urine cultures
• C&S; drug may be given as soon as culture is obtained
• Skin eruptions

Administer:
• With full glass of water

Perform/provide:
• Storage in tight, light-resistant container

Side effects: *italics* = common; **bold italics** = life-threatening

• Adequate intake of fluids (2 L) to decrease bacteria in bladder

Evaluate:

• Therapeutic response: absence of pain in bladder area, negative C&S

Teach patient/family:

• All aspects of drug therapy: need to complete entire course of medication to ensure organism death (10-14 days); culture may be taken after completed course of medication

• That drug must be taken in equal intervals around clock to maintain blood levels

• To notify nurse of nausea, vomiting, rash, severe fatigue, sore throat

---

trimethoprim-sulfamethoxazole (℞)

(trye-meth'oh-prim–sul-fa-meth-ox'a-zole)

Apo-Sulfatrim*, Apo-Sulfatrim DS*, Bactrim, Bactrim IV, Bethaprim, Comoxol, Cotrim, Novo-Trimel*, Novo-Trimel DS*, Nu-Cotrimox*, Nu-Cotrimox DS*, Roubac*, Septra, Septra DS, SMZ/TMP, Sulfatrim

Func. class.: Antiinfective

Chem. class.: Miscellaneous sulfonamide

Action: Sulfamethoxazole (SMZ) interferes with bacterial biosynthesis of proteins by competitive antagonism of PABA when adequate levels are maintained; trimethoprim (TMP) blocks synthesis of tetrahydrofolic acid; combination blocks 2 consecutive steps in bacterial synthesis of essential nucleic acids, protein

Uses: UTI, otitis media, acute and chronic prostatitis, shigellosis, *Pneumocystis carinii* pneumonitis,

chronic bronchitis, chancroid, traveler's diarrhea

Dosage and routes: Based on TMP content

UTI

• *Adult:* **PO** 160 mg TMP q12h × 10-14 days

• *Child:* **PO** 8 mg/kg TMP qd in 2 divided doses q12h

Otitis media

• *Child:* **PO** 8 mg/kg TMP qd in 2 divided doses q12h × 10 days

Chronic bronchitis

• *Adult:* **PO** 160 mg TMP q12h × 14 days

Pneumocystis carinii *pneumonitis*

• *Adult and child:* **PO** 20 mg/kg TMP qd in 4 divided doses q6h × 14 days; **IV** 15-20 mg/kg/day (based on TMP) in 3-4 divided doses for up to 14 days

• Dosage reduction necessary in moderate to severe renal impairment (CrCl <30 ml/min)

Available forms: Tabs 80 mg trimethoprim/400 mg sulfamethoxazole, 160 mg trimethoprim/800 mg sulfamethoxazole; susp 40 mg/200 mg/5 ml; IV 16 mg/80 mg/ml

Side effects/adverse reactions:

CNS: Headache, insomnia, hallucinations, depression, vertigo, fatigue, anxiety, *convulsions, drug fever,* chills, *aseptic meningitis*

CV: Allergic myocarditis

GI: Nausea, vomiting, abdominal pain, stomatitis, *hepatitis,* glossitis, pancreatitis, diarrhea, *enterocolitis,* anorexia

GU: Renal failure, toxic nephrosis; increased BUN, creatinine; crystalluria

HEMA: Leukopenia, neutropenia, thrombocytopenia, agranulocytosis, hemolytic anemia, hypoprothrombinemia, Henoch-Schönlein purpura, methemoglobinemia, eosinophilia I

INTEG: Rash, dermatitis, urticaria,

= Nursing alert   = Herb-drug interaction   = Do not crush

Stevens-Johnson syndrome, erythema, photosensitivity, pain, inflammation at injection site, *toxic epidermal necrolysis, erythema multiforme*

RESP: Cough, shortness of breath

SYST: **Anaphylaxis, SLE**

Contraindications: Hypersensitivity to trimethoprim or sulfonamides, pregnancy at term, megaloblastic anemia, infants <2 mo, CrCl <15 ml/min, lactation, porphyria

Precautions: Pregnancy (C), renal disease, elderly, G6PD deficiency, impaired hepatic/renal function, possible folate deficiency, severe allergy, bronchial asthma

Pharmacokinetics:

PO: Rapidly absorbed, peak 1-4 hr; half-life 8-13 hr, excreted in urine (metabolites and unchanged), breast milk; crosses placenta; 68% bound to plasma proteins; TMP achieves high levels in prostatic tissue and fluid

Interactions:

• Increased hypoglycemic response: sulfonylurea agents

• Increased anticoagulant effects: oral anticoagulants

• Decreased hepatic clearance of phenytoin

• Decreased response: cyclosporine

• Increased bone marrow depressant effects: methotrexate

• Thrombocytopenia: thiazide diuretics

Lab test interferences:

Increase: Alk phosphatase, creatinine, bilirubin

False positive: Urinary glucose test

NURSING CONSIDERATIONS

Assess:

• Allergic reactions: rash, fever (AIDS patients more susceptible)

• I&O ratio; note color, character, pH of urine if drug administered for UTI; output should be 800 ml less than intake; if urine is highly acidic, alkalization may be needed

• Kidney function studies: BUN, creatinine, urinalysis (long-term therapy)

• Type of infection; obtain C&S before starting therapy

• Blood dyscrasias, skin rash, fever, sore throat, bruising, bleeding, fatigue, joint pain

• Allergic reaction: rash, dermatitis, urticaria, pruritus, dyspnea, bronchospasm

Administer:

PO

• Medication after C&S; repeat C&S after full course of medication

• With resuscitative equipment, epinephrine available; severe allergic reactions may occur

• With full glass of water to maintain adequate hydration; increase fluids to 2 L/day to decrease crystallization in kidneys

IV

• After diluting 5 ml of drug/125 ml D_5W, run over 1-1½ hr

Syringe compatibilities: Heparin

Y-site compatibilities: Acyclovir, aldesleukin, allopurinol, amifostine, amphotericin B cholesteryl, atracurium, aztreonam, cefepime, cyclophosphamide, diltiazem, doxorubicin liposome, enalaprilat, esmolol, filgrastim, fludarabine, gallium, granisetron, hydromorphone, labetalol, lorazepam, magnesium sulfate, melphalan, meperidine, morphine, pancuronium, perphenazine, piperacillin/tazobactam, remifentanil, sargramostim, tacrolimus, teniposide, thiotepa, vecuronium, zidovudine

Perform/provide:

• Storage in tight, light-resistant container at room temperature

Evaluate:

• Therapeutic response: absence of pain, fever, C&S negative

Teach patient/family:

• To take each oral dose with full glass of water to prevent crystalluria; drink 8-10 glasses of water/day; to take on an empty stomach 1 hr ac, 2 hr pc

• To complete full course of treatment to prevent superinfection

• To avoid sunlight or use sunscreen to prevent burns

• To avoid OTC medications (aspirin, vit C) unless directed by prescriber

• If diabetic, to use Clinistix or Tes-Tape

• To use alternative contraceptive measures; decreased effectiveness of oral contraceptives may result

• To notify prescriber if skin rash, sore throat, fever, mouth sores, unusual bruising, bleeding occur

---

trimipramine (℞)

(tri-mip′ra-meen)

Apo-Trimip*, Novo-Tripramine*, Rhotrimine, Surmontil

Func. class.: Antidepressant—tricyclic

Chem. class.: Tertiary amine

Action: Selectively inhibits serotonin uptake by brain; potentiates behavioral changes

Uses: Depression, enuresis in children

Dosage and routes:

• *Adult:* **PO** 75 mg/day in divided doses, may be increased to 200 mg/day

• *Geriatric:* **PO** 25 mg hs, increase by 25 mg q3-7 days, max 100 mg/day

• *Child >6 yr:* 25 mg hs, may increase to 50 mg in child <12 yr or 75 mg in child >12 yr

Available forms: Caps 25, 50, 100 mg

Side effects/adverse reactions:

*HEMA: **Agranulocytosis, thrombocytopenia, eosinophilia, leukopenia***

CNS: Dizziness, drowsiness, confusion, headache, anxiety, tremors, stimulation, weakness, insomnia, nightmares, EPS (elderly), increase in psychiatric symptoms

GI: Diarrhea, *dry mouth,* nausea, vomiting, ***paralytic ileus,*** increased appetite, cramps, epigastric distress, jaundice, ***hepatitis,*** stomatitis, *constipation*

*GU: Urinary retention, **acute renal failure***

INTEG: Rash, urticaria, sweating, pruritus, photosensitivity

*CV: Orthostatic hypotension, ECG changes, tachycardia, **hypertension,** palpitations*

EENT: Blurred vision, tinnitus, mydriasis

Contraindications: Hypersensitivity to tricyclics, recovery phase of MI, convulsive disorders, prostatic hypertrophy

Precautions: Suicidal patients, severe depression, increased intraocular pressure, narrow-angle glaucoma, urinary retention, cardiac disease, hepatic disease, hyperthyroidism, electroshock therapy, elective surgery, pregnancy (C), elderly

Pharmacokinetics: Metabolized by liver, excreted by kidneys, steady state 2-6 days; half-life 7-30 hr

Interactions:

• Decreased effects of: guanethidine, clonidine, indirect-acting sympathomimetics (ephedrine)

• Increased effects of direct-acting sympathomimetics (epinephrine), alcohol, barbiturates, benzodiazepines, CNS depressants

---

◆ = Nursing alert   ∥ = Herb-drug interaction   ⊘ = Do not crush

◆Hyperpyretic crisis, convulsions, hypertensive episode: MAOIs

🖊 Increased anticholinergic effect: belladonna, henbane

🖊 Increased antidepressant action: scopolia

Lab test interferences:
Increase: Serum bilirubin, blood glucose, alk phosphatase
False increase: Urinary catecholamines
Decrease: VMA, 5-HIAA

NURSING CONSIDERATIONS
Assess:
• B/P (lying, standing), pulse q4h; if systolic B/P drops 20 mm Hg, hold drug, notify prescriber; take vital signs q4h in patients with cardiovascular disease
• Blood studies: CBC, leukocytes, differential, cardiac enzymes if patient is receiving long-term therapy
• Hepatic studies: AST, ALT, bilirubin, creatinine
• Weight qwk; appetite may increase with drug
• ECG for flattening of T wave, bundle branch block, AV block, dysrhythmias in cardiac patients
• EPS primarily in elderly: rigidity, dystonia, akathisia
• Mental status changes: mood, sensorium, affect, suicidal tendencies, increase in psychiatric symptoms, depression, panic
• Urinary retention, constipation; constipation is more likely to occur in children, elderly
• Withdrawal symptoms: headache, nausea, vomiting, muscle pain, weakness; not usual unless drug is discontinued abruptly
• Alcohol consumption; hold dose until morning
Administer:
• Increased fluids, bulk in diet for constipation, urinary retention
• With food, milk for GI symptoms

• Dosage hs for oversedation during day; may take entire dose hs; elderly may not tolerate once/day dosing
• Gum, hard candy, or frequent sips of water for dry mouth
Perform/provide:
• Storage in tight, light-resistant container at room temperature
• Assistance with ambulation during beginning therapy for drowsiness/dizziness
• Safety measures, including side rails, primarily for elderly
• Checking to see if PO medication swallowed
Evaluate:
• Therapeutic response: decreased depression or enuresis
Teach patient/family:
• That therapeutic effects may take 2-3 wk
• To use caution in driving, other activities requiring alertness because of drowsiness, dizziness, blurred vision
• To avoid alcohol ingestion, other CNS depressants
• Not to discontinue medication quickly after long-term use; may cause nausea, headache, malaise
• To wear sunscreen or large hat, since photosensitivity occurs
Treatment of overdose: ECG monitoring; induce emesis; lavage, activated charcoal; administer anticonvulsant

triprolidine (OTC, ℞)
(trye-proe′li-deen)
Actidil, Myidil, triprolidine HCl
Func. class.: Antihistamine
Chem. class.: Alkylamine, H_1-receptor antagonist

Action: Acts on blood vessels, GI, respiratory system by competing with histamine for H_1-receptor site; decreases allergic response by blocking histamine

Uses: Rhinitis, allergy symptoms

Dosage and routes:
• *Adult:* **PO** 2.5 mg tid-qid
• *Child >6 yr:* **PO** 1.25 mg tid-qid
• *Child 4-6 yr:* **PO** 0.9 mg tid-qid
• *Child 2-4 yr:* **PO** 0.6 mg tid-qid
• *Child 4 mo-2 yr:* 0.3 mg tid-qid

Available forms: Tabs 2.5 mg; syr 1.25 mg/5 ml

Side effects/adverse reactions:

CNS: Dizziness, drowsiness, poor coordination, fatigue, anxiety, euphoria, confusion, paresthesia, neuritis

CV: Hypotension, palpitations, tachycardia

RESP: Increased thick secretions, wheezing, chest tightness

HEMA: **Thrombocytopenia, agranulocytosis, hemolytic anemia**

GI: Constipation, dry mouth, nausea, vomiting, anorexia, diarrhea

INTEG: Rash, urticaria, photosensitivity

GU: Urinary retention, dysuria, frequency

EENT: Blurred vision, dilated pupils, tinnitus, nasal stuffiness, dry nose, throat, mouth

Contraindications: Hypersensitivity to H_1-receptor antagonist, acute asthma attack, lower respiratory tract disease

Precautions: Increased intraocular pressure, renal disease, cardiac disease, hypertension, bronchial asthma, seizure disorder, stenosed peptic ulcers, hyperthyroidism, prostatic hypertrophy, bladder neck obstruction, pregnancy (C)

Pharmacokinetics:

PO: Onset 20-60 min, duration 8-12 hr; detoxified in liver, excreted by kidneys (metabolites/free drug), half-life 20-24 hr

Interactions:
• Increased CNS depressants: barbiturates, opioids, hypnotics, tricyclics, alcohol
• Decreased effect of oral anticoagulants, heparin
• Increased effect of triprolidine: MAOIs
• Increased anticholinergic effect: henbane

Lab test interferences:
False negative: Skin allergy tests

NURSING CONSIDERATIONS
Assess:
• I&O ratio; be alert for urinary retention, frequency, dysuria; drug should be discontinued
• CBC during long-term therapy; blood dyscrasias
• Respiratory status: rate, rhythm, increase in bronchial secretions, wheezing, chest tightness
• Cardiac status: palpitations, increased pulse, hypotension

Administer:
• With meals for GI symptoms; absorption may slightly decrease

Perform/provide:
• Hard candy, gum, frequent rinsing of mouth for dryness
• Storage in tight container at room temperature

Evaluate:
• Therapeutic response: decreased itching associated with pruritus

Teach patient/family:
• All aspects of drug use; to notify prescriber of confusion, sedation, hypotension
• To avoid driving, other hazardous activity if drowsiness occurs
• To avoid concurrent use of alcohol, other CNS depressants

Treatment of overdose: Administer ipecac syrup or lavage, diazepam, vasopressors, barbiturates (short-acting)

◆ = Nursing alert   ⬧ = Herb-drug interaction   ⊘ = Do not crush

triptorelin (R)

(trip-toe'rel-in)
Trelstar Depot
Func. class.: Gonadotropin-releasing hormone
Chem. class.: Synthetic decapeptide analog of LHRH

Action: Inhibitor of pituitary gonadotropin secretion; initially increases LH and FSH, with increases in testosterone, reduction in sex steroid levels

Uses: Advanced prostate cancer

Dosage and routes:
• *Adult:* **IM** 3.75 mg qmo

Available forms: Microgranules, depot inj 3.75 mg

Side effects/adverse reactions:

CNS: Headache, insomnia, dizziness, lability, fatigue

CV: Hypertension

ENDO: Gynecomastia, breast tenderness, hot flashes

GI: Nausea, vomiting, diarrhea

GU: Impotence, urinary retention, UTI

INTEG: Rash, pain on inj, pruritus, hypersensitivity

MS: Osteoneuralgia

Contraindications: Hypersensitivity to this product or other LHRH agonists or LHRH, pregnancy (X), lactation

Pharmacokinetics: Metabolism may be by CYP 450, eliminated by liver, kidneys; terminal half-life is 3 hr in healthy males

Lab test interferences:

Increase: Alk phosphatase, estradiol, FSH, LH, testosterone levels

Decrease: Testosterone levels, progesterone

NURSING CONSIDERATIONS

Assess:
• Severe hypersensitivity: discontinue drug and give antihistamines, have emergency equipment nearby
• I&O ratios; palpate bladder for distention in urinary obstruction
• For relief of bone pain (back pain)
• Assess levels of testosterone and PSA

Administer:
• IM using implant, inserted by qualified person
• Using syringe with 20G needle, withdraw 2 ml sterile water for inj, inject into vial, shake well, withdraw vial contents, inject immediately

Evaluate:
• Therapeutic response: more normal levels of prostate-specific antigen, acid phosphatase, alk phosphatase; testosterone level of <25 ng/dl

Teach patient/family:
• That postmenopausal symptoms may occur but will decrease after treatment is discontinued

tromethamine (R)

(troe-meth'a-meen)
Tham
Func. class.: Alkalinizer
Chem. class.: Amine

Action: Proton acceptor that corrects acidosis by combining with hydrogen ions to form bicarbonate and buffer; acts as diuretic (osmotic)

Uses: Acidosis (metabolic) associated with cardiac disease, COPD

Dosage and routes:
• *Adult:* **IV** 0.3 M required = kg of weight × HCO_3^- deficit (mEq/L)
• *Child:* **IV** same as above given over 3-6 hr, not to exceed 40 ml/kg

Available forms: Inj 18 g/500 ml

Side effects/adverse reactions:

CV: Irregular pulse, *cardiac arrest*

T

META: Alkalosis, hypoglycemia, ***hyperkalemia with oliguria***
RESP: Shallow, slow respirations, cyanosis, ***apnea***
GI: **Hepatic necrosis**
INTEG: Infection at inj site, extravasation, phlebitis

Contraindications: Hypersensitivity, anuria, uremia

Precautions: Severe respiratory disease/respiratory depression, pregnancy (C), cardiac edema, renal disease, infants

Pharmacokinetics:
IV: Excreted in urine

Interactions:
🌿 Decreased alkaline effect: oak bark

NURSING CONSIDERATIONS
Assess:
• Respiratory rate, rhythm, depth; notify prescriber of abnormalities that may indicate acidosis
• Electrolytes, blood glucose, chloride; CO_2, before, during treatment
• Urine pH, urinary output, urine glucose during beginning treatment
• I&O ratio, report large increase or decrease
• IV site for extravasation, phlebitis, thrombosis
• For signs of K depletion

Administer:
• IV slowly to avoid pain at infusion site and toxicity
• IV undiluted as inf or added to priming fluid or ACD blood; give 5 ml or less/min

Evaluate:
• Therapeutic response: decreased metabolic acidosis

Teach patient/family:
• To increase K in diet: bananas, oranges, cantaloupe, honeydew, spinach, potatoes, dried fruit

tubocurarine (℞)
(too-boe-kyoor-ar'een)
Tubarine*, Tubocuraine
Func. class.: Neuromuscular blocker
Chem. class.: Curare alkaloid

Action: Inhibits transmission of nerve impulses by binding with cholinergic receptor sites, antagonizing action of acetylcholine

Uses: Facilitation of endotracheal intubation, skeletal muscle relaxation during mechanical ventilation, surgery, or general anesthesia

Dosage and routes:
• *Adult:* **IV BOL** 0.4-0.5 mg/kg, then 0.08-0.10 mg/kg 20-45 min after 1st dose if needed for long procedures

Available forms: Inj 3 mg/ml, 20 U/ml

Side effects/adverse reactions:
CV: Bradycardia, tachycardia, increased, decreased B/P
RESP: ***Prolonged apnea, bronchospasm, cyanosis, respiratory depression***
EENT: Increased secretions
INTEG: Rash, flushing, pruritus, urticaria

Contraindications: Hypersensitivity

Precautions: Pregnancy (C), cardiac disease, lactation, children <2 yr, electrolyte imbalances, dehydration, neuromuscular disease, respiratory disease

Pharmacokinetics:
IV: Onset 15 sec, peak 2-3 min, duration ½-1½ hr; half-life 1-3 hr; degraded in liver, kidney (minimally); excreted in urine (unchanged) crosses placenta

Interactions:
• Increased neuromuscular blockade: aminoglycosides, clindamy-

---

◆ = Nursing alert   🌿 = Herb-drug interaction   🚫 = Do not crush

cin, lincomycin, quinidine, local anesthetics, polymyxin antiinfectives, lithium, opioid analgesics, thiazides, enflurane, isoflurane, trimethaphan, magnesium salts
Dysrhythmias: theophylline

NURSING CONSIDERATIONS
Assess:
• For electrolyte imbalances (K, Mg); may lead to increased action of this drug
• Vital signs (B/P, pulse, respirations, airway) q15min until fully recovered; rate, depth, pattern of respirations, strength of hand grip
• I&O ratio; check for urinary retention, frequency, hesitancy
• Recovery: decreased paralysis of face, diaphragm, leg, arm, rest of body; allow to recover fully before completing neurologic assessment
• Allergic reactions: rash, fever, respiratory distress, pruritus; drug should be discontinued
Administer:
• With diazepam or morphine when used for therapeutic paralysis; provides no sedation alone
• Using nerve stimulator by anesthesiologist to determine neuromuscular blockade
• Anticholinesterase to reverse neuromuscular blockade
• IV undiluted 3 mg/ml; give single dose over 1-1½ sec by qualified person; diluted to 4 ml in NS given 0.5 ml/2 min for myasthenia testing
Solution compatibilities: D₅, D₁₀W, 0.9% NaCl, 0.45% NaCl, Ringer's, LR, dextrose/Ringer's or dextrose/LR combinations
Syringe compatibilities: Pentobarbital, thiopental
Perform/provide:
• Storage in light-resistant area; use only fresh sol
• Reassurance if communication is difficult during recovery from neuromuscular blockade

Evaluate:
• Therapeutic response: paralysis of jaw, eyelid, head, neck, rest of body
Treatment of overdose: Edrophonium or neostigmine, atropine, monitor VS; may require mechanical ventilation

---

urea (℞)
(yoor-ee'a)
Ureaphil
Func. class.: Diuretic, osmotic
Chem. class.: Carbonic acid diamide salt

Action: Elevates plasma osmolality, increasing flow of water into plasma from ocular and cranial fluids
Uses: To decrease intracranial pressure, intraocular pressure
Dosage and routes:
• *Adult:* IV 1-1.5 g/kg of 30% sol over 1-3 hr, not to exceed 4 ml/min; do not exceed 120 g/day
• *Child >2 yr:* IV 0.5-1.5 g/kg, not to exceed 4 ml/min
• *Child <2 yr:* IV 0.1 g/kg, not to exceed 4 ml/min
Available forms: Inj 40 g/150 ml
Side effects/adverse reactions:
CNS: Dizziness, disorientation, fever, syncope, *headache*
GI: Nausea, vomiting
INTEG: Venous thrombosis, phlebitis, extravasation
Contraindications: Severe renal disease, active intracranial bleeding, marked dehydration, liver failure, sickle cell disease with CNS involvement
Precautions: Hepatic disease, renal disease, pregnancy (C), electrolyte imbalances, lactation
Pharmacokinetics:
IV: Onset ½-1 hr, peak 1 hr, duration 3-10 hr (diuresis), 5-6 hr (intraoc-

U

ular pressure); half-life 1 hr; excreted in urine, breast milk; crosses placenta

Interactions:

• Incompatible with whole blood, alkalies in sol or syringe

• Increased renal excretion of lithium

NURSING CONSIDERATIONS
Assess:

• Weight, I&O qd to determine fluid loss; effect of drug may be decreased if used qd; for hourly urinary output

• Rate, depth, rhythm of respiration, effect of exertion

• B/P lying, standing, postural hypotension may occur

• Electrolytes: K, Na, Cl; include BUN, blood sugar, CBC, serum creatinine, blood pH, ABGs, LFTs

• Fever, signs of extravasation

• Confusion, especially in elderly; take safety precautions if needed

• Hydration: skin turgor, thirst, dry mucous membranes

Administer:

• IV after diluting 30 g/100 ml diluent with D_5, D_{10}; run 30% sol over 1-2 hr; check for extravasation; do not exceed 4 ml/min; may cause bleeding; use IV filter

• Within minutes of reconstitution; sol becomes ammonia on standing

Evaluate:

• Therapeutic response: improvement in edema of feet, legs, sacral area daily in CHF

Teach patient/family:

• That drug will cause diuresis in ½ hr

Treatment of overdose: Lavage if taken orally; monitor electrolytes, administer IV fluids, monitor BUN, hydration, CV status

urokinase (℞)
(yoor-oh-kin'ase)
Abbokinase, Abbokinase
Open-Cath
Func. class.: Thrombolytic enzyme
Chem. class.: β-Hemolytic streptococcus filtrate (purified)

Action: Promotes thrombolysis by directly converting plasminogen to plasmin

Uses: Venous thrombosis, pulmonary embolism, arterial thrombosis, arterial embolism, arteriovenous cannula occlusion, lysis of coronary artery thrombi after MI

Dosage and routes:

Lysis of pulmonary emboli

• *Adult and child:* IV 4400 IU/kg/hr × 12-24 hr, not to exceed 200 ml; then **IV** heparin, then anticoagulants

Coronary artery thrombosis

• *Adult:* **INSTILL** 6000 IU/min into occluded artery for 1-2 hr after giving **IV BOL** of heparin 2500-10,000 U

• May also give as **IV INF** 2 million-3 million U over 45-90 min

Venous catheter occlusion

• *Adult and child:* **INSTILL** 5000 IU into line, wait 5 min, then aspirate, repeat aspiration attempts q5min × ½ hr; if occlusion has not been removed, cap line and wait ½-1 hr, then aspirate; may need 2nd dose if still occluded

Available forms: Pwd for inj, lyophilized: 250,000 IU/vial; pwd for catheter clearance

Side effects/adverse reactions:

*HEMA: Decreased Hct, **bleeding***
INTEG: Rash, urticaria, phlebitis at IV infusion site, itching, flushing
CNS: Headache, fever
GI: Nausea, vomiting

RESP: Altered respirations, SOB, ***bronchospasm,*** cyanosis
MS: Low back pain
CV: Hypertension, dysrhythmias
EENT: Periorbital edema
*SYST: **GI, GU, intracranial, retroperitoneal bleeding,*** surface bleeding, ***anaphylaxis*** (rare)

Contraindications: Hypersensitivity, active bleeding, intraspinal surgery, neoplasms of CNS, ulcerative colitis/enteritis, severe hypertension, renal disease, hepatic disease, hypocoagulation, COPD, subacute bacterial endocarditis, rheumatic valvular disease, cerebral embolism/thrombosis/hemorrhage, intraarterial diagnostic procedure or surgery (10 days), recent major surgery

Precautions: Arterial emboli from left side of heart, pregnancy (B)

Pharmacokinetics:
IV: Half-life 10-20 min; small amounts excreted in urine

Interactions:
• Bleeding potential: aspirin, indomethacin, phenylbutazone, anticoagulants, other NSAIDs, abciximab, eptifibatide, tirofiban, clopidogrel, ticlopidine, some cephalosporins, plicamycin, valproic acid

Lab test interferences:
Increase: PT, APTT, TT

NURSING CONSIDERATIONS
Assess:
• VS, B/P, pulse, resp, neurologic signs, temp at least q4h; temp >104° F (40° C) is an indicator of internal bleeding; cardiac rhythm following intracoronary administration
• For neurologic changes that may indicate intracranial bleeding
• Retroperitoneal bleeding: back pain, leg weakness, diminished pulses
• Peripheral pulses, lung sounds, respiratory function
• Hypersensitivity: fever, rash, itching, chills, facial swelling, dyspnea; mild reaction may be treated with antihistamines; notify prescriber of severe reactions, stop drug, keep resuscitative equipment nearby
• Bleeding during 1st hr of treatment (hematuria, hematemesis, bleeding from mucous membranes, epistaxis, ecchymosis)
• Blood studies (Hct, platelets, PTT, PT, TT, APTT) before starting therapy; PT or APTT must be less than 2 × control before starting therapy TT; or PT q3-4h during treatment
• ECG continuously, cardiac enzymes, radionuclide myocardial scanning/coronary angiography

Administer:
IV
• Using infusion pump, terminal filter (0.45 µm or smaller)
• Reconstituting only with 5.2 ml sterile water for inj (not bacteriostatic water), and roll (not shake) to enhance reconstitution; further dilute with 190 ml; give as intermittent inf or give to clear cannula by using 1 ml of diluted drug; inject into cannula slowly, clamp 5 min, aspirate clot; avoid excessive pressure when urokinase is injected into catheter; force could rupture catheter or expel clot into circulation
• As soon as thrombi identified; not useful for thrombi over 1 wk old
• Cryoprecipitate or fresh frozen plasma if bleeding occurs
• Loading dose at beginning of therapy; may require increased loading doses
• Heparin therapy after thrombolytic therapy is discontinued, TT or APTT less than 2 × control (about 3-4 hr)

Y-site compatibilities: TPN 55, 56
Perform/provide:
• Storage in refrigerator; use immediately after reconstitution

U

• Bed rest during entire course of treatment; use caution in handling patients
• Avoidance of venous, arterial puncture procedures, inj, rectal temp
• Treatment of fever with acetaminophen or aspirin
• Placement of sign above patient's bed stating urokinase therapy
• Pressure for 30 sec to minor bleeding sites; 30 min to sites of arterial puncture followed by pressure dressing; inform prescriber if hemostasis not attained, apply pressure dressing

Evaluate:
• Therapeutic response: decreased clotting, thrombosis, embolism

---

ursodiol (R)

(ur-soh-die'-ohl)
Actigall
Func. class.: Gallstone solubilizing agent
Chem. class.: Ursodeoxycholic acid

Action: Suppresses hepatic synthesis, secretion of cholesterol; inhibits intestinal absorption of cholesterol
Uses: Dissolution of radiolucent, noncalcified gallbladder stones (less than 20 mm in diameter) in which surgery is not indicated
Investigational uses: Severe pruritus
Dosage and routes:
• *Adult:* **PO** 8-10 mg/kg/day in 2-3 divided doses using gallbladder ultrasound q6mo; determine if stones have dissolved; if so, continue therapy, repeat ultrasound within 1-3 mo
Available forms: Caps 300 mg
Side effects/adverse reactions:
GI: Diarrhea, nausea, vomiting, abdominal pain, constipation, stoma-

titis, flatulence, dyspepsia, biliary pain
INTEG: Pruritus, rash, urticaria, dry skin, sweating, alopecia
CNS: Headache, anxiety, depression, insomnia, fatigue
MS: Arthralgia, myalgia, back pain
OTHER: Cough, rhinitis
Contraindications: Calcified cholesterol stones, radiopaque stones, radiolucent bile pigment stones, chronic liver disease, hypersensitivity
Precautions: Pregnancy (B), lactation, children
Pharmacokinetics: 80% excreted in feces, 20% metabolized, excreted into bile, lost in feces
Interactions:
• Reduced action of ursodiol: cholestyramine, colestipol, aluminum-based antacids
• Increased risk of stone formation: clofibrate, gemfibrozil, estrogens, oral contraceptives

NURSING CONSIDERATIONS
Assess:
• GI status: diarrhea, abdominal pain, nausea, vomiting; drug may have to be discontinued if side effects are severe
• Skin for pruritus, rash, urticaria, dry skin; provide soothing lotion to lesions
• Musculoskeletal status: aches or stiffness in joints
Administer:
• For up to 9-12 mo; if no improvement is seen, discontinue drug
Evaluate:
• Therapeutic response: decreasing size of stones on ultrasound
Teach patient/family:
• That anxiety, depression, insomnia are side effects and are reversible after discontinuing drug

---

⬥ = Nursing alert   🖋 = Herb-drug interaction   🚫 = Do not crush

valacyclovir (℞)

(val-a-sye′kloh-vir)

Valtrex

Func. class.: Antiviral

Chem. class.: Acyclic purine nucleoside analog

Action: Interferes with DNA synthesis by conversion to acyclovir, causing decreased viral replication, time of lesional healing

Uses: Treatment or suppression of herpes zoster, genital herpes

Investigational uses: Prevention of CMV in advanced HIV, posttransplant patients

Dosage and routes:

Genital herpes

• *Adult:* PO 1 g bid × 10 days initially; 1 g qd or 500 mg bid in those with <10 recurrences/yr

Recurrent episodes

• *Adult:* PO 500 mg bid × 3 days

Suppressive therapy

• *Adult:* PO 1 g qd if those ≤ recurrences/yr

Herpes zoster

• *Adult:* PO 1 g tid × 1 wk

Renal dose

• *Adult:* PO CrCl 30-49 ml/min 1 g q12h (herpes zoster); CrCl 10-29 ml/min 1 g q24h (genital herpes); 500 mg q24h (recurrent genital herpes); CrCl <10 ml/min 500 mg q24h (genital herpes), 500 mg q24h (recurrent genital herpes)

Available forms: Tabs 500 mg, 1 g

Side effects/adverse reactions:

CNS: Tremors, lethargy, *dizziness, headache,* weakness

GI: Nausea, vomiting, diarrhea, abdominal pain, constipation

INTEG: Rash

Contraindications: Hypersensitivity to this drug or acyclovir

Precautions: Lactation, hepatic disease, renal diseae, electrolyte imbalance, dehydration, pregnancy (B)

Pharmacokinetics:

PO: Onset unknown, terminal half-life 2½-3½ hr; converted to acyclovir that crosses placenta and enters breast milk

Interactions:

• Increased blood levels of valacyclovir: cimetidine, probenecid

NURSING CONSIDERATIONS

Assess:

• Signs of infection; characteristics of lesions

• C&S before drug therapy; drug may be taken as soon as culture is taken; repeat C&S after treatement; determine the presence of other sexually transmitted diseases

• Bowel pattern before, during treatment

• Skin eruptions: rash

• Allergies before treatment, reaction of each medication; place allergies on chart in bright red letters

Evaluate:

• Therapeutic response: absence of itching, painful lesions; crusting and healed lesions

Teach patient/family:

• To take as prescribed; if dose is missed, take as soon as remembered up to 1 hr before next dose; do not double dose

• That drug may be taken orally before infection occurs; drug should be taken when itching or pain occurs, usually before eruptions

• That partners need to be told that patient has herpes; they can become infected; condoms must be worn to prevent reinfections

• That drug does not cure infection. just controls symptoms and does not prevent infection of others

Treatment of overdose: Discontinue drug, hemodialysis, resuscitate if needed

valdecoxib
See appendix a—selected new drugs

valganciclovir
See appendix a—selected new drugs

valproate
(val′proh-ate)
Depacon
valproic acid
(val′proh-ik)
Depakene, Myproic acid
divalproex sodium
(dye-val′proh-ex)
Depakote, Depakote ER, Epival*
Func. class: Anticonvulsant
Chem. class: Carboxylic acid derivative

Action: Increases levels of γ-aminobutyric acid (GABA) in brain, which decreases seizure activity

Uses: Simple (petit mal), complex (petit mal) absence, mixed, manic episodes associated with bipolar disorder, prophylaxis of migraine
Investigational uses: Tonic-clonic (grand mal), myoclonic seizures, migraines; rectal (valproic acid)
Dosage and routes:
Epilepsy
• *Adult and child:* **PO** 15 mg/kg/day divided in 2-3 doses, may increase by 5-10 mg/kg/day qwk, not to exceed 60 mg/kg/day in 2-3 divided doses; **IV** ≤20 mg/min over 1 hr
Mania (divalproex sodium)
• *Adult:* **PO** 750 mg qd in divided doses, max 60 mg/kg/day

Migraine
• *Adult:* **PO** 250 mg bid, may increase to 1000 mg/day if needed
Available forms: Valproic acid: caps 250, 500 mg; syr 250 mg/5 ml; divalproex: tabs delayed rel 125, 250, 500 mg; 125 mg sprinkle cap; valproate: inj 100 mg/ml
Side effects/adverse reactions:
*HEMA: **Thrombocytopenia, leukopenia, lymphocytosis,** increased PT*
CNS: Sedation, drowsiness, dizziness, headache, incoordination, paresthesia, depression, hallucinations, behavioral changes, tremors, aggression, weakness
GI: Nausea, vomiting, constipation, diarrhea, heartburn, anorexia, cramps, **hepatic failure, pancreatitis, toxic hepatitis,** stomatitis
INTEG: Rash, alopecia, bruising
GU: Enuresis, irregular menses
EENT: Visual disturbances

Contraindications: Hypersensitivity, pregnancy (D), hepatic disease
Precautions: Lactation, child <2 yr
Pharmacokinetics:
PO: Onset 15-30 min, peak 1-4 hr, duration 4-6 hr
Metabolized by liver; excreted by kidneys, breast milk; crosses placenta; half-life 9-16 hr
Interactions:
• Increased CNS depression: alcohol, opioids, barbiturates, antihistamines, MAOIs
• Increased toxicity of valproic acid: salicylates
• Increased action of: phenytoin
• Increased bleeding: antiplatelets, NSAIDs, tirofiban, eptifibatide, abciximab, cefamandole, cefoperazone, cefotetan, heparin, thrombolytics
• Decreased metabolism of valproic acid: cimetidine
Lab test interferences:
False positive: Ketones
Interference: Thyroid function tests

 = Nursing alert   ◢ = Herb-drug interaction   ◯ = Do not crush

NURSING CONSIDERATIONS
Assess:
• Blood studies: Hct, Hgb, RBC, serum folate, PT, platelets, vit D if on long-term therapy
• Hepatic studies: AST, ALT, bilirubin, hepatic failure
• Blood levels: therapeutic level 50-100 µg/ml
• Mental status: mood, sensorium, affect, memory (long, short)
• Respiratory dysfunction: respiratory depression, character, rate, rhythm; hold drug if respirations are <12/min or if pupils are dilated
Administer:
PO
🚫 Tablets or capsules whole; do not break, crush, or chew
• Elixir alone; do not dilute with carbonated beverage; do not give syrup to patients on sodium restriction
• Give with food or milk to decrease GI symptoms
Evaluate:
• Therapeutic response: decreased seizures
Teach patient/family:
• That physical dependency may result from extended use
• To avoid driving, other activities that require alertness
• Not to discontinue medication quickly after long-term use; convulsions may result
• To report visual disturbances, rash, diarrhea, light-colored stools, jaundice, protracted vomiting to prescriber

valrubicin (Ŗ)
(val-roo'bih-sin)
Valstar
Func. class.: Antineoplastic, antibiotic
Chem. class.: Anthracycline glycoside

Action: A semisynthetic analog of doxorubicin that inhibits DNA synthesis primarily; replication is decreased by binding to DNA, which causes strand splitting; active throughout entire cell cycle; a vesicant
Uses: Bladder cancer
Dosage and routes:
• *Adult:* Intravesically 800 mg qwk × 6 wk, delay administration ≥2 wk after transurethral resection of fulguration
Available forms: Sol for intravesical instillation: 40 mg/ml
Side effects/adverse reactions:
HEMA: ***Thrombocytopenia, leukopenia,*** *anemia*
GI: Nausea, vomiting, anorexia, diarrhea
GU: UTI, urinary retention, hematuria
INTEG: Rash
CV: Chest pain
Contraindications: Hypersensitivity to anthracyclines or *Cremophor El,* urinary tract infection, small bladder
Precautions: Pregnancy (C), lactation, children
Pharmacokinetics: Penetrates into bladder wall, not metabolized
NURSING CONSIDERATIONS
Assess:
• I&O ratio; report fall in urine output to <30 ml/hr
• Monitor temperature q4h; fever may indicate beginning infection

V

• Local irritation, pain, burning at inj site

Administer:

• After urinary catheter is inserted under aseptic conditions, drain bladder and instill the diluted 75 ml valrubicin by gravity for several min, withdraw catheter, drug should be retained for 2 hr, then void

• Use procedure for handling and disposal of cytotoxic agents

• Do not use polyvinyl chloride (PVC) or IV tubing

• Prepare/store valrubicin sol in glass, polypropylene, or polyolefin tubing/containers

• For instillation, 5 ml vials (200 mg valrubicin/5 ml/vial) should be warmed to room temperature, withdraw 20 ml for the 4 vials and dilute with 55 ml 0.9% NaCl inj to 75 ml of diluted valrubicin sol

• Valrubicin sol is clear red, at lower temps a waxy precipitate may form, warm in hand until sol is clear

Perform/provide:

• Strict hand-washing technique, gloves, protective clothing

• Increased fluid intake to 2-3 L/day to prevent urate, calculi formation

• Storage at room temperature for 12 hr after reconstituting

Evaluate:

• Therapeutic response: decreased tumor size, spread of malignancy

Teach patient/family:

• To consume fluids 2 L/day unless contraindicated

• To report any complaints, side effects to nurse or prescriber

• That urine and other body fluids may be red-orange for 48 hr

• That contraceptive measures are recommended during therapy

valsartan (R)

(val′sahr-tan)

Diovan

Func. class.: Antihypertensive

Chem. class.: Angiotensin II receptor antagonist (Type AT_1)

Action: Blocks the vasoconstrictor and aldosterone-secreting effects of angiotensin II; selectively blocks the binding of angiotensin II to the AT_1 receptor found in tissues

Uses: Hypertension, alone or in combination

Dosage and routes:

• *Adult:* **PO** 80-160 mg qd alone or in combination with other antihypertensives

Available forms: Tabs 80, 160 mg

Side effects/adverse reactions:

CNS: Dizziness, insomnia, depression, drowsiness, vertigo

CV: Angina pectoris, 2nd-degree AV block, *cerebrovascular accident,* hypotension, *myocardial infarction, dysrhythmias*

EENT: Conjunctivitis

GI: Diarrhea, abdominal pain, nausea, *hepatotoxicity*

GU: Impotence, *nephrotoxicity*

HEMA: Anemia, neutropenia

MS: Cramps, myalgia, pain, stiffness

RESP: Cough

Contraindications: Hypersensitivity, pregnancy, severe hepatic disease, bilateral renal artery stenosis

Precautions: Hypersensitivity to ACE inhibitors: congestive heart failure, hypertrophic cardiomyopathy aortic/mitral valve stenosis, CAD; lactation, children, elderly

Pharmacokinetics:

Peak 2 hr, duration >24 hr, extensively metabolized, half-life 9 hr; excreted in feces, urine, breast milk

---

◆ = Nursing alert   ∥ = Herb-drug interaction   ⊘ = Do not crush

NURSING CONSIDERATIONS
Assess:
• B/P, pulse q4h; note rate, rhythm, quality
• Blood studies: BUN, creatinine, LFTs before treatment
• Electrolytes: K, Na, Cl, total CO_2
• Baselines in renal, LFTs before therapy begins
• Edema in feet, legs qd
• Skin turgor, dryness of mucous membranes for hydration status
Administer:
PO
• Without regard to meals
Evaluate:
• Therapeutic response: decreased B/P
Teach patient/family:
• To comply with dosage schedule, even if feeling better
• To notify prescriber of fever, swelling of hands or feet, irregular heartbeat, chest pain
• That excessive perspiration, dehydration, diarrhea may lead to fall in blood pressure; consult prescriber if these occur
• That drug may cause dizziness, fainting; light-headedness may occur
• To rise slowly to sitting or standing position to minimize orthostatic hypotension
• Not to take this medication if pregnant or breastfeeding, or have had an allergic reaction to this drug
• That if a dose is missed, to take it as soon as possible, unless it is within an hour before next dose

vancomycin (R)

(van-koe-mye′sin)
Lyphocin, Vancocin,
Vancoled, vancomycin HCl
Func. class.: Antiinfective, misc.
Chem. class.: Tricyclic glycopeptide

Action: Inhibits bacterial cell wall synthesis

Uses: Resistant staphylococcal infections, pseudomembranous colitis, staphylococcal enterocolitis, endocarditis prophylaxis for dental procedures, diphtheroid endocarditis

Dosage and routes:
Serious staphylococcal infections
• *Adult:* **IV** 500 mg q6h or 1 g q12h
• *Child:* **IV** 40 mg/kg/day divided q6-8h
• *Neonate:* **IV** 15 mg/kg initially followed by 10 mg/kg q8-24h
Pseudomembranous/staphylococcal enterocolitis
• *Adult:* **PO** 500 mg/day in divided doses for 7-10 days
• *Child:* **PO** 40 mg/kg/day divided q6h, not to exceed 2 g/day
Endocarditis prophylaxis
• *Adult:* **IV** 1 g over 1 hr, 1 hr before dental procedure
Available forms: Pulvules 125, 250 mg; pwd for oral sol 1, 10 g; pwd for inj 500 mg, 1, 5, 10 g

Side effects/adverse reactions:
*CV: **Cardiac arrest, vascular collapse** (rare)
*EENT: **Ototoxicity, permanent deafness,** tinnitus*
*HEMA: **Leukopenia, eosinophilia, neutropenia***
*GI: **Nausea, pseudomembranous colitis***
RESP: Wheezing, dyspnea
*SYST: **Anaphylaxis***
*GU: **Nephrotoxicity,** increased BUN, creatinine, albumin, **fatal uremia***

V

INTEG: Chills, fever, rash, thrombophlebitis at inj site, urticaria, pruritus, necrosis (red man syndrome)

Contraindications: Hypersensitivity, previous hearing loss

Precautions: Renal disease, pregnancy (C), lactation, elderly, neonates

Pharmacokinetics:

IV: Peak 5 min; half-life 4-8 hr; excreted in urine (active form); IV; feces PO crosses placenta

PO: Absorption: poor

Interactions:

• Ototoxicity or nephrotoxicity: aminoglycosides, cephalosporins, colistin, polymyxin, bacitracin, cisplatin, amphotericin B, nondepolarizing muscle relaxants

NURSING CONSIDERATIONS

Assess:

• I&O ratio; report hematuria, oliguria; nephrotoxicity may occur

◆ Any patient with compromised renal system; drug is excreted slowly in poor renal system function; toxicity may occur rapidly; BUN, creatinine

• Blood studies: WBC

• Serum levels: peak 1 hr after 1 hr inf 25-40 mg/ml, trough prior to next dose 5-10 mg/ml

• C&S; drug may be given as soon as culture is taken

• Auditory function during, after treatment

• B/P during administration; sudden drop may indicate red man syndrome

• Signs of infection

• Hearing loss, ringing, roaring in ears; drug should be discontinued

• Skin eruptions

• Respiratory status: rate, character, wheezing, tightness in chest

• Allergies before treatment, reaction of each medication

Administer:

• Antihistamine if red man syndrome occurs: decreased B/P, flushing of neck, face

• Dose based on serum concentration

IV

• After reconstitution with 10 ml sterile water for injection (500 mg/10 ml); further dilution is needed for IV, 500 mg/100 ml 0.9%NaCl, D_5W given as int inf over 1 hr; decrease rate of infusion if red man syndrome occurs

Additive compatibilities: Amikacin, atracurium, calcium gluconate, cefepime, cimetidine, corticotropin, dimenhydrinate, famotidine, hydrocortisone, meropenem, ofloxacin, potassium chloride, ranitidine, verapamil, vit B/C

Y-site compatibilities: Acyclovir, allopurinol, amifostine, amiodarone, amsacrine, atracurium, cisatracurium, cyclophosphamide, diltiazem, doxorubicin liposome, enalaprilat, esmolol, filgrastim, fluconazole, fludarabine, gallium, granisetron, hydromorphone, insulin (regular), labetalol, lorazepam, magnesium sulfate, melphalan, meperidine, meropenem, midazolam, morphine, ondansetron, paclitaxel, pancuronium, perphenazine, propofol, remifentanil, sodium bicarbonate, tacrolimus, teniposide, theophylline, thiotepa, tolazoline, vecuronium, vinorelbine, warfarin, zidovudine

Perform/provide:

• Storage at room temperature for up to 2 wk after reconstitution

• Adrenaline, suction, tracheostomy set, endotracheal intubation equipment on unit; anaphylaxis may occur

• Adequate intake of fluids (2 L/day) to prevent nephrotoxicity

---

◆ = Nursing alert   🌿 = Herb-drug interaction   🚫 = Do not crush

Evaluate:
• Therapeutic response: absence of fever, sore throat; negative culture

Teach patient/family:
• All aspects of drug therapy: need to complete entire course of medication to ensure organism death (7-10 days); culture may be taken after completed course of medication
• To report sore throat, fever, fatigue; could indicate superinfection
• That drug must be taken in equal intervals around clock to maintain blood levels

---

RARELY USED

vasopressin (℞)
(vay-soe-press'in)
Pitressin Synthetic
Func. class.: Pituitary hormone

Uses: Diabetes insipidus (nonnephrogenic/nonpsychogenic), abdominal distention postoperatively, bleeding esophageal varices

Dosage and routes:
Diabetes insipidus
• *Adult:* **IM/SC** 5-10 U bid-qid as needed; **IM/SC** 2.5-5 U q2-3d (Pitressin Tannate) for chronic therapy
• *Child:* **IM/SC** 2.5-10 U bid-qid as needed; **IM/SC** 1.25-2.5 U q2-3d (Pitressin Tannate) for chronic therapy

Abdominal distention: Adult: **IM** 5 U, then q3-4h, increasing to 10 U if needed (aqueous)

Contraindications: Hypersensitivity, chronic nephritis

vecuronium (℞)
(vek-yoo-roe'nee-um)
Norcuron
Func. class.: Neuromuscular blocker
Chem. class.: Monoquaternary analog of pancuronium

Action: Inhibits transmission of nerve impulses by binding with cholinergic receptor sites, antagonizing action of acetylcholine

Uses: Facilitation of endotracheal intubation, skeletal muscle relaxation during mechanical ventilation, surgery, general anesthesia

Dosage and routes:
• *Adult and child >9 yr:* **IV BOL** 0.08-0.10 mg/kg, then 0.01-0.015 mg/kg for prolonged procedures

Available forms: 10 mg/5 ml vial

Side effects/adverse reactions:
CNS: Skeletal muscle weakness or paralysis (rare)
*RESP: **Prolonged apnea, possible respiratory paralysis***

Contraindications: Hypersensitivity

Precautions: Pregnancy (C), cardiac disease, lactation, children <2 yr, electrolyte imbalances, dehydration, neuromuscular disease, respiratory disease, hepatic disease

Do not confuse:
Nocuron/Narcan

Pharmacokinetics:
IV: Onset 15 min, peak 3-5 min, duration 45-60 min; half-life 65-75 min; not metabolized; excreted in feces; crosses placenta

Interactions:
• Increased neuromuscular blockade: aminoglycosides, clindamycin, lincomycin, quinidine, local anesthetics, polymyxin antibiotics, lithium, opioid analgesics, thiazides,

---

enflurane, isoflurane, succinylcholine

Dysrhythmias: theophylline

NURSING CONSIDERATIONS
Assess:
• For electrolyte imbalances (K, Mg); may lead to increased action of this drug
• Vital signs (B/P, pulse, respirations, airway) q15min until fully recovered; rate, depth, pattern of respirations, strength of hand grip
• I&O ratio; check for urinary retention, frequency, hesitancy
• Recovery: decreased paralysis of face, diaphragm, leg, arm, rest of body; allow to recover fully before completing neurologic assessment
• Allergic reactions: rash, fever, respiratory distress, pruritus; drug should be discontinued

Administer:
• With diazepam or morphine when used for therapeutic paralysis; provides no sedation alone
• Using nerve stimulator by anesthesiologist to determine neuromuscular blockade
• Anticholinesterase to reverse neuromuscular blockade
• IV after diluting with diluent provided; give by direct IV over 1 min; may give as continuous inf 10-20 mg/100 ml; titrate to patient response (only by qualified person)

Y-site compatibilities: Aminophylline, cefazolin, cefuroxime, cimetidine, diltiazem, dobutamine, dopamine, epinephrine, esmolol, fentanyl, fluconazole, gentamicin, heparin, hydrocortisone, hydromorphone, isoproterenol, labetalol, lorazepam, midazolam, milrinone, morphine, nicardipine, nitroglycerin, norepinephrine, propofol, ranitidine, sodium nitroprusside, trimethoprim-sulfamethoxazole, vancomycin

Perform/provide:
• Storage in refrigerator; discard in 24 hr
• Reassurance if communication is difficult during recovery from neuromuscular blockade

Evaluate:
• Therapeutic response: paralysis of jaw, eyelid, head, neck, rest of body

Treatment of overdose: Edrophonium or neostigmine, atropine, monitor VS; may require mechanical ventilation

---

venlafaxine (℞)

(ven-la-fax′een)
Effexor, Effexor-XR
Func. class.: Antidepressant (misc)

Action: Potent inhibitor of neuronal serotonin and norepinephrine uptake, weak inhibitor of dopamine; no muscarinic, histaminergic, or α-adrenergic receptors in vitro

Uses: Prevention/treatment of depression, long-term treatment of general anxiety disorder (Effexor-XR)

Investigational uses: Hot flashes

Dosage and routes:
Renal dose
• Mild-moderate impairment, 75% of dose

Hepatic dose
• Moderate impairment, 50% of dose

Depression
• *Adult:* **PO** 75 mg/day in 2 or 3 divided doses; taken with food, may be increased to 150 mg/day; if needed, may be further increased to 225 mg/day; increments of 75 mg/day at intervals of no less than 4 days; some hospitalized patients may require up to 375 mg/day in 3 divided doses; ext rel 37.5-75 mg PO qd, max 225 mg/day; give XR qd

---

Hot flashes (off-label)
• *Adult:* **PO** 12.5 mg bid × 4 wk or ext rel 37.5 mg × 4 wk
Available forms: Tabs scored 25, 37.5, 50, 75, 100 mg; cap ext rel 37.5, 75, 150 mg
Side effects/adverse reactions:

CNS: Emotional lability, vertigo, apathy, ataxia, CNS stimulation, euphoria, hallucinations, hostility, increased libido, hypertonia, hypotonia, psychosis
CV: Migraine, angina pectoris, hypertension, extrasystoles, postural hypotension, syncope, thrombophlebitis
EENT: Abnormal vision, ear pain, cataract, conjunctivitis, corneal lesions, dry eyes, otitis media, photophobia
GI: Dysphagia, eructation, colitis, gastritis, gingivitis, **rectal hemorrhage,** stomatitis, stomach and mouth ulceration
GU: Anorgasmia, dysuria, hematuria, metrorrhagia, vaginitis, impaired urination, albuminuria, amenorrhea, kidney calculus, cystitis, nocturia, breast and bladder pain, polyuria, **uterine hemorrhage, vaginal hemorrhage,** moniliasis
INTEG: Ecchymosis, acne, alopecia, brittle nails, dry skin, photosensitivity
META: Peripheral edema, weight loss or gain, diabetes mellitus, edema, glycosuria, hyperlipemia, hypokalemia
MS: Arthritis, bone pain, bursitis, myasthenia tenosynovitis
RESP: Bronchitis, dyspnea, asthma, chest congestion, epistaxis, hyperventilation, laryngitis
SYST: Accidental injury, malaise, neck pain, enlarged abdomen, cyst, facial edema, hangover, hernia
Contraindications: Hypersensitivity

Precautions: Mania, pregnancy (C), lactation, children, elderly, hypertension, seizure disorder
Pharmacokinetics: Well absorbed, extensively metabolized in the liver to an active metabolite; 87% of drug recovered in urine; 27% protein binding; half-life 5-7, 11-13 hr (active metabolite) respectively
Interactions:

◆Hyperthermia, rigidity, rapid fluctuations of vital signs, mental status changes, neuroleptic malignant syndrome: MAOIs
• Increased CNS depression: alcohol, opioids, antihistamines, sedative/hypnotics
• Increased serotonin effect: lithium
NURSING CONSIDERATIONS
Assess:
• B/P lying, standing; pulse q/4 h; if systolic B/P drops 20 mm Hg, hold drug, notify prescriber; take VS q4h in patients with cardiovascular disease
• Blood studies: CBC, leukocytes, differential cardiac enzymes if patient is receiving long-term therapy
• Hepatic studies: AST, ALT, bilirubin
• Weight qwk; weight loss or gain; appetite may increase
• With food, milk for GI symptoms
• Gum, hard candy, frequent sips of water for dry mouth
• Mental status: mood, sensorium, affect, suicidal tendencies, increase in psychiatric symptoms; depression, panic
• Withdrawal symptoms: headache, nausea, vomiting, muscle pain, weakness; not usual unless drug is discontinued abruptly
Perform/provide:
• Storage in tight container at room temperature; do not freeze
• Assistance with ambulation dur-

ing beginning therapy, since drowsiness, dizziness occur

• Checking to see if PO medication swallowed

Evaluate:

• Therapeutic response; decreased depression

Teach patient/family:

• To dispense in small amounts because of suicide potential, especially in the beginning of therapy

• To use with caution when driving or other activities requiring alertness because of drowsiness, dizziness, blurred vision

• To avoid alcohol ingestion, other CNS depressants

• Not to discontinue medication quickly after long-term use; may cause nausea, headache, malaise

• To wear sunscreen or large hat, since photosensitivity occurs

Treatment of overdose: ECG monitoring; induce emesis; lavage, activated charcoal; administer anticonvulsant

---

verapamil (R)

(ver-ap′a-mill)

Apo-Verap*, Calan, Calan SR, Isoptin, Isoptin SR , verapamil HCl, verapamil HCl SR, Verelan

Func. class.: Calcium channel blocker; antihypertensive; antianginal

Chem. class.: Phenylalkylamine

Action: Inhibits calcium ion influx across cell membrane during cardiac depolarization; produces relaxation of coronary vascular smooth muscle; dilates coronary arteries; decreases SA/AV node conduction; dilates peripheral arteries

Uses: Chronic stable angina pectoris, vasospastic angina, dysrhythmias, hypertension

Investigational uses: Prevention of migraine headaches, ventricular outflow obstruction in hypertrophic cardiomyopathy

Research note: Grapefruit juice given with verapamil resulted in increased verapamil levels[39]

Dosage and routes:

• *Adult:* **PO** 80 mg tid or qid, increase qwk; **IV BOL** 5-10 mg >2 min, repeat if necessary in 30 min

• *Child 1-15 yr:* **IV BOL** 0.1-0.3 mg/kg >2 min, repeat in 30 min, not to exceed 10 mg in a single dose

Available forms: Tabs 40, 80, 120 mg; sus rel tabs 120, 180, 240 mg; inj 5 mg/ml; sus rel caps 120, 180, 240, 360 mg

Side effects/adverse reactions:

CV: Edema, CHF, bradycardia, hypotension, palpitations, AV block

GI: Nausea, diarrhea, gastric upset, *constipation,* increased liver function studies

GU: Nocturia, polyuria

CNS: Headache, drowsiness, dizziness, anxiety, depression, weakness, insomnia, confusion, light-headedness

*SYST: **Stevens-Johnson syndrome***

Contraindications: Sick sinus syndrome, 2nd- or 3rd-degree heart block, hypotension less than 90 mm Hg systolic, cardiogenic shock, severe CHF

Precautions: CHF, hypotension, hepatic injury, pregnancy (C), lactation, children, renal disease, concomitant β-blocker therapy

Pharmacokinetics:

IV: Onset 3 min, peak 3-5 min, duration 10-20 min

PO: Onset variable, peak 3-4 hr, duration 17-24 hr, half-life (biphasic) 4 min, 3-7 hr (terminal)

Metabolized by liver, excreted in urine (96% as metabolites)

🔷 = Nursing alert   🖋 = Herb-drug interaction   🚫 = Do not crush

Interactions:
• Increased hypotension: prazosin, quinidine
• Increased effects: β-blockers, antihypertensives, cimetidine, digoxin
• Decreased effects of lithium
• Increased levels of digoxin, theophylline, cyclosporine, carbamazepine, nondepolarizing muscle relaxants
• Food/drug: increased hypotensive effects: grapefruit juice
Lab test interferences:
Increase: LFTs
NURSING CONSIDERATIONS
Assess:
• Cardiac status: B/P, pulse, respiration, ECG intervals (PR, QRS, QT)
◆ I&O ratios, weight qd; CHF: rales, weight gain, dyspnea, jugular vein distention
Administer:
• Before meals, hs; sus rel give with food
IV
• Undiluted through Y-tube or 3-way stopcock of compatible sol; give over 2 min, or 3 min elderly
Additive compatibilities: Amikacin, amiodarone, ascorbic acid, atropine, bretylium, calcium chloride, calcium gluconate, cefamandole, cefazolin, cefotaxime, cefoxitin, cephapirin, chloramphenicol, cimetidine, clindamycin, dexamethasone, diazepam, digoxin, dopamine, epinephrine, erythromycin, gentamicin, heparin, hydrocortisone sodium phosphate, hydrocortisone, hydromorphone, insulin (regular), isoproterenol, lidocaine, magnesium sulfate, mannitol, meperidine, metaraminol, methicillin, methyldopa, methylprednisolone, metoclopramide, mezlocillin, morphine, moxalactam, multivitamins, naloxone, nitroglycerin, norepinephrine, oxytocin, pancuronium, penicillin G potassium, penicillin G sodium, pentobarbital, phenobarbital, phentolamine, phenytoin, piperacillin, potassium chloride, potassium phosphates, procainamide, propranolol, protamine, quinidine, sodium bicarbonate, sodium nitroprusside, theophylline, ticarcillin, tobramycin, tolazoline, vancomycin, vasopressin, vit B/C
Syringe compatibilities: Amrinone, heparin, milrinone
Y-site compatibilities: Amrinone, ciprofloxacin, dobutamine, dopamine, famotidine, hydralazine, meperidine, methicillin, milrinone, penicillin G potassium, piperacillin, propofol, ticarcillin
Evaluate:
• Therapeutic response: decreased anginal pain, decreased B/P, dysrhythmias
Teach patient/family:
• To increase fluids/fiber to counteract constipation
• How to take pulse before taking drug; to keep record or graph
• To avoid hazardous activities until stabilized on drug, dizziness no longer a problem
• To limit caffeine consumption; no alcohol products
• To avoid OTC drugs unless directed by prescriber
• To comply with all areas of medical regimen: diet, exercise, stress reduction, drug therapy
• To change positions slowly to prevent syncope
Treatment of overdose: Defibrillation, atropine for AV block, vasopressor for hypotension

verteporfin (℞)

(ver-tee-poor'fin)
Visudyne
Func. class.: Ophthalmic phototherapy

Action: A light-activated drug for photodynamic therapy, using a 2-step process with this drug and nonthermal red light

Uses: Predominantly, classic subfoveal choroidal neovascularization (CNV) related to age-related macular degeneration

Investigational uses: Psoriasis, psoriatic arthritis, rheumatoid arthritis

Dosage and routes:

• Initiate 689 nm wavelength laser light for 83 sec, 15 min after start of the 10 min infusion of verteporfin

Available forms: Lyophilized cake 15 mg

Side effects/adverse reactions:

CV: Hypertension, atrial fibrillation, peripheral vascular disorder, varicose veins

GI: Constipation, GI cancers, *nausea*

EENT: Cataracts, diplopia, dry eyes, ocular itching, severe vision loss

MS: Arthralgia, arthrosis, myesthenia

CNS: Hypesthesia, vertigo, *insomnia*

RESP: Pharyngitis, pneumonia

MISC: Asthenia, back pain, elevated LFTs, photosensitivity

Contraindications: Porphyria, hypersensitivity

Precautions: Elderly, hepatic disease, pregnancy (C), lactation, children

Pharmacokinetics: Half-life 5-6 hr, excreted in feces

Interactions:

• Increased photosensitivity: tetra-

cyclines, sulfonamides, phenothiazines, sulfonylureas, thiazides, griseofulvin

• Decreased action of verteporfin: anticoagulants, antiplatelets

NURSING CONSIDERATIONS

Assess:

• Ocular sensitivity: sensitivity to sun, bright lights, car headlights, patients should wear dark sunglasses with an average light transmittance of <4%

• For extravasation at inj site: take care to protect from light

Administer:

• After reconstitution of each vial with 7 ml sterile water for inj for 2 mg/ml; protect from light and use within 4 hr; solution is dark green

Perform/provide:

• Wiping of spills with damp cloth, avoid skin/eye contact, dispose of material in polyethylene bag according to policy

• Store between 68°-77° F

Teach patient/family:

• To report eye sensitivity

• To wear sunglasses with average white light transmittance of <4% for 5 days after treatment; also to use protective clothing

vinblastine (VLB) (℞)

(vin-blast'een)
Velban, Velbe*, vinblastine sulfate
Func. class.: Antineoplastic
Chem. class.: Vinca rosea alkaloid

Action: Inhibits mitotic activity, arrests cell cycle at metaphase; inhibits RNA synthesis, blocks cellular use of glutamic acid needed for purine synthesis; a vesicant

Uses: Breast, testicular cancer, lymphomas, neuroblastoma; Hodgkin's, non-Hodgkin's lymphomas; mycosis fungoides, histiocytosis, Kaposi's sarcoma

Dosage and routes:
• *Adult:* IV 0.1 mg/kg or 3.7 mg/m² qwk or q2wk, not to exceed 0.5 mg/kg or 18.5 mg/m² qwk
• *Child:* 2.5 mg/m² then 3.75, 5, 6.25, 7.5 at 7-day intervals
Available forms: Inj, pwd 10 mg for 10 ml IV

Side effects/adverse reactions:
*HEMA: **Thrombocytopenia, leukopenia, myelosuppression***
GI: Nausea, vomiting, ileus, *anorexia, stomatitis,* constipation, abdominal pain, **GI, rectal bleeding, hepatotoxicity,** pharyngitis
GU: Urinary retention, ***renal failure***
INTEG: Rash, alopecia, photosensitivity
*RESP: **Fibrosis, pulmonary infiltrate, bronchospasm***
CV: Tachycardia, orthostatic hypotension
CNS: Paresthesias, peripheral neuropathy, depression, headache, ***convulsions***
META: SIADH

Contraindications: Hypersensitivity, infants, pregnancy (D)
Precautions: Renal disease, hepatic disease

Do not confuse:
vinblastine/vincristine

Pharmacokinetics: Half-life (triphasic) 35 min, 53 min, 19 hr; metabolized in liver, excreted in urine, feces; crosses blood-brain barrier
Interactions:
• Increased action of methotrexate
• Do not use with radiation
• Synergism: bleomycin
• Decreased phenytoin level: phenytoin
• Bronchospasm: mitomycin

NURSING CONSIDERATIONS
Assess:
• CBC, differential, platelet count qwk; withhold drug if WBC is

<2000/mm³ or platelet count is <75,000/mm³; notify prescriber
• Pulmonary function tests, chest x-ray studies before, during therapy; chest x-ray film should be obtained q2wk during treatment
• Neurologic status: sensory-vibratory evaluation if side effects occur
• Renal function studies: BUN, serum uric acid, urine CrCl, electrolytes before, during therapy
• I&O ratio; report fall in urine output of 30 ml/hr
• Monitor temp q4h; may indicate beginning infection
• LFTs before, during therapy (bilirubin, AST, ALT, LDH) as needed or qmo
• RBC, Hct, Hgb, since these may be decreased
• Bleeding: hematuria, guaiac, bruising or petechiae, mucosa of orifices q8h
• Dyspnea, rales, unproductive cough, chest pain, tachypnea, fatigue, increased pulse, pallor, lethargy
• Effects of alopecia on body image; discuss feelings about body changes
• Sensitivity of feet/hands, which precedes neuropathy
• Jaundiced skin, sclera; dark urine, clay-colored stools, itchy skin, abdominal pain, fever, diarrhea
• Buccal cavity q8h for dryness, sores or ulceration, white patches, oral pain, bleeding, dysphagia
• Local irritation, pain, burning, discoloration at inj site
• Symptoms indicating severe allergic reaction: rash, pruritus, urticaria, purpuric skin lesions, itching, flushing
• Frequency of stools and characteristics: cramping; acidosis; signs of dehydration: rapid respirations,

V

poor skin turgor, decreased urine output, dry skin, restlessness, weakness

Administer:
• Antiemetic 30-60 min before giving drug and prn to prevent vomiting
• Transfusion for anemia

IV
• After diluting 10 mg/10 ml NaCl; give through Y-tube or 3-way stopcock or directly over 1 min
• Hyaluronidase 150 U/ml in 1 ml NaCl, warm compress for extravasation for vesicant activity treatment

Additive compatibilities: Bleomycin

Syringe compatibilities: Bleomycin, cisplatin, cyclophosphamide, droperidol, fluorouracil, leucovorin, methotrexate, metoclopramide, mitomycin, vincristine

Y-site compatibilities: Allopurinol, amifostine, amphotericin B cholesteryl, aztreonam, bleomycin, cisplatin, cyclophosphamide, doxorubicin, doxorubicin liposome, droperidol, filgrastim, fludarabine, fluorouracil, granisetron, heparin, leucovorin, melphalan, methotrexate, metoclopramide, mitomycin, ondansetron, paclitaxel, piperacillin/tazobactam, sargramostim, teniposide, thiotepa, vincristine, vinorelbine

Perform/provide:
• Deep-breathing exercises with patient 3-4 ×/day; place in semi-Fowler's position
• Liquid diet: cola, Jell-O; dry toast or crackers may be added if patient is not nauseated or vomiting
• Increase fluid intake to 2-3 L/day to prevent urate deposits, calculi formation
• Rinsing of mouth tid-qid with water

• Brushing of teeth bid-tid with soft brush or cotton-tipped applicators for stomatitis; use unwaxed dental floss
• Nutritious diet with iron, vitamin supplements
• HOB raised to facilitate breathing

Evaluate:
• Therapeutic response: decreased tumor size, spread of malignancy

Teach patient/family:
• To report any complaints or side effects to nurse or prescriber
• To report any changes in breathing or coughing
• That hair may be lost during treatment, a wig or hairpiece may make patient feel better; tell patient that new hair may be different in color, texture
• To report change in gait or numbness in extremities; may indicate neuropathy
• To avoid foods with citric acid, hot or rough texture
• To report any bleeding, white spots or ulcerations in mouth to prescriber; to examine mouth qd
• To wear sunscreen, protective clothing, sunglasses

---

vincristine (VCR) (℞)
(vin-kris'teen)
Oncovin, Vincasar PFS, vincristine sulfate
Func. class.: Antineoplastic-misc
Chem. class.: Vinca alkaloid

Action: Inhibits mitotic activity, arrests cell cycle at metaphase; inhibits RNA synthesis, blocks cellular use of glutamic acid needed for purine synthesis; a vesicant
Uses: Breast, lung cancer, lymphomas, neuroblastoma, Hodgkin's disease, acute lymphoblastic and

---

◆ = Nursing alert　　🖋 = Herb-drug interaction　　🚫 = Do not crush

other leukemias, rhabdomyosarcoma, Wilms' tumor, osteogenic and other sarcomas

Dosage and routes:
• *Adult:* **IV** 1-2 mg/m^2/wk, not to exceed 2 mg
• *Child:* **IV** 1.5-2 mg/m^2/wk, not to exceed 2 mg

Available forms: Inj 1 mg/ml; pwd for inj 5 mg/vial

Side effects/adverse reactions:
INTEG: Alopecia
HEMA: ***Thrombocytopenia, leukopenia, myelosuppression, anemia***
GI: Nausea, vomiting, anorexia, stomatitis, constipation, ***paralytic ileus,*** *abdominal pain,* ***hepatotoxicity***
CV: Orthostatic hypotension
CNS: Decreased reflexes, numbness, weakness, motor difficulties, CNS depression, cranial nerve paralysis, ***seizures***

Contraindications: Hypersensitivity, infants, pregnancy (D)
Precautions: Renal disease, hepatic disease, hypertension, neuromuscular disease
Do not confuse:
vincristine/vinblastine
Pharmacokinetics: Half-life (triphasic) 0.85 min, 7.4 min, 164 min; metabolized in liver; excreted in bile, feces; crosses placental barrier, blood-brain barrier

Interactions:
• Increased action of methotrexate, anticoagulants
• Do not use with radiation
• Neurotoxicity: peripheral nervous system drugs
• Decreased digoxin level: digoxin
• Decreased action of vincristine: L-asparaginase
• Acute pulmonary reactions: mitomycin-c

NURSING CONSIDERATIONS
Assess:
• CBC, differential, platelet count qwk; withhold drug if WBC is <4000/mm^3 or platelet count is <75,000/mm^3; notify prescriber
• Renal function studies: BUN, serum uric acid, urine CrCl, electrolytes before, during therapy
• I&O ratio, report fall in urine output of 30 ml/hr
• Monitor temp q4h; may indicate beginning infection
• LFTs before, during therapy (bilirubin, AST, ALT, LDH) as needed or monthly
• RBC, Hct, Hgb; may be decreased
• Deep tendon reflexes; drug is neurotoxic
• Sensitivity of feet/hands, which precedes neuropathy
• Bleeding: hematuria, guaiac, bruising or petechiae, mucosa of orifices q8h
• Effects of alopecia on body image, discuss feelings about body changes
• Jaundiced skin, sclera; dark urine, clay-colored stools, itchy skin, abdominal pain, fever, diarrhea
• Buccal cavity q8h for dryness, sores or ulceration, white patches, oral pain, bleeding, dysphagia
• Symptoms indicating severe allergic reaction: rash, pruritus, urticaria, purpuric skin lesions, itching, flushing
• Frequency of stools, characteristics: cramping, acidosis; signs of dehydration: rapid respirations, poor skin turgor, decreased urine output, dry skin, restlessness, weakness
Administer:
• Agents to prevent constipation
• Antiemetic 30-60 min before giving drug and prn
• Transfusion for anemia
• Antispasmodic for GI symptoms
IV
• After diluting with diluent provided or 1 mg/10 ml of sterile H$_2$O

or NaCl; give through Y-tube or 3-way stopcock or directly over 1 min

Hyaluronidase 150 U/ml in 1 ml NaCl; apply warm compress for extravasation

Additive compatibilities: Bleomycin, cytarabine, fluorouracil, methotrexate

Syringe compatibilities: Bleomycin, cisplatin, cyclophosphamide, doxapram, doxorubicin, droperidol, fluorouracil, heparin, leucovorin, methotrexate, metoclopramide, mitomycin, vinblastine

Y-site compatibilities: Allopurinol, amifostine, amphotericin B cholesteryl, aztreonam, bleomycin, cisplatin, cladribine, cyclophosphamide, doxorubicin, doxorubicin liposome, droperidol, filgrastim, fludarabine, fluorouracil, granisetron, heparin, leucovorin, melphalan, methotrexate, metoclopramide, mitomycin, ondansetron, paclitaxel, piperacillin/tazobactam, sargramostim, teniposide, thiotepa, vinblastine, vinorelbine

Perform/provide:
• Liquid diet: cola, Jell-O; dry toast or crackers may be added if patient is not nauseated or vomiting
• Rinsing of mouth tid-qid with water
• Brushing of teeth bid-tid with soft brush or cotton-tipped applicators for stomatitis; use unwaxed dental floss
• Nutritious diet with iron, vitamin supplements

Evaluate:
• Therapeutic response: decreased tumor size, spread of malignancy

Teach patient/family:
• To report change in gait or numbness in extremities; may indicate neuropathy
• To report any complaints or side effects to nurse or prescriber

• To report any bleeding, white spots or ulcerations in mouth to prescriber; to examine mouth qd
• To increase bulk, fluids, exercise to prevent constipation

---

vinorelbine (℞)

(vi-nor'el-bine)

Navelbine

Func. class.: Antineoplastic-misc

Chem. class.: Semisynthetic vinca alkaloid

Action: Inhibits mitotic activity, arrests cell cycle at metaphase; inhibits RNA synthesis, blocks cellular use of glutamic acid needed for purine synthesis; a vesicant

Uses: Unresectable advanced non-small cell lung cancer (NSCLC) stage IV; may be used alone or in combination with cisplatin for stage III or IV NSCLC breast cancer

Dosage and routes:
• *Adult:* IV 30 mg/m^2 qwk

Hepatic dose
• *Adult:* IV total bilirubin 2.1-3 mg/dl 15 mg/m^2 qwk; total bilirubin ≥3 mg/dl 7.5 mg/m^2 qd

Available forms: Inj 10 mg/ml

Side effects/adverse reactions:

CV: Chest pain

RESP: Shortness of breath

HEMA: **Neutropenia, anemia, thrombocytopenia, granulocytopenia**

GI: Nausea, vomiting, ileus, *anorexia, stomatitis,* constipation, abdominal pain, diarrhea, *hepatotoxicity*

INTEG: Rash, alopecia, photosensitivity

CNS: Paresthesias, peripheral neuropathy, depression, headache, *convulsions,* weakness, jaw pain

---

META: SIADH

MS: Myalgia

Contraindications: Hypersensitivity, infants, pregnancy (D), granulocyte count <1000 cells/mm³ pretreatment

Precautions: Renal, hepatic disease, elderly, lactation, children

Pharmacokinetics: Half-life 27-43 hr, peak 1-2 hr

Interactions:

• Possible increased toxicity: fluorouracil

NURSING CONSIDERATIONS

Assess:

• B/P (baseline and q15min) during administration

• CBC, differential, platelet count weekly; withhold drug if WBC is <4000/mm³ or platelet count is <75,000/mm³; notify prescriber of results, recovery will take 3 wk

• For dyspnea, rales, unproductive cough, chest pain, tachypnea

• Renal function studies: BUN, serum uric acid, urine CrCl before, during therapy; I&O ratio; report fall in urine output to <30 ml/hr; for decreased hyperuricemia

• For cold, fever, sore throat (may indicate beginning infection); notify prescriber if these occur

• For bleeding: hematuria, guaiac, bruising or petechiae, mucosa or orifices q8h, no rectal temps; avoid IM injections; use pressure to venipuncture sites

• Nutritional status: an antiemetic may be needed

◆ For symptoms of severe allergic reactions: rash, pruritus, urticaria, itching, flushing, bronchospasm, hypotension, epinephrine and crash cart should be nearby

Administer:

• Antiemetic 30-60 min before giving drug and prn to prevent vomiting

IV

• Hyaluronidase 150 U/ml in 1 ml NaCl, warm compress for extravasation for vesicant activity treatment

• By cont inf: 40 mg/m² q3wk after an IV bol of 8 mg/m²; may be given in combination with doxorubicin, fluorouracil, cisplatin

Y-site compatibilities: Amikacin, aztreonam, bleomycin, bumetanide, buprenorphine, butorphanol, calcium gluconate, carboplatin, carmustine, cefotaxime, ceftazidime, ceftizoxime, chlorpromazine, cimetidine, cisplatin, clindamycin, cyclophosphamide, cytarabine, dacarbazine, dactinomycin, daunorubicin, dexamethasone, diphenhydramine, doxorubicin, doxorubicin liposome, doxycycline, droperidol, enalaprilat, etoposide, famotidine, filgrastim, floxuridine, fluconazole, fludarabine, gallium, gentamicin, granisetron, haloperidol, heparin, hydrocortisone, hydromorphone, hydroxyzine, idarubicin, ifosfamide, imipenem-cilastatin, lorazepam, mannitol, mechlorethamine, melphalan, meperidine, mesna, methotrexate, metoclopramide, metronidazole, minocycline, mitoxantrone, morphine, nalbuphine, netilmicin, ondansetron, plicamycin, streptozocin, teniposide, ticarcillin, ticarcillin/clavulanate, tobramycin, vancomycin, vinblastine, vincristine, zidovudine

Perform/provide:

• Liquid diet: cola, Jell-O; dry toast or crackers if patient not nauseated or vomiting

• Brushing of teeth bid-tid with soft brush or cotton-tipped applicators for stomatitis; unwaxed dental floss

• Nutritious diet with iron, vitamin supplements

V

Evaluate:
• Therapeutic response: decreased tumor size, spread of malignancy
Teach patient/family:
• To report change in gait or numbness in extremities; may indicate neuropathy
• To report any complaints or side effects to nurse or prescriber
• To examine mouth qd for bleeding, white spots, ulcerations; notify prescriber
• To avoid crowds, people with infections, vaccinations

---

vitamin A (℞, ᴏᴛᴄ)
Aquasol A, Del-Vi-A, Vitamin A
Func. class.: Vitamin, fat soluble
Chem. class.: Retinol

Action: Needed for normal bone, tooth development, visual dark adaptation, skin disease, mucosa tissue repair, assists in production of adrenal steroids, cholesterol, RNA
Uses: Vit A deficiency
Dosage and routes:
• *Adult and child >8 yr:* **PO** 100,000-500,000 IU qd × 3 days, then 50,000 qd × 2 wk; dose based on severity of deficiency; maintenance 10,000-20,000 IU for 2 mo
• *Child 1-8 yr:* **IM** 5000-15,000 IU qd × 10 days
• *Infant <1 yr:* **IM** 5000-15,000 IU × 10 days
Maintenance
• *Child 4-8 yr:* **IM** 15,000 IU qd × 2 mo
• *Child <4 yr:* **IM** 10,000 IU qd × 2 mo
Available forms: Caps 10,000, 25,000, 50,000 IU; drops 5000 IU; inj 50,000 IU/ml; tabs 10,000, 25,000, 50,000 IU

Side effects/adverse reactions:
GI: Nausea, vomiting, anorexia, abdominal pain, ***jaundice***
CNS: Headache, ***increased intracranial pressure, intracranial hypertension,*** lethargy, malaise
EENT: Gingivitis, papilledema, exophthalmos, inflammation of tongue and lips
INTEG: Drying of skin, pruritus, increased pigmentation, night sweats, alopecia
MS: Arthralgia, retarded growth, hard areas on bone
META: Hypomenorrhea, hypercalcemia
Contraindications: Hypersensitivity to vit A, malabsorption syndrome (PO)
Precautions: Lactation, impaired renal function, pregnancy (C)
Pharmacokinetics: Stored in liver, kidneys, fat; excreted (metabolites) in urine, feces
Interactions:
• Decreased absorption of vit A: mineral oil, cholestyramine, colestipol
• Increased levels of vit A: corticosteroids, oral contraceptives
• Do not administer IV because of risk of anaphylactic shock
Lab test interferences:
False increase: Bilirubin, serum cholesterol
NURSING CONSIDERATIONS
Assess:
• Nutritional status: yellow and dark green vegetables, yellow/orange fruits, vit A–fortified foods, liver, egg yolks
• Vit A deficiency: decreased growth, night blindness, dry, brittle nails; hair loss; urinary stones; increased infection, hyperkeratosis of skin; drying of cornea

---

◆ = Nursing alert   🌿 = Herb-drug interaction   ⃠ = Do not crush

Administer:
PO
• With food (PO) for better absorption

Perform/provide:
• Storage in tight, light-resistant container

Evaluate:
• Therapeutic response: increased growth rate, weight; absence of dry skin and mucous membranes, night blindness

Teach patient/family:
• That if dose is missed, it should be omitted
• That ophthalmic exams may be required periodically throughout therapy
• Not to use mineral oil while taking this drug
• To notify prescriber of nausea, vomiting, lip cracking, loss of hair, headache
• Not to take more than the prescribed amount

Treatment of overdose: Discontinue drug

---

vitamin D (chole-calciferol, vitamin D₃ or ergocalciferol, vitamin D₂) (℞, OTC)
Calciferol, Delta-D, Drisdol, Radiostol*, Radiostol Forte*, Vitamin D, Vitamin D₃
Func. class.: Vit D
Chem. class.: Fat soluble

Action: Needed for regulation of calcium, phosphate levels, normal bone development, parathyroid activity, neuromuscular functioning
Uses: Vit D deficiency, rickets, renal osteodystrophy, hypoparathyroidism, hypophosphatemia, psoriasis, rheumatoid arthritis

Dosage and routes:
Deficiency
• *Adult:* **PO/IM** 12,000 IU qd, then increased to 500,000 IU/day
• *Child:* **PO/IM** 1500-5000 IU qd × 2-4 wk, may repeat after 2 wk or 600,000 IU as single dose
Hypoparathyroidism
• *Adult and child:* **PO/IM** 200,000 IU given with 4 g Ca tab
Available forms: Tabs 400, 1000, 50,000 IU; caps 25,000, 50,000 IU; liq 8000 IU/ml; inj 500,000 IU/ml, 500,000 IU/5 ml

Side effects/adverse reactions:
GI: Nausea, vomiting, anorexia, cramps, diarrhea, constipation, metallic taste, dry mouth
CNS: Fatigue, weakness, drowsiness, **convulsions,** headache, psychosis
GU: Polyuria, nocturia, **hematuria, albuminuria, renal failure,** decreased libido
CV: Hypertension, dysrhythmias
MS: Decreased bone growth, early joint pain, early muscle pain
INTEG: Pruritus, photophobia

Contraindications: Hypersensitivity, hypercalcemia, renal dysfunction, hyperphosphatemia
Precautions: Cardiovascular disease, renal calculi, pregnancy (C)
Do not confuse:
Calciferol/calcitriol
Pharmacokinetics: Half-life 7-12 hr; stored in liver, duration 2 mo; excreted in bile (metabolites) and urine
Interactions:
• Decreased effects of vit D: cholestyramine, colestipol, phenobarbital, phenytoin
• Increased toxicity: diuretics (thiazides), antacids, verapamil

NURSING CONSIDERATIONS
Assess:
• Vit D levels q2wk during treatment

V

- Ca, PO$_4$, Mg, BUN, alk phosphatase, urine Ca, creatinine
- In children, monitor height and weight
- Nutritional status: egg yolk, fortified dairy products, cod, halibut, salmon, sardines

Administer:
- IM inj deep in large muscle mass; administer slowly; aspirate carefully; rotate inj sites; avoid IV administration

Evaluate:
- Therapeutic response: absence of rickets/osteomalacia, adequate Ca/phosphate levels, decrease in bone pain

Teach patient/family:
- That if dose is missed, to omit
- The necessary foods in diet
- To avoid vitamin supplements unless directed by prescriber
- To keep appointments with health care providers; line between therapeutic and toxic doses is narrow
- To report weakness, lethargy, headache, anorexia, loss of weight
- To report nausea, vomiting, abdominal cramps, diarrhea, constipation, excessive thirst, polyuria, muscle and bone pain
- To decrease intake of antacids and laxatives containing Mg

---

vitamin E (OTC)

Amino-Opti-E, Aquasol E, Daltose*, E-Complex-600, E-Ferol, E-Vitamin Succinate, E-200 I.U. Softgels, Gordo-Vite E, Tocopherol, Vitamin E, Vita-Plus E Softgells, Vitec

Func. class.: Vit E
Chem. class.: Fat soluble

Action: Needed for digestion and metabolism of polyunsaturated fats, decreases platelet aggregation, decreases blood clot formation, promotes normal growth and development of muscle tissue, prostaglandin synthesis

Uses: Vit E deficiency, impaired fat absorption, hemolytic anemia in premature neonates, prevention of retrolental fibroplasia, sickle cell anemia, supplement in malabsorption syndrome

Dosage and routes:
Deficiency
- *Adult:* **PO** 60-75 IU qd
- *Child:* **PO** 1 mg/0.6 g of dietary fat

Prevention of deficiency
- *Adult:* **PO** 30 IU/day; **TOP** apply to affected areas
- *Infants:* **PO** 5 IU/day

Available forms: Caps 100, 200, 400, 500, 600, 1000 IU; tabs 100, 200, 400 IU; drops 50 mg/ml; chew tabs 400 U; ointment, cream, lotion, oil

Side effects/adverse reactions:
META: Altered metabolism of hormones: thyroid, pituitary, adrenal; altered immunity
MS: Weakness
CNS: Headache, fatigue
GI: Nausea, cramps, diarrhea
GU: Gonadal dysfunction
CV: Increased risk of thrombophlebitis
EENT: Blurred vision
INTEG: Sterile abscess, contact dermatitis

Contraindications: None significant

Precautions: Pregnancy (A)

Pharmacokinetics:
PO: Metabolized in liver, excreted in bile

Interactions:
- Increased action of oral anticoagulants
- Decreased absorption: cholestyramine, colestipol, mineral oil, sucralfate

---

 = Nursing alert   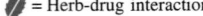 = Herb-drug interaction   ⊘ = Do not crush

NURSING CONSIDERATIONS
Assess:
- Vit E levels during treatment
- Nutritional status: wheat germ, dark green leafy vegetables, nuts, eggs, liver, vegetable oils, dairy products, cereals

Administer:
PO
- Administer with or after meals
- *Chewable tabs:* Chew well
- *Sol:* May be dropped in mouth or mixed with food

TOP
- To moisturize dry skin

Perform/provide:
- Storage in tight, light-resistant container

Evaluate:
- Therapeutic response: absence of hemolytic anemia, adequate vit E levels, improvement in skin lesions, decreased edema

Teach patient/family:
- The necessary foods in diet
- To omit if dose is missed
- To avoid vitamin supplements unless directed by prescriber

---

warfarin (℞)
(war′far-in)
Coumadin, warfarin sodium, Warfilone*

Func. class.: Anticoagulant

Action: Interferes with blood clotting by indirect means; depresses hepatic synthesis of vit K–dependent coagulation factors (II, VII, IX, X)

Uses: Pulmonary emboli, deep-vein thrombosis, MI, atrial dysrhythmias, postcardiac valve replacement

Research note: Nevirapine given with warfarin resulted in decreased warfarin action[40]

Dosage and routes:
- *Adult:* **PO/IV** 2.5-10 mg/day × 3 days, then titrated to prothrombin time or INR qd
- *Geriatric:* **PO/IV** 2-10 mg/day
- *Child:* 0.1 mg/kg/day titrated to INR

Available forms: Tabs 1, 2, 2.5, 5, 6, 7.5, 10 mg; inj 50 mg/2 ml

Side effects/adverse reactions:
GI: Diarrhea, nausea, vomiting, anorexia, stomatitis, cramps, ***hepatitis***
GU: ***Hematuria***
INTEG: Rash, dermatitis, urticaria, alopecia, pruritus
CNS: Fever
HEMA: ***Hemorrhage, agranulocytosis, leukopenia, eosinophilia***

Contraindications: Hypersensitivity, hemophilia, leukemia with bleeding, peptic ulcer disease, thrombocytopenic purpura, hepatic disease (severe), severe hypertension, subacute bacterial endocarditis, acute nephritis, blood dyscrasias, pregnancy (X), eclampsia, preeclampsia, lactation

Precautions: Alcoholism, elderly

Do not confuse:
Coumadin/Cardura
Coumadin/Compazine

Pharmacokinetics:
PO: Onset 12-24 hr, peak 1½-3 days, duration 3-5 days, half-life 1½-2½ days; metabolized in liver, excreted in urine/feces (active/inactive metabolites), crosses placenta, 99% bound to plasma proteins

Interactions:
- Increased action of warfarin: allopurinol, chloramphenicol, amiodarone, diflunisal, heparin, steroids, cimetidine, disulfiram, thyroid, glucagon, metronidazole, quinidine, sulindac, sulfinpyrazone, sulfonamides, clofibrate, salicylates, ethacrynic acids, indomethacin, mefenamic acid, oxyphenbutazones, phenylbutazone, cefamandole, chloral hydrate, cotrimoxazole, erythro-

---

w

mycin, quinolone antiinfectives, isoniazid, thrombolytic agents, tricyclics

Decreased action of warfarin: barbiturates, griseofulvin, ethchlorvynol, carbamazepine, rifampin, oral contraceptives, phenytoin, estrogens, vit K, cholestyramine, corticosteroids, mercaptopurine, sucralfate, vit K foods, vit supplements

Increased toxicity: oral sulfonylureas, phenytoin

Drug/food: grapefruit juice: may increase action of oral warfarin

🌿 Increased risk of bleeding: bromelain, cinchona, cayenne, feverfew, garlic, dan shen, ginkgo biloba, quinine, ginger, horse chestnut, papain, sweet clover, sweet vernal grass leaves, tonka bean seeds, vanilla leaf, woodruff

🌿 Decreased anticoagulation: ginseng, alfalfa, beet root/greens, broccoli flower buds, brussel sprout buds, cabbage leaves, Chinese cabbage leaves, collard leaves, corn silk, stigmas, kale, lettuce, parsley, plantain, shepherd's purse, smart weed plant, spinach, stinging nettle, turnip leaves, watercress

🌿 Increased metabolism of warfarin: crucifer

Lab test interferences:
Increase: T_3 uptake
Decrease: Uric acid

NURSING CONSIDERATIONS
Assess:
• Blood studies (Hct, platelets, occult blood in stools) q3mo
• Prothrombin time, which should be 1½-2 × control; PT often done qd initially or INR
• Bleeding gums, petechiae, ecchymosis, black tarry stools, hematuria
◆ Fever, skin rash, urticaria
• Needed dosage change q1-2wk; when stable, PT q3wk

Administer:
• At same time each day to maintain steady blood levels
• Tabs whole or crushed
• Avoiding all IM injections that may cause bleeding
IV
• After diluting with diluent provided (50 mg/2 ml); rotate vial, give through Y-tube or 3-way stopcock at [dH]25 mg/min
Y-site compatibilities: Amikacin, ascorbic acid, cefazolin, ceftriaxone, cephapirin, dopamine, epinephrine, heparin, lidocaine, metaraminol, morphine, nitroglycerin, oxytocin, potassium chloride, ranitidine
Perform/provide:
• Storage in tight container
Evaluate:
• Therapeutic response: decrease of deep-vein thrombosis
Teach patient/family:
• To avoid OTC preparations that may cause serious drug interactions unless directed by prescriber
• To use soft-bristle toothbrush to avoid bleeding gums, and to use electric razor
• To carry a Medic Alert ID identifying drug taken
• The importance of compliance
• To report any signs of bleeding: gums, under skin, urine, stools
• To avoid hazardous activities (football, hockey, skiing), dangerous work
• The importance of avoiding unusual changes in vitamin intake, diet or lifestyle
• To inform dentists and other physicians of anticoagulant intake
• That smoking increases dose requirements
• To limit foods high in vit K
Treatment of overdose: Administer vit K

◆ = Nursing alert   🌿 = Herb-drug interaction   🚫 = Do not crush

zafirlukast (℞)

(za-feer'loo-cast)
Accolate
Func. class.: Bronchodilator
Chem class: Leukotriene receptor antagonist

Action: Antagonizes the contractile action of leukotrienes (LTC_4, LTD_4, LTE_4) in airway smooth muscle; inhibits bronchoconstriction caused by antigens

Uses: Prophylaxis and chronic treatment of asthma in adults/children >12 yr

Dosage and routes:
• *Adult:* **PO** 20 mg bid, take 1 hr ac or 2 hr pc
Available forms: Tabs 20 mg
Contraindications: Hypersensitivity
Precautions: Pregnancy (B), elderly, lactation, children, hepatic disease
Interactions:
• Increased plasma levels of zafirlukast: aspirin
• Decreased plasma levels of zafirlukast: erythromycin, terfenadine, theophylline
• Increased PT: warfarin
• Drug/food: decreased bioavailability
Side effects/adverse reactions:
CNS: Headache, dizziness
GI: Nausea, diarrhea, abdominal pain, vomiting
OTHER: Infections, pain, asthenia, myalgia, fever, dyspepsia, increased ALT
Pharmacokinetics: Unknown
NURSING CONSIDERATIONS
Assess:
◆Adult patients carefully for symptoms of Churg-Strauss syndrome (rare), including eosinophilia, vasculitic rash, worsening pulmonary symptoms, cardiac complications, and/or neuropathy
• Respiratory rate, rhythm, depth; auscultate lung fields bilaterally; notify prescriber of abnormalities
Administer:
• PO after meals for GI symptoms; absorption may be affected
Evaluate:
• Therapeutic response: ability to breathe more easily
Teach patient/family:
• To check OTC medications, current prescription medications, which will increase stimulation
• To avoid hazardous activities; dizziness may occur
• That if GI upset occurs, to take drug with 8 oz water; avoid food if possible, absorption may be decreased
• To notify prescriber of nausea, vomiting, diarrhea, abdominal pain

zalcitabine (℞)

(zal-sit'a-bin)
ddC, dideoxycytidine, HIVID
Func. class.: Antiretroviral
Chem. class.: Synthetic pyrimidine nucleoside analog of 2'-deoxycytidine

Action: Inhibits HIV replication by the conversion of this drug by cellular enzymes to an active antiviral metabolite
Uses: Advanced HIV infections in combination in adults, children >13 yr who cannot use zidovudine or who do not respond to treatment
Dosage and routes:
• *Adult:* **PO** combined with other antiretrovirals in advanced HIV infection: 0.75 mg concomitantly with other antiretrovirals dosage reduction not necessary for patients weighing >30 kg; in presence of periph-

eral neuropathy initiate dose at 0.375 mg q8h of zalcitabine

Renal dose
• *Adult:* **PO** CrCl 10-40 ml/min 0.75 mg q12h; CrCl <10 ml/min 0.75 mg q24h

Available forms: Tabs 0.375, 0.75 mg

Side effects/adverse reactions:

GI: **Pancreatitis**, *diarrhea, nausea, vomiting,* abdominal pain, constipation, stomatitis, dysplasia, liver abnormalities, *oral ulcers,* flatulence, taste perversion, dry mouth, oral thrush, melena, *increased ALT, AST, alk phosphatase, amylase*

GU: Uric acid, **toxic nephropathy,** polyuria

CNS: Headache, peripheral neuropathy, seizures, confusion, anxiety, hypertonia, abnormal thinking, asthenia, insomnia, CNS depression, pain, *dizziness,* chills, *fever*

RESP: Cough, pneumonia, dyspnea, asthma, hypoventilation

ENDO: Hypoglycemia, hyponatremia, hyperbilirubinemia, hyperglycemia

INTEG: Rash, pruritus, alopecia, sweating, acne

MS: Myalgia, arthritis, myopathy, muscular atrophy

CV: Hypertension, vasodilation, dysrhythmia, syncope, palpitation, tachycardia

EENT: Ear pain, otitis, photophobia, visual impairment

HEMA: **Leukopenia, granulocytopenia, thrombocytopenia,** anemia

SYST: **Lactic acidosis**

Contraindications: Hypersensitivity

Precautions: Renal, hepatic disease, pregnancy (C), lactation, child <13 yr, peripheral neuropathy, heart failure

Pharmacokinetics:

PO: Elimination half-life 1.62 hr; administration within 5 min of food will decrease absorption; elimination via kidneys

Interactions:
• Increased risk of pancreatitis with agents that can cause pancreatitis
• Increased risk of peripheral neuropathy with other agents that can cause peripheral neuropathy: aminoglycosides, amphotericin B, chloramphenicol, cimetidine, cisplatin, dapsone, disulfiram, ethionamide, foscarnet, glutethimide, gold, hydralazine, iodoquinol, isoniazid, metronidazole, nitrofurantoin, phenytoin, probenecid, ribavirin, vincristine, other nucleoside analogs
• Decreased absorption: ketoconazole, dapsone, food, antacids, metoclopramide

NURSING CONSIDERATIONS
Assess:
• Neuropathy: tingling or pain in hands and feet, distal numbness
◆ Pancreatitis: abdominal pain, nausea, vomiting, elevated liver enzymes; drug should be discontinued, since condition can be fatal
◆ For lactic acidosis, severe hepatomegaly with steatosis that can be fatal, drug should be discontinued
• Children by dilated retinal exam q6mo to rule out retinal depigmentation
• Viral load CD4 baseline and throughout treatment
• CBC, differential, platelet count qwk; withhold drug if WBC is <4000/mm^3 or platelet count is <75,000/mm^3; notify prescriber
• Renal function studies: BUN, serum uric acid, urine CrCl before, during therapy
• Temp q4h; may indicate beginning infection
• LFTs before, during therapy (bilirubin, AST, ALT), triglycerides, amylase prn or qmo

---

◆ = Nursing alert   🖉 = Herb-drug interaction   Ⓢ = Do not crush

Perform/provide:
• Strict medical asepsis, protective isolation if WBC levels are low
Evaluate:
• Therapeutic response: absence of infection; symptoms of HIV
Teach patient/family:
• To report signs of infection: fever, sore throat, flulike symptoms
• To report signs of anemia: fatigue, headache, faintness, shortness of breath, irritability
• To report bleeding; avoid use of razors, commercial mouthwash
• That hair may be lost during therapy; a wig or hairpiece may make patient feel better

---

zaleplon (℞)

(zal'eh-plon)
Sonata
Func. class.: Sedative/hypnotic, antianxiety
Chem. class.: Pyrazolopyrimidine

Action: Binds selectively to omega-1 receptor of the GABA$_A$ receptor complex; results are sedation, hypnosis, skeletal muscle relaxation, anticonvulsant activity, anxiolytic action
Uses: Insomnia
Dosage and routes:
• *Adult:* PO 10 mg hs; may increase dose to 20 mg hs if needed; 5 mg may be used in low weight persons
Available forms: Caps 5, 10 mg
Side effects/adverse reactions:
CNS: Lethargy, drowsiness, daytime sedation, dizziness, confusion, anxiety, amnesia, depersonalization, hallucinations, hypesthesia, paresthesia, somnolence, tremor, vertigo
GI: Nausea, abdominal pain, constipation, anorexia, colitis, dyspepsia, dry mouth
EENT: Vision change, ear/eye pain, hyperacusis, parosmia
MISC: Asthenia, fever, headache, myalgia, dysmenorrhea
Contraindications: Hypersensitivity
Precautions: Hepatic disease, renal disease, elderly, psychosis, child <15 yr, pregnancy (C), lactation
Pharmacokinetics:
PO: Rapid onset, metabolized by liver extensively; excreted by kidneys (inactive metabolites); half-life 1 hr
Interactions:
• Increased effects of zaleplon: cimetidine
• Decreased effect of zaleplon: rifampin
• Food: prolonged absorption, sleep onset reduced: high-fat/heavy meal
NURSING CONSIDERATIONS
Assess:
• Mental status: mood, sensorium, affect, memory (long, short)
• Type of sleep problem: falling asleep, staying asleep
Administer:
• After removal of cigarettes to prevent fires
• After trying conservative measures for insomnia
• Immediately before hs for sleeplessness
• On empty stomach for fast onset
Perform/provide:
• Assistance with ambulation after receiving dose
• Safety measure: nightlight, call bell within easy reach
• Checking to see if PO medication has been swallowed
• Storage in tight container in cool environment
Evaluate:
• Therapeutic response: ability to

z

---

* = Canada only   Side effects: *italics* = common; ***bold italics*** = life-threatening

sleep at night, decreased amount of early morning awakening

Teach patient/family:
• To avoid driving or other activities requiring alertness until drug is stabilized
• To avoid alcohol ingestion or CNS depressants
• Alternative measures to improve sleep: reading, exercise several hr before hs, warm bath, warm milk, TV, self-hypnosis, deep breathing
• That drug may cause memory problems, dependence (if used for longer periods of time), changes in behavior/thinking
• That drug is for short-term use only
• To take immediately before going to bed
• Not to ingest a high-fat/heavy meal before taking

---

zanamivir (℞)

(zan'ah-mih-veer)
Relenza
Func. class.: Antiviral
Chem. class.: Neuramidase inhibitor

Action: Inhibits the enzyme needed for influenza virus replication

Uses: Treatment of influenza type A for those that have been symptomatic for no more than 2 days

Dosage and routes:
• *Adult and child >12 yr:* **INH** 2 inhalations (two 5 mg blisters) q12h × 5 days, on the 1st day 2 doses should be taken at least 2 hr between doses

Available forms: Blisters of powder for inhalation: 5 mg

Side effects/adverse reactions:
CNS: Headache, dizziness, fatigue
EENT: Ear, nose, throat infections
GI: Nausea, vomiting, diarrhea

RESP: Nasal symptoms, cough, sinusitis, bronchitis

Contraindications: Hypersensitivity

Precautions: Lactation, children <12 yr, respiratory disease, elderly, pregnancy (B)

Pharmacokinetics: Half-life 2½-5 hr, not metabolized, excreted in urine unchanged

Interactions:
• None known

NURSING CONSIDERATIONS

Assess:
• Bowel pattern before, during treatment
• Skin eruptions, photosensitivity after administration of drug
• Respiratory status: rate, character, wheezing, tightness in chest
• Allergies before initiation of treatment, reaction of each medication
• Signs of infection

Administer:
• Within 2 days of symptoms of influenza; continue for 5 days
• Give patient "Patient's Instruction for Use" and review all points before using delivery system

Perform/provide:
• Storage in tight, dry container

Evaluate:
• Therapeutic response: absence of fever, malaise, cough, dyspnea in infection

Teach patient/family:
• That this drug does not reduce transmission risk of influenza to others
• Patients with asthma or COPD to carry a fast-acting inhaled bronchodilator since bronchospasm may occur; to use scheduled inhaled bronchodilators before using this drug
• To avoid hazardous activities if dizziness occurs
• To take drug exactly as prescribed

◆ = Nursing alert   ✒ = Herb-drug interaction   ⊘ = Do not crush

zidovudine (R)

(zye-doe'-vue-deen)
Apo-Zidovudine*, Azidothymidine, AZT, Novo-AZT*, Retrovir

Func. class.: Antiviral
Chem. class.: Thymidine analog

Action: Inhibits replication of HIV virus by incorporating into cellular DNA by viral reverse transcriptase, thereby terminating the cellular DNA chain

Uses: Symptomatic/asymptomatic HIV infections (AIDS, ARC), confirmed *Pneumocystis carinii* pneumonia, absolute CD4 lymphocytes of <200/mm³, prevention of maternal-fetal HIV transmission

Dosage and routes:
• *Adult:* **PO** 200 mg q4h; may have to stop treatment if severe bone marrow depression occurs, and restart after bone marrow recovery; **IV** 1-2 mg/kg q4h, initiate **PO** as soon as possible
• *Child:* **PO** 90-180 mg/m²/dose q6h; **IV** same as adult
• *Neonates:* **PO** 2-3 mg/kg/dose q6h; **IV** same as adult

Prevention of maternal-fetal HIV transmission
• *Neonatal:* **PO** 2 mg/kg/dose q6h × 6 wk beginning 8-12 hr after birth; **IV** 1.5 mg/kg/dose over 30 min q6h until able to take **PO**
• *Maternal (>14 wk gestation):* **PO** 100 mg 5×/day until start of labor, then **IV** 2 mg/kg over 1 hr followed by **IV INF** 1 mg/kg/hr until umbilical cord clamped

Asymptomatic HIV infection
• *Adult:* **PO** 100 mg q4h while awake (5×/day)
• *Child 3 mo to 12 yr:* **PO** 90-180 mg/m² q6h (max 200 mg q6h); **IV** 1-2 mg/kg over 1 hr q4h

Symptomatic HIV infection
• *Adult:* **PO** 100 mg q4h; **IV** 1-2 mg/kg over 1 hr q4h
• *Child 3 mo to 12 yr:* **PO** 90-180 mg/m² q6h (max 200 mg q6h); **IV** 1-2 mg/kg over 1 hr q4h

Prevention of HIV following needlestick
• *Adult:* **PO** 200 mg tid plus lamivudine 150 mg bid, plus a protease inhibitor for high-risk exposure; begin within 2 hr of exposure

Available forms: Caps 100, 300 mg; inj 200 mg/20 ml; oral syr 50 mg/5 ml

Side effects/adverse reactions:
*HEMA: **Granulocytopenia, anemia***
CNS: Fever, headache, malaise, diaphoresis, *dizziness, insomnia,* paresthesia, somnolence, chills, tremor, twitching, anxiety, confusion, depression, lability, vertigo, loss of mental acuity
GI: Nausea, vomiting, diarrhea, anorexia, cramps, *dyspepsia,* constipation, dysphagia, *flatulence,* rectal bleeding, mouth ulcer
RESP: Dyspnea
EENT: Taste change, hearing loss, photophobia
INTEG: Rash, acne, pruritus, urticaria
MS: Myalgia, arthralgia, muscle spasm
GU: Dysuria, polyuria, urinary frequency, hesitancy

Contraindications: Hypersensitivity

Precautions: Granulocyte count <1000/mm³ or Hgb <9.5 g/dl, pregnancy (C), lactation, child, severe renal disease, impaired hepatic disease

Pharmacokinetics:
PO: Rapidly absorbed from GI tract, peak ½-1½ hr, metabolized in liver (inactive metabolites), excreted by kidneys

Z

Interactions:

• Toxicity: amphotericin B, dapsone, flucytosine, adriamycin, interferon, vincristine, vinblastine, pentamidine, probenecid, experimental nucleoside analogs, benzodiazepines, cimetidine, morphine, sulfonamides, acyclovir, ganciclovir, doxorubicin, acetaminophen, indomethacin, fluconazole, phenytoin, trimethoprim

• Granulocytopenia: acetaminophen, aspirin, indomethacin

NURSING CONSIDERATIONS
Assess:

• Blood counts q2wk; watch for decreasing granulocytes, Hgb; if low, therapy may have to be discontinued and restarted after hematologic recovery; blood transfusions may be required; viral load, CD4 counts baseline and throughout

Administer:

• By mouth; capsules should be swallowed whole

• Trimethoprim-sulfamethoxazole, pyrimethamine, or acyclovir as ordered to prevent opportunistic infections; if these drugs are given, watch for neurotoxicity

IV

• After diluting each 1 mg/0.25 ml or more D_5W to 4 mg/ml or less; give over 1 hr

Y-site compatibilities: Acyclovir, allopurinol, amifostine, amikacin, amphotericin B, amphotericin B cholesteryl, aztreonam, cefepime, ceftazidime, ceftriaxone, cimetidine, cisatracurium, clindamycin, dexamethasone, dobutamine, dopamine, doxorubicin liposome, erythromycin, filgrastim, fluconazole, fludarabine, gentamicin, granisetron, heparin, imipenem/cilastatin, lorazepam, melphalan, metoclopramide, morphine, nafcillin, ondansetron, oxacillin, paclitaxel, pentamidine, phenylephrine, piperacillin, piperacillin/tazobactam, potassium chloride, ranitidine, remifentanil, sargramostim, teniposide, thiotepa, tobramycin, trimethoprim-sulfamethoxazole, trimetrexate, vancomycin, vinorelbine

Perform/provide;

• Storage in cool environment; protect from light

Evaluate:

• Blood dyscrasias (anemia, granulocytopenia): bruising, fatigue, bleeding, poor healing

Teach patient/family:

• That GI complaints and insomnia resolve after 3-4 wk of treatment

• That drug is not cure for AIDS but will control symptoms

• To notify prescriber of sore throat, swollen lymph nodes, malaise, fever; other infections may occur

• That patient is still infective, may pass AIDS virus on to others

• That follow-up visits must be continued since serious toxicity may occur; blood counts must be done q2wk

• That drug must be taken q4h around clock, even during night; to take 30 min ac or pc

• That serious drug interactions may occur if OTC products are ingested; check with prescriber before taking aspirin, acetaminophen, indomethacin

• That other drugs may be necessary to prevent other infections

• That drug may cause fainting or dizziness

◆ = Nursing alert   ∥ = Herb-drug interaction   ⊘ = Do not crush

zileuton (℞)

(zye′loo-tahn)
Zyflo
Func. class.: Bronchodilator, leukotriene pathway inhibitor
Chem. class.: 5-Lipoxygenase inhibitor

Action: Inhibits leukotriene (LT) formation; leukotrienes exert their effects by increasing neutrophil, eosinophil migration; aggregation of neutrophils, monocytes; smooth muscle contraction, capillary permeability; these actions further lead to bronchoconstriction, inflammation, edema

Uses: Allergic rhinitis, asthma

Investigational uses: Ulcerative colitis, rheumatoid arthritis

Dosage and routes:

Asthma
• *Adult and child:* 12 yr: **PO** 600 mg qid, may be given with meal and hs

Ulcerative colitis
• *Adult:* **PO** 600 mg bid

Available forms: Tabs 600 mg

Side effects/adverse reactions:

CNS: Dizziness, insomnia, fatigue, paresthesias, headache

GI: Nausea, abdominal pain, dyspepsia, diarrhea, LFT abnormalities

INTEG: Hives

MS: Myalgia, asthenia

Contraindications: Hepatic disease, elevations in LFTs 3× upper limits, hypersensitivity

Precautions: Acute attacks of asthma, alcohol consumption, pregnancy (C)

Pharmacokinetics:

PO: Rapidly absorbed, peak 1-3 hr, half-life 2.1-2.5 hr, protein binding 93% (albumin); metabolized by liver, excretion in urine

Interactions:
• Increased action of zileuton: theophylline, propranolol
• May increase effects of anticoagulants

NURSING CONSIDERATIONS

Assess:
• CBC, blood chemistry during treatment
• LFTs before and qmo × 3 mo, then q2-3mo during treatment
• Respiratory rate, rhythm, depth; auscultate lung fields bilaterally; notify prescriber of abnormalities
• Allergic reactions: rash, urticaria; drug should be discontinued

Administer:

PO
• After meals for GI symptoms; absorption may be affected

Evaluate:
• Therapeutic response: ability to breathe more easily

Teach patient/family:
• To check OTC medications, current prescription medications for ephedrine, which will increase stimulation; to avoid alcohol
• To avoid hazardous activities; dizziness may occur
• That if GI upset occurs to take drug with 8 oz water or food; absorption may be decreased slightly
• To notify prescriber of nausea, vomiting, anxiety, insomnia

zinc (℞, OTC)

Orazinc, PMS Egozine*, Verazinc, Zinca-Pak, Zincate, Zinc 15, Zinc-220, zinc sulfate
Func. class.: Trace element; nutritional supplement

Action: Needed for adequate healing, bone and joint development (23% zinc)

Uses: Prevention of zinc deficiency, adjunct to vit A therapy

Investigational uses: Wound healing
Dosage and routes:
Dietary supplement
• *Adult:* **PO** 25-50 mg/day
Nutritional supplement (IV)
• *Adult:* **IV** 2.5-4 mg/day; may increase by 2 mg/day if needed
• *Child 1-5 yr:* **IV** 100 µg/kg/day
• *Infant <1.5-3 kg:* **IV** 300 µg/kg/day
Available forms: Tabs 66, 110 mg; caps 220 mg; inj 1 mg, 5 mg/ml
Side effects/adverse reactions:
GI: Nausea, vomiting, cramps, heartburn, ulcer formation
Overdose: Diarrhea, rash, dehydration, restlessness
Precautions: Pregnancy (A)
Interactions:
• Decreased absorption of other covalent cations
NURSING CONSIDERATIONS
Assess:
• Zinc levels during treatment
Administer:
• With meals to decrease gastric upset; avoid dairy products
Evaluate:
• Therapeutic response: absence of zinc deficiency
Teach patient/family:
• That element must be taken for 2 mo to be effective
• To report immediately nausea, diarrhea, rash, severe vomiting, restlessness, abdominal pain, tarry stools

ziprasidone (R)
(zi-praz'ih-dohn)
Geodon
Func. class.: Antipsychotic/neuroleptic
Chem. class.: Benzisoxazole derivative

Action: Unknown; may be mediated through both dopamine type 2 (D_2) and serotonin type 2 (5-HT_2) antagonism
Uses: Schizophrenia
Dosage and routes:
• *Adult:* **PO** 20 mg bid with food, adjust dosage every 2 days upward to max of 80 mg bid
Available forms: Tabs 20, 40, 60, 80 mg
Side effects/adverse reactions:
CNS: EPS, pseudoparkinsonism, akathisia, dystonia, tardive dyskinesia; drowsiness, insomnia, agitation, anxiety, headache, seizures, neuroleptic malignant syndrome
CV: Orthostatic hypotension, tachycardia, prolonged QT/QTc, sudden death
EENT: Blurred vision
GI: Nausea, vomiting, anorexia, constipation, jaundice, weight gain
RESP: Rhinitis
Contraindications: Hypersensitivity, lactation, seizure disorders
Precautions: Children, renal disease, pregnancy (C), hepatic disease, elderly, breast cancer
Pharmacokinetics:
PO: Extensively metabolized by liver to a major active metabolite, plasma protein binding 90%
Interactions:
• Increased sedation: other CNS depressants, alcohol
• Increased EPS: other antipsychotics, lithium
• Increased excretion of risperidone: carbamazepine
🍵 Increased CNS depression: kava
Lab test interferences:
Not known
NURSING CONSIDERATIONS
Assess:
• Mental status before initial administration
• Swallowing of PO medication; check for hoarding or giving of medication to other patients

◆ = Nursing alert   🍵 = Herb-drug interaction   Ⓢ = Do not crush

• I&O ratio; palpate bladder if urinary output is low
• Bilirubin, CBC, liver function studies qmo
• Urinalysis before, during prolonged therapy
• Affect, orientation, LOC, reflexes, gait, coordination, sleep pattern disturbances
• B/P standing and lying; also pulse, respirations; take these q4h during initial treatment; establish baseline before starting treatment; report drops of 30 mm Hg; watch for ECG changes
• Dizziness, faintness, palpitations, tachycardia on rising
• EPS, including akathisia (inability to sit still, no pattern to movements), tardive dyskinesia (bizarre movements of the jaw, mouth, tongue, extremities), pseudoparkinsonism (rigidity, tremors, pill rolling, shuffling gait)
◆ For neuroleptic malignant syndrome: hyperthermia, increased CPK, altered mental status, muscle rigidity
• Skin turgor qd
• Constipation, urinary retention qd; if these occur, increase bulk and water in diet

Administer:
• Reduced dose in elderly
• Antiparkinsonian agent on order from prescriber, to be used for EPS

Perform/provide:
• Decreased stimulus by dimming lights, avoiding loud noises
• Supervised ambulation until patient is stabilized on medication; do not involve in strenuous exercise program because fainting is possible; patient should not stand still for a long time
• Increased fluids to prevent constipation
• Sips of water, candy, gum for dry mouth

• Storage in tight, light-resistant container

Evaluate:
• Therapeutic response: decrease in emotional excitement, hallucinations, delusions, paranoia; reorganization of patterns of thought, speech

Teach patient/family:
• That orthostatic hypotension may occur and to rise from sitting or lying position gradually
• To avoid hot tubs, hot showers, tub baths; hypotension may occur
• To avoid abrupt withdrawal of this drug; EPS may result; drug should be withdrawn slowly
• To avoid OTC preparations (cough, hay fever, cold) unless approved by prescriber, since serious drug interactions may occur; avoid use with alcohol, CNS depressants; increased drowsiness may occur
• To avoid hazardous activities if drowsy or dizzy
• Compliance with drug regimen
• To report impaired vision, tremors, muscle twitching
• In hot weather, that heat stroke may occur; take extra precautions to stay cool

Treatment of overdose: Lavage if orally ingested; provide airway; *do not induce vomiting*

---

zoledronic acid
See appendix a—selected new drugs

---

zolmitriptan (℞)

(zole-mih-trip′tan)
Zomig, Zomig-ZMT
Func. class.: Migraine agent
Chem. class.: 5-HT₁ receptor agonist

Action: Binds selectively to the vascular 5-HT₁ receptor subtype, exerts antimigraine effect; causes vasoconstriction in cranial arteries

Uses: Acute treatment of migraine with or without aura

Dosage and routes:
• *Adult:* PO Start on 2.5 mg or lower (tab may be broken), may repeat after 2 hr, max 10 mg/24 hr

Available forms: Tabs 2.5, 5 mg; orally disintegrating tab 2.5 mg

Side effects/adverse reactions:
CV: Palpitations
GI: Abdominal discomfort, nausea
MS: Weakness, neck stiffness, myalgia
NEURO: Tingling, hot sensation, burning, feeling of pressure, tightness, numbness, dizziness, sedation
RESP: Chest tightness, pressure

Contraindications: Angina pectoris, history of MI, documented silent ischemia, ischemic heart disease, concurrent ergotamine-containing preparations, uncontrolled hypertension, hypersensitivity, basilar or hemiplegic migraine, risk of CV events

Precautions: Postmenopausal women, men >40 yr, risk factors for CAD, hypercholesterolemia, obesity, diabetes, impaired hepatic or renal function, pregnancy (C), lactation, children, elderly

Pharmacokinetics: Duration 2-3½ hr, 25% plasma protein binding, half-life 3-3½ hr, metabolized in the liver (metabolite), excreted in urine, feces

Interactions:
◆ Extended vasospastic effects: ergot, ergot derivatives
◆ Do not use within 2 wk of MAOIs
• Increased half-life of zolmitriptan: cimetidine, oral contraceptives
◆ Weakness, hyperreflexia, incoordination: SSRIs (fluoxetine, fluvoxamine, paroxetine, sertraline)

NURSING CONSIDERATIONS
Assess:
• Tingling, hot sensation, burning, feeling of pressure, numbness, flushing
• For stress level, activity, recreation, coping mechanisms
• Neurologic status: LOC, blurring vision, nausea, vomiting, tingling in extremities preceding headache
• Ingestion of tyramine foods (pickled products, beer, wine, aged cheese), food additives, preservatives, colorings, artifical sweeteners, chocolate, caffeine, which may precipitate these types of headaches
• For serotonin syndrome, if also taking an SSRI

Administer:
• Take with fluids as soon as symptoms of migraine occur

Perform/provide:
• Quiet, calm environment with decreased stimulation for noise, bright light, excessive talking

Evaluate:
• Therapeutic response: decrease in frequency, severity of headache

Teach patient/family:
• To report any side effects to prescriber
• To use contraception while taking drug

◆ = Nursing alert   ∥ = Herb-drug interaction   ⊘ = Do not crush

zolpidem (℞)

(zole'pih-dem)

Ambien

Func. class.: Sedative-hypnotic

Chem. class.: Nonbenzodiaz-epine of imidazopyridine class

Controlled Substance Schedule IV

Action: Produces CNS depression at limbic, thalamic, hypothalamic levels of CNS; may be mediated by neurotransmitter γ-aminobutyric acid (GABA); results are sedation, hypnosis, skeletal muscle relaxation, anticonvulsant activity, anxiolytic action

Uses: Insomnia, short-term treatment

Dosage and routes:

• *Adult:* **PO** 10 mg hs × 7-10 days only; total dose should not exceed 10 mg

• *Geriatric:* **PO** 5 mg hs

Available forms: Tabs 5, 10 mg

Side effects/adverse reactions:

HEMA: **Leukopenia, granulocytopenia** (rare)

CNS: Headache, lethargy, drowsiness, daytime sedation, dizziness, confusion, light-headedness, anxiety, irritability, amnesia, poor coordination

GI: Nausea, vomiting, diarrhea, heartburn, abdominal pain, constipation

CV: Chest pain, palpitation

Contraindications: Hypersensitivity to benzodiazepines

Precautions: Anemia, hepatic disease, renal disease, suicidal individuals, drug abuse, elderly, psychosis, child <18 yr, seizure disorders, pregnancy (B), lactation

Pharmacokinetics:

PO: Onset 1.5 hr, metabolized by liver, excreted by kidneys (inactive metabolites), crosses placenta, excreted in breast milk; half-life 2-3 hr

Interactions:

• Increased action of both drugs: alcohol, CNS depressants

🥢 Increased CNS depression: kava

Lab test interferences:

Increase: ALT, AST, serum bilirubin

Decrease: RAI uptake

False increase: Urinary 17-OHCS

NURSING CONSIDERATIONS

Assess:

• Blood studies: Hct, Hgb, RBC, if blood dyscrasias are suspected (rare)

• Hepatic studies: AST, ALT, bilirubin if liver damage has occurred

• Mental status: mood, sensorium, affect, memory (long, short)

• Blood dyscrasias: fever, sore throat, bruising, rash, jaundice, epistaxis (rare)

• Type of sleep problem: falling asleep, staying asleep

Administer:

• After removal of cigarettes to prevent fires

• After trying conservative measures for insomnia

• ½-1 hr before hs for sleeplessness

• On empty stomach for fast onset but may be taken with food if GI symptoms occur

Perform/provide:

• Assistance with ambulation after receiving dose

• Safety measures: side rails, nightlight, call bell within easy reach

• Checking to see if PO medication has been swallowed

• Storage in tight container in cool environment

Evaluate:

• Therapeutic response: ability to sleep at night, decreased amount of early morning awakening if taking drug for insomnia

Teach patient/family:
• That dependence is possible after long-term use
• To avoid driving or other activities requiring alertness until drug is stabilized
• To avoid alcohol ingestion, CNS depressants; serious CNS depression may result
• That effects may take 2 nights for benefits to be noticed
• Alternative measures to improve sleep: reading, exercise several hours before hs, warm bath, warm milk, TV, self-hypnosis, deep breathing
• That hangover is common in elderly but less common than with barbiturates; rebound insomnia may occur for 1-2 nights after discontinuing drug

Treatment of overdose: Lavage, activated charcoal; monitor electrolytes, vital signs

---

zonisamide (Ŗ)
(zone-is′a-mide)
Zonegran
Func. class.: Anticonvulsant
Chem. class.: Sulfonamides

Action: May act through action at sodium and calcium channels, but exact action is unknown
Uses: Epilepsy, adjunctive therapy of partial seizures
Dosage and routes:
• *Adults and child >16 yr:* 100 mg qd, may increase after 2 wk to 200 mg/day, may increase q2 wk, maximum dose >600 mg/day
Available forms: Caps 100 mg
Side effects/adverse reactions:
CNS: Dizziness, insomnia, paresthe-sias, depression, fatigue, headache, confusion
EENT: Diplopia, verbal difficulty, speech abnormalities, taste perversion
GI: Nausea, constipation, anorexia, weight loss, diarrhea, dyspepsia
INTEG: Rash
Contraindications: Hypersensitivity to this drug or sulfonamides, psychiatric condition, hepatic failure
Precautions: Allergies, hepatic disease, renal disease, elderly, pregnancy (C), lactation, child <16 yr
Pharmacokinetics: Peak 2-6 hr, half-life 63 hr
Metabolized by liver, excreted by kidneys
Interactions:
• Increased half-life of zonisamide: drugs inducing CYP 450 enzymes
NURSING CONSIDERATIONS
Assess:
• For seizures: duration, type, intensity precipitating factors
• Blood studies: CBC, platelets q2wk until stabilized, then qmo × 12, then q3mo; discontinue drug if neutrophils <1600/mm^3; renal function: albumin conc
• Mental status: mood, sensorium, affect, memory (long, short)
Evaluate:
• Therapeutic response; decreaase in severity of seizures
Teach patient/family:
• Not to discontinue drug abruptly; seizures may occur
• To avoid hazardous activities until stabilized on drug
• To carry Medic Alert ID stating drug use

References for Research Notes

[1]Hervey PS et al: Abacavir: a review of its clinical potential in patients with HIV infection, *Drugs* 60(2):447, 2000.

[2]Ziermann R et al: A mutation in human immunodeficiency virus type 1 protease, N88S, that causes in vitro hypersensitivity to amprenavir, *J Virol* 74(9):4414, 2000.

[3]Duvic M et al: Bexarotene is effective and safe for treatment of refractory advanced-stage cutaneous T-cell lymphoma: multinational phase II-III trial results, *J Clin Oncol* 19(9):2456, 2001.

[4]Chang SA et al: The effect of cilostazol on glucose tolerance and insulin resistance in a rat model of non–insulin dependent diabetes mellitus, *Korean J Intern Med* 16(2):87, 2001.

[5]Olsen E et al: A high-fat meal does not activate blood coagulation factor VII in minipigs, *Blood Coagul Fibrinolysis* 12(2):117, 2001.

[6]Olsen E et al: Pivotal phase III trial of two dose levels of denileukin diftitox for the treatment of cutaneous T-cell lymphoma, *J Clin Oncol* 19(2):376, 2001.

[7]Coursin DB et al: Dexmedetomidine, *Curr Opin Crit Care* 7(4):221, 2001 (review).

[8]Pedersen OD et al: Efficacy of dofetilide in the treatment of atrial fibrillation-flutter in patients with reduced left ventricular function: a Danish investigation of arrhythmia and mortality on dofetilide (diamond) substudy, *Circulation* 104(3):292, 2001.

[9]Maung HM et al: Efficacy and side effects of intermittent intravenous and oral doxercalciferol (1alpha-hydroxyvitamin D[2]) in dialysis patients with secondary hyperparathyroidism: a sequential comparison, *Am J Kidney Dis* 37(3):532, 2001.

[10]Vaamonde J et al: Motor impairment, in patients with severe Parkinson's disease, associated with dopaminergic hyperstimulation (entacapone), *Neurologia* 16(2):81, 2001.

[11]Meinardi MT et al: Prospective evaluation of early cardiac damage induced by epirubicin-containing adjuvant chemotherapy and locoregional radiotherapy in breast cancer patients, *J Clin Oncol* 19(10):2746, 2001.

[12]Kanazawa S et al: The effects of grapefruit juice on the pharmacokinetics of erythromycin, *Eur J Clin Pharmacol* 56(11):799, 2001.

[14]Arafah BM: Increased need for thyroxine in women with hypothyroidism during estrogen therapy, *N Engl J Med* 344(23):1743, 2001.

[15]Van de Poll ME et al: The effect of atovaquone on etoposide pharmacokinetics in children with acute lymphoblastic leukemia, *Cancer Chemother Pharmacol* 47(6):467, 2001.

[16]Beltrame D et al: Reproductive toxicity of exemestane, an antitumoral aromatase inactivator, in rats and rabbits, *Reprod Toxicol* 15(2):195, 2001.

[17]Weigmann H et al: Fluvoxamine but not sertraline inhibits the metabolism of olanzapine: evidence from a therapeutic drug monitoring service, *Ther Drug Monit* 23(4):410, 2001.

[18]Conlin PN et al: Effect of indomethacin on blood pressure lowering by captopril and losartan in hypertensive patients, *Hypertension* 36(3):461, 2000.

[19]Keane J et al: Tuberculosis associated with infliximab, a tumor necrosis factor–alpha neutralizing agent, *N Engl J Med* 345(15):1098, 2001.

[20]Ferreira JJ et al: Levodopa monotherapy can induce "sleep attacks" in Parkinson's disease patients, *J Neurol* 248(5):426, 2001.

[21]Abena PA et al: Linezolid and reversible myelosuppression, *JAMA* 268(16):1973, 2001.

[22]Brown CH: Effect of rofecoxib on the antihypertensive activity of lisinopril, *Ann Pharmacother* 34(12):1486, 2000.

[23]Conlin PN et al: Effect of indomethacin on blood pressure lowering by captopril and losartan in hypertensive patients, *Hypertension* 36(3):461, 2000.

[24]Kusumoto M et al: Effect of fluvoxamine on the pharmacokinetics of mexiletine in healthy Japanese men, *Clin Pharmacol Ther* 69(3):104, 2001.

[25]Morii M et al: Impairment of mycophenolate mofetil absorption by iron ion, *Clin Pharmacol Ther* 68(6):613, 2000.

[26]Khan AY et al: Increase in plasma levels of clozapine and norclozapine after administration of nefazodone, *J Clin Psychiatry* 62(5):375, 2001.

[27]Dionisio D et al: Need for increased dose of warfarin in HIV patients taking nevirapine, *AIDS* 15(2):277, 2001.

[28]Knopp RH: Evaluating niacin in its various forms, *Am J Cardiol* 86(12A):51L, 2000.

[29]Uno T et al: Effects of grapefruit juice on the stereoselective disposition of nicardipine in humans: evidence for dominant presystemic elimination at the gut site, *Eur J Clin Pharmacol* 56(9-10):643, 2000.

[30]Vaamonde J et al: Writer's cramp induced by olanzapine, *J Neurol* 248(5):422, 2001.

[31]Spina E et al: Plasma concentrations of risperidone and 9-hydroxyrisperidone during combined treatment with paroxetine, *Ther Drug Monit* 23(3):223, 2001.

[32]Konig F et al: Effect of paroxetine on thyroid hormone levels in severely depressed patients, *Neuropsychobiology* 42(3):135, 2000.

[33]Wong YW et al: The effects of concomitant phenytoin administration on the steady-state pharmacokinetics of quetiapine, *J Clin Psychopharmacol* 21(1):89, 2001.

[34]Wong YW et al: The effects of concomitant phenytoin administration on the steady-state pharmacokinetics of quetiapine, *J Clin Psychopharmacol* 21(1):89, 2001.

[35]Niemi M et al: Rifampin decreases the plasma concentrations and effects of repaglinide, *Clin Pharmacol Ther* 68(5):495, 2000.

[36]Niemi M et al: Rifampin decreases the plasma concentrations and effects of repaglinide, *Clin Pharmacol Ther* 68(5):495, 2000.

[37]Spina E et al: Plasma concentrations of risperidone and 9-hydroxyrisperidone during combined treatment with paroxetine, *Ther Drug Monit* 23(3):223, 2001.

[38]Stangier J et al: The effect of telmisartan on the steady-state pharmacokinetics of digoxin in healthy male volunteers, *J Clin Pharmacol* 40(12 Pt 1):1373, 2000.

[39]Ho PC et al: Effect of grapefruit juice on pharmacokinetics and pharmacodynamics of verapamil enantiomers in healthy volunteers, *Eur J Clin Pharmacol* 56(9-10):693, 2000.

[40]Dionisio D et al: Need for increased dose of warfarin in HIV patients taking nevirapine, *AIDS* 15(2):277, 2001.

Appendixes

Appendix a

Selected new drugs

alemtuzumab (R)
(al-em-tuz′uh-mab)
Campath
Func. class.: Misc. antineoplastic

Chem. class.: Monoclonal antibody

Action: Composed of recombinant DNA-derived humanized monoclonal antibody (campath-1H), binds to CD52 antigen that is present on surface of B and T lymphocytes, causes lysis of leukemic cells

Uses: B-cell chronic lymphocytic leukemia that has been treated with alkylating agents

Dosage and routes:
• *Adult:* IV 3 mg over 2 hr daily; when tolerated, increase to 10 mg; when 10 mg tolerated increase to 30 mg qd, maintenance is 30 mg/day 3×/wk on alternate days

Available forms: Sol for inj 30 mg/3 ml

Side effects/adverse reactions:
CNS: Dizziness, insomnia, depression, headache, tremor, somnolence, fatigue
CV: Hypotension, tachycardia, hypertension
GI: Anorexia, diarrhea, constipation, nausea, stomatitis, vomiting, abdominal pain, dyspepsia
HEMA: Anemia, neutropenia, thrombocytopenia, pancytopenia, purpura, epistaxis
INTEG: Rash, local reaction, pruritus
META: Hypokalemia, hypomagnesemia
MISC: Rigors, fever
RESP: Cough, pneumonia, rhinitis, ***bronchospasm***, dyspnea, pharyngitis
Contraindications: Hypersensitivity, active systemic infection, immunodeficiency
Precautions: Pregnancy (C), lactation, children
Pharmacokinetics: Steady state 6 wk
Interactions:
• Do not give live virus vaccines
Lab test interferences:
• *Interference:* Diagnostic tests using antibodies
NURSING CONSIDERATIONS
Assess:
• CBC, platelets qwk or more often if myelosuppression occurs; CD4$^+$ after therapy until recovery of >200 cells/µL
• For symptoms of infection; chills, fever, headache, may be masked by drug fever
• CNS reaction: LOC, mental status, dizziness, confusion
• Cardiac status: lung sounds; ECG before and during treatment, especially in those with cardiac disease
• Bone marrow depression: bruising, bleeding, blood in stools, urine, sputum, emesis
Administer:
• Do not give IV push or bolus
• Withdraw amount needed, use 5 µm filter before dilution, check for particulate matter and discoloration; inject into 100 ml sterile 0.9% NaCl

◆ = Nursing alert   ✎ = Herb-drug interaction   ⊘ = Do not crush or D_5W, invert to mix; do not add other drugs or infuse in same IV tubing

Perform/provide:
• Storage of reconstituted sol for ≤8 hr at room temperature, do not freeze; protect from light

Evaluate:
• Therapeutic response: decrease in production of malignant lymphocytes

Teach patient/family:
• To take acetaminophen for fever
• To avoid hazardous tasks, because confusion, dizziness may occur
• To report signs of infection: sore throat, fever, diarrhea, vomiting

---

almotriptan (R)
(al-moh-trip′tan)
Axert

Func. class.: Antimigraine agent
Chem. class.: 5-HT₁-Receptor agonist

Action: Binds selectively to the vascular 5-HT₁-receptor subtype, exerts antimigraine effect; causes vasoconstriction in cranial arteries

Uses: Acute treatment of migraine with or without aura

Dosage and routes:
• *Adult:* **PO** may use the 6.25-mg dose initially, but 12.5 mg is more effective; may repeat dose after 2 hr; do not give more than 2 doses/ 24 hr

Available forms: Tabs 6.25, 12.5 mg

Side effects/adverse reactions:
CV: Flushing, palpitations, tachycardia, coronary artery vasospasm
EENT: Throat, mouth, nasal discomfort; vision changes
GI: Abdominal discomfort
INTEG: Sweating
MS: Weakness, neck stiffness, myalgia
NEURO: Tingling, hot sensation, burning, feeling of pressure, tightness, numbness, dizziness, sedation, headache, anxiety, fatigue, cold sensation
RESP: Chest tightness, pressure

Contraindications: Concurrent use of ergotamine-containing preparations, uncontrolled hypertension, hypersensitivity, basilar or hemiplegic migraine; concurrent MAO inhibitor therapy or within 2 wk

Precautions: Postmenopausal women, men >40 yr, risk factors for CAD, hypercholesterolemia, obesity, diabetes, impaired hepatic or renal function, pregnancy (C), lactation, children, elderly

Pharmacokinetics: Onset of pain relief 2 hr; metabolized in the liver (metabolite); excreted in urine, feces

Interactions:
• Extended vasospastic effects: ergot, ergot derivatives, other 5-HT₁ agonists
• Increased almotriptan effect: MAOIs
• Increased plasma concentration of almotriptan: ketoconazole

NURSING CONSIDERATIONS
Assess:
• B/P; signs/symptoms of coronary vasospasms
• Tingling, hot sensation, burning, feeling of pressure, numbness, flushing
• For stress level, activity, recreation, coping mechanisms
• Neurologic status: LOC, blurring vision, nausea, vomiting, tingling in extremities preceding headache
• Ingestion of tyramine foods (pickled products, beer, wine, aged cheese), food additives, preservatives, colorings, artificial sweeteners, chocolate, caffeine, which may precipitate these types of headaches

Administer:
🚫 PO, swallow whole

Perform/provide:
• Quiet, calm environment with decreased stimulation from noise, bright light, excessive talking
Evaluate:
• Therapeutic response: decrease in severity of migraine
Teach patient/family:
• To report any side effects to prescriber
• To use contraception while taking drug
• To provide dark, quiet environment
• That drug does not prevent or reduce number of migraine attacks

---

anakinra (℞)
(an-ah-kin'rah)
Kineret
Func. class.: Antirheumatic agent (disease modifying), immunomodulator
Chem. class.: Recombinant form of human interleukin-1 receptor antagonist (IL-1Ra)

Action: A form of human interleukin-1 receptor antagonist (IL-1Ra) produced by DNA technology; blocks activity of IL-1, resulting in decreased cartilage degradation and decreased bone resorption
Uses: Reduction in signs and symptoms of moderate to severe active rheumatoid arthritis in patients ≥18 years of age who have not responded to other disease-modifying agents
Dosage and routes:
• *Adult:* **SC** 100 mg qd
Available form: Sol for inj 100 mg
Side effects/adverse reactions:
CNS: Headache
EENT: Sinusitis
GI: Abdominal pain, nausea, diarrhea
INTEG: Rash, *inj site reaction*

MISC: Flulike symptoms
RESP: URI
Contraindications: Hypersensitivity to *Escherichia coli*–derived proteins or this product, sepsis
Precautions: Pregnancy (B), lactation, children, renal impairment, elderly
Pharmacokinetics: Terminal half-life 4-6 hr
Interactions:
• Do not give concurrently with vaccines, immunizations should be brought up to date before treatment
NURSING CONSIDERATIONS
Assess:
• Pain, stiffness, ROM, swelling of joints during treatment
• For inj site pain, swelling; usually occur after 2 inj (4-5 days)
• For infections, stop treatment if present
Administer:
• Do not use if cloudy or discolored or if particulate is present
• Do not admix with other sol or medications, do not use filter
Evaluate:
• Therapeutic response: decreased inflammation, pain in joints
Teach patient/family:
• About self-administration if appropriate: inj should be made in thigh, abdomen, upper arm; rotate sites at least 1 inch from old site

---

bosentan (℞)
(boh'sen-tan)
Tracleer
Func. class.: Vasodilator
Chem. class.: Endothelin receptor antagonist

Action: Peripheral vasodilation occurs via antagonism of the effect of endothelin on endothelium and vascular smooth muscle
Uses: Pulmonary arterial hyperten-

 = Nursing alert   = Herb-drug interaction   ⃠ = Do not crush

sion with WHO class III, IV symptoms
Dosage and routes:
• *Adult >40 kg/>12 yr:* **PO** 62.5 mg bid × 4 wk, then 125 mg bid
• *Adult <40 kg/>12 yr:* **PO** 62.5 mg bid
Available forms: Tabs 62.5, 125 mg
Side effects/adverse reactions:
CNS: Headache, flushing, fatigue
CV: Hypotension, palpitations, edema of lower limbs
GI: Abnormal liver function, dyspepsia
INTEG: Pruritus
Contraindications: Pregnancy (X), hypersensitivity, CVA, CAD
Precautions: Mitral stenosis, elderly, lactation, hepatic function impairment
Pharmacokinetics: Induces CYP2C9, CYP3A4, and possibly CYP2C19, metabolized by the liver, terminal half-life 5 hr, steady state 3-5 days
Interactions:
• Increased bosentan level: ketoconazole
• Do not coadminister cyclosporine A and bosentan; bosentan is increased, cyclosporine is decreased
• Do not coadminister glyburide with bosentan; glyburide is decreased significantly, bosentan also is decreased
• Decreased effects of: simvastatin, other statins, hormonal contraceptives
NURSING CONSIDERATIONS
Assess:
• B/P, pulse during treatment until stable
• Hepatic tests: AST, ALT, bilirubin; liver enzymes may increase; if ALT/AST >3 and ≤5 × ULN, confirm lab value, decrease dose or interrupt treatment and monitor AST/ALT q2wk; if >8 × ULN, stop treatment

• Blood studies: Hct, Hgb may be decreased
• Hepatic involvement: vomiting, jaundice; drug should be discontinued
Perform/provide:
• Storage at room temperature
Evaluate:
• Therapeutic response: decrease in pulmonary hypertension
Teach patient/family:
• To report jaundice, dark urine, joint pain, fatigue, malaise, bruising, easy bleeding; may indicate blood dyscrasias
• To avoid pregnancy; to use non-hormonal form of contraception

---

cefditoren pivoxil (℞)
(sef-dit′oh-ren pih-vox′il)
Spectracef
Func. class.: Antiinfective
Chem. class.: Cephalosporin (2nd generation)

Action: Inhibits bacterial cell wall synthesis, rendering cell wall osmotically unstable, leading to cell death by binding to cell wall memberane
Uses: Acute bacterial exacerbation of chronic bronchitis caused by *Haemophilus influenzae, Haemophilus parainfluenzae, Streptococcus pneumoniae, Moraxella catarrhalis*; pharyngitis/tonsillitis caused by *Streptococcus pyogenes*; uncomplicated skin and skin structure infections caused by *Staphylococcus aureus, S. pyogenes*
Dosage and routes:
Acute bacterial exacerbation of chronic bronchitis
• *Adult:* **PO** 400 mg bid × 10 days
Pharyngitis/tonsillitis
• *Adult:* **PO** 200 mg bid × 10 days

Uncomplicated skin and skin structure infections
• *Adult:* **PO** 200 mg bid × 10 days
Renal dose
• CrCl 30-49 ml/min give ≤200 mg bid × 10 days
• CrCl <30 ml/min give 200 mg qd × 10 days
Available form: Tabs 200 mg
Side effects/adverse reactions:
CNS: Dizziness, headache, fatigue, paresthesia, fever, chills, confusion
GI: Diarrhea, nausea, vomiting, anorexia, dysgeusia, glossitis, bleeding; increased AST, ALT, bilirubin, LDH, alk phosphatase; abdominal pain, loose stools, flatulence, heartburn, stomach cramps, colitis, jaundice
INTEG: Rash, urticaria, dermatitis, ***Stevens-Johnson syndrome,*** diaphoresis, flushing
GU: Vaginitis, pruritus, candidiasis, increased BUN, ***nephrotoxicity, renal failure,*** pyuria, dysuria, reversible interstitial nephritis
HEMA: ***Leukopenia, thrombocytopenia, agranulocytosis,*** anemia, *neutropenia, lymphocytosis,* ***eosinophilia, pancytopenia, hemolytic anemia, leukocytosis, granulocytopenia***
RESP: Dyspnea
SYST: ***Anaphylaxis, serum sickness***
Contraindications: Hypersensitivity to cephalosporins or related antibiotics, carnitine deficiency, inborn errors of metabolism, milk protein hypersensitivity
Precautions: Pregnancy (B), lactation, children, renal disease, penicillin sensitivity
Pharmacokinetics: Peak 1-1½ hr, half-life ½-1 hr; 60%-75% bound by plasma proteins; crosses placenta; excreted in breast milk; poor penetration into CSF

Interactions:
• Increased renal toxicity: aminoglycosides
• Increased plasma level of cefditoren: probenecid
• Decreased plasma level of cefditoren: antacids, H$_2$-receptor antagonists
NURSING CONSIDERATIONS
Assess:
◆ Nephrotoxicity: increased BUN, creatinine
• I&O ratio
• Blood studies: AST, ALT, CBC, Hct, bilirubin, LDH, alk phosphatase, Coombs' test qmo if patient is on long-term therapy
• Electrolytes: K, Na, Cl qmo if patient is on long-term therapy
• Bowel pattern qd; if severe diarrhea occurs, drug should be discontinued; may indicate pseudomembranous colitis
• Urine output; if decreasing, notify prescriber (may indicate nephrotoxicity)
◆ Anaphylaxis: rash, flushing, urticaria, pruritus, dyspnea
• Bleeding: ecchymosis, bleeding gums, hematuria, stool guaiac daily
◆ Overgrowth of infection: perineal itching, fever, malaise, redness, pain, swelling, drainage, rash, diarrhea, change in cough, sputum
Administer:
• For 10 days to ensure organism death, prevent superinfection
• With food if needed for GI symptoms
• After C&S completed
Evaluate:
• Therapeutic response: Decreased symptoms of infection, negative C&S
Teach patient/family:
• Not to drink alcohol or take medications containing alcohol; reaction may occur

---

◆ = Nursing alert   ⦸ = Herb-drug interaction   ⊘ = Do not crush

• To complete full course of drug therapy
• To report persistent diarrhea or any side effects
• To notify prescriber if breastfeeding

Treatment of anaphylaxis: Epinephrine, antihistamines; resuscitate if needed

---

darbepoetin alfa (℞)
(dar'bee-poh'eh-tin al'fah)
Aranesp
Func. class.: Hematopoietic agent
Chem. class.: Recombinant human erythropoietin

Action: Stimulates erythropoiesis by the same mechanism as endogenous erythropoietin; in response to hypoxia, erythropoietin is produced in the kidney and released into the bloodstream, where it interacts with progenitor stem cells to increase red cell production

Uses: Anemia associated with chronic renal failure, in patients on and not on dialysis

Dosage and routes:
Correction of anemia
• *Adult:* **SC/IV** 0.45 µg/kg as a single inj, titrate not to exceed a target Hgb of 12 g/dl
Conversion from epoetin alfa to darbepoetin
• *Adult:* **SC/IV** estimate starting dose based on weekly epoetin alfa dose; because of longer serum half-life, darbepoetin must be administered less frequently than epoetin alfa; if epoetin was given 2-3×/wk, give darbepoetin 1×/wk; if epoetin was given 1×/wk, give darbepoetin 1× q2wk; do not increase doses more often than 1×/mo

Available forms: Sol 25, 40, 60, 100, 200 µg/ml
Side effects/adverse reactions:
*CNS: **Seizures**,* sweating, headache, dizziness
*CV: **Hypertension**,* hypotension, ***cardiac arrest,*** angina pectoris, ***thrombosis, CHF***
GI: Diarrhea, vomiting, nausea, abdominal pain, constipation
MISC: Infection, fatigue, fever, ***death***, chest pain, fluid overload, vascular access hemorrhage
MS: Bone pain, myalgia, limb pain
RESP: URI, dyspnea, cough, bronchitis
Contraindications: Hypersensitivity to mammalian cell-derived products or human albumin, uncontrolled hypertension
Precautions: Seizure disorder, porphyria, pregnancy (C), hypertension
Pharmacokinetics: **IV:** Onset of increased reticulocyte count 1-6 wk; distributed to vascular space; absorption slow and rate-limiting; terminal half-life 49 hr; peak concentration at 34 hr; increased Hgb levels not generally observed until 2-6 wk after treatment initiated
Interactions:
Unknown
NURSING CONSIDERATIONS
Assess:
• Renal studies: urinalysis, protein, blood, BUN, creatinine
• Blood studies: ferritin, transferrin qmo; transferrin sat ≥20%, ferritin ≥100 ng/ml; Hgb 2×/wk until stabilized in target range (30%-33%), then at regular intervals; those with endogenous erythropoietin levels of <500 U/L respond to this agent
• B/P; check for rising B/P as Hgb rises, antihypertensives may be needed

---

* = Canada only   Side effects: *italics* = common; ***bold italics*** = life-threatening

• CV status: hypertension may occur rapidly leading to hypertensive encephalopathy
• I&O; report drop in output to <50 ml/hr
• For seizures if Hgb is increased within 2 wk by 4 pts
• CNS symptoms: sweating, pain in long bones
• Dialysis patients: thrill, bruit of shunts, monitor for circulation impairment
Administer:
IV/ SC
• Without shaking; check for discoloration, particulate matter, do not use if present; do not dilute, do not mix with other drugs or solutions
Evaluate:
• Therapeutic response: increase in reticulocyte count, Hgb/Hct; increased appetite, enhanced sense of well-being
Teach patient/family:
• To avoid driving or hazardous activity during beginning of treatment
• To monitor B/P
• To take iron supplements, vit B_{12}, folic acid as directed

---

desloratadine (℞)
(des′lor-at′ah-deen)
Clarinex
Func. class.: Antihistamine, 2nd generation
Chem. class.: Selective histamine (H_1)-receptor antagonist

Action: Binds to peripheral histamine receptors, providing antihistamine action without sedation
Uses: Seasonal allergic rhinitis
Dosage and routes:
• *Adult and child ≥12 yr:* **PO** 5 mg qd
Hepatic/renal dose
• *Adult:* **PO** 5 mg qod
Available form: Tabs 5 mg

Side effects/adverse reactions:
CNS: Sedation (more common with increased doses), headache
Contraindications: Hypersensitivity, acute asthma attacks, lower respiratory tract disease
Precautions: Pregnancy (C), bronchial asthma, liver or renal impairment
Pharmacokinetics: Peak 1½ hr, elimination half-life 8½-28 hr; metabolized in liver to active metabolites, excreted in urine
Interactions:
• None significant
NURSING CONSIDERATIONS
Assess:
• Allergy: hives, rash, rhinitis; monitor respiratory status
Administer:
• Without regard to meals
Perform/provide:
• Storage in tight container at room temperature
Evaluate:
• Therapeutic response: absence of running or congested nose, other allergy symptoms
Teach patient/family:
• To avoid driving, other hazardous activities if drowsiness occurs; observe caution until drug's effects on the patient are known
• That drug may cause photosensitivity; use sunscreen or stay out of the sun to prevent burns

---

dexmethyl-phenidate (℞)
(dex′meth-ul-fen′ih-dayt)
Focalin
Func. class.: Central nervous system (CNS) stimulant

Controlled Substance Schedule II
Action: Increases release of norepinephrine and dopamine into the ex-

---

◆ = Nursing alert   *▯* = Herb-drug interaction   ⃠ = Do not crush traneuronal space, also blocks re-uptake of norepinephrine and do-pamine into the presynaptic neuron; mode of action in treating attention deficit hyperactivity disorder (ADHD) is unknown

Uses: ADHD

Dosage and routes:

• *Child >6 yr:* **PO** 2.5 mg bid with doses at least 4 hr apart, gradually increase to a maximum of 20 mg/day (10 mg bid); for those taking methylphenidate, use ½ of methylphenidate dose initially, then increase as needed to a maximum of 20 mg/day

Available forms: Tabs 2.5, 5, 10 mg

Side effects/adverse reactions:

CNS: Dizziness, headache, drowsiness, *toxic psychosis, neuroleptic malignant syndrome (rare)*, Gilles de la Tourette's syndrome

CV: Palpitations, B/P changes, angina, *dysrhythmias*

GI: Nausea, anorexia, abnormal liver function, *hepatic coma*, abdominal pain

INTEG: Exfoliative dermatitis, urticaria, rash, erythema multiforme

HEMA: Leukopenia, anemia, thrombocytopenic purpura

MISC: Fever, arthralgia, scalp hair loss

Contraindications: Hypersensitivity to methylphenidate, anxiety, history of Gilles de la Tourette's syndrome; children <6 yr, glaucoma, concurrent treatment with MAOIs or within 14 days of discontinuing treatment with MAOIs

Precautions: Hypertension, depression, pregnancy (C), seizures, lactation, drug abuse, psychosis, cardiovascular disorders

Pharmacokinetics: Readily absorbed, peak 1-1½ hr, elimination half-life 2.2 hr, onset ½-1 hr, duration 4 hr, metabolized by liver, excreted by kidneys

Interactions:

• Hypertensive crisis: MAOIs or within 14 days of MAOIs, vasopressors

• Increased sympathomimetic effect: decongestants, vasoconstrictors

• Decreased effects of: antihypertensives

• Increased effects of: anticonvulsants, tricyclics, SSRIs, coumarin anticoagulants (warfarin)

NURSING CONSIDERATIONS

Assess:

• VS, B/P; may reverse antihypertensives; check patients with cardiac disease more often for increased B/P

• CBC, urinalysis in diabetes; blood sugar, urine sugar; insulin changes may have to be made, because eating will decrease

• Height, growth rate q3mo in children; growth rate may be decreased

• Mental status: mood, sensorium, affect, stimulation, insomnia, aggressiveness

◆ Withdrawal symptoms: headache, nausea, vomiting, muscle pain, weakness

• Appetite, sleep, speech patterns

• For attention span, decreased hyperactivity in persons with ADHD

Administer:

• Twice daily at least 4 hr apart

• Without regard to meals

Evaluate:

• Therapeutic response: decreased hyperactivity or ability to stay awake

Teach patient/family:

• To decrease caffeine consumption (coffee, tea, cola, chocolate); may increase irritability, stimulation

• To avoid OTC preparations unless approved by prescriber

• To taper off drug over several wk to avoid depression, increased sleeping, lethargy

• To avoid alcohol ingestion

• To avoid hazardous activities until stabilized on medication
• To get needed rest; patients will feel more tired at end of day

Treatment of overdose: Administer fluids; hemodialysis or peritoneal dialysis; antihypertensive for increased B/P; administer short-acting barbiturate before lavage

---

drotrecogin alfa (℞)
(droh'treh-koh-jin al'fah)
Xigris
Func. class.: Thrombolytic agent
Chem. class.: Recombinant human activated protein C

Action: Activated protein C exerts an antithrombotic effect by inhibiting factor Va/VIIIa

Uses: Severe sepsis

Dosage and routes:
• *Adult:* IV INF 24 µg/kg/hr × 96 hr
Available forms: Pwd for inj, lyophilized, 5, 20 mg

Side effects/adverse reactions:
HEMA: Decreased Hct, *bleeding*
SYST: GI, GU, intracranial, intraabdominal, intrathoracic, retroperitoneal bleeding; surface bleeding

Contraindications: Hypersensitivity, active bleeding, intraspinal surgery, CNS neoplasms, ulcerative colitis, enteritis, hepatic disease, hypocoagulation, hemorrhagic stroke, epidural catheter in place, cerebral embolism/thrombosis/hemorrhage, recent major surgery

Precautions: Recent GI bleeding, prothrombin time – INR >3, pregnancy (C), lactation, children

Pharmacokinetics: Inactivated by endogenous plasma protease inhibitors

Interactions:
• Bleeding potential: aspirin, indomethacin, phenylbutazone, anticoagulants, thrombolytics, glycoprotein IIb/IIIa inhibitors

NURSING CONSIDERATIONS
Assess:
◆ For bleeding during treatment; hematuria, hematemesis, bleeding from mucous membranes, epistaxis, ecchymosis; may require transfusion (rare), continue to assess for bleeding
• Blood studies (Hct, platelets, PTT, PT, TT, aPTT) before starting therapy; PT or aPTT must be less than 2× control before starting therapy; PTT or PT q3-4h during treatment
• VS, B/P, pulse, respirations, neurologic signs, temp at least q4h; temp >104° F (40° C) indicates internal bleeding; cardiac rhythm following intracoronary administration; systolic pressure increase >25 mm Hg should be reported to prescriber
◆ For neurologic changes that may indicate intracranial bleeding
◆ Retroperitoneal bleeding: back pain, leg weakness, diminished pulses

Administer:
IV
• Reconstitute 5 mg vial/2.5 ml; 20 mg vial/10 ml sterile water for inj to a concentration of 2 mg/ml; slowly add sterile water for inj, do not shake or invert, gently swirl until dissolved
• Further dilute with 0.9% NaCl, slowly withdraw prescribed amount and add to bag of 0.9% NaCl, direct stream to side of bag, gently invert bag; do not transport infusion bag between locations using mechanical delivery systems
• Use immediately after reconstituting, may be held for only 3 hr at controlled room temperature 59°-86° F; must complete infusion within 12 hr after preparation

◆ = Nursing alert   🍃 = Herb-drug interaction   🚫 = Do not crush

• Do not use if discolored or if particulate is present
• If using an infusion pump, usual concentration is 100-200 µg/ml; if using a syringe pump, usual concentration is 100-1000 µg/ml
• Use a dedicated IV line, or dedicated lumen of central venous catheter; may use only 0.9% NaCl, LR, dextrose, or dextrose/saline mixtures through same line
• Do not expose to heat or direct sunlight

Perform/provide:
• Refrigerated storage at 2° to 8° C (36° to 46° F); do not freeze
• Protect unreconstituted vials from light; keep in carton until time of use

Evaluate:
• Therapeutic response: Decreasing symptoms of sepsis, lack of mortality

---

dutasteride (Ŗ)
(doo-tass'ter-ide)
Duagen
Func. class.: 5α-Reductase inhibitor
Chem. class.: Synthetic 4-azasteroid compound

Action: Inhibits both types 1 and 2 forms of a steroid enzyme that converts testosterone to 5α-dihydrotestosterone (DHT), which is responsible for the initial growth of prostatic tissue
Uses: Treatment of benign prostatic hyperplasia (BPH) in men with an enlarged prostate gland
Dosage and routes:
• *Adult:* **PO** 0.5 mg qd
Available form: Caps 0.5 mg
Side effects/adverse reactions:
GU: Decreased libido, impotence,

gynecomastia, ejaculation disorders (rare)
Contraindications: Hypersensitivity, pregnancy (X), lactation, women, children
Precautions: Hepatic disease
Pharmacokinetics: Peak 2-3 hr, protein binding 99%; metabolized in liver by CYP3A4, excreted in feces; half-life 5 wk at steady state
Interactions:
• Increased dutasteride concentrations: ritonavir, ketoconazole, verapamil, diltiazem, cimetidine, ciprofloxacin, or other drugs metabolized by the CYP3A4 pathway
Lab test interferences:
Increase: TSH
Decrease: PSA

NURSING CONSIDERATIONS
Assess:
• For decreasing symptoms in BPH: decreasing urinary retention, frequency, urgency, nocturia
• PSA levels, urinary obstruction; determine the absence of urinary cancer before starting treatment
• Liver function studies: ALT, AST, bilirubin
Administer:
• Without regard to meals
🚫 Caps whole; do not break, open, or chew
Evaluate:
• Therapeutic response: Decreasing symptoms of BPH—decreased urinary frequency, retention, urgency, nocturia
Teach patient/family:
• To notify prescriber if therapeutic response decreases; if edema occurs
• Not to discontinue drug abruptly
• About changes in sex characteristics
• That men taking dutasteride should not donate blood for at least 6 mo after last dose, to prevent blood administration to pregnant female

---

Side effects: *italics* = common; ***bold italics*** = life-threatening

• That caps should not be handled by a pregnant woman because this drug can be absorbed through the skin

• That ejaculate volume may decrease during treatment; that drug rarely interferes with sexual function

---

eprosartan mesylate/ hydrochlorothiazide (Rx)

(ep-roh-sar′tan)
Teveten HCT

Func. class.: Antihypertensive
Chem. class.: Angiotensin II–receptor antagonist (Subtype AT₁)

Action: Blocks the vasoconstrictor and aldosterone-secreting effects of angiotensin II; selectively blocks the binding of angiotensin II to the AT_1 receptor found in tissues

Uses: Hypertension, alone or in combination with other antihypertensives

Dosage and routes:
• *Adult:* **PO** 600 mg qd; dose may be divided and given bid with total daily doses ranging from 400-800 mg

Available forms: Tabs 600 mg/12.5, 600 mg/25

Side effects/adverse reactions:
CNS: Dizziness, depression, fatigue, headache
CV: Chest pain
EENT: Sinusitis
GI: Diarrhea, dyspepsia, abdominal pain
GU: UTI
META: Hypertriglyceridemia
MS: Myalgia, arthralgia
RESP: Cough, upper respiratory infection, rhinitis, pharyngitis, viral infection

Contraindications: Hypersensitivity, pregnancy (D) 2nd and 3rd trimesters

Precautions: Hypersensitivity to ACE inhibitors; pregnancy (C) 1st trimester, lactation, children, elderly; renal, hepatic disease

Pharmacokinetics: Peak 1-2 hr, food delays absorption, protein binding 98%, moderate renal impairment increases drug levels by 30%, hepatic impairment increases levels by 40%, excreted in urine and feces

Interactions:
Unknown

Lab test interferences:
Decrease: Hgb
Increase: ALAT, ASAT, alk phosphatase

NURSING CONSIDERATIONS
Assess:
• B/P with position changes, pulse q4h; note rate, rhythm, quality
• Electrolytes: K, Na, Cl
• Baselines in renal, LFTs before therapy begins
• Edema in feet, legs qd
• Skin turgor, dryness of mucous membranes for hydration status

Administer:
• Without regard to meals

Evaluate:
• Therapeutic response: decreased B/P

Teach patient/family:
• To comply with dosage schedule, even if feeling better
• To notify prescriber of fever, swelling of hands or feet, chest pain
• That excessive perspiration, dehydration, diarrhea may lead to fall in blood pressure; consult prescriber if these occur
• That drug may cause dizziness, avoid hazardous activities until effect is known
• Not to take this medication if pregnant or breastfeeding, or have had an allergic reaction to this drug

---

◆ = Nursing alert   🌿 = Herb-drug interaction   🚫 = Do not crush

• To take missed dose as soon as possible, unless within 1 hr before next dose

---

ertapenem (Rx)
(er-tah-pen'em)
Invanz
Func. class.: Antiinfective-misc.
Chem. class.: Carbapenem

Action: Interferes with cell wall replication of susceptible organisms; osmotically unstable cell wall swells, bursts from osmotic pressure

Uses: Adult patients with moderate to severe infections caused by the following organisms: intraabdominal infections—*Escherichia coli, Clostridium clostridioforme, Eubacterium lentum, Peptostreptococcus* sp., *Bacteroides fragilis, Bacteroides distasonis, Bacteroides ovatus, Bacteroides thetaiotaomicron, Bacteroides uniformis;* complicated skin/skin structure infections—*Staphylococcus aureus* (methicillin-susceptible), *Streptococcus pyogenes, E. coli, Peptostreptococcus* sp.; community-acquired pneumonia—*Streptococcus pneumoniae* (penicillin-susceptible), *Haemophilus influenzae* (β-lactamase-negative), *Moraxella catarrhalis;* complicated UTI—*E. coli, Klebsiella pneumoniae;* acute pelvic infections—*Streptococcus agalactiae, E. coli, B. fragilis, Porphyromonas asaccharolytica, Peptostreptococcus* sp., *Prevotella bivia*

Dosage and routes:
Complicated intraabdominal infections
• *Adult:* **IV/IM** 1 g qd × 5-14 days
Complicated skin/skin structure infections
• *Adult:* **IV/IM** 1 g qd × 7-14 days

Community-acquired pneumonia
• *Adult:* **IV/IM** 1 g qd × 10-14 days
Complicated UTI
• *Adult:* **IV/IM** 1 g qd × 10-14 days
Acute pelvic infections
• *Adult:* **IV/IM** 1 g qd × 3-10 days
Available form: Pwd, lyophilized, 1 g
Side effects/adverse reactions:
CNS: Insomnia, *seizures*, dizziness, headache
GI: Diarrhea, nausea, vomiting, *pseudomembranous colitis*
GU: Vaginitis
INTEG: Rash, urticaria, *pruritus,* pain at inj site, *infused vein complication,* phlebitis/thrombophlebitis, erythema at inj site
RESP: Dyspnea, cough, pharyngitis, rales, respiratory distress
SYST: **Anaphylaxis**
Contraindications: Hypersensitivity to this drug or its components, to amide-type local anesthetics (IM only); anaphylactic reactions to β-lactams
Precautions: Pregnancy (B), lactation, elderly, children, renal disease
Pharmacokinetics:
IV: Onset immediate, peak dose dependent, half-life 4 hr, metabolized by liver, excreted in urine, feces, breast milk
Interactions:
• Increased ertapenem plasma levels: probenecid; do not coadminister
NURSING CONSIDERATIONS
Assess:
• Sensitivity to carbapenem antibiotics, other β-lactam antibiotics, penicillins
• Renal disease: lower dose may be required
• Bowel pattern qd: if severe diarrhea occurs, drug should be discontinued; may indicate pseudomembranous colitis
• For infection: temp, sputum, char-

---

acteristics of wound before, during, after treatment

◆ Allergic reactions, anaphylaxis; rash, urticaria, pruritus; may occur a few days after therapy begins

• Overgrowth of infection: perineal itching, fever, malaise, redness, pain, swelling, drainage, rash, diarrhea, change in cough or sputum

Administer:

• By IV or IM

• After C&S is taken

IM route

• Reconstitute 1 g vial of ertapenem with 3.2 ml of 1% lidocaine HCl without epinephrine, shake well

• Withdraw contents, administer deep IM in large muscle mass, use within 1 hr

IV route

• Do not coinfuse or mix with other medications; do not use diluents containing dextrose

• Reconstitute 1 g vial of ertapenem with either 10 ml of water for inj, 0.9% NaCl, or bacteriostatic water for inj

• Shake well to dissolve, transfer contents of reconstituted vial to 50 ml 0.9% NaCl inj

• Complete inf within 6 hr

Evaluate:

• Therapeutic response: negative C&S, absence of signs and symptoms of infection

Teach patient/family:

• To report severe diarrhea; may indicate pseudomembranous colitis

• To report overgrowth of infection: black, furry tongue, vaginal itching, foul-smelling stools

• To avoid breastfeeding; drug is excreted in breast milk

Treatment of overdose: Epinephrine, antihistamines; resuscitate if needed (anaphylaxis)

---

esomeprazole (℞)
(es'oh-mep'rah-zohl)
Nexium
Func. class.: Antiulcer, proton pump inhibitor
Chem. class.: Benzimidazole

Action: Suppresses gastric secretion by inhibiting hydrogen/potassium ATPase enzyme system in gastric parietal cell; characterized as gastric acid pump inhibitor, because it blocks final step of acid production

Uses: Gastroesophageal reflux disease (GERD), severe erosive esophagitis; treatment of active duodenal ulcers in combination with antiinfectives for *Helicobacter pylori* infection

Dosage and routes:

Active duodenal ulcers associated with **H. pylori**

• *Adult:* **PO** 40 mg qd × 10 days in combination with clarithromycin 500 mg bid × 10 days and amoxicillin 1000 mg bid × 10 days

GERD

• *Adult:* **PO** 20 or 40 mg qd × 4-8 wk

Available forms: Caps 20, 40 mg

Side effects/adverse reactions:

CNS: Headache, dizziness

GI: Diarrhea, flatulence, anorexia, dry mouth

RESP: Cough

INTEG: Rash, dry skin

GU: UTI, urinary frequency

MISC: Fatigue

Contraindications: Hypersensitivity

Precautions: Pregnancy (B), lactation, children, elderly

Pharmacokinetics: Eliminated in urine as metabolites and in feces; in elderly, elimination rate decreased, bioavailability increased

---

◆ = Nursing alert   🌿 = Herb-drug interaction   🚫 = Do not crush

Interactions:
• Increased serum levels of esomeprazole: flurazepam, triazolam
• Possible increased bleeding: warfarin
• Possible decreased diazepam clearance resulting in increased diazepam serum concentrations

NURSING CONSIDERATIONS
Assess:
• GI system: bowel sounds q8h, abdomen for pain, swelling, anorexia
• Hepatic enzymes: AST, ALT, alk phosphatase during treatment

Administer:
• At least 1 hr before eating
🚫 Capsule swallowed whole; do not break, crush, or chew

Evaluate:
• Therapeutic response: absence of epigastric pain, swelling, fullness

Teach patient/family:
• To report severe diarrhea; drug may have to be discontinued
• That diabetic patient should know hypoglycemia may occur
• To avoid hazardous activities; dizziness may occur
• To avoid alcohol, salicylates, ibuprofen; may cause GI irritation

---

fondaparinux (Ⓡ)
(fon-dah-pair′ih-nux)
Arixtra
Func. class.: Anticoagulant, antithrombotic
Chem. class.: Synthetic, selective factor Xa inhibitor

Action: Acts by antithrombin III (ATIII)-mediated selective inhibition of factor Xa; neutralization of factor Xa interrupts blood coagulation and inhibits thrombin formation; does not inactivate thrombin (activated factor II) or affect platelets

Uses: Prevention of deep-vein thrombosis, pulmonary emboli in hip and knee replacement, hip fracture surgery

Dosage and routes:
• *Adult:* **SC** 2.5 mg qd; after hemostasis established, initial dose is given 6-8 hr after surgery
Available forms: Inj 2.5 mg/0.5 ml single-dose syringe

Side effects/adverse reactions:
CNS: Fever, confusion, headache, dizziness, *insomnia*
INTEG: Local reaction—*rash,* pruritus, inj site bleeding
GI: Nausea, vomiting, diarrhea, dyspepsia, *constipation,* increased AST, ALT
GU: UTI, urinary retention
HEMA: Anemia, minor bleeding, purpura, hematoma, ***thrombocytopenia, major bleeding (intracranial, cerebral, retroperitoneal hemorrhage), postoperative hemorrhage***
INTEG: Increased wound drainage, bullous eruption
META: Hypokalemia
OTHER: Hypotension, pain, *edema*

Contraindications: Hypersensitivity to this drug, heparin, or pork; hemophilia, leukemia with bleeding, peptic ulcer disease, hemorrhagic stroke, surgery, thrombocytopenic purpura, weight <50 kg, severe renal disease (CrCl <30 ml/min), children

Precautions: Alcoholism, hepatic disease (severe), blood dyscrasias, heparin-induced thrombocytopenia, severe hypertension, subacute bacterial endocarditis, acute nephritis, lactation, pregnancy (B), elderly

Pharmacokinetics: Rapidly, completely absorbed; peak steady state 3 hr; distributed primarily in blood, does not bind to plasma proteins except 94% to ATIII; metabolism

---

* = Canada only   Side effects: *italics* = common; ***bold italics*** = life-threatening

unknown; eliminated unchanged in 72 hr in normal renal function

Interactions:

• Do not mix with other drugs or infusion fluids

• Discontinue use of other drugs that may increase the risk of hemorrhage before starting fondaparinux; monitor closely if coadministration is essential

NURSING CONSIDERATIONS

Assess:

• Blood studies (Hct, CBC, coagulation studies, platelets, occult blood in stools), anti-Xa; thrombocytopenia may occur

• For bleeding: gums, petechiae, ecchymosis, black tarry stools, hematuria; notify prescriber

• For neurologic symptoms in patients who have received spinal anesthesia

Administer:

• Alone; do not mix with other drugs or solutions

• For 5-9 days

• Only after screening patient for bleeding disorders

• SC only; do not give IM

SC route

• Check for discolored sol or sol with particulate; if present, do not give

• Begin 2 hr before surgery

• Administer to recumbent patient, rotate inj sites (left/right anterolateral, left/right posterolateral abdominal wall)

• Wipe surface of inj site with alcohol swab, twist plunger cap and remove, remove rigid needle guard by pulling straight off needle, do not aspirate, do not expel air bubble from surface

• Insert whole length of needle into skinfold held with thumb and forefinger

• When drug is injected, a soft click may be felt or heard

• Give at same time each day to maintain steady blood levels

• Avoid all IM injections that may cause bleeding

◆ Administer only this drug when ordered; not interchangeable with heparin

Perform/provide:

• Storage at 25° C (77° F); do not freeze

Evaluate:

• Therapeutic response: Prevention of deep vein thrombosis

Teach patient/family:

• To use soft-bristle toothbrush to avoid bleeding gums, to use electric razor

• To report any signs of bleeding: gums, under skin, urine, stools

• To avoid OTC drugs containing aspirin

---

formoterol fumarate (℞)

(for-moh'ter-ahl fyoo'mah-rayt)
Foradil Aerolizer
Func. class.: β-Adrenergic agonist
Chem. class.: Sympathomimetic catecholamine

Action: Has β_1 and β_2 action; relaxes bronchial smooth muscle and dilates the trachea and main bronchi by increasing levels of cAMP, which relaxes smooth muscles; causes increased contractility and heart rate by acting on β-receptors in heart

Uses: Maintenance treatment of asthma, prevention of exercise-induced bronchospasm

Dosage and routes:

Maintenance treatment of asthma

• *Adult/child ≥5 yr:* INH AM and PM long term 1 cap q12h using aerolizer inhaler

---

◆ = Nursing alert　　🖊 = Herb-drug interaction　　🚫 = Do not crush

Prevention of exercise-induced bronchospasm

• *Adult/child ≥12 yr:* prn occasionally 1 cap at least 15 min before exercise

Available form: INH pwd in cap 12 µg

Side effects/adverse reactions:

CNS: Tremors, anxiety, insomnia, headache, dizziness, stimulation

CV: Palpitations, tachycardia, hypertension

GI: Nausea, vomiting

RESP: Bronchial irritation, dryness of oropharynx, ***bronchospasms*** (overuse)

Contraindications: Hypersensitivity to sympathomimetics, narrow-angle glaucoma

Precautions: Pregnancy (C), cardiac disorders, hyperthyroidism, diabetes mellitus, prostatic hypertrophy, elderly

Pharmacokinetics:

INH: Onset 15 min

Metabolized in liver, lungs, GI tract

Interactions:

• Increased effects of both drugs: other sympathomimetics

• Decreased action when used with β-blockers

NURSING CONSIDERATIONS

Assess:

• Respiratory function: B/P, pulse, lung sounds

• I&O ratio; check for urinary retention, frequency, hesitancy

• For paresthesias and coldness of extremities; peripheral blood flow may decrease

Perform/provide:

• Storage at room temperature, protection from heat, moisture; do not use discolored solution

Evaluate:

• Therapeutic response: ease of breathing

Teach patient/family:

• To rinse mouth after use

• Correct use of inhaler; review package insert with patient; to avoid getting aerosol in eyes; to wash inhaler in warm water and dry qd

• Use of spacer device in elderly or children

• About all aspects of drug; to avoid smoking, smoke-filled rooms, persons with respiratory infections

Treatment of overdose: Administration of a β-blocker

---

frovatriptan (R)

(froh-vah-trip′tan)

Frova

Func. class.: Antimigraine agent

Chem. class.: 5-HT₁-Receptor agonist

Action: Binds selectively to the vascular 5-HT₁B, 5-HT₁D receptor subtypes, exerts antimigraine effect; binds to benzodiazepine receptor sites

Uses: Acute treatment of migraine with or without aura

Dosage and routes:

• *Adult:* **PO** 2.5 mg, a 2nd dose may be taken after ≥2 hr; max 3 tabs (7.5 mg/day)

Available form: Tabs 2.5 mg

Side effects/adverse reactions:

CNS: Hot sensation, paresthesia, *dizziness,* headache, fatigue, cold sensation

CV: Flushing, MI, chest pain

GI: Dry mouth, dyspepsia

INTEG: Photosensitivity

MS: Skeletal pain

Contraindications: Angina pectoris, history of MI, documented silent ischemia, Prinzmetal's angina, ischemic heart disease; concurrent ergotamine-containing preparations; uncontrolled hypertension; hypersensitivity; basilar or hemiplegic migraine; ischemic bowel disease; peripheral vascular disease

Precautions: Postmenopausal women, men >40 yr, risk factors for CAD, hypercholesterolemia, obesity, diabetes, impaired hepatic function, pregnancy (C), lactation, children, elderly

Pharmacokinetics: Onset of pain relief 10 min–2 hr, terminal half-life 25-29 hr, protein binding 15%

Interactions:

• Extended vasospastic effects: ergot, ergot derivatives, other 5-HT$_1$ agonists

• Increased frovatriptan effect: oral contraceptives, propranolol

• Weakness, incoordination, hyperreflexia: SSRIs

NURSING CONSIDERATIONS

Assess:

• B/P; signs/symptoms of coronary vasospasms

• For stress level, activity, recreation, coping mechanisms

• Neurologic status: LOC, paresthesia, hot/cold sensations, dizziness, headache, fatigue

• Ingestion of tyramine-containing foods (pickled products, beer, wine, aged cheese), food additives, preservatives, colorings, artificial sweeteners, chocolate, caffeine, which may precipitate these types of headaches

Administer:

🚫 PO, swallow whole

Perform/provide:

• Quiet, calm environment with decreased stimulation from noise, bright light, excessive talking

Evaluate:

• Therapeutic response: decrease in frequency, severity of migraine

Teach patient/family:

• To report any side effects to prescriber

• To use sunscreen, wear protective clothing because of increased photosensitivity

• To use contraception while taking drug

• To have dark, quiet environment available

---

galantamine (℞)

(gah-lan'tah-meen)
Reminyl
Func. class.: Cholinesterase inhibitor

Action: May enhance cholinergic functioning by increasing acetylcholine

Uses: Alzheimer's dementia

Dosage and routes:

• *Adult:* **PO** 4 mg bid; after 4 wk or more may increase to 8 mg bid; may increase to 12 mg bid after another 4 wk

Available forms: Tabs 4, 8, 12 mg

Side effects/adverse reactions:

CNS: Tremors, insomnia, depression, dizziness, headache, somnolence, fatigue

CV: Bradycardia, anemia, hematuria

GI: Nausea, vomiting, anorexia, abdominal distress, flatulence, diarrhea

GU: Urinary incontinence

META: Weight decrease

MS: Asthenia

RESP: URI, rhinitis

Contraindications: Hypersensitivity to this drug

Precautions: Renal disease, hepatic disease, respiratory disease, seizure disorder, peptic ulcer, pregnancy (B), asthma, lactation, children

Pharmacokinetics: Rapidly and completely absorbed, metabolized by CYP450 enzyme, excreted via kidneys, clearance is lowered in the

---

🔶 = Nursing alert   🖊 = Herb-drug interaction   🚫 = Do not crush

APPENDIX

elderly, hepatic disease; clearance is 20% lower in females
Interactions:
• Synergistic effect: cholinomimetics, other cholinesterase inhibitors
• Increased galantamine bioavailability: cimetidine, paroxetine, ketoconazole, erythromycin
NURSING CONSIDERATIONS
Assess:
• Liver function enzymes: AST, ALT, alk phosphatase, LDH, bilirubin, CBC
• For severe GI effects: nausea, vomiting, anorexia, weight loss
• B/P, respiration during initial treatment
• Mental status: affect, mood, behavioral changes, depression
Administer:
• With meals; take with morning and evening meal
Perform/provide:
• Assistance with ambulation during beginning therapy
• Complete suicide assessment
Evaluate:
• Therapeutic response: decreased confusion
Teach patient/family:
• Correct procedure for giving oral solution, using instruction sheet provided
• To notify prescriber of severe GI effects
• To report hypo/hypertension

---

imatinib (℞)
(im-ah-tin′ib)
Gleevec
Func. class.: Antineoplastic, misc.
Chem. class.: Protein-tyrosine kinase inhibitor

Action: Inhibits Bcr-Abl tyrosine kinase created in chronic myeloid leukemia (CML)
Uses: Treatment of CML
Dosage and routes:
• *Adult:* **PO** 400 mg/day (chronic phase); 600 mg/day (accelerated phase/blast crisis); give with meal or large glass of water, continue as long as response is good, may increase by 200 mg/day as needed
Available form: Cap 100 mg
Side effects/adverse reactions:
CV: Hemorrhage
*CNS: **CNS hemorrhage,** headache*
*GI: Nausea, **hepatotoxicity,** vomiting, dyspepsia, **GI hemorrhage,** anorexia*
*HEMA: **Neutropenia, thrombocytopenia***
INTEG: Rash, pruritus
META: Fluid retention, hypokalemia, weight increase, edema
MISC: Fatigue, epistaxis, pyrexia, night sweats
MS: Cramps, pain, arthralgia, myalgia
RESP: Cough, dyspnea, nasopharyngitis, pneumonia
Contraindications: Hypersensitivity, pregnancy (D)
Precautions: Lactation, children, elderly
Pharmacokinetics: Half-life 18-40 hr
Interactions:
• Increased imatinib concentrations: ketoconazole, itraconazole, erythromycin, clarithromycin

---

• Decreased imatinib concentrations: dexamethasone, phenytoin, carbamazepine, rifampin, phenobarbital
• Increased plasma concentrations of simvastatin and dihydropyridine calcium channel blockers
• Increased plasma concentration of warfarin; avoid use with warfarin, use low-molecular-weight anticoagulants instead

🌿 Decreased imatinib concentration: St. John's wort

NURSING CONSIDERATIONS
Assess:
• ANC and platelets; in chronic phase if ANC <1 ×10⁹/L and/or platelets <50× 10⁹/L, stop until ANC >1.5 × 10⁹/L and platelets >75 × 10⁹/L; in accelerated phase/blast crisis if ANC <0.5 × 10⁹/L and/or platelets <10 × 10⁹/L, determine whether cytopenia is related to biopsy/aspirate, if not, reduce dose by 200 mg, if cytopenia continues, reduce dose by another 100 mg; if cytopenia continues for 4 wk, stop drug until ANC ≥1 × 10⁹/L
• For hepatotoxicity: monitor LFTs, before treatment and qmo
• CBC, differential, platelet count weekly; withhold drug if WBC is <3500/mm³, or platelet count <100,000/mm³; notify prescriber of these results; drug should be discontinued
• Food preferences: list likes, dislikes
• GI symptoms: frequency of stools
• Signs of fluid retention, edema: weigh, monitor lung sounds, assess for edema
Administer:
• With meal and large glass of water
Perform/provide:
• Nutritious diet with iron, vitamin supplement, low fiber, few dairy products
• Storage at 25° C (77° F)

Evaluate:
• Therapeutic response: decrease in spread of cancer
Teach patient/family:
• To report adverse reactions immediately: SOB, swelling of extremities, bleeding

---

nesiritide (℞)
(neh-seer'ih-tide)
Natrecor
Func. class.: Vasodilator
Chem. class.: Human B-type natriuretic peptide

Action: Uses DNA technology; human B-type natriuretic peptide binds to the receptor in vascular smooth muscle and endothelial cells, leading to smooth muscle relaxation
Uses: Acutely decompensated CHF
Dosage and routes:
• *Adult:* **IV** 2 µg/kg, then **IV INF** 0.01 µg/kg/min
Available forms: Pwd for inj, 1.5 mg single-use vial
Side effects/adverse reactions:
CNS: Headache, insomnia, dizziness, anxiety, confusion, paresthesia, tremor
*CV: Hypotension, **tachycardia,** dysrhythmias, bradycardia, ventricular tachycardia, ventricular extrasystoles, atrial fibrillation
GI: Vomiting, nausea
INTEG: Rash, sweating, pruritus, inj site reaction
MISC: Abdominal pain, back pain
RESP: Increased cough, hemaptysis, apnea
Contraindications: Hypersensitivity, cardiogenic shock or B/P <90 mm Hg as primary therapy
Precautions: Pregnancy (C); mitral stenosis; significant valvular stenosis, restriction, or obstructive car-

◆ = Nursing alert 🌿 = Herb-drug interaction 🚫 = Do not crush

diomyopathy, or any condition that is dependent upon venous return; renal disease, lactation, children
Pharmacokinetics: Half-life 18 min
Interactions:
• Increased symptomatic hypotension with ACE inhibitors
NURSING CONSIDERATIONS
Assess:
• PCWP, RAP, cardiac index, MPAP
• B/P, pulse during treatment until stable
Administer:
• Do not administer nesiritide through a central heparin-coated catheter; heparin should be administered through a separate catheter
• Prime IV fluid with infusion of 25 ml before connecting to patient's vascular access port and before bolus dose or IV infusion
• Reconstitute one 1.5 mg vial/5 ml of diluent from prefilled 250-ml plastic IV bag with diluent of choice (D$_5$, 0.9% NaCl, D$_5$/½ NaCl, D$_5$/0.2% NaCl); do not shake vial, roll gently; use only clear sol
• Withdraw all contents of reconstituted vial and add to the 250-ml plastic IV bag (6 μg/ml), invert bag several times
• Use within 24 hr of reconstituting
Evaluate:
• Therapeutic response: improvement in CHF with improved PCWP, RAP, MPAP

RARELY USED

perflutren lipid microsphere (℞)
(per-flu'tren)
Definity
Func. class.: Diagnostic drug

Uses: Contrast enhancement during echocardiographic procedures
Dosage and routes:
Use only after activation in the Vialmix apparatus
• *Adult:* **IV BOL** 10 μl/kg of the activated product within 30-60 sec, followed by 10-ml saline flush, may repeat
• *Adult:* **IV INF** 1.3 ml/50 ml preservative-free saline, give at 4 ml/min, not to exceed 10 ml/min
Contraindications: Hypersensitivity to octafluoropropane, known cardiac shunts, administration by direct intraarterial inj

tenofovir disoproxil fumarate (℞)
(ten-oh-foh'veer dis-oh-prox'il fyoo'mah-rate)
Viread
Func. class.: Antiretroviral
Chem. class.: Nucleoside analog reverse transcriptase inhibitor

Action: Inhibits replication of HIV virus by competing with the natural substrate and then incorporating into cellular DNA by viral reverse transcriptase, thereby terminating cellular DNA chain
Uses: HIV-1 infection with other antiretrovirals
Dosage and routes:
• *Adult:* **PO** 300 mg with meal; if

used with didanosine, give tenofovir 2 hr before or 1 hr after
didanosine
Available form: Tabs 300 mg: (300
mg of fumarate salt equivalent to
245 mg tenofovir disoproxil)
Side effects/adverse reactions:
CNS: Headache
GI: Nausea, vomiting, diarrhea, anorexia, *flatulence, abdominal pain*
SYST: Change in body fat distribution
Contraindications: Hypersensitivity
Precautions: Pregnancy (B), lactation, children, elderly, renal disease,
hepatic insufficiency
Pharmacokinetics: Rapidly absorbed, distributed to extravascular
space, excreted unchanged in urine
Interactions:
• Increased level of tenofovir: cidofovir, acyclovir, valacyclovir, gan-
ciclovir, valganciclovir
• Increased level of didanosine when
given with tenofovir
• Increased level of tenofovir: any
drug that decreases renal function
NURSING CONSIDERATIONS
Assess:
• Liver studies: AST, ALT, biliru-
bin; amylase, lipase, triglycerides
periodically during treatment
• For bone, renal toxicity: if bone
abnormalities are suspected, obtain
tests; serum phosphorus, creatinine
• For lactic acidosis, severe hepa-
tomegaly with steatosis
Administer:
• PO qd with meal
Perform/provide:
• Storage at 25° C (77° F)
Evaluate:
• Therapeutic response: Decrease in
signs/symptoms of HIV
Teach patient/family:
• To take this drug 2 hr before or 1
hr after taking didanosine (if used)
• To take with meal

• That GI complaints resolve after
3-4 wk of treatment
• Not to breastfeed while taking this
drug
• That drug must be taken qd even
if patient feels better
• That follow-up visits must be continued because serious toxicity may
occur; blood counts must be done
q2wk
• That drug will control symptoms
but is not a cure for HIV; patient is
still infectious, may pass HIV virus
on to others
• That other drugs may be necessary to prevent other infections
• That changes in body fat distribution may occur

---

valdecoxib (℞)
(val-deh-cock′sib)
Bextra
Func. class.: Nonsteroidal anti-
inflammatory
Chem. class.: COX-2 inhibitor

Action: Inhibits prostaglandin synthesis by decreasing COX-2 en-
zyme needed for biosynthesis; an-
algesic, antiinflammatory, antipy-
retic properties
Uses: Acute, chronic rheumatoid ar-
thritis, osteoarthritis, primary dys-
menorrhea
Dosage and routes:
*Osteoarthritis/adult rheumatoid ar-
thritis*
• *Adult:* **PO** 10 mg
Primary dysmenorrhea
• *Adult:* **PO** 20 mg bid, prn
Available forms: Tabs 10, 20 mg
Side effects/adverse reactions:
*CNS: Fatigue, anxiety, depression,
nervousness, paresthesia,* dizziness,
insomnia
*CV: **Tachycardia**, angina, **MI**,* pal-

◆ = Nursing alert   🖉 = Herb-drug interaction   🚫 = Do not crush

pitations, dysrhythmias, hypertension, fluid retention

EENT: Tinnitus, hearing loss, blurred vision, glaucoma, cataract, conjunctivitis, eye pain

GI: Nausea, anorexia, vomiting, constipation, dry mouth, diverticulitis, gastritis, gastroenteritis, hemorrhoids, hiatal hernia, stomatitis, *GI bleeding*

GU: Nephrotoxicity: dysuria, hematuria, oliguria, azotemia, cystitis, UTI

HEMA: Blood dyscrasias, epistaxis, bruising, anemia

INTEG: Purpura, rash, pruritus, sweating, erythema, petechiae, photosensitivity, alopecia

RESP: Pharyngitis, shortness of breath, pneumonia, coughing

Contraindications: Hypersensitivity to this drug, aspirin, iodides, other NSAIDs, sulfonamides; 3rd trimester of pregnancy, asthma triad, asthma, pregnancy 3rd trimester (D)

Precautions: Pregnancy 1st/2nd trimester (C), lactation; bleeding; GI, cardiac, renal, hepatic disorders; hypersensitivity to other antiinflammatory agents, glucocorticoids, anticoagulants; hypertension, severe dehydration, elderly, children <18 yr

Pharmacokinetics: Well absorbed; peak 3 hr, delayed 1-2 hr by high-fat meal; 98% bound to plasma proteins; half-life 8-11 hr; metabolized in liver by P450 and non-P450 systems, excreted in urine (metabolites, 70%)

Interactions:
• Increased effect of: anticoagulants
• Decreased effect of: aspirin, ACE inhibitors, thiazide diuretics, furosemide
• Increased adverse reactions: glucocorticoids, NSAIDs, aspirin
• Increased toxicity: lithium, antineoplastics
• Increased valdecoxib blood level: fluconazole, ketoconazole

NURSING CONSIDERATIONS
Assess:
• For pain of rheumatoid arthritis, osteoarthritis; check ROM, inflammation of joints, characteristics of pain
• Blood counts during therapy; watch for decreasing platelets; if low, therapy may need to be discontinued, restarted after hematologic recovery
◆ For blood dyscrasias (thrombocytopenia): bruising, fatigue, bleeding, poor healing

Administer:
PO
• With food or milk to decrease gastric symptoms, do not increase dose

Evaluate:
• Therapeutic response: decreased pain, inflammation in arthritic conditions, decreased dysmenorrhea

Teach patient/family:
• To check with prescriber to determine when drug should be discontinued before surgery
• That drug must be continued for prescribed time to be effective; to avoid other NSAIDs, aspirin, sulfonamides
• To notify prescriber if pregnancy is planned or suspected
• To notify prescriber of GI symptoms: black, tarry stools; cramping or rash; edema of extremities, weight gain
• To report bleeding, bruising, fatigue, malaise because blood dyscrasias do occur
• To take with a full glass of water to enhance absorption

valganciclovir (℞)
(val-gan-sy'kloh-veer)
Valcyte
Func. class.: Antiviral
Chem. class.: Synthetic nucleo-side analog

Action: Valganciclovir is metabo-lized to ganciclovir; inhibits repli-cation of human cytomegalovirus in vivo and in vitro by selective inhi-bition of viral DNA synthesis

Uses: Cytomegalovirus (CMV) ret-initis in immunocompromised per-sons, including those with AIDS, after indirect ophthalmoscopy con-firms diagnosis

Dosage and routes:
• *Adult:* **PO** induction 900 mg bid × 21 days with food; maintenance 900 mg qd with food

Renal dose
• Reduce dose; CrCl ≥60 ml/min same as above; CrCl 40-59 ml/min 450 mg bid, then 450 mg qd; CrCl 25-39 ml/min 450 mg qd, then 450 mg q2 days; CrCl 10-24 ml/min 450 mg q2 days, then 450 mg 2×/ week

Available form: Tab 450 mg

Side effects/adverse reactions:
CNS: Fever, chills, ***coma,*** convul-sion, *confusion,* abnormal thoughts, dizziness, bizarre dreams, *headache,* psychosis, tremors, somnolence, *paresthesia, weakness, seizures*
EENT: Retinal detachment in CMV retinitis
GI: Abnormal LFTs, nausea, vom-iting, anorexia, diarrhea, abdomi-nal pain, ***hemorrhage***
GU: ***Hematuria,*** increased creati-nine; BUN
HEMA: ***Granulocytopenia, throm-bocytopenia, irreversible neutrope-nia, anemia, eosinophilia***
INTEG: Rash, alopecia, *pruritus,* ur-ticaria, pain at site, phlebitis

MISC: Local and systemic infec-tions and sepsis
Contraindications: Hypersensitiv-ity to acyclovir or ganciclovir, ab-solute neutrophil count <500, plate-let count <25,000, hemodialysis
Precautions: Preexisting cytope-nias, renal function impairment, pregnancy (C), lactation, children <6 mo, elderly
Pharmacokinetics: Metabolized to ganciclovir, which has a half-life of 3-4½ hr, excreted by kidneys (un-changed); crosses blood-brain bar-rier, CSF

Interactions:
• Decreased renal clearance of val-ganciclovir: probenecid
• Increased toxicity: dapsone, pent-amidine, flucytosine, vincristine, vinblastine, adriamycin, doxorubi-cin, amphotericin B, trimethoprim-sulfamethoxazole combinations or other nucleoside analogs, cyclospor-ine
• Severe granulocytopenia: zidovu-dine, antineoplastics, radiation; do not give together
• Increased seizures: imipenem/ cilastatin

NURSING CONSIDERATIONS
Assess:
• For leukopenia/neutropenia/throm-bocytopenia: WBCs, platelets q2d during 2×/day dosing and then q1wk
• For leukopenia with qd WBC count in patients with prior leukopenia with other nucleoside analogs or for whom leukopenia counts are <1000 cells/mm^3 at start of treatment
• Serum creatinine or CrCl ≥q2wk
Administer:
PO
• With food
Evaluate:
• Therapeutic response: decreased symptoms of CMV

◆ = Nursing alert   ∥ = Herb-drug interaction   ⊘ = Do not crush

Teach patient/family:

• That drug does not cure condition, that regular ophthalmologic examinations are necessary

• That major toxicities may necessitate discontinuing drug

• To use contraception during treatment and that infertility may occur; men should use barrier contraception for 90 days after treatment

• To take with food

◆ To report infection: fever, chills, sore throat; blood dyscrasias: bruising, bleeding, petechiae

• To avoid crowds, persons with respiratory infections

• To use sunscreen to prevent burns

---

zoledronic acid (℞)

(zoh'leh-drah'nick ass'id)

Zometa

Func. class.: Bone-resorption inhibitor, electrolyte modifier

Chem. class.: Bisphosphonate

Action: Potent inhibitor of osteoclastic bone resorption; inhibits osteoclastic activity, reduces bone resorption and inhibits skeletal calcium release caused by stimulating factors released by tumors; reduction of abnormal bone resorption is responsible for therapeutic effect in hypercalcemia; may directly block dissolution of hydroxyapatite bone crystals; inhibits normal and abnormal bone resorption, apparently without inhibiting bone formation and mineralization

Uses: Moderate to severe hypercalcemia associated with malignancy

Dosage and routes:

• *Adult:* **IV INF** 4 mg, given as a single infusion over ≥15 min, may re-treat with 4 mg if serum calcium does not return to normal within 1 wk

Available form: Pwd for inj 4 mg

Side effects/adverse reactions:

CV: Hypertension

GI: Abdominal pain, anorexia, constipation, nausea, diarrhea

GU: UTI, fluid overload, possible reduced renal function

INTEG: Redness, swelling, induration, pain on palpation at site of catheter insertion

META: Anemia, hypokalemia, hypomagnesemia, hypophosphatemia

MISC: Fever, chills, arthralgias, myalgias, flulike symptoms

MS: Bone pain

Contraindications: Hypersensitivity to bisphosphonates

Precautions: Children, nursing mothers, pregnancy (C), renal dysfunction, asthma-sensitive asthmatic patients

Pharmacokinetics: Rapidly cleared from circulation and taken up mainly by bones, not metabolized, eliminated primarily by kidneys; approximately 50% is eliminated in urine within 24 hr of administration

Interactions:

• Hypomagnesemia, hypokalemia: digoxin

• Decreased effect of zoledronic acid: calcium, vit D

• Decreased serum calcium, increased potential for renal toxicity: aminoglycosides

• Do not mix with Ca-containing infusion sol such as lactated Ringer's sol

NURSING CONSIDERATIONS

Assess:

• Renal studies and Ca, P, Mg, K

• For hypercalcemia: paresthesia, twitching, laryngospasm; Chvostek's, Trousseau's signs

Administer:

• Saline hydration must be performed before administration; urine output should be 2 L/day during treatment, do not overhydrate

---

IV

• Administer after reconstituting by adding 5 ml of sterile water for inj to each vial, then add to ≥100 ml of sterile 0.9% NaCl, D$_5$, run over ≥5 min

• Administer in separate IV line from all other drugs

Perform/provide:

• Sol reconstituted with sterile water may be stored under refrigeration for up to 24 hr

Evaluate:

• Therapeutic response: decreased Ca levels

Teach patient/family:

• To report hypercalcemic relapse: nausea, vomiting, bone pain, thirst

• To continue with dietary recommendations including calcium and vit D

◆ = Nursing alert ◢ = Herb-drug interaction ⊘ = Do not crush

Appendix b

Recent FDA drug approvals

Generic name	Trade name	Use
pegfilgrastin	Neulasta	Decreasing infection in febrile neutropenia
pimecrolimus	Elidel	Atopic dermatitis
thyrotropin alfa	Thyrogen	Diagnostic tool for serum Tg testing

Appendix C

Ophthalmic, otic, nasal, and topical products

OPHTHALMIC PRODUCTS

α-ADRENERGIC BLOCKER
dapiprazole (R)
(da-pip'ra-zole)
Rev-Eyes

ANESTHETICS
proparacaine (R)
(proe-par'a-kane)
AK-Taine, Alcaine, Diocane*,
Ocu-Caine, Ophthaine,
Ophthestic, Spectro-Caine
tetracaine (R)
(tet'ra-kane)
Minims Tetracaine,
Pontocaine Eye, Pontocaine
HCl, tetracaine

ANTIHISTAMINES
emedastine (R)
(ee-med'ah-steen)
Emadine
levocabastine (R)
(lee-voh-cab'ah-steen)
Livostin
olopatadine (R)
(oh-loh-pat'ah-deen)
Patanol

ANTIINFECTIVES
bacitracin (R)
(bass-i-tray'sin)
AK-Tracin, Bacitracin
Ophthalmic

brimonidine (R)
(bri-moe'ni-deen)
Alphagan
chloramphenicol (R)
(klor-am-fen'i-kole)
AK-Chlor, Chloramphenicol,
Chloramphenicol
Ophthalmic, Chloromycetin
Ophthalmic, Chloroptic,
Chloroptic S.O.P., Fenicol*,
Isopto Fenical*, Pentamycin*
ciprofloxacin (R)
(sip-ro-floks'a-sin)
Ciloxan
erythromycin (R)
(er-ith-roe-mye'sin)
AK-Mycin, Erythromycin,
Ilotycin
gentamicin (R)
(jen-ta-mye'sin)
Garamycin Ophthalmic,
Genoptic Ophthalmic,
Genoptic S.O.P., Gentacidin,
Gent-AK, gentamicin,
Gentamicin Ophthalmic
Liquifilm, Gentak
idoxuridine-IDU (R)
(eye-dox-yoor'i-deen)
Herplex, Stoxil
levofloxacin (R)
(lee-voh-floks'a-sin)
Quixin
natamycin (R)
(nat-a-mye'sin)
Natacyn

◆ = Nursing alert   ⫽ = Herb-drug interaction   ⊘ = Do not crush

norfloxacin (R)
(nor-floks'a-sin)
Chibroxin, Ofloxacin, Ocuflox

ofloxacin (R)
(oh-flox'a-sin)
Ocuflox

polymyxin B (R)
(pol-ee-mix'in)
Aerosporin, polymyxin B
sulfate

silver nitrate 1% (R)
sulfacetamide
sodium (R)
(sul-fa-seet'a-mide)
AK-Sulf, Bleph-10 Liquifilm,
Bleph-10 S.O.P., Isopto
Cetamide, Ophthacet,
Sodium Sulamyd, sodium
sulfacetamide 10%, sodium
sulfacetamide 15%, sodium
sulfacetamide 30%, SOSS-10,
Sulfair 15

tetracycline (R)
(tet-ra-sye'kleen)
Achromycin Ophthalmic

tobramycin (R)
(toe-bra-mye'sin)
Tobrex

trifluridine (R)
(trye-floor'i-deen)
Viroptic

vidarabine (R)
(vye-dare'a-been)
Vira-A

β-ADRENERGIC BLOCKERS
betaxolol (R)
(beh-tax'oh-lole)
Betoptic, Betoptic 5

carteolol (R)
(kar-tee'oh-lole)
Ocupress

levobetaxolol (R)
(lee-voh-beh-tax'oh-lole)
Betaxon

levobunolol (R)
(lee-voe-byoo'no-lole)
Betagen

metipranolol (R)
(met-ee-pran'oh-lole)
Optipranolol

timolol (R)
(tye'moe-lole)
Apo-Timop*, Betimol,
Timoptic

CHOLINERGICS
(Direct-acting)
carbachol (R)
(kar'ba-kole)
Iosopto Carbachol, Miostat

pilocarpine (R)
(pye-loe-kar'peen)
Adsorbocarpine, Akarpine,
Isopto Carpine, Ocu-Carpine,
Ocusert-Pilo, Pilagan, Pilocar,
pilocarpine, Pilopine HS,
Piloptic-1, Piloptic-2, Pilostat,
Pilopto-Carpine

CHOLINESTERASE
INHIBITORS
demecarium (R)
(dem-e-kare'ee-um)
Humorsol

ecothiophate (R)
(ek-oh-thye'eh-fate)
Ecostigmine Iodide,
Phospholine Iodide

isoflurophate (R)
(eye-soe-floor'oh-fate)
Floropryl

physostigmine (R)
(fi-zoe-stig'meen)
Eserine Salicylate, Isopto
Eserin

CYCLOPLEGIC MYDRIATICS

atropine (Ŗ)
(a'troe-peen)
Atropine-1, Atropine Care Ophthalmic, Atropine Sulfate Ophthalmic, Atropine Sulfate S.O.P., Atropisol, Isopto Atropine

cyclopentolate (Ŗ)
(sye-kloe-pen'toe-late)
AK-Pentolate, Cyclogly, I-Pentolate

homatropine (Ŗ)
(home-a'troe-peen)
AK-Homatropine, I-Homatrine, Isopto Homatropine, Minims Homatropine*, Spectro-Homatropine

physostigmine (Ŗ)
(fi-zoe-stig'meen)
Fisostin, Isopto Eserine Solution/Eserine Sulfate Ointment

scopolamine (Ŗ)
(skoe-pol'a-meen)
Isopto-Hyoscine

tropicamide (Ŗ)
(troe-pik'a-mide)
Mydriacyl, Tropicacyl, I-Piramide

GLUCOCORTICOIDS

dexamethasone (Ŗ)
(dex-a-meth'a-sone)
AK-Dex, Decadron Phosphate, Dexamethasone Ophthalmic Suspension, Maxidex

fluorometholone (Ŗ)
(flure-oh-meth'oh-lone)
Flarex, Fluor-Op, FML, FML Forte, FML Liquifilm

medrysone (Ŗ)
(me'dri-sone)
HMS

prednisolone (Ŗ)
(pred-niss'oh-lone)
Econopred, Econopred Plus, AK-Pred, Inflamase Forte, Inflamase Mild Ophthalmic, Metreton Ophthalmic, Pred-Forte, Pred-Mild

rimexolone (Ŗ)
(ri-mex'a-lone)
Vexol

NONSTEROIDAL ANTIINFLAMMATORIES

diclofenac (Ŗ)
(dye-kloe'fen-ak)
Voltaren

flurbiprofen (Ŗ)
(flure-bih-proh'fen)
Ocufen

ketorolac (Ŗ)
(kee-toe'role-ak)
Acular

suprofen (Ŗ)
(soo-proe'fen)
Profenal

SYMPATHOMIMETICS

apraclonidine (Ŗ)
(a-pra-klon'i-deen)
Lopidine

brimonidine (Ŗ)
(brih-moh'nih-deen)
Alphagan

dipivefrin (Ŗ)
(dye-pi'vef-rin)
Propine

epinephrine bitartrate/epinephrine HCl/epinephryl borate (Ŗ)
(ep-i-nef'rin)
Epitrate, Mytrate/Epifrin, Glaucon/Epinal, Eppy*

◆ = Nursing alert　　〃 = Herb-drug interaction　　🚫 = Do not crush

OPHTHALMIC DECONGESTANTS/ VASOCONSTRICTORS

naphazoline (OTC, R̥)

(naf-az'oh-leen)

AK-Con Ophthalmic, Albalon Liquifilm Ophthalmic, Allerest Eye Drops, Clear Eyes, Comfort Eye Drops, Degest 2, Nafazair, naphazoline HCl, Naphcon, Naphcon Forte, Opcon, Vasoclear, Vasocon Regular, Estivin II

oxymetazoline (R̥)

(ox-i-meth'oh-lone)

OcuClear, Visine, LR

phenylephrine (OTC)

(fen-ill-ef'rin)

AK-Dilate Ophthalmic, AK-Nefrin Ophthalmic, Isopto Frin, Neo-Synephrine 2.5%, Neo-Synephrine 10% Plain, Neo-Synephrine Viscous, phenylephrine HCl, 2.5% Mydfrin Ophthalmic, Phenoptic Relief, Prefrin

tetrahydrozoline (OTC)

(tet-ra-hye-dro'zoe-leen)

Collyrium Fresh Eye Drops, Eyesine, Murine Plus Eye Drops, Optigene 3 Eye Drops, Soothe Eye Drops, tetrahydrozoline HCl, Tyzine HCl, Tyzine Pediatric, Visine Eye Drops

MISCELLANEOUS OPHTHALMICS

bimatoprost

(by-mat'oh-prahst)

Lumigan

brinzolamide (R̥)

(brin-zoh'la-mide)

Azopt

latanoprost

(la-tan'oh-proest)

Xalatan

dorzolamide (R̥)

(dor-zol'a-mide)

Trusopt

ketotifen (R̥)

(kee-toh-tif'en)

Zaditor

lodoxamide

(loe-dox'a-mide)

Alomide

travoprost

(trav'oh-prahst)

Travatan

unoprostone (R̥)

(un-oh-proe'stone)

Rescula

Pregnancy categories: Demecarium, isoflurophate (X); apraclonidine, cyclopentolate, ecothiophate, glucocorticoids, levobunalol, metipranolol, pilocarpine, proparacaine, suprofen, tetracaine (C); dapiprazole, dipivefrin (B)

β-*Adrenergic blockers*

Action: Reduces production of aqueous humor by unknown mechanism

Uses: Ocular hypertension, chronic open-angle glaucoma

Anesthetics

Action: Decreases ion permeability by stabilizing neuronal membrane

Uses: Cataract extraction, tonometry, gonioscopy, removal of foreign objects, corneal suture removal, glaucoma surgery (ophth); pruritus, sunburn, toothache, sore throat, cold sores, oral pain, rectal pain and irritation, control of gagging (top)

Antiinfectives

Action: Inhibits folic acid synthesis by preventing PABA use, which is necessary for bacterial growth

---

Uses: Conjunctivitis, superficial eye infections, corneal ulcers, prophylaxis against infection after removal of foreign matter from the eye

Antiinflammatories

Action: Decreases inflammation, resulting in decreased pain, photophobia, hyperemia, cellular infiltration

Uses: Inflammation of eye, eyelids, conjunctiva, cornea; uveitis, iridocyclitis, allergic conditions, burns, foreign bodies, postoperatively in cataract

Carbonic anhydrase inhibitor

Action: Converted to epinephrine, which decreases aqueous production and increases outflow

Uses: Open-angle glaucoma, ocular hypertension

Direct-acting miotic

Action: Acts directly on cholinergic receptor sites; induces miosis, spasm of accommodation, fall in intraocular pressure, caused by stimulation of ciliary, pupillary sphincter muscles, which leads to pulling away of iris from filtration angle, resulting in increased outflow of aqueous humor

Uses: Primary glaucoma, early stages of wide-angle glaucoma (less useful in advanced stages), chronic open-angle glaucoma, acute narrow-angle glaucoma before emergency surgery; also neutralizes mydriatics used during eye exam; may be used alternately with mydriatics to break adhesions between iris and lens

Side effects/adverse reactions:

CNS: Headache

CV: Hypertension, tachycardia, dysrhythmias

EENT: Burning, stinging

GI: Bitter taste

Contraindications: Hypersensitivity

Precautions: Pregnancy, lactation, children, aphakia, hypersensitivity

to carbonic anhydrase inhibitors, sulfonamides, thiazide diuretics, ocular inhibitors, hepatic and renal insufficiency

NURSING CONSIDERATIONS

Assess:

• Ophth exams and intraocular pressure readings

• Blood counts; liver, renal function tests and serum electrolytes during long-term treatment

Perform/provide:

• Storage at room temperature away from light

Evaluate:

• Positive therapeutic response

• Absence of increased intraocular pressure

Teach patient/family:

• How to instill drops

• That drug may cause burning, itching, blurring, dryness of eye area

NASAL AGENTS

NASAL DECONGESTANTS

azelastine (℞)

(ay-zell'ah-steen)

Astelin

desoxyephedrine (OTC)

(des-oxy-e-fed'rin)

Vicks Inhaler

ephedrine (OTC)

(e-fed'rin)

Kondon's Nasal Jelly, Pretz-D, Vicks Vatronol

epinephrine (OTC)

(ep-i-neff'rin)

Adrenalin

naphazoline (OTC)

(naff-a-zoe'leen)

Privine

oxymetazoline (OTC)

(ox-i-met-az'oh-leen)

Afrin, Afrin Children's Nose

◆ = Nursing alert   ∥ = Herb-drug interaction   ⊘ = Do not crush

Drops, Allerest 12-Hour Nasal, Chlorphed-LA, Coricidin Nasal Mist, Dristan Long Lasting, Duramist Plus, Duration, Genasal, NTZ Long-Acting Nasal, Nafrine*, Neo-Synephrine 12 Hour, Nostrilla, oxymetazoline HCl, Sinarest 12-Hour, Sinex Long-Acting, Twice-A-Day Nasal, 4-Way Long Acting Nasal

phenylephrine (OTC)
(fen-ill-eff'rin)
Alconefrin 12, Children's Nostril, Neo-Synephrine, Sinex

propylhexadrine (OTC)
(proe-pil-hex'a-dreen)
Benzedrex Inhaler

tetrahydrozoline (OTC)
(tet-ra-hye-dro'zoe-leen)
Tyzine

xylometazoline (OTC)
(zye-loh-meh-tazz'oh-leen)
Otrivin, Otrivin Pediatric Nasal Drops, xylometazoline HCl

NASAL STEROIDS
beclomethasone (R)
(be-kloe-meth'a-sone)
Beconase AQ Nasal, Beconase Inhalation, Vancenase AQ Nasal, Vancenase Nasal

dexamethasone (R)
(dex-a-meth'a-sone)
Decadron Phosphate Turbinaire

Pregnancy category: C
Action: Produces vasoconstriction (rapid, long acting) of arterioles, thereby decreasing fluid exudation, mucosal engorgement by stimulation of α-adrenergic receptors in vascular smooth muscle
Uses: Nasal congestion

Dosage and routes:
Desoxyephedrine
• *Adult and child >6 yr:* 1-2 **INH** in each nostril q2h or less
Ephedrine
• *Adult:* Fill dropper to the level marked, then use in each nostril q4h or less
Epinephrine
• *Adult and child >6 yr:* Apply with swab, drops, spray prn
Naphazoline
• *Adult and child >6 yr:* 1-2 drops/spray q6h or less
Oxymetazoline
• *Adult and child >6 yr:* **INSTILL** 2-3 gtt or sprays to each nostril bid
• *Child 2-6 yr:* **INSTILL** 2-3 gtt or sprays 0.025 sol bid, not to exceed 3 days
Phenylephrine
• *Adult and child >12 yr:* 2-3 drops/spray (0.25-0.5) in each nostril q3-4h or less; or 2-3 drops/spray (1%) in each nostril q4h or less
• *Child 6-12 yr:* 2-3 drops/spray (0.25%) in each nostril q3-4h
• *Infant >6 mo:* 1-2 drops (0.16%) in each nostril q3h
Propylhexadrine
• *Adult and child >6 yr:* 1-2 **INH** in each nostril q2h or less
Tetrahydrozoline
• *Adult and child >6 yr:* 2-4 drops (0.1%) q3-4h prn or 3-4 sprays in each nostril q4h prn
• *Child 2-6 yr:* 2-3 drops (0.05%) in each nostril q4-6h prn
Xylometazoline
• *Adult and child >12 yr:* 2-3 drops/spray (0.1%) in each nostril q8-10h
• *Child 2-12 yr:* 2-3 drops (0.05%) in each nostril q8-10h
Available forms: Nasal sol 0.025%, 0.05%
Side effects/adverse reactions:
CNS: Anxiety, restlessness, tremors, weakness, insomnia, dizziness, fever, headache

---

* = Canada only   Side effects: *italics* = common; ***bold italics*** = life-threatening

EENT: Irritation, burning, sneezing, stinging, dryness, rebound congestion

GI: Nausea, vomiting, anorexia

INTEG: Contact dermatitis

Contraindications: Hypersensitivity to sympathomimetic amines

Precautions: Children <6 yr, elderly, diabetes, cardiovascular disease, hypertension, hyperthyroidism, increased intracranial pressure, prostatic hypertrophy, pregnancy (C), glaucoma

NURSING CONSIDERATIONS

Assess:

• For redness, swelling, pain in nasal passages before and during treatment

• For syst absorption; hypertension, tachycardia; notify prescriber; syst absorption occurs at high doses or after prolonged use

Administer:

• Having patient tilt head back, squeeze bulb to create a vacuum, and draw correct amount of sol into dropper; insert 2 gtt of sol into nostril; repeat in other nostril

• Store in light-resistant container; do not expose to high temp or let sol come into contact with aluminum

• For <4 consecutive days

• Environmental humidification to decrease nasal congestion, dryness

Evaluate:

• Therapeutic response: decreased nasal congestion

Teach patient/family:

• That stinging may occur for several applications; drying of mucosa may be decreased by environmental humidification

• To notify prescriber if irregular pulse, insomnia, dizziness, or tremors occur

• Proper administration to avoid syst absorption

• To rinse dropper with very hot water to prevent contamination

TOPICAL GLUCOCORTICOIDS

alclometasone (R)
(al-kloe-met'a-sone)
Adovate

amcinonide (R)
(am-sin'oh-nide)
Cyclocort

betamethasone (R)
(bay-ta-meth'a-sone)
Alphatrex, Beben*,
Betacort*, Betaderm,
Betatrex, Beta-Val,
Bethovate*, Betmethacort,
Celestoderm*, Dermabet,
Diprolene, Diprosone,
Ectosonel*, Maxivate,
Metaderm*, Novobetamet,
Psorion, Uticort, Valisone,
Valnac

clobetasol (R)
(kloe-bay'ta-sol)
Dermovate*, Temovate

clocortolone (R)
(kloe-kore'toe-lone)
Cloderm

desonide (R)
(dess'oh-nide)
Des Owen, Tridesilon

desoximetasone (R)
(dess-ox-i-met'a-sone)
Topicort

dexamethasone (R)
(dex-a-meth'a-sone)
Aeroseb-Dex, Decaderm,
Decaspray

diflorasone (R)
(dye-flor'a-sone)
Florone, Maxiflor, Psorcon

fluocinolone (R)
(floo-oh-sin'oh-lone)
Fluocin, Licon, Lidemol*,
Lidex, Lyderm*, Topsyn*,
Vasoderm

◆ = Nursing alert   ⚫ = Herb-drug interaction   ⊘ = Do not crush

flurandrenolide (℞)
(flure-an-dren'oh-lide)
Cordran, Cordran SP,
Cordran Tape, Drenison
1/4*, Drenison Tape*

fluticasone (℞)
(floo-tik'a-sone)
Cutivate

halcinonide (℞)
(hal-sin'oh-nide)
Halog, Halog-E

halobetasol (℞)
(hal-oh-bay'ta-sol)
Ultravate

hydrocortisone (℞)
(hye-droe-kor'ti-sone)
Actiocort, Aeroseb-HC, Ala-
Cort, Allercort, Alphaderm,
Anusol HC, Bactine, Barriere-
HC*, Calde-CORT Anti-Itch,
Carmol HC, Cetacort, Corta-
cet*, Cortaid, Cortate*, Cort-
Dome, Cortef*, Corticaine,
Corticreme*, Cortifair, Corti-
zone, Cortoderm*, Cortril,
Delcort, Dermacort,
DemiCort, Dermtex HC,
Emo-Cort, Epifoam,
FoilleCort, Gly-Cort, Gyne-
cort, Hi-Cor, Hycort, Hy-
derm*, Hydro-Tex, Hytone,
Lacti-Care-HC, Lanacort,
Lemoderm, Locoid, My Cort,
Novoehydrocort*, Nutracort
Pharm, Pharmacort, Penta-
cort, Rederm, Rhulicort S-T
Cort, Synacort, Sarna HC*,
Texa-Cort, Unicort*, Westcort

methylprednisolone
(℞)
(meth-ill-pred-niss'oh-lone)
Depo-Medrol

mometasone (℞)
(moe-met'a-sone)
Elocon

prednicarbate (℞)
(pred-ni-kar'bate)
Dermatop

triamcinolone (℞)
(trye-am-sin'oh-lone)
Aristocort, Flutex, Kenac,
Kenalog, Kenonel,
Triaderm*, Trianide*,
Triderm, Trymex

Pregnancy category: C
Action: Antipruritic, antiinflamma-
tory
Uses: Psoriasis, eczema, contact der-
matitis, pruritus; usually reserved
for severe dermatoses that have not
responded to less potent formula-
tion
Dosage and routes:
• *Adult and child:* Apply to affected
area
Side effects/adverse reactions:
*INTEG: Acne, atrophy, epidermal
thinning, purpura, striae*
Contraindications: Hypersensitivity, viral infections, fungal infections
Precautions: Pregnancy (C)
NURSING CONSIDERATIONS
Assess:
• Temp; if fever develops, drug
should be discontinued
• For systemic absorption, increased
temp, inflammation, irritation
Administer:
• Only to affected areas; do not get
in eyes
• Leaving site uncovered or lightly
covered; occlusive dressing is not
recommended—systemic absorption
may occur
• Use only on dermatoses; do not
use on weeping, denuded, or infected area
• Cleansing before application of
drug
• Continuing treatment for a few
days after area has cleared

---

* = Canada only   Side effects: *italics* = common; ***bold italics*** = life-threatening

• Store at room temperature
Evaluate:
• Therapeutic response: absence of severe itching, patches on skin, flaking
Teach patient/family:
• To avoid sunlight on affected area, burns may occur
• To limit treatment to 14 days

TOPICAL ANTIFUNGALS

amphotericin B (OTC)
(am-foe-ter'i-sin)
Fungizone

butenafine (℞)
(byoo-tin'a-feen)
Mentex

ciclopirox (OTC)
(sye-kloe-peer'ox)
Loprox

clioquinol (OTC)
(klye-oh-kwin'ole)
Vioforim

clotrimazole (OTC)
(kloe-trye'ma-zole)
Canestew*, Clotrimaderm*, Lotrimin, Lotrimin AF, Mycelex, Mycelex OTC, Myclo*, Neozol*

econazole (OTC)
(ee-kon'a-zole)
Spectazole

haloprogin (OTC)
(hal-oh-proe'jin)
Halotex

ketoconazole (OTC)
(kee-toe-kon'a-zole)
Nizoral

miconazole (OTC)
(mye-kon'a-zole)
Micatin, Monistat-Derm

naftifine (OTC)
(naff'ti-feen)
Naftin

nystatin (OTC)
(nye-stat'in)
Mycostatin, Nodostine*, Nilstat, Nyoderm*, Nystex

oxiconazole (OTC)
(ox-i-kon'a-zole)
Oxistat

selenium (OTC)
(see-leen'ee-um)
Exsel, Head and Shoulders Intensive Treatment, Selenium Sulfide, Selsun, Selsun Blue

terbinafine (OTC)
(ter-bin'a-feen)
Lamisil

tolnaftate (OTC)
(tole-naf'tate)
Absorbine Antifungal, Absorbine Jock Itch, Absorbine Jr. Antifungal, Aftate For Athlete's Foot, Aftate for Jock Itch, Desenex Spray, Genaspor, NP-27, Quinsana Plus, Tinactin, Ting, tolnaftate, Zeasorb-AF

undecylenic acid (OTC)
(un-deh-sih-len'ik)
Caldesene, Cruex, Decylenes, Desenex, Desenex Maximum Strength, Protectol

Pregnancy category: B
Action: Interferes with fungal cell membrane permeability
Uses: Tinea cruris, tinea pedis, diaper rash, minor skin irritations; amphotericin B is used for *Candida* infections
Dosage and routes:
• Massage into affected area, surrounding area qd or bid, con-

---

⬥ = Nursing alert   📕 = Herb-drug interaction   🚫 = Do not crush tinue for 7-14 days, not to exceed 4 wk

Side effects/adverse reactions:

INTEG: Burning, stinging, dryness, itching, local irritation

Contraindications: Hypersensitivity

Precautions: Pregnancy (B), lactation, children

Interactions: None

NURSING CONSIDERATIONS

Assess:

• Skin for fungal infections; peeling, dryness, itching before and throughout treatment

• For continuing infection; increased size, number of lesions

Administer:

Topical route

• To affected area, surrounding area; do not cover with occlusive dressings

• Store below 30° C (86° F)

Evaluate:

• Therapeutic response: decrease in size, number of lesions

Teach patient/family:

• To apply with glove to prevent further infection; not to cover with occlusive dressings

• That long-term therapy may be needed to clear infection (2 wk-6 mo depending on organism); compliance is needed even after feeling better

• Proper hygiene; hand-washing technique, nail care, use of concomitant top agents if prescribed

• To avoid use of OTC creams, ointments, lotions unless directed by prescriber

• To use medical asepsis (hand washing) before, after each application; to change socks and shoes once a day during treatment of tinea pedis

• To report to health care prescriber

if infection persists or recurs; if blisters, burning, oozing, swelling occur

• To avoid alcohol because nausea, vomiting, hypertension may occur

• To use sunscreen or avoid direct sunlight to prevent photosensitivity

• To notify health-care prescriber of sore throat, fever, skin rash, which may indicate overgrowth of organisms

TOPICAL ANTIINFECTIVES

bacitracin (OTC)
(bass-i-tray′sin)
Baciguent, Bacitin*, Bacitracin

chloramphenicol (℞)
(klor-am-fen′i-kole)
Chloromycetin

erythromycin (OTC)
(er-ith-roe-mye′sin)
A/T/S, Akne-Mycin, C-Solve 2, Erycette, Eryderm, Erygel, Erymax, Erythromycin, E-Solve 2, ETS-2%, Staticin, Theramycin Z, T-Statd

gentamicin (℞)
(jen-ta-mye′sin)
G-Myticin, Garamycin, gentamicin

mafenide (℞)
(ma′fe-nide)
Sulfamylon

mupirocin (℞)
(myoo-peer′oh-sin)
Bactroban, Pseudomonic Acid A

neomycin (OTC)
(nee-oh-mye′sin)
Myciguent, Neomycin Sulfate

nitrofurazone (℞)
(nye-troe-fyoor′a-zone)
Furacin, Nitrofurazone

silver sulfadiazine (℞)
(sul-fa-dye'a-zeen)
Flamazine*, Silvadene, SSD,
SSD AF, Thermazene

sodium sulfacetamide lotion 10% (℞)
(sul-fa-see'ta-mide)

Klaron

tetracycline (℞)
(tet-ra-sye'kleen)
Achromycin, Topicycline

Pregnancy category: C
Action: Interferes with bacterial protein synthesis
Uses: Skin infections, minor burns, wounds, skin grafts, primary pyodermas, otitis externa
Side effects/adverse reactions:
INTEG: Rash, urticaria, scaling, redness
Contraindications: Hypersensitivity, large areas, burns, ulcerations
Precautions: Pregnancy (C), lactation, impaired renal function, external ear or perforated eardrum
NURSING CONSIDERATIONS
Assess:
• Allergic reaction: burning, stinging, swelling, redness
• For signs of nephrotoxicity or ototoxicity
Administer:
• Enough medication to cover lesions completely
• After cleansing with soap, water before each application; dry well
• To less than 20% of body surface area when patient has impaired renal function
Perform/provide:
• Storage at room temperature in dry place
Evaluate:
• Therapeutic response: decrease in size, number of lesions

TOPICAL ANTIVIRALS

acyclovir (℞)
(ay-sye'kloe-ver)
Zovirax

penciclovir (℞)
(pen-sye'kloe-ver)
Denavir

Pregnancy category: C
Action: Interferes with viral DNA replication
Uses: Simple mucocutaneous herpes simplex, in immunocompromised clients with initial herpes genitalis
Side effects/adverse reactions:
INTEG: Rash, urticaria, stinging, burning, pruritus, vulvitis
Contraindications: Hypersensitivity
Precautions: Pregnancy (C), lactation
NURSING CONSIDERATIONS
Assess:
• Allergic reaction: burning, stinging, swelling, redness, rash, vulvitis, pruritus
Administer:
• Using finger cot or rubber glove to prevent further infection
• Enough medication to cover lesions completely
• After cleansing with soap, water before each application; dry well
Perform/provide:
• Storage at room temperature in dry place
Evaluate:
• Therapeutic response: decrease in size, number of lesions
Teach patient/family:
• Not to use in eyes or when there is no evidence of infection
• To apply with glove to prevent further infection
• To avoid use of OTC creams, oint-

◆ = Nursing alert   🖊 = Herb-drug interaction   ⊘ = Do not crush

ments, lotions unless directed by prescriber

• To use medical asepsis (hand washing) before, after each application and avoid contact with eyes

• To adhere strictly to prescribed regimen to maximize successful treatment outcome

• To begin taking drug when symptoms arise

TOPICAL ANESTHETICS

benzocaine (OTC)
(ben'zoe-kane)
Anbesol Maximum Strength, Baby Anbesol, Children's Chloraseptic, Medamint, Orabase Baby, Oracin, Ora-Jel, Oratect, Spec-T Anesthetic, T-Caine, Tyrobenz

dibucaine (OTC)
(dye'byoo-kane)
dibucaine, Nupercainal

lidocaine (OTC, ℞)
(lye'doe-kane)
Aloe Extra, Anestacon, Burn Relief, Derma Flex, lidocaine HCl topical, lidocaine viscous, Solarcaine, Xylocaine, Xylocaine Viscous, Zilactin-L

pramoxine (OTC)
(pra-mox'een)
Fleet Relief, Prax, ProctoFoam, Tronolane, Tronothane

tetracaine (OTC)
(tet'ra-cane)
Pontocaine

Pregnancy category: C
Action: Inhibits conduction of nerve impulses from sensory nerves
Uses: Oral irritation, sore throat, toothache, cold sore, canker sore,

sunburn, minor cuts, insect bites, pain, itching

Dosage and routes:
• *Adult and child:* **TOP** apply qid as needed; **RECT** insert tid and after each BM

Side effects/adverse reactions:
INTEG: Rash, irritation, sensitization

Contraindications: Hypersensitivity, infants <1 yr, application to large areas

Precautions: Child <6 yr, sepsis, pregnancy (C), denuded skin

NURSING CONSIDERATIONS
Assess:
• Pain: location, duration, characteristics before and after administration

• For infection: redness, drainage, inflammation; this drug should not be used until infection is treated
Perform/provide:
• Storage in tight, light-resistant container; do not freeze, puncture, or incinerate aerosol container
Evaluate:
• Therapeutic response: decreased redness, swelling, pain
Teach patient/family:
• To avoid contact with eyes

• Not to use for prolonged periods: use for <1 wk; if condition remains, prescriber should be contacted

TOPICAL MISCELLANEOUS

docosanol (OTC)
(doe-koe'san-ole)
Abreva

pimecrolimus (℞)
(pim-eh-croh'lim-us)
Elidel

VAGINAL ANTIFUNGALS

butoconazole (OTC)
(byoo-toh-kone'ah-zole)
Femstat

clotrimazole (OTC)
(kloe-trye'ma-zole)
Canesten*, Gyne-Lotrimin, Mycelex G, Mycelex Twin Pak, Myclo*

miconazole (OTC)
(mye-kon'a-zole)
Monistat, Monistat 3, Monistat 7, Monistat Dual Pak

nystatin (OTC)
(nye-stat'in)
mycostatin, Nadostine*, Nilstat, Nyoderm*, O-V Statin

terconazole (OTC)
(ter-kone'ah-zole)
Terazol

tioconazole (OTC)
(tye-oh-kone'ah-zole)
Gyne-Trosyd*, Vagistat

Pregnancy category: Nystatin (A); clotrimazole (B); butoconazole, terconazole, tioconazole (C)

Action: Interferes with fungal DNA replication; binds sterols in fungal cell membranes, which increases permeability, leaking of nutrients

Uses: Vaginal, vulval, vulvovaginal candidiasis (moniliasis)

Dosage and routes:
Butoconazole
• *Adult:* **VAG** 5 g (1 applicator) hs × 3-6 days
Clotrimazole
• *Adult:* 100 mg (1 vag tab, 100 mg) hs × 1 wk, or 200 mg (2 vag tab, 100 mg) hs × 3 nights, or 500 mg (1 vag tab, 500 mg); or 5 g (1 applicator) hs × 1-2 wks

Miconazole
• *Adult:* 200 mg supp hs × 3 days or 100 mg supp × 1 wk
Nystatin
• *Adult:* 100,000 U qd × 2 wk
Terconazole
• *Adult:* **VAG** 5 g (1 applicator) hs × 7 days
Tioconazole
• *Adult:* 1 applicator hs × 1 wk

Side effects/adverse reactions:
GU: Vulvovaginal burning, itching, pelvic cramps
INTEG: Rash, urticaria, stinging, burning
MISC: Headache, body pain

Contraindications: Hypersensitivity

Precautions: Children <2 yr, pregnancy, lactation

Interactions: None

NURSING CONSIDERATIONS
Assess:
• For allergic reaction: burning, stinging, itching, discharge, soreness

Administer:
Topical route
• One full applicator every night high into the vagina
• Store at room temperature in dry place

Evaluate:
• Therapeutic outcome: decrease in itching or white discharge (vaginal)

Teach patient/family:
• About asepsis (hand washing) before, after each application
• To apply with applicator only; to avoid use of any other vaginal product unless directed by prescriber; sanitary napkin may prevent soiling of undergarments
• To abstain from sexual intercourse until treatment is completed; reinfection and irritation may occur
• To notify prescriber if symptoms persist

◆ = Nursing alert   ✔ = Herb-drug interaction   🚫 = Do not crush

OTIC STEROIDS

hydrocortisone
(hye-droe-kor'ti-sone)
Cortamed*, Otall (℞)

Pregnancy category: C
Action: Antiinflammatory, antipruritic
Uses: Ear canal inflammation
Side effects/adverse reactions:

EENT: Itching, irritation in ear
INTEG: Rash, urticaria
Contraindications: Hypersensitivity, perforated eardrum
Precautions: Pregnancy (C)
NURSING CONSIDERATIONS
Assess:

• For redness, swelling, fever, pain in ear, which indicates infection
Administer:

• After removing impacted cerumen by irrigation
• After cleaning stopper with alcohol
• After restraining child if necessary
• After warming sol to body temp
Evaluate:

• Therapeutic response: decreased ear pain, inflammation
Teach patient/family:

• The correct method of instillation using aseptic technique, including not touching dropper to ear
• That dizziness may occur after instillation

OTIC ANTIINFECTIVES

chloramphenicol (℞)
(klor-am-fen'i-kole)
Chloromycetin Otic,
Sopamycetin*
neomycin (℞)
(nee-oh-mye'sin)
Drotic, Otocort

Pregnancy category: C
Action: Inhibits protein synthesis in susceptible microorganisms
Uses: Ear infection (external), short-term use
Side effects/adverse reactions:

EENT: Itching, irritation in ear
INTEG: Rash, urticaria
Contraindications: Hypersensitivity, perforated eardrum
Precautions: Pregnancy (C)
NURSING CONSIDERATIONS
Assess:

• For redness, swelling, fever, pain in ear, which indicates superinfection
Administer:

• After removing impacted cerumen by irrigation
• After cleaning stopper with alcohol
• After restraining child if necessary
• After warming sol to body temp
Evaluate:

• Therapeutic response: decreased ear pain
Teach patient/family:

• The correct method of instillation using aseptic technique, including not touching dropper to ear
• That dizziness may occur after instillation

---

* = Canada only   Side effects: *italics* = common; ***bold italics*** = life-threatening

Appendix d

Commonly used antiinfectives in adults and children

amoxicillin
Adult: **PO** 750 mg-1.5 g qd in divided doses q8h
Child: **PO** 20-40 mg/kg/day in divided doses q8h
ampicillin
Adult: **PO** 1-2 g qd in divided doses q6h
IM/IV 2-8 g qd in divided doses q4-6h
Child: **PO** 50-100 mg/kg/day in divided doses q6h
IM/IV 100-200 mg/kg/day in divided doses q6h
cefaclor
Adult: **PO** 250-500 mg q8h
Child: **PO** 24-40 mg/kg/day in divided doses q8h
cephalexin
Adult: **PO** 250-500 mg q6h
Child: **PO** 25-50 mg/kg/day in 4 equal doses
chloramphenicol
Adult and child >3 mo: 50-100 mg/kg/day in divided doses q6h
clindamycin
Adult: **PO** 150-450 mg q6h
IM/IV 300 mg q6-12h
Child >1 mo: **PO** 8-25 mg/kg/day in divided doses q6-8h
IM/IV 15-40 mg/kg/day in divided doses q6-8h
erythromycin
Adult: 250-500 mg q6h
Child: 30-50 mg/kg/day in divided doses q6h
gentamicin
Adult: **IV INF** 3-5 mg/kg/day in divided doses q8h
Child: **IV/IM** 2-2.5 mg/kg q8h
Neonate and infant: **IV/IM** 2.5 mg/kg q8h
kanamycin
Adult and child: **IV INF/IM** 15 mg/kg/day in divided doses
q8-12h
methicillin
Adult: **IM/IV** 4-12 g/day in divided doses q4-6h
Child: **IM/IV** 50-300 mg/kg/day in divided doses q4-12h
PO 25-50 mg/kg/day in divided doses q6h
Neonate: **IM** 10 mg/kg q12h

◆ = Nursing alert   ∅ = Herb-drug interaction   ⊘ = Do not crush

nafcillin
Adult: **PO/IM/IV** 2-6 g/day in divided doses q4-6h
Child: **IM** 25 mg/kg q12h

nitrofurantoin
Adult and child >12 yr: **PO** 50-100 mg qid pc

oxacillin
Adult: **PO** 2-6 g/day in divided doses q4-6h
        IM/IV 2-12 g/day in divided doses q4-6h
Child: **PO/IM/IV** 50-100 mg/kg/day in divided doses q6h

penicillin G benzathine
Adult: **IM** 1.2 million U

penicillin G potassium
Adult: **PO** 400,000-500,000 U q6-8h
Child <12 yr: **PO** 25,000-90,000 U/kg/day in 3-6 divided doses

penicillin G procaine
Adult and child: **IM** 600,000-1.2 million U in 1-2 doses/day
Neonate: **IM** 50,000 U/kg qd

sulfisoxazole
Adult: **PO** 2-4 g loading dose, then 1-2 g qid
Child >2 mo: **PO** 75 mg/kg or 2 g/m^2 loading dose, then 150
        mg/kg/day or 4 g/m^2/day in divided doses q6h

ticarcillin
Adult: **IV/IM** 12-24 g/day in divided doses q3-6h
Child: **IV/IM** 50-300 mg/kg/day in divided doses q4-8h
Neonate: **IV INF** 75-100 mg/kg q8-12h

Appendix e Vaccines and toxoids

GENERIC NAME	TRADE NAME	USES	DOSAGE AND ROUTES	CONTRAINDICATIONS
BCG vaccine	TICE BCG	TB exposure	Adult/child >1 mo: 0.2-0.3 ml Child <1 mo: Reduce dose by 50% using 2 ml of sterile water after reconstituting	Hypersensitivity, hypogammaglobulinemia, positive TB test, burns
cholera vaccine	No trade name	Immunization for cholera in other countries	Adult/child >10 yr: IM/SC 2× of 0.5 ml, 7-30 days before traveling to cholera areas Booster is used q6mo 0.5 ml prn	Hypersensitivity, acute febrile illness
diphtheria and tetanus toxoids, adsorbed	No trade name	Induces antitoxins to provide immunity to diphtheria and tetanus	Adult/child ≥7 yr: IM (adult strength) 0.5 ml q4-8 wk × 2 doses, then 3rd dose 6-12 mo after 2nd dose, booster IM 0.5 ml q10yr Child 1-6 yr: IM (pediatric strength) 0.5 ml q4wk × 2 doses, booster 6-12 mo after 2nd dose Infant 6 wk-1 yr: IM (pediatric strength) 0.5 ml q4wk × 3 doses, booster 6-12 mo after 3rd dose	Hypersensitivity to mercury, thimerosal; immunocompromised patients; radiation; corticosteroids; acute illness
diphtheria and tetanus toxoids and whole-cell pertussis vaccine (DPT, DTP)	DTwP, Tr-Immunol	Prevention of diphtheria, tetanus, pertussis	Adult: booster dose q10yr Child >6 wk-6 yr: IM 0.5 ml at 2, 4, 6 mo, 1½ yr; booster needed 0.5 ml at age 6	Hypersensitivity, active infection, poliomyelitis outbreak, immunosuppression, febrile illness
diphtheria and tetanus toxoids and acellular pertussis vaccine	Accl-Imune, DTaP, Tripedia			
haemophilus b conjugate vaccine, diphtheria CRM197 protein conjugate (HbOC)	HibTITTER	Polysaccharide immunization of children 2-6 yr against H. influenzae b, conjugate	HibTITTER (IM 0.5 ml) Child: IM 0.5 ml Child 2-6 mo: 0.5 ml q2mo × 3 inj	Hypersensitivity, febrile illness, active infection
haemophilus b conjugate vaccine (PedvaxHIB)	PedvaxHIB	Immunization of child 2, 4, 6 mo	Child 7-11 mo: Previously unvaccinated 0.5 ml q2mo inj Child 12-14 mo: Previously unvaccinated 0.5 ml × 1 inj PedvaxHIB (IM only) Child 2-14 mo: 0.5 ml × 2 inj at 2, 4 mo of age (6 mo dose not needed), then booster at 12-18 mo against invasive disease	
haemophilus b conjugate vaccine, meningococcal protein conjugate (PRP-OMP)				

			child ≥1 yr mo. Previously unvaccinated 0.5 ml inj	
hepatitis A vaccine, inactivated	Havrix, Vaqta	Active immunization against hepatitis A virus	Adults: IM 1440 EL U (Havrix) or 50 U (Vaqta) as a single dose; booster dose is the same given at 6, 12 mo) Child 2-18 yr: IM 720 EL U (Havrix) or 25 U (Vaqta) as a single dose, booster dose is the same given at 6, 12 mo	Hypersensitivity
hepatitis B vaccine, recombinant	Engerix-B, Recombivax HB	Immunization against all subtypes of hepatitis B virus	Varies widely	Hypersensitivity to this vaccine or yeast
influenza virus vaccine, trivalent A and B (whole virus/split virus)	Fluogen, FluShield, Fluviral*, Fluvirin, Fluzone, influenza virus vaccine, trivalent	Prevention of Russian, Chilean, Philippine influenza	Adult/child >12 yr: IM 0.5 ml in 1 dose Child 3-12 yr: IM 0.5 ml, repeat in 1 mo (split) unless 1978-1985 vaccine was given Child 6 mo to 3 yr: IM 0.25 ml, repeat in 1 mo (split) unless 1978-1985 vaccine was given	Hypersensitivity, active infection, chicken egg allergy, Guillain-Barré syndrome, active neurologic disorders
Japanese encephalitis virus vaccine, inactivated	JE-VAX	Active immunity against Japanese encephalitis (JE)	Adult/child ≥3 yr: SC 1 ml, days 0, 7, 30; booster SC 1 ml 2 yr after last dose Child 1-3 yr: SC 0.5 ml, days 0, 7, 30; booster SC 0.5 ml 2 yr after last dose	Hypersensitivity to murine, thimerosal; allergic reactions to previous dose
Lyme disease vaccine (recombinant OspA)	LYMErix	Immunization against Lyme disease	Adult and adolescent 15-70: IM 30 μg in deltoid, repeat at 1, 12 mo after first dose	Hypersensitivity, antibiotic refractory Lyme arthritis
measles and rubella virus vaccine, live attenuated	M-R-Vax II	Immunity to measles and rubella by antibody production	Adult/child ≥15 mo: SC 0.5 ml (1000 U)	Hypersensitivity, immunocompromised patients, active untreated TB, cancer, blood dyscrasias, radiation, corticosteroids, pregnancy; allergic reactions to neomycin, eggs
measles, mumps, and rubella vaccine, live	M-M-R-II	Prevention of measles, mumps, rubella	Adult: SC 1 vial; 2 vials separated by 1 mo, in person born after 1957 Child >15 mo and adult: SC 0.5 ml	Hypersensitivity, blood dyscrasias, anemia, active infection, immunosuppression; egg, chicken allergy; pregnancy, febrile illness, neomycin allergy, neoplasms

*Canada only.

Continued

Appendix e   Vaccines and toxoids—cont'd

GENERIC NAME	TRADE NAME	USES	DOSAGE AND ROUTES	CONTRAINDICATIONS
measles virus vaccine, live attenuated	Attenuvax	Immunity to measles by antibody production	Adult/child ≥15 mo: SC 0.5 ml (1000 U); 1 dose 15 mo, 2nd dose age 4-6 or 11, or 12	Hypersensitivity to eggs, neomycin; cancer, radiation, corticosteroids, pregnancy, immunocompromised patients, blood dyscrasias, active untreated TB
meningococcal polysaccharide vaccine	Menomune-A/C/Y/W-135	Prophylaxis to meningococcal meningitis	Adult/child ≥2 yr: SC 0.5 ml	Hypersensitivity to thimerosal, pregnancy, acute illness
mumps virus vaccine, live	Mumpsvax	Active immunity to mumps	Adult/child ≥1 yr: SC 0.5 ml (20,000 U)	Hypersensitivity to eggs, neomycin; cancer, radiation, corticosteroids, pregnancy, immunocompromised patients, blood dyscrasias, active untreated TB
plague vaccine	No trade name	Active immunity to *Yersinia pestis* plague	Adult: IM 1 ml, then 0.2 ml in 4-12 wk, then 0.2 ml 5-6 mo after 2nd dose; booster 0.1-0.2 ml q6mo when in plague area	Hypersensitivity to phenol, sulfites, formaldehyde, beef, soy, casein; pregnancy, coagulation disorders
pneumococcal 7-valent conjugate vaccine	Prevnar	Immunity against *Streptococcus pneumoniae*	Child: IM 0.5 ml x 3 doses (7-11 mo); x 2 doses (12-23 mo); x 1 dose >2-9 yr	Hypersensitivity to diphtheria toxoid or this product
pneumococcal vaccine, polyvalent	Pneumovax 23, Pnu-Imune 23	Pneumococcal immunization	Adult/child ≥2 yr: IM/SC 0.5 ml	Hypersensitivity, Hodgkin's disease, ARDS
poliovirus vaccine, live, oral, trivalent (TOPV) poliovirus vaccine (IPV)	Orimune, IPOL	Prevention of polio	Adult/child ≥2 yr: PO 0.5 ml, given q8wk x 2 doses, then 0.5 ml ½-1 yr after dose 2 Infant: PO 0.5 ml at 2, 4, 18 mo; booster at 4-6 yr; may also be given: IPV at 2, 4 mo, then TOPV at 12-18 mo, booster at 4-6 yr	Hypersensitivity, active infection, allergy to neomycin/streptomycin, immunosuppression, vomiting, diarrhea

rabies vaccine, adsorbed	No trade name	Active immunity to rabies	**Preexposure** Adult/child: IM 1 ml day 0, 7, 21, or 28 days (total 3 doses); booster IM 1 ml prn q2-5 yr **Postexposure** Adult/child not vaccinated: IM 20 IU/kg of human rabies immune globulin (HRIG), give 5 total doses of 1-ml inj of rabies vaccine on days 0, 3, 7, 14, 28	Severe hypersensitivity to previous inj of vaccine, thimerosol
rabies vaccine, human diploid cell (HDCV)	Imovax Rabies, Imovax Rabies I.D.	Active immunity to rabies	**Preexposure** Adult/child: IM 1 ml day 0, 7, 21 or 28 (total 4 doses) **Postexposure** Adult/child: IM 1 ml on day 0, 3, 7, 14, 28 (total 5 doses)	No contraindications
rubella and mumps virus vaccine, live	Biavax II	Immunity to rubella and mumps by antibody production	Adult/child ≥1 yr: SC 0.5 ml	Hypersensitivity to eggs, neomycin; cancer, radiation, corticosteroids, pregnancy, immunocompromised patients, blood dyscrasias, active untreated TB
rubella virus vaccine, live attenuated (RA 27/3)	Meruvax II	Immunity to rubella by antibody production	Adult/child ≥1 yr: SC 0.5 ml (1000 U)	Hypersensitivity to eggs, neomycin; cancer, radiation, corticosteroids
tetanus toxoid, adsorbed/tetanus toxoid	No trade name	Tetanus toxoid: used for prophylactic treatment of wounds	Adult/child: IM 0.5 ml q4-6wk × 2 doses, then 0.5 ml 1 yr after dose 2 (adsorbed); SC/IM 0.5 ml q4-8wk × 3 doses, then 0.5 ml ½-1 yr after dose 3, booster dose 0.5 ml q10yr	Hypersensitivity, active infection, poliomyelitis outbreak, immunosuppression

*Canada only.

Continued

Appendix e Vaccines and toxoids—cont'd

GENERIC NAME	TRADE NAME	USES	DOSAGE AND ROUTES	CONTRAINDICATIONS
typhoid vaccine, parenteral	No trade name	Active immunity to typhoid fever	Adult: PO 1 cap 1 hr before meals × 4 doses, booster q5yr	Parenteral: systemic or allergic reaction, acute respiratory or other acute infection, intensive physical exercise in high temperatures Oral: hypersensitivity, acute febrile illness, suppressive or antibiotic drugs
typhoid vaccine, oral	Vivotif Berna Vaccine		Adult/child >10 yr: SC 0.5 ml, repeat in 4 wk, booster q3yr Child 6mo–10yr: SC 0.25 ml, repeat in 4 wk, booster q3yr	
typhoid Vi polysaccharide vaccine	Typhim Vi	Active immunity to typhoid fever	Adult/child ≥2 yr: IM 0.5 ml as a single dose, reimmunize q2yr 0.5 ml IM, if needed	Hypersensitivity, chronic typhoid carriers
varicella virus vaccine	Varivax	Prevention of varicella-zoster (chickenpox)	Adult/child ≥13 yr: SC 0.5 ml, 2nd dose SC 0.5 ml 4-8 wk later	Hypersensitivity to neomycin; blood dyscrasias, immunosuppression, active untreated TB, acute illness, pregnancy, diseases of lymphatic system
yellow fever vaccine	YF-Vax	Active immunity to yellow fever	Adult/child ≥9 mo: SC 0.5 ml deeply, booster q10yr Child 6-9 mo: same as above if exposed	Hypersensitivity to egg or chicken embryo protein, pregnancy, child <6 mo, immunodeficiency

*Canada only.

Appendix f Antitoxins and antivenins

GENERIC NAME	TRADE NAME	USE	DOSAGE AND ROUTES	CONTRAINDICATIONS
Black widow spider antivenin (*Lactrodectus mactans*)	No trade name	Black widow spider bite	Adult/child: IM 2.5 ml, 2nd dose may be given if severe; give in anterolateral thigh, obtain test for sensitivity before inj	Hypersensitivity to this product or horse serum
Crotalidae antivenom, polyvalent	No trade name	Rattlesnake bite	Adult/child: IV 20-150 ml depending on seriousness of bite, may give additional doses based on response	Hypersensitivity
Diphtheria antitoxin, equine	No trade name	Diphtheria	Adult/child: IM/slow IV 20,000-120,000 U, may give additional doses after 24 hr	Hypersensitivity
Micrurus fulvius antivenin	No trade name	East/Texas coral snake bite	Adult/child: IV 30-50 ml, give through running IV line of normal saline, give 1st 1-2 ml over 4-5 min, watch for allergic reaction	Hypersensitivity

Appendix g

Combination products

*222:
aspirin 375 mg
codeine 8 mg
caffeine 30 mg
Uses: Narcotic analgesic

*282 MEP:
aspirin 375 mg
codeine 15 mg
caffeine 30 mg
Uses: Narcotic analgesic

*292:
aspirin 375 mg
codeine 30 mg
caffeine 30 mg
Uses: Narcotic analgesic

*692:
aspirin 375 mg
propoxyphene 65 mg
caffeine 30 mg
Uses: Narcotic analgesic

A-200 Shampoo:
0.33% pyrethrins
4% piperonyl butoxide
Uses: Scabicide, pediculicide

Aceta w/Codeine:
acetaminophen 300 mg
codeine 30 mg
Uses: Narcotic analgesic

Aceta-Gesic:
325 mg acetaminophen
30 mg phenyltoloxamine
Uses: Nonnarcotic analgesic

Acid-X:
acetaminophen 500 mg
calcium carbonate 250 mg
Uses: Analgesic, antacid

Actifed:
pseudoephedrine 60 mg
triprolidine 2.5 mg
Uses: Decongestant

Actifed, Allergy, Nighttime:
pseudoephedrine 30 mg
diphenhydramine 25 mg
Uses: Decongestant, antihistamine

Actifed Plus:
pseudoephedrine 30 mg
triprolidine 1.25 mg
acetaminophen 500 mg
Uses: Decongestant, antihistamine

Actifed Sinus Daytime:
pseudoephedrine 30 mg
acetaminophen 500 mg
Uses: Decongestant

Actifed Sinus Nighttime:
pseudoephedrine 30 mg
diphenhydramine 25 mg
acetaminophen 500 mg
Uses: Decongestant, antihistamine

Adderall 5 mg:
dextroamphetamine sulfate 1.25 mg
dextroamphetamine saccharate
    1.25 mg
amphetamine sulfate 1.25 mg
amphetamine aspartate 1.25 mg
Uses: CNS stimulant

Adderall 10 mg:
dextroamphetamine sulfate 5 mg
dextroamphetamine saccharate
    2.5 mg
amphetamine sulfate 2.5 mg
amphetamine aspartate 2.5 mg
Uses: CNS stimulant

Adderall 20 mg:
dextroamphetamine sulfate 5 mg
dextroamphetamine saccharate
    5 mg
amphetamine sulfate 5 mg

amphetamine aspartate 5 mg
Uses: CNS stimulant
Adderall 30 mg:
dextroamphetamine sulfate 7.5 mg
dextroamphetamine saccharate
  7.5 mg
amphetamine sulfate 7.5 mg
amphetamine aspartate 7.5 mg
Uses: CNS stimulant
Advil Cold & Sinus Caplets:
pseudoephedrine 30 mg
ibuprofen 200 mg
Uses: Decongestant
Aggrenox:
200 mg ext rel dipyridamole
25 mg aspirin
Uses: Antiplatelet
AK-Cide Ophthalmic Suspension/
  Ointment:
10% sulfacetamide sodium
0.5% prednisolone acetate
Uses: Ophth antiinfective,
  antiinflammatory
Alamast:
0.005% lauralkonium
glycerin
dibasic/monobasic sodium
  phosphate
phosphoric acid
Aldactazide 25/25:
spironolactone 25 mg
hydrochlorothiazide 25 mg
Uses: Diuretic
Aldactazide 50/50:
spironolactone 50 mg
hydrochlorothiazide 50 mg
Uses: Diuretic
Aldoclor-150:
methyldopa 250 mg
chlorothiazide 150 mg
Uses: Antihypertensive
Aldoclor-250:
methyldopa 250 mg
chlorothiazide 250 mg
Uses: Antihypertensive

Aldoril-15:
methyldopa 250 mg
hydrochlorothiazide 15 mg
Uses: Antihypertensive
Aldoril-25:
methyldopa 250 mg
hydrochlorothiazide 25 mg
Uses: Antihypertensive
Alka-Seltzer Effervescent,
  Original:
sodium bicarbonate 1916 mg
citric acid 1000 mg
aspirin 325 mg
Uses: Antacid, adsorbent,
  antiflatulent
Alka-Seltzer Gold:
sodium bicarbonate 958 mg
citric acid 832 mg
potassium bicarbonate 312 mg
Uses: Antacid, adsorbent
Alka-Seltzer Plus Allergy
  Liqui-Gels:
pseudoephedrine 30 mg
chlorpheniramine 2 mg
acetaminophen 325 mg
Uses: Decongestant, antihistamine
Alka-Seltzer Plus Night-Time
  Cold Liqui-Gels:
doxylamine 6.25 mg
dextromethorphan 10 mg
pseudoephedrine 30 mg
acetaminophen 250 mg
Uses: Antitussive, decongestant
Alka-Seltzer Plus Cold & Cough
  Liqui-Gels:
pseudoephedrine 30 mg
chlorpheniramine 2 mg
dextromethorphan 10 mg
acetaminophen 250 mg
Uses: Antitussive, decongestant
Alka-Seltzer Plus Cold Liqui-Gels:
pseudoephedrine 30 mg
chlorpheniramine 2 mg
acetaminophen 250 mg
Uses: Decongestant, antihistamine

Alka-Seltzer Plus Flu & Body Aches Non-Drowsy Liqui-Gels:
pseudoephedrine 30 mg
dextromethorphan 10 mg
acetaminophen 250 mg
Uses: Decongestant, antitussive, analgesic

Allerest Headache Strength Advanced Formula:
pseudoephedrine 30 mg
chlorpheniramine 2 mg
acetaminophen 325 mg
Uses: Decongestant, antihistamine

Allerest Maximum Strength Tablets:
pseudoephedrine 30 mg
chlorpheniramine 2 mg
Uses: Decongestant, antihistamine

Allerest No-Drowsiness:
pseudoephedrine 30 mg
acetaminophen 325 mg
Uses: Decongestant, analgesic

Allerest Sinus Pain Formula:
pseudoephedrine 30 mg
chlorpheniramine 2 mg
acetaminophen 500 mg
Uses: Decongestant, antihistamine, analgesic

All-Nite Cold Formula Liquid:
Per 5 ml:
pseudoephedrine 10 mg
doxylamine 1.25 mg
dextromethorphan 5 mg
acetaminophen 167 mg
Uses: Decongestant, antihistamine, analgesic

Alor 5/500:
hydrocodone 5 mg
aspirin 500 mg
Uses: Analgesic

Amaphen:
acetaminophen 325 mg
butalbital 50 mg
caffeine 40 mg
Uses: Analgesic, barbiturates

Ambenyl Cough Syrup:
Per 5 ml:
bromodiphenhydramine 12.5 mg
codeine 10 mg
5% alcohol
Uses: Antihistamine, opioid analgesic

Anacin:
aspirin 400 mg
caffeine 32 mg
Uses: Analgesic

Anacin Maximum Strength:
aspirin 500 mg
caffeine 32 mg
Uses: Analgesic

Anacin PM (Aspirin Free):
diphenhydramine 25 mg
acetaminophen 500 mg
Uses: Analgesic

Anacin w/Codeine:
aspirin 325 mg
codeine 8 mg
caffeine 32 mg
Uses: Narcotic analgesic

Anaplex HD Syrup:
Per 5 ml:
hydrocodone 1.7 mg
phenylephrine 5 mg
chlorpheniramine 2 mg
Uses: Analgesic, adrenergic, antihistamine

Anaplex Liquid:
Per 5 ml:
chlorpheniramine 2 mg
pseudoephedrine 30 mg
Uses: Antihistamine, decongestant

Anatuss DM:
guaifenesin 400 mg
pseudoephedrine 60 mg
dextromethorphan 20 mg
Uses: Expectorant, adrenergic, antitussive

Anatuss DM Syrup:
Per 5 ml:
guaifenesin 100 mg
pseudoephedrine 30 mg

dextromethorphan 10 mg
Uses: Expectorant, adrenergic, antitussive
Anatuss LA:
pseudoephedrine 120 mg
guaifenesin 400 mg
Uses: Adrenergic, expectorant
Anexsia 5/500:
hydrocodone 5 mg
acetaminophen 500 mg
Uses: Analgesic
Anexsia 5/500:
hydrocodone 5 mg
acetaminophen 500 mg
Uses: Narcotic analgesic
Anexsia 7.5/650:
hydrocodone 7.5 mg
acetaminophen 650 mg
Uses: Analgesic
Anexsia 10/660:
hydrocodone 10 mg
acetaminophen 660 mg
Uses: Analgesic
Anoquan:
acetaminophen 325 mg
caffeine 40 mg
butalbital 50 mg
Uses: Nonnarcotic analgesic, antipyretic
Antrocol Elixir:
Per 5 ml:
atropine 0.195 mg
phenobarbital 16 mg
alcohol 20%
Uses: Anticholinergic, barbiturate
Apresazide 25/25:
hydralazine 25 mg
hydrochlorothiazide 25 mg
Uses: Antihypertensive
Apresazide 50/50:
hydralazine 50 mg
hydrochlorothiazide 50 mg
Uses: Antihypertensive
Aprodine w/Codeine Syrup:
Per 5 ml:
pseudoephedrine 30 mg

triprolidine 1.25 mg
codeine 10 mg
Uses: Adrenergic, analgesic
Aprodine Syrup:
Per 5 ml:
pseudoephedrine 30 mg
triprolidine 1.25 mg
Uses: Adrenergic, analgesic
Arthritis Pain Formula:
aspirin 500 mg
aluminum hydroxide 27 mg
magnesium hydroxide 100 mg
Uses: Analgesic, antacid
Arthrotec:
diclofenac 50 or 75 mg
misoprostol 200 µg
Uses: NSAID, gastric protectant
Asbron G Elixir:
theophylline 150 mg
guaifenesin 100 mg
alcohol 15%
Uses: Bronchodilator, expectorant
Asbron G Inlay:
theophylline 150 mg
guaifenesin 100 mg
sucrose
Uses: Bronchodilator, expectorant
Ascriptin:
aspirin 325 mg
magnesium hydroxide 50 mg
aluminum hydroxide 50 mg
calcium carbonate 50 mg
Uses: Nonnarcotic analgesic, antipyretic
Ascriptin A/D:
aspirin 325 mg
aluminum hydroxide 75 mg
magnesium hydroxide 75 mg
calcium carbonate 75 mg
Uses: Analgesic
Aspirin-Free Bayer Select Allergy Sinus:
pseudoephedrine 30 mg
chlorpheniramine 2 mg
acetaminophen 500 mg

Uses: Adrenergic, antihistamine, analgesic

Aspirin-Free Bayer Select Head & Chest Cold:
pseudoephedrine 30 mg
guaifenesin 100 mg
dextromethorphan 10 mg
acetaminophen 325 mg
Uses: Adrenergic, antitussive, expectorant, analgesic

Aspirin Free Excedrin:
acetaminophen 500 mg
caffeine 65 mg
Uses: Analgesic

Aspirin Free Excedrin Dual:
acetaminophen 500 mg
calcium carbonate 111 mg
magnesium carbonate 64 mg
magnesium oxide 30 mg
Uses: Analgesic, antacid

Augmentin 250:
amoxicillin 250 mg
clavulanic acid 125 mg
Uses: Antiinfective

Augmentin 500:
amoxicillin 500 mg
clavulanic acid 125 mg
Uses: Antiinfective

Augmentin 875:
amoxicillin 875 mg
clavulanic acid 125 mg
Uses: Antiinfective

Augmentin 125 Chewable:
amoxicillin 125 mg
clavulanic acid 31.25 mg
Uses: Antiinfective

Augmentin 250 Chewable:
amoxicillin 250 mg
clavulanic acid 62.5 mg
Uses: Antiinfective

Augmentin 125 mg/5 ml Suspension:
Per 5 ml:
amoxicillin 125 mg
clavulanic acid 31.25 mg
Uses: Antiinfective

Augmentin 250 mg/5 ml Suspension:
Per 5 ml:
amoxicillin 250 mg
clavulanic acid 62.5 mg
Uses: Antiinfective

Auralgan Otic Solution:
5.4% antipyrine
1.4% benzocaine
Uses: Otic analgesic

Azo-Gantanol:
sulfamethoxazole 500 mg
phenazopyridine 100 mg
Uses: Sulfonamide

Azo-Gantrisin:
sulfisoxazole 500 mg
phenazopyridine 50 mg
Uses: Sulfonamide

Azo-Sulfamethoxazole:
sulfamethoxazole 500 mg
phenazopyridine 100 mg
Uses: Sulfonamide

Azo-Sulfisoxazole:
sulfisoxazole 500 mg
phenazopyridine 50 mg
Uses: Sulfonamide

B&O Supprettes No. 15A Supps:
belladonna extract 15 mg
opium 30 mg
Uses: Anticholinergic, narcotic analgesic

B&O Supprettes No. 16A Supps:
belladonna extract 16.2 mg
opium 60 mg
Uses: Anticholinergic, narcotic analgesic

Bactrim:
trimethoprim 80 mg
sulfamethoxazole 400 mg
Uses: Antiinfective

Bactrim DS:
trimethoprim 160 mg
sulfamethoxazole 800 mg
Uses: Antiinfective

Bactrim I.V.:
trimethoprim 80 mg

◆ = Nursing alert   ⫽ = Herb-drug interaction   ⊘ = Do not crush

sulfamethoxazole 400 mg
Uses: Antiinfective
Bancap HC:
acetaminophen 500 mg
hydrocodone 5 mg
Uses: Analgesic
Bayer Plus, Extra Strength:
aspirin 500 mg
calcium carbonate
magnesium carbonate
magnesium oxide
Uses: Analgesic, antacid
Bayer Select Chest Cold:
dextromethorphan 15 mg
acetaminophen 500 mg
Uses: Antitussive, analgesic
Bayer Select Flu Relief:
acetaminophen 500 mg
pseudoephedrine 30 mg
dextromethorphan 15 mg
chlorpheniramine 2 mg
Uses: Analgesic, adrenergic,
    antitussive, antihistamine
Bayer Select Head & Chest Cold,
  Aspirin Free Caplets:
pseudoephedrine 30 mg
dextromethorphan 10 mg
guaifenesin 100 mg
acetaminophen 325 mg
Uses: Adrenergic, antitussive,
    expectorant, analgesic
Bayer Select Head Cold:
pseudoephedrine 30 mg
acetaminophen 500 mg
Uses: Adrenergic, analgesic
Bayer Select Maximum Strength
  Headache:
acetaminophen 500 mg
caffeine 65 mg
Uses: Nonnarcotic analgesic
Bayer Select Maximum Strength
  Menstrual:
acetaminophen 500 mg
pamabrom 25 mg
Uses: Nonnarcotic analgesic

Bayer Select Maximum Strength
  Night-Time Pain Relief:
acetaminophen 500 mg
diphenhydramine 25 mg
Uses: Analgesic, antihistamine
Bayer Select Maximum Strength
  Sinus Pain Relief:
acetaminophen 500 mg
pseudoephedrine 30 mg
Uses: Analgesic, adrenergic
Bayer Select Night Time Cold:
acetaminophen 500 mg
pseudoephedrine 30 mg
dextromethorphan 15 mg
triprolidine 1.25 mg
Uses: Analgesic, adrenergic,
    antitussive, antihistamine
BC Powder Original Formula:
aspirin 650 mg
salicylamide 195 mg
caffeine 33.3 mg
Uses: Nonnarcotic analgesic
BC Powder Arthritis Strength:
aspirin 742 mg
salicylamide 222 mg
caffeine 38 mg
Uses: Nonnarcotic analgesic
Bellatal:
phenobarbital 16.2 mg
hyoscyamine sulfate 0.1037 mg
atropine sulfate 0.0194 mg
scopolamine hydrobromide
    0.0065 mg
Uses: Barbiturate, anticholinergic
Bellergal-S:
ergotamine 0.6 mg
belladonna alkaloids 0.2 mg
phenobarbital 40 mg
Uses: α-Adrenergic blocker,
    anticholinergic, barbiturate
Bel-Phen-Ergot-SR:
phenobarbital 40 mg
ergotamine tartrate 0.6 mg
belladonna alkaloids 0.2 mg
Uses: α-Adrenergic blocker,
    anticholinergic, barbiturate

Benadryl Allergy Decongestant Liquid:
Per 5 ml:
diphenhydramine 12.5 mg
pseudoephedrine 30 mg
Uses: Antihistamine, adrenergic

Benadryl Allergy/Sinus Headache Caplets:
diphenhydramine 12.5 mg
pseudoephedrine 30 mg
acetaminophen 500 mg
Uses: Antihistamine, adrenergic, analgesic

Benadryl Decongestant Allergy:
pseudoephedrine 60 mg
diphenhydramine 25 mg
Uses: Adrenergic, antihistamine

Benylin Expectorant Liquid:
Per 5 ml:
dextromethorphan 5 mg
guaifenesin 100 mg
5% alcohol
Uses: Expectorant, antitussive

Benylin Multi-Symptom Liquid:
Per 5 ml:
dextromethorphan 5 mg
pseudoephedrine 15 mg
guaifenesin 100 mg
Uses: Antitussive, adrenergic, expectorant

Betoptic-Pilo:
0.25% betaxolol
1.75% pilocarpine
Uses: Ophthalmic

Biohist-LA Tablets:
pseudoephedrine 120 mg
carbinoxamine 8 mg
Uses: Adrenergic

Blephamide Ophthalmic Suspension/Ointment:
0.2% prednisolone
10% sodium sulfacetamide
Uses: Ophthalmic antiinfective, antiinflammatory

Bromfed Capsules:
pseudoephedrine 120 mg
brompheniramine 12 mg
Uses: Antihistamine, adrenergic

Bromfed-PD Capsules:
pseudoephedrine 60 mg
brompheniramine 6 mg
Uses: Adrenergic, antihistamine

Bromfed Tablets:
pseudoephedrine 60 mg
brompheniramine 4 mg
Uses: Antihistamine, adrenergic

Bromfenex:
brompheniramine 12 mg
pseudoephedrine 120 mg
Uses: Antihistamine, adrenergic

Bromfenex PD:
brompheniramine 6 mg
pseudoephedrine 60 mg
Uses: Antihistamine, adrenergic

Bromo-Seltzer:
sodium bicarb 2781 mg
acetaminophen 325 mg
citric acid 2224 mg
Uses: Antacid, analgesic

Brondelate Elixir:
theophylline 192 mg
guaifenesin 150 mg
Uses: Bronchodilator, expectorant

Brontex:
codeine 10 mg
guaifenesin 300 mg
Uses: Analgesic, expectorant

Bufferin:
aspirin 325 mg
calcium carbonate 158 mg
magnesium oxide 63 mg
magnesium carbonate 34 mg
Uses: Analgesic, antacid

Bufferin AF Nite-Time:
acetaminophen 500 mg
diphenhydramine 38 mg
Uses: Analgesic, antihistamine

Butace:
acetaminophen 325 mg
caffeine 40 mg

◆ = Nursing alert   ⫻ = Herb-drug interaction   ⊘ = Do not crush

butalbital 50 mg
Uses: Nonnarcotic analgesic
Butibel:
belladonna extract 15 mg
butabarbital 15 mg
Uses: Anticholinergic, barbiturate
Cafatine PB:
ergotamine 1 mg
caffeine 100 mg
belladonna alkaloids 0.125 mg
pentobarbital 30 mg
Uses: Migraine agent
Cafergot:
ergotamine 1 mg
caffeine 100 mg
Uses: Adrenergic blocker
Cafergot Suppositories:
ergotamine 2 mg
caffeine 100 mg
Uses: Adrenergic blocker
Caladryl:
8% calamine, camphor
2.2% alcohol
1% pramoxine
Uses: Top antihistamine
Caladryl Clear:
1% pramoxine
0.1% zinc acetate
2% alcohol
camphor
Uses: Top antihistamine
Calcet:
calcium 152.8 mg
vitamin D 100 IU
Uses: Supplement
Calcidrine Syrup:
Per 5 ml:
codeine 8.4 mg
calcium iodide 152 mg
Uses: Analgesic
Caltrate 600+D:
vitamin D 200 IU
calcium 600 mg
Uses: Supplement
Cama Arthritis Pain Reliever:
aspirin 500 mg

magnesium oxide 150 mg
aluminum hydroxide 125 mg
Uses: Nonnarcotic analgesic,
    antacid
Capital w/Codeine:
Per 5 ml:
acetaminophen 120 mg
codeine 12 mg
Uses: Narcotic analgesic
Capozide 25/15:
captopril 25 mg
hydrochlorothiazide 15 mg
Uses: Antihypertensive
Capozide 25/25:
captopril 25 mg
hydrochorothiazide 25 mg
Uses: Antihypertensive
Capozide 50/15:
captopril 50 mg
hydrochlorothiazide 15 mg
Uses: Antihypertensive
Capozide 50/25:
captopril 50 mg
hydrochlorothiazide 25 mg
Uses: Antihypertensive
Cardec DM Syrup:
Per 5 ml:
pseudoephedrine 60 mg
carbinoxamine 4 mg
dextromethorphan 15 mg
Uses: Adrenergic, antitussive
Cetacaine Topical:
14% benzocaine
2% tetracaine
0.5% benzalkonium chloride
0.005% cetyl dimethyl ethyl
    ammonium bromide
Uses: Local analgesic
Ceta Plus:
hydrocodone 5 mg
acetaminophen 500 mg
Uses: Analgesic
Cetapred Ointment:
0.25% prednisolone
10% sodium sulfacetamide

Side effects: *italics* = common; ***bold italics*** = life-threatening

Uses: Ophthalmic antiinfective,
antiinflammatory

Cheracol Syrup:
Per 5 ml:
codeine 10 mg
guaifenesin 100 mg
Uses: Analgesic, expectorant

Children's Cepacol Liquid:
Per 5 ml:
acetaminophen 160 mg
pseudoephedrine 15 mg
Uses: Analgesic, adrenergic

**Chlor-Trimeton Allergy 4 Hour
Decongestant:**
pseudoephedrine 60 mg
chlorpheniramine 4 mg
Uses: Antihistamine, adrenergic

**Chlor-Trimeton 12 Hour Relief
Tablets:**
pseudoephedrine 120 mg
chlorpheniramine 8 mg
Uses: Antihistamine, adrenergic

Chromagen:
ferrous fumarate 66 mg
vitamin B_{12} 10 µg
vitamin C 250 mg
intrinsic factor 100 mg
Uses: Supplement

Claritin-D:
loratidine 5 mg
pseudoephedrine 120 mg
Uses: Antihistamine, adrenergic

Claritin-D 24-Hour:
loratidine 10 mg
pseudoephedrine 240 mg
Uses: Antihistamine, adrenergic

Clindex:
chlordiazepoxide 5 mg
clidinium 2.5 mg
Uses: Antianxiety, anticholinergic

Clomycin Ointment:
bacitracin 500 U
neomycin sulfate 3.5 g
polymyxin B sulfate 500 U
lidocaine 40 mg
Uses: Antiinfective, local anesthetic

Co-Apap:
pseudoephedrine 30 mg
chlorpheniramine 2 mg
dextromethorphan 15 mg
acetaminophen 325 mg
Uses: Adrenergic, antihistamine,
antitussive, analgesic

Co-Gesic:
acetaminophen 500 mg
hydrocodone 5 mg
Uses: Analgesic

Codehist DH Elixir:
Per 5 ml:
pseudoephedrine 30 mg
chlorpheniramine 2 mg
codeine 10 mg
Uses: Adrenergic, antihistamine,
analgesic

Codiclear DH Syrup:
Per 5 ml:
hydrocodone 5 mg
guaifenesin 100 mg
Uses: Analgesic, expectorant

Codimal:
pseudoephedrine 30 mg
chlorpheniramine 2 mg
acetaminophen 500 mg
Uses: Adrenergic, antihistamine,
analgesic

Codimal DH Syrup:
Per 5 ml:
hydrocodone 1.66 mg
phenylephrine 5 mg
pyrilamine 8.33 mg
Uses: Analgesic, adrenergic

Codimal DM Syrup:
Per 5 ml:
phenylephrine 5 mg
pyrilamine 8.33 mg
dextromethorphan 10 mg
Uses: Adrenergic, antitussive

Codimal-LA:
chlorpheniramine 8 mg
pseudoephedrine 120 mg
Uses: Antihistamine, adrenergic

◆ = Nursing alert   ✦ = Herb-drug interaction   ⊘ = Do not crush

Codimal PH Syrup:
Per 5 ml:
codeine 10 mg
phenylephrine 5 mg
pyrilamine 8.33 mg
Uses: Analgesic, adrenergic
Col-Probenecid:
probenecid 500 mg
colchicine 0.5 mg
Uses: Antigout agent
ColBenemid:
probenecid 500 mg
colchicine 0.5 mg
Uses: Antigout agent
Coldrine:
pseudoephedrine 30 mg
acetaminophen 500 mg
Uses: Decongestant, nonnarcotic
    analgesic
Coly-Mycin S Otic Suspension:
1% hydrocortisone
neomycin base 3.3 mg/ml
colistin 3 mg/ml
0.05% thonzonium bromide
Uses: Otic antiinfective
Combipres 0.1:
chlorthalidone 15 mg
clonidine 0.1 mg
Uses: Antihypertensive
Combipres 0.2:
chlorthalidone 15 mg
clonidine 0.2 mg
Uses: Antihypertensive
Combipres 0.3:
chlorthalidone 15 mg
clonidine 0.3 mg
Uses: Antihypertensive
Combivent:
ipratropium bromide 18 µg
albuterol 103 µg/actuation
Uses: Bronchodilator
Combivir:
lamivudine 150 mg
zidovudine 300 mg
Uses: Antiviral

Comhist Tablets:
phenylephrine 10 mg
chlorpheniramine 2 mg
phenyltoloxamine 25 mg
Uses: Adrenergic, antihistamine
Comhist LA:
phenylephrine 20 mg
chlorpheniramine 4 mg
phenyltoloxamine 50 mg
Uses: Adrenergic, antihistamine
Comtrex Liquid:
Per 5 ml:
chlorpheniramine 0.67 mg
acetaminophen 108.3 mg
dextromethorphan 3.3 mg
pseudoephedrine 10 mg
Uses: Antihistamine, analgesic,
    antitussive, decongestant
Comtrex Allergy-Sinus:
chlorpheniramine 2 mg
acetaminophen 500 mg
pseudoephedrine 30 mg
Uses: Antihistamine, analgesic,
    decongestant
**Comtrex Maximum Strength
    Caplets:**
acetaminophen 500 mg
pseudoephedrine 30 mg
chlorpheniramine 2 mg
dextromethorphan 15 mg
Uses: Analgesic, decongestant,
    antihistamine, antitussive
**Comtrex Maximum Strength
    Multi-Symptoms Cold, Flu
    Relief:**
pseudoephedrine 30 mg
dextromethorphan 15 mg
chlorpheniramine 2 mg
acetaminophen 500 mg
Uses: Analgesic, decongestant,
    antihistamine, antitussive
**Comtrex Maximum Strength
    Non-Drowsy Caplets:**
acetaminophen 500 mg
pseudoephedrine 30 mg

---

dextromethorphan 15 mg
Uses: Analgesic, decongestant,
  antitussive
Congess SR:
guaifenesin 250 mg
pseudoephedrine 120 mg
Uses: Expectorant, decongestant
Congestac:
guaifenesin 400 mg
pseudoephedrine 60 mg
Uses: Expectorant, decongestant
Contac Cough & Chest Cold
  Liquid:
Per 5 ml:
pseudoephedrine 15 mg
dextromethorphan 5 mg
guaifenesin 50 mg
acetaminophen 125 mg
Uses: Decongestant, antitussive,
  expectorant, analgesic
Contac Cough & Sore Throat
  Liquid:
Per 5 ml:
dextromethorphan 5 mg
acetaminophen 125 mg
Uses: Antitussive, analgesic
Contac Day Allergy/Sinus:
pseudoephedrine 60 mg
acetaminophen 650 mg
Uses: Decongestant, analgesic
Contac Day Cold and Flu:
pseudoephedrine 60 mg
dextromethorphan 30 mg
acetaminophen 650 mg
Uses: Decongestant, antitussive,
  analgesic
Contac Night Allergy Sinus:
pseudoephedrine 60 mg
diphenhydramine 50 mg
acetaminophen 650 mg
Uses: Decongestant, antihistamine,
  analgesic
Contac Night Cold and Flu
  Caplets:
pseudoephedrine 60 mg
diphenhydramine 50 mg

acetaminophen 650 mg
Uses: Decongestant, antihistamine,
  antitussive, analgesic
Contac Severe Cold & Flu
  Nighttime Liquid:
Per 5 ml:
pseudoephedrine 10 mg
chlorpheniramine 0.67 mg
dextromethorphan 5 mg
acetaminophen 167 mg
18.5% alcohol
Uses: Decongestant, antihistamine,
  antitussive, analgesic
Coricidin:
chlorpheniramine 2 mg
acetaminophen 325 mg
Uses: Antihistamine, analgesic
Coricidin D Tablets:
chlorpheniramine 2 mg
acetaminophen 325 mg
Uses: Antihistamine, analgesic
Coricidin D Cold, Flu & Sinus:
chlorpheniramine 2 mg
acetaminophen 325 mg
pseudoephedrine sulfate 30 mg
Uses: Antihistamine, analgesic, decongestant
Cortisporin Ophthalmic/Otic
  Suspension:
0.35% neomycin polymyxin B
  10,000 U/ml
1% hydrocortisone
Uses: Ophthalmic antiinfective,
  antiinflammatory
Cortisporin Ophthalmic
  Ointment:
0.35% neomycin base
bacitracin 400 U
polymyxin B 10,000 U
hydrocortisone 1%
Uses: Ophthalmic antiinfective
Cortisporin Topical Cream:
0.5% neomycin sulfate
polymyxin B 10,000 U
0.5% hydrocortisone
Uses: Topical antiinfective

$\Longleftrightarrow$ = Nursing alert $/\!\!/$ = Herb-drug interaction $\bigcirc\!\!\!\!\diagup$ = Do not crush

Cortisporin Topical Ointment:
0.5% neomycin sulfate
bacitracin 400 U
polymyxin B 5,000 U
1% hydrocortisone
Uses: Topical antiinfective

Corzide 40/5:
nadolol 40 mg
bendroflumethiazide 5 mg
Uses: Antihypertensive

Corzide 80/5:
nadolol 80 mg
bendroflumethiazide 5 mg
Uses: Antihypertensive

Cough-X:
dextromethorphan 5 mg
benzocaine 2 mg
Uses: Antitussive, local anesthetic

Creon:
lipase 8,000 U
amylase 30,000 U
protease 13,000 U
pancreatin 300 mg
Uses: Digestive enzyme

Cyclomydril Ophthalmic Solution:
0.2% cyclopentolate
1% phenylephrine
Uses: Mydriatic

Dallergy Caplets:
chlorpheniramine 8 mg
phenylephrine 20 mg
methscopolamine 2.5 mg
Uses: Antihistamine, adrenergic

Dallergy Syrup:
Per 5 ml:
chlorpheniramine 2 mg
phenylephrine 10 mg
methscopolamine 0.625 mg
Uses: Antihistamine, adrenergic

Dallergy Tablets:
chlorpheniramine 4 mg
phenylephrine 10 mg
methscopolamine 1.25 mg
Uses: Antihistamine, adrenergic

Dallergy-D Syrup:
Per 5 ml:
phenylephrine 5 mg
chlorpheniramine 2 mg
Uses: Antihistamine, adrenergic

Damason-P:
hydrocodone 5 mg
aspirin 500 mg
Uses: Analgesic

Darvocet-N50:
acetaminophen 325 mg
propoxyphene 50 mg
Uses: Analgesic

Darvocet-N 100:
propoxyphene-N 100 mg
acetaminophen 650 mg
Uses: Analgesic

Darvon Compound-65:
propoxyphene 65 mg
aspirin 389 mg
caffeine 32.4 mg
Uses: Analgesic

*Darvon-N Compound:
aspirin 375 mg
propoxyphene 100 mg
caffeine 30 mg
Uses: Analgesic

*Darvon-N w/A.S.A.:
aspirin 325 mg
propoxyphene 100 mg
Uses: Analgesic

Deconamine:
pseudoephedrine 60 mg
chlorpheniramine 4 mg
Uses: Antihistamine, decongestant

Deconamine CX:
hydrocodone 5 mg
pseudoephedrine 30 mg
guaifenesin 300 mg
Uses: Analgesic, decongestant,
expectorant

Deconamine SR:
pseudoephedrine 120 mg
chlorpheniramine 8 mg
Uses: Antihistamine, decongestant

---

* = Canada only   Side effects: *italics* = common; ***bold italics*** = life-threatening

Deconamine Syrup:
Per 5 ml:
pseudoephedrine 30 mg
chlorpheniramine 2 mg
Uses: Antihistamine, decongestant

Defen-LA:
pseudoephedrine 60 mg
guaifenesin 600 mg
Uses: Decongestant, expectorant

Demi-Regroton:
chlorthalidone 25 mg
reserpine 0.125 mg
Uses: Antihypertensive

Demulen 1/50:
ethinyl estradiol 50 µg
ethynodiol diacetate 1 mg
Uses: Oral contraceptive

**Dexacidin Ophthalmic Ointment/
  Suspension:**
Per ml:
0.1% dexamethasone
0.35% neomycin
polymyxin B 10,000 U/g
Uses: Ophth, antiinfective/antiinflam-
  matory

**Dexasporin Ophthalmic
  Ointment:**
Per gram:
0.1% dexamethasone
0.35% neomycin
polymyxin B 10,000 U
Uses: Ophth, antiinfective/antiinflam-
  matory

DHC Plus:
dihydrocodeine 16 mg
acetaminophen 356.4 mg
caffeine 30 mg
Uses: Analgesic

Dialose Plus:
docusate sodium 100 mg
yellow phenolphthalein 65 mg
Uses: Laxative

Di-Gel Advanced Formula:
magnesium hydroxide 128 mg
calcium carbonate 280 mg

simethicone 20 mg
Uses: Antacid, adsorbent,
  antiflatulent

Di-Gel Liquid:
Per 5 ml:
aluminum hydroxide 200 mg
magnesium hydroxide 200 mg
simethicone 20 mg
Uses: Antacid, adsorbent,
  antiflatulent

Dihistine DH Liquid:
Per 5 ml:
pseudoephedrine 30 mg
chlorpheniramine 2 mg
codeine 10 mg
Uses: Decongestant, antihistamine,
  analgesic

Dilaudid Cough Syrup:
Per 5 ml:
guaifenesin 100 mg
hydromorphone 1 mg
5% alcohol
Uses: Expectorant, analgesic

Dilor-G Liquid:
dyphylline 300 mg
guaifenesin 300 mg
Uses: Bronchodilator, expectorant

Dilor-G Tablets:
dyphylline 200 mg
guaifenesin 200 mg
Uses: Bronchodilator, expectorant

Dimetane Decongestant:
brompheniramine 4 mg
phenylephrine 10 mg
Uses: Antihistamine, adrenergic

Dimetane-DX Cough Syrup:
Per 5 ml:
brompheniramine 2 mg
pseudoephedrine 30 mg
dextromethorphan 10 mg
Uses: Antihistamine, decongestant,
  antitussive

Dimetapp Sinus:
pseudoephedrine 30 mg
ibuprofen 200 mg
Uses: Decongestant, analgesic

◆ = Nursing alert   ⫽ = Herb-drug interaction   ⊘ = Do not crush

Diurigen w/Reserpine:
chlorothiazide 250 mg
reserpine 0.125 mg
Uses: Antihypertensive
Diutensin-R:
methylclothiazide 2.5 mg
reserpine 0.1 mg
Uses: Antihypertensive
Doan's PM Extra Strength:
magnesium salicylate 500 mg
diphenhydramine 25 mg
Uses: Analgesic, antihistamine
Dolacet:
hydrocodone 5 mg
acetaminophen 500 mg
Uses: Analgesic
Donnatal:
phenobarbital 16.2 mg
hyoscyamine 0.1037 mg
atropine 0.0194 mg
scopolamine 0.0065 mg
Uses: Anticholinergic, barbiturate
Donnatal Elixir:
Per 5 ml:
phenobarbital 16.2 mg
hyoscyamine 0.1037 mg
atropine 0.0194 mg
scopolamine 0.0065 mg
23% alcohol
Uses: Anticholinergic, barbiturate
Donnatal Extentabs:
phenobarbital 48.6 mg
hyoscyamine 0.3111 mg
atropine 0.0582 mg
scopolamine 0.0195 mg
Uses: Anticholinergic, barbiturate
Donnazyme:
pancreatin 500 mg
lipase 1000 U
protease 12,500 U
amylase 12,500 U
Uses: Pancreatic enzymes
Dorcol Children's Cold Formula Liquid:
Per 5 ml:
pseudoephedrine 15 mg

chlorpheniramine 1 mg
Uses: Decongestant, antihistamine
Doxidan:
docusate calcium 60 mg
phenolphthalein 65 mg
Uses: Stool softener
Dristan Cold:
pseudoephedrine 30 mg
acetaminophen 500 mg
Uses: Decongestant, analgesic
Dristan Cold Maximum Strength Caplets:
pseudoephedrine 30 mg
brompheniramine 2 mg
acetaminophen 500 mg
Uses: Decongestant, antihistamine, analgesic
Dristan Cold Multi-Symptom Formula:
acetaminophen 325 mg
phenylephrine 5 mg
chlorpheniramine 2 mg
Uses: Analgesic, adrenergic, antihistamine
Dristan Sinus:
pseudoephedrine 30 mg
ibuprofen 200 mg
Uses: Decongestant, analgesic
Drixoral Allergy Sinus:
pseudoephedrine 60 mg
dexbrompheniramine 3 mg
acetaminophen 500 mg
Uses: Decongestant, antihistamine, analgesic
Drixoral Cold & Allergy:
pseudoephedrine 120 mg
dexbrompheniramine 6 mg
Uses: Decongestant, antihistamine
Drixoral Cold & Flu:
pseudoephedrine 60 mg
dexbrompheniramine 3 mg
acetaminophen 500 mg
Uses: Decongestant, antihistamine, analgesic

* = Canada only   Side effects: *italics* = common; ***bold italics*** = life-threatening

Drixoral Cough & Congestion Liquid Caps:
pseudoephedrine 60 mg
dextromethorphan 30 mg
Uses: Decongestant, antitussive

Drixoral Cough & Sore Throat Liquid Caps:
dextromethorphan 15 mg
acetaminophen 325 mg
Uses: Antitussive, analgesic

Drixoral Plus:
pseudoephedrine 60 mg
dexbrompheniramine 3 mg
acetaminophen 500 mg
Uses: Decongestant, antihistamine, analgesic

DT:
Per 5 ml dose:
diphtheria toxoid 2LfU
tetanus toxoid 5LfU
Uses: Vaccine

DTP:
Per 0.5 ml dose:
diphtheria toxoid 6.5LfU
tetanus toxoid 5LfU
pertussis 4LfU
Uses: Vaccine

Dura-Vent/DA:
phenylephrine 20 mg
chlorpheniramine 8 mg
methscopolamine 2.5 mg
Uses: Adrenergic, antihistamine

Dyazide:
hydrochlorothiazide 25 mg
triamterene 37.5 mg
Uses: Diuretic

Dylline-GG Liquid:
dyphylline 300 mg
quaifenesin 300 mg
Uses: Bronchodilator, expectorant

Dynafed Asthma Relief:
ephedrine 25 mg
guaifenesin 200 mg
Uses: Adrenergic, expectorant

Dynafed Plus Maximum Strength:
pseudoephedrine 30 mg
acetaminophen 500 mg
Uses: Decongestant, analgesic

Dyphylline-GG Elixir:
Per 5 ml:
dyphylline 100 mg
guaifenesin 100 mg
Uses: Bronchodilator, expectorant

E-Lor:
acetaminophen 650 mg
propoxyphene 65 mg
Uses: Analgesic

E-Pilo-1 Ophthalmic Solution:
1% epinephrine bitartrate
1% pilocarpine
Uses: Miotic

E-Pilo-2 Ophthalmic Solution:
1% epinephrine bitartrate
2% pilocarpine
Uses: Miotic

E-Pilo-4 Ophthalmic Solution:
1% epinephrine bitartrate
4% pilocarpine
Uses: Miotic

Elase-Chloromycetin Ointment:
Per gram:
fibrinolysin 1 U
desoxyribonuclease 666.6 U
chloramphenicol 10 mg
Uses: Enzyme, antiinfective

Elase Ointment:
Per gram:
fibrinolysin 1 U
desoxyribonuclease 666.6 U
Uses: Enzyme

Elixophyllin GG Liquid:
Per 5 ml:
theophylline 100 mg
guaifenesin 100 mg
Uses: Expectorant, bronchodilator

EMLA Cream:
lidocaine 2.5 mg
prilocaine 2.5 mg
Uses: Local anesthetic

◆ = Nursing alert   🥢 = Herb-drug interaction   ⃠ = Do not crush

Empirin w/Codeine #3:
aspirin 325 mg
codeine phosphate 30 mg
Uses: Analgesic

Empirin w/Codeine #4:
aspirin 325 mg
codeine phosphate 60 mg
Uses: Analgesic

*Empracet-60:
acetaminophen 300 mg
codeine 60 mg
Uses: Analgesic

Endocet:
acetaminophen 325 mg
oxycodone 5 mg
Uses: Analgesic

*Endodan:
aspirin 325 mg
oxycodone 5 mg
Uses: Analgesic

Endolor:
acetaminophen 325 mg
caffeine 40 mg
butalbital 50 mg
Uses: Nonnarcotic analgesic

Enduronyl:
methyclothiazide 5 mg
deserpidine 0.25 mg
Uses: Antihypertensive

Enduronyl Forte:
methyclothiazide 5.0 mg
deserpidine 0.5 mg
Uses: Antihypertensive

Entex PSE:
pseudoephedrine 120 mg
guaifenesin 600 mg
Uses: Adrenergic, expectorant

Epifoam Aerosol Foam:
1% hydrocortisone
1% pramoxine
Uses: Topical corticosteroid

Equagesic:
meprobamate 200 mg
aspirin 325 mg
Uses: Antianxiety

Eryzole:
Per 5 ml:
erythromycin 200 mg
sulfisoxazole 600 mg
Uses: Macrolide antiinfective

Esgic-Plus:
butalbital 50 mg
acetaminophen 500 mg
caffeine 40 mg
Uses: Barbiturate, analgesic

Esimil:
guanethidine 10 mg
hydrochlorothiazide 25 mg
Uses: Antihypertensive

Estratest:
esterified estrogens 1.25 mg
methyltestosterone 2.5 mg
Uses: Androgen, estrogen

Etrafon:
perphenazine 2 mg
amitriptyline 25 mg
Uses: Antipsychotic, antidepressant

Etrafon 2-10:
perphenazine 2 mg
amitriptyline 10 mg
Uses: Antidepressant

Etrafon A:
perphenazine 4 mg
amitriptyline 10 mg
Uses: Antidepressant

Etrafon Forte:
perphenazine 4 mg
amitriptyline 25 mg
Uses: Antipsychotic, antidepressant

**Excedrin Aspirin Free Caplets
and Geltabs:**
500 mg acetaminophen
65 mg caffeine
Uses: Nonnarcotic analgesic

Excedrin Extra Strength:
aspirin 250 mg
acetaminophen 250 mg
caffeine 65 mg
Uses: Nonnarcotic analgesic

---

* = Canada only   Side effects: *italics* = common; ***bold italics*** = life-threatening

Excedrin Migraine:
aspirin 250 mg
acetaminophen 250 mg
caffeine 65 mg
Uses: Migraine agent
Excedrin P.M.:
acetaminophen 500 mg
diphenhydramine citrate 38 mg
Uses: Analgesic, antihistamine
Excedrin P.M. Liquid:
Per 30 ml:
acetaminophen 1000 mg
diphenhydramine 50 mg
Uses: Analgesic, antihistamine
Excedrin P.M. Liquigels:
acetaminophen 500 mg
diphenhydramine 25 mg
Uses: Analgesic, antihistamine
Excedrin Sinus Extra Strength:
pseudoephedrine 30 mg
acetaminophen 500 mg
Uses: Decongestant, analgesic
Fansidar:
sulfidoxine 500 mg
pyrimethamine 25 mg
Uses: Antimalarial
Fedahist:
pseudoephedrine 60 mg
chlorpheniramine 4 mg
Uses: Decongestant, antihistamine
Fedahist Expectorant Syrup:
Per 5 ml:
guaifenesin 200 mg
pseudoephedrine 20 mg
Uses: Expectorant, decongestant
Fedahist Gyrocaps:
pseudoephedrine 65 mg
chlorpheniramine 10 mg
Uses: Decongestant, antihistamine
Fedahist Timecaps:
pseudoephedrine 120 mg
chlorpheniramine 8 mg
Uses: Decongestant, antihistamine
Feen-A-Mint Pills:
docusate sodium 100 mg

phenolphthalein 65 mg
Uses: Laxative
Fem-1:
acetaminophen 500 mg
pamabrom 25 mg
Uses: Nonnarcotic analgesic
FemBack Caplets:
150 mg acetaminophen
150 mg salicylamide
44 mg phenyltoloxamine
Uses: Nonnarcotic analgesic
Femcet:
acetaminophen 325 mg
caffeine 40 mg
butalbital 50 mg
Uses: Nonnarcotic analgesic
Ferro-Sequels:
docusate sodium 100 mg
ferrous fumarate 150 mg
Uses: Laxative, hematinic
Fiorgen:
aspirin 325 mg
caffeine 40 mg
butalbital 50 mg
Uses: Nonnarcotic analgesic
Fioricet:
acetaminophen 325 mg
caffeine 40 mg
butalbital 50 mg
Uses: Analgesic, barbiturate
Fioricet w/Codeine:
acetaminophen 325 mg
caffeine 40 mg
butalbital 50 mg
codeine 30 mg
Uses: Analgesic, barbiturate
Fiorinal:
aspirin 325 mg
caffeine 40 mg
butalbital 50 mg
Uses: Analgesic, barbiturate
Fiorinal w/Codeine:
aspirin 325 mg
caffeine 40 mg
butalbital 50 mg

◆ = Nursing alert   ∥ = Herb-drug interaction   ⊘ = Do not crush

codeine 30 mg
Uses: Analgesic, barbiturate
FML-S Ophthalmic Suspension:
0.1% flurometholone
10% sulfacetamide
Uses: Ophth, antiinfective/antiinflam-
matory
Gas-Ban:
calcium carbonate 500 mg
simethicone 40 mg
Uses: Antiflatulent, antacid
Gas-Ban DS Liquid:
Per 5 ml:
aluminum hydroxide 400 mg
magnesium hydroxide 400 mg
simethicone 40 mg
Uses: Antiflatulent, antacid
Gaviscon:
magnesium trisilicate 20 mg
aluminum hydroxide 80 mg
Uses: Antacid, adsorbent,
antiflatulent
Gaviscon Liquid:
Per 5 ml:
aluminum hydroxide 31.7 mg
magnesium carbonate 119.3 mg
Uses: Antacid, adsorbent,
antiflatulent
Gelprin:
acetaminophen 125 mg
aspirin 240 mg
caffeine 32 mg
Uses: Analgesic
Gelusil:
aluminum hydroxide 200 mg
magnesium hydroxide 200 mg
simethicone 25 mg
Uses: Antacid, adsorbent,
antiflatulent
Genatuss DM Syrup:
Per 5 ml:
guaifenesin 100 mg
dextromethorphan 10 mg
Uses: Expectorant, antitussive
Glucovance:
glyburide: 1.25 mg

metformin: 250 mg
Uses: Antidiabetic
Glucovance:
glyburide: 2.5 mg
metformin: 500 mg
Uses: Antidiabetic
Glucovance:
glyburide: 5 mg
metformin: 500 mg
Uses: Antidiabetic
**Goody's Extra Strength Headache
Powder:**
250 mg acetaminophen
520 mg aspirin
32.5 mg caffeine
Uses: Nonopiate analgesic
Goody's Body Pain Powder:
325 mg acetaminophen
500 mg aspirin
Granulex Aerosol:
Per 0.82 ml:
trypsin 0.1 mg
balsam peru 72.5 mg
castor oil 650 mg
Uses: Top enzyme
Guaifenex PSE 60:
pseudoephedrine 60 mg
guaifenesin 600 mg
Uses: Decongestant, expectorant
Guaifenex PSE 120:
pseudoephedrine 120 mg
guaifenesin 600 mg
Uses: Decongestant, expectorant
Haley's M-O Liquid:
Per 15 ml:
magnesium hydroxide 900 mg
mineral oil 3.75 ml
Uses: Laxative
**Halotussin-DM Sugar Free
Liquid:**
Per 5 ml:
guaifenesin 100 mg
dextromethorphan 10 mg
Uses: Expectorant, antitussive
Helidac:
In a compliance package:

---

bismuth subsalicylate 262.4 mg tabs
metronidazole 250 mg tabs
tetracycline 500 mg caps
Uses: Antiinfective
Humibid DM Sprinkle Caps:
dextromethorphan 15 mg
guaifenesin 300 mg
Uses: Expectorant, antitussive
Humibid DM Tablets:
dextromethorphan 30 mg
guaifenesin 600 mg
Uses: Expectorant, antitussive
Hycodan:
hydrocodone 5 mg
homatropine 1.5 mg
Uses: Analgesic, mydriatic
Hycodan Syrup:
Per 5 ml:
hydrocodone 5 mg
homatropine 1.5 mg
Uses: Analgesic, mydriatic
Hycomine Compound:
chlorpheniramine 2 mg
acetaminophen 250 mg
phenylephrine 10 mg
hydrocodone 5 mg
caffeine 30 mg
Uses: Antihistamine, analgesic,
adrenergic
Hycotuss Expectorant:
Per 5 ml:
guaifenesin 100 mg
hydrocodone 5 mg
10% alcohol
Uses: Expectorant
Hydergine:
dihydroergocornine 0.167 mg
dihydroergocristine 0.167 mg
dihydroergocryptine 0.167 mg
Uses: Adrenergic blocker
Hydro-Serp:
hydrochlorothiazide 50 mg
reserpine 0.125 mg
Uses: Antihypertensive
Hydrocet:
hydrocodone 5 mg

acetaminophen 500 mg
Uses: Narcotic, opioid analgesic
Hydrogesic:
hydrocodone 5 mg
acetaminophen 500 mg
Uses: Narcotic, opioid analgesic
Hydropres-50:
hydrochlorothiazide 50 mg
reserpine 0.125 mg
Uses: Antihypertensive
Hydroserpine:
hydrochlorothiazide 25 mg
reserpine 0.125 mg
Uses: Antihypertensive
Hydroserpine:
hydrochlorothiazide 50 mg
reserpine 0.125 mg
Uses: Antihypertensive
Hyzaar:
losartan potassium 50 mg
hydrochlorothiazide 12.5 mg
potassium 4.24 mg
Uses: Antihypertensive
Iberet Filmtab:
ferrous sulfate 105 mg
ascorbic acid 150 mg
B-complex vitamins
Uses: Supplement
Iberet Liquid:
Per 5 ml:
ferrous sulfate 78.75 mg
ascorbic acid 112.5 mg
B-complex vitamins
Uses: Supplement
Imodium Advanced:
loperamide 2 mg
simethicone 125 mg
Uses: Antidiarrheal, antiflatulent
Inderide 40/25:
propranolol 40 mg
hydrochlorothiazide 25 mg
Uses: Antihypertensive
Inderide 80/25:
propranolol 80 mg
hydrochlorothiazide 25 mg
Uses: Antihypertensive

 = Nursing alert   = Herb-drug interaction   ⊘ = Do not crush

Inderide LA 80/50:
propranolol 80 mg
hydrochlorothiazide 50 mg
Uses: Antihypertensive
Inderide LA 120/50:
propranolol 120 mg
hydrochlorothiazide 50 mg
Uses: Antihypertensive
Inderide LA 160/50:
propranolol 160 mg
hydrochlorothiazide 50 mg
Uses: Antihypertensive
Innovar:
Per ml:
droperidol 2.5 mg
fentanyl 0.05 mg
Uses: Narcotic analgesic, general
  anesthetic
Iofed:
brompheniramine 12 mg
pseudoephedrine 120 mg
Uses: Antihistamine, adrenergic
Iofed PD:
brompheniramine 6 mg
pseudoephedrine 60 mg
Uses: Antihistamine, adrenergic
Iophen-C Liquid:
Per 5 ml:
iodinated glycerol 30 mg
codeine 10 mg
Uses: Expectorant, analgesic
Iophen-DM Liquid:
Per 5 ml:
iodinated glycerol 30 mg
dextromethorphan 10 mg
Uses: Expectorant, antitussive
Isollyl:
aspirin 325 mg
caffeine 40 mg
butalbital 50 mg
Uses: Nonnarcotic analgesic
Isopap:
isometheptene 65 mg
APAP 325 mg
dicloral-phenazone 100 mg
Uses: Migraine agent

Kaletra:
lopinavir 133.3 mg
ritonavir 33.3 mg
Uses: HIV
Kondremul w/Phenolphthalein:
Per 15 ml:
phenolphthalein 150 mg
55% mineral oil
Irish moss
Uses: Laxative
Lactinex:
Mixed culture of:
Lactobacillus acidophilus and
Lactobacillus bulgaricus
Uses: Supplement
Lanorinal:
aspirin 325 mg
caffeine 40 mg
butalbital 50 mg
Uses: Nonnarcotic analgesic
Lenoltec w/Codeine No. 1:
acetaminophen 650 mg
hydrocodone 10 mg
Uses: Analgesic
Levsin PB Drops:
Per ml:
hyoscyamine 0.125 mg
phenobarbital 15 mg
5% alcohol
Uses: Anticholinergic, barbiturate
Levsin w/Phenobarbital:
hyoscyamine 0.125 mg
phenobarbital 15 mg
Uses: Anticholinergic, barbiturate
Lexxel:
enalapril 5 mg
felodipine 5 mg
Uses: Antihypertensive
Librax:
chlordiazepoxide 5 mg
clidinium 2.5 mg
Uses: Antianxiety, anticholinergic
Lida-Mantel-HC-Cream:
0.5% hydrocortisone
3% lidocaine
Uses: Antiinflammatory, analgesic

---

* = Canada only   Side effects: *italics* = common; ***bold italics*** = life-threatening

Limbitrol DS:
chlordiazepoxide 10 mg
amitriptyline 25 mg
Uses: Antidepressant, antianxiety
Lobac:
salicylamide 200 mg
phenyltoloxamine 20 mg
acetaminophen 300 mg
Uses: Skeletal muscle relaxant,
  analgesic
Loestrin Fe 1.5/30:
norethindrone acetate 1.5 mg
ethinyl estradiol 30 μg
Uses: Oral contraceptive
Lomotil:
diphenoxylate 2.5 mg
atropine 0.025 mg
Uses: Antidiarrheal, anticholinergic
Lomotil Liquid:
Per 5 ml:
diphenoxylate 2.5 mg
atropine 0.025 mg
Uses: Antidiarrheal, anticholinergic
Lo Ovral:
ethinyl estradiol 30 μg
norgestrel 0.3 mg
Uses: Oral contraceptive
Lopressor HCT 50/25:
metoprolol 50 mg
hydrochlorothiazide 25 mg
Uses: Antihypertensive
Lopressor HCT 100/25:
metoprolol 100 mg
hydrochlorothiazide 25 mg
Uses: Antihypertensive
Lopressor HCT 100/50:
metoprolol 100 mg
hydrochlorothiazide 50 mg
Uses: Antihypertensive
Lorcet 10/650:
acetaminophen 650 mg
hydrocodone 10 mg
Uses: Analgesic
Lorcet Plus:
acetaminophen 650 mg

hydrocodone 7.5 mg
Uses: Analgesic
Lortab 2.5/500:
hydrocodone 2.5 mg
acetaminophen 500 mg
Uses: Analgesic
Lortab 5/500:
hydrocodone 5 mg
acetaminophen 500 mg
Uses: Analgesic
Lortab 7.5/500:
hydrocodone 7.5 mg
acetaminophen 500 mg
Uses: Analgesic
Lortab 10/500:
hydrocodone 10 mg
acetaminophen 500 mg
Uses: Analgesic
Lortab ASA:
aspirin 500 mg
hydrocodone 5 mg
Uses: Analgesic
Lortab Elixir:
Per 5 ml:
hydrocodone 2.5 mg
acetaminophen 167 mg
Uses: Analgesic
Lotensin HCT 5/6.25:
benazepril 5 mg
hydrochlorothiazide 6.25 mg
Uses: Antihypertensive
Lotensin HCT 10/12.5:
benazepril 10 mg
hydrochlorothiazide 12.5 mg
Uses: Antihypertensive
Lotensin HCT 20/12.5:
benazepril 20 mg
hydrochlorothiazide 12.5 mg
Uses: Antihypertensive
Lotensin HCT 20/25:
benazepril 20 mg
hydrochlorothiazide 25 mg
Uses: Antihypertensive
Lotrel 2.5/10:
amlopidine 2.5 mg

◆ = Nursing alert   ∥ = Herb-drug interaction   Ⓢ = Do not crush

benazepril 10 mg
Uses: Antihypertensive
Lotrel 5/10:
amlodipine 5 mg
benazepril 10 mg
Uses: Antihypertensive
Lotrel 5/20:
amlodipine 5 mg
benazepril 20 mg
Uses: Antihypertensive
Lotrisone Topical:
0.05% betamethasone
1% clotrimazole
Uses: Local antiinfective,
    antiinflammatory
Lufyllin-EPG Elixir:
Per 5 ml:
dyphylline 150 mg
ephedrine 24 mg
guaifenesin 300 mg
phenobarbital 24 mg
Uses: Bronchodilator, expectorant
Lufyllin-EPG Tablets:
dyphylline 100 mg
ephedrine 16 mg
guaifenesin 200 mg
phenobarbital 16 mg
Uses: Bronchodilator, adrenergic,
    expectorant, barbiturate
Lufyllin-GG:
dyphylline 200 mg
guaifenesin 200 mg
Uses: Bronchodilator, expectorant
Lufyllin-GG Elixir:
dyphylline 100 mg
guaifenesin 100 mg
alcohol 17%
Uses: Bronchodilator, expectorant
Lunelle:
25 mg medroxyprogesterone
5 mg estradiol cypionate/0.5 ml
Uses: Contraceptive
M-M-R-II:
measles
mumps

rubella
Uses: Vaccine, toxoid
M-R Vax II:
measles
rubella
Uses: Vaccine, toxoid
Maalox:
aluminum hydroxide 200 mg
magnesium hydroxide 200 mg
Uses: Antacid, adsorbent,
    antiflatulent
Maalox Plus:
aluminum hydroxide 200 mg
magnesium hydroxide 200 mg
simethicone 25 mg
Uses: Antacid, adsorbent, antiflatulent
Maalox Plus Extra Strength
Suspension:
Per 5 ml:
aluminum hydroxide 500 mg
magnesium hydroxide 450 mg
simethicone 40 mg
Uses: Antacid, adsorbent, antiflatulent
Maalox Suspension:
Per 5 ml:
aluminum hydroxide 225 mg
magnesium hydroxide 200 mg
Uses: Antacid, adsorbent,
    antiflatulent
Macrobid:
nitrofurantoin macrocrystals 25 mg
nitrofurantoin monohydrate 75 mg
Uses: Antiinfective
Magnaprin:
aspirin 325 mg
magnesium hydroxide 50 mg
aluminum hydroxide 50 mg
calcium carbonate 50 mg
Uses: Nonnarcotic analgesic
Magnaprin Arthritis Strength:
aspirin 325 mg
magnesium hydroxide 75 mg
aluminum hydroxide 75 mg
calcium carbonate 75 mg
Uses: Nonnarcotic analgesic

---

* = Canada only   Side effects: *italics* = common; ***bold italics*** = life-threatening

Malarone:
250 mg atovaquone
100 mg proguanil
Uses: Malaria

Malarone Pediatric:
62.5 mg atovaquone
25 mg proguanil
Uses: Malaria

Mapap Cold Formula:
acetaminophen 325 mg
chlorpheniramine 2 mg
pseudoephedrine 30 mg
dextromethorphan 15 mg
Uses: Bronchodilator, expectorant

Marax:
ephedrine 25 mg
theophylline 130 mg
hydroxyzine 10 mg
Uses: Bronchodilator, sedative/
  hypnotic

Marnal:
aspirin 325 mg
caffeine 40 mg
butalbital 50 mg
Uses: Nonnarcotic analgesic

Maxzide 1:
polythiazide 0.5 mg
prazosin 1 mg
Uses: Antihypertensive

Maxzide 2:
polythiazide 0.5 mg
prazosin 2 mg
Uses: Antihypertensive

**Maxitrol Ophthalmic Suspension/
  Ointment:**
Per ml:
0.35% neomycin
0.1% dexamethasone
polymyxin B 10,000 U
Uses: Ophthalmic antiinfective,
  antiinflammatory

Maxzide:
hydrochlorothiazide 50 mg
triamterene 75 mg
Uses: Antihypertensive, diuretic

Maxzide-25 MG:
hydrochlorothiazide 25 mg
triamterene 37.5 mg
Uses: Diuretic

Medi-Flu Liquid:
Per 5 ml:
pseudoephedrine 10 mg
chlorpheniramine 0.67 mg
dextromethorphan 5 mg
acetaminophen 167 mg
18.5% alcohol
Uses: Decongestant, antihistamine,
  antitussive, analgesic

Medigesic:
acetaminophen 325 mg
caffeine 40 mg
butalbital 50 mg
Uses: Nonnarcotic analgesic

Mepergan Fortis:
meperidine 50 mg
promethazine 25 mg
Uses: Analgesic, antihistamine

Mepergan Injection:
meperidine 25 mg
promethazine 25 mg
Uses: Analgesic

**Metimyd Ophthalmic Suspension/
  Ointment:**
0.5% prednisolone
10% sodium sulfacetamide
Uses: Ophthalmic antiinfective,
  antiinflammatory

**Midol Maximum Strength
  Multi-Symptom Menstrual
  Gelcaps:**
acetaminophen 500 mg
pyrilamine 15 mg
caffeine 60 mg
Uses: Analgesic

Midol PM:
acetaminophen 500 mg
diphenhydramine 25 mg
Uses: Analgesic, antihistamine

**Midol PMS Maximum Strength
  Caplets:**
acetaminophen 500 mg

 = Nursing alert   = Herb-drug interaction   = Do not crush

pyrilamine 15 mg
pamabrom 25 mg
Uses: Analgesic
Midol, Teen:
acetaminophen 400 mg
pamabrom 25 mg
Uses: Analgesic
Midrin:
isometheptene 65 mg
acetaminophen 325 mg
dichloralphenazone 100 mg
Uses: Analgesic
Minizide 1:
prazosin 1 mg
polythiazide 0.5 mg
Uses: Antihypertensive
Minizide 2:
prazosin 2 mg
polythiazide 0.5 mg
Uses: Antihypertensive
Minizide 5:
prazosin 5 mg
polythiazide 0.5 mg
Uses: Antihypertensive
Modane Plus:
docusate sodium 100 mg
phenolphthalein 65 mg
Uses: Laxative
Moduretic:
hydrochlorothiazide 50 mg
amiloride 5 mg
Uses: Diuretic
Motrin IB Sinus:
pseudoephedrine 30 mg
ibuprofen 200 mg
Uses: Adrenergic, analgesic
Murocoll-2 Ophthalmic Drops:
0.3% scopolamine
10% phenylephrine
Uses: Ophth anticholinergic,
 mydriatic
Mycolog II Topical:
Per gram:
0.1% triamcinolone acetonide
nystatin 100,000 U

Uses: Local antiinfective,
 antiinflammatory
Mylanta:
aluminum hydroxide 200 mg
magnesium hydroxide 200 mg
simethicone 20 mg
Uses: Antacid, adsorbent,
 antiflatulent
Mylanta Double Strength Liquid:
Per 5 ml:
aluminum hydroxide 400 mg
magnesium hydroxide 400 mg
simethicone 40 mg
Uses: Antacid, adsorbent,
 antiflatulent
Mylanta Gelcaps:
calcium carbonate 311 mg
magnesium carbonate 232 mg
Uses: Antacid, adsorbent,
 antiflatulent
Naldecon Tablets:
phenylpropanolamine 40 mg
phenylephrine 10 mg
phenyltoloxamine 15 mg
chlorpheniramine 5 mg
Uses: Antihistamine, decongestant
Naldecon Senior DX Liquid:
Per 5 ml:
dextromethorphan 10 mg
guaifenesin 200 mg
Uses: Expectorant, antitussive
**Naphcon-A Ophthalmic
 Solution:**
0.25% naphazoline
0.3% pheniramine
Uses: Ophth vasoconstrictor
Nasatab LA:
guaifenesin 500 mg
pseudoephedrine 120 mg
Uses: Expectorant, decongestant
**NeoDecadron Ophthalmic
 Ointment:**
0.35% neomycin
0.05% dexamethasone
Uses: Ophth antiinfective,
 antiinflammatory

---

* = Canada only   Side effects: *italics* = common; ***bold italics*** = life-threatening

NeoDecadron Ophthalmic Solution:
0.35% neomycin
0.1% dexamethasone
Uses: Ophth antiinfective, antiinflammatory

NeoDecadron Topical:
neomycin 0.5%
dexamethasone 0.1%
Uses: Top antiinfective, antiinflammatory

Neosporin Cream:
Per gram:
polymyxin B 10,000 U
neomycin 3.5 mg
Uses: Top antiinfective

Neosporin G.U. Irrigant:
Per ml:
neomycin 40 mg
polymyxin B 200,000 U
Uses: Antiinfective

Neosporin Ointment:
Per gram:
polymyxin B 5000 U
bacitracin zinc 400 U
neomycin 3.5 mg
Uses: Top antiinfective

Neosporin Ophthalmic Solution:
Per ml:
neomycin 1.75 mg
polymyxin B 10,000 U
gramicidin 0.025 mg
Uses: Ophthalmic antiinfective

Neosporin Ophthalmic Ointment:
Per gram:
neomycin 3.5 mg
polymyxin B 10,000 U
bacitracin zinc 400 U
Uses: Ophthalmic antiinfective

Neosporin Plus Cream:
polymyxin B 10,000 U
neomycin 3.5 mg
lidocaine 40 mg
Uses: Top antiinfective

Niferex-150 Forte:
ferrous sulfate 150 mg
vitamin B_{12} 25 μg
folic acid 1 mg
Uses: Supplement

Norgesic:
orphenadrine 25 mg
aspirin 385 mg
caffeine 30 mg
Uses: Skeletal muscle relaxant, analgesic

Norgesic Forte:
orphenadrine 50 mg
aspirin 770 mg
caffeine 60 mg
Uses: Skeletal muscle relaxant, analgesic

Novacet Lotion:
sodium sulfacetamine 10%
sulfur 5%
Uses: Acne agent

Novafed A:
pseudoephedrine 120 mg
chlorpheniramine 8 mg
Uses: Adrenergic, antihistamine

Novahistone Elixir:
Per 5 ml:
phenylephrine 5 mg
chlorpheniramine 2 mg
alcohol 5%
Uses: Antihistamine

Novo-Gesic* C8:
acetaminophen 300 mg
codeine 8 mg
caffeine 15 mg
Uses: Analgesic

NuLytely:
PEG 3350/420 g
sodium bicarbonate 5.72 g
sodium chloride 11.2 g
potassium chloride 1.48 g
Uses: Laxative

◆ = Nursing alert   🖊 = Herb-drug interaction   🚫 = Do not crush

NyQuil Hot Therapy:
Per packet:
acetaminophen 1000 mg
pseudoephedrine 60 mg
dextromethorphan 30 mg
doxylamine 12.5 mg
Uses: Analgesic, adrenergic,
antitussive
**NyQuil Nightime Cold/Flu
Medicine Liquid:**
Per 5 ml:
pseudoephedrine 10 mg
doxylamine 1.25 mg
dextromethorphan 5 mg
acetaminophen 167 mg
25% alcohol
Uses: Adrenergic, antitussive,
analgesic
Octicair Otic Suspension:
hydrocortisone 1%
neomycin 5 mg/ml
polymyxin B 10,000 U/ml
Uses: Otic antiinflammatory,
antiinfective
Opcon-A Ophthalmic Solution:
0.027% naphazoline
0.315% pheniramine
Uses: Ophth vasoconstrictor
Ornade Spansules:
phenylpropanolamine 75 mg
chlorpheniramine 12 mg
Uses: Antihistamine, decongestant
Ornex:
pseudoephedrine 30 mg
acetaminophen 500 mg
Uses: Adrenergic, analgesic
Ornex No Drowsiness Caplets:
acetaminophen 325 mg
pseudoephedrine 30 mg
Uses: Adrenergic, analgesic
Ortho-cept:
ethinyl estradiol 30 µg
desogestrel 0.15 mg
Uses: Oral contraceptive
Ortho-Novum 7/7/7:
Phase I:

0.5 mg norethindrone
35 µg ethinyl estradiol
Phase II:
0.75 mg norethindrone
35 µg ethinyl estradiol
Phase III:
1 mg norethinidrone
35 µg estradiol
Uses: Oral contraceptive
Otocort Otic Suspension:
hydrocortisone 1%
neomycin 5 mg/ml
polymyxin B 10,000 U
Uses: Otic antiinflammatory,
antiinfective
*Oxycocet:
acetaminophen 325 mg
oxycodone 5 mg
Uses: Analgesic
P-A-C Analgesic:
aspirin 400 mg
caffeine 32 mg
Uses: Nonnarcotic analgesic
Pain-X Topical:
0.05% capsaicin
5% menthol
4% camphor
Uses: Top analgesic
Pamprin Maximum Pain Relief:
acetaminophen 250 mg
pamabrom 25 mg
magnesium salicylate 250 mg
Uses: Analgesic
Pamprin Multi-Symptom:
acetaminophen 500 mg
pamabrom 25 mg
pyrilamine 15 mg
Uses: Analgesic
Panacet 5/500:
hydrocodone 5 mg
acetaminophen 500 mg
Uses: Analgesic
Panasal 5/500:
hydrocodone 5 mg
aspirin 500 mg
Uses: Analgesic

* = Canada only   Side effects: *italics* = common; ***bold italics*** = life-threatening

Pancrease Capsules:
amylase 20,000 U
protease 25,000 U
lipase 4500 U (microspheres)
Uses: Digestive enzyme

Pedia Care Cold-Allergy Chewable:
pseudoephedrine 15 mg
chlorpheniramine 1 mg
Uses: Adrenergic, antihistamine

Pedia Care Cough-Cold Liquid:
Per 5 ml:
pseudoephedrine 15 mg
chlorpheniramine 1 mg
dextromethorphan 5 mg
Uses: Adrenergic, antihistamine, antitussive

Pedia Care NightRest Cough-Cold Liquid:
Per 5 ml:
pseudoephedrine 15 mg
chlorpheniramine 1 mg
dextromethorphan 7.5 mg
Uses: Adrenergic, antihistamine, antitussive

Pediacof Syrup:
Per 5 ml:
codeine 5 mg
phenylephrine 2.5 mg
chlorpheniramine 0.75 mg
potassium iodide 75 mg
5% alcohol
Uses: Opioid, narcotic analgesic, antihistamine

Pediazole Suspension:
Per 5 ml:
erythromycin 200 mg
sulfisoxazole 600 mg
Uses: Antiinfective

Percocet:
oxycodone 5 mg
acetaminophen 325 mg
Uses: Analgesic

Percodan:
oxycodone 4.88 mg

aspirin 325 mg
Uses: Analgesic

Percodan-Demi:
aspirin 325 mg
oxycodone HCl 2.25 mg
oxycodone terephthalate 0.19 mg
Uses: Analgesic

*Percodan-Demi:
aspirin 325 mg
oxycodone 2.5 mg
Uses: Analgesic

Percogesic:
phenyltoloxamine 30 mg
acetaminophen 325 mg
Uses: Analgesic

Perdiem Granules:
Per teaspoon:
senna 0.74 g
psyllium 3.25 g
sodium 1.8 mg
potassium 35.5 mg
Uses: Laxative

Peri-Colace Capsules:
docusate sodium 100 mg
casanthranol 30 mg
Uses: Laxative

Peri-Colace Syrup:
Per 15 ml:
docusate sodium 60 mg
casanthranol 30 mg
Uses: Laxative

Phenaphen w/Codeine No. 3:
aspirin 325 mg
codeine 30 mg
Uses: Analgesic

Phenaphen w/Codeine No. 4:
aspirin 325 mg
codeine 60 mg
Uses: Analgesic

Phenerbel-S:
ergotamine tartrate 0.6 mg
belladonna alkaloids 0.2 mg
phenobarbital 40 mg
Uses: α-Adrenergic blocker, anticholinergic

◆ = Nursing alert   ∅ = Herb-drug interaction   ⊘ = Do not crush

Phenergan VC Syrup:
Per 5 ml:
phenylephrine 5 mg
promethazine 6.25 mg
Uses: Adrenergic, antihistamine

Phenergan VC w/Codeine Syrup:
Per 5 ml:
phenylephrine 5 mg
promethazine 6.25 mg
codeine 10 mg
Uses: Adrenergic, antihistamine,
  opioid analgesic

Phenergan w/Codeine Syrup:
Per 5 ml:
promethazine 6.25 mg
codeine 10 mg
Uses: Antihistamine, analgesic

Pherazine DM Syrup:
Per 5 ml:
dextromethorphan 15 mg
promethazine 6.25 mg
7% alcohol
Uses: Antitussive, antihistamine

Phillips' Laxative Gelcaps:
docusate sodium 83 mg
phenolphthalein 90 mg
Uses: Laxative

Phrenilin:
acetaminophen 325 mg
butalbital 50 mg
Uses: Nonnarcotic analgesic

Phrenilin Forte:
acetaminophen 650 mg
butalbital 50 mg
Uses: Nonnarcotic analgesic

PMB-400:
conjugated estrogens 0.45 mg
meprobamate 400 mg
Uses: Oral contraceptive

Polaramine Expectorant Liquid:
Per 5 ml:
guaifenesin 100 mg
dexchlorpheniramine 2 mg
pseudoephedrine 20 mg
7.5% alcohol
Uses: Expectorant

Polycillin-PRB Oral Suspension:
Per single dose:
ampicillin 3.5 g
probenecid 1 g
Uses: Antiinfective

Polycitra Syrup:
Per 5 ml:
potassium citrate 550 mg
sodium citrate 500 mg
citric acid 334 mg
Uses: Laxative

Poly-Histine Elixir:
Per 5 ml:
pheniramine 4 mg
pyrilamine 4 mg
phenyltoloxamine 4 mg
4% alcohol
Uses: Antihistamine

Poly-Pred Ophthalmic Suspension:
Per ml:
0.5% prednisolone acetate
0.35% neomycin
polymyxin B 10,000 U
Uses: Ophth antiinflammatory,
  antiinfective

Polysporin Ointment:
Per gram:
polymyxin B 10,000 U
bacitracin zinc 500 U
Uses: Top antiinfective

Polysporin Ophthalmic Ointment:
Per gram:
polymyxin B 10,000 U
bacitracin zinc 500 U
Uses: Ophthalmic antiinfective

Polytrim Ophthalmic:
Per ml:
trimethoprim 1 mg
polymyxin B 10,000 U
Uses: Ophthalmic antiinfective

Premphase:
In a compliance package:
conjugated estrogens 0.625 mg
medroxyprogesterone 5 mg
Uses: Oral contraceptive

---

* = Canada only   Side effects: *italics* = common; ***bold italics*** = life-threatening

Prempro:
In a compliance package:
conjugated estrogens 0.625 mg
medroxyprogesterone 2.5 mg
Uses: Oral contraceptive

Premsyn PMS:
acetaminophen 500 mg
pamabrom 25 mg
pyrilamine 15 mg
Uses: Analgesic

Prevpac:
In a compliance package:
amoxicillin 500 mg caps
clarithromycin 500 mg tabs
lansoprazole 30 mg caps
Uses: Antiinfective

Primatene:
theophylline 130 mg
ephedrine 24 mg
phenobarbital 7.5 mg
Uses: Bronchodilator, barbiturate

Primatene Dual Action:
theophylline 60 mg
ephedrine 12.5 mg
guaifenesin 100 mg
Uses: Bronchodilator, expectorant,
adrenergic

Primaxin 250 mg
IV for Injection:
imipenem 250 mg
cilastatin sodium 250 mg
Uses: Antiinfective

Primaxin 500 mg
IV for Injection:
imipenem 500 mg
cilastatin sodium 500 mg
Uses: Antiinfective

Prinzide 10-12.5:
lisinopril 10 mg
hydrochlorothiazide 12.5 mg
Uses: Antihypertensive

Prinzide 12.5:
lisinopril 20 mg
hydrochlorothiazide 12.5 mg
Uses: Antihypertensive

Prinzide 25:
lisinopril 20 mg
hydrochlorothiazide 25 mg
Uses: Antihypertensive

Probampacin Oral Suspension:
Per single dose:
ampicillin 3.5 g
probenecid 1 g
Uses: Antiinfective

Proben-C:
colchicine 0.5 mg
probenecid 500 mg
Uses: Antigout agent

Proctofoam-HC Aerosol Foam:
1% hydrocortisone
1% pramoxine
Uses: Topical corticosteroid

Propacet 100:
propoxyphene-N 100 mg
acetaminophen 650 mg
Uses: Analgesic

Pseudo-Chlor:
pseudoephedrine 120 mg
chlorpheniramine 8 mg
Uses: Antihistamine

Pseudo-Gest Plus:
pseudoephedrine 60 mg
chlorpheniramine 4 mg
Uses: Antihistamine

P-V-Tussin:
phenindamine 25 mg
guaifenesin 200 mg
hydrocodone 5 mg
Uses: Antihistamine, analgesic

P-V-Tussin Syrup:
Per 5 ml:
chlorpheniramine 2 mg
phenindamine 5 mg
phenylephrine 5 mg
pyrilamine 6 mg
Uses: Antihistamine, decongestant

Quadrinal:
ephedrine 24 mg
theophylline 65 mg
potassium iodide 320 mg
phenobarbital 24 mg

Uses: Adrenergic, bronchodilator, barbiturate

Quelidrine Cough Syrup:
Per 5 ml:
dextromethorphan 10 mg
phenylephrine 5 mg
ephedrine 5 mg
chlorpheniramine 2 mg
ammonium chloride 40 mg
ipecac 0.005 ml
Uses: Expectorant, adrenergic, antihistamine

Quibron-300:
theophylline 300 mg
guaifenesin 180 mg
Uses: Bronchodilator, expectorant

Quibron:
theophylline, 150 mg
guaifenesin 90 mg
Uses: Bronchodilator, expectorant

R&C Shampoo:
0.3% pyrethrins
3% piperonyl butoxide
Uses: Scabicide, pediculicide

Rauzide:
bendroflumethiazide 4 mg
powdered Rauwolfia serpentina 50 mg
Uses: Diuretic, antihypertensive

Regroton:
chlorthalidone 50 mg
reserpine 0.25 mg
Uses: Diuretic, antihypertensive

Regulace:
docusate sodium 100 mg
casanthranol 30 mg
Uses: Laxative

Renese-R:
polythiazide 2 mg
reserpine 0.25 mg
Uses: Diuretic, antihypertensive

Repan:
acetaminophen 325 mg
caffeine 40 mg
butalbital 50 mg
Uses: Nonnarcotic analgesic

Respahist:
pseudoephedrine 60 mg
brompheniramine 6 mg
Uses: Adrenergic, antihistamine

Respaire-60:
guaifenesin 200 mg
pseudoephedrine 60 mg
Uses: Expectorant, adrenergic

RID Shampoo:
0.3% pyrethrins
3% piperonyl butoxide
Uses: Scabicide, pediculicide

Rifamate:
isoniazid 150 mg
rifampin 300 mg
Uses: Antitubercular, antileprotic

Rifater:
rifampin 120 mg
isoniazid 50 mg
pyrazinamide 300 mg
Uses: Antitubercular

Rimactane/INH Dual Pack:
isoniazid 300 mg (30 tabs)
rifampin 300 mg (60 caps)
Uses: Antitubercular

Riopan Plus Suspension:
Per 5 ml:
magaldrate 540 mg
simethicone 40 mg
Uses: Antacid, adsorbent, antiflatulent

Robaxisal:
methocarbamol 400 mg
aspirin 325 mg
Uses: Skeletal muscle relaxant, analgesic

Robitussin A-C Syrup:
Per 5 ml:
codeine 10 mg
guaifenesin 100 mg
3.5% alcohol
Uses: Analgesic, expectorant

Robitussin Cold & Cough Liqui-Gels:
pseudoephedrine 30 mg
guaifenesin 200 mg

---

dextromethorphan 10 mg
Uses: Antitussive, expectorant
Robitussin-DAC Syrup:
Per 5 ml:
codeine 10 mg
guaifenesin 100 mg
pseudoephedrine 30 mg
1.4% alcohol
Uses: Analgesic, expectorant,
  adrenergic
Robitussin-DM Liquid:
Per 5 ml:
guaifenesin 100 mg
dextromethorphan 10 mg
Uses: Expectorant, antitussive
**Robitussin Maximum Strength
  Cough and Cold Liquid:**
dextromethorphan 15 mg
pseudoephedrine 30 mg
Uses: Antitussive, adrenergic
Robitussin Night Relief Liquid:
dextromethorphan 5 mg
pyrilamine 8.3 mg
pseudoephedrine 10 mg
acetaminophen 108.3 mg
Uses: Antitussive, adrenergic
**Robitussin Pediatric Cough &
  Cold Liquid:**
Per 5 ml:
pseudoephedrine 15 mg
dextromethorphan 7.5 mg
Uses: Antitussive, adrenergic
Robitussin-PE Syrup:
guaifenesin 100 mg
pseudoephedrine 30 mg
1.4% alcohol
Uses: Expectorant, adrenergic
**Robitussin Severe Congestion
  Liqui-Gels:**
guaifenesin 200 mg
pseudoephedrine 30 mg
Uses: Expectorant, adrenergic
Rolaids Calcium Rich:
magnesium hydroxide 80 mg
calcium carbonate 412 mg
Uses: Antacid, adsorbent,
  antiflatulent
Rondec:
pseudoephedrine 60 mg
carbinoxamine 4 mg
Uses: Adrenergic
Rondec DM Drops:
Per ml:
pseudoephedrine 25 mg
carbinoxamine 2 mg
dextromethorphan 4 mg
Uses: Adrenergic, antitussive
Rondec DM Syrup:
Per 5 ml:
pseudoephedrine 60 mg
carbinoxamine 4 mg
dextromethorphan 15 mg
Uses: Adrenergic, antitussive
Rondec Oral Drops:
Per 5 ml:
pseudoephedrine 25 mg
carbinoxamine 2 mg
Uses: Adrenergic
Roxicet:
Per 5 ml:
acetaminophen 325 mg
oxycodone 5 mg
Uses: Opioid analgesic
Roxicet 5/500:
oxycodone 5 mg
acetaminophen 500 mg
Uses: Opioid analgesic
Roxiprin:
aspirin 325 mg
oxycodone HCl 4.5 mg
oxycodone terephthalate 0.38 mg
Uses: Analgesic
Roxicet Oral Solution:
Per 5 ml:
acetaminophen 325 mg
oxycodone 5 mg
Uses: Analgesic
Ru-Tuss DE:
pseudoephedrine 120 mg
guaifenesin 600 mg
Uses: Adrenergic, expectorant

◆ = Nursing alert　　　　∥ = Herb-drug interaction　　　　⊘ = Do not crush

Ru-Tuss Expectorant Liquid:
Per 5 ml:
guaifenesin 100 mg
pseudoephedrine 30 mg
dextromethorphan 10 mg
10% alcohol
Uses: Adrenergic, expectorant,
antitussive
Ryna-C Liquid:
Per 5 ml:
pseudoephedrine 30 mg
chlorpheniramine 2 mg
codeine 10 mg
Uses: Adrenergic, antihistamine,
analgesic
Ryna Liquid:
Per 5 ml:
pseudoephedrine 30 mg
chlorpheniramine 2 mg
Uses: Adrenergic, antihistamine
Rynatan:
phenylephrine 25 mg
chlorpheniramine 8 mg
pyrilamine 25 mg
Uses: Adrenergic, antihistamine
Rynatan Pediatric Suspension:
Per 5 ml:
phenylephrine 5 mg
chlorpheniramine 2 mg
pyrilamine 12.5 mg
Uses: Adrenergic, antihistamine
Rynatuss:
ephedrine 10 mg
carbetapentane 60 mg
chlorpheniramine 5 mg
phenylephrine 10 mg
Uses: Adrenergic, antihistamine
Saleto Tablets:
115 mg acetaminophen
210 mg aspirin
65 mg salicylamide
16 mg caffeine
Uses: Nonnarcotic analgesic
Salutensin:
hydroflumethiazide 50 mg

reserpine 0.125 mg
Uses: Antihypertensive
Salutensin Demi:
hydroflumethiazide 25 mg
reserpine 0.125 mg
Uses: Antihypertensive
Scot-Tussin DM Liquid:
Per 5 ml:
chlorpheniramine 2 mg
dextromethorphan 15 mg
Uses: Antihistamine, antitussive
**Scot-Tussin Original 5-Action
Liquid:**
phenylephrine 4.2 mg
pheniramine 13.3 mg
sodium citrate 83.3 mg
sodium salicylate 83.3 mg
caffeine citrate 25 mg
Uses: Adrenergic, analgesic
Scot-Tussin Senior Clear Liquid:
Per 5 ml:
guaifenesin 200 mg
dextromethorphan 15 mg
Uses: Antitussive, expectorant
Sedapap-10:
acetaminophen 650 mg
butalbital 50 mg
Uses: Analgesic, barbiturate
Semprex-D:
acrivastine 8 mg
pseudoephedrine 60 mg
Uses: Adrenergic, bronchodilator
Senokot-S:
docusate 50 mg
senna concentrate 187 mg
Uses: Laxative
Septra:
sulfamethoxazole 400 mg
trimethroprim 80 mg
Uses: Antiinfective
Septra DS:
sulfamethoxazole 800 mg
trimethroprim 160 mg
Uses: Antiinfective

Septra I.V. for Injection:
Per 5 ml:
trimethoprim 80 mg
sulfamethoxazole 400 mg
Uses: Antiinfective

Septra Suspension:
Per 5 ml:
trimethoprim 40 mg
sulfamethoxazole 200 mg
Uses: Antiinfective

Ser-A-Gen:
hydrochlorothiazide 15 mg
hydralazine 25 mg
reserpine 0.1 mg
Uses: Antihypertensive

Ser-Ap-Es:
hydrochlorothiazide 15 mg
reserpine 0.1 mg
hydralazine 25 mg
Uses: Diuretic, antihypertensive

Seralazide:
hydrochlorothiazide 15 mg
hydralazine 25 mg
reserpine 0.1 mg
Uses: Antihypertensive

Serpazide:
hydrochlorothiazide 15 mg
hydralazine 25 mg
reserpine 0.1 mg
Uses: Antihypertensive

Silafed Syrup:
Per 5 ml:
pseudoephedrine 30 mg
triprolidine 1.25 mg
Uses: Adrenergic, antihistamine

Sinarest Extra Strength:
pseudoephedrine 30 mg
chlorpheniramine 2 mg
acetaminophen 500 mg
Uses: Adrenergic, antihistamine,
  analgesic

Sinarest No Drowsiness:
pseudoephedrine 30 mg
acetaminophen 500 mg
Uses: Adrenergic, analgesic

Sinarest Sinus:
pseudoephedrine 30 mg
chlorpheniramine 2 mg
acetaminophen 325 mg
Uses: Adrenergic, antihistamine,
  analgesic

Sine-Aid IB:
pseudoephedrine 30 mg
ibuprofen 200 mg
Uses: Adrenergic, analgesic

Sine-Aid Maximum Strength:
pseudoephedrine 30 mg
acetaminophen 500 mg
Uses: Adrenergic, analgesic

Sinemet 10/100:
carbidopa 10 mg
levodopa 100 mg
Uses: Antiparkinsonian

Sinemet 25/100:
carbidopa 25 mg
levodopa 100 mg
Uses: Antiparkinsonian

Sinemet 25/250:
carbidopa 25 mg
levodopa 250 mg
Uses: Antiparkinsonian

Sinemet CR 25-100:
carbidopa 25 mg
levodopa 100 mg
Uses: Antiparkinsonian

Sinemet CR 50-200:
carbidopa 50 mg
levodopa 200 mg
Uses: Antiparkinsonian

**Sine-Off Maximum Strength No
  Drowsiness Formula Caplets:**
pseudoephedrine 30 mg
acetaminophen 500 mg
Uses: Adrenergic, analgesic

Sine-Off Sinus Medicine:
pseudoephedrine 30 mg
chlorpheniramine 2 mg
acetaminophen 500 mg
Uses: Adrenergic, antihistamine,
  analgesic

◆ = Nursing alert   ▨ = Herb-drug interaction   ⊘ = Do not crush

Sinus Excedrin Extra Strength:
acetaminophen 500 mg
pseudoephedrine 30 mg
Uses: Nonnarcotic analgesic

Sinus-Relief:
acetaminophen 325 mg
pseudoephedrine 30 mg
Uses: Nonnarcotic analgesic

Sinutab:
acetaminophen 325 mg
chlorpheniramine 2 mg
pseudoephedrine 30 mg
Uses: Nonnarcotic analgesic

Sinutab without Drowsiness:
acetaminophen 325 mg
pseudoephedrine 30 mg
Uses: Nonnarcotic analgesic

Sinutab Maximum Strength Sinus Allergy:
acetaminophen 500 mg
pseudoephedrine 30 mg
chlorpheniramine 2 mg
Uses: Analgesic, adrenergic, antihistamine

Sinutab Maximum Strength Without Drowsiness:
acetaminophen 500 mg
pseudoephedrine 30 mg
Uses: Analgesic, adrenergic

Sinutab Non-Drying:
pseudoepedrine 30 mg
guaifenesin 200 mg
Uses: Adrenergic, expectorant

Slo-Phyllin GG Syrup:
theophylline 150 mg
guaifenesin 90 mg
Uses: Bronchodilator, expectorant

Soma Compound w/Codeine:
carisoprodol 200 mg
aspirin 325 mg
codeine 16 mg
Uses: Skeletal muscle relaxant

Synophylate-GG Syrup:
theophylline 150 mg
guaifenesin 100 mg

alcohol 15%
Uses: Bronchodilator, expectorant

Soma Compound:
carisoprodol 200 mg
aspirin 325 mg
Uses: Skeletal muscle relaxant, analgesic

Spec-T Lozenge:
dextromethorphan 10 mg
benzocaine 10 mg
Uses: Antitussive, topical anesthetic

Sudafed Cold & Cough Liquicaps:
pseudoephedrine 30 mg
dextromethorphan 10 mg
guaifenesin 100 mg
acetaminophen 250 mg
Uses: Adrenergic, antitussive, expectorant, analgesic

Sudafed Plus:
pseudoephedrine 60 mg
chlorpheniramine 4 mg
Uses: Adrenergic, antihistamine

Sudafed Severe Cold:
pseudoephedrine 30 mg
dextromethorphan 15 mg
Uses: Adrenergic, antitussive

Sudafed Sinus Maximum Strength:
pseudoephedrine 30 mg
acetaminophen 500 mg
Uses: Adrenergic, analgesic

Sudal 60/500:
pseudoephedrine 60 mg
guaifenesin 500 mg
Uses: Adrenergic, expectorant

Sudal 120/600:
pseudoephedrine 120 mg
guaifenesin 600 mg
Uses: Adrenergic, expectorant

Sulfimycin:
Per 5 ml:
erythromycin 200 mg
sulfisoxazole 600 mg
Uses: Macrolide antiinfective

---

* = Canada only　　　　Side effects: *italics* = common; ***bold italics*** = life-threatening

Sultrin Triple Sulfa Vaginal Cream:
3.42% sulfathiazole
2.86% sulfacetamine
3.7% sulfabenzamide
Uses: Antiinfective

Sultrin Triple Sulfa Vaginal Tablets:
sulfathiazole 172.5 mg
sulfacetamide 143.75
sulfabenzamide 184 mg
Uses: Antiinfective

Synalgos-DC:
aspirin 356.4 mg
caffeine 30 mg
dihydrocodeine 16 mg
Uses: Analgesic

Synercid:
quinupristin 150 mg
dalfopristin 350 mg
Uses: Antiinfective

Talacen:
acetaminophen 650 mg
pentazocine 25 mg
Uses: Analgesic

Talwin Compound:
aspirin 325 mg
pentazocine 12.5 mg
Uses: Analgesic

Talwin NX:
pentazocine 50 mg
naloxone 0.5 mg
Uses: Analgesic, opioid antagonist

Tarka 182:
trandolapril 2 mg (immed rel)
verapamil 180 mg (sus rel)
Uses: Antihypertensive, calcium channel blocker

Tarka 241:
trandolapril 1 mg (immed rel)
verapamil 240 mg (sus rel)
Uses: Antihypertensive, calcium channel blocker

Tarka 242:
trandolapril 2 mg (immed rel)
verapamil 240 mg (sus rel)
Uses: Antihypertensive, calcium channel blocker

Tarka 244:
trandolapril 4 mg (immed rel)
verapamil 240 mg (sus rel)
Uses: Antihypertensive, calcium channel blocker

Tavist Sinus:
acetaminophen 500 mg
pseudoephedrine 30 mg
Uses: Analgesic, adrenergic

*Tecnal:
aspirin 330 mg
caffeine 40 mg
butalbital 50 mg
Uses: Nonnarcotic analgesic

Teczem:
enalapril 5 mg (extended release)
diltiazem 180 mg (extended release)
Uses: Antihypertensive, calcium channel blocker

Tedrigen:
ephedrine 22.5 mg
theophylline 120 mg
phenobarbital 7.5 mg
Uses: Adrenergic, bronchodilator, barbiturate

Tegrin-LT Shampoo:
0.33% pyrethrins
3.15% piperonyl butoxide
Uses: Scabicide, pediculicide

Tencet:
acetaminophen 325 mg
caffeine 40 mg
butalbital 50 mg
Uses: Nonnarcotic analgesic

Tenoretic 50:
atenolol 50 mg
chlorthalidone 25 mg
Uses: Antihypertensive

Tenoretic 100:
atenolol 100 mg
chlorthalidone 25 mg
Uses: Antihypertensive

= Nursing alert   = Herb-drug interaction   = Do not crush

Terra-Cortril Ophthalmic Suspension:
1.5% hydrocortisone acetate
0.5% oxytetracycline
Uses: Ophth antiinflammatory, antiinfective

Terramycin w/Polymycin B Sulfate Ophthalmic Ointment:
Per gram:
polymyxin B 10,000 units
oxytetracycline 5 mg
Uses: Ophth antiinfective

T-Gesic:
hydrocodone 5 mg
acetaminophen 500 mg
Uses: Analgesic

Theodrine:
ephedrine 22.5 mg
theophylline 120 mg
Uses: Adrenergic, bronchodilator

Theolate Liquid:
theophylline 150 mg
guaifenesin 90 mg
Uses: Bronchodilator, expectorant

Theophylline Kl Elixir:
theophylline 80 mg
potassium iodide 130 mg
Uses: Bronchodilator, expectorant

Thera-Flu, Flu & Cold Medicine Powder:
Per packet:
pseudoephedrine 60 mg
chlorpheniramine 4 mg
acetaminophen 650 mg
Uses: Adrenergic, antihistamine, analgesic

Thera-Flu, Flu, Cold & Cough Powder:
Per packet:
pseudoephedrine 60 mg
chlorpheniramine 4 mg
dextromethorphan 20 mg
acetaminophen 650 mg
Uses: Adrenergic, antihistamine, antitussive, analgesic

Thera-Flu NightTime Powder:
Per packet:
pseudoephedrine 60 mg
chlorpheniramine 4 mg
dextromethorphan 30 mg
acetaminophen 1000 mg
Uses: Adrenergic, antihistamine, antitussive, analgesic

Thera-Flu Non-Drowsy Flu, Cold & Cough Maximum Strength Powder
Per packet:
pseudoephedrine 60 mg
dextromethorphan 30 mg
acetaminophen 1000 mg
Uses: Adrenergic, antitussive, analgesic

Thera-Flu Non-Drowsy Formula Maximum Strength Caplets:
pseudoephedrine 30 mg
dextromethorphan 15 mg
acetaminophen 500 mg
Uses: Adrenergic, antitussive, analgesic

Timentin for Injection:
Per 3.1-g vial:
ticarcillin 3 g
clavulanic acid 0.1 g
Uses: Antiinfective

Timolide 10/25:
timolol 10 mg
hydrochlorothiazide 25 mg
Uses: Antihypertensive

Titralac Plus:
calcium carbonate 420 mg
simethicone 21 mg
Uses: Antacid, adsorbent, antiflatulent

Tobra Dex Ophthalmic Suspension/Ointment:
tobramycin 0.3%
dexamethasone 0.1%
Uses: Ophth antiinfective, antiinflammatory

---

* = Canada only   Side effects: *italics* = common; ***bold italics*** = life-threatening

Triacin-C Cough Syrup:
Per 5 ml:
codeine 10 mg
pseudoephedrine 30 mg
triprolidine 1.25 mg
Uses: Analgesic, adrenergic,
  antihistamine

Triad:
acetaminophen 325 mg
caffeine 40 mg
butalbital 50 mg
Uses: Nonnarcotic analgesic

Triaminic-12:
phenylpropanolamine 75 mg
chlorpheniramine 12 mg
Uses: Antihistamine

Tri-Hydroserpine:
hydralazine 25 mg
hydrochlorothiazide 15 mg
reserpine 0.1 mg
Uses: Antihypertensive

Tri-Levlen:
Phase I:
levonorgestrel 0.05 mg
ethinyl estradiol 30 μg
Phase II:
levonorgestrel 0.075 mg
ethinyl estradiol 40 μg;
Phase III:
levonorgestrel 0.125 mg
ethinyl estradiol 30 μg
Uses: Oral contraceptive

**Triaminic AM Cough & Decon-
  gestant Formula Liquid:**
Per 5 ml:
pseudoephedrine 15 mg
dextromethorphan 7.5 mg
Uses: Adrenergic, antitussive

Triaminic Nite Light Liquid:
Per 5 ml:
pseudoephedrine 15 mg
chlorpheniramine 1 mg
dextromethorphan 7.5 mg
Uses: Adrenergic, antihistamine,
  antitussive

**Triaminic Sore Throat Formula
  Liquid:**
Per 5 ml:
pseudoephedrine 15 mg
dextromethorphan 7.5 mg
acetaminophen 160 mg
Uses: Adrenergic, antitussive

Triavil 2-10:
perphenazine 2 mg
amitriptyline 10 mg
Uses: Antidepressant, antipsychotic

Triavil 4-10:
perphenazine 4 mg
amitriptyline 10 mg
Uses: Antidepressant, antipsychotic

Triavil 2-25:
perphenazine 2 mg
amitriptyline 25 mg
Uses: Antidepressant, antipsychotic

Trinalin Repetabs:
azatadine maleate 1 mg
pseudoephedrine 120 mg
Uses: Antihistamine

Triphasil:
Phase I:
levonorgestrel 0.05 mg
ethinyl estradiol 30 μg
Phase II:
levonorgestrel 0.075 mg
ethinyl estradiol 40 μg
Phase III:
levonorgestrel 0.125 mg
ethinyl estradiol 30 μg
Uses: Oral contraceptive

**Triple Antibiotic Ophthalmic
  Ointment:**
Per gram:
polymyxin B 10,000 U
neomycin 3.5 mg
bacitracin 400 U
Uses: Antiinfective

Trizivir:
300 mg abacavir
150 mg lamivudine
300 mg zidovudine
Uses: HIV

◆ = Nursing alert   ∥ = Herb-drug interaction   ⊘ = Do not crush

Tuinal 100 mg:
amobarbital 50 mg
secobarbital 50 mg
Uses: Sedative-hypnotic
Tuinal 200 mg:
amobarbital 100 mg
secobarbital 100 mg
Uses: Sedative-hypnotic
Tusibron-DM Syrup:
Per 5 ml:
guaifenesin 100 mg
dextromethorphan 15 mg
Uses: Expectorant, antitussive
**Tussionex Pennkinetic
  Suspension:**
Per 5 ml:
chlorpheniramine 8 mg
hydrocodone 10 mg
Uses: Antihistamine, analgesic
Tussi-Organidin NR Liquid:
Per 5 ml:
codeine 10 mg
guaifenesin 100 mg
Uses: Analgesic, expectorant
Tussi-Organidin DM NR Liquid:
Per 5 ml:
guaifenesin 100 mg
dextromethorphan 10 mg
Uses: Expectorant, antitussive
Two-Dyne:
acetaminophen 325 mg
caffeine 40 mg
butalbital 50 mg
Uses: Nonnarcotic analgesic
**Tylenol Allergy Sinus, Maximum
  Strength Gelcaps:**
acetaminophen 500 mg
chlorpheniramine 2 mg
pseudoephedrine 30 mg
Uses: Antihistamine, adrenergic,
  analgesic
Tylenol Children's Cold:
acetaminophen 80 mg
chlorpheniramine 0.5 mg
pseudoephedrine 7.5 mg

Uses: Antihistamine, adrenergic,
  analgesic
Tylenol Children's Cold Liquid:
Per 5 ml:
acetaminophen 160 mg
chlorpheniramine 1 mg
pseudoephedrine 15 mg
Uses: Antihistamine, adrenergic,
  analgesic
**Tylenol Children's Cold Multi-
  Symptom Plus Cough Liquid:**
Per 5 ml:
acetaminophen 160 mg
dextromethorphan 5 mg
chlorpheniramine 1 mg
pseudoephedrine 15 mg
Uses: Antihistamine, adrenergic,
  analgesic
**Tylenol Children's Cold Plus
  Cough Chewable:**
acetaminophen 80 mg
pseudoephedrine 7.5 mg
dextromethorphan 2.5 mg
chlorpheniramine 0.5 mg
Uses: Antihistamine, adrenergic,
  analgesic
Tylenol Cold Multi-Symptom:
acetaminophen 325 mg
chlorpheniramine 2 mg
pseudoephedrine 30 mg
dextromethorphan 15 mg
Uses: Antihistamine, adrenergic,
  analgesic
Tylenol Cold No Drowsiness:
acetaminophen 325 mg
pseudoephedrine 30 mg
dextromethorphan 15 mg
Uses: Analgesic, adrenergic,
  antitussive
**Tylenol Flu Maximum Strength
  Gelcaps:**
dextromethorphan 15 mg
pseudoephedrine 30 mg
acetaminophen 500 mg
Uses: Analgesic, adrenergic,
  antitussive

---

* = Canada only   Side effects: *italics* = common; ***bold italics*** = life-threatening

Tylenol Flu NightTime Maximum Strength Gelcaps:
pseudoephedrine 30 mg
chlorpheniramine 2 mg
acetaminophen 500 mg
Uses: Adrenergic, antihistamine, analgesic

Tylenol Flu NightTime Maximum Strength Powder:
pseudoephedrine 60 mg
diphenhydramine 50 mg
acetaminophen 1000 mg
Uses: Adrenergic, antihistamine, analgesic

Tylenol Headache Plus, Extra Strength:
acetaminophen 500 mg
calcium carbonate 250 mg
Uses: Analgesic, antacid

Tylenol Multi-Symptom Cough Liquid:
Per 5 ml:
dextromethorphan 10 mg
acetaminophen 216.7 mg
5% alcohol
Uses: Antitussive, analgesic

Tylenol Multi-Symptom Cough w/Decongestant Liquid:
Per 5 ml:
dextromethorphan 10 mg
acetaminophen 200 mg
pseudoephedrine 20 mg
Uses: Antitussive, analgesic, adrenergic

Tylenol Multi-Symptom Hot Medication:
Per packet:
acetaminophen 650 mg
chlorpheniramine 4 mg
pseudoephedrine 60 mg
dextromethorphan 30 mg
Uses: Analgesic, antihistamine, adrenergic, antitussive

Tylenol PM, Extra Strength:
acetaminophen 500 mg
diphenhydramine 25 mg
Uses: Analgesic, antihistamine

Tylenol Severe Allergy:
diphenhydramine 12.5 mg
acetaminophen 500 mg
Uses: Analgesic, antihistamine

Tylenol Sinus Maximum Strength:
pseudoephedrine 30 mg
acetaminophen 500 mg
Uses: Adrenergic, analgesic

Tylenol w/Codeine Elixir:
Per 5 ml:
acetaminophen 120 mg
codeine 12 mg
Uses: Analgesic

Tylenol w/Codeine No. 1:
acetaminophen 300 mg
codeine 7.5 mg
Uses: Analgesic

Tylenol w/Codeine No. 2:
acetaminophen 300 mg
codeine 15 mg
Uses: Analgesic

Tylenol w/Codeine No. 3:
acetaminophen 300 mg
codeine 30 mg
Uses: Analgesic

Tylenol w/Codeine No. 4:
acetaminophen 300 mg
codeine 60 mg
Uses: Analgesic

Tylox:
oxycodone 5 mg
acetaminophen 500 mg
Uses: Analgesic

Tyrodone Liquid:
Per 5 ml:
hydrocodone 5 mg
pseudoephedrine 60 mg
5% alcohol
Uses: Analgesic, adrenergic

Unasyn for Injection 1.5 g:
ampicillin 1 g
sulbactam 0.5 g
Uses: Antiinfective

◆ = Nursing alert   ✍ = Herb-drug interaction   ⃠ = Do not crush

Unasyn for Injection 3 g:
ampicillin 2 g
sulbactam 1 g
Uses: Antiinfective

Uniretic:
moexipril 7.5 mg
hydrochlorothiazide 12.5 mg
or moexipril 15 mg
hydrochlorothiazide 25 mg
Uses: Antihypertensive, diuretic

Unituss HC Syrup:
hydrocodone 2.5 mg
phenylephrine 5 mg
chlorpheniramine 2 mg
Uses: Analgesic, adrenergic,
   antihistamine

Urised:
methenamine 40.8 mg
phenylsalicylate 18.1 mg
atropine 0.03 mg
hyoscyamine 0.03 mg
benzoic acid 4.5 mg
methylene blue 5.4 mg
Uses: Antiinfective

Urobiotic 250:
oxytetracycline 250 mg
sulfamethizole 250 mg
phenazopyridine 50 mg
Uses: Antiinfective

Ursinus Inlay:
pseudoephedrine 30 mg
aspirin 325 mg
Uses: Adrenergic, analgesic

Vanquish:
aspirin 227 mg
acetaminophen 194 mg
caffeine 33 mg
aluminum hydroxide 25 mg
magnesium hydroxide 50 mg
Uses: Nonnarcotic analgesic

Vaseretic 10-25:
enalapril 10 mg
hydrochlorothiazide 25 mg
Uses: Antihypertensive, diuretic

Vasocidin Ophthalmic Ointment:
sulfacetamide 10%

prednisolone 0.5%
Uses: Ophthalmic antiinfective,
   antiinflammatory

Vasocidin Ophthalmic Solution:
sulfacetamide 10%
prednisolone 0.25%
Uses: Ophthalmic antiinfective,
   antiinflammatory

Vasocon-A Ophthalmic Solution:
naphazoline 0.05%
antazoline 0.5%
Uses: Ophthalmic vasoconstrictor

**Vicks 44D Cough & Head
   Congestion Liquid:**
Per 5 ml:
dextromethorphan 10 mg
pseudoephedrine 20 mg
Uses: Antitussive, adrenergic

Vicks 44E Liquid:
Per 5 ml:
dextromethorphan 6.7 mg
guaifenesin 66.7 mg
Uses: Antitussive, expectorant

**Vicks 44M Cold, Flu, & Cough
   LiquiCaps:**
dextromethorphan 10 mg
pseudoephedrine 30 mg
chlorpheniramine 2 mg
acetaminophen 250 mg
Uses: Antitussive, adrenergic,
   antihistamine, analgesic

**Vicks 44 Non-Drowsy Cold &
   Cough LiquiCaps:**
dextromethorphan 30 mg
pseudoephedrine 60 mg
Uses: Antitussive, adrenergic

**Vicks Children's NyQuil Night-
   time Cough/Cold Liquid:**
Per 5 ml:
pseudoephedrine 10 mg
chlorpheniramine 0.67 mg
dextromethorphan 5 mg
Uses: Adrenergic, antihistamine,
   antitussive

Vicks Cough Silencers:
dextromethorphan 2.5 mg

---

* = Canada only   Side effects: *italics* = common; ***bold italics*** = life-threatening

benzocaine 1 mg
Uses: Antitussive, top anesthetic

Vicks DayQuil Liquid:
Per 5 ml:
dextromethorphan 3.3 mg
pseudoephedrine 10 mg
acetaminophen 108.3 mg
guaifenesin 33.3 mg
Uses: Antitussive, adrenergic,
   analgesic, expectorant

**Vicks DayQuil Sinus Pressure
   & Pain Relief:**
pseudoephedrine 30 mg
acetaminophen 500 mg
Uses: Adrenergic, analgesic

Vicks NyQuil Liquicaps:
pseudoephedrine 30 mg
doxylamine 6.25 mg
dextromethorphan 10 mg
acetaminophen 250 mg
Uses: Adrenergic, antihistamine,
   antitussive, analgesic

**Vicks NyQuil Multi-Symptom
   Cold Flu Relief Liquid:**
pseudoephedrine 10 mg
doxylamine 2.1 mg
dextromethorphan 5 mg
acetaminophen 167 mg
Uses: Adrenergic, antihistamine,
   antitussive, analgesic

**Vicks Pediatric Formula 44e
   Liquid:**
Per 5 ml:
dextromethorphan 3.3 mg
guaifenesin 33.3 mg
Uses: Expectorant, antitussive

**Vicks Pediatric Formula 44 m
   Multi-Symptom Cough & Cold
   Liquid**
pseudoephedrine 10 mg
chlorpheniramine 0.67 mg
dextromethorphan 5 mg
Uses: Adrenergic, antihistamine,
   antitussive

Vicodin:
acetaminophen 500 mg

hydrocodone 5 mg
Uses: Analgesic

Vicodin ES:
acetaminophen 750 mg
hydrocodone 7.5 mg
Uses: Analgesic

Vicodin HP:
hydrocodone 10 mg
acetaminophen 660 mg
Uses: Analgesic

VicodinTuss:
Per 5 ml:
hydrocodone 5 mg
guaifenesin 100 mg
Uses: Analgesic, expectorant

Vicoprofen:
hydrocodone 7.5 mg
ibuprofen 200 mg
Uses: Analgesic

Wigraine Suppositories:
ergotamine 2 mg
caffeine 100 mg
Uses: α-Adrenergic blocker

Yasmin:
ethinylestadiol 30 μg
dropirenone 3 mg
Uses: Oral contraceptive

Zestoretic 10/12.5:
lisinopril 10 mg
hydrochlorothiazide 12.5 mg
Uses: Antihypertensive

Zestoretic 20/12.5:
lisinopril 20 mg
hydrochlorothiazide 12.5 mg
Uses: Antihypertensive

Zestoretic 20/25:
lisinopril 20 mg
hydrochlorothiazide 25 mg
Uses: Antihypertensive

Ziac 2.5:
bisoprolol 2.5 mg
hydrochlorothiazide 6.25 mg
Uses: Antihypertensive

Ziac 5:
bisoprolol 5 mg

hydrochlorothiazide 6.25 mg
Uses: Antihypertensive
Ziac 10:
bisoprolol 10 mg
hydrochlorothiazide 6.25 mg
Uses: Antihypertensive

Zydone:
hydrocodone 5 mg
acetaminophen 500 mg
Uses: Analgesic

Appendix h Less frequently used antihistamines

GENERIC NAME	TRADE NAME(S)	USES	DOSAGES AND ROUTES	AVAILABLE FORMS	INTERACTIONS	CONTRAINDICATIONS
acrivastine/ pseudoephedrine (B)	Semprex-D	• Rhinitis • Allergy symptoms • Chronic idiopathic urticaria	• Adult, child >12 yr: PO 8 mg q4-6h	• Caps 8 mg/60 mg	• Increased CNS depression: alcohol, narcotics, sedatives, hypnotics • Hypertensive crisis: MAOIs • May increase CNS depression: kava • May increase anticholinergic effect: henbane leaf	• Hypersensitivity to this drug or triprolidine • Severe hypertension • Cardiac disease
azatadine (B)	Optimine	• Allergy symptoms • Rhinitis • Chronic urticaria	• Adult: PO 1-2 mg bid, not to exceed 4 mg/day • Geriatric: PO 1 mg qd-bid	• Tabs 1 mg	• Increased CNS depression: barbiturates, narcotics, hypnotics, tricyclics, alcohol • Decreased effect of: oral anticoagulants • Increased effect of azatadine: MAOIs • Increased CNS depression: kava • Increased anticholinergic effect: henbane leaf	• Hypersensitivity to H₁-receptor antagonists • Acute asthma attack • Lower respiratory tract disease • Child <12 yr
buclizine (B)	Bucladin-S, Softabs	• Motion sickness • Dizziness • Nausea • Vomiting • Antihistamine	• Adult: PO 25-50 mg prn ½ hr before travel; may be repeated q4-6h prn	• Tabs 50 mg	• Increased anticholinergic effect: henbane leaf • Increased CNS depression: kava	• Hypersensitivity to cyclizines • Shock
clemastine (B)	Contac Allergy 12 Hour, Tavist, Antihist-1	• Allergy symptoms • Rhinitis • Angioedema • Urticaria • Common cold	• Adult and child >12 yr: PO 1.34-2.68 mg bid-tid, not to exceed 8.04 mg/day	• Tabs 1.34, 2.68 mg; Syr 0.67 mg/ml	• Increased CNS depression: barbiturates, opioids, hypnotics, tricyclics, alcohol	• Hypersensitivity to H₁-receptor antagonists • Acute asthma attack

	Uses	Dosage	Interactions	Contraindications
cyclizine (OTC, ℞)	Marezine • Motion sickness • Prevention of postoperative vomiting • Antihistamine	*Vomiting* • Adult: IM 25-50 mg ½ hr before termination of surgery, then q4-6h prn (lactate) • Child: IM 3 mg/kg divided in 3 equal doses *Motion sickness* • Adult: PO 50 mg then q4-6h prn, not to exceed 200 mg/day (HCl) • Child: PO 25 mg q4-6h prn • Tabs 50 mg • Inj 50 mg/ml	• Increased effect of clemastine: MAOIs • Increased CNS depression: kava ◊ Increased anticholinergic effect: henbane leaf • May increase CNS effect: alcohol, tranquilizers, narcotics • Increased CNS depression: kava	• Lower respiratory tract disease • Hypersensitivity to cyclizines • Shock
dexchlorpheniramine (℞)	Dexchlor, dexchlorpheniramine maleate, Poladex, Polaramine • Allergy symptoms • Rhinitis • Pruritus • Contact dermatitis	• Adult: PO 1-2 mg tid-qid; repeat action 4-6 mg bid-tid • Child 6-11 yr: PO 1 mg q4-6h, or time rel 4 mg hs • Child 2-5 yr: PO 0.5 mg q4-6h; do not use repeat action form • Tabs 2 mg • Repeat action tabs 4, 6 mg • Syr 2 mg/5 ml	• Increased CNS depression: barbiturates, narcotics, hypnotics, tricyclics, alcohol • Decreased effect: oral anticoagulants, heparin • Increased effect of dexchlorpheniramine: MAOIs ◊ Increased anticholinergic effect: henbane leaf	• Hypersensitivity to H$_1$-receptor antagonists • Acute asthma attack • Lower respiratory tract disease

Continued

KEY: * = Canada only; ◊ = herb/drug interaction

Appendix h Less frequently used antihistamines—cont'd

GENERIC NAME	TRADE NAME(S)	USES	DOSAGES AND ROUTES	AVAILABLE FORMS	INTERACTIONS	CONTRAINDICATIONS
trimeprazine (℞)	Panectyl* , Temaril	• Pruritus	• Adult: PO 2.5 mg qid; time-rel 5 mg bid • Geriatric: PO 2.5 mg bid • Child 3-12 yr: PO 2.5 mg tid or hs • Child 6 mo-1 yr: PO 1.25 mg tid or hs	• Tabs 2.5 mg • Time-rel spanules 5 mg • Syr 2.5 mg/5 ml	• Increased CNS depression: barbiturates, narcotics, hypnotics, tricyclics, alcohol • Decreased effect of oral anticoagulants, heparin • Increased effect of trimeprazine: MAOIs 🍃 Increased anticholinergic effect: henbane leaf	• Hypersensitivity to H₁-receptor antagonists • Acute asthma attack • Lower respiratory tract disease
tripelennamine (℞)	PBZ, PBZ-SR, Pelamine, tripelennamine HC1	• Rhinitis • Allergy symptoms	• Adults: PO 25-50 mg q4-6h, not to exceed 600 mg/day; time-rel 100 mg bid-tid, not to exceed 600 mg/day • Child >5 yr: PO time-rel 50 mg q8-12h, not to exceed 300 mg/day • Child <5 yr: PO 5 mg/kg/day in 4-6 divided doses, not to exceed 300 mg/day	• Tabs 25, 50 mg • Time-rel tabs 100 mg • Elix 37.5 mg/5 ml	• Increased CNS depression: barbiturates, narcotics, hypnotics, tricyclics, alcohol • Decreased effect of oral anticoagulants, heparin • Increased effect of tripelennamine: MAOIs 🍃 Increased anticholinergic effect: henbane leaf	• Hypersensitivity to H₁-receptor antagonists • Acute asthma attack • Lower respiratory tract disease

KEY: * = Canada only; 🍃 = herb/drug interaction

Appendix I

High alert drugs

The Joint Commission on Accreditation of Healthcare Organizations recently released a list of medications with the highest risk of injury when misused. Based upon a study performed by the Institute for Safe Medication Practices, these high-alert medications were divided into six groups: insulins, opiates, antineoplastics, injectable potassium chloride or phosphate, intravenous anticoagulants, and sodium chloride solutions stronger than 9%. To help nurses identify these drugs, each specific drug monograph has been identified with a light color screen throughout the book. A complete list of high-alert drugs located in this book follows.

abciximab
adenosine
aldesleukin
alteplase
amiodarone
anistreplase
antihemophilic factor
antithrombin III
ardeparin
argatroban
arsenic trioxide
asparaginase
atropine
basiliximab
bivalirudin
bleomycin
bretylium
busulfan
calfactant
carboplatin
carmustine
cisplatin
coagulation factor VIIa,
    recombinant
cyclophosphamide
cytarabine
dacarbazine
daclizumab
dactinomycin
dalteparin
danaparoid

daunorubicin
dezocine
digoxin
diltiazem
dopamine
doxacurium
doxorubicin
droperidol
enoxaparin
ephedrine
epinephrine
epirubicin
eptifibatide
etoposide
factor IX complex/factor IV
fentanyl
fentanyl/droperidol
fluorouracil
gallamine
gemtuzumab
heparin
hydromorphone
ibutilide
idarubicin
ifosfamide
inamrinone
insulin
irinotecan
ketamine
lepirudin
leuprolide

lidocaine
magnesium sulfate
melphalan
meperidine
methadone
methotrexate
milrinone
mitomycin
mitoxantrone
mivacurium
morphine
nalbuphine
nitroprusside
norepinephrine
oxycodone
oxymorphone
oxytocin
pancuronium
pegaspargase
pentazocine
pentobarbital IV
pentostatin
phenobarbital IV
pipecuronium

plicamycin
poractant alfa
potassium chloride inj concentrate
propofol
propoxyphene
remifentanil
rocuronium
secobarbital IV
streptokinase
succinylcholine
sufentanil
tenecteplase
thiopental
tinzaparin
topotecan
trastuzumab
tubocurarine
urokinase
vecuronium
vinblastine
vincristine
vinorelbine
warfarin

1. Cohen MR, Kilo CM: High-alert medications: safeguarding against errors. In Cohen MR, editor: *Medication errors*, Washington, DC, 1999 American Pharmaceutical Association.
2. High-alert medications and patient safety, *Sentinel Event Alert* 11, Nov 1999.

Appendix j

Look-alike/sound-alike drug names

acetohexamide	acetazolamide
Adriamycin	Aredia
Adriamycin	Idamycin
albuterol	atenolol
allopurinol	Apresoline
alprazolam	lorazepam
Altace	alteplase
Ambien	Amen
Amikin	Amicar
amitriptyline	nortriptyline
amoxapine	amoxicillin
amoxapine	Amoxil
amoxicillin	Amoxil
Artane	Altace
Asacol	Ansaid
Asacol	Os-Cal
Atrovent	Alupent
Bactocil	Pathocil
Bentyl	Aventyl
Betalin	Benylin
Brethine	Banthine
Brevital	Brevibloc
Bumex	Buprenex
Cafergot	Carafate
calcitriol	Calciferol
carboplatin	cisplatin
Cardene	Cardizem
Cardene SR	Cardizem SR
Cardizem CD	Cardizem SR
Cardura	Coumadin
Cataflam	Catapres
cefaclor	cephalexin
Cefotan	Ceftin
cefprozil	cefuroxime
ceftazidime	ceftizoxime
cefuroxime	cefotaxime
cefuroxime	deferoxamine
Cefzil	Ceftin
Cefzil	Kefzol
cephapirin	cephradine
chlorpromazine	chlorpropamide
chlorpromazine	prochlorperazine
Clinoril	Clozaril
Clinoril	Oruvail
clomipramine	clomiphene
clomipramine	Norpramin (desipramine)
clonidine	Klonopin (clonazepam)
Cordarone	Inocor
Corgard	Cognex
Coumadin	Compazine
Cozaar	Zocor
cyclobenzaprine	cyproheptadine
cyclophosphamide	cyclosporine
cyclosporine	cycloserine
Cytovene	Cytosar
Cytoxan	Cytosar (cytarabine)
Cytoxan	Cytotec
Dantrium	danazol
daunorubicin	doxorubicin
Decadron	Percodan
Depo-Medrol	Solu-Medrol
Diabeta	Zebeta
Dialose Plus (docusate potassium/ casanthranol)	Dialose Plus (docusate sodium/ phenolphthalein)
diazepam	Ditropan
Diflucan	Diprivan
Dilaudid	Demerol
Diphenatol	diphenidol
diphenhydramine	dicyclomine
Diupres	Daypro
Dobutrex	Diamox
dopamine	dobutamine
doxorubicin	idarubicin
Edecrin	Eulexin
Elavil	Mellaril
Eldepryl	enalapril
enalapril	ramipril
Estratest	Estratab
etidronate	etretinate
etomidate	etidronate
Fioricet	Fiorinal
Flumadine	fludarabine
fluorouracil	flucytosine
FUDR	Fludara

Gamulin Rh	MICRhoGAM
Garamycin	kanamycin
Glucotrol	glyburide
Halotestin	haloperidol
Hycodan	Vicodin
hydrocodone	hydrocortisone
hydromorphone	meperidine
hydromorphone	morphine
Imferon	Roferon-A
imipenem	Omnipen
imipramine	Desipramine
Imuran	Imferon
Inderal LA	IMDUR
Klonopin	clonidine
Lamictal	Lomotil
Lanoxin Lasix	Lomotil
leucovorin Leukine	Leukeran
Levsin	Levoxine
Librium	Librax
Lodine	codeine
Lortab	Lorabid
Lotensin	Lioresal
Lotensin	Loniten
Lotrimin	Otrivin
Lupron	Lopurin
Luvox	Lasix
Mazicon	Mivacron
Mepron	Mepron
(atovaquone	(meprobamate
in U.S.)	in Australia)
methyldopa	L-Dopa (levodopa)
methylphenidate	methadone
methylprednisolone	medroxypro-
	gesterone
metolazone	methotrexate
metolazone	metoclopramide
metoprolol	misoprostol
Monopril	minoxidil
Mylanta Gas	Mylicon
Narcan	Norcuron
Nasalide	Nasalcrom
Nicobid	Nitro-Bid
Norflex	Noroxin
	(norfloxacin)
Norpramin	nortriptyline
Norvasc	Navane
Novolin 70/30	Novolin 70/30
Penfill Prefilled	
Nuprin	Lupron
Ocufen	Ocuflox
	(ofloxacin)
Ocufen	Ocupress
Oruvail	Elavil
paroxetine	paclitaxel

Paxil	paclitaxel
Paxil	Taxol
pentobarbital	phenobarbital
Phenergan	Theragran
phenobarbital	pentobarbital
pindolol	Parlodel
Plendil	pindolol
Plendil	Prinivil
Pravachol	Prevacid
prednisone	methylprednisolone
prednisone	prednisolone
Premarin	Primaxin
Prepidil	bepridil
Prilosec	prednisone
Prilosec	Prozac
Prinivil	Prilosec
Prinivil	Proventil
Prokine	Proleukin
Provera	Premarin
Prozac Proscar	Prosom
Psorion	Psorcon
quinidine	quinine
ranitidine	amantadine
Reglan	Megace
Regroton	Hygroton
reserpine	Risperdal
	(risperidone)
Ridaura	Cardura
rifampin	rifabutin
rimantadine	amantadine
Roxanol	Roxicet
Sinequan	Serentil
Soma	Soma Compound
Stadol	Haldol
sulfasalazine	sulfisoxazole
Symmetrel	Synthroid
Taxol	Paxil
Tegretol	Toradol
Temaril	Demerol
thiamine	Tenormin
Thyrar	Thyrolar
Timoptic	Viroptic
Tobrex	TobraDex
Toradol	Inderal
Toradol	Torecan
Toradol	tramadol
torsemide	furosemide
trifluoperazine	trihexyphenidyl
Trimox	Diamox
Trimox	Tylox
Tronothane	Tronolane
Uridon	Vicodin
Urispas	Urised
Vantin	Ventolin

Versed	Vistaril	Xanax	Zantac
Versed	Vepesid	Zantac	Xanax
vincristine	vinblastine	Zinacef	Zithromax
Viroptic	Timoptic	Zocor	Zoloft
Wymox	Tylox	Zofran	Zantac
Xanax	Lanoxin	Zosyn	Zofran
Xanax	Tylox	Zyvox	Vioxx

Appendix k

Herbal products

agrimony

Uses: Mild diarrhea, gastroenteritis, intestinal mucous secretion, inflammation of the mouth and throat, cuts and scrapes, amenorrhea

alfalfa

Uses: Poor appetite, hay fever and asthma, high cholesterol, nutrient source

aloe

Uses of aloe vera gel:
• *External:* Minor burns, skin irritations, minor wounds, frostbite, radiation-caused injuries
• *Internal:* To heal intestinal inflammation and ulcers, as a digestive aid to stimulate bile secretion

angelica

Uses: Heartburn, indigestion, gas, colic, poor blood flow to the extremities, bronchitis, poor appetite, psoriasis, vitiligo, as an antiseptic

arnica

Uses: Topical application for muscle and joint inflammation and swelling; in homeopathic preparations as a remedy for shock, injury, pain

astragalus

Uses: Immune stimulant, viral infections, HIV/AIDS, cancer, vascular disorders, improve circulation, lower blood pressure, possible efficacy in myasthenia gravis

bilberry

Uses: Diabetic retinopathy, macular degeneration, glaucoma, cataract, capillary fragility, varicose veins, hemorrhoids, mild diarrhea

black cohosh

Uses:
• *Menopause:* Hot flashes, nervous conditions associated with menopause
• *Dysmenorrhea:* Menstrual cramps, pain, inflammation

Adapted from: Debusk, Ruth, and Treadwell, Phillip. *Serious Drug/Herb Interactions.* Skidmore-Roth Publishing, Inc. 1999.

black haw (cramp bark)

Uses: Dysmenorrhea, menstrual cramps and pain, menopausal metrorrhagia, hysteria, asthma, lower blood pressure, heart palpitations

blessed thistle

Uses: Loss of appetite, indigestion, intestinal gas

blue cohosh

Uses: Menopausal symptoms, uterine and ovarian pain, improve flow of menstrual blood, antiinflammatory, antirheumatic, popular remedy in black ethnic medicine

borage

Uses: Antiinflammatory for premenstrual syndrome, rheumatoid arthritis, Raynaud's disease, other inflammatory conditions, atopic dermatitis, infant cradle cap, cystic fibrosis, high blood pressure, diabetes

burdock root

Uses: Skin diseases, inflammation, rashes, cold and fever, cancer, gout, arthritis

calendula

Uses:
• *External:* Minor skin ailments
• *Internal:* Inflammation throughout the gastrointestinal tract, toxic liver and gallbladder, menstrual bleeding and pain, yeast infections

capsicum (cayenne)

Uses: Muscle spasms, pain of inflammation, neuromas, psoriasis, dry mouth, as an antioxidant food, as a food seasoning

cascara

Uses: Chronic constipation, hepatitis, gallstones

cat's claw

Uses: Cancer, herpes, HIV/AIDS, rheumatoid arthritis, gastritis, gout, wounds, gastric ulcers

chamomile

Uses:
• *External:* As an antiseptic and soothing agent for inflamed skin and minor wounds
• *Internal:* As an antispasmodic, gas-relieving, and antiinflammatory agent for the treatment of digestive problems; light sleep aid and sedative for adults and children; possible anticancer agent

---

* = Canada only   Side effects: *italics* = common; ***bold italics*** = life-threatening

chaparral

Uses: Not recommended—potentially toxic to the liver and kidneys

chicory

Uses: Coffee substitute, source of fructo-oligosaccharides, mild laxative for children, gout, rheumatism, loss of appetite, digestive distress

comfrey

Uses: Bruises, sprains, broken bones, acne, boils

cranberry

Uses: Urinary tract infections (UTIs); susceptibility to kidney stones

dong quai

Uses: To restore vitality to tired women; for a variety of gynecologic, menstrual, and menopausal symptoms; cirrhosis of the liver

echinacea

Uses: Low immune status, hard-to-heal superficial wounds, sun protection

elder (elderberry)

Uses: Susceptibility to colds, flu, yeast infections; nasal and chest congestion; earache associated with chronic congestion; hay fever

eleuthero (See siberian ginseng)

ephedra (ma huang)

Uses: Seasonal and chronic asthma, nasal congestion, cough

evening primrose

Uses: Premenstrual syndrome, arthritis and inflammatory disorders in general, dry skin, eczema, asthma, diabetes, migraines, chronic fatigue syndrome, heart disease and stroke, circulatory disorders, Raynaud's disease, NSAID use, multiple sclerosis

fenugreek

Uses: Loss of appetite, inflamed areas of the skin, water retention, cancer, constipation, diarrhea, high cholesterol, high blood sugar, calcium oxalate stones

◆ = Nursing alert   ✏ = Herb-drug interaction   ⊘ = Do not crush

feverfew

Uses: Migraines, cluster headaches, fever, psoriasis, inflammation

flaxseed

Uses: Constipation, as a source of omega-3 fatty acids

fo-ti

Uses: Tiredness, constipation, elevated cholesterol

garcinia cambogia

Uses: Appetite control, weight loss, high cholesterol

garlic

Uses: Vascular disease, elevated LDL, elevated triglycerides, low HDL, high blood pressure, poor circulation, risk of cancer, inflammatory disorders, childhood ear infection, yeast infection

ginger

Uses: Nausea, motion sickness, indigestion, inflammation

ginkgo

Uses: Poor circulation; age-related decline in cognition, memory; diabetes; vascular disease; cancer; inflammatory disorders; impotence; degenerative nerve conditions

ginseng

Uses: Physical and mental exhaustion, stress, viral infections, diabetes, sluggishness, fatigue, weak immunity, convalescence

goldenseal

Uses: High blood pressure, poor appetite, infections, menstrual problems, minor sciatic pain, muscle spasms, eye washes

gotu kola

Uses: Chronic wounds, psoriasis

grape seed

Uses: Antioxidant, chronic disease prevention, inflammation

green tea

Uses: Cancer prevention, heart disease prevention, hypercholesterolemia, diarrhea

guggul

Uses: High LDL cholesterol, elevated triglycerides, weight loss

gymnema sylvestre

Uses: High blood sugar levels

hawthorn

Uses: Poor circulation, chest pain, irregular heartbeat, high blood fats, high blood pressure

hops

Uses: Mild sedative, diuretic, weak antibiotic, insomnia, hyperactivity, pain, fever, jaundice, improve appetite

horse chestnut

Uses: Fever, fluid retention, frostbite, hemorrhoids, inflammation, lower extremity swelling, phlebitis, varicose veins, wounds

horsetail

Uses: Diuretic, genitourinary astringent, anti-hemorrhagic, Bell's Palsy, healing broken bones

kava

Uses: Nervous anxiety, restlessness, sleep disturbances, stress

khat

Uses: Obesity, gastric ulcers, stimulant

kombucha

Uses: Numerous claims for a wide variety of ills; none has been substantiated to date

konjac

Uses: Blood sugar control, constipation, high blood fats, high blood pressure, excessive appetite

kudzu

Uses: Alcohol cravings, menopausal symptoms

lapacho (pau d'arco)

Uses: Cancer, inflammation, infection

lemon balm (melissa)

Uses: Abdominal gas and cramping, cold sores

licorice

Uses: Allergies, arthritis, asthma, constipation, esophagitis, gastritis, hepatitis, inflammatory conditions, peptic ulcers, poor adrenal function, poor appetite

maitake

Uses: Immunostimulant activity, diabetes, hypertension, high cholesterol, obesity

maté

Uses: Diuretic, depurative

melatonin

Uses: Jet lag, insomnia, cancer protection, oral contraceptive

milk thistle

Uses: Protection for alcoholic cirrhosis and hepatitis, antiinflammatory

monascus

Uses: Maintaining acceptable cholesterol levels

morinda

Uses: Headache, digestive, heart and liver conditions, arthritis

nettle

Uses: Diuretic, hay fever

octacosanol

Uses: Herpes, inflammation of the skin, physical endurance

passionflower

Uses: Antifungal, hypertension, sedative, group A hemolytic streptococcus

peppermint

Uses: GI disorders

pygeum

Uses: Benign prostate hypertrophy, antiinflammatory

raspberry leaves

Uses: Facilitation of childbirth, dysmenorrhea, uterine tonic, fever, vomiting

red clover

Uses: Antispasmodic, expectorant, sedative, psoriasis, eczema, amenorrhea

rose hips

Uses: Source of vit C, cold, fever, mild infections

st. john's wort

Uses: Depression, antiviral

sarsaparilla

Uses: Antiinflammatory, antiseptic, syphilis, skin diseases, rheumatism, necrosis, mercury poisoning

sassafras

Uses: Banned in the United States

saw palmetto

Uses: Benign prostatic hypertrophy

schisandra

Uses: GI disorders, liver protection, tonic

scull cap

Uses: Antibacterial, sedative

senna

Uses: Laxative

siberian ginseng (eleuthero)

Uses: Improve appetite, memory loss, hypertension, insomnia, rheumatism, improve circulation, heart ailments, diabetes, headache

tea tree oil

Uses: Topical use for infections; inhaled for respiratory disorders

uva ursi

Uses: Diuretic, urinary tract infections, contact dermatitis, arthritis

valerian

Uses: Sedative

vitex

Uses: Premenstrual and menstrual disorders, spasms, estrogen gestagen imbalance

yarrow

Uses: To decrease bleeding, Gi disorders, hypertension, thrombi, to improve circulation

yohimbine

Uses: Male organic impotence

◆ = Nursing alert   ⫽ = Herb-drug interaction   ⊘ = Do not crush

Appendix I

FDA pregnancy categories

A   No risk demonstrated to the fetus in any trimester

B   No adverse effects in animals, no human studies available

C   Only given after risks to the fetus are considered; animal studies have shown adverse reactions, no human studies available

D   Definite fetal risks, may be given in spite of risks if needed in life-threatening conditions

X   Absolute fetal abnormalities; not to be used anytime during pregnancy

Note: **UK** = Unknown fetal risk (used in this text but not an official FDA pregnancy category).

Appendix m

Controlled substance chart

Drugs	United States	Canada
Heroin, LSD, peyote, marijuana, mescaline	Schedule I • High abuse potential • No currently accepted medical use	Schedule H
Opium (morphine), meperidine, amphetamines, cocaine, short-acting barbiturates (secobarbital)	Schedule II • High abuse potential; potentially severe psychologic or physical dependence • Currently accepted medical use but may be severely restricted • Telephone orders only in emergencies if written Rx follows promptly • No refills	Schedule G
Glutethimide, paregoric, phendimetrazine	Schedule III • Abuse potential less than the drugs/substances in Schedules I and II; potentially moderate or low physical dependence or high psychologic dependence • Currently accepted medical use • Telephone orders permitted • Prescriber may authorize limited refills	Schedule F

Drugs	United States	Canada
Chloral hydrate, chlordiazepoxide, diazepam, mazindol, meprobamate, phenobarbital (Canada—G)	Schedule IV • Low abuse potential relative to drugs/substances in Schedule III; potentially limited physical or psychologic dependence • Currently accepted medical use • Telephone orders permitted • Prescriber may authorize limited refills	Schedule F
Antidiarrheals with opium (Canada—G), antitussives	Schedule V • Lowest abuse potential; potentially very limited physical or psychologic dependence • Currently accepted medical use • Prescriber determines refills • Some products containing limited amounts of Schedule V substances (e.g., cough suppressants) available OTC to patients >18 yr	Schedule F

Appendix n

Abbreviations

AAS	argininosuccinic acid synthetase
abd	abdomen
ABG	arterial blood gas
ac	before meals
ACE	angiotensin-converting enzyme
ADA	American Diabetes Association
ADH	antidiuretic hormone
ALT	alanine aminotransferase
ANA	antinuclear antibody
AP	anteroposterior
APTT	activated partial thromboplastin time
ASA	acetylsalicylic acid, aspirin
ASHD	arteriosclerotic heart disease
AST	aspartate aminotransferase (SGOT)
AV	atrioventricular
bid	twice a day
BM	bowel movement
BMR	basal metabolic rate
B/P	blood pressure
BPH	benign prostatic hypertrophy
BPM	beats per minute
BS	blood sugar
BUN	blood urea nitrogen
C	Celsius (centigrade)
Ca	cancer
CAD	coronary artery disease
cap	capsule
Cath	catheterization or catheterize
CBC	complete blood cell count
CC	chief complaint
cc	cubic centimeter
CHF	congestive heart failure
cm	centimeter
CNS	central nervous system
CO_2	carbon dioxide
CONT	continuous
COPD	chronic obstructive pulmonary disease
CPAP	continuous positive airway pressure
CPK	creatine phosphokinase
CPR	cardiopulmonary resuscitation
CPS	carbamoyl phosphate synthetase
CrCl	creatinine clearance
C&S	culture and sensitivity
C sect	cesarean section
CSF	cerebrospinal fluid
CV	cardiovascular
CVA	cerebrovascular accident
CVP	central venous pressure
D&C	dilatation and curettage
DIC	diffuse intravascular coagulation
DIR INF	direct infusion
dr	dram
D_5W	5% glucose in distilled water
ECG	electrocardiogram (EKG)
EDTA	ethylenediamine tetraacetic acid
EEG	electroencephalogram
EENT	ear, eye, nose, and throat
EPS	extrapyramidal symptom
ESR	erythrocyte sedimentation rate
EXT REL	extended release
EXTRA STREN SUSP	extra strength suspension
FBS	fasting blood sugar
FHT	fetal heart tones
FSH	follicle-stimulating hormone
g	gram
GABA	γ-aminobutyric acid
GI	gastrointestinal

gr	grain	**MAC**	monitored anesthesia care
GT	glucose tolerance test	**MAOI**	monoamine oxidase inhibitor
gtt	drops	**mEq**	milliequivalent
GU	genitourinary	**mg**	milligram
H₂	histamine₂	**µg**	microgram
HCG	human chorionic gonado-tropin	**µm**	micron
		MI	myocardial infarction
Hct	hematocrit	**min**	minute
HDCV	human diploid cell rabies vaccine	**ml**	milliliter
		mm	millimeter
Hgb	hemoglobin	**mo**	month
H & H	hematocrit and hemoglobin	**Na**	sodium
5-HIAA	5-hydroxyindoleacetic acid	**neg**	negative
HIV	human immunodeficiency virus (AIDS)	**ng**	nanogram
		NOS	not otherwise specified
H₂O	water	**NPO**	nothing by mouth (Lat. *nulla per os*)
HOB	head of bed		
HR	heart rate	**NS**	normal saline
hr	hour	**O₂**	oxygen
hs	at bedtime	**OBS**	organic brain syndrome
IgG	immunolobulin G	**od**	right eye
IM	intramuscular	**OR**	operating room
INF	infusion	**os**	left eye
INH	inhalation	**OTC**	over-the-counter
inj	injection	**OU**	each eye
I&O	intake and output	**oz**	ounce
INT	intermittent	**p̄**	after
IPPB	intermittent positive-pressure breathing	**P56**	plasma-lyte 56
		PaCO₂	arterial carbon dioxide tension (pressure)
ITP	idiopathic thrombocytopenic purpura		
		PaO₂	arterial oxygen tension (pressure)
IUD	intrauterine device		
IV	intravenous	**PAT**	paroxysmal atrial tachy-cardia
IVP	intravenous pyelogram		
K	potassium	**PBI**	protein-bound iodine
kg	kilogram	**pc**	after meals
L	liter	**PCWP**	pulmonary capillary wedge pressure
lb	pound		
LDH	lactic dehydrogenase	**PEEP**	positive end-expiratory pressure
LE	lupus erythematosus		
LFT	liver function test	**PERRLA**	pupils equal, round, react to light and accommodation
LH	luteinizing hormone		
LLQ	left lower quadrant	**pH**	hydrogen ion concentration
LMP	last menstrual period	**PO**	by mouth
LOC	level of consciousness	**postop**	postoperative
LR	lactated Ringer's solution	**PP**	postprandial
LT	leukotriene	**preop**	preoperative
LUQ	left upper quadrant	**prn**	as required
M	meter	**PT**	prothrombin time
m	minim	**PTT**	partial thromboplastin time
m²	square meter		

PVC	premature ventricular contraction
pwd	powder
qAM	every morning
qd	every day
qh	every hour
q2h	every 2 hours
q3h	every 3 hours
q4h	every 4 hours
q6h	every 6 hours
q12h	every 12 hours
qid	four times daily
qod	every other day
qPM	every night
qs	sufficient quantity
qt	quart
R	right
RAIU	radioactive iodine uptake
RBC	red blood cell count or red blood cell
RECT	rectal
RLQ	right lower quadrant
ROM	range of motion
RUQ	right upper quadrant
SC	subcutaneous
SIMV	synchronous intermittent mandatory ventilation
SL	sublingual
SLE	systemic lupus erythematosus
SOB	shortness of breath
sol	solution
ss	one half
suppos	suppository

SUS REL	sustained release
syr	syrup
T&A	tonsillectomy and adenoidectomy
tab	tablet
tbsp	tablespoon
temp	temperature
tid	three times daily
tinc	tincture
TPN	total parenteral nutrition
top	topical
TRANS	transdermal
TSH	thyroid-stimulating hormone
tsp	teaspoon
TT	thrombin time
U	unit
UA	urinalysis
UTI	urinary tract infection
UV	ultraviolet
vag	vaginal
VMA	vanillylmandelic acid
vol	volume
VS	vital sign
WBC	white blood cell count
wk	week
wt	weight
yr	year
>	greater than
<	less than
=	equal
°	degree
%	percent
α	alpha
β	beta
γ	gamma

Appendix o

Weights and equivalents

METRIC SYSTEM

Weight

kilogram	= kg	=	1000 grams
gram	= g	=	1 gram
milligram	= mg	=	0.001 gram
microgram	= µg	=	0.001 milligram

Volume

liter	= L	=	1 L
milliliter	= ml	=	0.001 L

AVOIRDUPOIS WEIGHT

1 ounce (oz) = 437.5 grains

1 pound (lb) = 16 ounces = 7000 grains

METRIC AND APOTHECARY EQUIVALENTS

Exact weight equivalents

Metric	Apothecary
1 mg	1/64.8 grain
64.8 mg	1 grain
324 mg	5 grains
1 g	15.432 grains
31.103 g	1 ounce = 480 grains

Exact volume equivalents

Metric	Apothecary		
1.00 ml	16.23 minims		
3.69 ml	1 fluidram	=	60 minims
29.57 ml	1 fluid ounce	=	480 minims
473.16 ml	1 pint	=	7680 minims
946.33 ml	1 quart	=	15,360 minims

Appendix p

Formulas for drug calculations

Surface area rule:

$$\text{Child dose} = \frac{\text{Surface area (m}^2)}{1.73\text{m}^2} \times \text{Adult dose}$$

Calculating strength of a solution:

Solution Strength: *Desired Solution:*

$$\frac{x}{100} = \frac{\text{Amount of drug desired}}{\text{Amount of finished solution}}$$

Calculating flow rate for IV:

$$\textbf{Rate of flow} = \frac{\text{Amount of fluid} \times \text{Administration set calibration}}{\text{Running time}}$$

$$\frac{x}{1} = \frac{\text{(ml) (gtt/min)}}{\text{min}}$$

Calculation of medication dosages:

Formula method:

$$\frac{\text{Amount ordered}}{\text{Amount on hand}} \times \text{Vehicle} = \text{Number of tablets, capsules, or amount of liquid}$$

Vehicle is the drug form or amount of liquid containing the dosage. Amounts used in calculation by formula must be in same system.

Ratio—proportion method:

1 tablet:tablet in mg on hand::x tablet order in mg
        Know or have::Want to know or order

Multiply means and extremes, divide both sides by known amount to get x. Amounts used in equation must be in same system.

Dimensional analysis method:

$$\textbf{Order in mg} \times \frac{\text{1 tablet or capsule}}{\text{What 1 tablet or capsule is in mg}}$$

$$= \text{Tablets or capsules to be given}$$

If amounts are in different systems:

$$\textbf{Order in mg} \times \frac{\text{1 tablet or capsule}}{\text{What 1 tablet or capsule is in g}} \times \frac{1}{1000 \text{ mg}}$$

$$= \text{Tablets or capsules to be given}$$

Appendix q

Nomogram for calculation of body surface area

Place a straight edge from the patient's height in the left column to the patient's weight in the right column. The point of intersection on the body surface area column indicates the body surface area (BSA). (Reproduced from Behrman RE, and Vaughn VC (editors): *Nelson's textbook of pediatrics,* ed 12, Philadelphia, 1983, WB Saunders.)

Appendix r

Bibliography

Blumenthal M: *The complete German Commission E monographs: Therapeutic guide to herbal medicines,* Austin, 1998, American Botanical Council.

Clark JB, Queener SF, Karb VB: *Pharmacological basis of nursing practice,* ed 5, St Louis, 1998, Mosby.

Drug information: Bethesda, American Hospital Formulary Service.

Facts and comparisons: St Louis, updated monthly.

Gahart BL: *Intravenous medications,* ed 15, St Louis, 2001, Mosby.

Goodman A and others: *Goodman and Gilman's the pharmacological basis of therapeutics,* ed 10, New York, 1998, Pergamon Press.

McKenry LM, Salerno E: *Mosby's pharmacology in nursing,* ed 18, St Louis, 1996, Mosby.

Mediphor Editorial Group: *Drug interaction facts,* Philadelphia, updated quarterly, JB Lippincott.

Review of natural products: Philadelphia, updated monthly, *Facts and Comparisons.*

Entries can be identified as follows: *Combination Products,* DISEASES/DISORDERS, *DRUG CATEGORIES,* generic names, Trade Names.

Entries can be identified as follows: *Combination Products,* DISEASES/DISORDERS, *DRUG CATEGORIES,* generic names, Trade Names.

Entries can be identified as follows: *Combination Products,* DISEASES/DISORDERS,
DRUG CATEGORIES, generic names, Trade Names.

Entries can be identified as follows: *Combination Products,* DISEASES/DISORDERS, *DRUG CATEGORIES,* generic names, Trade Names.

Entries can be identified as follows: *Combination Products,* DISEASES/DISORDERS,
DRUG CATEGORIES, generic names, Trade Names.

Argesic-SA, 877-878
Aricept, 362-363
Arimidex, 131-132
Aristocort, 979-981, 1071-1072
Aristocort Forte, 979-981
Aristocort Intralesional,
    979-981
Aristospan Intra-Articular,
    979-981
Aristospan Intralesional,
    979-981
Arixtra, 1051-1052
Arm-A-Med, 624-625
Arm & Hammer Pure Baking
    Soda, 894-896
Armour Thyroid, 948-949
arnica, 1136
Aromasin, 412-413
Arrestin, 988-989
ARSENIC POISONING
    dimercaprol, 349
arsenic trioxide, 27, 138, 1131
Artane, 987-988, 1133
Artane Sequels, 987-988
ARTERIOVENOUS CANNULA
        OCCLUSION
    streptokinase, 905
Arthra-G, 877-878
Arthrinol, 142-144
Arthrisin, 142-144
ARTHRITIS
    indomethacin, 522
    magnesium salicylate, 600
    OSTEOARTHRITIS. *See*
        OSTEOARTHRITIS
    RHEUMATOID. *See*
        RHEUMATOID
        ARTHRITIS
    sulindac, 920
Arthritis Foundation Pain
    Reliever Aspirin-Free,
    71-73
Arthritis Pain Formula, 1089
Arthropan, 256-257
Arthrotec, 1089
Articulose-50, 808-810

Articulose L.A., 979-981
Artria S.R., 142-144
A.S.A., 142-144
Asacol, 621-622, 1133
Asbron G Elixir, 1089
Asbron G Inlay, 1089
ascorbic acid, 66, 139-140
Ascorbicap, 139-140
Ascriptin, 1089
Ascriptin A/D, 1089
Asendin, 115-117
A-200 Shampoo, 1086
Asmalix, 940-941
asparaginase, 27, 140-142, 1131
Aspergum, 142-144
ASPHYXIA NEONATORUM
    naloxone, 689
ASPIRATION PNEUMONITIS
    cimetidine, 262
aspirin, 61, 142-144
Aspirin Free Anacin, 71-73
*Aspirin-Free Bayer Select Allergy
    Sinus,* 1089-1090
*Aspirin-Free Bayer Select Head
    & Chest Cold,* 1090
Aspirin Free Excedrin, 1090
Aspirin Free Excedrin Dual,
    1090
Aspirin Free Pain Relief, 71-73
Aspir-Low, 142-144
Aspirtab, 142-144
Astelin, 1068-1070
ASTHMA
    beclomethasone, 159-160
    bitolterol, 174
    cromolyn, 293
    epinephrine, 389
    formoterol fumarate, 1052
    isoproterenol, 544
    montelukast, 673
    prednisolone, 808-809
    theophylline, 940
    triamcinolone, 980
    zileuton, 1029
AsthmalHaler Mist, 389-391
AsthmaNefrin, 389-391

Entries can be identified as follows: *Combination Products,* DISEASES/DISORDERS, *DRUG CATEGORIES,* generic names, Trade Names.

Entries can be identified as follows: *Combination Products,* DISEASES/DISORDERS, *DRUG CATEGORIES,* generic names, Trade Names.

Entries can be identified as follows: *Combination Products,* DISEASES/DISORDERS,
DRUG CATEGORIES, generic names, Trade Names.

Entries can be identified as follows: *Combination Products,* DISEASES/DISORDERS,
DRUG CATEGORIES, generic names, Trade Names.

Entries can be identified as follows: *Combination Products,* DISEASES/DISORDERS, *DRUG CATEGORIES,* generic names, Trade Names.

Entries can be identified as follows: *Combination Products,* DISEASES/DISORDERS, *DRUG CATEGORIES,* generic names, Trade Names.

Entries can be identified as follows: *Combination Products,* DISEASES/DISORDERS, *DRUG CATEGORIES,* generic names, Trade Names.

Entries can be identified as follows: *Combination Products,* DISEASES/DISORDERS, *DRUG CATEGORIES,* generic names, Trade Names.

Entries can be identified as follows: *Combination Products,* DISEASES/DISORDERS, *DRUG CATEGORIES,* generic names, Trade Names.

Entries can be identified as follows: *Combination Products,* DISEASES/DISORDERS,
DRUG CATEGORIES, generic names, Trade Names.

Entries can be identified as follows: *Combination Products,* DISEASES/DISORDERS, *DRUG CATEGORIES,* generic names, Trade Names.

Entries can be identified as follows: *Combination Products,* DISEASES/DISORDERS,
DRUG CATEGORIES, generic names, Trade Names.

Entries can be identified as follows: *Combination Products,* DISEASES/DISORDERS,
DRUG CATEGORIES, generic names, Trade Names.

Entries can be identified as follows: *Combination Products,* DISEASES/DISORDERS, *DRUG CATEGORIES,* generic names, Trade Names.

Entries can be identified as follows: *Combination Products,* DISEASES/DISORDERS, *DRUG CATEGORIES,* generic names, Trade Names.

Entries can be identified as follows: *Combination Products,* DISEASES/DISORDERS, *DRUG CATEGORIES,* generic names, Trade Names.

Entries can be identified as follows: *Combination Products,* DISEASES/DISORDERS, *DRUG CATEGORIES,* generic names, Trade Names.

Entries can be identified as follows: *Combination Products,* DISEASES/DISORDERS,
DRUG CATEGORIES, generic names, Trade Names.

Entries can be identified as follows: *Combination Products,* DISEASES/DISORDERS,
DRUG CATEGORIES, generic names, Trade Names.

Entries can be identified as follows: *Combination Products,* DISEASES/DISORDERS, *DRUG CATEGORIES,* generic names, Trade Names.

Entries can be identified as follows: *Combination Products,* DISEASES/DISORDERS, *DRUG CATEGORIES,* generic names, Trade Names.

Entries can be identified as follows: *Combination Products,* DISEASES/DISORDERS, *DRUG CATEGORIES,* generic names, Trade Names.

Entries can be identified as follows: *Combination Products,* DISEASES/DISORDERS, *DRUG CATEGORIES,* generic names, Trade Names.

Entries can be identified as follows: *Combination Products,* DISEASES/DISORDERS,
DRUG CATEGORIES, generic names, Trade Names.

Entries can be identified as follows: *Combination Products,* DISEASES/DISORDERS, *DRUG CATEGORIES,* generic names, Trade Names.

Entries can be identified as follows: *Combination Products*, DISEASES/DISORDERS, *DRUG CATEGORIES*, generic names, Trade Names.

Entries can be identified as follows: *Combination Products,* DISEASES/DISORDERS,
DRUG CATEGORIES, generic names, Trade Names.

Entries can be identified as follows: *Combination Products,* DISEASES/DISORDERS,
DRUG CATEGORIES, generic names, Trade Names.

Entries can be identified as follows: *Combination Products,* DISEASES/DISORDERS,
DRUG CATEGORIES, generic names, Trade Names.

Entries can be identified as follows: *Combination Products,* DISEASES/DISORDERS,
DRUG CATEGORIES, generic names, Trade Names.

Entries can be identified as follows: *Combination Products,* DISEASES/DISORDERS, *DRUG CATEGORIES,* generic names, Trade Names.

Entries can be identified as follows: *Combination Products,* DISEASES/DISORDERS, *DRUG CATEGORIES,* generic names, Trade Names.

Entries can be identified as follows: *Combination Products,* DISEASES/DISORDERS,
DRUG CATEGORIES, generic names, Trade Names.

Entries can be identified as follows: *Combination Products,* DISEASES/DISORDERS, *DRUG CATEGORIES,* generic names, Trade Names.

Entries can be identified as follows: *Combination Products,* DISEASES/DISORDERS, *DRUG CATEGORIES,* generic names, Trade Names.

Entries can be identified as follows: *Combination Products,* DISEASES/DISORDERS,
DRUG CATEGORIES, generic names, Trade Names.

Entries can be identified as follows: *Combination Products,* DISEASES/DISORDERS, *DRUG CATEGORIES,* generic names, Trade Names.

Entries can be identified as follows: *Combination Products,* DISEASES/DISORDERS, *DRUG CATEGORIES,* generic names, Trade Names.

Entries can be identified as follows: *Combination Products,* DISEASES/DISORDERS,
DRUG CATEGORIES, generic names, Trade Names.

Entries can be identified as follows: *Combination Products,* DISEASES/DISORDERS,
DRUG CATEGORIES, generic names, Trade Names.

Entries can be identified as follows: *Combination Products*, DISEASES/DISORDERS, *DRUG CATEGORIES*, generic names, Trade Names.

Entries can be identified as follows: *Combination Products,* DISEASES/DISORDERS, *DRUG CATEGORIES,* generic names, Trade Names.

Entries can be identified as follows: *Combination Products,* DISEASES/DISORDERS,
DRUG CATEGORIES, generic names, Trade Names.

Entries can be identified as follows: *Combination Products,* DISEASES/DISORDERS, *DRUG CATEGORIES,* generic names, Trade Names.

Entries can be identified as follows: *Combination Products,* DISEASES/DISORDERS,
DRUG CATEGORIES, generic names, Trade Names.

Entries can be identified as follows: *Combination Products,* DISEASES/DISORDERS, *DRUG CATEGORIES,* generic names, Trade Names.

Entries can be identified as follows: *Combination Products,* DISEASES/DISORDERS, *DRUG CATEGORIES,* generic names, Trade Names.

Entries can be identified as follows: *Combination Products,* DISEASES/DISORDERS,
DRUG CATEGORIES, generic names, Trade Names.

Entries can be identified as follows: *Combination Products,* DISEASES/DISORDERS, *DRUG CATEGORIES,* generic names, Trade Names.

Entries can be identified as follows: *Combination Products,* DISEASES/DISORDERS, *DRUG CATEGORIES,* generic names, Trade Names.

Entries can be identified as follows: *Combination Products,* DISEASES/DISORDERS,
DRUG CATEGORIES, generic names, Trade Names.

Entries can be identified as follows: *Combination Products,* DISEASES/DISORDERS,
DRUG CATEGORIES, generic names, Trade Names.

Entries can be identified as follows: *Combination Products,* DISEASES/DISORDERS, *DRUG CATEGORIES,* generic names, Trade Names.

Entries can be identified as follows: *Combination Products,* DISEASES/DISORDERS, *DRUG CATEGORIES,* generic names, Trade Names.

Entries can be
DRUG CATEGORY follows: *Combination Products,* DISEASES/DISORDERS, names, Trade Names.

Entries can be identified as follows: *Combination Products,* DIS
DRUG CATEGORIES, generic names, Trade Names.

Entries can be identified as follows: *Combination Products,* DISEASES/DISORDERS, *DRUG CATEGORIES,* generic names, Trade Names.

Mosby's DrugPro CD-ROM to accompany Mosby's 2003 Nursing Drug Reference

Use *Mosby's DrugPro to Accompany Mosby's 2003 Nursing Drug Reference* to find drug information fast! This three-in-one CD-ROM provides you with alternative remedies, a drug interaction tool, and English and Spanish patient teaching handouts.

Mosby's DrugPro includes:

● **Herbal Remedies** by Steve Blake, ND, MH, DSc, MT
Use this electronic encyclopedia to search for reliable, up-to-date information and photos on more than 30 of the most commonly used herbal remedies. *Herbal Remedies* allows you to search by alternative names, actions, constituents, body systems and health conditions.

● **Drug Master Plus** (from *Mosby's Drug Consult*)
Use this powerful drug interaction tool for instant access to drug-drug interactions, drug-diet interactions, and drug-lab test interactions.

● **Patient Drug Consult** (from *Mosby's Drug Consult*)
Select up-to-date English and Spanish patient teaching handouts for more than 100 of the most commonly used drugs.

Contact Us
For further information, visit us at *www.mosby.com* or call us at (800) 545-2522.

Mini CD-ROM
This mini CD-ROM will work in your CD-ROM drive. Place it on the inner ring of the tray, as shown, and follow the on-screen installation instructions.

This mini-CD does not work in:
    Floppy Drives
    Slot Drives
    Zip Drives
    Stereos
Insert this mini-CD into your CD-ROM drive as shown at left.

Important
No credit or refund will be issued on this book if the CD envelope has been opened, torn, or otherwise tampered with.